Pathology of
Domestic Animals

THIRD EDITION   Volume 2

Pathology of Domestic Animals

THIRD EDITION   Volume 2

K. V. F. JUBB
School of Veterinary Science
University of Melbourne
Victoria, Australia

PETER C. KENNEDY
Department of Pathology
School of Veterinary Medicine
University of California
Davis, California

NIGEL PALMER
Veterinary Services Laboratory
Ministry of Agriculture and Food
Guelph, Ontario, Canada

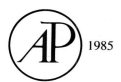 1985

ACADEMIC PRESS, INC.
Harcourt Brace Jovanovich, Publishers
Orlando   San Diego   New York
Austin   Boston   London   Sydney
Tokyo   Toronto

ACADEMIC PRESS, INC.
Orlando, Florida 32887

United Kingdom Edition published by
ACADEMIC PRESS INC. (LONDON) LTD.
24–28 Oval Road, London NW1 7DX

Library of Congress Cataloging in Publication Data

Jubb, K. V. F.
    Pathology of domestic animals.

    Includes index.
    1. Veterinary pathology. I. Kennedy, Peter C.
(Peter Carleton), date   . II. Palmer, Nigel.
III. Title.
SF769.J82 1985   636.089'607   84-2960
ISBN 0-12-391602-X (v. 2 : alk. paper)

PRINTED IN THE UNITED STATES OF AMERICA

86 87 88   9 8 7 6 5 4 3 2

Contents

CHAPTER 2
The Liver and Biliary System

CHAPTER 3
The Pancreas

CHAPTER 4
The Peritoneum, Retroperitoneum, and Mesentery

CHAPTER 5
The Urinary System

CHAPTER 6

The Respiratory System

Preface to the Third Edition

Much has been happening in veterinary pathology between editions of this work. We had, from the time of the first edition, an expectation and a hope that as the number of scientists dedicated to this field of study grew, so also would the variety of publications to serve the diversity of interests. This anticipation has only partly been realized. We still have few books that address themselves to diseases of a single domestic species or to a single organ system of domestic animals. The need for a comprehensive treatment of diseases of domestic species, from the viewpoint of the pathologist, remains. The reception of earlier editions and the interest of our colleagues around the world have influenced us to try for the third time to produce a work of some universal usefulness.

The amount of information available on the pathology of animal disease has grown enormously, and the task of integrating so much new information into a coherent statement has grown on an equal or larger scale. Changes have become necessary in this book. This edition introduces the new generation of veterinary pathologists to a literary task that has grown much beyond what the original authors could handle. We take great satisfaction in this growth and in our colleagues' willingness to join us in the project. The contributors are identified with those chapters or parts of chapters for which they have been individually responsible, although this method does understate the contribution and the dedicated commitment of our coauthors to what has been very much a cooperative effort.

We have retained the original style and format. It was established as the medium for what were personal statements by the authors. We hope that we have been able to maintain some of that flavor. Some features of the style and the format have proven to be awkward in use by the busy working pathologist, and in recognition of this we have given attention to subdivisions in the text, to an expansion of tables of content, to details in indexation (including addition of a cumulative index, in Volume 3), and to an expanded selection of illustrations. The wish to preserve the original style has presented to us and to our contributing authors challenges on content and balance. We hope that these have reasonably been met. Inevitably, we have had to make choices in blending the contributions of our contributing authors into a whole. We have had to reduce excellent sections to keep these volumes within reasonable size, and we have expanded other sections for the sake of completeness. Inevitably too, some of our editorial judgments will be imperfect, and responsibility remains with us for deficiencies in the final compilation.

It is not possible adequately to acknowledge the many people who have contributed to this work; most of them will in this prefatory statement remain unnamed. The contributors, all of whom volunteered effort without which this work could not have been completed, will find that the uses to which these volumes are put in the next few years will be a fuller tribute to their work than can be written here. The support of our many other colleagues in veterinary pathology is perhaps best indicated by their generosity in providing illustrative material. We have brought forward many of the plates or figures from the earlier editions and have added many new ones. Those brought forward or added are acknowledged in the legends, but many more excellent photographs were received than could be used. We are deeply grateful to those colleagues who offered them.

The institutions with which we are individually affiliated have made time and other resources available to us. The several chapters contain acknowledgments for assistance received, but we must here acknowledge Sandy Brown, Jean Middlemiss, and Edward W. Eaton of the University of Guelph for preparing most of the draft manuscript and many illustrations, Denise Heffernan, Lynette Magill, and Frank Oddi of the University of Melbourne for the preparation of final copy and illustrations, and Tammie Goates of that university for editing the bibliographies. We gratefully acknowledge a generous donation from Syntex Agribusiness toward the costs of preparation of the manuscript. We are grateful again to receive the courtesy and cooperation of Academic Press in this shared contribution to the study of animal disease.

Melbourne, Australia   K. V. F. JUBB
1984   PETER C. KENNEDY
                                                           NIGEL PALMER

Preface to the Second Edition

The first edition of "Pathology of Domestic Animals" went to press, not without some sense of satisfaction, with a philosophic acceptance of the many imperfections and a tentative hope that any future edition would provide an opportunity to refine our knowledge, understanding, and technique of communication. Alas, imperfections remain, different ones perhaps, inevitable products of the interaction of limited time, limited intellect, and unlimited supplies of scientific data.

We are impressed by the masses of data that weekly flood our libraries and by the short half-life of much of it, by the exponential increase in knowledge and the splintering of disciplines that proliferate therefrom, and by the inability of many disciplines relevant to medical science to be completely self-sustaining. More and more it is evident that the theme of pathology provides the central and connecting link in medical education and practice and the basis on which a multidisciplined structure can be supported. This is a difficult role for pathologists, but one which they will fill, not by virtue of superior intellects and capacious memories, desirable though these attributes may be, but rather by the proper application of the logic of the scientific method.

Therefore, in preparing this second edition we have attempted to incorporate new knowledge on the specific diseases of animals and, more earnestly, to find a theme of organ susceptibility and responsiveness. We do not doubt the validity of the approach even if we are unable as yet to apply it feasibly to all organs and systems. The format of this edition remains the same as for the first and for the same reasons; the logistics of suitable alternatives are too formidable.

Once again we must express our gratitude to the many people who have contributed in some way to the preparation of this edition. Especially, we are indebted to Professor T. J. Hulland of the University of Guelph for revising the chapter on muscle, to Dr. Anne Jabara, University of Melbourne for the section on mammary tumours, and to Dr. N. C. Palmer and Dr. J. S. Wilkinson of the University of Melbourne for material assistance and many fruitful conversations. As always, a heavy burden falls on those who convert our notes to manuscript and arrange the bibliography, a task shared and cheerfully and devotedly performed by Mrs. Sylvia Lewis and Miss Frances Douglas. We hope that we have done justice to those who have contributed illustrative material: Dr. A. Seawright, University of Queensland; Dr. D. Kradel, Pennsylvania State University; Dr. E. Karbe, University of Zurich; Dr. B. C. Easterday, National Animal Disease Laboratory at Ames; Mr. J. D. J. Harding, Central Veterinary Laboratory, Weybridge; Dr. J. Morgan, University of California; Miss Virginia Osborne, University of Sydney.

Melbourne, Australia
October, 1969

K. V. F. JUBB
PETER C. KENNEDY

Preface to the First Edition

The preface offers the opportunity to an author to present his excuses for having written the book and his justification of the content and mode of presentation. Our reasons for writing ''Pathology of Domestic Animals'' are as insubstantial but as compelling as those which committed Captain Ahab to the pursuit of Moby Dick, and we offer no excuses. Neither shall we attempt justification because a bad book cannot be justified and a good book is its own justification.

These volumes are based on our experience and on as much of the relevant literature of the world as we have been able to find and evaluate and we offer them to our colleagues and to all students of pathology in the hope that they will contribute to an understanding of animal disease. We anticipate some criticism in offering these as student texts but in doing so we indicate our confidence in teachers of pathology to guide students in the use of such volumes and in the ability of the student to profit from the exposure. Moreover, these volumes represent, it seems to us, a fair assessment of the needs of veterinary students in these times, since we realize as we should, that the knowledge of pathology possessed by most graduating students must serve them for the rest of their lives.

We should have preferred to write at greater length and in more detail of our chosen field, but practicality and economics have dictated that we can present here no more than a précis of the wealth of information that is the gift of our predecessors and contemporaries to the veterinary profession. In compensation, we have appended to each chapter an extensive but selected bibliography by the proper use of which the earnest seeker after further knowledge will be richly rewarded. Many valuable contributions from old and foreign literature will not be listed in our bibliographies, perhaps because we have failed to appreciate their significance but largely because we have not obtained access to them.

We wish to emphasize to our younger colleagues that there exist vast gaps in our present knowledge, and we hope future work will do much to fill these gaps. For any errors of established fact that appear and for errors of interpretation of published information we tender, with our apologies, a request that they be drawn to our attention. We have not always attempted to distinguish between what we know and what we think we know, and in stating our position on many matters of controversy it is inevitable that we are sometimes in error; but we do prefer to state our positions while reserving our right to change our opinions when necessary.

The aim of the scientific method is to provide understanding, and the ultimate aim in all study of disease is to understand well enough to preserve the organism and prevent the disease. But disease and the temper of the community do not wait upon the languid spirit of most scientific enquiry; in the annals of veterinary science there are many endemic and epidemic diseases concerning which a broad search for understanding is necessarily postponed in the interests of quickly finding a way to avoid the disease or to face and exert some measure of control over it. Such hastily constructed controls are often satisfactory, but seldom enough, and usually they merely stem the tide while further enquiry can be made and understanding sought. It is from pathology, viewed broadly, that understanding comes and the need is great because there are old diseases still to be contended with, others now in existence but still to be recognized, and new ones to be anticipated. The pathologist is necessarily concerned with all matters pertaining to disease and we would enjoin him to remember this and meet his responsibilities in an age when urgency disturbs the spirit of the Groves of the Academy.

We have departed somewhat from tradition in the arrangement of these volumes. General pathology is well covered in many existing textbooks and we have not taken space for it, but have restricted our discussions to systemic or special pathology. Almost all we have to say on a particular subject or specific disease is said in one place under the organ system in which it appears most appropriate, although we have waived this general rule in an attempt to make the sections devoted to genitalia and special senses self-sufficient. A few diseases which resisted our systemic classification are relegated to an appendix in Volume 2. Detailed tables of contents are included for each volume to indicate the organization of the text and our classification of the diseases of the systems.

Guelph, Ontario   K. V. F. JUBB
January, 1963   P. C. KENNEDY

Contents of
Other Volumes

CHAPTER 1

The Alimentary System

IAN K. BARKER
Ontario Veterinary College, Canada

A. A. VAN DREUMEL
Ontario Ministry of Agriculture and Food, Canada

Oral Cavity

Examination of the oral cavity should be standard procedure during any postmortem examination. To obtain a clear view of the mucous membranes, teeth, tongue, gums, and tonsils, it is essential to split the mandibular symphysis and separate the mandibles as far as possible. A thorough examination of all structures will reveal not only local lesions but often those that may be due to systemic disease. Lesions may be associated with congenital anomalies, trauma (physical and chemical), bacterial, mycotic, viral, and parasitic infections, metabolic and toxic diseases, and dysplastic and neoplastic disease. The poor nutritional state of an animal may be directly related to oral lesions that result in difficulties of prehension, mastication, or swallowing of food.

Congenital Anomalies

The development of normal facies and the oral cavity depends on the integrated development of a large number of embryonic processes. The complexity and protracted period of this development may lead to a great variety of aberrations. These are usually expressed in the newborn in the form of clefts resulting from failures of integrated growth and fusion. A common failure of fusion is that of the maxillary processes to the frontonasal process. This may leave facial fissures, uni- or bilateral primary cleft palate (formerly called harelip), or secondary cleft palate (formerly called cleft palate).

Facial clefts may involve the skin only or the deeper tissues as well. They are variously located, and not all are obviously related to normal lines of fusion. All are rare. The least uncommon is a complete cleft from one angle of the mouth to the ear of that side. This results from failure of fusion of the lateral portions of the maxillary and mandibular processes. A defect extending from a harelip to the eye results from failure of fusion of the maxillary and frontonasal processes; its least expression is superficial and a failure of closure of the nasolacrimal duct.

Primary cleft palate (harelip) includes developmental anomalies of the lips anterior to the nasal septum, columella, and premaxilla. They may be uni- or bilateral and superficial or extend into the nostril. The defect arises from incomplete fusion of the frontonasal process with the maxillary processes.

Secondary cleft palate (cleft palate, palatoschisis) (Fig. 1.1B) is often associated with primary cleft palate. The hard palate is formed, except for a small anterior contribution from the frontonasal process, by the bilateral ingrowth of the palatine shelves from the maxillary processes. At the midline, they fuse with each other and the nasal septum, except in their posterior part, which becomes the soft palate. Inadequate growth of either palatine shelf leaves a central defect that communicates between the oral and nasal cavities.

Cleft palates have been reported in most species of domestic animals. Secondary cleft palate and arthrogryposis frequently occur together in Charolais calves and appear to be hereditary (probably simple autosomal recessive). In calves, cleft palate is one of the most common anomalies. The defect is uncommon in lambs, in which it may be genetic in origin (possibly simple recessive) or associated with ingestion of *Veratrum californicum*. In swine, primary cleft palate is less common than secondary cleft palate, although the two anomalies often occur together. The defects are probably polygenic or multifactorial

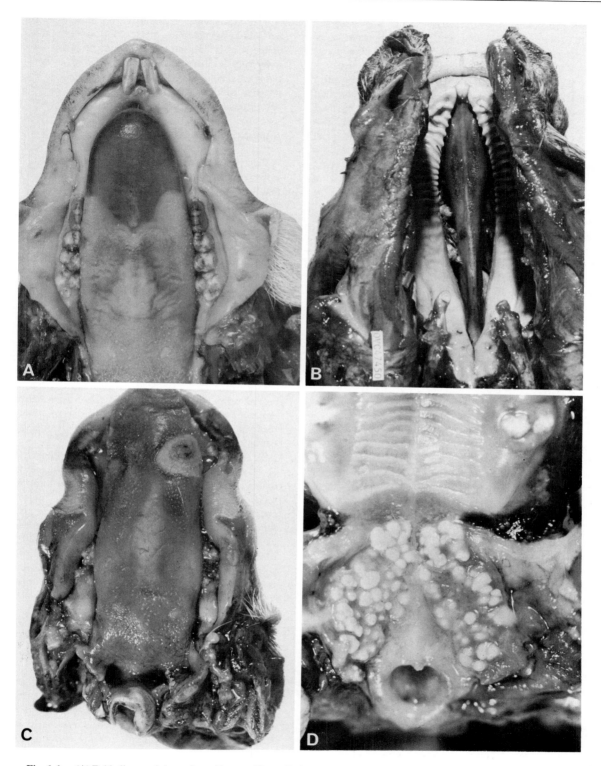

Fig. 1.1. (**A**) Epitheliogenesis imperfecta. Tongue. Pig. (**B**) Secondary cleft palate exposing the nasal cavity. Pig. (**C**) Necrotic glossitis and stomatitis. Pig. *Fusobacterium necrophorum* infection associated with trauma by needle teeth. (**D**) Suppurative tonsillitis. Piglet. Streptococci and *Escherichia coli*.

developmental anomalies in this species and also may be associated with *Crotalaria* intoxication. Secondary cleft palate occurs in Siamese cats and is thought to be hereditary in this breed, although the mode of inheritance has not been determined.

Anomalies of the growth of jaws are quite common. **Brachygnathia superior**, shortness of the maxillae, is an inherited breed characteristic among dogs and swine. It has been reported in the Large White or Yorkshire breed. The condition is progressive with age, resulting in malapposition of the incisor and cheek teeth, which interferes with prehension and mastication. In swine, brachygnathia superior may be confused with atrophic rhinitis. In Jersey cattle, brachygnathia superior occurs as a simple autosomal recessive trait. It may, in any species, be associated with chondrodysplasia.

Brachygnathia inferior or micrognathia, shortness of the mandibles, may be a mild to lethal defect in cattle and sheep and is a breed characteristic of long-nosed dogs. Micrognathia is a common defect in calves. It is inherited, probably as a simple autosomal recessive trait. There is a higher incidence in males. In Aberdeen Angus calves the defect may occur concurrently with cerebellar hypoplasia, and with osteopetrosis in this and other breeds (see Bones and Joints, Volume 1). Mild brachygnathia inferior, termed "parrot mouth," is a common conformational defect in horses.

Prognathism refers to an abnormal prolongation of the mandibles. It too is rather common especially in sheep. It may develop with recovery from calcium deficiency in this species (see Bones and Joints, Volume 1). The malformation is relative, and it is not always easy to determine whether the jaw is absolutely long or merely apparently so, relative to a mild brachygnathia superior.

Agnathia is a mandibulofacial malformation characterized by absence of the lower jaw, due to failure of development of the first branchial arch and associated structures. The defect is one of the most common anomalies in lambs but is rare in cattle. Associated malformations in lambs may include ateloprosopia (incomplete development of the face), microglossia or aglossia, and atresia of the oral pharynx. Concurrent anomalies affecting other body systems may also be evident.

Epitheliogenesis imperfecta is an anomaly causing widespread defects in cutaneous epithelium that also affects the epithelial lining of the oral cavity, especially the tongue (Fig. 1.1A) (see diseases of Skin and Appendages, Volume 1). The condition is characterized by irregular, well-demarcated, red, ulcerated areas in the oral mucosa. Histologically, these consist of abruptly ulcerated areas in the squamous mucosa with inflammation of the submucosal connective tissues. The anomaly occurs in most species and is inherited as a simple autosomal recessive character in cattle, horses, and pigs; the mode of inheritance is unknown in the other species.

A lethal glossopharyngeal hereditary defect, termed "bird tongue" and caused by a simple recessive autosomal gene has been reported in dogs. The breed in which the condition occurred was not revealed. The affected pups have a narrow tongue, especially the anterior half where the margins are folded medially onto the dorsal surface. The pups are unable to swallow. The muscle fibers of the affected tongues are normal histologically.

There are several hereditary skin conditions in animals that have minor involvement of the lips and oral mucosa, such as epidermolysis bullosa simplex in collie dogs, ovine epidermolysis bullosa in Suffolk and South Dorset Down sheep, and familial acantholysis of Aberdeen Angus calves. The reader is referred to the Skin and Appendages (Volume 1) for detailed descriptions of these conditions.

Diseases of Teeth and Dental Tissues

Dental examinations in animals are usually cursory, except to assess age, but dental disease is common and often is the factor that limits the useful life span, especially of sheep. The "borderland of embryology and pathology" is never more nebulous than it is for teeth, and the comments on dental development and anatomy given below are intended to assist the understanding of dental disease.

Teeth develop from horseshoe-shaped thickenings in the oral ectoderm called dental laminae. Neural crest cells beneath the laminae induce formation of tooth buds, which generate the enamel organs. These epithelial structures grow into the underlying ectomesenchyme and organize it to form dental papillae, which they enclose like a cap. Surrounding both is another mesenchymal condensation, the dental sac. The inner enamel epithelium of the enamel organ induces differentiation of odontoblasts from the mesenchyme of the papilla. They produce dentin, which in turn induces enamel formation by the inner enamel epithelium. Formation of dentin is essential for formation of enamel. These inductive interactions of epithelium and mesenchyme are considered to be important in the histodifferentiation of some tumors of dental tissues.

The free edge of the enamel organ extends beyond the enamel–dentin junction, and this extension is called Hertwig's epithelial root sheath. It molds dental papilla to form the root or apex of the tooth. Subsequently it fragments, allowing mesenchymal cells from the dental sac to contact the root dentin, differentiate into cementoblasts, and deposit cementum on the dentin. Remnants of the root sheath are called epithelial rests of Malassez. They persist in the periodontal ligament and may give rise to tumors or cysts. They may be important in the induction or repair of cementum, and in periodontal reattachment following injury. If cells of the root sheath adhere to the dentin, they may produce enamel pearls.

Once the dental lamina has produced the buds of the permanent teeth, it degenerates. Epithelial remnants persist as epithelial pearls or islands in the gingiva and jaws. These remnants also may give rise to tumors and cysts.

There are important differences between the brachydont teeth of humans, carnivores, and swine, in which the enamel is restricted to the tooth crown, and the hypsodont teeth of herbivores. In hypsodont teeth, enamel extends far down on the roots and is invaginated into the dentin to form infundibula. Also, the hypsodont teeth of herbivores, except the mandibular premolars of ruminants, are covered by cementum that more or less fills the infundibula. Exceptions to these rules are provided by the tusks of boars, which are hypsodont but not covered by cementum, and by ruminant incisors, which are brachydont but do have enamel covering part of the root dentin.

The three hard tissues of teeth are dentin, enamel, and cementum. **Dentin** is light yellow and constitutes most of the tooth. It consists of about 35% organic matter and 65% mineral. Thus its composition is similar to bone, and like bone it contains type I collagen. Dentin is produced by columnar cells with basal nuclei called odontoblasts, which differentiate from mesenchyme of the dental papilla. Initially it is unmineralized (predentin), but later mineralized. The odontoblasts move away from the dentin–enamel junction, gradually encroaching on the pulp cavity as they produce dentin. Each odontoblast has a process extending into the dentin, encased in a dentinal tubule, that arborizes at the dentin–enamel junction. The process also anastomoses with the processes of other odontoblasts. Dentinal tubules are visible in histologic sections, but the anastomoses are not. Except for the processes, and nerve endings in the dentin near the pulp, dentin is acellular.

Normal dentin contains incremental or imbrication lines of von Ebner, which are fine basophilic lines running at right angles to the dentinal tubules. They represent normal variations in the structure and mineralization of dentin. Sublethal injury caused by certain infections, metabolic stresses, or toxic states may injure the odontoblasts, which then produce accentuated incremental lines known as the contour lines of Owen. Sometimes, irregular zones of unmineralized or poorly mineralized dentin form between foci of normal mineralization. These are zones of interglobular dentin, which may be caused by hypophosphatemia.

Odontoblasts normally are active throughout life, producing layers of secondary dentin that often contain fewer dentinal tubules than primary dentin. Reparative dentin is produced locally in response to injury and contains a limited number of twisted tubules and sometimes a few odontoblasts, which soon die. Sclerotic (transparent) dentin is formed when dentinal tubules are occluded by calcium salts. The junctions between primary, secondary, and reparative dentin are usually demarcated by basophilic lines.

Enamel has about 5% organic matter and 95% mineral. It is produced by the tall, columnar ameloblasts of the inner enamel epithelium. Enamel is produced in the form of prisms or rods, cemented together by a matrix. Mineralization begins as soon as it is formed and is a two-stage process, somewhat similar to that in bone but much more rapid. The cells of the inner enamel epithelium also move away from the dentin–enamel junction as the tooth is formed, but unlike odontoblasts, they do not have processes. Enamel is hard, dense, brittle, and permeable and is translucent and white. Mature enamel is not present in demineralized sections, but some of the matrix of immature enamel may be visible near ameloblasts of developing teeth.

Ameloblasts are very sensitive to environmental changes. Normal enamel contains incremental lines of Retzius, which are analogous to the incremental lines of von Ebner in dentin and also reflect variations in structure and mineralization. The incremental lines are accentuated during periods of metabolic stress. More severe injury, in fluorosis or infections by some viruses (Fig. 1.2A,B), can produce focal hypoplasia or aplasia of enamel.

Formation of enamel ends before tooth eruption. The inner enamel epithelium then merges with the cells of the underlying stratum intermedium and the outer enamel epithelium to form the reduced enamel epithelium. It protects the enamel of the formed tooth prior to eruption and digests the connective tissue separating it from the gingival epithelium. Fusion of the two epithelia is necessary for eruption to occur. Degeneration of this protective layer permits connective tissue to contact the enamel, and there may be resorption of enamel or deposition of a layer of cementum on it. This normally occurs during odontogenesis in horses.

Cementum is an avascular, bonelike substance, produced by cementoblasts; it contains about 55% organic and 45% inorganic matter. In general, the dentin of brachydont teeth is covered by cementum wherever it is not covered by enamel. When dentin formation has begun in the root, degeneration of Hertwig's epithelial root sheath begins and permits mesenchymal cells from the dental sac to contact dentin. They differentiate into cementoblasts, which produce cementoid and later mineralize it. Some layers of cementum do not contain cells (acellular cementum), but in other layers cementocytes are enclosed in lacunae. Sharpey's fibers from alveolar bone are embedded in the cementum. Cementum is more resistant to resorption than bone, and unlike bone, normally is not resorbed and replaced as it ages; instead, a new layer of cementum is deposited on top of the old layer. In some pathologic conditions cementum is resorbed; subsequently, cellular or acellular cementum is deposited, more or less repairing the defect.

Hypercementosis is abnormal thickening of cementum and may involve part or all of one or many teeth. When extra cementum improves the functional properties of teeth, it is called cementum hypertrophy; if not, it is called cementum hyperplasia. Extensive hyperplasia often is associated with chronic inflammation of the dental root.

The periodontal ligament is a very cellular, well-vascularized connective tissue that develops from the dental sac. The **periodontium** comprises the periodontal ligament, gingival lamina propria, cementum, and alveolar bone. The ligament supports the tooth and adjusts to its movement during growth. It is well supplied with nerves and lymphatics, which drain into alveolar bone. The periodontal ligament also is a source of the cells that remodel alveolar bone and, in disease, cementum.

Epithelial rests of Malassez are present in the periodontal ligament and are particularly numerous in the incisor region of sheep. In all species, they may proliferate and become cystic when there is inflammation of the periodontium. The periodontium is also a site of origin of tumors. The periodontal ligament normally is visible in radiographs as a radiolucent line between tooth and alveolar bone. In prolonged hyperparathyroidism, alveolar bone is resorbed and the ligament is no longer outlined radiographically, a change referred to as "loss of the lamina dura."

Developmental Anomalies of Teeth

Anodontia, absence of teeth, is inherited in calves, probably as a sex-linked recessive trait in males, and is associated with skin defects. **Oligodontia**, fewer teeth than normal, occurs sporadically in horses, cats, and dogs, and also as an inherited trait in dogs. In brachycephalic breeds, the cheek teeth are deficient; in toy breeds, the incisors are deficient. **Pseudooligodontia** and

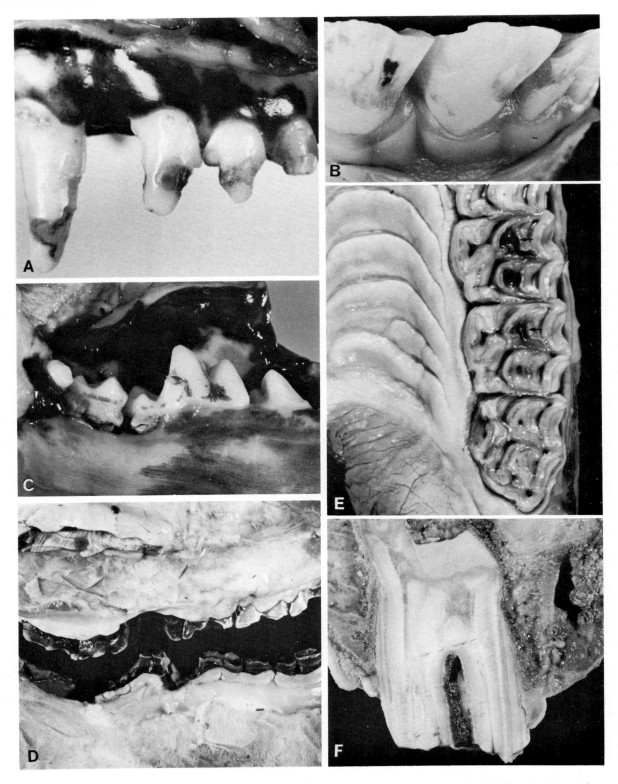

Fig. 1.2.   (**A**) Focal enamel hypoplasia, sequel to canine distemper. Dog.   (**B**) Enamel hypoplasia. Calf. Sequel to intrauterine infection by bovine virus diarrhea virus. (Courtesy of R. B. Miller.)   (**C**) Periodontal disease. Dog. Marked gingival recession with exposure of roots of the molar teeth.   (**D**) Irregular wear of teeth. Horse.   (**E**) Infundibular necrosis of first and second maxillary molars (arrows). Horse. Necrosis confined to cement lakes.   (**F**) Section through (**E**), showing black discoloration of infundibulum.

pseudoanodontia result from failed eruption. These defects may be associated with bone modeling defects in *grey* lethal mice with osteopetrosis. Delayed eruption of permanent teeth occurs in Lhasa Apso and Shih Tsu dogs. **Polyodontia**, excessive teeth, occurs in brachycephalic dogs; the incisors are involved, and the defect is probably related to breeding for broad muzzles. A high incidence of canine polyodontia, involving particularly an extra maxillary premolar, has been reported from the Netherlands. Polyodontia also occurs in horses and cats, involving either incisors or cheek teeth. **Pseudopolyodontia** is retention of deciduous teeth after eruption of the permanent dentition. It occurs in horses, cats, and dogs, especially in the miniature breeds.

Heterotopic polyodontia is an extra tooth, or teeth, outside the dental arcades. The best known example is the "ear tooth" of horses, which develops in a branchiogenic cyst. The cysts originate from failure of closure of the first branchial cleft, or from the inclusion of cellular rests in this area. They are lined by a stratified mucous- or cutaneous-type epithelium and may contain one or more teeth, either loosely attached in the cyst wall or deeply embedded in the petrous temporal bone. The tooth is derived from misplaced tooth germ of the first branchial arch, which is displaced toward the ear with the first branchial cleft. The cysts form in the parotid region and may fistulate to the exterior. They are occasionally bilateral, and rarely the tooth may form a pedunculated mass enclosed by skin and attached by a pedicle to the skin of the head. Heterotopic polyodontia also occurs in cattle, dogs, pigs, and sheep.

Malformation and malpositioning of teeth accompany abnormalities of the jaw bones. Aberdeen Angus and Hereford calves with congenital osteopetrosis have brachygnathia inferior, malformed mandibles, and impacted cheek teeth (see Bones and Joints, Volume 1). Impacted molars occur as an inherited lethal in shorthorns; an association with osteopetrosis apparently has not been investigated in this breed.

Odontogenic cysts are epithelium-lined cysts derived from cell rests of Malassez, cell rests of dental laminae, reduced enamel epithelium, or malformed enamel organs. **Dentigerous cysts** are, by definition, cysts that contain part or all of a tooth, which often is malformed. Of the odontogenic cysts just listed, all except those derived from cell rests of Malassez are potentially dentigerous. (The rests of Malassez are the probable source of periodontal cysts.) Dentigerous cysts originating in malformed enamel organs should include malformed teeth, since development of enamel is incomplete until the organ degenerates. Those teeth in cysts of reduced enamel epithelium or rests of dental laminae are not necessarily abnormal. The affected teeth probably "erupt" into the preformed cysts. Dentigerous cysts enclose at least the crown of the tooth, but may include it all. The most common form of odontogenic dentigerous cysts in animals are those involving the vestigial wolf teeth of horses and the vestigial canines, especially of mares. The smaller cysts appear as tumors of the gums, while some of the larger ones may cause swelling of the jaw or adjacent maxillary sinus. Dentigerous cysts of animals are not as destructive as those in humans, in which they are regarded as the most common benign destructive lesion of the skeleton.

The ear tooth of horses is probably the most common nono-dontogenic dentigerous cyst (see heterotopic polyodontia, above). Occasionally, true dentigerous cysts form when a tumor prevents normal eruption or when there is maleruption due to odontodystrophy.

Cystic dental inclusions about vestigial supernumerary teeth also occur in the juxtamolar positions in cattle but are insignificant. These too may be dentigerous, or they may be primordial cysts developed before the stage of enamel formation, and hence containing no mineralized tooth structures. Either type of cyst may give rise to ameloblastomas.

A high incidence of dentigerous cysts involving incisors occurs in some sheep flocks in Scotland and New Zealand.

Permanent teeth are unique in that their development continues for a long time after birth. Thus inflammatory and metabolic disease of postnatal life can produce hypoplasia of dentin and enamel. Hypoplasia of enamel of deciduous teeth occurs in some calves with intrauterine bovine virus diarrhea infection. Extreme fragility of deciduous teeth is a feature of bovine osteogenesis imperfecta, but the variety of inherited dentinal dysplasias and enamel anomalies that occur in humans is not recognized in domestic animals.

Degenerative Conditions of Teeth and Dental Tissue

PIGMENTATION OF TEETH. Normal enamel is white and shiny, but normal cementum is off-white to light yellow and normal dentin is slightly darker yellow. Depending on the tooth, or the part of the tooth being examined, the normal color may be any one of these. Normal enamel is never discolored. Hypoplastic enamel of chronic fluorosis is discolored yellow through brown to almost black. Discoloration of brachydont teeth results from pigmentation of dentin, which is then visible through the semitransparent enamel, or pigmentation of the cementum of the root. Dentin may be colored red-brown by pulpal hemorrhages or inflammation, gray-green in putrid pulpitis, and yellow in icterus. Congenital erythropoietic porphyrias of calves, cats, and swine discolor the dentin red in young animals (pink tooth) and darker brown in adults, although in swine the discoloration may disappear with aging. Transient porphyria with pink discoloration of teeth has been reported in a dog.

Yellow to brown discoloration of teeth, and bright yellow fluorescence in ultraviolet light, due to deposition of tetracycline antibiotics in mineralizing dentin, enamel, and probably cementum, occurs in all species. Treatment of the pregnant dam may cause staining of deciduous teeth in the offspring. Tetracyclines are toxic to ameloblasts in the late differentiation and early secretion stages and, at high dose rate, may produce enamel hypoplasia.

Black discoloration of ruminant cheek teeth is extremely common and is caused by impregnation of mineral salts with chlorophyll and porphyrin pigments from herbage.

DENTAL ATTRITION. The mature conformation of teeth is largely the outcome of opposed growth and wear, and the degree of wear depends on the type of tooth, the species of animal, and the matter chewed. Wear is most evident in herbivores, and irregularities of wear are perhaps the most common dental abnormalities. In general, with normal occlusion and use, the extraalveolar portion of the tooth does not shorten; instead, its length is maintained initially by growth (the period of growth depending on the species) then by hypertrophy of the root cementum and proliferation of alveolar bone (which serves to push the tooth out), and finally by senile atrophy of the alveolar processes. Cementum hypertrophy and alveolar atrophy may result in loss of teeth in senility, or if combined with subnormal wear, produce teeth that in old age are excessively long. Normal wear of the complicated cheek teeth of horses and cattle causes smoothing of the occlusal surfaces. As soon as wear of enamel exposes the dentin, which being softer wears more rapidly, secondary dentin is deposited to protect the pulp. In time, this may fill the pulp cavity and cause death of the tooth.

Abnormalities of wearing are most common in herbivores (Fig. 1.2D). Subnormal wear, due to loss of the opposing tooth, occurs in oligodontia, abnormal spacing of adjacent teeth, and acquired loss of teeth; it results in abnormal lengthening. Such elongated teeth may grow against the opposing gum or, if deviated, into an adjacent soft structure such as cheek or lip. These teeth usually wear in abnormal places because complete loss of antagonism is unusual, because the upper and lower arcades do not coincide exactly, and the coincidence is further reduced by the displacement of chewing. Incomplete longitudinal coincidence of the molar arcades allows irregular wear and hook formation on the first and last cheek teeth. Abnormal wear due to abnormal chewing is caused by voluntary, as in painful conditions, or mechanical impairment of jaw movement. Lateral movements of the jaws without the normal rotary grinding movements allow the ridges of the teeth of herbivores to become accentuated. Steep angulation of the occlusal surfaces results from inadequate lateral movement of the jaws, and sharp edges form on the buccal aspect of the maxillary teeth and the lingual aspect of the mandibular teeth. This may be unilateral when the animal chews with only one side of its mouth, the other side then being affected. The teeth wear progressively sharper and pass each other like shear blades, hence the term ''shear mouth.'' Subnormal resistance to wear on the part of the molar teeth is common and results in ''weave mouth'' or ''step mouth,'' in which successive teeth in an arcade wear at different rates. The weave or step form of the antagonistic arcade is reversed so that the teeth of the two arcades interdigitate. This pattern of attrition is caused by variation in the hardness of opposing teeth, and usually is caused by intermittent odontodystrophy. Opposing teeth of the upper and lower jaws do not develop at the same time, thus discontinuous nutritional deficiencies often result in unequal wear. Certain vices, such as crib biting, also produce abnormal wear. In severely worn ruminant incisors a central black core may be visible, which is secondary dentin deposited in the pulp cavity. It is not carious but stains darker than the surrounding primary dentin.

ODONTODYSTROPHIES. Odontodystrophies are diseases of teeth caused by nutritional, metabolic, and toxic insults. They are manifest by changes in the hard tissues of the teeth and their supporting structures. Lesions of enamel and dentin are emphasized here. The most prominent affects of odontodystrophies appear in enamel, and lesions of enamel are most significant because they are irreparable.

Formation of enamel occurs in a set pattern. It begins at the occlusal surface and progresses toward the root. Mineral maturation occurs in the same sequence, but for each level it begins at the dentin–enamel junction and moves toward the ameloblast. Deleterious influences have their most severe affects on those ameloblasts that are forming and mineralizing enamel. Depending of the severity of the insult, ameloblasts may produce no enamel, a little enamel, or poorly mineralized enamel. Removal of the insult permits those ameloblasts not yet active to begin making normal enamel. Thus enamel defects vary in severity from isolated opaque spots or pits on the surface to deep and irregular, horizontal indentations. These defects are most clearly seen on the incisor teeth and canine teeth and are usually bilaterally symmetric. Similar lesions are also produced by infectious agents that injure ameloblasts, such as the viruses of canine distemper and bovine virus diarrhea (Fig. 1.2A,B).

Odontoblasts are susceptible to many of the same influences as ameloblasts, but they can be replenished from the undifferentiated cells of the dental pulp. Thus lesions in actively forming dentin may be repaired, while those in enamel are permanent.

Because of their close anatomic association with the jaws, teeth are very susceptible to disruption in the harmony of growth. This harmonious arrangement often is upset in the odontodystrophies and osteodystrophies and leads to malocclusion and anomalous development of teeth.

There are several nutritional and toxic conditions that produce odontodystrophy. Fluorine poisoning is exemplary (see metabolic diseases of bone, in Bones and Joints, Volume 1). In vitamin A deficiency, ameloblasts do not differentiate normally, and their organizing ability is disturbed. As a result, odontoblastic differentiation is abnormal. Several lesions develop, including enamel hypoplasia and hypomineralization, cellular, vascularized dentin (osteodentin), and retarded or obviated eruption.

Calcium deficiency retards eruption and causes enamel hypoplasia and mild dentin hypoplasia. Teeth formed during the period of deficiency are very susceptible to wear. Recovery from prolonged calcium deficiency results in malocclusion due to inferior prognathia in sheep. This reflects inadequate maxillary, but normal mandibular repair during the recovery phase.

Phosphorus deficiency, combined with vitamin D deficiency, depresses dentin formation slightly but has virtually no effect on enamel, at least not in sheep. Hypophosphatemia is associated with formation of interglobular dentin in humans. Malocclusion and abnormalities of bite in rachitic sheep are secondary to mandibular deformity.

Severe, experimental malnutrition also produces malocclusion. Recovery from malnutrition does not correct the lesion and in addition is associated with misshapen, malformed teeth, oligodontia, and polyodontia.

The major effects of odontodystrophies in herbivores are malocclusion and/or accelerated attrition. Sometimes a high incidence of these abnormalities is attributable to one of the causes discussed above, but often they are idiopathic. Most of the lesions described in experimental odontodystrophies also occur in natural diseases. A syndrome of dental abnormalities of sheep on the North Island of New Zealand is characterized by excessive wear of deciduous teeth, maleruption and excessive wear of permanent teeth, periodontal disease involving permanent teeth, and development of dentigerous cysts involving permanent incisors. Mandibular osteopathy is also present. All animals more than 5 years old are culled for dental problems. The odontodystrophy (and osteodystrophy) possibly is caused by deficiencies of calcium and copper, and perhaps other nutrients such as protein and energy. Sheep from an affected flock, pastured elsewhere, have minimal lesions.

This syndrome exemplifies the naturally occurring odontodystrophies in that it probably has a complex pathogenesis and is associated with an osteodystrophy. The latter association is to be expected since bones and teeth usually are susceptible to the same insults.

Infectious and Inflammatory Diseases of Teeth and Periodontium

The role of viruses in enamel hypoplasia is mentioned above. Bacterial plaque is discussed below along with other tooth-accumulated materials.

Tooth enamel is covered by a translucent pellicle, which is formed by selective adsorption of salivary constituents and which is essential to the development of plaque. **Dental plaque** is a dense, nonmineralized, bacterial mass, firmly adherent to tooth surfaces, that resists removal by salivary flow. Formation of plaque involves adhesion of bacteria to the pellicle and adhesion of bacteria to each other. Only organisms with the ability to adhere to pellicle can initiate the formation of plaque; those that cannot are removed by oral secretions and mechanical action.

The bacteria in plaque are usually Gram-positive. Most are streptococci and *Actinomyces* spp., which form an organized array on the tooth surface. Some plaque-forming bacteria synthesize extracellular polymers that constitute the matrix of the plaque and permit adhesion between organisms of the same species. Some utilize polymers derived from host secretions to adhere to the pellicle, while others attach to bacteria of a different species already fixed to the tooth. Plaque increases in mass with time, and its composition becomes more complex as Gramnegative bacteria join the streptococci and actinomycetes that initiated plaque formation.

Plaque is metabolically active. It utilizes dietary carbohydrates to produce the adhesive polymers and, as energy sources, for maintenance and the production of various enzymes and mediators of inflammation. Dental plaque is important because it initiates the development of dental caries and periodontal disease. Enamel may harbor extensive deposits of supragingival plaque that are virtually invisible unless treated with a disclosing solution.

Dental calculus (tartar) is mineralized plaque. The mineral mainly comes from saliva. In horses, it is predominantly calcium carbonate; in dogs, calcium phosphate. Calculus is often found in old dogs and cats, occasionally in horses and sheep, and rarely in other species. The distribution is often uneven, but it is most abundant next to the orifices of salivary ducts. Calculus on horses' teeth is chalky and easily removed. In dogs, it is hard, firmly attached, and often discolored. Red-brown to black calculus with a metallic sheen develops in pastured sheep and goats. It usually involves all the incisors, principally on the neck of the buccal surface. Minor amounts are common along the gum–tooth junction of the molar teeth, but occasionally, larger (up to 2.0 cm), hard, black, rounded concretions may protrude from between opposed surfaces of the premolars.

Materia alba is a mixture of salivary proteins, desquamated epithelial cells, disintegrating leukocytes, and bacteria that adheres to teeth. The bacteria are not organized, and materia alba is easily removed. It is distinct from dental plaque, and from food debris, which also accumulates between uncleaned teeth.

DENTAL CARIES.　Dental caries is a disease of the hard tissues of teeth, characterized by demineralization of the inorganic part and enzymatic degradation of the organic matrix. This definition permits the inclusion of equine infundibular necrosis as a form of caries (see below).

Dental caries is the principal disease of teeth in humans up to about the age of 30 years. It is then superseded by periodontal disease. Caries is common in horses and sheep but rare in dogs and cats.

There are two types of caries, "pit" or "fissure" caries and smooth-surface caries. The first type develops in irregularities or indentations, usually on the occlusal surface of the tooth, which trap food and bacteria. Plaque is not essential for initiation of this form of caries, of which equine infundibular necrosis is an example. Smooth-surface caries usually occurs on proximal (adjacent) surfaces of teeth, typically just below contact points or around the neck, and requires dental plaque for its initiation.

The organic acids, principally lactic, that initiate demineralization are produced by bacterial fermentation of dietary carbohydrates. In smooth-surface caries, plaque produces the acid and maintains a low pH on the surface of the tooth. Progression of lesions depends on various factors such as salivary pH and hardness and resistance to demineralization of enamel. The enzymes that lyse the organic matrix probably are produced by plaque but may be derived from leukocytes, for which plaque is chemotactic. Carious enamel loses its sheen and becomes dull, white, and pocked. When dentin is exposed, it becomes brown or black. Dentin is softer and more readily demineralized than enamel, and a pinpoint lesion in enamel may lead to a large defect when the carious process reaches the dentin.

In horses and dogs, caries develops most often on the occlusal surface of the maxillary first molar. In sheep, the proximal surfaces of mandibular teeth are usually affected, and caries is commonly accompanied by periodontitis. Cats, whose teeth do not have retaining centers where food can collect, sometimes develop caries-like lesions of the neck region of cheek teeth. In some cases they are associated with hypervitaminosis A. These lesions seem to be distinct from conventional caries, but their pathogenesis is not known.

The enamel invaginations (infundibula) in the cheek teeth of horses normally are filled with cementum before the teeth erupt. Filling proceeds from the occlusal surface toward the apex, but often is not completed before eruption. At this time the blood supply is cut off, and ischemic necrosis of any residual cementogenic tissue in the infundibula occurs. The deficiency of cementum is called hypoplasia. Anterior infundibula are affected more frequently than posterior, and the first molar more often than other teeth (Fig. 1.2E,F).

Teeth with incompletely filled infundibula may accumulate food material and bacteria, and in some animals the necrotic area expands to involve all the cementum and the adjacent enamel and dentin. Decay of the mineralized tissues sometimes progresses to coalescence of the cement lakes, fracture of the tooth, root abscess, and empyema of the paranasal sinuses. The incidence of infundibular necrosis increases with age, and 80–100% of horses more than 12 years old may have the lesion. Most are without signs, and in most the lesion does not progress. Inflammation of the dental pulp, in horses and in other species, may result from direct expansion of caries, or from penetration of bacteria and bacterial degradation products along the dentinal tubules. Production of reparative dentin in the pulp cavity is expected.

PULPITIS.   The dental pulp is derived from the dental papilla. It is surrounded by odontoblasts and dentin, except at the apical foramen, through which vessels and nerves pass. Pulp is a loose syncytium of stellate fibrocytes and contains histiocytes and undifferentiated mesenchymal cells. The latter are odontoblastic precursors.

The apical foramen is narrow, and this predisposes to vascular occlusion, ischemic necrosis of the pulp, and death of the tooth in pathologic processes. Production of abundant secondary dentin and reparative dentin can do this, but the usual cause is inflammation. Pulp is the only vascular tissue of the tooth, and along with the periodontium, the only site of conventional inflammation. Pulpitis is always related to infection, the effector bacteria or their products entering through fractures; carious perforations, especially in teeth with enamel defects; perforations resulting from abnormal wear; periodontitis; and possibly hematogenously. In herbivores the pulp is divided by enamel foldings, inflammation usually is limited to one division and is usually purulent. Very mild pulpitis may heal, but usually it terminates in necrosis, suppuration, or gangrene.

Inflammation of the pulp may extend to the periodontium and the jaws. Osteomyelitis of the jaws is a complication of clipping the tusks of piglets. Some chronic inflammations are confined to the periodontium and become slowly expansive, spherical granulomas about the root apex (root granulomas). Occasionally these granulomas are enclosed by an epithelial cyst (periodontal cyst) derived from cell rests of Malassez. The epithelium contains plasma cells, and the combination may have a protective role in periapical sepsis.

PERIODONTAL DISEASE.   Periodontal disease is the most common chronic disease of humans, the most common dental disease of sheep and dogs, and an important problem in horses, ruminants, and cats. Although there are minor differences between species, in general, periodontal disease begins as plaque-associated gingivitis and may progress through gingival recession and loss of alveolar bone to chronic periodontitis and exfoliation of teeth.

The gingival sulcus or crevice is an invagination formed by the gingiva as it joins with the tooth surface at the time of eruption. Clinically normal animals have a few lymphocytes, plasma cells, and macrophages under the crevicular epithelium of the gingiva, which forms the outer wall of the crevice, and under the junctional epithelium, which is apposed to the enamel of the tooth.

Clinical gingivitis usually is initiated by accumulation of plaque in the crevice, but may be associated with impaction of feed, especially seeds, between teeth. The gingivitis initially is characterized by increased leukocytes and fluid in the gingival crevice, then by acute exudative inflammation and accumulation of plasma cells, lymphocytes, macrophages, and neutrophils in the marginal gingiva. Marked loss of gingival collagen occurs in a few days due to the activity of enzymes from neutrophil lysosomes, or possibly from plaque. Grossly, the gingiva is red. Acute gingivitis may become quiescent, with lymphocyte aggregations beneath the junctional epithelium.

Continuation and exacerbations of the inflammation cause apical recession of the tooth–gingiva attachment, and resorption of alveolar bone. If gingival recession precedes bone loss, the sulcus is deepened to form a periodontal pocket, which is the site of chronic active inflammation (Fig. 1.2C). When gingival recession is accompanied by concomitant loss of alveolar bone and gingival collagen, pockets do not form. In either case, destruction of the periodontium and resorption of alveolar bone, cementum, and root dentin leads to exfoliation of teeth. In dogs, pocket formation is quite unpredictable and may be present on one root of a tooth and absent on the other. Gingivitis in dogs is unusually proliferative, the gingiva being replaced by collagen-poor, highly vascular granulation tissue, which appears as a red, rolled edge next to the tooth. Bone loss in dogs is often more severe at the bifurcation of two-rooted teeth than in interproximal areas. Resorption of bone is associated with osteitis as the inflammation extends from the periodontium into alveolar bone. In dogs, the premolars and, to a lesser extent, the first molars and central incisors are most severely affected, while the second molars and mandibular canines are quite resistant.

In sheep, periodontal disease may involve all teeth, but the effects are most severe on the incisors, and periodontal disease is a major cause of premature exfoliation. Sheep develop acute gingivitis during tooth eruption, in association with accumulation of subgingival plaque around the tooth. Chronic gingivitis ensues, and on farms with a high incidence of "broken mouth," this progresses to chronic active periodontal disease.

A major part of chronic periodontal disease is resorption of alveolar bone, which modifies the attachment site of the periodontal ligament. Evidence that periodontal disease in humans and other animals is primarily a nutritional disease, and that the bone resorption is caused by hyperparathyroidism, has been presented but is not generally accepted. It seems reasonable, however, that the less bone that is present when the disease is initiated, the more rapid the progression of this aspect of the disease.

The sequelae of suppurative periodontitis are many, being variations on a theme of osteomyelitis. The osteomyelitis frequently leads to the development of a fistula. If the mandible is involved, the fistula usually develops on the ventral margin. If the maxillary molars are involved, fistulation may occur into the maxillary sinus. If the premolars are involved, fistulation may develop into the nasal cavity or externally. In dogs, involvement of the canine teeth may produce internal or external fistulas, and involvement of the maxillary carnassials usually produces a fistula beneath the eye, and orbital inflammation. Fistulation may be prevented for some time or permanently by ossifying periostitis over the involved bone. Fistulas in the upper jaw tend to be persistent. In the lower jaw, they may heal, usually with extensive deposition of new bone. Occasionally, especially in horses, chronic mild periodontitis may be confined by the periodontium, which is, however, expanded by granulation tissue to form a root granuloma. Under the same circumstances there may be hyperplastic exostosis of the cementum.

Diseases of the Buccal Cavity and Mucosa

Pigmentation

Melanotic pigmentation is normal and common in most breeds of animals and increases with age. It may be irregular, or the mucosa may be entirely pigmented. Diffuse, yellow discoloration may be seen in icterus.

Circulatory Disturbances

Examination of the mucous membranes is an essential detail in any clinical or autopsy examination. Pallor may indicate anemia but is misleading in a cadaver. In cyanosis, the mucosa is a dark reddish blue color. The mucosae are muddy in methemoglobinemia. Congestion and edematous swelling of the tongue and buccal mucosa are specific lesions of bluetongue of sheep. An acute congestion and cyanosis associated with ulceration is common in dogs and sometimes in cats in chronic uremia. Hemorrhages are indicative of septicemia, and larger ones may accompany local inflammation, trauma, and the hemorrhagic diatheses. Petechiae on the ventral surface of the tongue and frenulum in horses are consistent with equine infectious anemia or other thrombocytopenic or purpuric conditions. The active hyperemia that gives the diffuse, pink coloration to the mucosa in diffuse stomatitis disappears immediately at death, so that at autopsy the inflamed mucosa is disappointingly blanched.

Foreign Bodies in the Oral Cavity

The presence of feed in the mouth of a cadaver is abnormal. In most cases it is attributable to disease that results in paralysis of deglutition or semiconsciousness. It is common in horses with encephalitis, leukoencephalomalacia, and hepatic encephalopathy. The food in such cases is usually poorly masticated and readily differentiated from that refluxed postmortem. Bones or other large foreign bodies lodged in the pharynx of cattle suggest pica of phosphorus deficiency. They may cause asphyxiation or pressure necrosis in the wall of the pharynx. Large portions of root crops may also lodge in the pharynx. In dogs, bones, sticks, or balls may be found. The bones and sticks tend to be wedged across the mouth behind the carnassial teeth. In this species, too, a foreign-body glossitis occurs, caused by plant fibers, burrs, or quills that become deeply embedded and provoke exuberant granulomas. These must be differentiated from neoplasms.

Sharp foreign bodies that cause laceration of the mucosa predispose to necrotic and deep stomatitis. Grass grains and awns frequently impact between the retracted gingival margin and teeth in periodontitis of ruminants and exacerbate the local initial lesion, perhaps predisposing to the development of osteomyelitis. Swine have a diverticulum of the pharynx in the posterior wall immediately above the esophagus, and barley awns and other rough plant fibers occasionally lodge here and penetrate the pharynx. This occurs mainly in young pigs, and death follows pharyngeal cellulitis. Similar problems occur in sheep, following improper use of drenching guns.

Inflammations of the Oral Cavity

Inflammatory processes of the oral cavity may be diffuse (stomatitis) or localized predominantly in certain regions to produce, if the pharynx is involved, pharyngitis; the tongue, glossitis; the gums, gingivitis; the tonsils, tonsillitis (Fig. 1.1D); and the soft palate, angina. Lesions limited to the mucosa of the oral cavity are termed superficial stomatitides. Processes seated in connective tissues of the mouth, the deep stomatitides, are usually sequelae to transient superficial lesions.

Superficial Stomatitis

Inflammatory changes may be associated with ingestion of irritating chemicals such as caustic or toxic compounds. An example is paraquat, a herbicide, which may cause a severe erosive stomatitis in dogs. Electrical burns are occasionally seen in puppies or kittens that chew through electrical wires. It is often not possible to differentiate the cause of diffuse stomatitides, but an attempt to do so is important because it may indicate a systemic disease state. Viral diseases causing stomatitis will be considered in detail under Infectious and Parasitic Diseases of the Gastrointestinal Tract.

Inflammatory disease, localized to the buccal cavity and not part of systemic viral disease, is also common and important. It is generally due to the indigenous bacterial flora. The oral microbiota ordinarily contains many microbial species, mainly anaerobes, such as *Actinomyces, Fusobacterium,* and spirochetes, which exist in balance with each other and in harmony with the host. The oral mucosa is quite resistant to microbial invasion for several reasons. These include the squamous mucosal lining, antibacterial constituents of saliva (e.g., lysozyme), immunoglobulins (especially IgA) in oral secretions, and the presence of submucosal inflammatory cells. Factors altering the balance of indigenous organisms are not well delineated. Systemic illness, stress, and nutritional and hormonal imbalances may alter the microbial population by altering the amount, composition, and pH of saliva. The integrity of the oral epithelium depends on a high rate of epithelial regeneration to balance loss due to a high rate of abrasion and desquamation. Rapid epithelial replication promotes quick healing of superficial lesions.

The lamina propria of the oral epithelium is well vascularized, but generally dense and relatively inelastic. For this reason, there is little distention of lymphatics and tissue spaces with fluid exudate, and therefore, swelling due to edema is not a significant part of stomatitis involving gums and hard palate.

CATARRHAL STOMATITIS. Catarrhal stomatitis is a superficial inflammation of the oral mucosa that usually involves the posterior fauces and may be associated with mild gingivitis. It is a common nonspecific lesion that often develops in the course of debilitating diseases. The mucosae are hyperemic, and the loose texture of the submucosa in the fauces permits development of edema. The swelling is aggravated by edema and hyperplasia of the abundant lymphoid tissues of the soft palate, tonsil, and pharyngeal mucosa. The epithelium accumulates, producing a dull, gray mucosal surface. There is excessive mucus production by palatine glands. Catarrhal stomatitis resolves with the return of normal oral function.

Thrush, or oral candidiasis, occurs most commonly in foals, pigs, and dogs. It involves the proliferation of yeasts and hyphae in the parakeratotic superficial layers of the oral epithelium. It appears grossly as patchy, pale pseudomembranous material on the oral mucosa and back of the tongue and probably reflects alterations in epithelial turnover and oral flora. It is considered more fully under Infectious and Parasitic Diseases of the Gastrointestinal Tract.

VESICULAR STOMATITIDES. Stomatitis, characterized by the formation of vesicles, occurs in most species of domestic animals. The vesicles develop as accumulations of serous fluid within the epithelium or between the epithelium and the lamina propria. These may coalesce to form bullae, and the elevated epithelium is easily rubbed off during chewing to leave raw eroded patches with bits of epithelium still adherent. The transition from vesicle to erosion occurs rapidly so that in individual animals, vesicles may not be seen. This is especially so in dogs and cats because the oral mucosa is very thin. Because the basal epithelium or basement membrane remains intact, regeneration and healing are complete in a few days unless the local lesions are complicated by bacterial or mycotic infections. However, foci of previous erosion may be identifiable for some months by their slight depression and lack of pigmentation.

Vesicular stomatitides in animals have been associated with viral infections, and these are still the most common causes. In horses, cattle, and swine, oral vesicles should be regarded as indicating foot and mouth disease, vesicular stomatitis, swine vesicular disease, or vesicular exanthema until proven otherwise. These conditions are described in detail under Infectious and Parasitic Diseases of the Gastrointestinal Tract.

Since the early 1970s, the bullous immune skin diseases have been reported with increased frequency, especially in dogs, and some of these have severe oral lesions, which will be described in detail here; the reader is also referred to the Skin and Appendages (Volume 1).

Pemphigus vulgaris is a severe chronic, vesicular, bullous autoimmune disease. It is characterized by acantholysis of the epidermis, which results in formation of flaccid bullae and erosions involving mainly mucocutaneous junctions, oral mucosa, and to a lesser extent, skin. The disease is similar, if not identical, to pemphigus vulgaris in humans. Clinically, affected dogs and cats show excessive salivation, halitosis, and erosions and ulcerations of the oral mucosa. The oral lesions are generally more prominent than, and precede, the skin lesions. They are most obvious on the dorsal surface of the tongue, which is bright red with a few scattered pink raised areas representing islands of normal mucosa. The lesions vary greatly in severity and distribution, although the hard palate is often severely ulcerated. Bullae are rarely seen in the oral cavity because they ulcerate rapidly.

Microscopically, the earliest lesion consists of suprabasilar acantholysis, which is followed by the formation of clefts. These lead to ulceration of the mucosa. The basal cells of the epidermis remain attached to the basement membrane and form a so-called row of tombstones. A few neutrophils and eosinophils may infiltrate the epithelium. There is a variable lymphocytic and plasmacytic lichenoid reaction in the propria.

The presence of suprabasilar clefts and bullae due to acantholysis are considered to be diagnostic of pemphigus vulgaris. However, extensive erosion and ulceration of the mucosa and secondary bacterial infections frequently obscure these clefts and bullae. Several biopsies from different areas of the oral mucosa may be required to demonstrate the characteristic lesions. A presumptive histologic diagnosis should be supported by direct immunofluorescence tests showing autoantibodies (usually IgG) and complement in the intercellular spaces of stratified squamous epithelium.

Bullous pemphigoid is characterized by mucocutaneous, superficial vesicobullous or ulcerative disease of mucous membranes (including the oral mucosa) and skin. Clinically, the disease is often impossible to distinguish from pemphigus vulgaris. Bullous pemphigoid has been reported in humans and dogs. The characteristic microscopic lesions are subepidermal blisters, which may contain fibrinocellular exudate. Direct immunofluorescence of lesions shows autoantibody (IgG) and complement deposits along the basement membrane.

The oral lesions of pemphigus vulgaris and bullous pemphigoid must be differentiated from lesions due to trauma, toxic epidermal necrolysis, drug eruptions, chronic uremia, mucocutaneous candidiasis, and lymphoreticular malignancies, which are described in other sections of this chapter and with diseases of skin (in the Skin and Appendages, Volume 1).

Feline calicivirus belongs to the Picornaviridae and causes mainly a respiratory infection in cats. The disease is complicated by lingual and oropharyngeal ulcers, which start out as vesicles. They are 5–10 mm in diameter, smooth, and well demarcated from the surrounding normal mucosa. They occur mainly on the anterodorsal and lateral surfaces of the tongue and each side of the midline of the hard palate. The palatine lesions are apparently more severe in cats fed dry food. Microscopically, the earliest lesions consist of foci of pyknotic cells in the stratum corneum and superficial stratum spinosum. They progress to foci of necrosis with vesicle formation and subsequent erosion and ulceration of the mucosa. Regeneration of the oral mucosa in the ulcerated areas generally occurs within 10 to 12 days. A single layer of squamous epithelial cells extends from the margins of the ulcer beneath a layer of exudate. Active viral replication also takes place in the tonsillar crypt epithelial cells, and virus may be recovered from these areas for weeks postinfection. Inclusions have not been observed in oral epithelial cells.

EROSIVE AND ULCERATIVE STOMATITIDES. Erosive and ulcerative stomatitides are characterized by local epithelial defects of the oral mucosa and nasolabium and usually associated with acute diffuse stomatitis and pharyngitis. Erosions are circumscribed areas of loss of epithelium that leave the stratum germinativum and basement membrane more or less intact. They are usually associated with acute inflammation in the underlying propria. The erosions vary in size and shape, and although they are often a nonspecific development in a wide variety of conditions, they are also an essential part of a number of important diseases. They heal cleanly and quickly, but if secondarily infected or complicated, may develop into ulcers.

Ulcers, in contrast to erosions, are deeper deficiencies that extend into the substantia propria. They too vary greatly in size and shape, the edges tend to be elevated and ragged, and when they heal it is with scar formation.

The causes of ulcerative stomatitis are in general those of erosive stomatitis. There are, however, a number of recognized syndromes and specific diseases in which the predominant change is ulcerative. Viral diseases causing erosive–ulcerative stomatitis in ungulates are described under Infectious and Parasitic Diseases of the Gastrointestinal Tract. Erosive–ulcerative conditions in other species are discussed below.

Ulcerative stomatitis and **glossitis** in cats is an ulcerative and chronic inflammation of the mucosa of the fauces, the angle of the jaws, and less commonly, the hard palate, gingiva, and tongue, occurring particularly in older cats. These lesions may comprise the largest group of feline oral clinical conditions. The cause is unknown but is probably multifactorial, involving imbalance in the oral microbial flora, with predominance of spirochetes.

Eosinophilic ulcer (eosinophilic granuloma, lick granuloma, labial ulcer, "rodent ulcer") is a chronic, superficial ulcerative lesion of the mucocutaneous junctions of the lips and to a lesser extent the oral mucosa and skin, in cats of all ages. The cause is unknown, but the lesions may respond to corticosteroid or radiation therapy, although recurrences are common.

Typically, well-demarcated, red-brown, shallow ulcers, often with elevated margins, occur on the upper lip on either side of the midline. They are usually a few millimeters wide and several centimeters long. Occasionally, ulcers are present elsewhere in the mouth, such as the gums, palate, pharynx, and tongue. Skin lesions are located in those areas that are frequently licked, such as the neck, lumbar area, and abdomen. Microscopically, eosinophilic ulcer is characterized by ulceration of the squamous mucosa, with large areas of necrosis of the underlying connective tissues, accompanied by a marked inflammatory cell reaction. The cellular reaction consists predominantly of neutrophils at the periphery of the ulcers, with a mainly mononuclear-cell reaction (plasma cells and mast cells) in the propria. Eosinophils and histiocytes may be seen occasionally. In our experience, the eosinophils and mast cells may predominate, but this difference may be only a reflection of the evolution of the lesion.

Eosinophilic ulcer is considered to be one of the three different types of lesion that have been associated with the so-called eosinophilic granuloma complex. The other two conditions, eosinophilic plaque and linear granuloma, cause mainly skin lesions, which are different clinically and morphologically from eosinophilic ulcer. The differences are discussed in the Skin and Appendages (Volume 1).

Oral eosinophilic granuloma (linear granuloma) in dogs occurs as a familial disease in young Siberian huskies. Affected dogs have single or multiple, firm, often ulcerated, raised plaques, which are covered by a yellow-brown exudate, on the lateral or ventral surfaces of the tongue. Lesions on the soft palate are less common, and there they tend to be oval to circular ulcers that have slightly elevated borders. Cytologic preparations made from scrapings of the oral lesions show many eosinophils, a few neutrophils, occasional macrophages, and epithelial cells.

Microscopically, the lesions are characterized by foci of collagen degeneration (necrobiosis), in the mid and deep zones of the lingual submucosa, surrounded by a granulomatous inflammatory reaction. The reaction consists mainly of histiocytes, including epithelioid macrophages, with fewer lymphocytes, plasma cells, and mast cells. Eosinophils are a constant feature, but their numbers vary from few to many. Multinucleated giant cells may also be present.

The lesions are identical to those seen in linear granuloma of cats. The cause is unknown, although the morphology of the lesion and the response to corticosteroid therapy are suggestive of hypersensitivity reaction. The familial tendency may indicate that hereditary factors are involved. Eosinophilic granuloma must be differentiated from oral mast-cell tumors, which also affect the tongue in dogs. Necrobiosis of collagen fibers is often a feature of mast-cell tumors; however, the characteristic mixture of mast cells and eosinophils infiltrate the tongue and connective tissues more diffusely. The mast cells may be in various stages of degranulation, and inflammation is minimal or absent in mast-cell tumors.

Feline viral rhinotracheitis is a common upper respiratory tract infection of cats caused by feline herpesvirus-1 (see the Respiratory System, this volume). This virus may cause ulcerative lesions in the mouth, especially on the tongue. Rarely, oral and skin ulcers may occur, without evidence of concurrent respiratory tract infection. Microscopic lesions are characterized by foci of cytoplasmic vacuolation in squamous epithelium that evolve into areas of necrosis and ulceration. The ulcers are often covered by a layer of fibrinocellular exudate. Herpetic inclusions may be present in epithelial cells at the periphery of the ulcers.

Ulcerative stomatitis in **uremia** occurs commonly in dogs and less commonly in cats; a fetid ulcerative stomatitis develops in the course of chronic renal disease. The buccal cavity, and especially the tongue, are deeply cyanotic. Dirty grayish brown ulcers occur on the gums, lateral surface and margin of the tongue (Fig. 1.3D), and inner surface of the lips and cheeks. The margins of the ulcers are swollen and hyperemic.

The pathogenesis of the oral lesions in uremia is still poorly understood. Urease-producing bacteria, normally present in the oral microflora, generate ammonia from salivary urea. Ammonia has a caustic effect on the oral mucous membranes. This may explain why the lesions are mainly located where salivary ducts enter the oral cavity. There is apparently a poor correlation between the levels of blood urea nitrogen and the development of uremic stomatitis, suggesting that other factors are involved in its pathogenesis.

Ulcerative glossitis and **stomatitis** in **swine** is commonly part of exudative epidermitis ("greasy-pig disease") of preweaning pigs (see bacterial diseases of skin, in the Skin and Appendages, Volume 1). In addition to the characteristic skin lesions, about a third of the piglets may develop ulcers on the

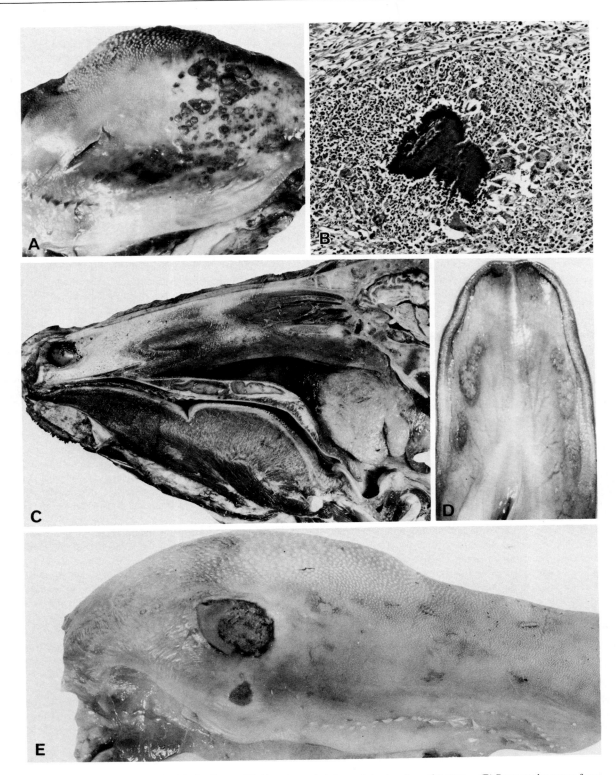

Fig. 1.3. (**A** and **B**) Actinobacillosis. Cow. (**A**) Granulomas bulging on lateral surface of tongue. (**B**) Pyogranulomatous focus containing club colony of *Actinobacillus lignieresi*. (**C**) Pharyngeal actinomycosis. Cow. Fleshy mass in pharynx, which resembles actinobacillosis. (**D**) Superficial necrotic lesions on the ventral aspect of the tongue. Dog with uremic stomatitis. (**E**) Oral necrobacillosis. Calf.

dorsum of the tongue. Erosions and ulcers of the hard palate occur in a small number of piglets. Microscopically, there is ulceration of the squamous mucosa with coagulation necrosis, and vesicle and pustule formation in the superficial epithelium of the rete pegs. A pleocellular inflammatory reaction is evident in the connective tissue below the ulcers.

Deep Stomatitides

Lesions of the oral mucosa may permit the entry of pyogenic bacteria, often normal oral flora, into the connective tissues of the submucosa and muscle. Purulent inflammation or cellulitis may develop in the lips, tongue, cheek, soft palate, and pharynx. Abscesses may form and may fistulate through the mucosa or skin. Abscesses in the wall of the pharynx may result from necrosis of retropharyngeal lymph nodes. Necrotic stomatitis with simple necrosis of the epithelium and lamina propria may be produced by thermal or chemical agencies, but in animals, it is usually caused by *Fusobacterium necrophorum* and other anaerobes.

ORAL NECROBACILLOSIS. *Fusobacterium necrophorum* is the principal cause of necrotic stomatitis in animals. It is also associated with necrotizing lesions elsewhere in the upper and lower alimentary tract and liver. Wherever it occurs, it is usually a secondary invader following previous mucosal damage. The organism produces a variety of exo- and endotoxins, whose exact role in the pathogenesis of the lesions has yet to be determined. The exotoxins include leukocidins, hemolysins, and a cytoplasmic toxin, all of which probably enhance the necrotizing ability of the organism. Once established in a suitable focus, *F. necrophorum* proliferates, causing extensive coagulation necrosis.

The best known form of necrobacillary stomatitis is **calf diphtheria**, an acute necrotizing ulcerative inflammation of the buccal and pharyngeal mucosa. The predisposing lesions may include trauma, infectious bovine rhinotracheitis, and papular stomatitis. Necrosis of palatine and pharyngeal tonsils may be seen. The incidence of diphtheria in slaughtered beef cattle may be as high as 1.4%. The same syndrome is rather common in housed lambs as a complication of contagious ecthyma. The infection also may be initiated in the gums about erupting teeth in any species, and by the trauma produced in baby pigs by removing the needle teeth. It is frequently fatal in young animals, in which extension often occurs to other organs. In adults, oral necrobacillosis tends to remain localized to the oral cavity, where it may complicate vesicular and ulcerative stomatitides. It is not unusual, however, for the infection to spread down the alimentary tract. In the lower alimentary tract, the Peyer's patches especially are involved, perhaps as a complication of bovine virus diarrhea.

The early lesions are large, well-demarcated, yellowish gray, dry areas of necrosis, surrounded by a zone of hyperemia (Fig. 1.1C and 1.3E). They are found on the sides or dorsal groove of the tongue and on the cheeks, gums, palate, and pharynx, especially the recesses beside the larynx. Primary foci may occur in the laryngeal ventricles. Death may be associated with asphyxia. The necrotic tissue projects slightly above the normal surface and is friable but adherent and is not easily detached. In

time it may slough and leave deep ulcers, which may heal by granulation. The necrotic tissues are histologically structureless and are surrounded at first by a zone of vascular reaction, later by a dense but narrow rim of leukocytes, and later still by thick, encapsulating granulation tissue. The bacteria are arranged in long filaments, particularly at the advancing edge of the lesions. The submucosal extension of the lesions may take them deeply into the underlying soft tissues and bone.

Spread from the oral foci occurs down the trachea (causing aspiration pneumonia), down the esophagus, and via blood vessels. Death may occur acutely in septicemia with only multiple small serosal hemorrhages as evidence, or metastases may occur in other tissue. Venous drainage from the face to the vascular sinuses of the meninges may lead to pituitary and cerebral abscessation.

More recently, *Fusobacterium necrophorum* has been associated with a syndrome of necrotic stomatitis, enteritis, and granulocytopenia in calves. Affected calves have a nonregenerative anemia, leukopenia, absolute neutropenia, hypoproteinemia, and increased fibrinogen levels. In addition to the characteristic oral lesions, there is marked depletion of lymphoid tissues and necrotic enteritis. *Fusobacterium*-like organisms are present in large numbers in a variety of organs, including the bone marrow. Possibly, very virulent strains of *F. necrophorum* produce enough leukotoxins, especially in immunodeficient calves, to suppress bone marrow activity.

A gross diagnosis of oral necrobacillosis is ordinarily possible but may be confirmed by a smear from the margin of the lesion. The organism is difficult to cultivate due to its strict anaerobiasis.

NOMA. Noma is a rapidly spreading pseudomembranous or gangrenous stomatitis; it is not caused by a specific pathogen but is associated with tissue invasion by the normal oral flora, particularly spirochetes and fusiforms. The predisposing factors are unknown, but they are probably nonspecific and associated with mucosal trauma and debility. The disease, which is observed occasionally in horses, dogs, and monkeys, is in many respects similar to oral necrobacillosis. In the lesions, the spirochetes can be found in large numbers at the advancing margins as well as in peripheral viable tissue. In the deep layers of necrosis, fusiforms predominate, and toward the surface there is a variety of other organisms, chiefly cocci.

The initial lesion is a small, tattered ulcer of the cheek or gum, which spreads rapidly and may involve much of the buccal surface of the gums and the mucosa of the cheek. It is intensely fetid and consists of a dirty necrotic pseudomembrane surrounded by a zone of acute inflammation. The necrotic tissue may slough to leave deep ulcers; the cheek may be perforated to leave a gaping defect, or gangrene may supervene.

ACTINOBACILLOSIS. Actinobacillosis is a deep stomatitis caused in cattle by *Actinobacillus lignieresi*, a member of the normal oral flora. When introduced into the submucosa it causes pyogranulomatous inflammatory foci centered on club colonies containing Gram-negative coccobacilli. Morphologically similar lesions may be caused by a variety of organisms (Fig. 1.3C). *Actinomyces bovis*, a Gram-positive filamentous organism, causes pyogranulomatous mandibular and maxillary osteomyelitis in cattle (see inflammatory diseases of bones, in Bones and Joints, Volume 1) and mastitis in sows. Staphylococci may cause pyogranulomatous lesions (botryomycosis) in any species, especially mastitis in sows (see the Skin and Appendages, Volume 1, and the Female Genital System, Volume 3). Less common causes of similar microscopic lesions include *Nocardia* and the various agents associated with mycetomas (see the Skin and Appendages).

Actinobacillosis is typically a disease of soft tissue, spreading as a lymphangitis and usually involving the regional lymph nodes. This distinguishes it from actinomycosis, which causes bone lesions. The tongue is often involved in actinobacillosis, and the chronic condition produces clinical "wooden tongue."

Entry of actinobacilli to the tongue may be gained through traumatic erosions along its sides, but often the primary lesion is in the lingual groove. Here, trapped grass grains and awns may provoke the initial trauma. Lesions elsewhere in the soft tissue of the mouth may be attributed to disruption of the mucosa by similar types of insults and eruption of, or abrasion by, teeth.

Microscopically, the lesion is a pyogranuloma, centered on a mass of coccobacilli, surrounded by radiating eosinophilic "clubs," probably made up of immune complexes (Fig. 1.3B). The club colonies, in turn, are surrounded by variable numbers of neutrophils and are invested by macrophages or giant cells. Lymphocytic and plasmacytic infiltrates are present in the surrounding reactive fibrous stroma or granulation tissue. An individual inflammatory focus appears grossly as a nodular, firm, pale, fibrous mass a few millimeters to 1.0 cm in diameter, containing in the center minute yellow "sulfur granules," which are the club colonies.

Actinobacillosis causes a lymphangitis, and lymphogenous spread is common. Affected lymphatics are thickened, and nodules are distributed along their course. This distribution is best seen beneath the mucosa of the dorsum and the lateral surface of the tongue and can often be traced through to the pharyngeal lymphoid tissue (Fig. 1.3A). Some of these more superficial nodules erode the overlying epithelium, and coalescence may produce quite large ulcers. The most common form of lingual actinobacillosis consists of granulation tissue in which are embedded many small abscesses surrounded by a dense connective-tissue capsule. The epithelium overlying these large granulomas may be intact or ulcerated. Diffuse sclerosing actinobacillosis of the tongue (wooden tongue) is characterized by firmness, the result of extensive proliferation of connective tissue that replaces the muscle fibers. Granulomatous nodules are sparsely scattered in the fibrous stroma.

Although actinobacillosis in cattle is best known as a disease of the tongue, the infection may occur in any of the exposed soft tissues, especially those of mouth and neck; occasionally it involves the wall of the forestomachs, any portion of skin, and the lungs. Lesions in these sites resemble those described for the tongue.

Actinobacillosis causes regional lymphadenitis. The cut surface of the node reveals small, soft yellow or orange granulomatous masses that project somewhat above the capsular contour and contain "sulfur granules." There is also sclerosing inflammation of the surrounding tissues, which may cause adhesion to overlying skin or mucous membranes. The retropharyngeal and submaxillary nodes are most often affected, as well as the lymphoid tissues of the submucosa of the soft palate and pharynx. Involvement of the pharynx and the retropharyngeal lymph nodes may cause dyspnea and dysphagia.

Oral actinobacillosis in swine causes lesions similar to those in cattle, including glossitis. Actinobacillosis may also occur sporadically or as outbreaks in sheep, but in this species the tongue seems to be exempt. The characteristic lesions in sheep occur in the subcutaneous tissue of the head, especially of the cheeks, nose, lips, submaxillary and throat regions, and on the nasal turbinates. They may also occur on the soft palate and pharynx as complications of wounds received at drenching.

ORAL DERMATOPHILOSIS IN CATS. *Dermatophilus congolensis* is a bacterium that commonly causes an exudative dermatitis in a wide variety of species (see bacterial diseases of skin, in the Skin and Appendages, Volume 1). In cats, the organism is uncommonly associated with oral granulomas affecting especially the tongue and tonsillar crypt. Large numbers of Gram-positive, filamentous, branching organisms, with longitudinal and transverse divisions, may be demonstrated in the necrotic centers of submucosal granulomas. The organisms most likely enter through damaged mucosa. The lesion must be differentiated from the more common squamous-cell carcinomas of the tongue. In cattle, cutaneous streptothricosis involving the muzzle may extend into the oral cavity.

Parasitic Diseases of the Oral Cavity

Parasitic disease of the oral cavity are of minor significance. Sarcosporidiosis and cysticercosis occur in the striated muscles of the tongue and produce the same lesions as they do elsewhere (see parasitic diseases of muscle, in Muscles and Tendons, Volume 1). *Trichinella spiralis* may be found in muscles of the tongue and mastication. *Gongylonema* spp. are found in the mucosal lining of the tongue, especially in swine allowed to graze, and less commonly in cattle and sheep. They evoke little or no inflammation of the mucosa, but a mild to moderate lymphocytic and eosinophilic reaction may be evident in the underlying lamina propria. The larvae of *Gasterophilus* spp. in the horse and of *Oestrus ovis* in sheep are found attached to the pharyngeal mucosa, where they may cause focal ulceration and excite mild inflammation. The larvae of *Gasterophilus nasalis* migrate from the lips and invade the gums around and between the teeth and behind the alveolar processes to cause small, suppurating pockets.

Tonsils

The tonsils are normally prominent and protrude slightly from the tonsillar fossa in the dog and cat. In swine, tonsillar lymphoid tissue is concentrated in the posterior soft palate. In other species, the tonsils are diffuse. They are subject to the usual conditions of lymphoid tissue and undergo progressive atrophy with age.

By virtue of their function in immune surveillance in the oropharynx, tonsils are constantly exposed to antigenic stimuli.

As a result, they are a usual site of functional lymphoid hyperplasia and physiologic inflammation. Many bacteria native to the oropharyngeal mucosa probably inhabit the tonsillar crypts. A significant percentage of swine may carry *Erysipelothrix rhusiopathiae* and *Salmonella* spp. in the tonsils. They consequently may serve as portal of entry for a variety of bacterial agents, including *Streptococcus suis* and intracellular organisms, and for viruses that are lymphotropic.

Desquamated epithelium, bacteria, necrotic debris, and neutrophils may normally be present to moderate degree in tonsillar crypts. This reaction is exaggerated and may be associated with ulceration of the crypt and suppuration of involuted tonsillar lymphoid tissue, in certain bacterial infections, causing the formation of visible yellowish nodules. Conditions in which such bacterial tonsillitis may occur include pasteurellosis in sheep and pigs, and necrobacillosis in all species. In porcine anthrax, hemorrhagic necrotizing tonsillitis is reported.

Involution of B-dependent tonsillar lymphoid follicles due to viral lymphocytolysis may occur during the early phase of a number of lymphotropic diseases such as feline panleukopenia, canine parvovirus infection, canine distemper, bovine virus diarrhea, rinderpest, and swine vesicular disease. Numerous karyorrhexic nuclei, lymphocyte depletion, and prominent histiocytes signal such damage. In distemper, involuted tonsils are susceptible to secondary bacterial invasion and suppuration. Compensatory lymphoid hyperplasia may occur during the postviremic phase of parvoviral infections and distemper.

Neoplastic and Like Lesions of the Oral Cavity

Many of the lumps, bumps, and cysts that develop in and around the oral cavity are malformations, hyperplasias, and neoplasias originating in tooth germs or teeth. The classification of these masses, especially those containing more than one tissue, is not established and must be arbitrary. Malformations of dental origin have been considered previously under Developmental Anomalies of Teeth. Gingival masses of all types, many of which are of tooth germ origin, are common in dogs and rarely occur in other species. The oral and pharyngeal mucosa is the fourth most common site of malignant tumors in the dog. It is also a common site of malignant tumors in cats; large domestic animals have a low prevalence of such tumors. When they do occur in ungulates, they usually are nonaggressive.

Regional geographic differences exist in the prevalence of certain oral tumors, especially in dogs and cattle. These differences may be related to types and levels of carcinogens in the environment and warrant further investigation from the point of view of comparative oncology.

The most common types of malignant oral tumors in dogs and cats are, in order of their frequency, squamous-cell carcinomas, malignant melanomas (in dogs only), and fibrosarcomas. They vary considerably in their behavior, depending on species and location. Dogs and cats 7 years of age or older are mainly affected. Typical clinical signs associated with these tumors are excessive salivation, halitosis, pain, dysphagia, loose teeth, oral bleeding, coughing, and a change in voice. All of these signs are determined by the location of the tumor. All malignant oral tumors in dogs and cats tend to follow a rapid course, and re-

gardless of the type of malignancy, the prognosis is poor. Radiography and exfoliative cytology are useful diagnostic aids in concert with histopathologic examination.

ORAL PAPILLOMATOSIS. Oral papillomas, benign epithelial tumors ("warts") in dogs and cattle, are caused by papovaviruses. In dogs, they occur mainly in young animals, but older dogs in close contact may become infected. The virus is host and site specific. It can be transmitted only to the scarified oral mucosa and not to other mucous membranes. The incubation period is generally 1 month. Spontaneous recovery, followed by solid immunity usually occurs within 2 to 3 months. The warts first develop on the lips as single, smooth, papular elevations that are pale or the color of the mucosa. These lesions progress to multiple, proliferative, cauliflower-like, firm, white to gray growths (Fig. 1.4F). Similar lesions develop on the inside of the cheeks and on the tongue, palate, and walls of the pharynx. The gingiva are usually not affected. The esophagus may be involved.

The microscopic structure is typically papillomatous with a very thick squamous epithelium covering thin, branching, often pedunculated cores of proprial papillae. Individual or small groups of epithelial cells in the upper areas of the stratum spinosum undergo hydropic or acidophilic degeneration with loss of intercellular bridges. There is also marked acanthosis. Intranuclear basophilic inclusions may be found in the cells in the outer spinose layers.

Oral papillomas, due to bovine papillomavirus type 4, occur commonly in cattle. Their morphology and distribution are similar to the papillomas of dogs, and they are considered more fully under Neoplasia of the Esophagus and Forestomachs.

PYOGENIC GRANULOMAS. Pyogenic granuloma is a bright red or blue mass on the gums. It is composed of extremely vascular chronic granulation tissue and ulcerates and bleeds easily. Pyogenic granuloma is probably an exaggerated response to local irritation.

GINGIVAL HYPERTROPHY. Hypertrophy of the gums is common in dogs and is either generalized or localized to one or more teeth. When localized, it is a discrete tumor-like mass and, whether local or general, may cover part of the crown (Fig. 1.4A). Local enlargement is caused by chronic, probably painless, inflammation. It may be associated with periodontal disease.

Diffuse gingival hypertrophy is familial in boxer dogs, and a more severe overgrowth, termed hyperplastic gingivitis, occurs as a recessive inherited disease in Swedish silver foxes. In the foxes, both jaws are affected and the hypertrophy causes displacement and malalignment of teeth, eventually reaching such proportions that the mouth cannot be closed. Diffuse gingival hypertrophy sometimes is associated with prolonged anticonvulsant therapy in humans.

EPULIDES. Epulis is the generic and clinical term for tumor-like masses on the gingiva. By common usage, however, it refers to the epulides of periodontal origin that are so numerous in dogs and develop occasionally in cats.

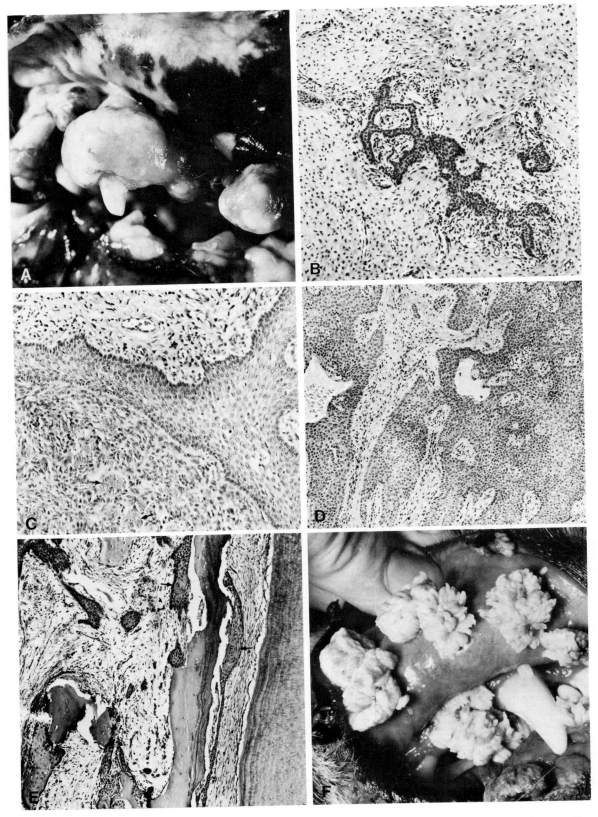

Fig. 1.4. (**A**) Epulis (gingival hypertrophy). Boxer dog. (**B**) Branching cords of epithelium in mesenchymal stroma. Epulis. Dog. (**C**) Acanthomatous epithelium in canine epulis with giant cells in stroma (arrows). (**D**) Acanthomatous epulis. Dog. (**E**) Acanthomatous epulis invading bone (arrows). Cementum (right), alveolar bone (center). (**F**) Oral papillomatosis. Dog. (Courtesy of W. R. Kelly.)

Epulides are firm to hard, gray-pink neoplasms, often projecting from between the teeth or from the hard palate near the teeth. They are most common around the carnassial and canine teeth of brachycephalic breeds (Fig. 1.4A). Often they are mushroom-shaped and have an irregular, smooth surface.

Epulides are stromal tumors, and the stromal tissue occasionally resembles periodontal membrane, comprising well-vascularized, interwoven bundles of cellular fibrous tissue; usually the stroma is mature, dense collagen. About 60% contain branching cords or islands of epithelium that usually are continuous with the gingiva. The epithelium is bordered by a row of cuboidal cells somewhat resembling odontogenic epithelium (Fig. 1.4B,C). Epulides sometimes are divided into fibromatous and ossifying types, depending on the abundance of hard tissue (osteoid, bone, cementum, etc.) that develops by stromal metaplasia in ~ 60% of affected dogs. There is no prognostic value in this distinction since these are all benign tumors that are cured by excision. Indeed, some authorities believe them to be hyperplasias.

Easily confused with these benign epulides is the epithelial tumor variously called oral adamantinoma and acanthomatous epulis. Clinically, these initially resemble epulis, but in many dogs recurrence and local invasion of alveolar bone (Fig. 1.4E) with loss of teeth follow conservative treatment. Histologically, the tumor is composed of sheets and anastomosing cords of epithelium bordered by a row of cuboidal to columnar cells. Prominent intercellular bridges are present between many of the central polyhedral cells. In some tumors there are intraepithelial cysts containing vacuolated, otherwise structureless, eosinophilic material and cellular debris (Fig. 1.4D). These cysts probably form from degenerate epithelium. Small areas of hard tissue may develop by metaplasia in the stroma between the epithelium.

Some of these neoplasms transform to squamous-cell carcinoma when they invade bone. Others have reported development of squamous-cell carcinoma at the site of irradiated acanthomatous epulis. The characteristic appearance of these tumors, and of the epithelial component of benign epulides, is probably a function of epithelial–mesenchymal interaction between tissues of dental origin.

The naming of these tumors is unsettled. "Adamantinoma" is an obsolete synonym for ameloblastoma and is therefore unsatisfactory. "Acanthomatous epulis" is morphologically more accurate for the superficial lesion and is used widely but does not disclose the behavioral characteristics of the tumor. Indeed, it is confusing, since epulis is widely recognized in veterinary medicine as a nonneoplastic or benign oral tumor. Nevertheless, until more of the invasive tumors have been studied and a suitable alternative established, "acanthomatous epulis" is likely to persist. Squamous-cell carcinoma, acanthomatous type, may prove to be more appropriate.

TUMORS OF DENTAL TISSUES. Tumors of dental tissues are classified as epithelial tumors, with or without inductive effects, and mesodermal tumors. The latter are very rare in animals. Some of the former are neoplasms, and others are probably malformations. Tooth development provides the classic example of epithelial–mesenchymal interactions, and it is generally accepted that inductive influences are active in certain mixed tumors. Familiarity with dental embryology assists an understanding of the origin, appearance, and classification of the tumors discussed below.

Most tumors of dental tissues are rare, nonmalignant, and infiltrative or expansive. Their location involves destruction of bone, however, and they are difficult to remove.

Ameloblastoma is an invasive tumor consisting of proliferating odontogenic epithelium in a fibrous stroma. The proportions of epithelium and stroma vary widely. *Ameloblastoma* is preferable to the synonyms adamantinoma and enameloblastoma. These tumors are more common in dogs and cattle than in cats and horses, and seem to occur more often in the mandible than the maxilla.

Ameloblastomas occur at any age and originate from the dental lamina, the outer enamel epithelium, the dental follicle around retained unerupted teeth, the oral epithelium, or odontogenic epithelium in extraoral locations. Because of their predominantly intraosseous location, they may destroy large amounts of bone and extend into the oral cavity or sinuses. Large tumors undergo central degeneration and become cystic.

The odontogenic epithelium, which is the criterion for diagnosis of ameloblastoma, may form any one of several patterns (Fig. 1.5D). Follicular and plexiform patterns are most common, consisting of discrete islands or irregular masses and strands of epithelium, respectively. Many tumors contain both patterns. In both, central masses of cells, often resembling the stellate reticulum of the enamel organ, but sometimes with an acanthomatous appearance, are surrounded by a single layer of cuboidal or columnar cells that resemble inner enamel epithelium. Cysts originate from degeneration of the centers of epithelial islands, or from stromal degeneration. Small cysts may coalesce to form gross cavities. Ameloblastomas occasionally undergo keratinization. In some there is stromal osteoid and bone. Stromal ossification may be an epithelial inductive effect.

Ameloblastic fibroma (fibroameloblastoma) is a rare tumor in calves and in the maxilla of young cats. It consists of cords of epithelium resembling dental lamina, intimately associated with spindle cells resembling dental pulp. It behaves like an ameloblastoma.

Ameloblastic fibroma corresponds to that stage of odontogenesis when dental epithelium invests the dental papilla but odontoblasts have not yet differentiated.

Ameloblastic odontoma (ameloblastic fibro-odontoma) resembles ameloblastic fibroma but contains dentin and enamel, and the epithelium is more typical of the enamel organ. It occurs in horses, cows, and dogs, often in immature animals.

Complex and **compound odontomas** are malformations in which all of the dental tissues are represented. In complex odontomas the tissues are disorganized, while in compound odontomas toothlike structures (denticles) are present, each one containing enamel, dentin, cementum, and pulp, arranged as in a normal tooth. Separation of the two may be arbitrary. Separate areas of ameloblastic epithelium are not present in complex and compound odontomas. A tumor that contains areas of ameloblastic epithelium and areas of complex or compound odontoma is an odontoameloblastoma.

Odontomas are usually located in the mandibular or maxillary

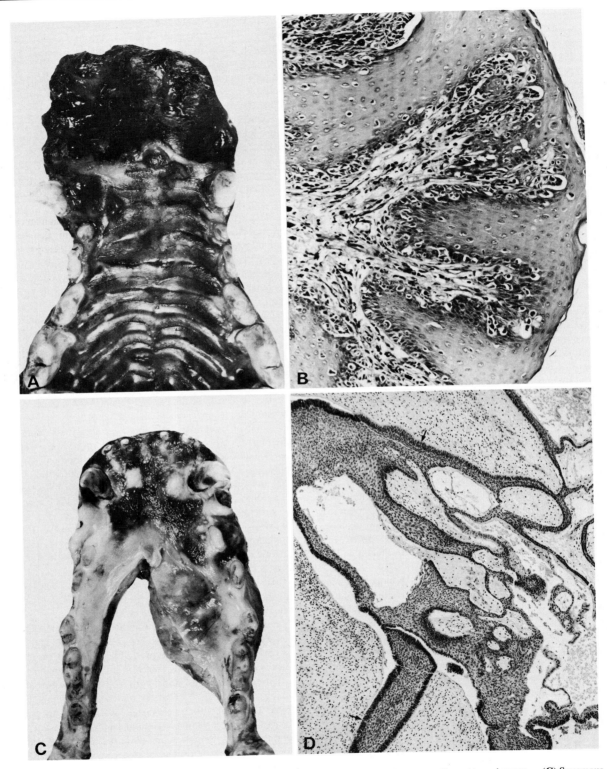

Fig. 1.5.   (A) Malignant melanoma of palate. Dog.   (B) Junctional activity in oral mucosa adjacent to melanoma.   (C) Squamous carcinoma arising from alveolus of right canine tooth and invading mandible. Dog.   (D) Ameloblastoma. Cow. Tall, enamel-type epithelium (arrows) and cyst formation.

arch and are less rare in cattle and horses than in other species. They are connected with existing dental alveoli and are detected when they bulge the contour of the host bone or interfere with other teeth. They may originate from normally or abnormally placed dental anlagen as well as from supernumerary dental anlagen.

SQUAMOUS-CELL CARCINOMA. Squamous-cell carcinoma is the most common oral malignancy of cats. It is most frequently located on the ventral lateral surface of the body of the tongue. The tonsils and gingiva are less common sites. Microscopically, the tumor is conventional in appearance. It is locally invasive and metastatic to regional lymph nodes and distant organs.

In the dog, this tumor is second to melanoma in prevalence in the oral cavity. It usually involves the tonsils, although the gingivae are common sites. Squamous-cell carcinoma is apparently more common in male than female dogs.

Grossly, tonsillar carcinoma usually appears unilateral. The earliest lesion appears as a small, slightly elevated, granular plaque on the mucosal surface. In the advanced stages, the affected tonsil is two to three times normal size, nodular, firm, and white, and the surface may be ulcerated. There is often extensive infiltration of the surrounding tissues. Histologic examination of the grossly unaffected tonsil frequently also shows early carcinoma. Squamous-cell carcinomas originating in the tongue and tonsils often metastasize to the regional nodes, with distant metastases to visceral organs, especially the lungs, in dogs. Tonsillar carcinoma must be differentiated from involvement of the tonsil in lymphosarcoma.

Gingival squamous-cell carcinomas may be associated with chronic periodontitis in dogs. It is not always clear whether they have predisposed to periodontitis or have resulted from chronic irritation of the gingiva. Their appearance is conventional, though often obscured by chronic active inflammation. They are most common about the incisor and canine teeth and are locally invasive, and may invade bone (Fig. 1.5C). However, they are less likely to metastasize than squamous-cell carcinoma of the tonsil. It is assumed that some originate in the gingiva and others in subgingival or periodontal epithelium (see also acanthomatous epulis, above).

In horses, squamous-cell carcinomas are rarely found on the gums and hard palate, possibly arising in chronically irritated hyperplastic alveolar epithelium in cases of chronic periodonitis. They are slow growing, exceedingly destructive, and metastatic only to the regional lymph nodes. Such tumors are large when first observed and may project from the palate or gums as grayish, extensively ulcerated masses, or appear as craterous ulcers. The large ones are extensively necrotic and putrid, and the teeth are lost or loosely embedded in the tumor. These tumors of the maxilla rapidly fill the adjacent sinuses and cause bulging of the face and may extend further into the nasal, orbital, and cranial cavities.

In cattle, oral squamous-cell carcinomas are very rare, with the exception of a few geographic foci where they are associated with oral papillomatosis and ingestion of bracken fern. A similar association is made in the etiology of squamous carcinomas of the esophagus and forestomachs in cattle and is considered more fully under Neoplasia of the Esophagus and Forestomachs.

MELANOMA. In contrast to cutaneous melanomas in the dog, which are usually benign, melanomas of the oral mucosa are almost always malignant. Melanomas are the most common malignant oral tumor in dogs. They are usually located on the gums, buccal mucosa, lips, and palate (Fig. 1.5A,B). The prevalence is higher in males than females. The degree of pigmentation of these tumors varies considerably, and there appears to be no relationship between the amount of pigment and biologic behavior, although the information supporting this last observation is quite controversial. They grow rapidly; necrosis and ulceration are common, and 70–90% metastasize to the regional lymph nodes, mainly the submandibular nodes. They may spread via hematogenous and lymphatic routes to more distant sites.

The histologic appearance of melanomas varies greatly from a fairly well differentiated, heavily pigmented type to a highly anaplastic amelanotic type. The diagnosis of the latter is often difficult. However, there are certain features that are evident in most of these tumors. Anaplastic melanocytes, which have large oval or elongated nuclei with distinct nucleoli and abundant cytoplasm, show junctional activity, infiltrating the junction between the basilar epithelial cells and the submucosa. Frequently there is a characteristic mixture of epithelial-like and spindle-shaped cells, which have a marked tendency to form nests extending deep into the submucosa. Multinucleated giant cells may also be present. About 75% of melanomas have melanin pigment, but detection of this pigment often requires careful examination of individual tumor cells.

Melanin, free and in macrophages, is often found in superficial areas of the submucosa in a variety of nonneoplastic lesions resulting from irritation to the mucosa. This so-called pigmentary incontinence must be differentiated from malignant melanoma.

Although cutaneous melanomas are common in horses and certain breeds of swine, these species have no tendency to develop oral melanomas. These tumors are also rare in cats.

FIBROSARCOMA. Fibrosarcoma is the most common sarcoma of the oral cavity in dogs. It occurs mainly on the gums of the upper molars and adjacent soft palate, and the anterior half of the lower mandible. Infiltration of maxillary and mandibular bone is common. It grows rapidly and frequently recurs after surgical removal. About 35% metastasize to regional nodes, and pulmonary metastases occur early in its course.

MAST-CELL TUMOR. Mast-cell tumor occurs occasionally in the oral cavity of the dog. It may be an extension of cutaneous tumors in the lip, or it may arise in submucosal areas, especially of the tongue. The tumor should be considered potentially malignant, with metastasis to regional lymph nodes a likely possibility. Mast-cell tumor should be considered in the differential diagnosis of oral lesions resembling granulation tissue or eosinophilic granuloma in dogs.

GRANULAR-CELL MYOBLASTOMA. Granular-cell myoblastoma, a rare tumor or tumor-like lesion probably of Schwann-cell origin, occurs mainly in the base of the tongue in the dog. It is elevated, red, and granular or smooth on the mucosal surface. The cut surface is white and firm. Microscopically, the mass consists of large, polyhedral to round, epithelioid cells that have abundant acidophilic granular cytoplasm. The cytoplasmic granules are strongly periodic acid–Schiff (PAS) positive. The nuclei are round to oval, centrally located, and have one or two nucleoli. Mitotic figures are rare. The tumor cells have a marked tendency to form nests, which are separated by a delicate network of reticulin fibers. None of these tumors in dogs has recurred after excision, nor has any metastasized. Similar tumors occur in humans, where they are most common in the skin but may occur in a variety of organs.

Salivary Glands

The most common affections of the salivary glands are functional, ptyalism being an increased secretion of saliva and aptyalism a reduced or ceased secretion. Ptyalism (to be differentiated from failure to swallow) is seen as abnormal accumulation of saliva in the mouth. It occurs in a variety of conditions, including heavy-metal poisoning, poisoning with organophosphates, encephalitis, and most often, stomatitis. Decreased secretion of saliva is less common but accompanies fever, dehydration, and salivary gland disease.

Ptyalism in cattle and horses may be an expression of a mycotoxicosis. *Rhizoctonia leguminicola,* which causes "black patch" disease of several legumes, is the offensive fungus. On well-cured legume hay, the mycelial growth is not visible grossly. The fungus has a wide geographic distribution. The toxic principle is a parasympathomimetic alkaloid called slaframine, which literally means "an amine that causes an animal to salivate." In addition to excessive salivation, other signs include anorexia, excessive lacrimation, diarrhea, frequent urination, and bloat. Milk production is reduced, and there is loss of body weight. No specific lesions have been associated with slaframine toxicosis. Guinea pigs are extremely sensitive to the toxin. Presumptive diagnosis may be based on feeding trials in that species, if chromatographic analysis for slaframine is not readily accessible.

Foreign bodies occasionally are present in the ducts, usually the parotid duct but sometimes the submaxillary. They are usually of plant origin, being awns or fiber. They invariably cause some degree of inflammation with secondary infection; if the duct epithelium is destroyed, a local cellulitis occurs. **Salivary calculi** (sialoliths) may also cause obstruction and inflammation. They are more common in horses than other species. Calculi are composed largely of calcium carbonate, possibly centered on a small foreign body and whitish, hard, and laminated. Calculi are usually single and cylindric, and they may be quite large. Most of them lodge at the orifice and cause some degree of salivary retention, glandular atrophy, and a predisposition to infection and further inflammation.

Dilations of the duct are due to stagnation of flow, and this in turn is a result of obstruction by foreign bodies, calculi, and inflammatory strictures. The dilated ducts appear as fluctuating cords, sometimes with local diverticula. Ranula is the term applied to a cystic distension of the duct in the floor of the mouth. These present as a smooth, rounded prominence with a bluish tinge and fluctuations. The contents may be serous or of thick, tenacious mucus. Rupture of a duct or a gland to an epithelial surface results in permanent fistulas as the continued flow of saliva prevents normal restoration, the duct epithelium fusing with that of the surface.

While ranula by definition is a dilation of a duct with its lining epithelium more or less intact, accumulation of salivary secretions in single or multiloculated cavities adjacent to ducts is now referred to as **salivary mucocele**. These cystic formations do not have an epithelial lining. Small mucoceles, seldom exceeding 0.5 cm in size, are occasionally observed on the side of the bovine tongue. Their origin is presumably from rupture of the fine tortuous ducts of the dorsal part of the sublingual gland.

Mucoceles in dogs are well known because they are large enough to be a surgical problem. They occur in dogs of any breed. There may be a history of an antecedent ranula-like swelling in the mouth. Many mucoceles are probably the result of trauma to the duct. They may be located anywhere, from the mandibular symphysis to the middle of the neck, the latter due to gravitational displacement. Most are ventrolateral, sometimes bilateral or midline, at the angle of the mandible. It appears that they arise most commonly from the sublingual salivary gland, either from individual units of the polystomatic portion or from the duct of the monostomatic portion. Zygomatic salivary mucoceles also occur, associated with local swelling and exophthalmos. Most mucoceles are subcutaneous and are up to 10 cm in diameter, the larger ones being pendulous. The wall is of soft, pliable connective tissue, well vascularized, with a glistening lining. The contents are brown and mucinous, becoming progressively inspissated and tenacious with time.

The histologic appearance of mucoceles varies greatly, apparently depending on the stage of development. Initially, the outer wall consists of an outer, highly vascularized layer of immature connective tissue and an inner zone of loosely arranged fibroblasts. A pleocellular inflammatory reaction is evident in the central area, which also contains much amorphous acidophilic or amphophilic debris. Collagenous connective tissue forms the wall in later stages. The inflammatory cells are mainly mononuclear, and plasma cells often predominate. The debris in the center becomes progressively more basophilic.

Cysts of other origins do occur in this region. Cysts of the thyroglossal duct are midline and distinguishable readily when they contain thyroid follicles. Cystic salivary adenomas are rare. Branchial cleft cysts may be located ventrolaterally, as are the salivary cysts, or dorsolaterally on the neck. Their distinction is probably valid when no demonstrable connection occurs with a salivary duct and a pseudostratified columnar or stratified squamous lining epithelium is present.

Sialoadenitis, inflammation of the salivary glands, is uncommon in animals though inflammation of the zygomatic gland in dogs is a cause of retrobulbar abscess. The infection usually gains entrance via the excretory duct, although the infection may be hematogenous or develops by local trauma. Inflammation of the duct results in its obstruction by exudate, desquamated epithelial cells, and mucus. Some of this may be expressed from the ductal orifice as pus; the orifice is usually acutely inflamed. Obstruction of the duct, whether partial or complete, produces secondary atrophic changes in the glands, although there is initial enlargement due to the combined effects of retained secretion and inflammation. The ducts throughout the gland dilate, and leukocytes infiltrate the lumen and stroma. The acini undergo compression atrophy or swell and rupture from retained secretion. In acute infections this often leads to suppuration, and in chronic ones only remnants of atrophic epithelium remain in a mass of inflamed scar tissue.

Specific inflammations of the salivary glands in domestic animals are unusual, although sialoadenitis does occur in rabies and malignant catarrhal fever. In rabies there is often focal lysis of acinar cells, a mononuclear infiltration, and uncommonly, Negri bodies in the ganglionic neurons. The lesions of malignant catarrhal fever, also specific in type, are described under Infectious and Parasitic Diseases of the Gastrointestinal Tract. Probably the most common associations with sialoadenitis in animals are strangles in horses and distemper in dogs. It is suggested that mumps virus may infect dogs. Sialoadenitis also occurs in vitamin A deficiency in calves and pigs and in cattle poisoned with highly chlorinated naphthalenes. In these latter conditions, the inflammations, often purulent, are secondary to squamous metaplasia of the ducts, with stasis of flow and secondary infection; squamous metaplasia of interlobular ducts is an early and rather specific lesion of vitamin A deficiency.

Neoplasms of the salivary glands are rare in all species but have been reported in cattle, sheep, pigs, horses, and cats. Local invasion by tumors originating in adjacent tissue is more common than primary neoplasia. Only in dogs do salivary tumors occur often enough to permit a general statement. They may arise from either the major or the minor salivary glands, involvement of the major glands being twice as frequent; of these the most susceptible is the parotid. The tumors develop almost exclusively in aged animals; the majority grow rapidly, become fixed to the overlying skin, and are painful.

Salivary tumors have two main sites of origin within the gland: the ducts and the glandular tissue. In most cases, the histogenesis can be recognized, the duct neoplasms being papillomatous if benign, and carcinomas squamous or mucoepidermoid if malignant. Tumors arising in the glandular tissue are usually adenomatous. Their malignant potential may be manifest only by carcinomatous areas at the periphery of the neoplasm.

The histologic structure of salivary tumors in animals is as diverse as in humans, and the accepted classifications apply. The most frequent variety in dogs is of acinar-cell origin, and although there are various structural patterns, an acinar arrangement is usually evident. This arrangement is emphasized by the common occurrence of pseudocystic dissolution, in which tumor cells with clear vesicular cytoplasm rupture, the secretion forming cystlike spaces. Mixed tumors, comparable to those of the mammary gland, occur. The mesenchymal component probably originates from myoepithelial cells. It is similar to that in mammary tumors, with areas of myoepithelial cells embedded in a mucinous matrix that also contains neoplastic epithelial cells. Bone and cartilage form in these areas.

Esophagus

The esophagus merits particular attention during the examination of animals with inadequate growth rate, cachexia, ptyalism, dysphagia, regurgitation, vomition, and aspiration pneumonia. In the ruminant, tympany may be a sequel to esophageal disease. The presence of a "bloat line" in the esophagus at the thoracic inlet may indicate a condition causing increased intraabdominal pressure, such as gastric dilatation or ruminal tympany. The squamous mucosa is frequently eroded or ulcerated in viral diseases, with similar lesions elsewhere in the upper alimentary tract. Conditions of striated muscle such as nutritional myodegeneration and eosinophilic myositis will occur in the esophageal muscle of the ruminant.

Anomalies, Epithelial Metaplasia, and Similar Lesions

Congenital anomalies of the esophagus are very rarely recorded, and their interpretation as such can be difficult, since some similar defects may develop as sequelae of esophageal trauma or inflammation.

Rare **segmental aplasia** of the proximal esophagus may be apparent in the neonate. A short, blind pouch communicates with the pharynx, and a thin, fibrous band connects it to the distal patent limb of the esophagus, which follows a normal course to the stomach. Esophageal aplasia and congenital esophagorespiratory communications result from anomalies occurring when the respiratory primordium buds from the embryonic foregut. **Esophagorespiratory fistulas** without esophageal atresia are more commonly recognized in animals, and in calves and dogs strong circumstantial evidence suggests that some of these are congenital. Short, fibrous bands with a narrow, mucosa-lined lumen connecting an esophagus of normal diameter with trachea or bronchus are reported, as are small apertures connecting the lining of esophageal diverticula with the respiratory tree. The lining of such defects changes from stratified squamous to columnar respiratory epithelium in the fistula or wall of the diverticulum. Gastric distention by air in calves, and pneumonia due to aspiration, have been associated with esophagorespiratory fistulas.

The diagnosis of esophagorespiratory fistulas and diverticula as congenital anomalies is best based on recognition early in life, since both may be acquired following esophageal obstruction. Gradual-pressure necrosis caused by an intraluminal mass and adhesion of esophagus to underlying trachea, or lung, with development of a fistula into the adjacent airway, creates the acquired communication. This may be lined eventually by epithelium of esophageal or respiratory origin.

Esophageal diverticula are irregular outpouchings or herniations of the esophageal mucosa through the muscularis, with a thin, fibrous wall. They communicate with the esophagus by variously sized, often slitlike apertures. Most are probably acquired. Increased intraluminal pressure associated with foreign bodies, obstruction, or stenosis is considered the cause of "pulsion" diverticula, in which the mucosa is forced out through the distended or ruptured muscularis. Such diverticula may be large in the horse and dog, where they are most common. Traction diverticulum is the result of maturation of a periesophageal fibrous adhesion, following perforation and inflammation, drawing with it a pouch of esophageal mucosa that is usually small and inconsequential. Ingesta and foreign bodies may accumulate in diverticula, causing gradual enlargement, with the potential for local esophagitis, ulceration, and perforation or fistula formation.

Rare **anomalies** of the **mucosa** include epithelial inclusion cysts, the presence of papillae resembling those of the rumen in the distal esophagus of cattle, and gastric heterotopia. The presence of gastric glands of the cardiac mucous type in the distal esophagus of dogs and cats is uncommon, and whether it is a developmental anomaly or a metaplastic response to mucosal injury, perhaps gastric reflux, is unclear. Hyperkeratosis and thickening of the epithelium may be signs of vitamin A deficiency or chlorinated naphthalene toxicity. Squamous metaplasia in the ducts of submucosal esophageal mucous glands and in ducts and glands elsewhere should be sought. Mild hyperkeratosis may be difficult to assess since in herbivores some degree of keratinization may be normal, and anorexia or failure to swallow results in loss of the abrasive effect of food passage, with accumulation of keratinized squames. Parakeratotic thickening and basal hyperplasia of the epithelium should be considered indicative of response to epithelial injury, and in the distal esophagus of pigs it is a concomitant of ulceration of the pars esophagea of the stomach. Parakeratosis of the esophagus occurs in pigs with cutaneous parakeratosis of zinc deficiency.

Esophagitis

Erosive and ulcerative esophagitis is a common finding associated with viral diseases causing similar lesions in the oropharynx or reticulorumen. Bovine virus diarrhea, rinderpest, and malignant catarrhal fever tend to produce longitudinal epithelial defects in cattle; bovine papular stomatitis, infectious bovine rhinotracheitis, the herpesviruses of small ruminants and calicivirus in cats may on occasion produce focal necrotizing esophageal lesions, which tend to be punctate or round, perhaps with a raised periphery. Healing focal esophageal ulcers repair by granulation. Local epithelial proliferation and thickening produce an opaque, pearly appearance of the edge of the lesion or surface of the scar.

Caustic or irritant chemicals, ionizing radiation, or hot ingesta may cause mucosal injury, the severity of which depends on the nature of the insult and duration of exposure. Mild acute insult may result in diffuse or local reddening of the mucosa. Deep sloughing of the mucosa, liquefactive necrosis associated with alkalis, and coagulation necrosis following acid and toxins such as paraquat reflect more severe insult and may result in ulceration extending to deeper layers of the esophagus. Superficial epithelial damage heals uneventfully, though repeated insult may cause thickening of the epithelium, with the development of prominent rete pegs. Ulcerated mucosa will granulate, and raised islands of surviving pearly proliferative epithelium may be present over the surface. The inflammatory reaction in ulceration frequently involves muscularis and adventitia. The ultimate development of a contracted fibrous scar causes stricture or stenosis if the original mucosal defect involved a significant portion of the esophageal circumference.

Reflux esophagitis results from the action on the esophageal mucosa of gastric acid, pepsin, probably regurgitated bile salts, and possibly pancreatic enzymes. Stratified squamous epithelium appears more susceptible to the corrosive effects of gastric secretion than other types of mucosa in the lower gastrointestinal tract. Relatively short duration of exposure to re-fluxed gastric content is required to induce epithelial damage, signaled by hyperemia or linear erosions and ulcers, perhaps with superficial fibrinonecrotic debris, and erythematous margins. Such damage is most common in the distal esophagus but may extend well forward, in some instances to the esophageal origin. The expected microscopic basal epithelial activation, rete-peg elongation, and epithelial transmigration of neutrophils occur in response to mild superficial epithelial necrosis. A thinned epithelium following recent moderate insult or granulation of an ulcerated surface may be evident. Reepithelialization with a columnar mucous cell type may occur in distal esophagus adjacent to the cardia. Papillomatous esophagitis of unknown etiology has been reported in the distal esophagus of the cat, which normally has a somewhat corrugated mucosa.

Functional integrity of the lower esophageal sphincter may be compromised or overwhelmed by airway occlusion and increased intraabdominal pressure, the pharmacologic effects of preanesthetic agents, or abnormality of the hiatus. Reflux esophagitis is thus most common in dogs and cats as a sequel to surgery involving general anesthesia, though it may follow chronic gastric regurgitation or vomition for any cause (Fig. 1.6D). In swine and horses, it may be associated with ulceration of the squamous esophageal portion of the stomach (Fig. 1.6E). In dogs, it is associated with rare hiatus herniation. Hiatus hernia usually involves sliding herniation of all or part of the abdominal esophagus, cardia, and stomach into the thoracic esophagus, rather than periesophageal herniation. It is usually self-reducing and associated with lower esophageal sphincter failure and reflux rather than gastric herniation and obstruction. Gastroesophageal intussusception is a very rare event, most reported in puppies of large breeds of dogs, and may be associated with congenital megaesophagus. The entire stomach everts into the esophagus, and occasionally the spleen and pancreas may be involved.

Thrush, or mycotic esophagitis caused by *Candida albicans*, is seen in piglets and weaner swine, where the lesions may involve squamous mucosa of the entire upper alimentary canal. The condition is probably secondary to other intercurrent problems, including antibiotic therapy, inanition, and possibly esophageal gastric reflux and is considered more fully under Mycotic Diseases of the Gastrointestinal Tract. Similarly, secondary zygomycotic granulomatous involvement of the esophagus is a rarely recorded complication of debilitating systemic disease states and heavy use of glucocorticoids and antibiotics.

Esophageal Obstruction, Stenosis, and Perforation

"Choke," obstruction, or impaction of the esophagus occurs when large or inadequately chewed and lubricated foods such as beets, potatoes, corncobs, apples, bones, or masses of grain or fibrous ingesta lodge in the lumen of the esophagus (Fig. 1.6C). Sites of lodgment are often where the esophagus deviates or is slightly restricted normally, and include the area over the larynx, the thoracic inlet, at the base of the heart, and immediately anterior to the diaphragmatic hiatus. Complications of obstruction include pressure necrosis and ulceration of the mucosa, which may progress to perforation. Usually, fatal cellulitis of the

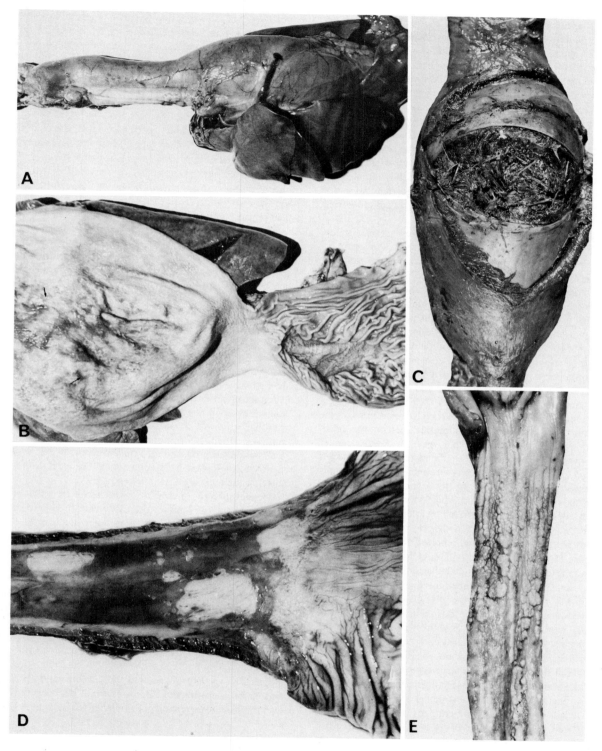

Fig. 1.6. **(A)** Megaesophagus. Dog. Congenital esophageal dilatation. Thoracic esophagus is particularly distended. **(B)** Congenital esophageal dilatation. Dog. Mucosal erosions (arrows). Capacity of distal esophagus exceeds that of stomach. **(C)** Impaction of esophagus with rupture of muscularis. Horse. **(D)** Reflux esophagitis following chronic vomition. Dog. Islands of squamous epithelium remain, surrounded by ulcerated mucosa. **(E)** Reflux esophagitis associated with esophagogastric ulceration. Pig.

periesophageal tissue ensues, which may involve the mediastinum directly or by extension along fascial planes from the cervical region, depending on the site of perforation. Alternatively, perforation of the thoracic esophagus may lead to sepsis of the pleural space, and pleuritis. Perforations of the pharyngoesophageal diverticulum above the cricoid cartilage, due to injuries caused by administration of medication by balling or drenching guns, or by passage of a stomach tube, probang, or endoscope may have similar consequences. Sharp objects, such as needles, quills, grass grains (seeds), awns, etc., may penetrate and track from the esophagus. Diverticulum or esophagorespiratory fistula may also ensue following obstruction by foreign bodies. The cervical esophagus may be perforated by sharp objects such as wire or needles, penetrating from the external surface of the skin.

Removal or dissolution of an obstructing object may be followed by scarring of the segmentally ulcerated esophagus, resulting in a narrowing of the lumen, stricture or stenosis. Esophagitis, especially due to gastric reflux, may have a similar sequel. Although hypertrophy of internal and external muscle layers is seen occasionally in the distal esophagus of cattle and horses (in which species the distal esophageal muscle is normally somewhat thickened), obstruction is not apparent. Stenosis may also result from rare intramural or intraluminal neoplasia, or commonly by external compression. Among causes of external compression may be enlarged hyperplastic or neoplastic thyroids, and neoplasia of the thymus and cervical and mediastinal lymph nodes.

The most common causes of external constriction of the esophagus are ''vascular ring'' anomalies, seen in dogs, occasionally in cats, and rarely in other species. Dextraaorta, or development of the aortic arch from the right instead of the left fourth arch, is the most common of these anomalies. This results in entrapment and constriction of the esophagus between the heart and pulmonary artery ventrally, the anomalous right-sided aortic arch dorsally, and the ligamentum arteriosum or remnant of the ductus arteriosus on the left. Other vascular anomalies that may constrict the esophagus, and reported only in the dog, are persistence of both right and left aortic arches; persistent right ductus arteriosus; aberrant left subclavian artery, in association with persistent right aortic arch; aberrant right subclavian artery, arising distal to the left subclavian artery and passing dorsally over the esophagus. Esophageal deviation and stenosis have been associated in English bulldogs with ''thoracic shortening'' due to hemivertebra and esophageal compression between the left subclavian artery and the brachiocephalic artery.

The site of stricture, with its narrowed esophageal lumen, is readily identified at autopsy. Constricting mural fibrosis or other causative internal or external obstructive lesions will be obvious. The mucosa at the site of stricture may be ulcerated, as the result of impaction of ingesta or as a sequel to antecedent esophagitis, pressure necrosis, or neoplasia. The esophagus anterior to the stenotic area is dilated, may contain retained ingesta, and itself may have evidence of esophagitis.

Dysphagia

Dysphagia, or disorder of swallowing, is a major sign of esophageal disease. Swallowing is a complex and highly coordinated physical act, which may be conveniently divided into three phases. **Oral-phase dysphagias** are the product of painful physical lesions of the oral cavity and tongue, such as stomatitis, glossitis, gingivitis, or lesions that limit movement of the tongue or delivery of the bolus to the pharynx. Loss of hypoglossal nerve function associated with hydrocephalus, trauma, or myasthenia gravis impairs lingual function. Cleft palate results in nasal regurgitation at this phase.

Pharyngeal dysphagia may be associated with painful pharyngitis, tonsillitis, retropharyngeal abscesses, and granulomas. Abscesses, granulomas, and neoplastic processes involving the tonsils and regional lymph nodes may physically intrude on the pharyngeal space. Encephalitis involving the medulla oblongata and the nuclei or tracts of the major cranial nerves involved in pharyngeal contraction and lingual function (V, IX, X, XII) should be sought in pharyngeal dysphagia, unexplained on physical grounds. Rabies and brain abscess in all species, infectious bovine rhinotracheitis, and listeriosis in cattle are candidate central causes of pharyngeal paralysis. Retropharyngeal abscesses and lesions of the equine guttural pouch may cause peripheral nerve damage and paralysis. Idiopathic myodegeneration and myasthenia gravis have been reported as causes of impaired pharyngeal muscle function. Bluetongue and Ibaraki disease cause necrosis of lingual, pharyngeal, and esophageal muscle, resulting in dysphagia and aspiration of ingesta.

Cricoesophageal incoordination or **achalasia** may impede the first stage of the esophageal phase of swallowing, the opening of the upper esophageal sphincter to accept the approaching bolus. This condition is recognized in the dog, but not the cat. It is probably a result of a neurologic rather than local physical or muscular deficit. Microscopic examination of the cricopharyngeal muscle has produced inconsistent observations, though either hypertrophy or degeneration might impede relaxation of the muscle and opening of the esophagus.

Megaesophagus or **esophageal ectasia** is the result of atony of the esophageal muscle, flaccidity, and luminal dilatation (Fig. 1.6A,B). This is the product of segmental or diffuse motor dysfunction of the body of the esophagus. This results in failure of peristaltic propulsion of the food bolus to, and through, the lower esophageal sphincter, or high-pressure zone, to the stomach. Ingesta accumulates in the esophageal lumen, with eventual regurgitation of undigested food. Retention of some ingesta in the esophagus may lead to putrefaction and esophagitis in dilated or dependent areas. The volume of the dilated thoracic and cervical esophagus may greatly exceed that of the stomach, and the intrathoracic trachea and heart may be displaced ventrally. Animals presenting with esophageal hypomotility or megaesophagus may have signs of marked malnutrition, including emaciation, dehydration, and osteopenia, often in association with rhinitis and aspiration pneumonia resulting from regurgitation.

Idiopathic megaesophagus is a relatively common congenital disease in dogs. It is considered to be a neuromuscular developmental disorder or immaturity, which may improve functionally to some extent with time. Megaesophagus in this manifestation is not secondary to physical obstruction or failure to open by the lower esophageal sphincter. Hence it is not comparable to esophageal achalasia in humans. No consistent reduction in number of ganglia in the esophageal myenteric plexus has been recognized. The functional defect in the dog has no basis in the vagal dorsal motor nucleus, since the external muscle layers of the entire esophagus are striated and are innervated directly by fibers arising from lower motor neurons in the nucleus ambiguus. These fibers are not parasympathetic, despite being carried in the vagus nerve. The striated esophageal muscle does not show consistent signs of neurogenic atrophy in idiopathic megaesophagus, and vagal stimulation causes contraction. Hence it is inferred that the lower motor unit is intact. The functional lesion may reside in the upper motor neurons of the central swallowing center or in the afferent sensory arm of the reflex controlling peristalsis, which arises in the esophagus. The pathogenesis of the lesion in megaesophagus in unknown.

Congenital idiopathic megaesophagus in dogs has its highest prevalence in Great Danes, followed by German shepherds, and Irish setters. The condition appears to be heritable, with a pattern in miniature schnauzers compatible with a simple autosomal dominant, or a 60% penetrance autosomal recessive mode of inheritance. Analogous idiopathic functional and morphologic defects may also develop in mature dogs. In addition, megaesophagus in older dogs may be secondary to myasthenia gravis, hypoadrenocorticism, canine giant axonal neuropathy, immune-mediated polymyositis and systemic lupus erythematosus, and Chagas' disease.

Megaesophagus in the cat may be congenital, with signs appearing about weaning time, and is associated particularly with Siamese breeding. The pathogenesis is unclear. Since the esophageal muscle of the cat is smooth in the distal half, dependent on the myenteric plexus for motor control and the vagus for coordination of peristalsis, the pathogenesis probably differs from that in the dog. One report associates megaesophagus in cats with functional pyloric stenosis. Neuronal degeneration or denervation atrophy of muscles are not recognized in the esophageal wall.

Several foals have been reported with esophageal dilatation or ectasia, apparently congenital. Dilation of the anterior portion, with a normal or thickened caudal thoracic esophagus, was found in two cases. Examination of the wall, which is smooth muscle in the caudal half, revealed equivocal muscle abnormalities, and no anomalies of the autonomic ganglia.

Parasitic Diseases of the Esophagus

Sarcosporidiasis occurs in the striated esophageal muscle of sheep. Esophageal sarcocysts appear as ovoid, white, thin-walled nodules ~1.0 cm long projecting from the esophageal muscle (Fig. 1.7A). The species producing large esophageal cysts and similar large cysts in skeletal muscle is spread by cats, where gametogony and sporogony occur in the lamina propria of the small intestine. Other species of microscopic sarcocysts also may be encountered in esophageal striated muscle. Sarcocysts in esophageal muscle normally incite little or no local inflammatory reaction and are of significance only in meat inspection, though lesions of eosinophilic myositis, possibly associated with rupture of cysts, are found in the esophageal muscle.

Larvae of *Gasterophilus* may be temporarily attached to the caudal pharyngeal and cranial esophageal mucosa, and to the mucosa cranial to the cardia, in horses. Insignificant focal ulceration may occur at the sites of attachment.

The larvae of the warble fly (*Hypoderma lineatum*) migrate to the dermis of the back following a period of residence in the submucosa or adventitia of the bovine esophagus. The easily overlooked translucent larvae may be only 2–4 mm in length, but they instigate local hemorrhage and neutrophil infiltration. *Hypoderma* assumes significance in a small proportion of animals treated with systemic organophosphate insecticides while larvae reside in the esophageal wall. An acute inflammatory reaction, probably an allergic response to products of dead larvae, develops in the esophageal submucosa. This leads to swelling, hemorrhage, and necrosis, causing usually fatal esophageal obstruction, tympany, and esophageal perforation.

Spirurid nematodes of the genus *Gongylonema* may be encountered in the stratified squamous mucosa of the upper alimentary tract, including the esophagus, in ruminants and swine. White, threadlike worms up to 10 to 15 cm long, they burrow in the epithelium, and occasionally the propria of the esophageal wall. They usually produce white or red, blood-filled zigzag tracks in the mucosa (Fig. 1.7B). Their presence is inconsequential to the host.

Spirocera lupi is a spirurid nematode that parasitizes the esophageal wall of Canidae and some other carnivores. It is most common in warm climatic zones where appropriate species of dung beetles are found to act as intermediate hosts and where the opportunity for dogs to obtain access to larvae in vertebrate transport hosts is high. The normal site for the adult nematode is in large, thick-walled cystic granulomas in the submucosa of the caudal portion of the esophagus, where one or more pink worms surrounded by purulent exudate are found (Fig. 1.7C,D). A fistulous tract to the esophageal lumen is usually present, through which the tail of the female worm may protrude, and which provides the outlet for ova to the gastrointestinal tract. Third-stage larvae, ingested with dung beetles or encysted in the insectivorous transport hosts, penetrate the gastric mucosa and migrate along arteries to the aorta. Here they migrate, often subintimally, forward to the caudal thoracic area, which they attain within several weeks of infection. Following 2–4 months in an inflammatory granuloma in the aortic adventitia, worms migrate to the subjacent esophagus, where they develop to adulthood in the submucosa and perforate the epithelium. Larvae that adopt aberrant migratory pathways may be found in granulomas in sites such as the subcutis, bladder, and kidney as well as stomach and intrathoracic locations.

Aortic lesions associated with *Spirocerca* are detailed under diseases of the Cardiovascular System (Volume 3) but include subintimal and medial hemorrhage and necrosis with eosinophilic inflammation, intimal roughening with thrombosis, aneurysm with rare aortic rupture, and subintimal and medial mineralization and heterotopic bone deposition. The presence of persistent aortic lesions in the dog, even in the absence of esophageal granuloma, is evidence for prior infection with *S. lupi*. Spondylosis of the ventral aspects of thoracic vertebral bodies 5–10 occurs in some cases. Exostoses or bony spurs arise from one or both ends of the vertebral bodies and presumably are instigated by the local irritant effects of migrating worms.

In some animals with *Spirocerca lupi*, mesenchymal neoplasms develop in the wall of the esophageal granuloma (Fig. 1.7E), and there is a report of a pulmonary fibrosarcoma associated with an ectopic worm. The granulomas around *Spirocerca*

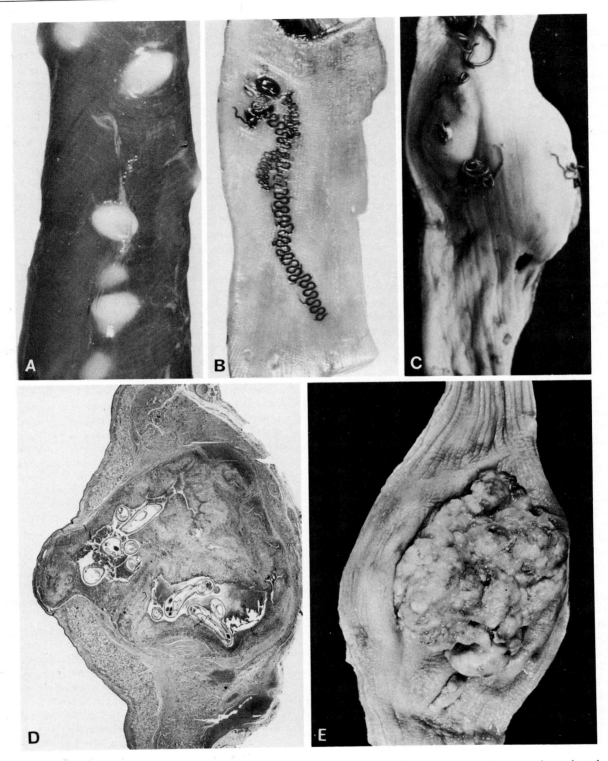

Fig. 1.7.   (**A**) Cysts of *Sarcocystis* sp. in esophageal muscle. Sheep.   (**B**) Blood-filled tracks and small hematoma in esophageal mucosa. *Gongylonema pulchrum*. Cow.   (**C**) *Spirocerca lupi* nodules in distal esophagus. Dog. Worms protrude through fistulas into esophageal lumen. (Courtesy of R. G. Thomson.)   (**D**) Section through esophageal nodule containing *Spirocerca lupi*. Dog. (**E**) Ulcerating fibrosarcoma associated with *Spirocerca* granuloma. Distal esophagus. Dog. (Courtesy of R. G. Thomson.)

contain highly reactive pleomorphic fibroblasts with large, open nuclei and numerous mitotic figures. Neoplasms arising from such lesions have cytologic characteristics typical of fibrosarcoma and osteosarcoma with local tissue invasion and, in many cases, pulmonary metastasis. The carcinogenic stimuli associated with the development of these tumors are unknown. Hypertrophic pulmonary osteopathy is a concomitant lesion found in animals with *Spirocerca*-associated sarcoma and, rarely, granuloma. Clinical disease, exclusive of that associated with neoplasia, is uncommon in animals with *S. lupi* and is restricted to aortic thrombosis, aneurysmal rupture, or occasionally, partial esophageal obstruction.

Forestomachs

The importance of closely examining the rumen contents is often overlooked during routine autopsy. The first, and sometimes only, indication of the presence of certain toxic substances may be provided by the odor and appearance of the rumen content. Urea toxicity may be indicated by an ammoniacal odor and alkaline pH. Organophosphates have a characteristic pungent insecticidal smell reminiscent of cooked turnip. *Taxus* toxicity is signified by an aromatic odor like cedar oil, and the presence of needles in the ingesta. In other suspected plant poisonings, characteristic foliage should be sought in rumen contents. The presence of paint flakes, pieces of metallic lead, and oily content and odor (from used crankcase oil) point to lead poisoning. Frothy voluminous rumen content will support a diagnosis of primary tympany. Porridge-like content with a fermentative odor and perhaps acid pH (<5.0) suggests grain overload.

Dystrophic Changes in the Ruminal Mucosa

The ruminal papillae in the newborn are rudimentary, which gives the mucosa a relatively smooth and pale appearance. Subsequent development of the ruminal papillae depends mainly on the type of diet fed. Little or no growth of papillae occurs in animals as long as they are fed milk. Animals on rations containing adequate levels of roughage develop long, slender, regular, white to gray, ruminal papillae. The ruminal pillars normally lack papillae. Microscopically, the normal papilli are covered by a thin layer of keratinized squamous epithelial cells.

Rations high in concentrate give rise to black, club- and tongue-shaped papillae that have a tendency to form clumps, nodules, and rosettes. They are distributed over the entire mucosa, except for a small area in the dorsal sac where the gas cap would be located. The most prominent changes are mainly in the atrium ruminis and ventral caudal sac, depending somewhat on the age of the animal and the type of concentrate. Microscopically, there is marked acanthosis, hyper- and parakeratosis, and hyperpigmentation of the papillary epithelial cells. Hyperplasia of secondary papillae is also prominent, which may explain the formation of clumps and rosettes seen grossly. The wall is thickened due to fibroplasia of the lamina propria and submucosa. Rumens in animals fed barley rations have similar changes. In addition, animal and vegetable hairs, from the rachillas of barley, adhere to the mucosa, especially in the interpapillary areas, giving it a distinct matted appearance (Fig. 1.8F). Large numbers of hairs are seen in sections of the mucosa. They penetrate the mucosa and lamina propria, where they evoke a leukocytic inflammatory reaction, often causing microabscesses. A diffuse pleocellular reaction is evident in the thickened fibrotic wall.

The pathogenesis of morphologic variations in the ruminal papillae depends on several factors. These include the level, type, and proportion of volatile fatty acids evolved in the ruminal contents, the pH, and the proportion and coarseness of the roughage fed. Other factors are probably involved. High concentrate rations result in increased levels of propionic and butyric acids and lower concentrations of acetic acid. The pH is also lowered, but not enough to cause chemical rumenitis. Hyper- and parakeratosis do not occur when ruminants are fed rations containing adequate levels (~15%) of coarse roughage. The dystrophic changes in the mucosa are reversible when high concentrates are replaced by such levels of roughage. Such a change in the ratio of roughage to concentrate in the diet results in a rise in pH and a shift in the proportions of fatty acids; acetic acid levels increase, and propionic and butyric acids decrease. Roughage is also thought to remove keratinaceous debris and food particles from the mucosal surface. The animal and vegetable hairs in barley rations may provide the portal of entry for bacteria that cause the mild rumenitis and microabscesses in the ruminal wall. Hyperkeratosis of the ruminal epithelium also occurs in calves deficient in vitamin A.

Postmortem Change

The ruminal mucosa usually sloughs within a few hours after death. It separates from the lamina propria in large gray patches, which cover the ingesta when the rumen is opened.

Persistent firm attachment of epithelium is abnormal. This undue adhesion occurs in dystrophic changes, described earlier, in acute rumenitis, especially if caused by fungi, and about healed lesions of necrobacillary rumenitis. Adhesion may not occur in the early stages of ruminal acidosis.

Dilation of the Rumen
(Tympany, Hoven, Bloat)

Tympanitic distension of the forestomachs may be acute, or chronic and recurrent, and there is a basic distinction between the two. The acute tympany of cattle fed legumes is characterized by foaming of the rumen contents, whereas in chronic or recurrent tympany the gas is free but retained because of some physical or functional defect of eructation.

Primary tympany is also called frothy bloat. Foam production in ruminal contents occurs normally. The amount of foam produced is small, however, and it is also unstable. There is apparently a delicate balance between pro- and antifoaming factors. These factors are multiple, and there is considerable controversy as to the extent each one influences the production of the foamy, viscous ruminal content so characteristic of frothy bloat.

The formation of foam is primarily dependent on soluble proteins, which are present in high levels (up to 4.5%) in bloat-inducing legumes. Legumes that are not associated with bloat, such as bird's-foot trefoil, have low levels of soluble protein, generally less than 1.0%. These soluble proteins are released

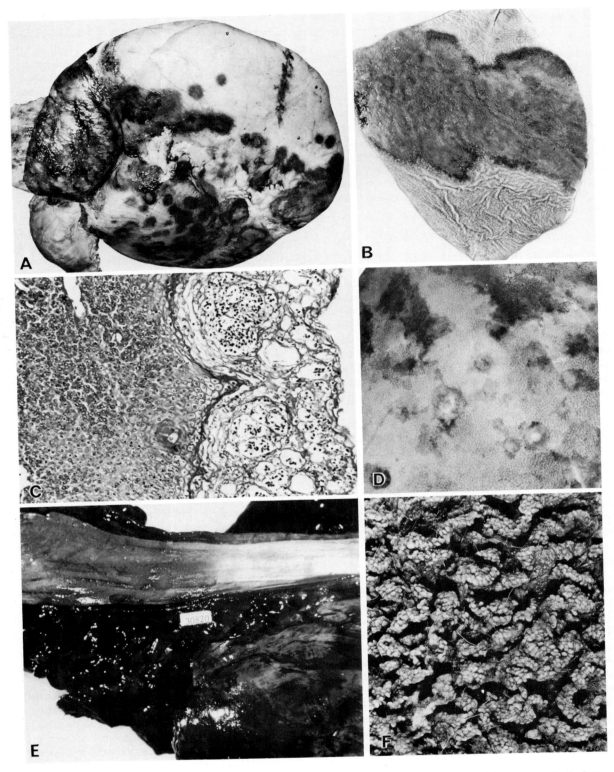

Fig. 1.8. (**A** and **B**) Mycotic rumenitis following acidosis. Cow.   (**A**) Dark areas of infarction involving rumen and reticulum. *Aspergillus* and *Rhizopus*.   (**B**) Appearance of mucosal surface of rumen.   (**C**) Vacuolation and neutrophil infiltration into superficial epithelium of rumen papilla. Chemical rumenitis (ruminal acidosis) due to excess carbohydrate intake.   (**D**) Necrosis in liver due to metastasis of fungi via portal circulation from primary foci of zygomycotic rumenitis.   (**E**) "Bloat line." Cow. Ruminal tympany. Congestion of esophagus and connective tissue cranial to thoracic inlet and blanching of esophagus caudal to thoracic inlet. (**F**) Clubbing and adhesion of rumen papillae with parakeratotic epithelium, associated with feeding a ration high in barley. Plant fibers and hairs are among the matted papillae.

from chloroplasts. When they are degraded by the rumen microflora, they rise to the surface, where they are denatured, become insoluble, and stabilize the foam. The optimum pH (isoelectric point) for foam production by soluble proteins ranges from 5.4 to 6.0. Pectins are considered to increase viscosity of ruminal fluid and may act as foam-stabilizing agents. Plant lipids may act as antifoaming agents by competing for metal ions with the soluble proteins, thus inhibiting the denaturation of these proteins and resulting in decreased foam production.

Animal factors that may contribute to bloat are less accessible to study, and rather little is known of them. Excessive foam production causes distension of the rumen because the animals are unable to eructate foam. Frothy ruminal contents prevents the clearing of the cardia, which is essential for normal eructation to take place. When foam enters the esophagus, it stimulates the swallowing reflex, which also interferes with normal eructation. There is a genetic predisposition to bloating in cattle. Certain sires are known to produce cows that have a high susceptibility to bloating. Monozygotic twins may have similar bloating tendencies.

The variation among animals in their susceptibility to bloat may be determined in part by variations in the amount and composition of saliva secreted. Saliva apparently has properties that may promote or prevent foaming in the rumen. When secretion of saliva decreases, the viscosity of ruminal contents increases, which in turn promotes foaming. Cows that have a high susceptibility to bloating produce less saliva than cows that have a low susceptibility. Succulent and high-concentrate feeds reduce salivary secretion, thus increasing viscosity of rumen contents. The composition of saliva affects foam production in several ways. Combination of salivary bicarbonate with organic acids such as citric, malonic, and succinic acids, which are present in high levels in legumes, results in the production of large amounts of carbon dioxide, enhancing bubble formation. Carbon dioxide accounts for 40 to 70% of the total gas produced in the rumen.

Salivary mucoproteins increase viscosity, while mucins reduce viscosity. The levels of the various pro- and antifoaming compounds in saliva are dependent on the gland of origin. The parotid and submaxillary glands produce saliva with a high concentration of mucins. These glands actively secrete saliva when the animal is eating and when ruminal pressure is high. The buffering action of saliva may raise the pH of the ruminal contents above the range at which soluble proteins are most likely to produce stable foam. The knowledge of the full role played by saliva in bloat is still incomplete, and more research in this area may show that other factors are involved.

Rations high in concentrate and low in roughage not only reduce saliva secretion, they also change the ruminal microflora. They promote the growth of large numbers of encapsulated bacteria, which increase the concentration of polysaccharides, and these in turn increase the viscosity. These bacteria are also often mucinolytic and may destroy the salivary mucins. Perhaps this explains the more gradual onset of feedlot bloat, since it takes time for the ruminal flora to change.

The cause of death in bloat is probably due to the combined effects of increased intraabdominal pressure on the diaphragm, inhibiting respiration, and the shunting of a large volume of blood away from the abdominal viscera. Anoxia may be caused by respiratory embarrassment. Increased intraabdominal pressure also has a marked effect on the hemodynamics of the abdominal viscera. There is compression of the posterior vena cava, which results in a redirection of blood flow from the caudal areas of the animal. The blood is shunted through the lumbar veins, into the longitudinal vertebral sinuses, from there to the intercostal veins, and into the hemiazygos or costocervical vein. There is considerable variation among animals, and in individual animals from day to day, in the ruminal pressures that can be tolerated.

The bloated animal is often found dead and distended with gas; blood exudes from the orifices, and because of the gaseous distension, the carcass often rolls on its back. The blood is dark and clots poorly; both features are indicative of death due to anoxia. Subcutaneous hemorrhages are prominent in the neck and trunk. There is marked edema, congestion, and hemorrhage of the cervical muscles and of the lymph nodes of the head and neck. An inconsistent, but significant, finding is the so-called bloat line in the esophageal mucosa (Fig. 1.8E). This lesion is formed due to congestion with petechial and ecchymotic hemorrhages in the mucosa of the cervical esophagus, which changes abruptly or gradually to a pale mucosa at the level of the thoracic inlet. The tracheal mucosa is hemorrhagic, especially anterior to the thoracic inlet. Blood clots are frequently seen in the bronchi and paranasal and frontal sinuses. The lungs are compressed into the anterior thorax by the bulging diaphragm. There is pressure ischemia of the abdominal viscera, especially the liver. The extreme margins of the hepatic lobes may be congested. Lymph nodes and the muscles of the hind legs are pale. There may be marked subcutaneous edema, particularly of the vulva and perineum. If the autopsy is done soon after death, the ruminal contents are bulky and foamy. The foam gradually disappears after death and is usually absent if the autopsy is delayed for 10 to 12 hr. Inguinal hernia and diaphragmatic rupture may occur after death.

Secondary tympany, or secondary bloat, may be acute but is usually chronic, with periods of acute exacerbation. It is usually the result of a physical or functional defect in eructation of gas produced by normal rumen fermentation. The more common physical problems include obstructions of the esophagus or esophageal groove by tumor, papilloma, or foreign body; reticular adhesions; and esophageal stenosis of any cause. Functional causes of secondary tympany include organophosphate intoxication and vagal damage due to adhesion or lymphosarcomatous infiltrates. It is a component of the syndromes collectively termed "vagus indigestion." Secondary tympany, sometimes fatal, occurs in bucket-fed calves. A diagnosis of secondary bloat at autopsy is based on physical findings like those described in primary bloat, but without frothy rumen content, and with the addition of any physical cause of impaired eructation.

Bloat must be differentiated from other causes of sudden death. These include hypomagnesemia, blackleg, malignant edema, anthrax, lightning stroke, and accidental electrocution. None of these conditions has lesions associated with the redistribution of abdominal blood flow, nor are the rumen contents foamy. The bacterial infections are characterized by typical muscle lesions in the case of blackleg and malignant edema, and there are septicemic lesions including an enlarged raspberry-like spleen in anthrax. Ruminal distention occurs with grain overload; however, the contents are watery and have a fermentative odor.

Postmortem distention of the rumen must not be mistaken for antemortem tympany. Extraruminal lesions must be present to establish a diagnosis of bloat.

Foreign Bodies in the Forestomachs

Cattle are notoriously lacking in alimentary finesse, a deficiency that allows an amazing variety of foreign bodies, prehended with the food, to be deposited in the forestomachs. Sheep are largely immune because of their more selective eating habits. Foreign bodies are rarely found in the rumen of goats, despite their reputation for indiscriminate feeding habits. In consequence, a large proportion of adult cattle, and very few goats or sheep, have foreign bodies in the rumen and reticulum but rarely in the omasum. It is possible that many of the lighter and smaller foreign bodies are regurgitated.

Foreign bodies consisting largely of hair or wool (**trichobezoars**), or plant fibers (**phytobezoars**) may also form in these compartments. Hair balls are most common in younger ruminants, the hair being swallowed after licking, particularly by animals deprived of dietary fiber. They may have some other foreign body as a nucleus and contain a proportion of plant fibers, the whole mass concreted by organic substances and inorganic salts. The same general comments apply to phytobezoars. Being smooth, neither are important unless regurgitated to lodge in the esophagus or passed on to obstruct the pylorus or intestine.

The important foreign bodies are those, such as lead, that when dissolved cause intoxication, and those that being abrasive or sharp, penetrate the mucosa. In calves on diets low in roughage, ingestion of wood shavings or straw may lead to diffuse cellulitis of the forestomachs and sometimes the abomasum. A mixed bacterial flora containing clostridia is responsible, presumably following mucosal trauma. The sequel to penetration by sharp objects in adult cattle is traumatic reticuloperitonitis.

TRAUMATIC RETICULOPERITONITIS AND ITS COMPLICATIONS. Perforation of the forestomachs by foreign bodies virtually always is a penetration of the reticular wall by a sharp foreign body, usually a piece of wire or a nail. Incomplete perforation of the wall is usually without significant effect, although in some cases a suppurative or granulomatous inflammation develops in the wall of the reticulum, with minor overlying peritonitis. There are no adequate answers as to why perforation occurs or why it is so frequently in the anteroventral direction. It is probably caused by forceful contraction of the reticulum, and many cases seem to be precipitated by the increased intraabdominal pressure of late pregnancy and parturition.

There is a rather uniform train of events when complete perforation occurs, but variations of the pattern are common. The perforation is usually in the anteroventral direction and is followed immediately by an acute local peritonitis. If the foreign body is short or bent, it may progress no further, and some foreign bodies are apparently withdrawn with the reticular

movement; in such instances a chronic local peritonitis with adhesions develops. The foreign body may advance to perforate the diaphragm and pericardium, resulting in traumatic pericarditis, but this advancement may be delayed.

A ventral penetration may result in subperitoneal and subcutaneous abscess near the xiphoid. Rare perforation of one of the larger regional arteries may result in sudden death from hemorrhage, and sudden death may also occur if there is penetration of the myocardium or rupture of a coronary artery. Penetration of the thoracic cavity may occur without perforation of the pericardium and cause pneumonia and pleuritis. Right lateral deviation of the penetrating agent causes involvement of the wall of the abomasum. It is unusual for the liver or spleen to be penetrated, but metastatic abscesses in the liver are common.

As soon as the foreign body penetrates the serosa, a local fibrinous peritonitis develops, leading later to dense adhesion of variable extent between the reticulum and adjacent structures. Further progression of the foreign body is ordinarily slow and produces a canal surrounded by chronic granulation tissue and containing, besides the foreign body, ingesta, purulent exudate, and detritus. The bacteria commonly active in the tract are *Corynebacterium pyogenes, Fusobacterium necrophorum,* and a variety of putrefactive types. In many cases, a foreign body cannot be found, perhaps because it has rusted away or been withdrawn into the reticulum.

Traumatic pericarditis is a less common sequel now, perhaps because so many of the initial penetrations are diagnosed and the foreign body removed surgically. The pericardial reaction is copious, fibrinopurulent, and putrid. There are usually additional lesions of traumatic pneumonia and pleurisy, with emphysema from rupture of the lung.

The prophylactic use of magnets has become common practice in many herds, and this probably contributes to the marked decrease in fatal cases. Frequently, these magnets are found incidentally in the reticulum, completely covered with metal foreign bodies, including nails and wires, which might otherwise have penetrated the reticular wall. The replacement of baling wire with binder twine is another reason for the apparent decline in the prevalence of this disease.

One of the variants in the usual pattern of migration of the foreign body is penetration of the side of the reticulum, leading to a suppurative inflammation in the grooves between the reticulum, omasum, and abomasum. Although the acute local peritonitis causes immediate cessation of ruminal movements, a persistent ruminal atony or inactivity may ensue. Clinically, this is referred to as "vagus indigestion," and at autopsy there are very characteristic changes in the stomachs.

In "vagus indigestion," the abomasum may be distended and impacted with dry ingesta presumably due to functional pyloric stenosis or abomasal stasis. The omasum in this condition can be very large and impacted with dehydrated ingesta. The rumen is distended with enough fluid to cause sloshing if the carcass is jolted. There is no ruminal fermentation or odor, and bits of unmacerated straw and food particles float on the watery fluid. The more normal ingesta has sedimented.

The question of the importance of vagal nerve damage in the pathogenesis of so-called vagus indigestion remains unresolved. The rumen and reticulum are dependent on intact vagi for normal movement, and a minority of cases of "vagus indigestion" appear to be associated with damaged nerves. Vagal lesions may be intrathoracic, such as in lymphosarcomatous infiltration, or abdominal. The latter are usually investment of the nerve in adhesions following reticular perforation, or trauma following abomasal volvulus. In other cases, degeneration of the vagus is not evident, and the dysfunction and lesions are more likely to be due to peritonitis and the subsequent abscessation or adhesions that interfere with normal motility of the forestomachs and the abomasum. A diagnosis of vagal indigestion at autopsy is orinarily dependent on evidence of abnormal abomasal, omasal, or reticuloruminal motility, in association with morphologic lesions of the vagus nerves, or adhesion involving the forestomachs and abomasum.

Rumenitis

Inflammatory lesions in the forestomachs occur in a number of viral diseases of the alimentary mucosae in ruminants. In neonatal calves, necrosis of ruminal mucosa is an important sequel to infectious bovine rhinotracheitis infection. Bovine papular stomatitis and contagious ecthyma will rarely cause rumen lesions. Rumenal erosions and ulcers are present in some cattle with bovine virus diarrhea; they are reportedly less frequently found in rinderpest. Extensive hemorrhage and ulceration of the reticuloruminal mucosa may be seen in bluetongue in sheep. Adenovirus infection occasionally causes a multifocal fibrinohemorrhagic rumenitis. Focal or diffuse rumenitis may be present in cattle with malignant catarrhal fever. These conditions are described under Infectious and Parasitic Diseases of the Gastrointestinal Tract.

A mild inflammation of the forestomachs occurs in some young calves fed milk from a pail, when, because of laxity of the esophageal groove reflex, the milk spills into the rumen and reticulum in large quantity. A similar problem occurs with feeding by stomach tube. Putrefaction in these compartments leads to mild rumenitis.

Accidental consumption of excessive quantitites of urea, in the form of nonprotein nitrogen supplement, or fertilizer, in liquid or powder form, results in the production of ammonia in the rumen. The toxic effect is accelerated by urease in soy-based rations and is based on the production of high blood levels of ammonia. A history of abdominal pain and central nervous signs such as incoordination and violent struggling may be available. Rumen contents smell ammoniacal when the organ is opened, the content is alkaline, and there may be congestion or coagulation necrosis of the anteroventral wall of the rumen.

A more common form of acute chemical rumenitis develops after overeating on rapidly fermentable carbohydrate, usually grain.

RUMENITIS AND ACIDOSIS CAUSED BY OVEREATING GRAIN. Ruminal acidosis and rumenitis associated with ingestion of excess carbohydrate is a problem mainly of intensive beef and dairy production. Sheep and, especially, goats are also susceptible to this problem. Its importance lies partly in loss of production and partly in mortality due to the acute disease, in which the rumenitis is of minor significance, and the lactic acidosis is the major cause of morbidity and mortality. Rumenitis assumes sig-nificance in subclinical disease or in survivors of acute episodes by providing a portal for the entry for fungi and *Fusobacterium necrophorum*. These complications are discussed below. There are other complications. Primary tympany (frothy bloat) may coexist and be the fatal partner of grain overload in feedlot cattle.

Ruminal acidosis usually follows the ingestion of excess carbohydrate in the form of grain or other fermentable feedstuffs occasionally used, such as bread, brewer's waste, and apples. There is a wide variation in the amount of carbohydrate necessary to kill an animal, because tolerance to rations high in starch does develop. Sudden increments in the amount of carbohydrate ingested are of more importance than the actual amount, provided this increases slowly. In sheep, for which some information is available, ~60 g of wheat per kilogram of body weight must be ingested to cause death; probably this figure is generally applicable to cattle also. Lesser amounts than this may cause illness but permit eventual recovery. Even after cattle are accustomed to high concentrate rations, they may still develop ruminal acidosis. Sudden changes from concentrates with lower energy values to those with higher values may predispose to acidosis. Extreme environmental temperature changes, either hotter or cooler, may result in temporary reductions in feed consumption, and acidosis may develop once animals return to full feed.

Shortly after the ingestion of a toxic amount of carbohydrate, the ruminal pH begins to fall. The decrease in pH during the first 8 hr is mainly due to an increase in dissociated volatile fatty acids, not lactic acid. The production of the latter increases after there has been a marked change in the ruminal flora, which is very responsive to the substrate available for fermentation. The normal pH of ruminal fluid in cattle and sheep varies between 5.5 and 7.5, depending on the diet fed.

The Gram-negative bacteria that predominate in the normal flora and the protozoa are very sensitive to changes in the pH. Most of these organisms die at a pH of 5.0 or less. Once the pH of the ruminal contents starts to fall, there is a rapid proliferation of streptococci, mainly *Streptococcus bovis*, and these bacteria are the main source of lactic acid. When the pH reaches 5.0–4.5, the numbers of streptococci decrease, with a concomitant increase in lactobacilli. The pH of rumen content may fall as low as 4.5 to 4.0 in fatal cases.

As the ruminal pH drops, ruminal atony develops, mainly as the result of an increase in the concentration of dissociated fatty acids, rather than of lactic acid, as was once thought. There is also a cessation of salivary secretion so that the buffering effect of saliva is absent. The increase in ruminal organic acids, mainly lactate, causes an increase in ruminal osmotic pressure. This results in movement of fluid from the blood into the rumen, producing bulky and liquid ruminal contents and severe dehydration. There is a reduction in plasma volume; hemoconcentration, anuria, and circulatory collapse follow. Serum protein levels, urea, inorganic phosphorus, lactate, pyruvate, and liver enzymes are all elevated. The osmotic pressure of the intestinal contents also increases when the ingesta with the high lactate concentration arrives there. Loss of fluid at this level probably contributes further to the dehydration, and it may also play a significant role in the development of the diarrhea that is commonly seen clinically.

In those animals that survive the acute phase of ruminal acidosis, complete recovery is delayed until a normal ruminal flora is reestablished through contact with other animals. A temporary recovery may be followed by what appears clinically to be a relapse in acidosis, but which is a developing mycotic rumenitis. If treatment of the initial fluid imbalance is delayed, death may occur in a week or so from ischemic renal cortical necrosis.

In addition to the osmotic effects, there is acidosis due to the absorption of lactate from the rumen, and possibly from the intestine. Almost equal concentrations of D and L isomers of lactic acid are produced in the rumen. However, the D isomer of lactic acid is poorly metabolized by the host and hence accumulates eventually to a much higher concentration in plasma than the L isomer. This is probably reinforced by endogenous lactate produced in the state of relative anaerobiosis of peripheral circulatory failure. The blood pH may drop as low as 7.0, which causes a marked depletion of alkali reserves. Absorption of D-lactate exceeds the rate of metabolic breakdown, and further aggravation of the acidosis may occur when the excretion of this isomer is impaired due to reduced renal function. Such a reduction in the plasma clearance of lactic acid occurs only after the blood pH drops to 7.14 or less and lactic acid levels have risen to ~25 ml/liter or higher. There are other toxic factors, including histamine, produced in this disease, but the amounts absorbed from an acid rumen are probably too low to have any effect.

The low ruminal pH that develops is lethal to much of the normal flora and fauna. The protozoa appear to be particularly sensitive, but many types of bacteria are also lost. Therefore, in animals that show signs of immediate recovery, with or without therapeutic aid, the reestablishment of normal fermentation reactions may be delayed.

The morbid anatomy of this metabolic disease is not specific, and a practical diagnosis requires knowledge of access to fermentable carbohydrate and a clinically observed circulatory failure. At autopsy, the eyes are sunken and the blood may be thick and dark due to dehydration and hypoxia, and there is general venous congestion. The appearance of the ruminal contents varies with the time interval between ingestion of the carbohydrate and the autopsy. In the early stages, there is a copious amount of porridge-like rumen contents, which has a distinct fermentative odor. The amount of grain or corn varies considerably and is an unreliable indication of acidosis, and the presence of finely ground concentrate may be overlooked. Ruminal pH is helpful only when it is low (<5.0), since it may rise in later stages of acidosis. Although the ruminal contents may appear relatively normal in more advanced cases of acidosis, the intestinal contents tend to remain very watery. Absence of protozoa is consistent with chemical rumenitis but is also influenced by the interval between death and the postmortem examination.

The diagnosis of ruminal acidosis at autopsy can be difficult. The most suggestive abnormality is the rumenitis. It is probably chemical and dependent on the low pH, and is not readily discerned grossly. There may be a slight, poorly defined bluish coloration in the ventral sac of the rumen and reticulum and in the omasum, visible through the serosa. When the epithelium is detached, the lamina propria is seen to be hyperemic in patches.

Microscopic examination of the ruminal mucosa is the most reliable way to confirm a diagnosis of chemical rumenitis. The ruminal papillae appear enlarged. There is marked cytoplasmic vacuolation of the epithelial cells, often leading to vesiculation. A mild to marked neutrophilic reaction is evident in the mucosa and submucosa (Fig. 1.8C). Focal areas of erosion and ulceration may or may not be present.

Fusobacterium necrophorum is a normal inhabitant of the anaerobic ruminal environment. This bacterium is usually responsible for the infective complications of ruminal acidosis, and it produces characteristic lesions in the forestomachs (Fig. 1.9A–C) and metastases in the liver. Invasion of the wall of the rumen probably does not occur with significant frequency unless a foothold is provided by the superficial necrosis and inflammation of acidosis. Necrobacillary rumenitis is common in feedlot cattle, probably a product of mild acidosis following a too rapid introduction to a high-concentrate ration. It is also an observed complication in other cattle, especially dairy cows, which gain access to unusual amounts of grain, and in sheep under the same circumstances.

Necrobacillary rumenitis affects the papillated areas of the ventral sac and occasionally the pillars. On the inner surface, the early lesions are visible as multiple, irregular patches from 2 to 15 cm across, in which the villi are swollen, dark, slightly mushy, and matted together by fibrinocellular inflammatory exudate. The affected villi are necrotic, but ulceration may be delayed if there is ruminal atony and stasis. If the animal recovers from the immediate effects of overeating, the necrotic epithelium sloughs, the ulcer contracts, and epithelial regeneration begins from the margins. The regenerated epithelium is flat and white, and the specialized villi do not completely return. A stellate scar remains, but many of the smaller lesions may disappear completely (Fig. 1.9C). Hepatic metastases are initially typical of necrobacillosis, consisting of coagulative necrosis, but in time they liquefy to form typical abscesses and these often persist long after the initial ruminal lesions have healed, cicatrized, and disappeared.

It is unusual for ruminal necrobacillosis in cattle to be more than a superficial infection, and although the muscle layers are involved in the inflammation, they are not ordinarily invaded by the organism. Infection of the omasum differs in that perforation of the omasal leaves is common. In sheep, the infection is more progressive than in cattle.

When inflammation in the wall of the forestomachs extends to the serosa and is hemorrhagic, mycotic infection should be suspected. The fungi, which are opportunists like *Fusobacterium necrophorum*, are usually members of the genera *Mucor, Rhizopus,* and *Absidia,* and these cannot be differentiated from each other in histologic sections. In the few cases cultured, the incriminated organism was *Rhizopus.*

Mycotic rumenitis is much more severe and extensive than necrobacillary rumenitis and is often fatal. The inflammation extends to the peritoneum, causing a hemorrhagic and fibrinous peritonitis that mats the omentum to the rumen. In fatal cases, most of the ventral sac and parts of the omasum are involved. The lesions are very striking and suggest on initial inspection that the walls have been massively infarcted, which in part they have (Fig. 1.8A,B). The margins are well demarcated, usually by a narrow zone of congestive swelling. The affected areas are red to black in color, thickened to a centimeter or more, firm,

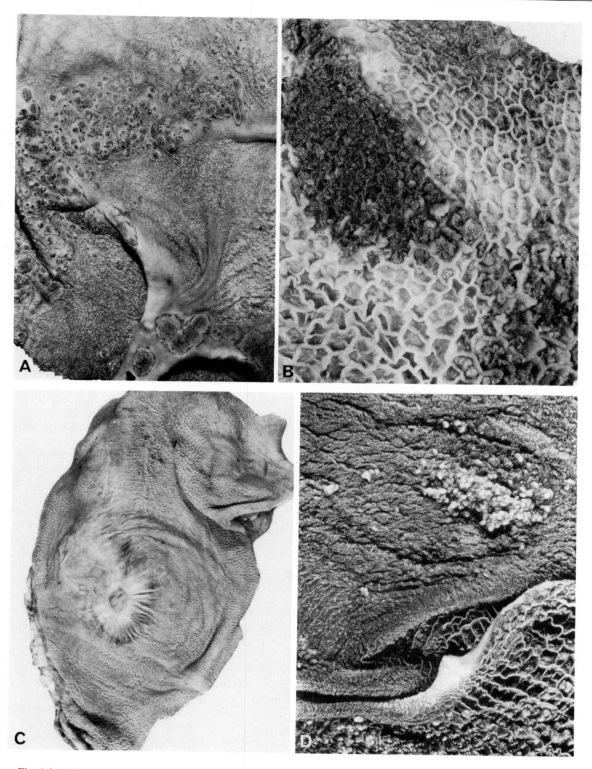

Fig. 1.9. (**A** and **B**) Acute necrobacillosis in rumen and reticulum. Cow. (**C**) Stellate scarring of incompletely healed ulcer in rumen mucosa in fusobacterial rumenitis. (**D**) *Paramphistomum* sp. flukes on the mucosa of the reticulorumen.

and leathery. There is acute fibrinohemorrhagic inflammation of the overlying peritoneum, and beneath it in the grooves there is a bloodstained, inflammatory edema. Thrombosis, as the result of vasculitis due to the invasion of the vessels by the fungus, is the basis for this lesion.

On the inner surface of the rumen, the lesions are more hemorrhagic than those of necrobacillosis, and often more irregular in outline, and the necrotic epithelium is difficult to detach. Histologically, the rumenitis is characterized by hemorrhagic necrosis of all structures in the wall, by copious fibrinous exudate, and by rather scant leukocytic reaction. A severely necrotizing vasculitis is characteristic, the fungus being readily visible in the necrotic tissues and the lumina of the blood vessels.

Metastases sometimes occur in the liver and cause a necrotizing thrombophlebitis of the portal radicles, visible as small irregular, tan areas of infarction surrounded by a deep red margin (Fig. 1.8D).

Other conditions that have been associated with ruminal acidosis are laminitis and an encephalopathy that morphologically resembles the lesions of early polioencephalomalacia. The pathogenesis of laminitis are discussed in the Skin and Appendages (Volume 1). The encephalopathy has been observed in experimental acidosis in sheep. Grossly, the brain is swollen due to edema. The cerebellar vermis prolapses into the fourth ventricle, and there is coning of the cerebellum into the foramen magnum. Microscopically, there is neuronal degeneration of the middle laminae of the cerebral cortex and perivascular edema. These lesions may be due to an induced thiamine deficiency. There is no storage of thiamine. In the normal ruminal flora, thiamine production depends on a delicate balance between thiamine and thiaminase-producing bacteria. In ruminal acidosis this balance may be disturbed by the proliferation of *Streptococcus bovis,* which is known to consume thiamine. In addition, the acid medium may be favorable for thiaminase-producing organisms such as *Clostridium sporogenes* and *Bacillus thiaminolyticus.* The prevalence of the cerebral lesions in spontaneous cases of ruminal acidosis is not known but warrants further investigation.

Parasitic Diseases of the Forestomachs

Gongylonema species occur in the epithelium of the rumen. They appear as described for the esophagus. They are insignificant as pathogens.

More important parasites are the conical flukes belonging to the family Paramphistomatidae. They are found in cattle and sheep in warm temperate, subtropical, and tropical regions. These reddish, plump, droplet-shaped flukes are about the size of the papillae between which they reside in the rumen, where they are nonpathogenic (Fig. 1.9D). Their significance lies in the potential for larval paramphistomes in the duodenum to cause disease. The biology and pathogenicity of paramphistomes is discussed under Infectious and Parasitic Diseases of the Gastrointestinal Tract.

Myiasis of the rumen caused by larvae of the ''screwworm'' fly *Cochliomyia hominivorax* is occasionally a cause of mortality in young calves in South America. The larvae are presumed to be licked from cutaneous wounds and swallowed. They lodge in the rumen and perforate it.

Neoplasia of the Esophagus and Forestomachs

Neoplasia of the esophagus and reticulorumen is, with the exception of papilloma, uncommon in domestic animals.

Papillomas of the esophagus in dogs are uncommon and may be associated with oral papilloma. In cattle, papillomas of the esophagus and reticulorumen may be common in some areas. They are caused by bovine papillomavirus type 4, which infects only squamous mucosa of the mouth, pharynx, and upper alimentary tract. Bovine alimentary papillomas are usually solitary, though a minority of infected animals may have multiple lesions. Most are small (<1.0 cm), broadly pedunculate, tapering, acuminate masses. They are composed of a number of closely packed fronds of squamous epithelium, each supported by a light core of fibrous stroma and arising from a common fibrous base. Some form flattened sessile hyperplastic epithelial plaques, while others, usually limited to the esophagus, form fibropapillomas. The latter are smooth, nodular masses comprised of acanthotic epithelium supported by a fibromatous stroma, occasionally found in close physical association with a more typical papilloma. In a low proportion of typical alimentary papillomas in cattle, but not in fibropapillomas, eosinophilic intranuclear inclusion bodies may be present in keratinizing cells. In these, and in vacuolate nuclei containing amphophilic material, papovaviruses may be found by electron microscopy. Papillomas are normally asymptomatic, though large lesions of the reticular groove and esophagus may interfere with eructation and deglutition.

Malignant neoplasms of the **esophagus** and **forestomachs** in ruminants are ordinarily extremely rare. In several localities, however, squamous-cell carcinoma is relatively commonly found in association with papilloma. It has been suggested that an interaction between viral papillomas and ingestion of carcinogens in bracken fern predisposes to the development of squamous-cell carcinomas of the esophagus and forestomachs in the hill country of Scotland and northern England. In Brazil a similar association is made with carcinomas of the oropharynx. A high prevalence of carcinoma of the esophagus and forestomachs also has been reported from a single valley in Kenya, in association with papillomas, not confirmed as viral, and with a carcinogen apparently ingested with or derived from native forest plants. Esophageal and ruminal carcinomas are associated with dysphagia or difficult deglutition, rumen tympany, and apparent abdominal pain with progressive cachexia. Concurrent papillomas, carcinomas, and hemangiomas of the bladder like those causing enzootic hematuria are often found in cattle with esophageal or ruminal cancer. In Scotland, intestinal adenomas or adenocarcinomas were also found in many cases.

Esophageal and **ruminal carcinoma** may be seen developing from recognizable papillomas, as brownish, irregular, roughened hyperplastic epithelium, or as ulcerated or irregular proliferative fungating lesions. The distal esophagus, reticular groove, and adjacent ruminal wall are the sites most commonly affected with carcinoma. Microscopically, they are typical squamous-cell carcinomas and invade locally, causing induration of the wall of the organ. They may metastasize to local lymph nodes and to distant sites such as liver and lung.

Squamous-cell carcinomas may also be encountered rarely in the esophagus of cats, where they develop in the distal portion, forming proliferative plaques of neoplastic cells that eventually ulcerate and invade the wall of the esophagus and adjacent mediastinum. In horses, squamous-cell carcinomas of the stomach may also involve the adjacent terminal esophagus.

Mesenchymal tumors of the esophagus, with the exception of the *Spirocerca*-associated fibrosarcomas and osteosarcomas in dogs, referred to previously, are very rare. Connective-tissue tumors of the rumen are similarly rare. Occasional involvement of the omasum and reticulum by direct extension from adjacent affected abomasum may occur in cattle with lymphosarcoma. Invasion of or metastasis to the canine esophagus by thyroid, respiratory, and gastric carcinomas is also reported.

Stomach and Abomasum

Normal Form and Function

Particular attention should be paid to the stomach in the examination of animals of any species with a history of inappetence or anorexia, cachexia, hypoproteinemia, diarrhea, regurgitation, or vomition. Abdominal distention may be associated with gastric dilatation or displacement. Hematemesis, melena, or anemia may signify gastric bleeding. Many infectious diseases with major systemic or alimentary tract signs elsewhere produce gastric lesions. Systemic states such as uremia and toxemia cause characteristic gastric lesions in some species.

In the horse and pig, an obvious smooth, white or yellowish esophageal region is present. It is covered by stratified squamous epithelium, with susceptibility to insult and reparative capacity similar to that of the esophageal lining. This area is most extensive in the horse, incorporating the cranial third of the stomach, including the saccus cecus. The pars esophagea of the stomach of the pig is a rectangular area around the cardia. Chronic inflammatory infiltrates and lymphoid follicles are normally present in the lamina propria and submucosa of the cardiac gland mucosa abutting the esophageal region, especially in the pig. The cardiac gland zone has a grayish color and is particularly well developed in this species, lining the gastric diverticulum, fundus, and about half the body of the stomach. In the dog, cat, and ruminant, cardiac glands are limited to a narrow zone at the cardia or omasal opening. Cardiac glands are branched tubular structures, lined almost exclusively by columnar mucous cells with a few endocrine cells interspersed, though chief cells may be present in the pig. These glands open into gastric pits or foveolae, which are lined by tall columnar mucous cells continuous with the covering of the gastric surface. The anterior portions of the equine and porcine stomach are so modified to permit bacterial fermentation and evolution of volatile fatty acids in an environment of relatively high pH (>5), buffered by saliva and cardiac gland secretions.

The fundic or oxyntic gland acid-secretory mucosa in the horse and pig is reddish brown and slightly irregular but not highly folded. More prominent longitudinally oriented rugae or plicae are present in the dog and cat, and in the abomasum. Gastric secretion undiluted by ingesta in the dog or cat normally should have a pH less than 4. Abomasal content should have a pH of 3.5 to 4.0. Tall columnar mucous cells cover the gastric surface and line pits or foveolae in this region of the stomach as well. Fundic glands contain several classes of cells. The junction of the base of the foveolus and the upper portion of the gland proper is termed the isthmus. Here the proliferative compartment of the gland is found. Cuboidal, or low columnar mucous neck cells in a narrow zone in this area undergo mitosis. Some daughter cells differentiate into foveolar mucous cells, migrating up onto the gastric surface, where they are lost, probably in about 4 to 6 days. The neck of the oxyntic gland below the isthmus is lined by pyramidal, peripherally located, acid- and intrinsic-factor-producing parietal cells. Interspersed are inconspicuous mucous neck cells, mainly in the upper neck, and scattered endocrine cells. In the base of the gland, pepsinogen-producing zymogen or chief cells are concentrated.

Mucous neck cells, like foveolar and surface mucous cells, stain PAS-positive. The cytoplasm of these cells contains, in addition to mucous granules, many polyribosomes and rough endoplasmic reticulum, suggesting poor specialization. Parietal cells differentiate from mucous neck cells proliferating at the isthmus and appear to be relatively long-lived, that is, of the order of weeks to months in the species studied. They contain many mitochondria, hence staining well with eosin. A complex tubulovesicular–canalicular structure opens at the luminal apex of the cell in the secretory state. A number of long-lived endocrine cells, probably derived from proliferative elements at the isthmus, are recognized in the oxyntic gland: ECL cells (histamine, serotonin), EC cells (serotonin, peptides), D cells (somatostatin), and A, D_1, and X cells (function unclear). Endocrine cells usually abut the basement membrane of the gland, lack exposure to the gland lumen, and have characteristic basal granules visible in thin, plastic-embedded sections. The chief cells are apparently long-lived cells, probably derived from stem cells at the isthmus, but possibly autonomously replicative at a slow rate. Ultrastructurally, they have extensive rough endoplasmic reticulum, a prominent Golgi zone, and numerous zymogen granules.

Under normal circumstances, mitotic figures are not commonly encountered in cells at the isthmus of fundic glands, and virtually never at any distance from the isthmus. The fundic mucosa of newborn ruminants and, especially, piglets may be relatively poorly differentiated and proliferative. The proliferative compartment is sensitive to radiomimetic insults. This is reflected in attenuation of the lining epithelium and narrowing of the isthmus and upper neck of oxyntic glands in dogs with parvovirus infection (Fig. 1.32A) and in animals treated with cytotoxic agents such as cyclophosphamide. *Spirillum*-like bacteria are considered normal in the fundic glands of dogs and cats. *Chlamydia* has been recognized in surface mucous cells of otherwise normal fundic mucosa in cats, with no specific signs of disease.

The pyloric mucosa is also covered by columnar mucous cells, which form a slightly pitted or irregular surface in the distal portion of the stomach, including the pyloric antrum. It extends further cranially along the lesser, compared to the greater, curvature. The knoblike torus pyloricus at the pylorus of the pig is a normal structure. The tubular glands of the pyloric mucosa open into deep gastric pits, which may extend half the thickness of the mucosa. The glands are lined by pale mucous cells, with interspersed endocrine elements, mainly G (gastrin) and D (somatostatin) cells. Scattered parietal cells may be present, especially in glands in the zone intergrading with fundic mucosa.

The stromal elements of the gastric lamina propria are relatively inconspicuous, in the fundic mucosa in particular. Normally, relatively few lymphocytes and plasma cells and scattered mast cells are present, mainly deep between glands. Occasional lymphocytic nodules or follicles may be present, usually near the muscularis mucosae. Lymphoid infiltrates are more common in the antral mucosa.

Regulation of Gastric Secretion

The major function of the stomach, hydrolysis of protein in preparation for subsequent intestinal digestion and absorption, is accomplished by acid and pepsin, activated by autocatalysis from pepsinogen at low pH. Secretion of acid (and intrinsic factor) is the function of the oxyntic or parietal cells, about one billion of which are present in the stomach of a 20-kg dog. Regulation of the volume and acidity of gastric secretion is physiologically complex and highly integrated, involving neurocrine, endocrine, and paracrine mechanisms.

The parietal cell secretes hydrochloric acid in response to stimulation by histamine, acetylcholine, and gastrin. Studies on isolated parietal cells suggest that receptors specific for each of these secretagogues are present on the cell membrane. All three agonists are probably continuously present and involved in basal acid secretion. However, the effects of acetylcholine and gastrin are largely dependent on concurrent stimulation by histamine. Potentiation or synergism of effect occurs when histamine–acetylcholine, histamine–gastrin, or all three agents together act on the cell. The mechanism of this synergism is unclear, but it involves intracellular metabolic events beyond the receptor, and probably beyond the second messenger.

Histamine, probably derived from mast cells in the lamina propria, and possibly from local enteroendocrine cells, is a paracrine permissive stimulant, continuously present in the environment of the oxyntic cells. Evidence for a stimulus causing a phasic increase in histamine effects on parietal cells is not available, though it is suggested that gastrin may promote histamine release in some species. The oxyntic cell has an H_2 histamine receptor, which, when occupied, causes, through the mediation of adenylcyclase, enhanced generation of the second messenger, cyclic adenosine monophosphate. This in turn stimulates, via poorly understood mechanisms, intracellular metabolic events culminating in acid secretion.

Acetylcholine, the neurocrine agonist, is released near the oxyntic cell from processes of parasympathetic postganglionic neurons. Its release is both background and phasic, being enhanced by vagal activity during the central stimulation of the cephalic phase—the Pavlovian response. Gastric distention also stimulates the parietal cell via vagovagal and short intramural reflex pathways. The effect of acetylcholine is associated with calcium-ion influx as second messenger.

Gastrin is a hormone released into the bloodstream by G cells, located mainly in the pyloric antrum. Stimuli for gastrin release are of two types. Direct action of calcium, amino acids, and peptides in ingesta, impinging on G cells, may stimulate gastrin release. In addition, vagal stimulation during the cephalic phase, and fundic–pyloric vagovagal reflexes, in concert with pyloric vagovagal and local intramural antral reflexes, initiated by distention, cause G cells to release gastrin. This stimulus is probably the product of removal of paracrine somatostatin inhibition of the G cell, coupled with neurocrine stimulatory effects of bombesin on the G cell. Gastrin alone appears to be a weak calcium-ion-dependent stimulator of acid production by isolated cells, but it contributes to the synergistic effects on secretion seen in cells exposed to histamine and acetylcholine. This probably explains its contribution to phasic acid secretion in the intact animal. In addition, gastrin has an important trophic effect on parietal cell mass, stimulating synthesis of nucleic acid and protein and increasing the number of parietal cells in fundic mucosa.

Inhibition of acid production during the gastric phase of secretion occurs as the result of the negative-feedback effect of acid in the antrum, possibly by paracrine somatostatin influence on the G cell, inhibiting gastrin release below pH 3. In addition, the presence of acid, fat, and hyperosmolal solutions in the proximal small intestine inhibit acid secretion, perhaps in part by the mediation of neural reflexes and secretin, gastric inhibitory polypeptide, or other enterogastrones. The effects of histamine on the parietal cell are central to its basal secretion and its susceptibility to the synergistic effects of cholinergic and gastrin stimulation.

The chief cell is probably susceptible to the same general stimuli for secretion as the parietal cell, with the exception that secretin stimulates, rather than inhibits, pepsinogen release.

Gastric Mucosal Barrier

The gastric mucosal barrier to acid back diffusion and autodigestion presumably resides largely in the single layer of foveolar and surface mucous cells, and their secretion. Gastric mucus is freely permeable to hydrogen ions and has little innate buffering capacity. Cardiac gland mucosa in the pig, and pyloric mucosa in several species, secretes bicarbonate in considerable quantities and normally resists acid attack. Fundic surface mucous cells also may actively secrete bicarbonate into a thin, unstirred layer of surface mucus. Here a sharp pH gradient is maintained, neutral on the cell-surface side, acid on the luminal side. By this means, bicarbonate secretion of relatively small magnitude in relation to total acid secretion may hypothetically protect the mucosa against attack by acid. Mucus is itself susceptible to enzymatic proteolysis but provides a good barrier to diffusion by these large molecules. Continual mucus secretion on the cell side of the layer presumably balances hydrolysis and loss on the luminal side.

Bicarbonate secretion by surface mucous cells is stimulated by PGE_2 and PGF_2 at low concentration in amphibians and similar phenomena may occur in mammals. Prostaglandins, ubiquitous in gastric mucosal lamina propria, may have protective effects other than by stimulation of bicarbonate secretion by mucous cells and by inhibition of histamine-stimulated acid secretion by parietal cells. In some species, prostacyclin (PGI_2) and prostaglandins of the E and A series cause vasodilation and increased blood flow in addition to inhibiting acid secretion. The high metabolic rate of the gastric mucosa requires a high blood flow to maintain an intact surface epithelium and experimentally, increased perfusion is protective against a number of significant mucosal insults.

Response of the Gastric Mucosa to Insult

Repair of acute erosive physical or chemical trauma to the mucosal surface, such as that caused by aspirin and, presumably, by abrasive foreign bodies, is by proliferation of cells in the isthmus, if the erosive lesion is superficial, and spares the progenitor cells. An acute inflammatory reaction demarcates eroded or superficially necrotic mucosa. Mitoses become common in the upper gland. During the early phase of repair, cells lining shallow foveolae and covering the surface are basophilic, poorly differentiated, and flattened, cuboidal, or low columnar. Sites of epithelial exfoliation and neutrophil transmigration or effusion into the lumen may be evident. Congestion, edema, mild neutrophilia, and fibroplasia are seen in the superficial lamina propria. The evolution and repair of gastric ulceration, to which erosion may be antecedent, is discussed later. The progenitor cells of the fundic mucosa have the potential to produce tall columnar mucous cells of the foveolar or surface type, to produce mucous neck cells, and presumably by further differentiation, to evolve parietal cells. **Atrophy** of **parietal cell mass** without extensive mucous-cell hyperplasia occurs in animals, particularly ruminants, that have signs of gastrointestinal disease including inappetence. The change is not evident grossly. Microscopically, fewer parietal cells are seen in the upper neck of fundic glands, and apparently, in the depth of the gland. This is accompanied by epithelial proliferation, indicated by moderate numbers of mitotic figures at the isthmus and in the neck of the gland. The PAS stain demonstrates the encroachment of increased numbers of such cells into the deeper portion of fundic glands. In extreme cases, mucous neck cells are present to the base of glands, and achlorhydria occurs.

The cause of this change is unclear. It has been demonstrated in sheep infected with intestinal nematodes, but similar findings occur in animals with a wide variety of syndromes involving loss of appetite. Starvation of moderate duration does not produce comparable lesions. Reduction in, or interference with, the trophic effect of gastrin on parietal cell mass, might be the mechanism in parietal-cell atrophy of this type.

Inflammatory infiltrates are unusual and mild in normal fundic mucosa. Chronic inflammation in the fundic stomach in all species is associated with the development of **mucous metaplasia** and **hyperplasia** of glands in the vicinity of inflammatory foci. As the lesion evolves, parietal cells are present only in the basal portion of the glands, and they appear to be progressively displaced by hyperplastic mucous cells.

Mitotic figures may be numerous throughout the neck of the gland, which elongates. The epithelium in early lesions tends to resemble mucous neck cells. In established lesions, columnar mucous cells with regular nuclear polarity, similar to foveolar mucous cells, may be present. When inflammatory infiltrates are local, the mucous change is limited to a few surrounding glands. More diffuse inflammation is associated with the development of widespread epithelial mucous metaplasia.

Mucous metaplasia and hyperplasia may be mediated in part by immune events or inflammation in the lamina propria. Interactions between immune processes in the stomach and epithelial differentiation are poorly explored. Secretion of lysozyme, and of secretory piece and IgA, are properties of mucous neck cells in gastritis in humans. Cell-mediated immune events in the lamina propria of the small intestine are increasingly implicated in altered proliferation and differentiation of enteric epithelium by as yet undefined mechanisms. It may be that similar phenomena in the stomach await recognition and investigation.

Such atrophy of the parietal cells and mucous metaplasia and hyperplasia apparently do not result from withdrawal of the trophic stimulus of gastrin. At least in *Ostertagia*-induced gastritis, it occurs in the face of gastrin concentrations many times above normal levels, which are not simply the result of achlorhydria and failure of suppression of G-cell secretion by antral acidification. Mucous metaplasia and hyperplasia are associated with focal or diffuse, superficial or mucosal, proprial infiltrates of plasma cells and lymphocytes. Often, neutrophils, eosinophils, and Russell-body cells will be present in the lamina propria, and lymphocytes may be between epithelial cells in glands. Globule leukocytes are present in the epithelium of glands, especially in the parasitized abomasum.

This mucous metaplasia, hyperplasia, and chronic inflammation are associated with a variety of causes, including chronic traumatic insults, such as those due to implanted foreign bodies, which may render the mucosa permeable to antigen present in the lumen. Abomasal involvement in bovine virus diarrhea or herpes rhinotracheitis is associated with mucosal lesions of this type. The specific agency most commonly recognized is gastric parasitism by nematodes such as *Ostertagia* spp., *Trichostrongylus axei*, and *Hyostrongylus rubidus*, where the distribution of the lesion is closely related to the physical presence of nematodes and to the interstitial inflammatory reaction they incite. Mucous metaplasia and hyperplasia are also typically present around the healing margins of chronic ulcers, perhaps in response to local inflammation.

The mucosa affected in these circumstances is grossly thickened, as on the overhanging margin of an ulcer or in an *Ostertagia* "nodule," with a pebbled or convoluted surface if the lesion is widespread. Gastric rugae or plicae are thickened, partially as a result of mucosal hypertrophy, perhaps with submucosal edema. The surface of the stomach is usually paler than normal in affected areas; however, local congestion or hyperemia may be evident. Though the surface may be glistening, profuse mucus secretion is not usually obvious. Achlorhydria is the consequence of widespread change of this type. Mucous metaplasia and hyperplasia are differentiated on the basis of the degree of mucous-cell hyperplasia and differentiation, and the presence of inflammatory cells, from fundic atrophy associated with loss of appetite.

Antral mucosa also undergoes hyperplasia and thickening in

antritis. Some chronic inflammatory infiltrate between antral glands and at the base of the mucosa is usual, and lymphoid follicles may be present in the lamina propria. Expansion of the proliferative compartment in the antral glands is recognized as mitotic figures scattered in the neck of the gland. Foveolar and glandular mucous cells increase in number, and the antral mucosa is thickened and superficially rugose, perhaps with local congestion or erythema. The stimulus for antritis is often unclear. Gastric reflux of duodenal contents containing bile may be of some significance in the dog. In ruminants, the pyloric mucosa may be colonized by abomasal nematodes, and by a few worms of species normally found in the small intestine if enteric populations are high.

The functional significance of gastric mucous metaplasia is unclear. Presumably, hyperplasia of cells is partly a response to soluble local immune-mediated stimuli or products of inflammation. Replacement of parietal cells by mucous neck cells, or an apparently more fully differentiated mucous cell in chronic gastritis, may be a protective response. It may eliminate the threat of local acid corrosion and promote the transfer into the lumen of protective soluble factors such as lysozyme and IgA or its analogs.

Achlorhydria ensues in severe chronic gastritis and mucous metaplasia. The pH of gastric secretion approaches or exceeds neutrality under some circumstances, as sodium ion replaces hydrogen ion in gastric content and bicarbonate is secreted. With diminished gastric acid concentration, progressive microbial colonization of the stomach and upper intestine ensues. Parietal-cell atrophy and replacement by mucous neck cells in ruminants with anorexia due to enteric disease may predispose to mycotic invasion of the mucosa. Mucous metaplasia and hyperplasia, as seen in chronic gastritis or conditions like ostertagiosis, does not seem to render the mucosa prone to mycosis. Loss of the hydrolytic effects of acid and pepsin, in achlorhydria, seems to have little effect on digestion of protein and uptake of nitrogen, at least in animals with ostertagiosis, and effects of atrophic gastritis in humans on protein digestion appear to be minimal.

Pyloric Stenosis

Pyloric stenosis is a functional and sometimes anatomic problem that, in part, represents probably the only anomaly of the stomach recognized in animals. It is apparently common in dogs and rare in cats and horses. It appears as a presumably congenital problem in many instances. Recurrent vomition and poor growth in recently weaned animals suggest the clinical diagnosis of a congenital lesion. Signs beginning later in life indicate an acquired problem. Contrast radiographic studies will confirm delayed gastric emptying. There is limited critical information on this problem. Clinical reports indicate that in some dogs there may be hypertrophy of pyloric muscle, which appears grossly thickened. Tonic stenosis of the pyloric sphincter may occur in dogs, perhaps due to unconfirmed lesions of the myenteric plexus or due to gastrin excess. In cats, no gross alteration in the diameter of the pylorus or the thickness of its muscle is recognized. An association with esophageal dilatation has been made in the cat. Congenital pyloric stenosis in a foal was associated with signs of abdominal pain and reluctance to consume solid feed. In all species the clinical problem is usually abolished by pyloromyotomy.

Acquired pyloric stenosis or obstruction occurs following ulceration and stricture of the pyloric canal in any species, due to hypertrophic antritis in dogs, and as a complication of polyps and tumors in the area.

Gastric Dilatation and Displacement

Gastric dilatation in the **horse** is often a secondary effect of obstruction of the small bowel or of colic with ileus and is also part of the syndrome "grass sickness," discussed elsewhere. Primary gastric dilation, and sometimes rupture, in horses is a sequel to consumption of excess fermentable carbohydrate or sudden access to lush pasture. The pathogenesis is analogous to that of grain overload in cattle. Ingesta may swell through absorption of saliva and gastric secretion. Evolution of gas and organic acids, including lactic acid, by bacterial fermentation of carbohydrate occurs in the cranial portion of the stomach. An influx of water follows as the result of increased osmotic pressure in the stomach, contributing to increased distention and systemic dehydration. Animals surviving for any time with acute gastric dilatation of this type may develop laminitis. The contents of the stomach in gastric dilation may be fluid, especially in secondary dilatation, and can smell fermented in primary dilation. Gastric rupture may ensue. Rupture usually occurs along the greater curvature parallel to the omental attachment, releasing gastric content into the omental bursa or the abdominal cavity. Death ensues acutely as the result of shock and peritonitis. The margins of the gastric laceration, which may be 10–15 cm long, show evidence of antemortem hemorrhage. Postmortem rupture of the dilated stomach is common and must be differentiated. There may be congestion of the cervical esophagus and blanching of the thoracic esophagus, producing a prominent "bloat line." This, and compression atelectasis of the lungs in some cases, attests to the tremendous increase in intraabdominal and intrathoracic pressure exerted by the dilated stomach prior to rupture. Congestion of cervical and cranial soft tissues and blanching of the abdominal organs also are found. Perforation, as distinct from rupture, of the stomach in the horse is rare and is associated with parasitism, peptic ulcer, or neoplasia.

Gastric dilatation and **volvulus** occur relatively commonly in the dog (Fig. 1.11D), and the condition has been reported in swine and a cat. In dogs, gastric dilatation and volvulus is usually a problem associated with overeating and probably aerophagia, especially in the deep-chested breeds such as Great Danes, St. Bernards, Irish setters, wolfhounds, borzois, and bloodhounds. Beyond that, hereditary factors, management, behavior, and type of feed may contribute in obscure ways to the development of dilation. The gas, which appears to play a large part in the development of dilation, is probably the result of aerophagia and evolution of carbon dioxide by physiologic mechanisms, rather than the product of intragastric clostridial fermentation. Inability to relieve the accumulation of food, fluid, and gas in the stomach causes the organ to dilate and alter its intraabdominal position, so that its long axis rotates from a transverse left–right orientation to one paralleling that of the abdomen. In simple dilation, the esophagus is not physically completely occluded, the spleen remains on the left side, and the duodenum is only slightly displaced dorsally and toward the midline. The gastric mucosa at this stage is usually not infarcted, though the effects of dilation on venous return from the abdomen and on the systemic circulation may be substantial.

For reasons that are unclear, gastric dilatation may be converted to gastric volvulus. Perhaps this is related to laxity or laceration of the gastrohepatic ligament, or to the development of violent antiperistalsis and abdominal contraction in vain attempts by the dog to vomit against a functionally or physically obstructed cardia. The stomach rotates about the esophagus in a clockwise direction, as viewed from the ventrocaudal aspect. The greater curvature of the distended organ moves ventrally and caudally, and then rotates dorsally and to the right. This forces the pylorus and terminal duodenum cranially to the right and clockwise around the esophagus. Ultimately, they lie to the left of midline across and ventral to the esophagus, compressed between the esophagus and the dilated stomach. Depending on the degree of volvulus, the spleen, which follows the gastrosplenic ligament, usually ends up lying in a right ventral position, between the stomach and liver or diaphragm. It is bent into a V shape by tension on its ligaments, becomes extremely congested, and may undergo torsion, infarction, and rupture. The esophagus becomes completely occluded in volvulus, which may involve rotation of up to 270 to 360°. Venous infarction of the gastric mucosa ensues as volvulus progressively constricts venous outflow from the stomach. The mucosa and, usually, the full thickness of the gastric wall are edematous and dark red to black, and there is bloody content in the lumen of the stomach. Necrosis of ischemic mucosa occurs, and the stomach may rupture.

Obstruction of veins by volvulus and pressure exerted by the distended stomach result in decreased venous return via the portal vein and posterior vena cava, causing reduced cardiac output and circulatory shock. Endotoxemia is implicated speculatively in disseminated intravascular coagulation and may contribute to shock. A variety of acid–base and electrolyte abnormalities ensue in dogs with gastric dilatation and volvulus, contributing to the physiologically precarious state. Cardiac arrhythmias as a sequel to gastric dilatation and volvulus have been associated with putative release of "myocardial depressant factor" from an ischemic pancreas, and with myocardial necrosis, possibly the result of ischemia. Death is inevitable in dogs not treated early.

Abomasal displacement and **volvulus** is a common clinical problem in high-producing, intensively managed, dairy cattle, particularly around the time of parturition. The displacement usually is ventrally and to the left of the rumen. Many affected animals have concurrent problems, including ketosis, hypocalcemia, metritis, and retained placenta. Abomasal atony and increased gas production are believed to be prerequisites for displacement of the organ. Influx of high concentrations of volatile fatty acids from the rumen, and hypocalcemia, may play a part in instigating hypomotility, while evolution of gas in the abomasum is directly related to the amount of concentrate in the ration. Left displacement of the gas-filled abomasum is amenable to treatment and is rarely encountered at autopsy. Handling of an affected animal postmortem may correct displacements in any case. Other than possible scarring of the lesser omentum, the abomasum may be unremarkable. Simple right displacement, which accounts for 9 to 15% of abomasal displacements, is probably caused by similar agencies. But right displacement may be complicated in about a fifth of cases by progression to abomasal volvulus, which is clinically serious.

Abomasal volvulus is probably the sequel to rotation of a loop formed by a distended abomasum and attached omasum and duodenum, counterclockwise about a transverse axis through the lesser omentum when viewed from the right side. Rotation, buoyed by the gas-filled body of the abomasum, may be in the sagittal plane. With a 360° volvulus, the pylorus ends in the anterior right portion of the abdomen dorsal to the twisted omasum, with the duodenum trapped medial to the omasum and lateral to the partially rotated reticulum. Alternative modes of displacement and rotation are possible, but all may end in this relationship. Obstruction of duodenal outflow in volvulus results in sequestration of chloride in the abomasal content and the development of metabolic alkalosis. Severe volvulus causes obstruction of blood vessels at the neck of the omasum, as well as causing trauma to the vagus nerves in the region. The abomasum becomes distended with bloodstained fluid and gas. Infarction of the deeply congested mucosa may result in ultimate abomasal rupture, often near the omaso–abomasal orifice, and peritonitis. Damage to the vagal branches may prohibit return of normal abomasal motility in animals successfully withstanding surgery.

Gastric Foreign Bodies and Impaction

A variety of foreign bodies may be encountered in the stomach and, rarely, in the abomasum. Most are incidental findings, or at worst, associated with vomition, mild acute or chronic gastritis, or occasionally ulceration. Rarely, obstruction of the pyloric outlet ensues. Hair balls are often found in the stomach of longhaired cats, and in calves reared on diets low in roughage, where most are in the rumen, with a few in the abomasum. Accumulation of considerable amounts of fine sand may occur in the abomasum, apparently with little ill effect.

Gastric impaction by inspissated content is reported in the horse as a clinical problem of unknown cause. It causes severe abdominal pain and is to be differentiated clinically and at autopsy from gastric dilation secondary to intestinal obstruction, and from primary gastric dilation due to ingestion of excess fermentable carbohydrate.

Primary abomasal impaction is the product of a regime of restricted water intake and coarse, high-roughage feed, such as wheat stubble or straw, as may occur in winter feeding of cattle in northern prairie areas. Secondary abomasal impaction may follow pyloric stenosis, physical or functional, of any cause. Rarely, foreign bodies such as ingested placenta or hair balls block the pylorus. It is perhaps most common as a functional abomasal stasis in one of the manifestations of "vagus indigestion," which is discussed more fully under Traumatic Reticuloperitonitis and Its Complications. Loss of abomasal motility may be the product of intrathoracic inflammatory or neoplastic vagal lesions, vagal involvement in adhesions following traumatic reticuloperitonitis, vagal trauma in surgically corrected abomasal volvulus, or adhesions of the abomasum and omasum, which may physically impair motility. The abomasum is impacted with inspissated coarse ingesta, despite an apparently patent pylorus. Metabolic derangement due to sequestration of chloride in the rumen following regurgitation from the obstructed abomasum, and hypokalemia due to decreased intake in feed in the face of continued normal renal excretion, place these animals in perilous physiologic circumstances before inanition becomes a significant factor.

Circulatory Disturbances

Hyperemia of the gastric mucosa is a concomitant of the ingestion of chemicals such as arsenic, thallium, and aspirin. It usually coexists in these circumstances with superficial erosion, which is discussed later with gastric ulcer. Focal hyperemia may be related to local irritation of the mucosa by foreign bodies, and with focal acute viral lesions of the abomasum in cattle. Congestion of the mucosa can occur in conditions causing portal hypertension, including cirrhosis and shock in the dog.

Uremic "gastritis" presents as severe congestion of the body of the stomach, associated with signs of hematemesis and melena, is found in some dogs with chronic renal disease. In such animals, the mucosa is thickened and deep red-black. Lesions vary in severity from case to case, and premonitory changes without severe hemorrhage and necrosis are present in animals euthanized earlier in the course of disease. In such dogs there may be no gross gastric lesion, or variable edema and thickening of rugal mucosa, perhaps with focal ulceration.

Microscopically, the lamina propria between glands is edematous, and there are increased numbers of mast cells. Deposits of basophilic ground substance and mineral are found, especially on the basement membrane of vessels and glands, or on collagen fibrils and in degenerative smooth muscle. These changes occur particularly in the middle and deeper portions of the mucosa. Parietal cells in this area are usually mineralized as well. Such mineral deposits may be appreciated at autopsy in gross cross sections of mucosa. More extensive mineral deposition also involves arterioles of the submucosa and serosa. Such vessels also show evidence of endothelial damage, medial necrosis, and in some cases, thrombosis. Severe mucosal congestion, edema, and necrosis are possibly related to ischemia secondary to the vascular lesions, though perhaps not directly associated with arterial thrombosis and obstruction, which is often not readily found. Microvascular lesions in the lamina propria and systemic states in uremia may be contributory. Impaired renal degradation and excretion of gastrin may promote hyperchlorhydria and exacerbate mucosal damage.

The cause of the vascular lesions may be a poorly characterized circulating toxic peptide associated with uremia. Mineral deposition is probably the product of altered systemic metabolism of calcium in renal failure, perhaps coupled with the local microenvironment resulting from bicarbonate moving across the basal border of secreting parietal cells. Membrane lesions in metabolically compromised parietal cells may also act as foci of mineral deposition (see the Urinary System, this volume, for discussion of uremia).

Gastric venous infarction is a common lesion in swine and is also encountered in ruminants and horses. It is related to endothelial damage and thrombosis in venules, usually associated with endotoxemia or other bacterial or toxic damage. Salmonellosis and *Escherichia coli* septicemia in all species and, in addition, in swine, postweaning coliform gastroenteritis, erysipelas, swine dysentery, Glasser's disease, and hog cholera are associated with the lesion. The fundic mucosa is bright red or deep red-black and may have some excess mucus or perhaps fibrin on the surface (Fig. 1.34D). Occasionally, the superficial mucosa is obviously necrotic and may lift off with the ingesta. In section there is thrombosis of venules in the mucosa and often at the mucosal–submucosal junction, usually with prominent fibrin plugs. Thrombosed capillaries and venules may be present at any level of the mucosa, along the base of the ischemic zone of superficial coagulation necrosis, with local hemorrhage and edema. There may be an acute inflammatory reaction delineating the necrotic area in the mucosa. Sometimes the full thickness of the gastric mucosa, focally or diffusely, may be necrotic.

Edema of the gastric rugae occurs with hypoproteinemia in any species and is found in the abomasum of cattle poisoned by arsenic. Edema fluid collects in the submucosa of the folds and is particularly obvious in the normally thin abomasal plicae. Edema may contribute to the thickening of rugae seen in gastritis. Edema of the submucosa of the stomach is a common and important lesion in gut edema of swine (Fig. 1.34C). It is best appreciated by making several slices through the serosa and external muscle to the submucosa over the body of the stomach. Gut edema is considered fully under Infectious and Parasitic Diseases of the Gastrointestinal Tract.

Gastritis

Gastritis is a poorly defined term often applied to acute gastric injury with grossly visible hemorrhage or erosion, when inflammatory processes, strictly speaking, are scarcely present. The differential considerations in diffuse gastric hemorrhage, and the etiopathogenesis of mucosal erosion will be considered later, with ulcer. Microscopic acute inflammatory infiltrates in the gastric wall are usually associated with subacute superficial erosion, the floor of a stable gastric ulcer, gastric venous infarction, clostridial and mycotic gastritis, chronic active interstitial inflammation, and some acute systemic viral infections.

Chronic gastritis, as it is seen in humans, is rarely recognized in domestic animals. **Chronic superficial gastritis** is a term applied in humans to a lesion with a chronic inflammatory infiltrate confined to the interfoveolar propria; normal gastric glands with minimal interstitial infiltrate are present. Such an entity might occur in animals sporadically, with no etiologic connotation. Chronic atrophic gastritis, as it is defined in human beings, is very rarely encountered. Atrophy of parietal cell mass, associated with autoimmune phenomena and the development of pernicious anemia, does not occur spontaneously in animals, though it can be induced in dogs by immunization with gastric juice. Chronic antritis with reduced gastrin secretion theoretically might result in atrophy of parietal cell mass. Duodenal reflux in dogs has been associated with a syndrome of vomition and gastric hyposecretion. Mononuclear-cell infiltrates and follicle formation in the lamina propria of the antrum and fundus are found, with subjective atrophy of parietal cell mass.

Intestinal metaplasia of the gastric mucosa, considered to be a sequel to chronic gastritis in humans, is rarely, if ever, found in domestic animals. The stomach in dogs is involved very uncommonly in eosinophilic gastroenteritis. Eosinophils may infiltrate the mucosa and submucosa in large numbers, in association with a syndrome of protein loss, eosinophilia, and eosinophilic infiltrates in more distal gut (see diseases of the intestine, below). Even rarer cases of scirrhous eosinophilic gastritis and arteritis, and of histiocytic gastritis in association with amyloidosis in dogs, are on record.

Chronic hypertrophic gastritis, similar to Menetrier's disease of humans, occurs in dogs. Vomition and weight loss, in some cases associated with inappetence or diarrhea, are described in the history. The characteristic lesion is marked gastric rugal hypertrophy involving part or most of the fundic mucosa in the greater curvature. Grossly thickened folds of gastric mucosa over an area 4–10 or 12 cm in diameter are thrown up in a convoluted pattern that may resemble cerebral gyri. Microscopically, these areas are composed of hyperplastic mucosa, which may or may not include secondary folds of muscularis mucosa and submucosa. Findings are variable in the few cases reported. There may be foveolar and glandular hyperplasia with progressive or total loss of parietal cells, which are replaced by mucous cells of varying degrees of differentiation. Cystic dilatation of mucous glands may occur. Mononuclear cells infiltrate the lamina propria between glands and near the muscularis mucosa, and the propria may be edematous.

The lesion is to be differentiated from adenomatous polyps, Zollinger–Ellison syndrome, and infiltrating lymphoid tumors. Its cause is unknown. The condition in humans is associated with protein-losing gastropathy. Perhaps significantly, chronic gastritis and chronic hypertrophic gastritis have been reported a number of times in the basenji, a breed in which a syndrome of protein-losing gastroenteritis and diarrhea is well recognized. This syndrome, and the enteric lesions associated with it, will be discussed with diseases of the intestine. Hypertrophic antritis, producing a thickened, sometimes convoluted mucosa in the antrum, has been associated with pyloric stenosis in dogs, considered earlier. Its cause is unknown but may be related to chronic irritation by duodenal reflux.

Braxy, or bradsot, is an acute abomasitis of sheep and, rarely, cattle, due to infection with *Clostridium septicum* (Fig. 1.41B). It is a sporadic disease of young animals, usually occurring in cooler climates. It is reported from Iceland, Scandinavia, Scotland, Canada, the northern United States, and Tasmania. The factors initiating bacterial invasion are unknown. Cold weather is usually associated with the disease, but it is difficult to imagine feed being cold enough, by the time it attains the abomasum, for significant mucosal hypothermia and necrosis to occur. Evolution of exotoxin by *C. septicum* causes the signs and death, which usually ensues acutely.

At autopsy there may be blood-tinged abdominal fluid, and the serosa of the abomasum may be congested or fibrin covered. Mucosal lesions may be diffuse or involve demarcated foci of variable size and shape. Abomasal folds may be thickened, reddened, occasionally hemorrhagic, or necrotic. Most notable is the presence of extensive gelatinous edema and emphysema in the submucosa. Diffuse edema, and extensive areas of suppurative infiltrate demarcating areas of coagulation necrosis, with prominent pockets of emphysema, are evident in tissue

sections. These involve mainly submucosa and extend into adjacent mucosa and external muscle. There may be venous thrombosis and hemorrhage. Gram-positive bacilli are usually evident as individuals or colonies in affected tissue. They may be identified as *Clostridium septicum* by fluorescent antibody reaction or culture. Such lesions are occasionally complicated by other clostridia. Braxy must be differentiated from cellulitis of the abomasal wall due to mixed anaerobic flora without *C. septicum*.

Abomasitis associated with **viral infection** occurs in a number of the systemic viral diseases affecting the gastrointestinal tract, including infectious bovine rhinotracheitis in calves and, rarely, older animals, herpesvirus infections of small ruminants, bovine virus diarrhea, rinderpest, malignant catarrhal fever, and bluetongue. Abomasal lesions are rarely the sole manifestation of these diseases but form part of a picture at autopsy that may suggest an etiologic diagnosis. The appearance and pathogenesis of abomasitis in these diseases varies with the conditions, which are discussed in detail under Infectious and Parasitic Diseases of the Gastrointestinal Tract.

Mycotic gastritis is a sporadic problem almost invariably secondary to insults that cause achlorhydria (or focal atrophy), necrosis, or ulceration under conditions where mycotic colonization can occur. Compromised resistance, perhaps associated with neoplasia, endogenous or exogenous steroids, lympholytic viral disease, and altered gastrointestinal flora due to antiobiotic therapy, may further promote mycosis. Fungal hyphae attaining the submucosa typically invade venules and arterioles, causing thrombosis and a hemorrhagic infarct. The agents involved are usually zygomycetes (phycomycetes) such as *Rhizopus, Absidia,* or *Mucor;* rarely, *Aspergillus* may be implicated.

Mycotic abomasitis in calves is secondary to gastrointestinal infectious bovine rhinotracheitis and to venous infarction of the mucosa in endotoxemia or septicemia with *E. coli* or *Salmonella.* Bovine virus diarrhea and, occasionally, gastric ulcer provide conditions for mycotic invasion of the abomasum in older cattle. The lesions are areas of necrosis, with an intensely congested or hemorrhagic periphery, ranging in diameter from 1 to 2 cm, to confluence over much of the body of the stomach (Fig. 1.11A). Affected mucosa is thickened, red or pale in the necrotic zone, and may be covered by hemorrhage. Edema and hemorrhage are evident in the submucosa. The lesion may penetrate to the serosa, where it is typically seen as a roughly circular area of hemorrhage in the external muscle and subserosa. Hyphae, usually broad and nonseptate zygomycotic in type, are present in sections of the necrotic mucosa, submucosa, and invading vessels, where they initiate thrombosis (Fig. 1.11B,C). The associated inflammatory infiltrate is usually consistent with acute or subacute insult.

In dogs, rare cases of acute multifocal **infarctive** or **granulomatous gastritis** are reported, associated with zygomycetes. **Mycosis** of the glandular stomach of horses and pigs is virtually unknown. **Candidiasis** of the pars esophagea may occur in swine, often in association with preulcerative epithelial hyperplasia and parakeratosis. An overview of mycosis of the digestive system, and its sequelae, is provided under Infectious and Parasitic Diseases of the Gastrointestinal Tract.

Parasitic gastritis is generally of little significance in small animals. Members of the genera *Physaloptera* and *Gnathostoma* are found in dogs, where the former cause focal ulceration and the latter are the cause of submucosal inflammatory cysts containing suppurative exudate and worms. In cats, *Physaloptera* spp. may attach to mucosal ulcers, while *Gnathostoma* spp. and *Cylicospirura felineus* are found in nodules in the gastric wall. *Ollulanus tricuspis* is found on the mucosa of the stomach in cats, where it may cause mild to, rarely, severe chronic gastritis.

In the horse, *Draschia megastoma* is found in inflammatory nodules in the submucosa of the cardiac zone, especially along the margo plicatus. *Habronema muscae* and *H. majus* (formerly *microstoma*) are found on the mucosa and have been associated with mild ulceration. *Trichostrongylus axei* may cause chronic gastritis in the horse. Bots of the genus *Gasterophilus* are found attached to small erosions and ulcers in the esophageal and glandular mucosa.

In swine, the spirurids *Ascarops* spp., *Physocephalus* spp., and *Simondsia* spp. are associated with mild gastritis in heavy infections. *Gnathostoma* may be embedded in inflammatory cysts in the submucosa. *Ollulanus tricuspis* may be encountered. *Hyostrongylus rubidus* can cause chronic gastritis and wasting in pigs.

In cattle, sheep, and goats, members of the genera *Haemonchus* and *Mecistocirrus* are large, abomasal, bloodsucking trichostrongyles, capable of causing severe anemia and hypoproteinemia. *Ostertagia* spp. and related genera, including *Camelostrongylus*, *Teladorsagia*, *Marshallagia*, and *Trichostrongylus axei* in various ruminants cause chronic abomasitis with mucous metaplasia, achlorhydria, diarrhea, and plasma protein loss. Large schizonts of undetermined coccidia in sheep produce harmless, pinpoint, pale foci in the abomasal mucosa; formerly the obsolete name *Globidium gilruthi* was applied. The pathology and pathogenesis of the significant gastric parasitisms is considered in greater detail under Infectious and Parasitic Diseases of the Gastrointestinal Tract.

Gastroduodenal Ulceration

Gastroduodenal ulcer produces signs of disease much less often in animals than in humans. The pathogenesis of peptic ulcer in humans or animals is by no means clear. It resolves into a relative imbalance between the necrotizing effects of gastric acid and pepsin on one hand, and the ability of the mucosa to maintain its integrity on the other. Hypersecretion of acid, or impairment of mucosal integrity in the face of normal acid secretion, may be invoked as general mechanisms. Some suggest that peptic ulceration of the duodenum, pylorus, or combined gastric and duodenal ulcers in humans reflect mainly hypersecretion, while ulcers in the body of the stomach mainly are a result of deficient mucosal resistance.

Factors implicated in hypersecretion of acid include abnormally high basal secretion, possibly associated with an expanded parietal cell mass, perhaps the result of increased trophic stimulation by gastrin. Gastrinomas cause the Zollinger–Ellison syndrome, characterized by elevated gastric acid secretion and severe gastroduodenal ulceration. Increased histamine levels associated with mastocytosis or mastocytoma also cause acid hypersecretion and ulceration.

Ulceration due to compromise of mucosal protective mechanisms is attributed to nonsteroidal antiinflammatory agents such as aspirin, phenylbutazone, and indomethacin. The therapeutic and ulcerogenic properties of these drugs reside largely in their effects on prostaglandin metabolism. This they block by interfering with the cyclooxygenase-catalyzed conversion of arachidonic acid to the prostaglandin endoperoxides PGG_2 and PGH_2. In the stomach, prostaglandin-mediated vasodilatation, modulation of histamine-induced acid secretion, and stimulation of bicarbonate secretion by mucous cells may be impaired. In addition to the effect of ionized aspirin on prostaglandin synthesis, in the acid gastric environment un-ionized, lipid-soluble acetylsalicylic acid readily crosses the surface-cell membrane. It damages the cell metabolically, permitting back-diffusion of acid and incipient ulceration.

Reflux of duodenal contents containing bile salts has been implicated in the induction of gastritis and gastric ulcer. Under some experimental conditions, acid back diffusion into the gastric mucosa, and morphologic damage, have been caused by application of bile salts. The effects are dependent on the pK_a of the bile salt, which must be soluble at acid pH, and on the concentration of hydrogen ion. Lipid solubility of bile salts, and associated damage to surface-cell membranes, may mediate these effects. Alcohols, also lipid-soluble compounds, alter permeability of gastric mucosa and permit back diffusion of acid. Lysolecithin, formed when pancreatic lipase hydrolyzes lecithin in bile, increases gastric mucosal permeability too.

Glucocorticoids and "stress" have been implicated in the genesis of ulcer, though the role of steroids is controversial. Experimentally, gastroduodenal hemorrhage and ulceration occur in some species of animals stressed by restraint or social factors, and they are a feature of "trap-death syndrome" in small mammals. Severe gastric hemorrhage or ulceration may occur following neurosurgery, trauma to the spinal cord, and burns, and it is considered by some to be stress related. Administration of steroids may cause increased gastrin and acid secretion. Steroids decrease reparative gastric epithelial-cell turnover and, by stabilizing membranes, decrease the availability of arachidonic acid for prostaglandin synthesis. These effects may predispose to development of ulcer when combined with other insults.

Reduced mucosal perfusion or ischemia may be a principal factor interacting in stress-associated ulceration, and in that initiated by other modalities discussed previously. Reduced blood flow to the mucosa in local areas has been suspected, under a number of circumstances, to precede mucosal hemorrhage or erosion. Ischemia will result in hypoxemic compromise of surface cells. In combination with the effects of other insults, this may cause reduced bicarbonate secretion and initiate mucosal permeability and back diffusion of acid. Mechanisms of mucosal ischemia are obscure. Reduction in local prostaglandin concentration may contribute, as may local or systemic hypotension. Following mucosal damage and back diffusion of hydrogen ions, vasodilatation and hyperemia develop, perhaps the result of liberation of mucosal histamine. Microvascular disruption then results in hemorrhage.

Whatever the cause, the results of a breach of the gastric mucosa have the potential to follow a **common pathway** to **ulceration** in all species. Acute superficial lesions such as those associated with stress or following administration of aspirin are often seen as areas of reddening and hemorrhage, especially along the margins of rugae in the fundic mucosa. Acid treatment of hemoglobin gives blood on the surface or in the gastric lumen a red-brown or black color. In some species, severe "stress-associated" gastric hemorrhage may occur diffusely over the entire congested gastric mucosa, resulting in hypovolemic shock and anemia, with melena. In some instances, melena, presumably the result of a recent episode of gastric bleeding, may be present in the lower intestine, with minimal gross evidence of hemorrhage or ulceration in the stomach. The microscopic lesion associated with hemorrhage of this type is often subtle, bleeding seemingly resulting from diapedesis, with minimal mucosal damage. Usually there is superficial erosion of the mucosa, often difficult to differentiate from autolysis, with granules of brown, acid hematin in debris on the surface. Inflammation is usually absent. Evidence for healing mild gastric erosion is the presence of basophilic, poorly differentiated, flattened, cuboidal or low columnar cells on the mucosal surface, with mitotic cells in the upper neck of the glands.

Lesions of any genesis proceeding to gastric ulcer do so by progressive coagulation necrosis of the gastric wall. Ulcers vary in microscopic appearance depending on their aggression, and the point in their development at which they are intercepted. Acute gastric lesions appear as erosions with superficial eosinophilic necrotic debris and loss of mucosal architecture to the depths of the foveolae, or as a depression in the mucosal surface with necrotic debris at the base. Necrosis usually extends rapidly to the muscularis mucosae, causing ulceration. Once the superficial portion of the mucosa is destroyed, natural local buffering by surface cells is lost, and the proliferative compartment of the gland, which is near the surface, is obliterated, preventing a local epithelial reparative response. Ulcers attaining the submucosa impinge on arterioles of increasing diameter, multiplying the risk of significant gastric hemorrhage. The ulcer may progress through the muscularis and serosa, culminating in perforation of the gastric wall. Severe gastric hemorrhage and perforation are relatively common sequelae of gastroduodenal ulceration in domestic animals.

Ulcers that come into equilibrium with reparative processes may do so at any level of the gastric wall below the mucosa, but usually at the submucosa. Subacute to chronic ulcers are typified by a base and sides composed of granulation tissue of varying thickness and maturity, infiltrated by a mixed inflammatory cell population, and overlain by a usually thin layer of necrotic debris. Chronic ulcers wax and wane. Depending on the relative dominance of reparative processes and aggressive ulceration, the layer of granulation tissue may be thick and mature, or thinner, less mature, and with superficial evidence of recent necrosis. There is mucous metaplasia and hyperplasia in glands at the periphery of the ulcer, which, with time, overhang the edge of the lesion. Under favorable conditions they gradually fill in the mucosal defect from the margins. Healed ulcers are usually depressed and may be somewhat puckered, with a scirrhous submucosa on cut section. The mucosa of healed ulcers, even in the fundic zone, is comprised of mucous glands. Excessive scarring of healed ulcers strategically located near the pylorus may lead to pyloric obstruction in any species.

Duodenal ulcers, which usually occur proximal to the open-ing of the pancreatic and bile ducts, resemble gastric ulcer in their pathogenesis, microscopic appearance (allowing for their intestinal location), evolution, and sequelae.

Peptic ulcer occurs commonly in cattle, uncommonly in dogs, rarely in cats, and is unusual in horses and swine, where ulceration of the esophageal, rather than glandular, gastric mucosa is the rule. In most species the prevalence of ulcer is probably underestimated, since only lesions producing severe signs associated with pain, hemorrhage, or perforation come to attention.

Peptic ulcer in **dogs** is relatively infrequently reported in the literature but is seen on a regular basis in university clinics, usually in adult animals. Signs associated with peptic ulcer include variable appetite, abdominal pain, vomition, melena, and anemia. Ulcers, a few millimeters to 3 to 4 cm in diameter, are found most commonly in the pyloric antrum or proximal duodenum. The gross and microscopic appearance of ulcers vary with their aggressiveness and duration, as previously described. Thrombosed arterioles and venules cut by the ulcerative process are often seen and should be sought in the bed of gastric and duodenal lesions associated with anemia or obvious hemorrhage.

Perforation of **gastric** or **duodenal ulcers** may lead to massive hemorrhage or release of gastric contents into the abdomen. Perforating duodenal ulcer may instigate pancreatitis. Some ulcers perforate silently, the serosal lesion healing by granulation, or adhesion by, and fibroplasia in, the omentum. The irritant nature of gastric contents released in these circumstances may lead to chronic inflammation, granulation, and thickening of the serosa, even when previous perforation cannot be appreciated. A search for microscopic particles of food such as plant material or muscle fibers in the serosal inflammatory response confirms perforation in this circumstance. Chronic peptic ulcers with thickened mucosal margins, scirrhous bases, and perhaps serosal thickening associated with perforation or near perforation must be differentiated from gastric adenocarcinoma in the dog.

Syndromes clearly the result of **hypersecretion** of **acid** occur in dogs. Mastocytoma has been associated with peptic ulcer, presumably due to histamine-stimulated acid hypersecretion and microvascular effects. The tumor and mastocytosis do not involve the stomach directly, and ulcers may occur in animals with solitary skin tumors. In one series of 24 dogs with recurrent or metastatic mastocytoma, gastric and duodenal erosions or ulcers, frequently multiple, were present in 20. In many cases such lesions are clinically silent, and they should be sought at autopsy in animals with mastocytoma. Mast-cell tumors have been associated rarely with gastric ulceration in the cow, and in the cat, where gastric ulcer is very uncommon.

Zollinger–Ellison syndrome, peptic ulcer due to gastrin-secreting pancreatic islet-cell tumors or gastrinomas, has been reported in a few dogs. The history usually includes inappetence, vomition, weight loss, and possibly diarrhea or melena. Reflux esophagitis and gastric or duodenal ulcer are present in most cases. Small, nodular masses histologically confirmed as islet-cell tumors may be found in the pancreas with, in most animals, metastases to the liver or hepatic lymph nodes. Hypertrophy of the fundic mucosa has been associated with a subjective increase in parietal cell mass. Peptic ulcer and reflux esophagitis in such cases result from gastrin-stimulated acid hypersecretion. Firm diagnosis rests on demonstration of elevated serum gastrin levels by radioimmunoassay, by identification of gastrin-bearing cells in fixed or frozen tumor tissue by immunocytochemistry, or by demonstration of gastrin in extracts of frozen tumor. Other peptide hormones may also be present. The microscopic appearance of these islet-cell tumors is not diagnostic for gastrinoma, nor is the ultrastructural appearance of tumor cells necessarily characteristic of the G cell. Pancreatic islet-cell neoplasms may be difficult to find and should be sought assiduously in suspect cases. In humans, some gastrinomas arise in the wall of the stomach or duodenum. The usual therapy in humans is removal of the target tissue, the fundic mucosa, by gastric resection, rather than attempted ablation of often occult and disseminated islet-cell tumor.

The cause in dogs of gastroduodenal ulcer possibly associated with decreased resistance to back diffusion of acid is less clear. Hepatic disease is often present in dogs with gastric ulcer, but the basis for a causal association is obscure. Some ulcers are obviously associated with administration of glucocorticoids in high doses as antiinflammatory, immunosuppressive, or antineoplastic therapy. Nonsteroidal antiinflammatory drugs such as aspirin, naproxen, or indomethacin, sometimes given by the owner in excessive quantity, are also associated with spontaneous ulcers. Gastric hemorrhage and gastroduodenal ulceration are occasionally seen in dogs following trauma or major surgery. A syndrome of gastric hemorrhage, pancreatitis, and colonic ulceration and perforation is recognized in dogs following spinal trauma. The pathogenesis of this problem is obscure and undoubtedly complex. Endogenous and exogenous hyperglucocorticoidism appear to be implicated, in association with the stress of trauma and surgery and putative neurogenic influences initiated by damage to the spinal cord. In dogs, diffuse gastric hemorrhage due to reduced mucosal resistance to acid must be differentiated from the effects of heavy-metal ingestion, uremic gastritis, coagulopathy (especially due to warfarin or disseminated intravascular coagulation), and canine hemorrhagic gastroenteritis, among others.

Peptic ulcer in **cattle** is confined largely to the abomasum, where it is common (Fig. 1.10C); duodenal ulcer is rarely encountered in this species. Acute ulcers or erosions considered to be the result of stress are frequently seen incidentally in animals, of any age, dying of a variety of causes. They are present usually as linear areas of brown or black hemorrhage or erosion along the margins of abomasal rugae, or as punctate hemorrhages and erosions scattered over the mucosa, especially of the fundus. Such lesions must be differentiated from foci of acute necrosis and ulceration due to systemic viral infections.

In feedlot animals in one study, a prevalence of abomasal ulcer of about 3 to 4% was described, with about half the cases having clinical signs. Bleeding abomasal ulcer or perforation and septic peritonitis are the usual cause of death due to abomasal ulcers. Most ulcers are in the pyloric region in feedlot cattle, and it is in this area that perforations commonly occur. Frequently more than one ulcer is present. Most are 2–4 cm in diameter and approximately circular, though some may be irregular and up to 15 cm in size. Active ulcers may have a dirty brown or gray necrotic floor with some fibrin. Arteries may be visible in the base of bleeding lesions. Older ulcers are puckered, with an overhanging periphery. Abomasal rugae or plicae may be scalloped along their margins or perforated by active or healed ulcers, and in a study of pastured dairy cattle most ulcers and scars were found in the fundic area.

The causes of abomasal ulcer are usually unclear. Some appear to occur under stressful circumstances, as in weaned calves or after transportation. Lactic acid and histamine entering the abomasum from the forestomachs in animals poorly adapted to high-concentrate rations may contribute to mucosal damage. Abomasal stasis may play a part in animals with physical or physiologic abomasal obstruction. Ulceration of the abomasal mucosa infiltrated by lymphosarcoma will occur.

Bleeding abomasal ulcer should be sought in cattle with melena or anemia, and perforating abomasal ulcer in animals presenting with septic peritonitis, especially if digesta is in the abdominal cavity. Some points of perforation will be adherent to the abdominal wall or occluded by superficially adherent omentum.

Abomasal ''stress'' ulcer in calves must be differentiated from lesions associated with infectious bovine rhinotracheitis, and mycotic abomasitis must be differentiated from ulcer in calves and older animals. Mycosis is a rare complication of peptic ulcer. In juvenile and adult cattle, focal abomasal lesions due to bovine virus diarrhea must be differentiated.

Gastric ulcer in **swine** is usually restricted to the pars esophagea (Fig. 1.10D–F); in a small proportion of affected pigs lesions extend into the contiguous esophagus. Rarely are significant ulcers of the cardiac, fundic, or pyloric mucosa encountered in swine, sometimes in association with ulcer of the pars esophagea, occasionally with gastric parasitism or systemic disease. Venous infarcts in the body of the stomach in swine are not to be confused with gastric ulcer. There is little disagreement over the pathology of ulceration of the pars esophagea; its etiopathogenesis remains unresolved.

Under conditions of modern pig husbandry, the prevalence of ulcer and associated abnormalities of the pars esophagea is high. Weaned growers and feeders are commonly affected. Most lesions are subclinical; however, some prove fatal. Pigs die without premonition, or with a short history that may include anemia, weakness, inappetence, vomition, and melena. Other animals are affected chronically, with signs of anorexia, intermittent melena, and weight loss, which may culminate in death or slow recovery with runting. Despite its high subclinical prevalence, and occasional outbreaks of clinical disease or loss of individual valuable pigs, most studies indicate that the economic significance of gastric ulceration is marginal. Little or no effect on growth rate or feed efficiency is evident in most subclinically affected animals.

Lesions of the pars esophagea may involve only a small part, or virtually all, of the gastric squamous mucosa. The lesion evolves through parakeratosis, to fissuring and erosion, with ultimate ulceration in severe cases. All stages in this progression will be encountered at autopsy in pigs. The milder lesions are incidental findings. The epithelium of the pars esophagea often appears yellowish and is thickened, irregular, roughened, and may flake or peel off readily. This gross change is the result of microscopic thickening and parakeratosis, with nucleated cells present at the irregular mucosal surface. *Candida* may be present over the epithelial surface, with hyphae invading the parakeratotic epithelium, perhaps due to favorable cystine or glycogen levels. Rete pegs and proprial papillae are elongate. Neutrophils and eosinophils may be present at the tips of proprial papillae, infiltrating into the epithelium, which appears hydropic and may erode over the tips of papillae.

Erosion of the epithelium progresses to ulceration and exposure of papillae and deeper propria, which bleed as small vessels are disrupted. Such lesions begin as fissures in the hyperplastic parakeratotic epithelium but advance to ulcerate the entire pars esophagea. They usually spare only a microscopically visible margin of squamous epithelium adjacent to the cardiac gland mucosa. Ulcers of the pars esophagea, like peptic ulcer, have a floor or necrotic debris overlying exposed connective tissue (Fig. 1.10F). Depending on the stage and aggression of the ulcer, there may be a well-developed inflammatory margin to the necrosis and a bed of granulation tissue. Fatal gastric hemorrhage often occurs, and thrombosed arterioles and venules cut by ulceration are exposed in the floor of the acute ulcer, which is often overlain by a blood clot. Ulcers of the pars esophagea usually involve only the submucosa, but they may advance to the muscularis externa and occasionally to the serosa. They rarely perforate.

Grossly, fully developed ulceration of the pars esophagea is apparent as a punched-out lesion with elevated rolled edges, obliterating the entire pars esophagea and obscuring the esophageal opening (Fig. 1.10D). Pigs with gastric ulcer at any stage of evolution tend to have fluid content in the stomach. Those with hemorrhagic ulcer may have red-brown gastric content, or massive hemorrhage into the stomach with large blood clots in the lumen, and thrombosed blood adherent to the base of the ulcer and its exposed bleeding points. Melenic content will often be in the intestine, and the colon may contain firm, black, pelleted feces. The carcasses of animals that bleed out with gastric ulcer are very pale. Blood in the intestine associated with gastric ulcer in pigs must be differentiated from mesenteric torsion and proliferative hemorrhagic enteropathy due to *Campylobacter*. A few pigs with parakeratosis, erosion, and ulceration of the pars esophagea have esophageal lesions suggestive of gastric reflux.

Gastric ulcers in some pigs resolve by granulation, and they may become reepithelialized. Such lesions usually become scirrhous, puckered, and contracted as the ulcer closes from the periphery, and scarring may be visible from the serosa (Fig. 1.10E). In these circumstances occlusion of the esophageal opening into the stomach may occur, and pigs with this problem can develop muscular hypertrophy of the distal esophagus. Swine that have suffered chronic gastric hemorrhage may have an enlarged spleen due to extramedullary hematopoiesis.

Factors implicated in the etiology of ulceration of the pars esophagea are many, and their mode of involvement, if any, is usually obscure. Stressful husbandry practices have been considered to contribute to development of ulcer, though glucocorticoid administration causes lesions of the fundus, not pars esophagea, in pigs. High dietary copper levels, feeding of whey, starchy diets low in protein, and high levels of dietary unsatu-

rated fatty acids have been associated. Experimental infection with *Ascaris suum* has been implicated with ulcer, but natural infection is not considered causally associated. Experimentally, factors stimulating acid secretion, especially histamine, consistently cause ulcers of the pars esophagea, suggesting that gastric acidity may play an etiologic role. Repeatedly, finely ground rations have been found to be ulcerogenic and are the single most important contributing factor.

Squamous epithelium has no innate buffering capacity, and it is highly susceptible to attack by gastric acid, as occurs in reflux esophagitis. Similar events may initiate ulceration of the pars esophagea. Swine with gastric ulcer often have abnormally fluid stomach contents. In experimental studies there is slow gastric emptying with progressive declines in pH with time. Feeding of finely divided rations is associated experimentally with increased water in stomach content. There is loss of partitioning of gastric content, and the pH gradient from esophagus to pylorus that occurs in the normal porcine stomach is not established. Relatively low pH occurs at the esophageal end of the stomach, while the pH at the pylorus is higher than normal. Under these conditions of prolonged gastric distention and relatively high antral pH, gastrin-stimulated acid secretion may be excessive. Fluidity and increased mixing of content may expose the pars esophagea, which should normally be in contact with material buffered to pH 5 or greater, to excess acid. This may initiate the epithelial changes described, which culminate in ulceration. Whey may in itself be acid, and would presumably cause an abnormally fluid gastric environment. This could explain its association with ulcer in swine. How other factors mentioned above might be implicated in ulcerogenesis is less clear.

In **horses**, **ulcers** in the **stomach** of foals and adults are often found at autopsy incidental to some other disease process. Gastric ulcer as a clinical entity is less commonly recognized, though a syndrome of abdominal pain, in some cases associated with gastric reflux, has been described. Ulcers in horses are most common in foals more than 2 weeks of age, are often multiple, and can simultaneously involve all four mucosal zones of the stomach and the duodenum.

Ulcers of the esophageal zone are common. They are frequently most severe at or adjacent to the margo plicatus, sometimes involving the edge of the squamous epithelium. They are often large and irregular in shape. There may be extensive fissuring, erosion, and ulceration of the bulk of the squamous mucosa. Often, islands of thickened white proliferative mucosa are scattered as plaques on a predominantly ulcerated mucosa (Fig. 1.10A,B). Ulcers in the secretory stomach are also often large and multiple, though a full range from focal punctate to extensive deep lesions may be seen. Microscopically, gastric ulcers in horses follow the typical pattern previously described. *Candida* may colonize hyperkeratotic squamous mucosa of the esophageal portion of the stomach in some horses with ulcers.

Perforation may occur at any site of ulceration and in one series represented 1% of 600 autopsies on foals. Pyloric and duodenal stenosis have been associated with healing ulcers in horses. Severe esophagitis occurs in foals with ulcer and gastric reflux. Lesions of the margo plicatus have been reported as a site colonized with *Clostridium botulinum* type B, implicated in toxicoinfectious botulism of horses.

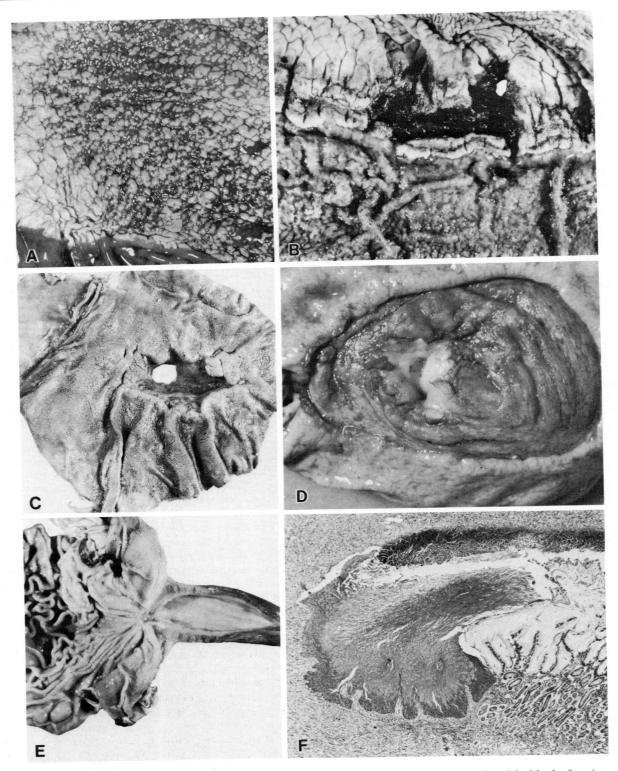

Fig. 1.10. (A) Stomach. Foal. Multiple confluent areas of ulceration of the squamous mucosa. Smooth nodular islands of surviving hyperplastic mucosa are scattered over the ulcerated area. (B) Ulceration with perforation of squamous gastric mucosa. Foal. (C) Perforated abomasal ulcer. Calf. (D) Ulceration of the pars esophagea. Pig. Squamous mucosa is ulcerated, but adjacent cardiac glandular mucosa is unscathed. (E) Scarring of distal esophagus and pars esophagea following ulceration. Pig. (F) Margin of ulcer. Pars esophagea. Pig. Cardiac glandular mucosa and normal remnant of squamous mucosa overhang margin of ulcer.

The pathogenesis of gastric ulcers in horses is unclear. Many cases are associated with enteric disease, ileus, surgery, or other circumstances that can be considered stressful. Administration of steroids and analgesics such as flunixin meglamine and phenylbutazone is commonly associated. *Candida* is considered contributory to ulceration by some, but it is often not present. Esophageal reflux and the severity of lesions in the esophageal portion of the stomach suggest that altered partitioning of abnormally fluid gastric content, and access of acid to squamous mucosa, may explain lesions in the nonglandular gastric mucosa and esophagus. Hypersecretion of acid has not been confirmed, but some cases show subjective clinical response to the histamine-receptor-blocking agent, cimetidine.

Gastric Neoplasia

Gastric neoplasms are uncommon in all species and are very rare in some.

Adenocarcinoma of the **stomach** is most frequently reported in dogs, usually in animals less than 10 years of age, and it comprises the majority of the gastric neoplasms found in that species. Males predominate in the population with gastric cancer, and more than half of gastric adenocarcinomas in dogs occur in the pyloric region. Grossly, some gastric neoplasms appear as nonulcerating, firm thickenings involving most of the gastric wall and causing loss of the normal rugal pattern on the mucosal surface. Others are more localized, plaquelike thickenings, which tend to obliterate rugae and ulcerate centrally. Ulceration is expected in more than half of canine gastric adenocarcinomas. Surface proliferation or irregularity other than ulceration is very uncommon in gastric carcinoma in dogs. Cut sections through the stomach wall invaded by carcinoma reveal edema and pale, firm, fibrous tissue. Induration or plaquelike pale masses may be evident on the serosa, where the outline of infiltrated lymphatics may be prominent. Widespread gastric mural fibrosis and thickening causes ''linitis plastica'' or the so-called leather-bottle appearance. The scirrhous nature of most gastric carcinomas in the dog is the result of desmoplasia induced by the malignant epithelium.

These tumors adopt two basic microscopic forms. Most gastric adenocarcinomas in dogs are of the diffuse type. Most of these consist of widespread random infiltrates of neoplastic cells in small clusters or dispersed singly between supporting stromal elements. The cell type is usually relatively uniform within a single neoplasm, commonly consisting of poorly differentiated, round or angular, mucus-secreting epithelial cells. In many of these tumors, some cells adopt the hollow, mucus-filled ''signet ring'' appearance, and extracellular mucin may be present. Occasional tumors of this type have a more variable cell population, with some cells containing little cytoplasm, others with extensive eosinophilic cytoplasm, and large atypical nuclei. Other tumors will have scattered, irregular, glandlike structures. Desmoplasia is typically heavy in diffuse gastric carcinomas.

Adenocarcinomas of the tubular or intestinal type are encountered less commonly in the canine stomach. They are characterized by tubular glandular structure, with a lumen, and a relatively well differentiated and polarized lining epithelium. They retain this form with some variation as they infiltrate and metastasize, and they are relatively less scirrhous than the diffuse type. There may be papilliform infoldings of the epithelium of tubular adenocarcinomas; some form smaller acinar structures; others rarely adopt a more solid form of growth, with occasional acinar structures and a more anaplastic cytologic appearance. Cells may have eosinophilic cytoplasm, and many contain mucin. The better differentiated tubular tumors resemble pyloric glands. Infiltrates of lymphocytes and plasma cells, sometimes with follicle formation, may occur in the primary site of all types of gastric carcinoma.

A single squamous-cell carcinoma has been reported arising from the pyloric gland mucosa in a dog, and carcinoids develop, very rarely, in the gastric mucosa.

Gastric carcinomas in dogs infiltrate the stomach wall aggressively, invading lymphatics, and they have usually metastasized to the local lymph nodes, and often to distant organs, particularly lung, liver, and adrenal, by the time they are diagnosed.

Benign ''adenomatous'' polyps or sessile proliferative lesions occur uncommonly in the pyloric stomach in dogs. These have been alluded to previously as a potential cause of pyloric stenosis or obstruction and as a possible hyperplastic sequel to chronic antritis. Their exact status, whether inflammatory hyperplasia or benign neoplasia, is unclear. Although there are reports of malignant polypoid adenocarcinoma, it seems, on the basis of the relative frequency of ''adenomas'' *vis-à-vis* adenocarcinoma, that they are unlikely to be common precursors of gastric cancer. Grossly, these lesions appear as solitary or multiple, raised, convoluted, nodular, sessile or sometimes pedunculate, polypoid masses, usually 1–2 cm in size. Microscopically, there is foveolar and glandular hyperplasia, with well-differentiated columnar mucous cells on the surface and in glands. Some mucus-filled glandular cysts may be present, and mononuclear-cell infiltrates are often in the mucosal propria.

Mesenchymal tumors of the stomach in dogs are less common than adenocarcinomas. Most are typical leiomyomas, which may produce nodular, sometimes polypoid, masses several centimeters in size that project into the gastric lumen or protrude from the serosa. Leiomyosarcomas, lymphosarcomas, and rare anaplastic sarcomas are also found in the canine stomach. These tumors may ulcerate the mucosa and, to that extent, mimic the behavior of adenocarcinoma. Their microscopic appearance is typical.

Tumors other than lymphosarcoma are rarely encountered in the stomach of cats, and even that is uncommon. Several cases of gastric adenocarcinoma have been described, adopting tubular and diffuse patterns.

Gastric adenocarcinoma in **cattle** is exceptionally uncommon, but when it occurs it resembles patterns adopted by similar tumors in other species, being scirrhous, invading the wall, and capable of ulceration. Much more important in cattle is **lymphosarcoma** of the abomasum. Involvement of this organ is common in adult cattle. Diffuse submucosal and mucosal lymphocytic infiltrates or nodular proliferations may occur. Strategically placed pyloric tumor may cause obstruction. Diffuse lesions, thickening the gastric wall, frequently ulcerate and hemorrhage from such ulcers, producing melena. The lymphoid infiltrates are recognizable as firm, gray-white tissue in the submucosa and mucosa. Involvement of abomasal lymph nodes is dispropor-

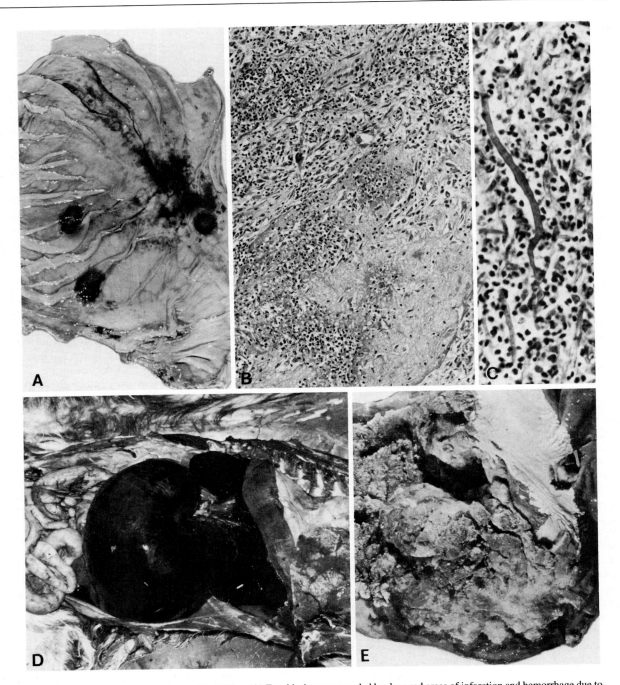

Fig. 1.11. (A–C) Mycotic abomasitis. Calf. (A) Focal lesions surrounded by deep red areas of infarction and hemorrhage due to thrombosis of mucosal and submucosal vessels. (B) Thrombosis of a venule in submucosa of abomasum due to hyphal invasion. (C) Nonseptate hyphae of zygomycete invading the submucosa. (D) Gastric volvulus in a dog. The stomach has undergone venous infarction due to strangulation of its vascular outflow and is extremely distended and congested. (E) Fungating and ulcerative squamous-cell carcinoma arising from the gastric squamous mucosa. Horse.

tionately slight. Gastric lymphosarcoma also occurs in swine, where it is usually diffuse. The wall of the stomach is thickened by submucosal lymphocytic infiltrates, which sometimes invade the mucosa locally in many areas, producing nodular elevations that may ulcerate.

In the horse, most gastric neoplasms are **squamous-cell carcinomas** derived from the esophageal mucosa; occasional adenocarcinomas, originating in glandular epithelium, and leiomyomas are also reported. Squamous-cell carcinomas occur in middle-aged horses. They usually present in an advanced state, with a history of unexplained anorexia, occasionally dysphagia, and weight loss sometimes progressing rapidly to emaciation. At autopsy there may be peritoneal effusion, and there is usually evidence of the neoplasm on the serosa of the stomach. There also may be peritoneal implants, especially on intestine, testes, omentum, parietal abdominal surfaces, and diaphragm; direct extension to adjacent organs, including liver, spleen, and diaphragm, with progression to the pleural space; and sometimes distant metastases, usually in liver and lung. The appearance of the tumor on serosal surfaces resembles mesothelioma, with smooth, creamy plaques or nodules up to 2 to 4 cm in diameter.

The origin of these lesions is in a fungating, cauliflower-like mass 10–40 cm in diameter, with superficial fissures, usually projecting above the surface of the pars esophagea (Fig. 1.11E). Sometimes these lesions are superficially more ulcerative than proliferative. Necrosis and hemorrhage are evident in the tumor mass, which is usually well demarcated from adjacent normal squamous mucosa. Occasionally the tumor extends into the distal esophagus and may obstruct it. Microscopically, these neoplasms are typical squamous-cell carcinomas, invading in cords or nests of cells through the gastric wall. They induce desmoplasia, imparting a scirrhous, firm texture and appearance to the thickened gastric wall and to the peritoneal and pleural implants. One such tumor has been reported as a cause of pseudohyperparathyroidism in a horse.

Intestine

Normal Form and Function

Small Intestine

The microtopography of the small bowel is extensively modified, to increase its surface area, by spiral mucosal folds in some species, and by villi projecting into the lumen. The villi, projections of lamina propria covered by a layer of epithelium one cell thick, are calculated to expand the absorptive surface of the small bowel 7- to 14-fold. In most species, villi are tallest in the duodenum and decline somewhat in height toward the ileum. The length and shape of villi in "normal" animals varies with the species, age, intestinal microflora, and immune status. In general, villi in dogs, cats, and neonatal piglets and ruminants tend to be tall and cylindric; those in horses and young ruminants tend to be moderately tall and cylindric; villi in weaned ruminants and swine may be cylindric, leaf- or tongue-shaped or, rarely, ridgelike, with their broad surface at right angles to the long axis of the gut.

Opening onto the mucosal surface around the base of each villus are several crypts of Lieberkühn. These are straight or somewhat coiled (depending on the species and the proliferative status), glandlike structures, lined by a single layer of epithelium. The progenitor compartment of the enteric epithelium resides here, producing cells that differentiate and move up onto the surface of villi, mainly as absorptive enterocytes, ultimately to be extruded as effete cells from the tips of villi.

Primordial stem cells are present at the base of the crypts, and they divide to produce cells of four main types. Poorly differentiated cuboidal or low columnar cells with relatively few, short microvilli are the predominant type of cell lining crypts; especially in the lower half of crypts, these cells form a population that cycles rapidly, undergoing amplification division. One of the ensuing daughter cells usually differentiates and moves into the functional compartment of absorptive enterocytes on the villus.

Oligomucous cells, derived by mitosis from the basal stem cells, are also a population undergoing amplification division. They contain mucous granules and are intermediate in structure between undifferentiated crypt epithelium and goblet cells, into which they mature. Well-differentiated goblet cells are present in crypts and on the surface of villi, with varying prevalence and distribution at various levels of the intestine, and in the different species. They have basal nuclei and secrete mucus, apparently by exocytosis, from the luminal border of the cell. The precise function of intestinal mucus, which stains strongly for neutral and sialic acid–rich mucosubstances, is uncertain. It probably serves to "insulate" the surface from organisms, which it may entrap or immobilize. It contains lysozyme, and IgA secreted into it by epithelium. Mucus secretion appears to be promoted by a variety of noxious stimuli and by immune events in the gut.

Paneth cells, a population of cells turning over slowly in the base of crypts, are not found in dogs, cats, or swine, and they are not prominent in the intestine of ruminants. Among domestic animals they are most obvious in horses. Eosinophilic secretory granules are present in the apical cytoplasm of Paneth cells; though the function of the granules is unclear, it seems that they may be lysozyme, which could have an antimicrobial function in the crypt and in mucus.

The fourth type of cell found in intestinal crypts is the **enteroendocrine cell**. They too are derived from crypt stem cells and comprise a heterogenous population of about a dozen amine- or peptide-secreting endocrine/paracrine cells. These are the cells variously recognized as enterochromaffin, argentaffin, or argyrophil; the specific cell type is defined by immunocytochemistry and the ultrastructure of secretory granules. Enteroendocrine cells are scattered singly among other cells on villi and, more commonly, in crypts. They tend to be located peripherally in the epithelial layer, with little luminal exposure, and contain scattered small secretory granules in the basal cytoplasm. Hormones with relatively clearly understood functions, such as secretin and cholecystokinin, as well as peptides or amines, whose endocrine or paracrine implications are less certain, are secreted. Some probably integrate in function with similar neurohormones secreted by the submucosal nervous plexus. With the exception of carcinoid tumors of serotonin-secreting cell origin, and rare functional neoplasms of other enteroendocrine cells in humans, the pathologic implications of this class of cells are still very poorly defined.

Scattered among the cells of the crypt and villus are specialized **caveolated** or "**tuft**" **cells**. These are flask-shaped cells tapering toward the luminal border, also found in other gastrointestinal and respiratory epithelial surfaces. They are characterized by the presence of an apical tubulovesicular system, from which they derive their name, but the function of these cells is not known. Specialized "cup" epithelial cells, of unknown function also, have been described on villi in the ileum of several species.

The **enterocytes**, which are responsible for the final digestion and absorption of nutrients, electrolytes, and water, are by far the predominant cells on intestinal villi. They are normally tall columnar cells, hexagonal in cross section, with a regular basal nuclear polarity. A tight junction, which is nevertheless "leaky" to small ions and water, joins the apical margins of adjacent cells. Basal to the tight junction, the lateral cell membranes interdigitate loosely, and a long, narrow potential space exists between enterocytes. The basolateral cell membrane is the site of (Na^+, K^+)-ATPase activity, driving the sodium pump, and of carrier systems exporting monosaccharides from the cell. Absorptive epithelial cells lie on a basal lamina, which they may produce.

The apical surface of normal enterocytes is highly modified into microvilli, about $0.5–1.5$ μm long and 0.1 μm wide, which are regularly arrayed in close apposition to each other at right angles to the surface of the cell. They are visible as the "brush border" by conventional microscopy. Microvilli increase the surface area of absorptive epithelium by a factor of about 15 to 40. The plasmalemma of microvilli is studded with massive numbers of enzyme molecules, including aminopeptidases and disaccharidases involved in terminal digestion of peptides and carbohydrates. These protrude as minute knoblike structures into the glycoprotein "glycocalyx," which coats the surface of microvilli. Proteins binding calcium ions, vitamin B_{12} and water-soluble vitamins, and proteins involved in the transport into the cell of peptides, amino acids, glucose, galactose, and triglyceride, coupled with transport of sodium ion, are also embedded in the plasmalemma of microvilli. Clines in the distribution of microvillus-associated functions are present along the small intestine. The activities of alkaline phosphatase and most disaccharidases are greater in the anterior small bowel, while the receptor for vitamin B_{12}:intrinsic factor is concentrated in the ileum.

In neonatal swine and ruminants, vacuolation of absorptive enterocytes is normal, and the nucleus is often also displaced into the apical cytoplasm. In piglets, vacuolation is usual in the ileum (Fig. 1.34B), not in the duodenum, and seems to be a function of cell age. Such vacuolation should be differentiated from the presence of eosinophilic colostrum present in cytoplasmic vacuoles in the epithelial cells of neonates (Fig. 1.14A). The cytoplasm of absorptive enterocytes is stabilized at the apical border by the filaments of the terminal web. Smooth endoplasmic reticulum is most prominent in the upper half of cells, while cisternal elements of rough endoplasmic reticulum are more uniformly distributed. The Golgi zone lies above the nucleus. Free ribosomes and polyribosomes are numerous in differentiating cells of the upper crypt and lower villus and are relatively fewer in mature absorptive enterocytes.

The complex of endoplasmic membranes and Golgi apparatus is active particularly in handling absorbed lipid, which diffuses from micelles at the cell surface, through the apical membrane, in the form of long-chain fatty acids or monoglyceride. These are reesterified to triglyceride, appearing in the smooth endoplasmic reticulum, and are complexed with apoproteins produced in the rough endoplasmic reticulum, to be excreted via the Golgi apparatus through the basolateral cell membrane as chylomicrons. Chylomicrons enter the extracellular space and leave the villus via the lacteal. Mitochondria are numerous in the metabolically active absorptive enterocyte. Vacuoles formed by endocytosis of macromolecules at the base of microvilli fuse with lysosomes in the subapical cytoplasm, and by this process of heterophagia, potentially noxious material is destroyed. In addition to lysosomes, acid phosphatase–containing vesicular bodies, and peroxisomes containing catalase but of uncertain function, are also found in intestinal epithelium.

The epithelium of the small intestinal mucosa is supported by a highly plastic mesenchymal stroma, the **lamina propria**. This is composed of loose, fibrous tissue, through which course blood vessels and in which smooth muscle, inflammatory, and immune-active cells are interspersed. Surrounding the crypt of Lieberkühn and underlying the basal lamina of the epithelium of the villi is a fibroblast sheath. Proliferation of elements of this sheath has been demonstrated around the crypt, and [³H]thymidine-labeled mesenchymal cells appear to move in concert with overlying epithelium up onto villi, ultimately undergoing degeneration in the lamina propria at the villus tip. There, histiocytes containing nuclear fragments may be found, presumably phagocytosing effete sheath cells.

Scattered in the lamina propria of villi and between crypts are lymphocytes, neutrophils, and eosinophils. The latter are particularly common in the intestine of ruminants and horses, with no specific pathologic connotation. Intraepithelial lymphocytes (theliolymphcytes) are frequently found between epithelial cells on villi and, less commonly, in crypt lining. Globule leukocytes may be found in the epithelium of crypts and low on villi, or sometimes in the lamina propria between crypts. Plasma cells normally are not numerous in villi but are concentrated in the lamina propria between the upper portions of crypts. Few attempts at quantitative assessment of the distribution of the various cell types in the lamina propria of "normal" animals have been undertaken in domestic species.

The **vascular supply** to the **mucosa** arises in submucosal arteries, which give off arterioles at right angles, some of which send branches to a capillary plexus around crypts of Lieberkühn. The majority pass up the centers of villi, arborizing near the villus tip into a dense capillary plexus that lies immediately beneath the basal lamina of the epithelium. Capillaries in villi have fenestrations facing the basal lamina, which may be more permeable than the remainder of the endothelium. One or more venules drain blood from the capillaries in villi and between crypts and flow into larger veins in the submucosa, which drain into mesenteric veins and the hepatic portal circulation. At least in swine there appear to be anastamoses between the capillary plexi of villus and crypt. The lacteal, or central lymphatic vessel of the villus is sufficiently permeable to permit the entry of macromolecules and chylomicrons and is the main route of lipid transport from the villus.

It is suggested that the juxtaposition of arteriole and venule in the villus may result in a countercurrent multiplier system in the villus, establishing an increasing gradient of sodium concentration and a decreasing oxygen gradient toward the tip of the villus. Anastomoses between capillary plexuses surrounding the villi and crypts might provide a mechanism for shunting electrolytes and water, just absorbed in the villi, into the vicinity of crypts, where secretion is occurring. Thus a putative crypt–villus fluid and electrolyte circuit would be provided with a direct vascular arm.

Large Intestine

The anatomy and size of the cecum and colon vary widely among domestic animals, depending largely on the significance of microbial fermentation of carbohydrate in the hindgut. Production of volatile fatty acid from carbohydrate by colonic flora occurs in all species. In the horse, this is a primary source of energy, and it is significant in swine and ruminants as well. Extensive movement of electrolytes and water occurs across the colonic wall. In the horse, a volume of fluid up to one-third that of the extracellular fluid space of the animal may be in the large bowel, which must maintain a fluid medium for microbial fermentation; daily fluid absorption from the hindgut may equal the extracellular fluid volume. Absorption of electrolytes and water, an electrolyte-conserving mechanism, is probably the major function of the colon in dogs and cats, and of the distal colon of herbivores.

The mucosa of the cecum and colon in all domestic species lacks villi, though there are ridges or folds on the mucosal surface. The surface of the hindgut is lined by a single layer of tall columnar absorptive epithelial cells with basal nuclei. These cells have sparser and fewer regular microvilli in comparison with absorptive cells of the small bowel, and numerous glycoprotein-laden vesicles are in the apical cytoplasm. Typical goblet cells are also interspersed on the colonic surface in variable numbers, depending on the species and a variety of other factors.

Colonic crypts or glands are straight, tubular structures. The architecture of colonic glands and their cell population resemble somewhat those of small intestinal crypts. Stem cells are present in the base of the gland, and poorly differentiated mitotic columnar epithelium may be present in the basal two-thirds of the gland, though its extent may vary considerably. These cells differentiate progressively toward absorptive epithelium as they approach the surface. Oligomucous cells, derived from basal stem cells, form a second proliferative population in the lower half of the colonic gland. Well-differentiated goblet cells are usually present in the upper half of glands in the large bowel as well as on the surface. Spirochetes have been found in colonic goblet cells in apparently normal dogs and cats and in some laboratory animals. Enteroendocrine cells of about a half dozen types have been recognized, scattered in the cell column lining glands in the large bowel.

The lamina propria of the colon is minimal between closely packed glands. It contains a cell population similar to that in the small bowel. A fibroblast sheath encloses the colonic glands and appears to migrate with the epithelium. Normally, relatively few inflammatory and immune-active cells are present in the superficial mucosa; most plasma cells and lymphocytes are between deeper portions of glands.

Electrolyte and Water Transport in the Intestine

The small intestinal mucosa is highly permeable to the passive movement of small ions and water and is therefore considered "leaky," despite the presence of "tight" junctions at the apical margins of absorptive enterocytes. Epithelia of this type, which also include gallbladder and renal proximal tubule, are specialized for the absorption of large volumes of salts and water in isotonic concentrations and for separating compartments similar in osmolality and ion composition. The leakiness of the epithelium of the small bowel ensures that the intestinal content is approximately isosmolal with the interstitial fluid space. The leaks in the small intestinal epithelium are paracellular, at the tight junctions, and act as water-filled spaces 0.4–0.8 nm in diameter. The permeability of junctional complexes appears to be sensitive to Starling forces, influenced by intravascular hydrostatic and oncotic pressure, so that fluid and solute actively absorbed may leak back into the lumen, thus modulating net absorption by the mucosa.

Sodium absorption takes place by three active transcellular mechanisms. Chloride ion moves independently via a paracellular route, or coupled with sodium by a transcellular route. Fundamentally, sodium absorption depends on electrochemical forces established by the ATP-dependent sodium pump on the basolateral cell membrane of the enterocyte. This pump moves Na^+ up a concentration gradient from the cell in the lateral intercellular space. The first mechanism involves independent, or uncoupled, electrogenic Na^+ absorption. Sodium ion enters the cell from the luminal solution down an electrostatic and concentration gradient established by the sodium pump, which exchanges K^+ for Na^+, but not at an equal rate. Absorption of Na^+ is also coupled to that of organic solutes such as amino acids and glucose. Sodium moves into the cell down the electrochemical gradient established by the sodium pump, but it does so coupled to movement of the organic solute. Sodium is then pumped out across the basolateral membrane, while the organic solute moves via carrier-mediated facilitated diffusion out of the cell. Most sodium and chloride is probably absorbed together by a neutral process, involving transcellular route for both ions. Sodium ion moving into the cell at the apical margin, as a result of the gradient established by the sodium pump, is coupled with Cl^-, carrying it "uphill" into the cell, whence it moves passively to the interstitium, while Na^+ is pumped out. An alternate hypothesis suggests that Na^+ and Cl^- are absorbed into the epithelium by processes that exchange them for H^+ and HCO_3^-, which enter the gut lumen.

The concentration by these mechanisms of solute, especially sodium and chloride ion, in the lateral intercellular space, causes water to follow from the intestinal lumen down an osmotic gradient. Since cell membranes and junctional complexes are highly permeable to water, movement is rapid via both transcellular and paracellular routes, and differences in osmotic pressure between lumen and lateral intercellular space are small. Absorbed solute and water in isotonic proportions move into the interstitium of the villus, where within a few micrometers, they encounter a subepithelial capillary or lacteal. The dilated lateral intercellular space is readily seen in sections of villus epithelium in mucosa that was actively absorbing when fixed.

The colon of carnivores, the spiral colon of ruminants and swine, and the small colon of horses are charged with the task of reducing the volume of electrolyte and water lost to the animal in the feces. This process is relatively poorly understood. In contrast to the small intestine, the colonic epithelium is moderately restrictive to the free movement of sodium and chloride, though not potassium. Therefore it is capable of maintaining differences is osmotic pressure, ionic composition, and electrical potential between luminal and proprial surfaces, which make it more efficient than the small bowel in absorbing some electrolytes and water. Ultimately, fecal water may be hypotonic with respect to plasma. Absorption of volatile fatty acids also accounts for considerable water absorption from the colon. Potassium increases in concentration in colonic content as sodium concentration declines; this may be due to an active secretory process, or involve mainly paracellular flux down an electrochemical gradient. Colonic sodium, chloride, and water absorption and potassium secretion are stimulated significantly by aldosterone.

In pathologic states, both the small intestinal mucosa and that of the large bowel secrete sodium chloride and water. There is accumulating evidence that this process, which appears to be a function mainly of the crypts, also may be physiologic and perhaps segmental, involved in maintaining the fluidity of the intestinal content. Intestinal secretion will be considered more fully later as part of the pathogenesis of diarrhea.

Immune Elements of the Gastrointestinal Tract

The gastrointestinal tract is continually presented with food antigens, ingested toxins, viruses, bacteria and their products, and parasites and their excretions and secretions. The epithelial barrier of the gut is but one cell thick and has enormous surface area. Therefore, it is not surprising that the epithelium and associated lymphoid and inflammatory cells in the mucosa and submucosa have evolved a complex system for sampling, blocking, neutralizing, and eliminating antigens. Lymphoid tissue has been estimated to constitute 25% of the intestinal mucosal mass and to exceed that of the spleen in volume.

The epithelial cell of the neonate is capable of uptake and transport of macromolecules from the intestinal lumen to the basolateral cell surface. In all species of domestic animals, **colostral transfer** of **immunoglobulins** by this route provides the neonate with passive humoral immunity during the early postnatal period. The selectivity of macromolecular transfer varies with the species, being least specific in neonatal ruminants, piglets, and foals, which take up most macromolecules contacting the epithelium. Permeability of the gut to macromolecules is the result of energy-dependent pinocytosis by the apical cell membrane at the base of microvilli. Colostral protein is transferred in membrane-bound vacuoles in the cytoplasm to the basolateral membrane, where, by exocytosis, the contents are extruded, to find their way via the lacteal and lymphatics to the general circulation. The period of active uptake of macromolecules is short, usually only 24–48 hr in ungulates, and "closure" precludes further bulk transport of macromolecules. Closure is probably at least partly related to "maturity" of the epithelium and involves failure of intracellular transport or exocytosis, possibly due to replacement of surface enterocytes by cells incapable of export of proteins. Cells containing eosinophilic protein-filled cytoplasmic vacuoles (Fig. 1.14A), which may displace the nucleus toward the surface, persist longest in the distal small bowel.

Although bulk transport does not occur, experimental data suggest that nutritionally inconsequential amounts of macromolecules continue to be transferred by enterocytes in mature animals, via mechanisms analagous to those occurring in the neonate. For significant uptake to occur, molecules must escape intraluminal hydrolysis, and pinocytosis must exceed the rate of lysosomal degradation to permit molecules to be exported from the cell. This is presumably one mechanism by which antigens encounter immune-active cells in the mucosa. Macromolecules

gaining entry to the portal circulation are largely phagocytosed by Kupffer cells in the liver. Certainly, these cells form a second line of defense against absorbed macromolecules from the gut and are particularly important in clearing endotoxin from the portal blood.

In addition to the pinocytotic activity of absorptive enterocytes, specific epithelial cells called **M cells**, associated with Peyer's patches and intestinal lymphoid follicles, actively "sample" particulate matter and macromolecules impinging on the mucosal surface. The M cells are called so because of the presence of microfolds, rather than microvilli, on their apical surface in humans, though this characteristic seems to be restricted to that species. The M cells are present, interspersed among cells resembling absorptive enterocytes, on the surface of the "dome" in the mucosa overlying lymphoid aggregates in the submucosa. In the neonatal calf, M cells cover the dome completely. These cells often adopt an inverted "cup" shape, with one or more lymphocytes and occasional macrophages in the basal concavity, in intimate contact with the membrane of the M cell. Macromolecular and particulate material taken up by M cells is transmitted to the associated lymphocytes or macrophages. The M cell is a likely portal of entry to the mucosa for bacteria, perhaps including *Salmonella, Yersinia,* and *Listeria* in some species, and some viruses. Neutrophils are seen transmigrating the epithelium of the dome and in the lumen over the dome, in enteric bacterial infections of calves in particular. Neutrophils may also play a role in phagocytosis in the enteric lumen in pigs under some conditions.

The **aggregated lymphoid follicles**, or **Peyer's patches**, and solitary lymphoid follicles are scattered in the mucosa of the small intestine of all species, and solitary lymphoid follicles stud the colonic mucosa. Peyer's patches are present throughout the length of the small intestine in all species, though they tend to be larger distally. They are grossly visible, usually as oval or elongate structures up to several centimeters wide, thickening the antimesenteric wall of the intestine. They may project slightly above the mucosal surface or appear as depressions, which must not be mistaken for ulcers, especially in dogs. In neonates of some species, including swine, they may be poorly developed and not visible grossly. Continuous, elongate Peyer's patches have been described in the distal 1 to 1.5 m of ileum in calves and piglets. Peyer's patches in sheep are reported to involute as the animal matures.

Peyer's patches are comprised of follicular aggregates of B lymphocytes in the submucosa, underlying a discontinuous muscularis mucosae. Between the upper borders of adjacent lymphoid follicles are aggregates of T lymphocytes. Overlying the lymphoid follicles is a mixed population of T and B lymphocytes, extending into the lamina propria in rounded mucosal projections, the domes, which lie between villi. Short crypts provide epithelium to domes and adjacent villi. Cell populations of Peyer's patches in newborns and gnotobiotes of most species tend to be sparser than those in older or bacterially colonized animals, though those in neonatal calves appear relatively well developed. The microscopic organization of solitary lymphoid follicles and associated mucosa essentially resembles that of the Peyer's patch.

The **B** and **T immunoblasts** gain access to Peyer's patches via permeable postcapillary venules. The major cell populations in Peyer's patches appear to be B lymphocytes committed mainly to IgA production, while among the T cells is a large proportion of T-helper-cell precursors. How or whether antigen is processed in Peyer's patches is unclear; macrophages apparently are present in lower concentration in Peyer's patches than in lamina propria, and their place in the interaction among M cells and T and B lymphocytes is uncertain. They probably play an effector role in cell-mediated reactions to bacteria entering via Peyer's patches, and certainly in response to agents such as *Mycobacterium paratuberculosis* and *Histoplasma capsulatum* found in the lamina propria.

Macrophages scattered in the lamina propria may play a role in presenting antigen to sensitize lymphocytes present in the propria. In addition to functioning in defense against microorganisms, macrophages phagocytose inert particulate matter reaching the lamina propria from the lumen. They also may accumulate iron pigment under some circumstances and, by loss at the villus tip, may have some function in its excretion. Bile pigment, perhaps derived from meconium, is seen sometimes in macrophages in the tips of villi in neonates. The involvement of macrophages in the phagocytosis of cells (enterocytes, theliolymphocytes, fibroblast sheath) in the subepithelial lamina propria at the tips of villi or between the openings of colonic glands has been alluded to previously. This process is most obvious in equine large and small intestine, where it should be distinguished from necrotic foci in the lamina propria. Its pathologic significance is uncertain.

The **IgA lymphoblasts** leave the Peyer's patch for the mesenteric lymph node and, via the thoracic duct, the general circulation, whence they home in on the intestinal mucosa and other mucosal surfaces, including the respiratory tract, mammary gland, and salivary glands. In the lamina propria of the intestine they differentiate into IgA-secretory plasma cells, found mainly in close apposition to columnar epithelium of the upper crypt. Dimeric IgA may bind to glycoprotein "secretory component" present on the basolateral border of columnar crypt epithelial cells, though this is not certain. With secretory component, it is transported in vesicles through the cytoplasm to be released from the apical border of the cell into the lumen of the crypt. It then spreads over the intestinal surface, at least partly bound to mucus. Dimeric IgA entering the circulation is selectively taken up by hepatocytes and is secreted into bile, at least in some nonruminant species.

IgA-secreting cells are the predominant class of plasma cell in the lamina propria in most species. However, IgM-secreting plasma cells are prevalent in young calves, swine, and dogs. IgM is also taken up by secretory component in some species and transported to the intestinal lumen. This may be significant in the young piglet and calf. Although IgA and IgM are secreted, IgG_1 is the major antibody class in intestinal secretion in cattle; it appears to be selectively secreted by the gut and in the bile in that species. The situation in sheep is less clear.

The function of IgA in the gut lumen probably lies mainly in blocking attachment by bacteria and viruses to epithelial cells, neutralizing intraluminal toxins, and limiting absorption of antigens originating in food and produced by microorganisms in the gut. It thereby reduces the likelihood of reaginic and other forms of immune response in the propria. Secretion into the bile, by hepatocytes, of IgA complexed with antigen may, in the species in which it occurs, be a significant means of clearing the circulation of antigen absorbed from the gut.

Plasma cells containing IgG are relatively uncommon in the intestinal lamina propria in species other than ruminants. However, locally produced and systemically circulating IgG may assume significance when vascular permeability and inflammation occur, due to its ability to fix complement, facilitate antibody-dependent cell-mediated cytotoxicity, and opsonize.

Plasmacytes producing IgE are present in the lamina propria, and this class of immunoglobulin has been implicated particularly in immune responses to some intestinal parasites. Its significance may be in IgE-dependent cytotoxicity by eosinophils and perhaps by mast cells, as well as in mediating reaginic reactions in the mucosa.

Intestinal mast cells differ histochemically and physiologically from mast cells in most other tissues. They are not readily demonstrable after formalin fixation; Carnoy's fixative is best. The proliferation of intestinal mast cells (probably of bone marrow origin) appears to be dependent on factors derived from T cells and is a prominent feature of some parasitisms.

Globule leukocytes are visible in hematoxylin- and eosin-stained tissue sections as mononuclear cells with large, eosinophilic cytoplasmic granules, in the epithelium of the crypt and lower villus, and sometimes in the lamina propria. Possibly they are derived from intestinal mast cells. The effects of histamine, serotonin, and other mediators released by mast cells on vascular tone and permeability, motility, chemotaxis, and effector function of leukocytes, on immune-active cells, and possibly in mucus release are many and complex. Intestinal eosinophils probably do not differ functionally from eosinophils in other sites, being cytotoxic effector cells and modulators of local inflammation.

The T cells are present in Peyer's patches and are distributed throughout the mucosa, in the lamina propria, and are the great majority of the **intraepithelial lymphocyte population**. Lymphocytes may comprise in excess of 10 to 20% of cells present in the epithelial layer of the small intestine. A significant proportion of the intraepithelial lymphocytes contain granules resembling those in mast cells; these "large granular lymphocytes" may be natural killer cells. Many of the other intraepithelial lymphocytes may be suppressor T cells. In contrast, a lower proportion of proprial T lymphocytes have markers characteristic of suppressor cells, and some may also be T-helper cells or pluripotential stem T cells. As might be expected, B lymphocytes are numerous in the lamina propria and are most highly concentrated in Peyer's patches, where the greatest numbers of T-helper cells are also found.

The T immunoblasts from the gut seem to follow a pathway similar to that of B lymphocytes, through mesenteric lymph nodes and the systemic circulation before homing in on the lamina propria or intraepithelial intercellular space. Increased numbers of intraepithelial lymphocytes are associated with cell-mediated immune reactions in the intestinal mucosa. Understanding of the mechanisms of cell-mediated immunity in the intestine is still poor. They may be mediated by T-helper-cell-promoted antibody production, by local direct cytotoxic effects, and by release of lymphokines. In some circumstances (intestinal parasitism, probably some food allergies, celiac disease in humans), soluble factors associated with cell-mediated immune events cause alterations in epithelial proliferation and differentiation that may culminate in villus atrophy.

Immunoinflammatory events in the large bowel are less well understood than those in the small intestine. Presumably, similar principles prevail. Lymphoglandular complexes, consisting of homogeneous submucosal lymphoid aggregates penetrated by glands extending from the mucosa, occur in the cecum and proximal colon of the dog and at the cecocolic junction in ruminants. Epithelium lining glands is in close contact with lymphocytes. Solitary submucosal lymphoid nodules, normally without penetrating glands, are also scattered throughout the cecum and colon in all species. Plasma cells in the lamina propria are principally IgA producing. Depending on the species, their location varies. In dogs, most tend to be in the deeper portion of the lamina propria between glands. Intraepithelial lymphocytes are present.

Gastrointestinal Microflora

After birth, no part of the gastrointestinal tract is sterile. The species of bacteria inhabiting the stomach and intestine are several hundred in number, forming an ecosystem of enormous complexity. Generally speaking, bacterial populations are least in the stomach and upper small intestine of ruminants and carnivores, being limited by the acid gastric environment and by peristalsis. The anaerobes and facultative anaerobes, mainly *E. coli*, increase to $\sim 10^7$ per gram of content in the lower small intestine, and total bacterial populations in excess of 10^{10} or 10^{11} per gram of content are present in the cecum and colon. Prominent among colonic bacteria are coliforms, *Lactobacillus*, and strict anaerobes, including *Bacteroides*, *Fusobacterium*, *Clostridium*, *Eubacterium*, *Bifidobacterium*, and *Peptostreptococcus*. Spirochetes are found in swine and dogs. Anaerobic bacteria outnumber facultative anaerobes by a thousandfold in the large bowel.

The complex ecology of the gut flora imparts on it a considerable stability, and if disturbed it tends to return toward the original state. It is relatively resistant to the intrusion of new inhabitants, and this is one of the major factors protecting against the establishment of pathogenic bacteria. It is no coincidence that bacterial diarrhea occurs most commonly in the neonate with a poorly established flora, or after changes in husbandry or antibiotic therapy that may disturb the enteric bacterial population.

Normal flora acts as a barrier to colonization by pathogens through several means. The secretion of proteins such as colicins has little significance in modulating enteric bacterial populations; more important is the production of acetic and butyric acids by the anaerobes. Under the pH and anaerobic conditions in the large bowel, fatty acids are highly detrimental to members of the Enterobacteriaceae. The high population of lactobacilli in the gut of milk-fed animals probably reduces establishment of Enterobacteriaceae by this means. Facultative anaerobes are important in maintaining the redox environment for strict anaerobes, by scavenging oxygen. Competition for energy, and

the effect of metabolites other than short-chain fatty acids produced by the native flora, militate against establishment by exogenous bacteria. Host factors influencing gut flora include composition of the diet; peristalsis, which continually flushes the small intestine of a large proportion of its bacterial population; lysozyme; lactoferrin; gastric acidity if unbuffered or undiluted; and in the abomasum of suckling calves, perhaps a lactoperoxidase–thiocyanide–hydrogen peroxide system.

The enteric microbial flora promotes the development of a population of immune and inflammatory cells in the lamina propria, by antigenic stimulation. Mucosal epithelial kinetics are also speeded up in conventional animals, in comparison with those that are germ free. In germ-free gut, the proliferative compartment in the crypts is smaller and less active, and epithelial transit times to the tips of villi are slower than in conventional animals. The effects of altered intestinal epithelial turnover and immune activity on normal flora are poorly defined and probably minor as far as luminal bacteria are concerned. IgA secretion into the lumen probably influences populations close to the mucosa, and immune activity as a whole must limit establishment on and ingress by microorganisms and their products into the mucosa. Colostrum has an inhibitory effect on enteric organisms if it contains specific antibodies against those organisms.

Mechanisms of Bacterial Disease Arising in the Intestine

Disequilibrium of the normal microflora, or a competitive advantage, may permit the establishment in the intestine of pathogenic strains of bacteria, or the abnormal proliferation by opportunistic pathogens of the resident flora.

An abnormal microflora, colonic in character, may develop in the small intestine. This bacterial overgrowth is due to achlorhydria and physical or physiologic derangements resulting in gut stasis or loss of normal peristaltic flushing. Deconjugation of bile salts and fat malabsorption result in steatorrhea and other complications considered more fully later, with malabsorption and diarrhea.

Availability of abnormally large amounts of nutrient substrate may permit the proliferation of strains of toxigenic *Clostridium perfringens*. The toxins produced can have a local necrotizing effect in the gut, as occurs in lambs, piglets, and calves, and may be implicated in canine intestinal hemorrhage syndrome and perhaps colitis X in horses. *Clostridium perfringens* type D produces ε toxin. It has no physical effect in the gut but exemplifies the principle of enterotoxemic diseases by being absorbed and acting at a site or sites distant from the intestine. The soluble factor released by strains of *E. coli* causing edema disease (gut edema), also falls into this category.

Certain strains of *E. coli* have the capacity to attach to the epithelium of the small intestine by pili, permitting colonization. Production of secretory diarrhea by the local effect of a toxin that has a physiologic, but little or no physical, effect on the gut is characteristic of these strains; some strains of *Salmonella* may also be **enterotoxic**. *Salmonella*, however, is generally considered to be **enteroinvasive**, traversing the epithelium at a number of sites, perhaps including solitary or aggregated lymphoid follicles. Enteroinvasive bacteria often stimulate acute inflammation and cause extensive mucosal damage, including erosion and effusion of tissue fluid. Some strains of *E. coli* may also have this capability.

Changes interpreted as increased epithelial proliferation, associated with superficial erosion, are characteristic of *Treponema* infection in swine dysentery and some *Campylobacter* infections, particularly intestinal adenomatosis complex in pigs. The organisms penetrate the epithelial cells in the latter condition; spirochetes are essentially noninvasive in swine dysentery. The effect in both these diseases is to cause loss of absorptive function and to permit effusion of tissue fluid. In intestinal adenomatosis complex, severe mucosal damage, by unknown mechanisms, may culminate in hemorrhage.

Mucosal invasion by mycobacteria will produce granulomatous enteritis, lymphangitis, and lymphadenitis, associated with villus atrophy and intestinal protein loss in **Johne's disease**. Localization of *Corynebacterium equi* largely in local lymphoid tissue in the gut, with ulceration, may progress to suppurative lymphadenitis. Rarely in domestic animals, *Yersinia* may follow a similar route, which may culminate in caseous lymphadenitis and/or bacteremia.

The intestinal mucosa can be a site for embolic establishment by circulating bacteria, and subsequent ulceration, as occurs in *Haemophilus somnus* septicemia of cattle and *Pasteurella* septicemia in lambs. More often, bacteria originating in the gut enter the lymphatics or portal drainage, gaining access to the circulation and causing bacteremia or septicemia. Bacteria causing Tyzzer's disease in foals, septicemic salmonellosis in some species, and probably some cases of *E. coli* septicemia in calves and lambs arise in the gut. For details of the pathogenesis and pathology of disease caused by these agents, see Infectious and Parasitic Diseases of the Gastrointestinal Tract.

Congenital Anomalies of the Intestine

Congenital **enzyme deficiencies** of the intestinal absorptive epithelium, such as the specific disaccharidase deficiencies of humans, have not been reported in domestic animals. Membranous cytoplasmic bodies have been reported in duodenal epithelial cells and in various cell types in the lamina propria in cats with generalized congenital gangliosidosis (see the Nervous System, Volume 1).

Segmental anomalies of the tubular intestine are commonly encountered. In early embryonal life the intestine consists of a simple tube, the lumen of which is lined by epithelial cells of endodermal origin. An outer layer of connective tissue from the splanchnic ectoderm surrounds and supports the tube. As the intestines grow with the developing fetus, they form coiled loops that herniate into the umbilicus. In the later stages of fetal development, the intestines withdraw, in an anterior to posterior direction, from the umbilicus into the abdomen. Although several theories have been proposed on the cause of segmental developmental anomalies, the most plausible is that there is impairment of blood supply to a segment of gut during early fetal life, resulting in ischemic necrosis of the affected area.

The segmental anomalies of the intestine may be divided into two types: **stenosis** implies incomplete occlusion of the lumen;

complete occlusion is referred to as **atresia**. Atresia is further subdivided into membrane atresia, when the obstruction is formed by a simple membrane or diaphragm; cord atresia, in which the blind ends of the gut are joined by a cord of connective tissue; and blind-end atresia, in which a segment of gut and the corresponding mesentery are missing, leaving two blind ends.

Atresia ilei is the most common segmental anomaly in the small intestine. It is most prevalent in calves, and rare in lambs, piglets, and pups. **Atresia jejuni** in Jersey cattle and atresia ilei in Swedish highland cattle are inherited as autosomal recessive traits. **Atresia coli** is also commonly encountered, particularly in Holstein calves and in foals, in which it may be hereditary. These obstructions prevent the normal movement of gut content and meconium in the fetus. Therefore, they lead to dilation of the anterior segment, with abdominal distention that may be so marked as to produce fetal dystocia.

Congenital **colonic agangliosis** has been reported in white foals that are the offspring of overo spotted parents. Clinically, the foals, which are predominantly white with a few pigmented dots on the muzzle, abdomen, and hindquarters, develop colic and die generally within 48 hr after birth. There is stenosis mainly of the small colon, but the entire colon and rectum may be involved. The intestine anterior to the stenotic segment is distended with gas and meconium. The descending colon is contracted but patent. Microscopically, ganglia of the myenteric plexus are absent in the walls of the ileum, cecum, and colon. Except for the few pigmented spots in the skin mentioned earlier, melanocytes are absent in the skin. The condition is similar in many respects to aganglionic colon in *piebald* and *spotted* mutant mouse strains. Cutaneous melanoblasts and the myenteric plexus are both derived from the neural crest, which may explain the association between unpigmented skin and lack of the myenteric ganglia.

Atresia ani, overall, is the most common congenital defect of the lower gastrointestinal tract. It may affect all species and is most frequently encountered in calves and pigs, in which it is hereditary. The defect may consist only of failure of perforation of the membrane separating the endodermal hindgut from the ectodermal anal tissue, or both anus and rectum may be atretic. Atresia ani may be an isolated abnormality, or it may be associated with other malformations, especially of the distal spinal column and the genitourinary tract; in this case the terminal portion of the intestine may empty into the vagina or urinary bladder.

Persistent Meckel's diverticulum is an uncommon anomaly of the lower small bowel, mainly in swine and horses. It is derived from the omphalomesenteric duct, which is the stalk of the yolk sac. This duct is normally obliterated before the end of the first third of pregnancy. Rarely, it may be retained in postnatal life as a patent tube extending from the antimesenteric side of the intestine to the umbilicus. More commonly, only that portion immediately adjacent to the intestine remains patent. This pouch or tubelike remnant is Meckel's diverticulum. Its mucosal lining is similar to that of the ileum. In swine it usually occurs as a tube the width of the ileum, 5–30 cm in length (Fig. 1.12A). In horses it is present as a short, cone-shaped sac ~10 cm in diameter, which may be attached by mesodiverticular

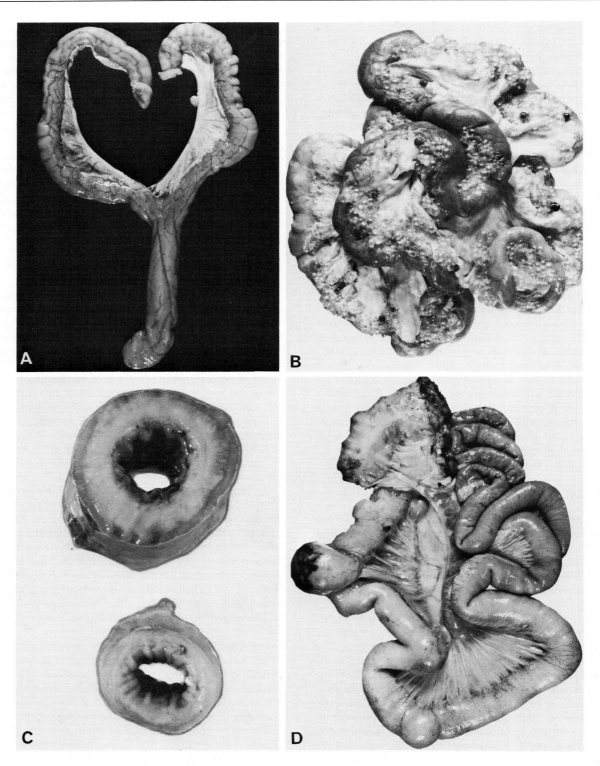

Fig. 1.12. (**A**) Persistent Meckel's diverticulum. Midjejunum. Pig. (**B**) Intestinal emphysema. Pig. (**C**) Ileal muscular hypertrophy. Horse. Normal equine ileum below. (**D**) Multiple saccular dilatations with impending perforation in muscular hypertrophy of ileum. Pig. (Courtesy of S. W. Nielsen and the *Journal of the American Veterinary Medical Association.*)

bands to the mesentery. It is usually an incidental finding, although in horses it has been associated with strangulation of the intestine herniating through the mesodiverticular bands.

Miscellaneous Conditions of the Intestinal Tract

INTESTINAL LIPOFUSCINOSIS. Intestinal lipofuscinosis is characterized grossly by brown discoloration of the intestinal serosa. It may involve all areas from the stomach to the rectum but is most commonly present in the lower small intestine. The bladder and mesenteric and peripheral lymph nodes may also be affected grossly. Although the lesion is usually an incidental finding, it has more commonly been associated with chronic enteric and pancreatic disease. Lipofuscinosis has been reported in boxer dogs with histiocytic ulcerative colitis, but a definite correlation between the two conditions has not been established. A high prevalence of lipofuscinosis has also been reported in dogs that were fed rations high in polyunsaturated fats with a relative deficiency of vitamin E. Feeding of high levels of vitamin E has prevented the condition. It appears that any condition causing a reduction in the absorption of fats and consequently of the fat-soluble vitamins, especially in the presence of polyunsaturated fatty acids in the diet, may predispose to lipofuscinosis.

The microscopic lesions of brown gut are characterized by gray to brown granules in the perinuclear regions of smooth muscle cells in both inner and outer layers of the gut wall. The granules stain as lipofuscin.

MUSCULAR HYPERTROPHY OF THE ILEUM. Formerly a common finding in swine, muscular hypertrophy of the ileum appears to have diminished in prevalence in most areas. It may be found in apparently healthy animals at slaughter as a uniform thickening of the muscular coats of the terminal ileum. The segment involved always includes the most caudal portion, but it may extend a variable distance forward, usually between 25 and 50 cm. The affected area is thickened and has the turgid feel of a rubber hose. The lumen is small, and the mucosa is thrown into thick, convoluted folds suggestive of Johne's disease, but it is apparent that the major component of the increase in thickness of the wall is in the muscular layers. This condition must be differentiated from adenomatosis and necrotic ileitis, manifestations of enteropathy associated with *Campylobacter* spp. in swine.

The outcome of the condition is not always benign, and impaction and rupture are important and disastrous sequelae. It is probable that diet and intercurrent disease contribute to the tendency to rupture, as it may be associated with the impaction of dehydrated feed in the hypertrophic segment. The actual rupture may be a result of violent peristaltic contractions, or diverticula may develop (Fig. 1.12D), the mucosa undergoing necrosis with secondary bacterial inflammation. Perforation occurs at these weakened areas.

While the underlying basis of this condition is obscure, it is likely that the muscular hypertrophy is secondary to a functional obstruction of the ileocecal valve.

Muscular hypertrophy of the small intestine, of unknown cause, also occurs in horses (Fig. 1.12C). The lesions are similar to those described in swine, except that the affected segment may occur at any point along the small intestine, although the ileum is the most common site. Horses with this condition may have chronic mild colic or intermittent diarrhea with progressive loss of weight. Unlike pigs, perforation is an unusual complication in the horse.

DIVERTICULOSIS OF THE SMALL INTESTINE. Diverticulosis of the small intestine is sometimes, but not necessarily, associated with muscular hypertrophy in pigs and horses. It is characterized by the presence of cystic structures, which are lined by intestinal mucosa, in the muscularis and subserosa of the small intestine. The diverticula tend to follow the pathway of blood vessels and are mainly located adjacent to the mesenteric attachment. Rupture of the diverticula causes peritonitis.

In sheep, diverticulosis occurs independently from muscular hypertrophy, and the most common sites are the duodenum and ileum.

INTESTINAL EMPHYSEMA IN PIGS. Intestinal emphysema is a rare condition found mainly in postweaning pigs. The lesion is usually an incidental finding in slaughtered animals and has no economic significance. It is characterized by numerous thin-walled, gas-filled cystic structures, a few millimeters to several centimeters in diameter, in the gut wall and on the serosal surface (Fig. 1.12B). These are located mainly in the small intestine, although the large intestine, mesentery, and mesenteric lymph nodes may be involved. Microscopically, the cystic structures appear to be dilated lymphatics located in the lamina propria, submucosa, muscularis, subserosa, mesentery, and mesenteric lymph nodes. A pleocellular inflammatory reaction may be evident in the walls of the cysts. Although production of gas by bacteria has been implicated, the cause remains obscure.

RECTAL PROLAPSE. Rectal prolapse most commonly occurs in swine, sheep, and cattle. It may occur in any animal that has prolonged episodes of tenesmus or straining, usually associated with colitis or urinary infection or obstruction. In pigs, rectal prolapse occurs as a herd problem when the ration contains zearalenone, an estrogenic mycotoxin produced by fungi of the genus *Fusarium*. The toxin causes marked swelling and congestion of the vulva and vaginal mucosa, which may be followed by vaginal prolapse. Affected pigs strain continuously, and rectal prolapse is a common complication. Rectal prolapse in sheep may be the consequence of ingestion of estrogenic pastures and is accompanied by other signs of hyperestrogenism (see the Female Genital System, Volume 3).

The prolapsed rectum is edematous, congested, and there may be necrosis and ulceration of the everted mucosa. These lesions are ischemic in origin due to interference with venous blood flow from the prolapsed section. Only the mucosa, or all layers, may be involved in the prolapse. In swine surviving slough or amputation of the prolapsed tissue, rectal stricture may ensue. Rectal strictures are discussed further with salmonellosis.

Intestinal Obstruction

Clinically acute obstruction typically involves the upper or middle small intestine; chronic blockage usually involves the ileum and large bowel. Intestinal obstruction may be the sequel to a physical blockage of the lumen resulting from **stenosis** due to an intrinsic lesion involving the intestinal wall, **obturation** by an intraluminal mass, or extrinsic **compression**. Failure of the intestinal circular smooth muscle to contract (paralytic ileus) blocks the peristaltic wave, causing **functional obstruction**. Ileus is a common sequel to peritoneal irritation and occurs proximal to any form of mechanical obstruction. Circulatory embarrassment of a segment of bowel, through embolism or venous infarction, will also cause functional obstruction without a physical blockage. Many of the displacements of gut that produce obstruction, such as volvulus, strangulation of a hernia, or intussusception, may cause ischemia. Mucosal hypoxia may also be a sequel to venous occlusion, resulting from distention of gut proximal to a site of obstruction, or it may result from local pressure caused by an adjacent mass. Ischemia in any circumstance is a serious complication, the pathogenesis of which is dealt with later.

We shall consider first the evolution of the sequelae to intestinal obstruction, then return for a closer look at the various types of blockage. Proximal to the point of obstruction there is accumulation of fluid, derived from ingesta and gastric, biliary, pancreatic, and intrinsic intestinal secretion, and gas, swallowed or originating with bacterial activity in the gut. Intestinal distention results in sequestration of water and electrolyte in the intestinal lumen, further secretion into the gut, edema of the mucosa, and in extreme cases, transudation from the peritoneal surface. Upper small bowel obstruction progresses rapidly to cause vomiting in those species that can vomit, with dehydration, hypochloremia, hypokalemia, and metabolic alkalosis due to loss of acid in vomitus, or sequestration of fluid in the forestomachs.

Obstruction of the lower small intestine may result in distention with dehydration. But there is usually less acute electrolyte and acid–base imbalance, since vomition is less severe and absorption of fluid proximal to the obstruction may prevent serious distention and its associated secretion for some time. Secretion into obstructed gut is mainly stimulated by distention but may partially be related to bacterial overgrowth of the stagnant intestinal content. Metabolic acidosis eventually ensues following dehydration and catabolism of fat and muscle due to cessation of food consumption and assimilation. Incomplete or slowly developing obstruction may be associated with compensatory muscular hypertrophy proximal to the offending lesion. Incomplete obstruction often becomes total due to progress of the primary lesion or the accumulation of solid digesta. Colonic obstruction may result in accumulation of large quantities of content in the bowel, with considerable abdominal distention.

If ischemia and its complications do not ensue, the animal with acute obstruction succumbs to the systemic effects of hypovolemia and electrolyte and acid–base disturbance. Lower intestinal or colonic obstruction may result in eventual metabolic acidosis and starvation following a chronic course.

In obstruction, the outstanding gross alteration in the bowel is distention proximal to the point of blockage due to paralytic ileus and the accumulation of fluid contents and gas. The location, degree, and duration of the obstruction determines the segment and length of bowel involved and the degree of distention. As distention increases, interference with venous return may develop and the mucosa and submucosa become congested. Devitalization of severely dilated gut, or pressure necrosis of the mucosa at the site of lodgment of intraluminal foreign bodies, may occur, leading to gangrene or perforation and peritonitis. Distal to the point of obstruction the bowel is collapsed and empty.

Stenosis and Obturation

Intrinsic obstruction due to congenital segmental atresia and imperforations is considered under Congenital Anomalies of the Intestine, above. Acquired stenosis due to pathologic processes arising within the wall of the intestine may be partial or complete. The primary lesions include intramural abscesses, primary neoplasms (Fig. 1.19A), and scarring following ulceration. Many of these develop slowly, with a course as described above for simple chronic obstruction.

All kinds of **foreign bodies** are commonly found. Small, rounded foreign bodies and even some sharp-edged objects may pass through the intestines uneventfully, but for these and many large foreign bodies the course is unpredictable. Some may reside in the intestine for long periods and produce no disturbance until they act as a nucleus for the development of an enterolith. Sand may remain sedimented in the colon of horses that have grazed on poorly covered sandy soils. It may cause a chronic colitis and, in some cases, obstruction. Sharp-pointed foreign bodies may become impacted in the intestine and cause pressure necrosis with ulceration and possibly perforation. Blunt foreign bodies that become impacted cause acute or chronic obstruction depending on their size and often too are the cause of local pressure necrosis, perforation occurring in some cases. Strips of cloth or string, which are not infrequently ingested by dogs and cats, may pass through the intestine. When they become impacted, however, they produce a typical lesion; one portion of a string becomes fixed and then is stretched taut distally by peristaltic movements. It progressively cuts into the lesser curvature of intestinal loops, causing first a puckering of the mesentery and finally perforation and peritonitis.

Enteroliths (mineral concrements) were common in the colon of horses in the past, are less so now, and are rare in other species. They vary greatly in size, some weighing as much as 10 kg, and in number, there being one or more large ones or many small ones. They are smooth and usually spherical, but contact and abrasion may smoothly flatten some surfaces. The stones are composed largely of phosphate. The concrement is deposited in concentric lamellae, and at the center there is a nucleus, comprising a foreign body or particle of feed. The development of an enterolith depends on the presence of soluble ingredients and a nidus for precipitation. The source of the magnesium phosphate is probably grain. Normally it is ionized in the acid gastric juice, and the phosphate is absorbed in the small intestine. Unsplit salt escaping to the colon combines with ammonia, produced as a result of bacterial digestion of protein, to form magnesium ammonium phosphate (triple phosphate).

Fiber balls (**phytotrichobezoars**) consist largely of plant fibers impregnated with some phosphate salt. They are not as heavy as enteroliths, are moist, and have a velvety surface. They are usually round and smooth, but some are convoluted like the surface of the cerebrum. Hair balls (**trichobezoars**) sometimes occur in dogs and cats and in ruminants; in the latter they occur in the forestomachs and abomasum. Enteroliths and bezoars in horses are often without significance. Apparently they are moved about enough by peristalsis to avoid pressure necrosis. They become important when they are impacted, usually in the pelvic flexure. Small enteroliths may pass in the feces without consequence.

Parasites are capable of causing intestinal obstruction when they form ropelike, tangled masses in the lumen. This is not uncommon in pigs and foals infected with large numbers of ascarids. It also occurs rarely in sheep heavily infested with tapeworms.

Impaction of the colon, by feces in dogs and cats and by digesta in horses, is not uncommon and causes a simple intestinal obstruction, complicated in the horse by intestinal tympany from fermentative gases. In dogs, it may be the result of voluntarily suppressed painful defecation, as in prostatic enlargement and inflammation of the anal sacs. Occasionally it is due to an impaction with foreign bodies, especially fine bones in the colon or rectum. It may also complicate paralyzing lesions of the spinal cord.

Impaction of the cecum or colon in horses is largely a disease of older animals in which probably there is some degree of motor and secretory insufficiency. It is often precipitated by a change of diet from something soft and lush to hay or chaff, which because of the dental attrition of old age is poorly masticated and salivated. In these animals, impaction of the cecum may be recurrent. Ingestion of rope or pieces of conveyor belt has been associated with colonic impaction caused by indigestible synthetic fibers. Ingestion of large numbers of acorns and leaves may also cause impaction of the intestinal tract in ruminants.

Extrinsic Obstruction

Compression of intestine causing obstruction is rather common and is caused by tumors, abscesses, peritonitis, and fibrous adhesions. Neoplasms involve the intestine by extension from adjacent viscera, particularly pancreas. Therefore, most of them involve the anterior–dorsal part of the abdominal cavity and impinge on the duodenum. Inflammatory peritoneal adhesions are common, and fibrous bands may stretch from the wall of the bowel to some fixed point or between two or more points along the bowel or mesentery; the obstruction develops gradually as cicatrization ties the bowel down or puts kinks in the mesentery. Large, firm masses of abdominal fat necrosis cause compression stenosis of small intestine, coiled colon, and particularly, descending colon and rectum of cattle. Peduncles of some tumors, especially mesenteric lipomas in older horses, occasionally become wound about loops of intestine and cause obstruction and strangulation. Incarceration in hernias, discussed elsewhere, is also a common cause of compression obstruction of the gut.

Functional Obstruction

Paralytic ileus is in itself not of specific interest to the pathologist but is a rather common condition. It frequently follows abdominal surgery in transient episodes, especially when the intestines are handled roughly or traumatized. It also occurs in peritoneal irritation of any cause, especially in peritonitis. It probably is the result of a variety of neurogenic and reflex factors that interfere with the networks controlling the inhibitory neurons of the myenteric plexus. Continual tonic discharge by these neurons inhibits contraction of circular smooth muscle and prevents peristalsis.

The intestines are distended with a mixture of gas and fluid, and the wall is flaccid. The defect may be segmental, involving less than a meter of the intestinal length, but there may be many such segments involved, especially in diffuse peritonitis. Gastric rupture may occur in the horse as a complication of obstructive or postoperative ileus of the small intestine.

Grass sickness in **horses**, for which there is as yet no good pathologic definition, occurs chiefly in parts of the United Kingdom and western Europe, with few exceptions in animals at pasture. Although horses of any age may be afflicted, the disease is more common in those 3–6 years of age. Affected animals are dull but show occasional bouts of colicky restlessness. In the acute disease, there is progressively severe tympany, swallowing is avoided, and saliva drools freely. Any attempt to swallow is apparently painful and stimulates reverse peristalsis in the esophagus. Fine muscular tremors develop over the shoulders, and there is sweating. The course in acute cases is from 12 to 72 hr. Some survive the acute phase to live much longer, but most usually die in due course.

Lesions are confined to the alimentary tract. The esophageal wall is sometimes edematous, and the mucosa may show longitudinal bands of congestion and ulceration. The stomach is distended with fluid (up to 22 liters have been measured), often of khaki color and pea-soup consistency, although sometimes more watery with fibrous material. This fluid is alkaline and mucinous. Some stomachs are ruptured. There is also a great excess of fluid in the small intestine, but except for some hemorrhage and edema at the mesenteric junction, there is no other change. The large intestine is impacted with dry contents, and the fecal pellets in the colon are small and dry. These masses may have a surface blackened by a small amount of exuded blood. In chronic cases, the volume of alimentary content is reduced to scant amounts in the stomach and small intestine, and the content of the large intestine is soupy.

The cause of grass sickness is speculative. In Europe and Britain, degenerative lesions have been described in the autonomic ganglia, especially the celiacomesenteric, but these are difficult structures to work with histologically and claims for ganglion-cell degeneration must be very critically evaluated. Specific neutralizing antibodies to *Clostridium perfringens* type A have been demonstrated in horses that survived a disease claimed to resemble grass sickness in Colombia. Sera from recovered horses in Scotland did not contain such antibodies, suggesting that the diseases in these areas are not the same or that they have a different cause. Transfusion of whole blood from donor horses that show clinical signs of grass sickness, into ponies, results in lesions in the autonomic ganglia that are similar to those present in spontaneous cases. However, the ponies remain clinically normal. The putative neurotoxic factor is in the plasma protein fraction of the blood and has a molecular weight of 30,000 or greater. Intraperitoneal injection of the neurotoxic factor into ponies produces characteristic lesions but not clinical disease. These observations suggest that the neurotoxic factor may be the result, rather than the cause, of grass sickness, or that relatively high plasma concentrations are required to cause clinical signs.

It is, however, difficult to avoid the conclusion that this disease is, in the final analysis, neurogenic ileus. Its differentiation from primary colonic impaction may be difficult.

Displacements of the Intestines

Eventration

Eventration is displacement of a portion of the intestine, usually the small intestine, outside the abdominal cavity. These are commonly congenital as in schistosomus reflexus, patent umbilicus, and congenital diaphragmatic hernia. Acquired eventrations result from trauma and therefore are varied. In some cases, the displaced intestine herniates into the abdominal muscle or subcutis, or it may be completely exteriorized.

Cecal Dilatation and Torsion in Cattle

Cecal dilatation and torsion is a rare condition that occurs mainly in animals fed high-concentrate rations. About 30% of the carbohydrates in the ration are digested in the cecum of ruminants. Normally, the volatile fatty acids produced by fermentation are absorbed through the cecal mucosa by passive diffusion. Sudden change from a diet consisting mainly of roughage to a grain-based ration results in an increase in the concentration of volatile fatty acids, with only a slight decrease in pH in the cecal contents. When the increase in the concentration of dissociated volatile fatty acids, especially butyric acid, is severe, the cecum becomes atonic and dilation follows. Once the cecum is dilated and distended with watery ingesta, various degrees of clockwise or counterclockwise torsion can occur, which may incorporate adjacent viscera, particularly a loop of distal jejunum.

Left Dorsal Displacement of the Colon

Left dorsal displacement of the colon is encountered as a cause of obstruction and colic in horses. The cecum, small intestine, and stomach are distended as a result of compression of the displaced colon, and the stomach and spleen are displaced caudally and ventromedially. The altered gastric location is the result of displacement of the sternal and diaphragmatic flexures into the space cranial to the stomach, in apposition with the left lobe of the liver. The left dorsal and ventral colon move dorsally and are trapped between the suspensory ligament of the spleen and the dorsal abdominal wall. Pelvic flexure may double back on itself and become wedged between stomach and liver as well. Compression of the colon may cause partial ischemia of the displaced organ. The cause is unknown. Surgical intervention is necessary for resolution.

Abnormal flexion of the cecum and/or colon may occur in the horse. The pelvic flexure may be displaced medially, laterally, or dorsally. The tip of the cecum may similarly bend upon itself. In displacement of both organs there is the risk of vascular embarrassment and infarction due to kinking of the bowel.

Internal Hernia

Internal hernia is a displacement of intestine through normal or pathologic foraminae within the abdominal cavity without the formation of a hernial sac. It is uncommon.

Herniation through a **natural foramen** occurs in horses in two locations. A portion of small intestine may pass down into the omental bursa and become incarcerated if the normally short and slitlike epiploic foramen of Winslow is dilated for any reason. Occasionally the small intestine, small colon, or left large colon is incarcerated in the nephrosplenic space formed by the dorsal end of the spleen, its renal ligament, the left kidney, and the ventral spinal muscles.

Omental hernia occurs when a loop of intestine passes through a tear in the greater or lesser omentum. **Mesenteric hernia** is due to passage of intestine through a tear in the mesentery. These are probably traumatic defects and usually involve the mesentery of the small intestine and, in horses, that of the colon.

Herniation through a **natural foramen** occurs in horses in young ruminants and, more rarely, in other species following castration. During the operation, excessive traction on the spermatic cord may tear the peritoneal fold of the ductus deferens, which fixes the duct to the pelvic wall. A hiatus is formed between the ductus deferens and the lateral abdominal or pelvic walls, and through it, loops of intestine may become incarcerated.

External Hernia

External hernia typically consists of a hernial sac formed as a pouch of parietal peritoneum; a covering of skin and soft tissues; depending on the location of the hernia, a hernial ring; and the hernial contents. The hernial ring is an opening in the abdominal wall, and this may be acquired, or it may be natural as, for example, the inguinal ring. The hernia usually contains a portion of omentum, the more freely mobile portions of the intestine, and occasionally, one or more of the other viscera. Unless the sac is obliterated by adhesions, it contains a small amount of peritoneal fluid.

Ventral hernia occurs in horses, less commonly in cattle, and exceptionally in other species. These hernias may be apparently spontaneous in pregnant females or be a consequence of blunt trauma, horn injuries, surgical scars, or inflammations that cause weakening or perforation of the supporting musculature. They may attain very large size in herbivores because of the weight of the alimentary viscera and pregnant uterus.

Umbilical hernia is common and is often present as a congenital and inherited defect. It is most frequent in pigs, foals, calves, and pups and depends on persistent patency of the umbilical ring. The hernial sac is formed by peritoneum and skin, and the contents depend on the size of the ring and of the sac.

Scrotal hernia is an exaggerated degree of inguinal herniation in which the viscera pass down the inguinal canal and come to lie in the cavity of the tunica vaginalis. The internal inguinal ring remains patent in male animals, but its diameter and the tendency to herniation is inherited. If the hernia is scrotal, there may be degeneration of the testicles. Routine castration of such animals may lead to eventration through the scrotal incision, and closed castration may cause infarction of the herniated loop of gut. The bitch differs from females of other species in having a patent inguinal ring and canal through which the round ligament, the omentum, and the uterus may pass. The herniated uterus may become incarcerated when pregnant or if pyometra develops. False inguinal hernias may also develop in males, the displaced viscus passing not within the cavity of the tunica vaginalis but outside it in a subcutaneous position in a true peritoneal hernial sac.

Femoral hernias develop as an outpouching of peritoneum through the femoral triangle along the course of the femoral artery. They contain omentum and small intestine.

Perineal hernias occur principally in old male dogs in association with prostatic enlargements and obstipation. They are precipitated by undue abdominal straining and are probably predisposed to by weakening of perineal fascia and muscles from some unknown cause, possibly hormonal. They are very unusual in females. The weakening of the pelvic diaphragm takes place between the coccygeus medialis muscle and the anterior border of the anal sphincter. Through this defect bulges the retroperitoneal pelvic fat. Usually this is the only tissue to prolapse, and the lesion consists essentially of a loss of support on one side of the anal ring. Concomitantly with the loss of pelvic support, the rectum deviates and diverticula may form, and the prostate and the bladder may move into the pelvis. Further displacement may occur occasionally, and then the latter organs are forced through the ruptured perineal fascia. Retroflexion of the bladder kinks the urethra and leads to an acute obstruction. Perineal hernias are most commonly unilateral, but the perineal fascia may fail bilaterally, and the anus, having lost its support on both sides, is forced directly back at each attempt at defecation. The bulging is then symmetric.

Diaphragmatic hernias are common. The defect in the diaphragm may be congenital, but most often it is acquired. In dogs and cats, acquired rupture of the diaphragm is a result of acute abdominal compression, usually from automobile accidents. Omentum and small intestine pass through the smaller clefts; liver, stomach, and other viscera may pass through the larger defects. The herniation is usually into one or other pleural sac, and only exceptionally into the pericardial sac. In cattle, diaphragmatic hernia is usually a consequence of traumatic reticuloperitonitis. Horses with diaphragmatic hernias often have a chronic history of intermittent colic that terminates with an acute fatal episode. The congenital form is often located in the left dorsal quadrant, and it may be associated with arthrogryposis and scoliosis. Acquired hernias mainly involve the tendinous portion of the diaphragm.

The **sequelae** of **hernias** depend largely on their location and content, but there are some generalities that are applicable to all. As long as the hernial contents remain freely movable and the hernia is reducible there may be no untoward sequelae. Fixation of the hernial contents (incarceration) is a serious development. It is most important when the small intestine is incarcerated because of the liability to intestinal obstruction and perforation, with death occurring from paralytic ileus or peritonitis. Incarceration may result from progressive stenosis of the hernial ring, adhesion between the contents and the sac, or distention of the herniated viscus. This distention may be due to accumulated gas or ingesta in the intestine, urine in a herniated bladder, and fetuses or pus in a herniated uterus. With some herniations, incarceration is the result of only slight pressure by the neck of the pouch, by which venous drainage is impaired and a vicious cycle is initiated; the edema caused by the venous stasis increases the bulk of the contents so that they become incarcerated.

Intestinal Ischemia and Infarction

Inadequate or interrupted circulation of blood to the gut is a common problem, particularly in the horse. Obstruction of the efferent veins, blockage of afferent arteries, and reduced flow through an open circulation cause hypoxic damage to the intestine. Whatever the initiating agency, the effect of hypoxia at the level of the mucosa is the same.

In the small intestine, within 5 to 10 min of the onset of ischemia, changes are observed at the tips of villi in tissue sections examined under the light microscope, and lesions are well advanced by 30 min. Separation of the epithelium from the basement membrane, beginning at the tip of the villus and progressing with time toward the base, causes the formation of the so-called Gruenhagen's space. Epithelial cells appear relatively normal but may separate from the villus in sheets. Within 1 to 2 hr, the villus is completely denuded of epithelium and the mesenchymal core is disintegrating or collapsed and stumpy, with hemorrhage from capillaries. That the lesion is largely a function of hypoxia is indicated by the mitigating effects of intraluminal oxygen perfusion. The putative countercurrent exchange of oxygen between the afferent arteriole and efferent venules in the villus, and an associated progressive decline in oxygen tension distally in the villus, may render the tip prone to early damage in hypoxia. Intraluminal enzymes, especially elastase, may contribute to epithelial damage by altering glycoproteins in the vicinity of the brush border, perhaps opening the way for further damage by other pancreatic enzymes.

Dissociation and necrosis of cells in the crypts of Lieberkühn begins ~2 hr after the initiation of ischemia, and within 4 to 5 hr the mucosal epithelium appears completely necrotic or has sloughed, leaving a mesenchymal ghost of the mucosa. The muscularis mucosae may undergo necrosis, but the muscularis externa remains viable for 6 to 7 hr.

The colon, of the dog at least, seems less sensitive to ischemia than the small intestine. Mild morphologic damage is found after 1 hr, but severe mucosal lesions are evident by 3 hr.

If hypoxia is only partial, or ischemia is transient, with reflow occurring, the outcome may be variable. Short-term ischemia with preservation of at least the base of the crypts of Lieberkühn will permit resolution, as proliferation of cells in the crypts reepithelializes the mucosal surface within 1 to 3 days. Normal architecture is reestablished after up to 1 to 2 weeks, though necrotic muscularis mucosae is not replaced. Effusion of tissue fluid and acute inflammatory cells prevail until epithelium extends to fully cover the eroded surface. Partial damage to the proliferative compartment results in dilation of crypts, lined by flattened epithelium resembling that seen after radiation injury.

Ischemic necrosis of the full thickness of the mucosa will be bounded by an acute inflammatory reaction in the submucosa, which under favorable conditions evolves into a granulating ulcerated surface. Neutrophilic infiltration and effusion may be considerable if bacterial contamination of the lumen is heavy. Focal ulcerative lesions may ultimately heal by epithelial migration, over the bed of granulation tissue, from surviving crypts within the lesion and around the periphery.

Extensive mucosal ulcers that form following ischemia with vascular reflow have little chance of resolution, due to their large surface area. Chronic ischemic ulcers in the small bowel tend to develop a depressed, fairly clean, granulating surface, occasionally with some fibrinous exudate. Many ulcers in the large bowel, especially of horses, develop a dirty yellow-gray fibrinonecrotic surface, perhaps due to the effects of anaerobic bacteria. If the animal does not succumb to the effects of malabsorption and protein loss from the defect, or to transmural bacterial invasion, scarring and stricture may occur.

The sequelae of ischemia with reflow are seen mainly in strangulated segments of gut that have been reduced without, or with inadequately extensive, resection, and in some cases of presumed thromboembolic infarction of the equine colon.

Persistent ischemia results in necrosis involving all mural elements. The full thickness of the gut wall ultimately becomes gangrenous, green-brown or black, flaccid, and friable.

The consequences of ischemic lesions are partly a function of the species and of the level of bowel affected. Strangulation, volvulus, and similar lesions cause physical obstruction at the site, and ileus proximal to it. Reduced arterial perfusion or thromboembolism causes functional obstruction and ileus. Loss of mucosal integrity results in cessation of electrolyte and water absorption, and ultimately in effusion of tissue fluid and blood into the lumen. Proliferation of anaerobes occurs in the lumen of the stagnant ischemic area, with accumulation of gas and extreme distention of the closed loop in strangulation obstruction. Toxin production by anaerobes, particularly clostridia, plays a large part in gangrene and ultimate rupture of ischemic gut, as well as having systemic effects. Absorption of endotoxin or endotoxin-like molecules from the lumen may occur through devitalized mucosa via the portal flow, lymphatic return, or peritoneum. These compounds have a severe detrimental effect on cardiovascular function, contributing to the circulatory failure. If death from some other cause does not supervene, transmural invasion by enteric bacteria or perforation of the devitalized wall results in septic peritonitis, which is ultimately fatal.

Venous Infarction

Obstruction of efferent veins is by far the most common cause of intestinal ischemia. This is a sequel to incarceration of herniated loops of bowel, strangulation by pedunculated masses, torsion (twist about long axis of the viscus), volvulus (twist across the long axis of the gut), and intussusception. In these circumstances, compression of thin-walled veins tends to occur before the influx of arterial blood is obstructed. Primary thrombosis of the mesenteric veins is a rare cause of infarction in domestic

animals. Local invasion of the mucosa by mycotic agents may result in focal or segmental lesions, however, due to hyphal invasion of submucosal veins. The affected tissue field, sometimes including involved mesentery, becomes intensely edematous, congested, and hemorrhagic, so that the hypoxic bowel wall is thickened and eventually assumes a deep red-black appearance. Bloody fluid content and gas distend the lumen of the infarcted segment. As gangrene of the intestinal wall proceeds, the tissue becomes green-black and septic peritonitis eventually ensues, with or without perforation of the bowel.

Advanced venous infarction involves the full thickness of the intestinal wall, and the initiating intestinal accident is commonly evident, except in cases subjected to surgery. Even if a displacement, volvulus, or strangulation has been reduced, the limits of the infarcted segment are generally sharply demarcated. Microscopically, severe edema, congestion, distention of veins, sometimes venous thrombosis, and hemorrhage are present, initially most severe in the mucosa and submucosa. With time, the full thickness of the mucosa becomes necrotic, and the deeper layers of the muscular wall are also devitalized, with invading enteric flora present throughout.

Displacements of intestine that may progress to incarceration or strangulation and infarction have been discussed in the previous section. **Torsion** of the **long axis** of the **mesentery** occurs commonly in suckling ruminants, in swine, uncommonly in horses, and rarely in dogs and cats. In all species, the result is rapid death. The abdomen is distended, and on opening the cavity, the tensely dilated deep red to black loops of bowel are immediately apparent. In swine, the mesentery of the small intestine and sometimes the large bowel is often involved in a torsion that usually is counterclockwise, when viewed from the ventrocaudal aspect. In torsion involving the small and large intestines, the apex of the cecum may be pointing cranial in the anterior right quadrant of the abdomen, reflecting the rotation of ~180°. In swine, mesenteric torsion may be due to gas production from a highly fermentable substrate in the colon, and its subsequent displacement, with progression to mesenteric torsion. Mesenteric torsion is a common cause of sporadic sudden death in swine but may occur as a herd problem. Many cases of so called intestinal hemorrhage syndrome in that species are probably misdiagnosed mesenteric torsion (Fig. 1.13B). The presence of red-black or bloody content in the intestine of feeder swine, without torsion, may also signal bleeding gastric ulcer or proliferative hemorrhagic enteropathy associated with *Campylobacter*.

Death due to mesenteric torsion is common in suckling or artificially reared calves and lambs. In these species, vigorous ingestion of large amounts of feed over a short period may predispose to gas formation in the gut, or perhaps hypermotility, which induces torsion. Usually only the mucosa of the proximal duodenum and terminal ileum, cecum, and colon is spared the effects of infarction. Similar lesions are occasionally encountered in other species.

Volvulus of varying lengths of the small intestine may occur in any species but is perhaps most prevalent in the horse, where it is a common cause of strangulation obstruction of the bowel. Volvulus of the left large colon of the horse is predisposed to by its lack of mesenteric anchorage, and potential mobility. It usually occurs as the left dorsal colon moves mesially on the left

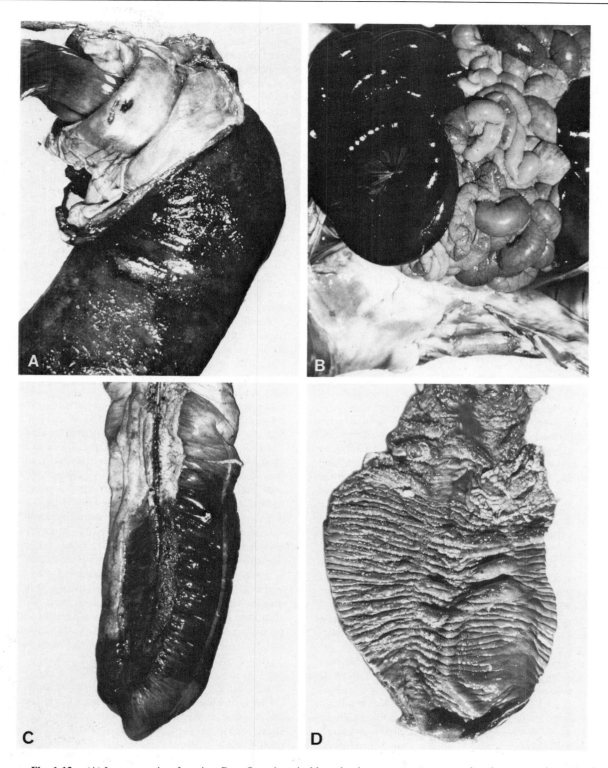

Fig. 1.13. (**A**) Intussusception. Intestine. Dog. Outer intestinal layer has been cut away to expose the edematous and congested infarcted mucosa of strangulated portion of the intussusception. (**B**) Deeply congested segment of small intestine, infarcted as a result of volvulus or mesenteric torsion. Pig. (**C**) Equine cecum. Infarction of distal half. Cecal artery contains a thrombus. Congestion and edema of serosa and musculature suggest that reflow and hemorrhage have occurred. (**D**) Mucosa of cecum in (**C**). Surface of infarcted mucosa is covered by a fibrinonecrotic membrane. Ulcerated areas along proximal margin of lesion are covered by fibrinous exudate.

ventral colon, progressing to volvulus at the sternal and diaphragmatic flexures. At autopsy, the usual signs of strangulation obstruction are evident, including dilatation and devitalization of the infarcted segment, distention of the cecum, and perhaps, postmortem rupture of the diaphragm or abdominal wall due to tympany.

Intussusception involves the telescoping of one segment of bowel into an outer sheath formed by another, usually distal segment of gut. Any level of the gut with sufficient mesenteric mobility may be involved. The cause is usually not apparent, though linear foreign bodies, heavy parasitism, previous intestinal surgery, enteritis, and intramural lesions such as abscesses and tumors may be associated. It also may be a terminal, agonal, or postmortem event. The history is that of partial or complete intestinal obstruction, perhaps with bloody feces. Intussusception is common in dogs (Fig. 1.13A), where most frequently it is ileocolic. It is much less common in cats. Intussusception is also moderately common in lambs, calves, and young horses, where it may involve small intestine, cecum, and colon.

The progressive invagination of the leading edge of the intussusceptum into the posterior segment is limited by the increasing tension on the mesentery drawn into the lesion, to about 10 to 12 cm in small animals, and about 20 to 30 cm in large animals. This tension along one edge of the gut causes the mass to become bowed or spiraled. Tension and compression of mesenteric veins cause the intussusceptum, or a portion of it, to undergo venous infarction. It swells, with edema and congestion, and the adjacent apposed serous surfaces become adherent as fibrin and inflammatory cells effuse from the affected bowel. Adhesion quickly renders the intussusception irreducible. Necrosis and gangrene of the invaginated intestine usually develop, but sometimes the intussusceptum will slough, and the remaining viable segments will maintain continuity of the gut, or rarely, will form two adjacent blind ends. Incidental terminal, agonal, or postmortem intussusception is recognized by the relative absence of congestion, edema, and adhesion of the involuted segment of gut.

Arterial Thromboembolism

Ischemia due to arterial thrombosis and embolism is rare in domestic animals other than the horse. Mucosal and occasionally transmural focal or segmental infarctive lesions are seen in *Pasteurella* septicemia in lambs and in *Haemophilus somnus* bacteremia in cattle. In horses it is associated with endarteritis, mainly at the root of the cranial mesenteric circulation, in animals less than ~3 years of age, caused by migrating larvae of *Strongylus vulgaris* (see the Cardiovascular System, Volume 3). Suffice it to say here that endarteritis due to this worm is most common in the cranial mesenteric circulation, sometimes at a number of sites a considerable distance distal to the usual location at the root of the artery. Although endarteritis is common, in only a small minority of horses dying of intestinal accidents can the infarction be confidently attributed to *S. vulgaris*.

Candidates for a diagnosis of arterial thromboembolism are animals in which the anatomic distribution of an infarctive lesion is incomptabile with volvulus or strangulation, or where physical evidence for incarceration or strangulation obstruction is not present in the surgical history or at autopsy. In the horse, animals

in this category may have relatively localized mucosal or transmural damage, or extensive transmural lesions of the distal small intestine, cecum, and large colon, that is, in the circulatory field of the cranial mesenteric artery. Lesions limited essentially to the mucosa appear usually to be subacute and are ulcerative or fibrinonecrotic. They may vary in area from tens to many hundreds of square centimeters. Transmural lesions are of two types. The least common is a large, irregular area of devitalized gut, sometimes involving most of the cecum or colon, with a dirty khaki-colored, flaccid, friable wall, which is not markedly thickened. Along the poorly defined margin of the necrotic tissue there may be transmural congestion, hemorrhage, and edema. The fluid content in the affected gut is foul-smelling, but not particularly blood tinged. More commonly, irregularly demarcated areas of infarcted intestine have a thickened, edematous, congested wall, which appears deep red-black or green-black on both mucosal and serosal aspects. Gut content is blood tinged. The peritoneal cavity may contain an excessive quantity of turbid yellow or blood-tinged fluid, and animals with both types of transmural lesions may progress to rupture of the bowel, with distribution of content throughout the abdomen.

We interpret devitalized gray-brown intestine of normal thickness to represent arterial obstruction without subsequent reflow, except along the boundary with viable tissue. Large edematous, congested, or hemorrhagic full-thickness lesions, physically or anatomically inconsistent with strangulation, we interpret as severe arterial obstruction of some duration, with subsequent reflow either by relief of the obstruction or by way of collaterals. Ischemic damage to the mucosa, submucosa, and perhaps, deeper structures results in hemorrhage and edema when blood flow returns (Fig. 1.13C,D). Ulcerative or fibrinonecrotic mucosal lesions are probably the result of transient ischemia and superficial or mucosal damage, with subsequent reflow. Similar lesions may occur following relief of strangulation of short duration, and in salmonellosis, which itself may be in part the result of mucosal microthrombosis.

Evidence of reflow, and failure to find thrombi lodged in arteries in the infarcted area, may be explained in several ways. Fibrinolysis may have removed the obstructing thrombi; thrombi may be multiple and microscopic (sometimes they are found in arteries in tissue sections of infarcted tissue); or the lesions may be the result of diminished tissue perfusion due to obstructed flow caused by verminous endarteritis (but not thromboembolism) or by vascular spasm. In the latter case they may be the result of "slow flow," discussed further below.

Reduced Perfusion

Ischemia due to reduced perfusion of the intestinal vascular bed is a difficult and uncommon diagnosis. Circumstances under which it may be expected to occur include severe hypovolemic states, such as hemorrhagic shock in the dog, cat, and possibly other species; in animals, particularly dogs, with disseminated intravascular coagulation; in dogs with hepatic fibrosis and portal hypertension; as a result of hypotensive shock due to heart failure; and in animals with reduced mesenteric arterial perfusion, mainly horses with severe verminous endarteritis obstructing flow. In "shock gut" in dogs and, rarely, other species, associated terminally with heart failure, hemorrhage, hypovolemia, and disseminated intravascular coagulation, part or all of the mucosa of the small intestine is deeply congested and the content hemorrhagic. The pathogenesis of the lesion is related to reflex vasoconstriction in the mucosa and submucosa, shunting of blood away from the mucosa, dilation of mucosal capillaries, and reduction in rate of flow of blood through the villus. Countercurrent transfer of oxygen from the afferent to efferent vessels in the villus aggravates hypoxemia in the villus by increased shunting of oxygen to the efferent venule. Splanchnic pooling of blood, systemic arterial hypotension, and intestinal vasoconstriction occur in endotoxic shock in dogs, causing similar mucosal lesions. Microthrombosis associated with sluggish flow, disseminated intravascular coagulation, and endotoxemia may contribute to mucosal ischemia by obstructing capillaries in the villi, and mucosal and submucosal venules; microthrombi in these vessels in association with hemorrhagic mucosal necrosis suggest the possibility of ischemia due to slow flow.

Acute acorn poisoning in the horse may cause severe gastrointestinal edema and focal hemorrhage, with infarction and ulceration in the cecum and colon. Microscopic lesions in the small and large intestine are consistent with an ischemic pathogenesis, and microthrombi have been associated with mucosal infarcts in the large bowel as well as in other organs.

Transient or incomplete reduction in perfusion due to obstruction of the arterial blood supply has a similar effect on the mucosa. Mucosa devitalized by hypoxia will become hemorrhagic with continued blood flow. Since the primary problem may not involve a systemic state as complicated as severe shock, the animal may survive long enough to develop an effusive ulcerated or pseudomembranous mucosa, with some prospect of stabilization or repair if the lesion is not widespread. Slow flow due to reduced arterial perfusion with inadequate collateral flow may be expected to affect the ''watershed'' of a circulatory field preferentially. In the horse, this may be the explanation for mucosal lesions at the pelvic flexure and apex of the cecum in which thromboembolism cannot be implicated, but in which mural thrombi in the cranial mesenteric root could have caused significantly reduced perfusion. Ischemia at the periphery of the circulatory field of the caudal mesenteric artery may possibly predispose to rectal perforation in horses. The precarious perfusion of the mucosa at this site may contribute to ischemic ulceration and the development of rectal stricture in swine. This condition in many cases appears to be associated with *Salmonella* infection, and it is discussed further under Salmonellosis, in Swine.

Transient or noninfarctive slow flow has been proposed as a cause of intermittent colic due to verminous arteritis. It may also play a role in the development of functional obstruction and volvulus in horses with cranial mesenteric arterial lesions.

Epithelial Renewal in Health and Disease

Small Intestine

The intestinal mucosa is lined by an extremely labile population of cells, ultimately derived from stem cells at the base of crypts or glands but with its proximate source in amplifier populations of undifferentiated columnar or oligomucous cells in the lower half of the crypts. These cells differentiate into goblet cells and the functional population of enterocytes as they move from the crypt to the villus, losing their ability to undergo mitosis. In most species, they are shed from the tips of villi in about 2 to 8 days. Relatively little definitive information is available on the transit time of epithelium moving from crypt to tip of villus in domestic animals. Generally, cells move off the villus more quickly in the ileum than in the duodenum; presumably this is related to the decline in height of villi with distance down the gut in most species. As well, in some species the number of crypts contributing cells to a single villus is lower in the ileum than in the duodenum.

Under normal circumstances, the mass and topography of the mucosa are quite stable. This steady state is the product of a dynamic equilibrium between the rate of movement of cells out of crypts and onto villi, and the rate at which they are lost from the tips of villi. The stability of this equilibrium suggests that local feedback exists between the functional compartment on villi and the proliferative compartment in the crypts. Soluble chalones released from the functional compartment have been proposed as the effectors of a negative-feedback mechanism acting on crypt cells, but they are poorly characterized. Experimental destruction of the functional epithelium on villi by transient local ischemia stimulates hyperplasia in the proliferative compartment serving affected villi, however, confirming that local feedback control is real.

In the young animal the intestine grows by generation of new crypts, and with them, new villi. As the bowel attains mature size, the number of villi stabilizes and apparently remains relatively constant. The number of crypts also stabilizes, but some adaptive variation in the ratio of crypts to villi may occur. Adaptive responses to a variety of factors alter the size and rate of turnover of the proliferative and functional epithelial-cell populations and with them the microtopography of the gut. The ''normal'' appearance of the small intestinal mucosa is a compromise, achieved by the equilibrium between the rate of cell production and rate of loss. At one extreme lies the intestine of the germ-free animal, with a short crypt containing a small proliferative compartment, and tall villi supporting a large functional compartment with a low rate of cell loss. At the other end of the spectrum is the animal suffering from severe intestinal helminthosis, with long crypts reflecting an increased proliferative compartment, yet a flat mucosal surface with relatively few functional enterocytes and an apparently high rate of cell loss.

In the diagnostic situation, it is necessary to make subjective or semiquantitative assessment of the status of the proliferative and functional compartments in tissue sections. The size of the proliferative compartment is reflected in the length and diameter of the crypts; no inferences can be drawn about the proportion of the crypt-cell population that is replicating, or the duration of the cell cycle. There is obviously also some correlation between the length and profile of villi and the functional surface area, though the three-dimensional structure of an abnormal mucosa is often poorly reflected in section. Hence, it is highly desirable to correlate the histologic appearance with the microtopography of the mucosa as seen under the dissecting or scanning electron microscope. The degree of differentiation, and therefore, the functional status of enterocytes on villi, can be inferred from their appearance. Cytoplasmic basophilia, loss of regular basal nuclear polarity, low columnar, cuboidal, or squamous shape, and an ill-defined brush border all point to a poorly differentiated population of surface enterocytes, which is possibly turning over more rapidly than normal.

Fasting reduces the mucosal epithelial mass, the atrophy being related to prolongation of the postmitotic phase of the cell cycle in the proliferative compartment. Villi do not regress severely, however, since cells on the surface persist for twice as long, moving off the villus more slowly. The effect is reversed immediately by refeeding. Total parenteral nutrition does not abolish the effect of starvation. Surgical removal of a loop of bowel from the flow of digesta also causes atrophy of the epithelial population, which is reversed by restoration of continuity with the rest of the gut. Resection of a segment of gut causes hypertrophy of the mucosa remaining distal to the surgical site, which is reflected in dilation of the bowel and thickening of the mucosa due to longer crypts and villi. Postresectional hypertrophy also occurs in the mucosa of separated loops of gut and in cross-circulated animals, suggesting a hormonal influence. Diversion of the opening of the pancreatic and bile ducts to the distal small bowel causes hypertrophy of the ileal mucosa but does not result in atrophy of more proximal mucosa.

Many of these adaptive changes in experimental or surgical situations are interpreted as supporting the concept that stimulation of enterocytes by nutrients is trophic and an important factor in maintaining mucosal mass. The direct role of pancreatic secretion and bile is uncertain. Hormonal and, possibly, paracrine factors are also active. Gastrin appears to be trophic for duodenal mucosa; glucocorticoids also have trophic effects on intestine under some circumstances. Enteroglucagon is the prime candidate as a hormone trophic for the intestinal mucosa and is apparently elevated in calves with neonatal diarrhea, suggesting that it has a role in the adaptive response to mucosal damage. Such also appears to be the case in celiac sprue in humans, where crypt-cell proliferation is high and enteroglucagon levels are concurrently elevated. There is speculation that paracrine effects of other peptides released from enteroendocrine cells in the gut, in response to a variety of luminal stimuli, may also influence epithelial proliferation.

VILLUS ATROPHY.   Atrophy of villi is a common pathologic change in the intestine of domestic animals. It results in malabsorption of nutrients and sometimes is associated with increased plasma protein loss in the gut. Mucosa with atrophic villi can be categorized morphologically into two broad types, recognition of which has implications with respect to pathogenesis and prognosis. The first category includes intestine with atrophy of villi to varying degrees, associated with apparently normal or hypertrophic crypts. The second category is comprised of gut with variable villus atrophy and some evidence of damage to the proliferative compartment. The recognition, evolution, and interpretation of each will be considered in turn.

Villus atrophy with an **intact** or **hypertrophic proliferative compartment** is seen in a wide variety of circumstances in domestic animals. A primary increase in rate of loss of epithelium from the surface of villi is one mechanism initiating such a lesion. This is the major pathogenetic action of transient ischemia, in which the effect is limited to the functional compart-

ment; of a number of important virus diseases, including coronavirus (Fig. 1.30) and rotavirus (Fig. 1.31A–C) infection; of some coccidial infections that may damage surface enterocytes predominantly (Fig. 1.49A); of some enteroinvasive bacteria; and in some circumstances, of necrotizing toxins released by clostridia in the lumen of the bowel. The effect of these agents is to cause significantly increased loss of surface epithelium over a relatively short period of time. Villi contract as the size of the functional compartment is diminished, and they may become very stubby. If the animal survives the metabolic sequelae to the reduced absorptive function, which results from the usually transient damage to surface cells, compensatory expansion of the proliferative compartment in crypts permits complete recovery. New epithelium emerging from crypts causes regeneration of villi, resulting in a normal mucosal topography within a few days, and full function returns.

The microscopic appearance of the mucosa in section depends partly on the number of functional cells lost, which determines the initial degree of villus atrophy, and partly on the amount of regeneration that has occurred by the time the animal dies or the gut is sampled. During the early phase of cell loss, damaged epithelium may be seen exfoliating into the lumen of the gut, and villi are shorter or blunter than normal. Subsequently, the atrophic villi are covered by poorly differentiated, low columnar, cuboidal, or squamous cells (Fig. 1.30B). There may be fusion of the lateral surfaces or tips of villi in some areas (Fig. 1.30D). In severe atrophy there may be mild erosion if inadequate epithelium is available to cover even the much reduced mucosal surface area. In the acute phase, crypts appear of normal size, but within 12 to 24 hr, proliferative activity is noticeably increased. Crypts enlarge in diameter and length to accommodate more mitotic epithelial cells, which are basophilic, crowded, and obviously dividing, sometimes very close to the surface of the mucosa. The lamina propria appears moderately hypercellular, perhaps due to condensation, possibly due to a mild mononuclear-cell infiltrate. As regeneration occurs, progressively longer villi with increasingly well differentiated epithelium are evident, and hypertrophy of the proliferative compartment gradually subsides.

Atrophy of villi and hypertrophy of crypts in the small intestine are also associated with nematode parasitism (Fig. 1.45B,C); chronic coccidial infection of surface epithelium: giardiasis in some species; response to dietary antigens in some species, including that to soybean protein in calves; chronic inflammatory reactions in the lamina propria, such as Johne's disease (Fig. 1.42D) and histoplasmosis; and idiopathic granulomatous enteritis or chronic enteritis characterized by heavy lymphocytic and plasmacytic infiltrates in the mucosa. The epithelial kinetics have not been investigated in most of these situations in domestic animals. They all have in common a chronic antigenic exposure, parasitism, or an infectious process in the lumen, epithelium, or lamina propria, however, usually associated with a significant lymphocytic and plasmacytic infiltrate in the mucosa.

Experimental evidence is accumulating that cell-mediated immune events in the mucosa initiate villus atrophy and cryptal hypertrophy in graft-versus-host reaction, intestinal trichinellosis, and giardiasis in mice. These observations are being extrapolated in humans to intestinal allergy to some dietary antigens, and to celiac disease; similar phenomena are likely to be active in domestic animals. In these conditions, villus atrophy and loss of cells from the mucosal surface persist despite obvious hyperplasia in the proliferative compartment.

Studies of the kinetics of experimental mucosal lesions induced by cell-mediated immunity show that hypertrophy of the proliferative compartment precedes the development of villus atrophy and is not a response to it. This also occurs in *Nippostrongylus*-infected rats and *Eimeria acervulina*–infected chickens. In experimental intestinal trichostrongylosis, hypertrophy of crypts appears to be an early event, preceding villus atrophy; the epithelium emerging from hypertrophic crypts exfoliates soon after reaching the surface, rather than moving up the villus.

Evidence now points to a local effect on the proliferative compartment, and perhaps, the associated fibroblast sheath by soluble mediators (lymphokines) released by lymphocytes engaging in cell-mediated immune reactions in the mucosa. Cytotoxicity or damage to the functional compartment is apparently not a necessary precursor to hyperplasia by crypt cells, though it is not ruled out. Epithelial cells leaving the crypts usually do not differentiate fully; they slough prematurely, and as preexisting enterocytes are shed, villi undergo atrophy. Surface epithelium is subsequently rapidly lost into the lumen, matching the rate of cell production. In experimental intestinal trichinellosis, fewer surface receptors for lectins are present on enterocytes, suggesting an altered cell membrane.

In villus atrophy of this type, the microtopography of the gut may vary from moderately short, cylindric villi, through short leaf or tongue shapes, to ridges on the mucosa. These would be interpreted in section as villi of varying height. More severely attenuated mucosal projections form convoluted intercrypt ridges, which in section may be misinterpreted as stumpy villi, with crypts opening directly onto the surface (subtotal villus atrophy; Fig. 1.45B). In extreme cases the mucosa becomes virtually flat, and crypt mouths project above the surface (total villus atrophy; Fig. 1.45C). In cases with moderate villus atrophy, the surface epithelium may appear relatively normal by light microscopy; enterocytes that appear poorly differentiated are usually present on more severely atrophic mucosa. In severe atrophy, the epithelium may become squamous, and the surface may be eroded.

Hypertrophy of crypts is the early and outstanding change in this lesion and is consistently present. In its milder forms, the lesion may be better characterized by elongate crypts than by obvious atrophy of villi. The proliferative compartment is expanded and active, and mitotic figures are numerous. Elongation of crypts may be so great that even with severe atrophy of villi the total mucosal thickness will not be much reduced from normal. The lamina propria often has a prominent population of lymphocytes, plasmacytes, and associated inflammatory cells, and intraepithelial lymphocytes are common. The etiologic agent, in the form of parasites, intracellular bacteria, or yeast, may be evident. Removal of the causal stimulus usually results in a return to "normal" within several weeks.

However induced, atrophy of villi with hypertrophy of crypts is associated with local malabsorption of nutrients and water; elongate crypts and, perhaps, poorly differentiated surface epithelium may secrete electrolyte and water; and if there is proprial inflammation and microerosion of the mucosa, effusion of tissue fluid may ensue. Increased turnover of epithelium may contribute to enteric loss of endogenous protein.

Villus atrophy associated with **damage** to the **proliferative compartment** is also seen commonly in domestic animals. It is the sequel to insults that cause necrosis of cells in crypts or impair their mitotic capacity. The agents that produce these lesions usually have a propensity for damaging dividing cells in any tissue; since ionizing radiation was recognized early as a cause of such lesions, they are often termed "radiomimetic." Other causative agencies include cytotoxic chemicals (Fig. 1.32E), mitotic poisons and viruses that infect proliferating cells, particularly the parvoviruses, bovine virus diarrhea, and rinderpest. Ischemia of duration sufficient to cause necrosis of some or all cells lining the crypts causes a lesion that may be included in this category also (Fig. 1.32F).

The microscopic appearance of affected mucosa depends on the severity and extent of the insult, and the interval since it occurred. The primary event is damage to the proliferative compartment, and except in ischemia, lesions will be evident in crypts well before significant atrophy of villi occurs. Necrotic or exfoliated epithelial cells and polymorphs may be present in the lumen of damaged crypts, which tend to dilate. If crypt-cell necrosis is severe, remaining cells become extremely flattened in the course of attempting to maintain the integrity of the crypt lining. Following radiation, cytotoxic damage, and parvovirus infection, bizarre irregular epithelial cells with large nuclei and nucleoli may be present in crypts and will migrate onto the surface. Preexisting surface epithelium continues to move off the tips of villi at an apparently normal rate even though few or no new cells emerge from crypts. Villi eventually become atrophic or collapse as the surface cell population shrinks. If most proliferative and stem cells have been damaged, crypts stripped of epithelium will also collapse or "drop out," perhaps leaving a few scattered cystic remnants, lined by attenuated epithelium, in the deeper lamina propria. The overlying surface will be covered by squamous epithelial cells derived from surviving crypts or will be eroded and may eventually ulcerate. Crypts that have not been so severely damaged will hypertrophy as compensatory hyperplasia of lining cells occurs within a week or so of the original insult (Fig. 1.32D).

In viral diseases the severity and appearance of the lesion often vary considerably at different sites in the gut and even within an individual tissue section. Lesions due to ischemia tend to be uniform in severity but may be localized; acute or subacute lesions are often hemorrhagic. Cytotoxic and radiation damage tend to be relatively uniform and more widespread, though some variation occurs due to differences in the proliferative activity, and therefore susceptibility, of the epithelium at the time of insult. The inflammatory reaction depends on the availability of leukocytes, which may also have been diminished by the same insult that caused the epithelial necrosis. In the early stages, neutrophils and eosinophils may be in and around damaged crypts. Extensive lesions of the gut lead to severe malabsorption and to effusion of tissue fluid and hemorrhage. The mucosa is often invaded by the enteric flora because the animal frequently is immunosuppressed. Local ulceration may lead to persistent plasma loss, and if circumferential, to stricture and stenosis. Small ulcers in areas where a few crypts have dropped out will heal as epithelium from adjacent crypts moves over the surface, but crypts may not regenerate, and local villus atrophy will persist.

Villus atrophy occurs commonly in association with **alimentary lymphosarcoma**. Diffuse or focal infiltration of the lamina propria by neoplastic lymphocytes appears to separate and crowd out crypts. It also distorts the shape of villi, which become stubby and covered by low columnar or cuboidal epithelium. Presumably the atrophy of villi is related at least partially to a reduced density of crypts in the mucosa, and therefore fewer cells moving onto the surface per unit area. In severe cases, erosion of the epithelium will occur over lymphosarcomatous infiltrates.

Large Intestine

Epithelial turnover in the cecum and colon is fundamentally similar to that in the small intestine, though villi are not present on the surface. Cells lose the ability to divide after leaving the proliferative compartment in the lower part of the gland. In the upper portion of the gland they differentiate into goblet cells or columnar absorptive cells that emerge and move out over the surface. They are lost into the lumen, probably within about 4 to 8 days of being produced, though no studies of colonic epithelial turnover have been made in domestic animals. Fasting reduces, and refeeding restores, proliferative activity in colonic glands in experimental animals, and physical distention and dietary bulk in the colon also appear to be trophic for the mucosa. The colon of gnotobiotic animals has a small number of proliferative cells, limited to the lower portion of the glands.

Lesions presumed to be associated with increased epithelial turnover in large bowel include alteration in both surface and glandular epithelium. The number of goblet cells on the surface and in the upper portion of glands is diminished, and epithelium in these areas appears poorly differentiated, is more basophilic than normal, and may be low columnar, cuboidal, or squamous. In severe diseases, microerosion of the surface is present. The proliferative compartment in the gland may hypertrophy, causing glands to elongate and dilate. Crowded mitotic cells are present over a greater proportion of the length of the gland, sometimes virtually to the surface of the mucosa. Such changes may be associated with acute, chronic, or chronic active inflammation of the lamina propria. It is uncertain whether such changes are caused both by primary damage to surface epithelium and by primary immune-mediated stimulation to the proliferative compartment. Experimentally, cell-mediated immune reactions increase crypt-cell production, but not length of glands. Colonic lesions consistent with increased epithelial cell turnover occur mainly in swine dysentery, intestinal adenomatosis complex in swine, trichuriasis, canine histiocytic ulcerative colitis, granulomatous colitis due to a variety of agents, and idiopathic colitis of dogs.

The proliferative compartment in the cecal and colonic glands is damaged by the same insults that attack cells in the crypts of the small bowel. Cytotoxins and parvoviruses tend not to produce severe lesions so commonly in large bowel as they do in small intestine, however, perhaps because a lower proportion of the proliferative compartment is in mitosis at the time of maximum availability of drug or virus. Additions to the list of agents damaging the proliferative compartment in the large intestine include coronavirus in calves and several species of coccidia in ruminants, which develop in the cells lining glands in the large bowel.

The evolution and sequelae of lesions resulting from damage to proliferative epithelium in the large intestine are similar to those in small bowel. Dilatation of crypts containing necrotic debris, and lined by attenuated epithelium, indicates such damage. Severe lesions will lead to loss of glands and erosion and ulceration of the mucosa, perhaps with hemorrhage. Stricture and stenosis may ensue. Following milder damage, which spares some stem cells in each gland, the mucosa has the potential to recover fully after a period of reparative hyperplasia.

Pathophysiology of Enteric Disease

The detrimental effects of gastrointestinal diseases are mediated by a number of often interacting mechanisms. Common consequences of enteric disease include inability to eat or loss of appetite; reduced growth rate, weight loss, or cachexia; hypoproteinemia; and anemia, perhaps with obvious hemorrhage into the gut. Dehydration and acid–base imbalance are associated with reduced water consumption, obstruction, vomition, or diarrhea. Dysfunction of systemic homeostasis, and of other organs, may be caused by toxins, parasites, bacteria, or viruses originating in the gut.

The consequences of diseases of the upper alimentary system, of enteric obstruction, and of ischemia have already been considered. Malabsorption of nutrients occurs commonly in animals with gastrointestinal disease. Failure to assimilate nutrients may result in a reduced growth rate and in emaciation and cachexia if nutrient requirements for maintenance are not met. Malabsorption often occurs concurrently with enteric protein loss, and the contribution of these two factors, along with loss of appetite, to reduced growth rate or to cachexia must be recognized and differentiated. Diarrhea is a common sign of malabsorption, but its pathogenesis is only partly explained by this mechanism.

Malabsorption

Digestion and assimilation of nutrients have an intraluminal phase, mediated by the biliary and pancreatic secretions, and an epithelial phase, carried out by enzyme systems on the surface and in the cytoplasm of absorptive enterocytes. The final step is delivery of the nutrient by the enterocyte to the interstitial fluid, and its uptake into the blood or lymph.

Pancreatic exocrine insufficiency is the major cause of intraluminal maldigestion, and it is usually due to pancreatic hypoplasia in dogs or to pancreatic fibrosis following repeated episodes of pancreatic necrosis (see the Pancreas, this volume). Bile salt deficiency as a cause of intraluminal maldigestion is rarely seen in domestic animals. The epithelial phase of digestion is impaired by loss of functional epithelial surface area. This occurs in short bowel syndrome following intestinal resection and, more commonly, in villus atrophy. Congenital deficiencies of enzymes normally present on the microvilli are not recognized in domestic animals. However, neonates and ruminants have low levels of maltase; ruminants lack sucrase. In most species, lactase levels decline with age, and malabsorption in dogs fed milk has been attributed to low levels of lactase. The poorly differentiated surface epithelium present on atrophic villi may lack the full complement of enzymes on the brush border and in the cytoplasm necessary for nutrient digestion and assimilation. Delivery of nutrients, especially lipid, to the circulation may be impaired in lymphangiectasia. The pathogenesis of malabsorption of the major classes of nutrients will be considered briefly.

Assimilation of **fat** is susceptible to interference at all three phases of digestion and absorption. Lipolysis is impaired if insufficient lipase is available. Most commonly this is a result of pancreatic atrophy or fibrosis. It may be due to failure by atrophic intestinal mucosa to release the cholecystokinin/pancreozymin necessary for pancreatic secretion. The availability of bile salts for micelle formation is reduced in intrahepatic cholestasis or biliary obstruction and by depletion of the bile salt pool due to reduced ileal absorption following resection or atrophy. As a result, fatty acid and monoglyceride are not incorporated onto micelles and emulsified; they are therefore not as accessible to absorptive enterocytes. Reduced surface area for lipid uptake will contribute to malabsorption of fat. Poorly differentiated enterocytes on atrophic gut may be less able than normal epithelium to reesterify long-chain fatty acids to triglyceride and produce chylomicrons for export from the cell. In lymphangiectasia, granulomatous enteritis, and intestinal lymphosarcoma, lymphatic drainage may be obstructed, and with it the flow of chylomicrons to the systemic circulation.

Steatorrhea (excess fat in the feces) is the sequel to malabsorption of lipids. It is seen in monogastric animals, especially dogs, in which fat often forms a large proportion of the daily caloric intake. Severe fat malabsorption may result in deficiencies of fat-soluble vitamins. Malabsorption of calcium, magnesium, and zinc occurs due to their sequestration in soaps formed by combination with malabsorbed luminal fatty acids. Increased absorption of oxalate may be a sequel to reduced concentrations of calcium in the lumen due to soap formation. Malabsorbed lipid may cause colonic diarrhea, by mechanisms that will be discussed subsequently.

Maldigestion of **polysaccharides** occurs if levels of pancreatic amylase are reduced; this is encountered most commonly in dogs with pancreatic disease in which very little functional exocrine tissue remains. Calves and older ruminants normally lack significant amounts of pancreatic amylase and digest starch poorly in the small intestine. Mucosal oligosaccharidase deficiency occurs in villus atrophy, with reduced mucosal surface area. Poor differentiation of enterocytes results in irregular, short, and sparse microvilli and a reduced complement of oligosaccharidases. The result is impaired membrane digestion of disaccharide and malabsorption of carbohydrate, much of which is subsequently fermented by colonic flora. The osmotic effect of malabsorbed disaccharide augments intraluminal fluid accumulation in the small intestine, and this may be compounded by hydrolysis in the colon. Carbohydrate malabsorption is an important component of disease in neonatal diarrhea due to rotavirus and coronavirus, and in other conditions in which there is extensive villus atrophy in the small intestine.

Protein digestion in the lumen is reduced if pancreatic protease activity is decreased to ~10% of normal, as may occur with exocrine pancreatic insufficiency. Loss of gastric proteolytic activity is of little nutritional significance. In conditions with villus atrophy, reduced mucosal surface area and poor differentiation of enterocytes result in malabsorption of small peptides and particularly of amino acids by mechanisms similar to those involved in carbohydrate malabsorption. It is conceivable that atrophy of duodenal villi may result in reduced availability of the brush-border enzyme enterokinase, which is necessary for the activation of pancreatic trypsinogen to trypsin, initiating the subsequent activation of other pancreatic proteases by trypsin. Some dogs with mucosal malabsorption do appear to have partial pancreatic insufficiency, perhaps for this reason. The influence of reduced protein digestion and assimilation on energy metabolism and anabolic activity must be differentiated from the effects of the loss of plasma and other endogenous protein into the lumen of the gut.

A reduction in absorption of **minerals** and **vitamins** may be intuitively expected in animals with reduced absorptive surface in villus atrophy, above and beyond specific mechanisms alluded to previously. If villus atrophy is relatively localized, the reserve capacity of more distal small bowel may offset the effects of local nutrient malabsorption, and there may not be net malabsorption over the full length of the small intestine.

Diarrhea

Diarrhea is the presence in feces of water in relative excess in proportion to fecal dry matter. Diarrhea usually reflects increased absolute fecal loss of water, but may not if absolute fecal dry matter excretion is markedly reduced. Loss of solute and water in diarrhea may lead to severe electrolyte depletion, acid–base imbalance, and dehydration, which are life threatening if not corrected.

Large volumes of fluid derived from ingesta and secretion from the stomach, bile, pancreas, and the gut itself enter the small bowel; in addition, considerable passive movement of water occurs into the upper small bowel from the circulation in response to osmotic effects. Absorption by enterocytes of osmotically active nutrient molecules and electrolyte draws water from lumen into the interstitial space. Overall, the bulk of the fluid entering the small intestine is absorbed, so that the volume leaving the ileum and entering the colon is but a small fraction of the total fluid flux through the small bowel. The large size of this flux implies that relatively small perturbations in unidirectional movement of electrolyte and water may have large effects on the net movement of fluid.

The colon, in addition to its fermentative function, has the ultimate responsibility for conserving electrolyte and water by absorption from the digesta, thereby minimizing fecal losses. It has a finite capacity for absorption of electrolyte and fluid, and if this is exceeded by the rate at which content enters from the small bowel, diarrhea occurs. This is thought to be important in "small bowel diarrheas," where the lesion is in the small intestine. Since the colon has a large reserve capacity for absorption, the excess volume entering from the ileum must be considerable for diarrhea to occur. The large absorptive capacity and fermentative function of the equine colon may mitigate to some extent the expression of small bowel diarrhea in mature animals of that species, even when malabsorption occurs in the small intestine.

SMALL INTESTINE. Small bowel diarrhea is classed as secretory, malabsorptive, and effusive, but the mechanisms are not mutually exclusive.

Secretory diarrhea is due to an excess of secretion over absorption of fluid in the small intestine and is probably the result of derangement of normal secretory and absorptive mechanisms in the mucosa. It is best exemplified by the effects of diarrheagenic bacterial enterotoxins. *Vibrio cholerae* and *E. coli* are the most important sources of such toxins, though only the latter occurs in domestic animals; some *Salmonella* serotypes, *Yersinia enterocolitica,* and perhaps *Shigella* also produce enterotoxin. Cholera and heat-labile *E. coli* enterotoxin act through the mediation of cyclic AMP. In surface enterocytes, toxin-stimulated cAMP shuts down sodium chloride cotransport at the luminal cell membrane, reducing passive water absorption. Meanwhile, in crypt epithelium, cAMP-stimulated chloride secretion is promoted, and water follows. The resultant increase in secretion by crypts and decrease in absorption by villi increases the solute and water load passing from the small bowel for the colon. Heat-stable *E. coli* and *Y. enterocolitica* enterotoxins apparently stimulate cGMP-mediated secretion by the mucosa.

Malabsorptive diarrhea is exemplified by the osmotic retention of water in the gut lumen by poorly absorbed magnesium sulfate, used therapeutically as a cathartic. Malabsorption commonly results from villus atrophy, no matter what the cause. Electrolyte and nutrient solute, malabsorbed as the result of reduced villous and microvillous surface area, are retained in the lumen of the bowel in abnormal amounts, along with osmotically associated water. If compensatory absorption does not occur in more distal small intestine, the additional solute and water is passed on to the colon. A secretory component probably contributes to diarrhea due to villus atrophy, at least in transmissible gastroenteritis in pigs. Here, since the "villous" limb of the postulated crypt–villus fluid circuit is diminished or missing, fluid secreted by the crypts may not be absorbed. However, it is not clear if crypts are abnormally secretory. Poorly differentiated cells emerging onto the intestinal surface from crypts also may retain some secretory capacity.

Increased permeability of the mucosa may contribute to diarrhea by permitting increased retrograde movement of solute and fluid from the lateral intercellular space to the lumen, or by facilitating transudation of tissue fluid. "Filtration secretion" is characterized by increased fluid movement through the epithelial membrane via the paracellular route; the force for secretion is provided by the transepithelial hydrostatic pressure gradient. Portal hypertension or right-sided heart failure, hypoalbuminemia, and expansion of plasma volume establish such conditions. Effusion may occur similarly in lymphatic obstruction or lymphangiectasia, and in inflamed lamina propria, with increased vascular permeability, proprial edema, and enteric plasma protein loss. Increased exfoliation of epithelium and transient microerosions provide further potential sites for effusion of interstitial fluid.

LARGE INTESTINE. Large bowel diarrhea is the product of a reduced innate capability of the colon to handle the solute and fluid presented by the more proximal bowel. A change in net absorption by the colon that is relatively small in absolute terms may be sufficient to cause fluid feces. Colonic diarrhea is characterized by frequent passage of small amounts of fluid feces. Colonic dysfunction has not received the same attention as small bowel disease, but secretory, malabsorptive, and effusive mechanisms are implicated here as well, and they frequently appear to act concurrently.

The colonic mucosa is not as innately "leaky" as the small intestinal mucosa due to the nature of the tight junctions between epithelial cells. As a result, it resists alterations in permeability due to increased hydrostatic pressure in the propria, when compared with the small intestine. Ulceration or erosion may be expected to result in reduced colonic function due to loss of absorptive surface epithelium. Although effusion is anticipated in these states, abnormal macromolecular permeability was not demonstrated in *Salmonella* colitis or swine dysentery. In swine dysentery, however, net electrolyte and water absorption ceases.

Bile acids mediate diarrhea associated with ileal disease, and fatty acids are the cause of diarrhea in steatorrhea. The mechanism of action of these agents appears to be similar; though both may affect the small bowel, the major effect is in the colon. Moderate ileal damage or resection results in the escape of excess bile acids to the colon. This loss is compensated by increased hepatic synthesis to maintain the size of the bile salt pool. But the increased load of bile salts entering the colon is converted to secondary bile acids by the colonic flora. Fatty acids enter the colon in increased quantities in steatorrhea resulting from bile salt depletion, or from other mechanisms in which lipolysis by pancreatic lipase is not severely inhibited. Both dihydroxy bile acids and long-chain fatty acids, especially hydroxy fatty acids produced by bacterial action, alter mucosal permeability and cause mild damage to the surface epithelium. They both also stimulate cAMP-mediated secretion by the colonic mucosa, perhaps by causing local prostaglandin release. The result is net fluid secretion by the colon, and diarrhea. This also is the mode of action of a number of laxatives, including senna and castor oil, which contains the hydroxy fatty acid ricinoleic acid.

Although colonic secretion stimulated by bacterial enterotoxin is not clearly implicated in diarrhea, alterations in the flora in the large bowel may be detrimental to normal function. Absorption of volatile fatty acids produced by bacterial fermentation is responsible for considerable concurrent absorption of water in the large intestine. Reduced production and absorption of volatile fatty acids, secondary to imbalance of the bacterial flora in the cecum and colon, may explain some problems of wasting and diarrhea in horses in which no morphologic abnormality of the mucosa can be found.

Osmotic overload of the large bowel results from the delivery by the small bowel of a large volume of fermentable substrate. This may be due to an excess of dietary carbohydrate or, more commonly, malabsorption in the small intestine. Of the malabsorbed nutrients, carbohydrate is the only one of significance in initiating colonic osmotic overload. Bacterial fermentation of carbohydrate results in the production of an increased number of molecules of volatile fatty acid. They are readily handled by the colon under normal circumstances, by rapid absorption, and by bicarbonate buffering. A heavy carbohydrate load may overwhelm the colonic buffering capacity, however, and cause a reduced pH. This results in an altered gut flora dominated by organisms producing lactic acid, which is absorbed at a slower rate than the volatile fatty acids. Further acidification causes mucosal permeability, permitting an influx of water and solute into the lumen from the tissue, as a result of the increased osmotic pressure generated by lactic acid in the lumen. Diarrhea follows.

MOTILITY AND DIARRHEA. Increased intestinal motility probably does not have a primary role in the pathogenesis of diarrhea. Often the small intestine of animals with diarrhea is flaccid and fluid filled rather than hypermotile. Increased colonic motor activity is often segmental and antiperistaltic, and probably unrelated to increased transit. Hypermotility, if it does occur, may be in response to, rather than a cause of, increased volumes of fluid in the gut.

Ileus or hypomotility, partial small bowel obstruction, and radiation injury may set up conditions conducive to bacterial overgrowth in the small bowel. Achlorhydria or hypochlorhydria in the dog may also predispose to this problem. "Stagnant loop" or "blind loop" syndrome ensues, as anaerobes in particular proliferate in the lumen of the small intestine to levels approaching those in the large bowel. Mild or moderate villus atrophy may develop in the affected area, and bacteria will be seen on the mucosal surface in tissue sections, an unusual finding in the small bowel. Ultrastructural lesions and cytoplasmic lipid accumulation can be present in surface enterocytes, though the brush border may be intact. Deconjugation of bile acids by anaerobes results in free bile acids, many of which precipitate at the pH of the gut content and are lost to the recirculating pool. Some are absorbed passively, but dihydroxy secondary bile salts may be the cause of damage to enterocytes. Fat malabsorption occurs when conjugated bile acids fall below critical micellar concentrations, reducing emulsion and absorption. Malabsorption is further exacerbated by the toxic damage to cells. Steatorrhea results.

Protein digestion and absorption may not be affected by bacterial overgrowth; however, some amino acids may be deaminated by anaerobes and metabolized to ammonia which is absorbed, converted to urea in the liver, and largely lost through the kidneys. Plasma protein loss into the gut can also occur, as may impaired uptake of disaccharides. Binding of vitamin B_{12} by enteric flora prevents absorption in the ileum and may lead to deficiency. Dihydroxy bile acids and malabsorbed fatty acids promote secretion by the small bowel and colon, resulting in diarrhea.

Protein Metabolism in Enteric Disease

Disorders of protein metabolism attributable to enteric disease are responsible for significant economic loss in the form of reduced weight gain, wool growth, and milk production. Severe derangement in any species may lead to cachexia, hypoproteinemia, and death. Nitrogen economy may be affected at three main points: nitrogen intake may be reduced; there may be decreased protein digestion and assimilation; or increased cata-

bolism and loss of endogenous nitrogen may occur. The metabolism and distribution of nitrogen in the body may vary, depending on the way in which its economy is disrupted.

Decreased protein intake is the most obvious threat to the nitrogen economy, and it is probably the most important in many chronic gastrointestinal diseases. Subclinical inefficiency in production, reduced growth, and emaciation may be the products of varying degrees of inappetence. If the quality of the feed available is poor, the effect of reduced intake on production will be compounded. Painful prehension or mastication, dental attrition, chronic dysphagia, or recurrent vomition are all obvious causes of reduced feed intake. A sharp decline in appetite, or anorexia, is a common sign of indigestion, obstruction, or systemic disease. In ruminants, loss of appetite to varying degrees is an important component of the pathogenicity of gastrointestinal parasites, including those infecting the abomasum (*Ostertagia*), small intestine (*Trichostrongylus*), and large bowel (*Oesophagostomum*). About 40–90% of the inefficiency in production in these parasitisms is attributable to reduced feed intake. The factors influencing satiety in animals are uncertain and deserve greater attention. Among them may be the hormones gastrin and cholecystokinin, which are elevated in association with inappetence in parasitized sheep. The bulk and particle size of the feed consumed influences distention of the reticulorumen and rate of throughput of digesta. Altered gastrointestinal motility or stasis may also detrimentally influence feed intake, as may reduced absorption of amino acids from the small intestine.

Malabsorption of peptides and amino acids may occur locally in the small intestine as a result of significant villus atrophy. Unless the lesion is widespread, or low in the small bowel, however, net absorption of nitrogen over the length of the small intestine may not be reduced, due to the compensatory capacity of more distal normal mucosa. Overall, the contribution of malabsorption to disordered nitrogen metabolism appears to be minor in most situations.

Protein-losing gastroenteropathy, increased catabolism, and loss of endogenous nitrogen via the gastrointestinal tract are important in many diseases. Excess endogenous protein entering the intestine is derived from two main sources, namely, increased turnover of cells lining the gut and effusion of plasma protein into the lumen of the bowel. The contribution to endogenous nitrogen loss by increased turnover of enterocytes and secretion of mucoprotein has not been well defined. In conditions causing chronic villus atrophy, such as intestinal parasitism by *Trichostrongylus* and *Strongyloides*, however, it may be substantial.

Plasma protein loss into the gut presupposes abnormal permeability of the mucosa to large molecules. This may be the product of the bloodsucking activity of nematodes such as *Haemonchus*, *Ancylostoma*, and *Bunostomum* or hemorrhage from sites of trauma in the mucosa caused by the feeding activity of worms such as *Oesophagostomum columbianum*, *Chabertia*, and *Strongylus*. Erosive lesions result in considerable loss of red blood cells and plasma protein. Such lesions may be due to infarction, severe cryptal necrosis, or acute inflammatory damage to the mucosa associated with bacteria, viruses, and coccidia, causing fibrinohemorrhagic enteritis. Microscopic "leaks" in the mucosa also permit plasma loss into the gut. These may result from increased exfoliation of enterocytes into the lumen in villus atrophy, as transient gaps in the mucosa at the site where the cells sloughs. In villus atrophy with a high rate of enterocyte turnover, temporary microerosions may develop when flattened cells fail to maintain the integrity of the surface epithelium. The permeability of tight junctions between epithelial cells may be sufficiently altered to permit transit of plasma protein molecules when the hydrostatic pressure in the proprial interstitium is elevated in congestive heart failure, by increased vascular permeability in acute or chronic inflammation, and in lymphatic obstruction or lymphangiectasia.

Plasma protein loss into the gut is nonselective. Albumin, immunoglobulins, clotting factors, and a variety of transport or carrier proteins, including transferrin, ceruloplasmin, and transcortin, are lost. The physiologic consequences of protein-losing enteropathy may reflect increased catabolism of any of these molecules but are most obviously related to increased turnover of the albumin pool. Plasma albumin lost into the gut, when expressed as a proportion of the total body pool, will vary in absolute terms, depending on the size of the pool. This concept of *fractional catabolic rate* is essential to understanding the kinetics of plasma protein turnover.

In protein-losing enteropathy, albumin turnover may pass through three phases. During the first phase, the fractional catabolic rate increases, and with it, the absolute amount of protein lost into the bowel; as the size of the circulating pool of albumin shrinks, so does the absolute rate of loss of protein, even though the fractional rate remains the same. During the second phase, the size of the circulating pool stabilizes as the rate of albumin synthesis by the liver increases to match in absolute terms the rate of loss. The plasma albumin pool is then in a state of hyperkinetic equilibrium; the pool is smaller, with a higher than normal fractional catabolic rate compensated by an increased rate of hepatic synthesis. Provided that the size of the loss does not exceed the synthetic capacity of the liver, this equilibrium may persist for a considerable period. In the third phase, hypoalbuminemia develops as the fractional catabolic rate continues to increase so that it exceeds in absolute terms the synthetic capacity of the liver, or if the rate of synthesis declines, it develops as a result of deficiency in amino acids derived from the diet and by catabolism of other body protein. The hypoalbuminemia in enteric plasma loss is often associated with hyperglobulinemia, since compensatory synthesis of immunoglobulin is remarkable. Several times more immunoglobulin than albumin may be lost into the gut as a result.

The progress and clinical manifestations of protein-losing enteropathy vary with the rate of onset of plasma loss and the fractional catabolic rate. A sudden onset of severe plasma protein loss may cause death during the first phase, before there is time for compensatory synthesis. If the fractional catabolic rate is gradually and only slightly increased, so that compensation occurs with the albumin pool in equilibrium in only a marginally reduced state (perhaps near or within the "normal" range), subclinical protein loss occurs. Though the fractional catabolic rate is only slightly elevated, the relatively large size of the albumin pool may mean that the absolute loss of protein exceeds

that in a hypoalbuminemic animal with a higher fractional catabolic rate but a smaller albumin pool.

Plasma protein leaking from the stomach or upper small intestine, and protein derived from exfoliated cells in villus atrophy with increased epithelial turnover, may be digested and absorbed in the small intestine. This is dependent on luminal proteolysis by pancreatic enzymes, and compensatory membrane digestion and absorption, making up for any malabsorption by proximal atrophic mucosa. But the efficiency of protein digestion, even if it is not reduced, is not total. Therefore, a proportion of the increased endogenous protein entering the lumen will be added to the protein escaping digestion in the small bowel and will enter the large intestine. There, most of this protein may be converted to ammonia by the colonic flora and absorbed, so that in animals losing protein high in the gut, there may be little or no increase in fecal nitrogen excretion. On the other hand, much of the protein lost into the colon from lesions at that level is passed in the feces, often as protein, and is lost. Ammonia nitrogen absorbed from the colon is converted in the liver mainly to urea. Animals with increased endogenous protein loss into the stomach or small intestine tend to have slightly raised levels of blood urea nitrogen and an elevated rate of urinary urea excretion.

Elevated hepatic synthesis of albumin due to increased turnover of the plasma albumin pool, and increased enteric protein synthesis in support of elevated epithelial turnover in conditions with chronic villus atrophy, is at the expense of anabolic processes elsewhere. Dietary amino acid is "diverted" to synthesis of enteric and plasma protein preferentially. If protein intake is poor due to inappetence or a low-quality ration, or if the rate of protein loss is high, the animal moves into negative nitrogen balance. Catabolism of peripheral protein then assumes an increasingly important role in maintaining the pool of amino acids available for plasma and intestinal protein synthesis. This explains in part the reduced growth rate, decreased muscle mass, and depressed deposition of bone matrix in sheep with subclinical or mild parasitism and the cachexia of severe parasitism. The additional metabolic cost of increased protein synthesis also causes inefficiency in energy utilization. These principles probably hold for all syndromes causing enteric loss of endogenous protein in any species.

Loss of enteric protein and, especially, plasma, should be suspected in cachectic or hypoproteinemic animals. Diarrhea is often, but not invariably, present. The two major routes of occult abnormal plasma protein loss are the kidney in glomerular disease and the gastrointestinal tract. Weeping skin lesions are another source. Anemia and hypoproteinemia may be due to hemorrhage externally or into the gastrointestinal tract. Advanced liver disease may cause hypoalbuminemia; other signs of hepatic failure will likely be concurrent (see the Liver and Biliary System, this volume). Inability to eat, inadequate nutrition, or starvation also cause emaciation, usually without profound hypoalbuminemia. The cachexia of malignancy must also be differentiated. Provided it is adequately hydrated, the hypoalbuminemic animal shows evidence of subcutaneous, mesenteric, or gastric submucosal edema, perhaps with hydrothorax or ascites. Wasting of muscle mass may be marked if the protein loss has been severe and of some standing. Unlike starvation, protein-losing gastroenteropathy may be associated with the presence of internal fat depots, since assimilation of energy is not necessarily severely impaired.

Anemia

The principles discussed in the kinetics of plasma albumin during enteric plasma loss may be applied also to the kinetics of the erythron following loss of blood into the gastrointestinal tract. Blood loss of any origin, including that due to hematophagous parasites, may cause anemia. Erythroid hyperplasia in the marrow or in extramedullary sites may not compensate for the continued bleeding. Resolution of the hemorrhage results in eventual restoration of normal red cell numbers and an ultimate decline in erythrocyte production. Chronic blood loss may culminate in depletion of iron stores and development of a nonresponsive hypochromic microcytic anemia.

Syndromes Associated with Malabsorption and/or Protein Loss in the Small Intestine

Malabsorption of nutrients, electrolyte, and water is at the root of disease in animals caused by rotavirus, coronavirus, *Cryptosporidium,* and rarely, *E. coli;* significant loss of protein probably does not occur in these conditions. Intestinal nematode parasitism due to *Trichostrongylus* in ruminants, and *Strongyloides* in all species, causes malabsorption and plasma loss. Hookworms suck blood, causing anemia, hypoproteinemia, and perhaps, wasting. Johne's disease in ruminants, and probably intestinal adenomatosis in swine, are associated with plasma loss into the gut and malabsorption. Erosion, ulceration, and villus atrophy due to coccidiosis, enteroinvasive bacteria, parvoviruses, bovine virus diarrhea, and some other viruses cause malabsorption and increased mucosal permeability.

In dogs and horses, and to a lesser extent in other species, there may be idiopathic, sporadic or breed-related disease variably signaled clinically by chronic diarrhea, weight loss, hypoproteinemia, and often malabsorption, as defined by tests of carbohydrate and lipid assimilation. Intestinal biopsy is usually necessary to make a diagnosis, permitting the establishment of a prognosis and course of therapy. These syndromes are usually characterized by abnormal infiltrates in the lamina propria, perhaps associated with some degree of villus atrophy. Eosinophils, lymphocytes, and plasma cells, granulomatous inflammation, or amyloid are the infiltrates most commonly implicated. Lymphangiectasia may also produce a similar syndrome.

Lymphangiectasia

Lymphangiectasia has been described in the dog, where it appears to be among the more common causes of malabsorption/protein-losing enteropathy. It is associated with a syndrome variably characterized by chronic diarrhea, wasting, hypoproteinemia, lymphopenia, hypocalcemia, and hypocholesterolemia. Peripheral edema, ascites, and hydrothorax result from hypoalbuminemia. The intestinal lesion is dilation of the lacteals, and often lymphatics of the submucosa, intestinal wall, serosa, and mesentery (Fig. 1.14D). Villi containing di-

lated chyle-filled lacteals may stand out grossly as white papillate foci in a thickened, transversely folded edematous mucosa (Fig. 1.14C). Serosal and mesenteric lymphatics may be prominent, white, and dilated. Small nodular white masses may be present on the serosa at the mesenteric border and along lymphatics.

In section, villi may be of normal length or somewhat blunt or stubby. The surface epithelium may appear normal or perhaps slightly attenuated, and lateral interepithelial spaces are often dilated. The lacteals in many villi are distended, and lymphatics in deeper portions of the mucosa may be also. Occasional lipid-laden macrophages are present in and around lacteals and lymphatics; large focal accumulations of lipophages form the grossly visible white masses sometimes present. The lamina propria is edematous, and the submucosa and deeper portions of the gut wall may be. The proprial inflammatory cell population may be normal, or the numbers of lymphocytes and plasma cells may be increased.

The cause of lymphangiectasia is presumably usually lymphatic obstruction. Many cases appear to be acquired, and some may be due to lymphosarcomatous or granulomatous infiltrates obstructing flow in mesenteric lymph nodes. Usually, no congenital or acquired obstruction of the lymphatic drainage is obvious. Experimental obstruction of mesenteric lymphatics produces hypoproteinemia and lymphangiectasia but not diarrhea and weight loss, suggesting that the etiology of the clinical syndrome may be more complex than simple lymphatic obstruction.

Moderate malabsorption of lipid, and plasma protein loss into the gut, cause the signs associated with lymphangiectasia. Malabsorbed lipid may contribute to diarrhea via the effects of fatty acids on colonic secretion. Mucosal permeability associated with increased proprial hydrostatic pressure may cause net intestinal secretion and contribute to plasma protein loss. It has been proposed that dilated lacteals may rupture, releasing lymph into the lumen of the intestine. Hypocalcemia may be related to loss of the mineral bound to plasma albumin, and perhaps to formation of soaps with malabsorbed lipid in the gut lumen. Hypocholesterolemia is due to lipid malabsorption and effusion of plasma. Lymphopenia is thought to be the result of the loss of lymphocyte-rich lymph into the gut.

In cattle, dilated lacteals and lymphatics in the small intestine have been associated with Johne's disease and hypoalbuminemia due to abomasal parasitism. In Johne's disease, the lesion may be the result of local edema due to inflammation in the propria and mesenteric lymphatics combined with hypoproteinemia. In the second situation, dilated lacteals may be secondary to edema resulting from reduced plasma oncotic pressure, rather than the cause of such a problem.

Chronic Inflammatory Disease

EOSINOPHILIC GASTROENTERITIS. Eosinophilic gastroenteritis has been well described but is rarely encountered. Conditions typified by abnormally heavy eosinophilic infiltrates of the gastrointestinal mucosa occur in dogs, cats, and horses.

In **dogs,** eosinophilic gastroenteritis is a segmental or region-

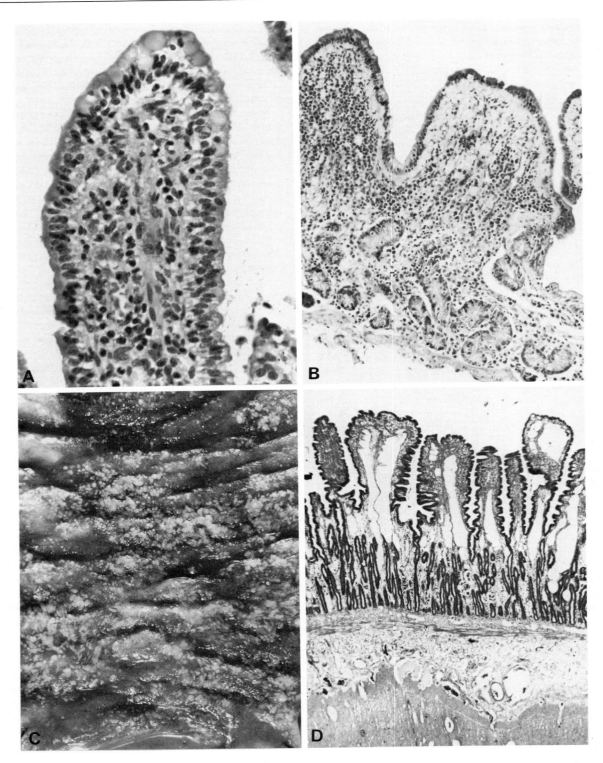

Fig. 1.14. (A) Distended vacuoles containing eosinophilic colostral protein in apical cytoplasm of enterocytes at the tip of the villus of a 2-day-old calf. (B) Intestine. Goat. Deposits of pale amorphous amyloid beneath the epithelium on villi, and scattered in the lamina propria. (Courtesy of J. R. Duncan.) (C) Lymphangiectasia. Small intestine. Dog. Mucosa, thickened by edema, is thrown in folds. Many villi contain white, chyle-filled lacteals. (D) Lymphangiectasia. Dog. Lacteals are dilated, lamina propria and submucosa are edematous, and lymphatics in submucosa and muscularis are open.

al affliction, affecting one or more areas of the alimentary tract from stomach to rectum. Signs may vary from vomition associated with gastritis, to chronic small bowel diarrhea, or chronic large bowel diarrhea with hematochezia resulting from ulcerative eosinophilic colitis. Diarrhea and weight loss suggest malabsorption and protein-losing enteropathy, and circulating eosinophilia is often present. The disease is best known in German shepherds, but it may occur in any breed.

At autopsy or laparotomy, aside from lesions attributable to cachexia and hypoproteinemia, there may be enlarged mesenteric lymph nodes. The affected segment of the alimentary tract is thickened, or the mucosa may be irregularly folded or nodular and perhaps hemorrhagic, eroded, or ulcerated. Gross lesions are associated with heavy infiltrates of normal eosinophils in the mucosa, submucosa, and often transmurally, involving muscularis and serosa. Villi may be mildly to severely atrophic; the epithelium can appear relatively normal, or enterocytes may be low columnar or cuboidal. In the colon the epithelium may be eroded or the mucosa ulcerated in areas with heavy infiltrates of eosinophils. Eosinophils may be present in sinusoids throughout affected lymph nodes.

In one series of German shepherds, eosinophilic granulomas were present in gastrointestinal tissues and other organs, and larvae of *Toxocara canis* were implicated. Granulomas are not reported in other cases, which probably represent a separate condition. Scirrhous eosinophilic gastritis and arteritis is also pathologically unique. The etiology of eosinophilic gastroenteritis in dogs may be related to a reaginic response to antigens in the lumen or wall of the gastrointestinal tract, with infiltration by immunomodulating eosinophils.

Eosinophilic enteritis in **cats** is rare and appears to be one manifestation of a hypereosinophilic syndrome that may involve many organs. Diarrhea, sometimes bloody, vomition, loss of appetite, and loss of condition may be represented in the history. Clinically, intestinal thickening, hepato- and splenomegaly, and enlarged mesenteric lymph nodes may be present, in association with circulating eosinophilia and hyperplasia of the eosinophil series in the marrow.

The postmortem picture reflects the clinical findings. Enlargment of the various organs, including liver, spleen, lymph nodes in many locations, and tan nodularities on the kidneys, are associated with heavy infiltrates of usually well differentiated eosinophils. In the small intestine the eosinophilic infiltrate may be transmural and is accompanied by hypertrophy of the muscle layers, causing a thickened appearance grossly. Lymph nodes may have hyperplastic follicles and many mature eosinophils in sinusoids, or they may vary through eosinophilic lymphadenitis with fibrosis to complete obliteration of normal architecture and replacement by eosinophils in a fibrillar stroma extending through the capsule into surrounding tissue.

Chronic eosinophilic enteritis in **horses** has been described in Australia as a distinct syndrome, and it occurs elsewhere. Affected animals have weight loss and diarrhea or unformed feces, associated with hypoalbuminemia, suggesting enteric loss of plasma protein. Reduced absorption of glucose occurs, but peripheral eosinophilia is absent. At autopsy, mucosal and sometimes transmural thickening may occur at any level of the alimentary tract from esophagus to rectum. Thickened mucosa is

thrown into turgid, transverse folds, or occasionally is fissured and roughened. Focal caseous ulcers 1–15 mm in diameter may be present on the surface or in the mucosa and submucosa of the small and large intestine and common bile duct.

Microscopically, there is diffuse infiltration of the mucosa, submucosa, and often, deeper layers of the enteric wall by eosinophils, mast cells, macrophages, lymphocytes, and some plasma cells. Moderate to severe villus atrophy, fibroplasia in the lamina propria, and hypertrophy of the muscularis mucosae occur. Caseous foci in the mucosa and submucosa consist of central masses of eosinophils, sometimes surrounded by macrophages, giant cells, and occasionally, fibrous tissue. Eosinophilic granulomas have been described in the biliary and pancreatic ducts, pancreas, capsule and outer cortex of enlarged firm mesenteric lymph nodes, and near portal tracts in the liver. The skin may be thickened and hyperkeratotic, and the limbus of the hoof thickened and ulcerated. Acanthotic epithelium in affected areas is infiltrated by eosinophils, as is the underlying dermis.

Villus atrophy is common, but where large bowel lesions are absent, there is no diarrhea. Chronic inflammation in the mucosa may explain protein loss and hypoalbuminemia. The cause of this syndrome is unknown, though the involvement of a reaction to ingested allergens is suggested.

LYMPHOCYTIC–PLASMACYTIC ENTERITIS. Some animals, mainly dogs, showing signs consistent with malabsorption and/or plasma loss into the gut, have microscopic lesions in the small intestine described as lymphocytic–plasmacytic enteritis.

The cardinal finding is abnormally intense infiltrates of well-differentiated lymphocytes and plasma cells in the lamina propria of villi, between crypts, and sometimes in the submucosa. Normally, plasma cells are uncommon in the lamina propria of villi. A layer of lymphocytes, plasma cells, eosinophils, and histiocytes may be present along the proprial–submucosal junction above the muscularis mucosae. Villi may be normal, clubbed, or moderately atrophic, and occasionally fusion of villi may be prevalent (Fig. 1.15A,B). The surface epithelium may appear relatively normal, or low columnar to cuboidal with an indistinct brush border; theliolymphocytes may be common. Crypts may be hypertrophic. In this and other conditions with increased inflammatory infiltrates or edema in the lamina propria, some crypts may be obstructed and dilated and contain mucus and a few exfoliated epithelial cells. Occasionally, evidence of rupture of such crypts will been seen; lakes of mucus, reactive histiocytes, and occasional giant cells are present in the lamina propria (Fig. 1.15C,D). Other crypts may contain casts of eosinophilic glycoprotein. There may be edema of the lamina propria and dilatation of lacteals, suggesting concurrent lymphangiectasia.

Lymphocytic–plasmacytic enteritis must be differentiated from giardiasis, bacterial overgrowth, granulomatous enteritis, and intestinal lymphosarcoma.

In the Lundehund and in the basenji, syndromes of hypoalbuminemia, chronic diarrhea, and wasting occur with high prevalence. They seem primarily attributable to the development of lymphocytic–plasmacytic enteritis, perhaps with lymphangiectasia in some dogs. In the basenji, chronic gastritis

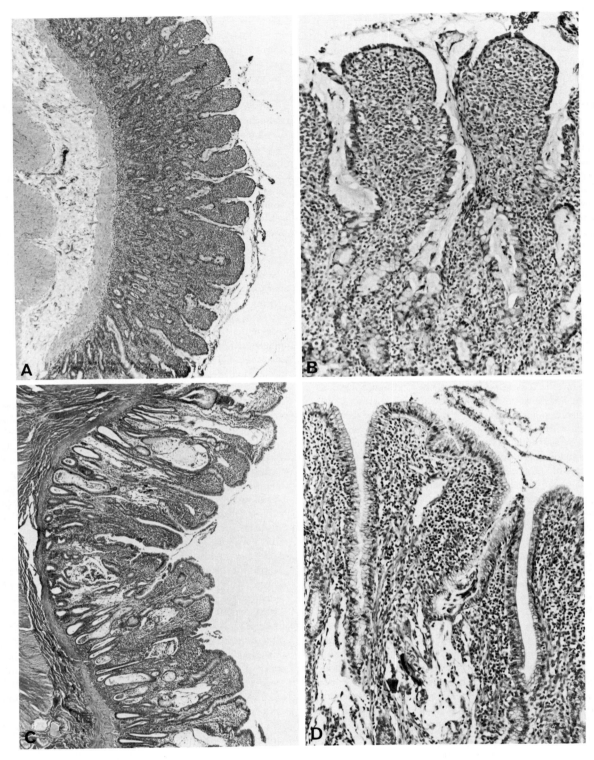

Fig. 1.15. (A and B) Lymphocytic–plasmacytic enteritis. Dog. (A) Villi are stumpy, club-shaped, or fused. Excessive mononuclear infiltrate at all levels of the mucosa, including between the base of crypts and the muscularis mucosae. (B) Blunt and club-shaped villi, cuboidal and attenuated surface epithelium, excess mucus secreted from crypts, and abnormal infiltrate of lymphocytes, plasma cells, and histiocytic cells in lamina propria. (C) Small intestine. Dog with malabsorption and intestinal protein loss. Blunt and occasionally fused villi, mononuclear cells in lamina propria, and elongate, dilated, and mucus-filled crypts. Some distended crypts have ruptured, releasing mucus into lamina propria. (D) Detail of (C), showing mucus in lamina propria due to rupture of a dilated crypt. Leak of cells and mucus from lamina propria and abnormal numbers of bacteria in lumen.

or hypertrophic gastritis may be associated. Hypergamma-globulinemia occurs commonly in the late stages of the syndrome in basenjis, and lymphosarcoma develops in some affected animals. Animals with the gray collie syndrome (cyclic hematopoiesis) also may have lymphocytic–plasmacytic enteritis (see the Hematopoietic System, Volume 3).

The cause of lymphocytic–plasmacytic enteritis is not known in any species. Though it may represent an abnormal response to antigen entering from the lumen, no dietary or other antigen has been conclusively implicated.

GRANULOMATOUS ENTERITIS. The presence of chronic inflammatory infiltrates including aggregates of histiocytes, and perhaps giant cells, in the lamina propria is the criterion for a diagnosis of granulomatous enteritis. Johne's disease, intestinal tuberculosis, and *Histoplasma* enteritis are specific examples, but usually the cause is not identified. Granulomatous enteritis occurs in all species. Transmural granulomatous enteritis is seen rarely in **dogs**. It is usually segmental and perhaps discontinuous in distribution, affecting the lower ileum, colon, and draining lymph nodes; the term ''regional enteritis'' is often applied. Idiopathic granulomatous enteritis as a cause of wasting and protein-losing enteropathy is most commonly seen as a sporadic problem in **horses**.

Depending on the duration of the disease, animals may be markedly cachectic, have subcutaneous edema especially of dependent areas, and there may be hydrothorax, hydropericardium, and ascites. Lesions in the horse usually affect the small intestine; stomach and large bowel are occasionally involved also. There may be thickened pale plaques or prominent lymphatics on the serosa of the bowel. The mucosa of the small intestine may be irregularly granular or thickened; there may be transverse corrugations of the mucosa, or raised firm gray areas with hyperemic foci may be evident. Linear ulcers of small and large bowel have been described. Mesenteric lymph nodes are usually enlarged, edematous, with mottled firm gray areas, fibrotic nodules, or rarely, caseous or mineralized foci on the cut surface. Granulomatous pale, caseous, or calcified foci may be scattered in the liver.

The microscopic lesion may be patchy, regional, or diffuse, and it may be mucosal, or transmural, ultimately gaining the draining lymph nodes. Villi are mildly to markedly atrophic with hypertrophy of crypts. The epithelium may vary from apparently normal to low columnar or cuboidal with an indistinct brush border. There may be leaks between cells on the surface, or microerosions may be present, through which neutrophils and proteinaceous exudate pass into the lumen. The lamina propria is edematous and contains scattered aggregates of histiocytes and perhaps giant cells, or less commonly, more organized granulomatous foci. Neutrophils and eosinophils are distributed diffusely throughout the lamina propria and may be concentrated in or near granulomatous foci. A heavy population of lymphocytes and plasma cells inhabits the lamina propria, and the infiltrate and edema may separate crypts abnormally from each other. The inflammatory reaction may follow lymphatics into the submucosa and through the muscularis to the serosa. The submucosa is usually edematous, and lymphatics are prominent. Granulomas may be present in the submucosa or at intervals

along lymphatics. The affected lymph nodes are hyperplastic, usually with prominent sinus histiocytosis. Giant cells may be present in sinusoids, or granulomatous foci of varying sizes may be evident. Sinusoids contain numerous neutrophils and perhaps eosinophils, and neutrophils may accumulate in the center of granulomas.

Rarely are agents isolated or identified in such lesions in horses and dogs. *Mycobacterium avium* or environmental mycobacteria are incriminated occasionally. *Mycobacterium paratuberculosis* will also cause granulomatous enteritis rarely in horses. In **cats**, focal pyogranulomatous aggregates associated with blood vessels are found in the submucosa and especially subserosa of the intestine of animals with feline infectious peritonitis.

AMYLOIDOSIS. Amyloid deposition in the small intestine may be encountered occasionally, in animals with systemic amyloidosis. Sometimes the gastrointestinal lesions predominate and contribute to the clinical syndrome. Significant intestinal amyloidosis leads to signs consistent with malabsorption and enteric protein loss. Usually there is no gross indication of the deposition of amyloid in the intestine. Occasionally, however, focal ulceration or hemorrhage may be noted. Microscopically, amyloid is seen as the typical acellular, amorphous, eosinophilic, fibrillar deposit, beneath the epithelium or throughout the propria in villi, and perhaps around vessels in the submucosa (Fig. 1.14B). It must not be mistaken for collagen deposition, which is most unusual in these locations, though a band of collagenous material is sometimes present at the base of the mucosa in cats. The pathogenic effects of amyloid in the intestine seem to involve either impaired movement of interstitial fluid into lacteals or perhaps increased permeability of capillaries, possibly explaining protein loss into the lumen.

Inflammation of the Large Intestine

The general reaction to insult of the cecal and colonic epithelium was considered above under Epithelial Renewal in Health and Disease.

Ischemia, obliteration of the proliferative epithelium by viruses or coccidia, severe inflammation in the mucosa, and perhaps, necrotizing toxic insults from the lumen are responsible for the development of focal or diffuse ulceration of the large intestine. Inflammatory infiltrates in the lamina propria may be classified broadly as acute, chronic or chronic active, and granulomatous. They may be limited in distribution to the mucosa or be transmural, involving submucosa, muscularis, serosa, and frequently, the draining lymph nodes. **Typhlitis** and **colitis** may be manifestations of a generalized or systemic disease; they may be part of an enterocolitis involving both small and large intestine; or they may be regional and limited to a segment of the intestine, often terminal ileum, cecum, and colon or some shorter part of the large bowel.

The colonic mucosa may provide the portal of entry for systemic bacterial invasion and for uptake of toxins. Increased mucosal permeability in the colon may permit enteric loss of plasma protein or of blood. Disordered large bowel flora in hindgut fermenters may compromise uptake of volatile fatty acids and water. In any species, damage to the colonic mucosa may result in malabsorption of electrolytes and water, and perhaps net secretion. Colitis in each of the species will be considered in turn.

Colitis cystica profunda, the presence of dilated colonic glands protruding through the muscularis mucosae into the submucosa has been reported in several species. It is perhaps most often seen in swine, where it is an occasional finding (Fig. 1.39E). The dilated glands may be grossly visible through the serosa and muscularis as nodular masses a few millimeters in diameter. Microscopically, a single large, flask-shaped gland, lined by columnar epithelium and containing mucus and exfoliated cells or necrotic debris, may be present. Alternatively, a cluster of glands appears to herniate into the submucosa, where one or more may become dilated by mucus and debris. The cause is unknown; the lesion may be a sequel to colitis and local damage to the muscularis mucosae, or it may represent herniation into the space left by an involuted submucosal lymphoid follicle. Though the lesion has been seen with colitis in a variety of circumstances, it is usually found incidentally, and there is no specific etiologic association.

Typhlocolitis in Dogs

Inflammation of the large bowel in dogs is usually associated with signs of diarrhea, typically frequent, small in volume, mucoid or bloody, and often accompanied by tenesmus. More severe acute necrotizing colitis, perhaps leading to ulceration and perforation of the proximal descending colon, with subsequent peritonitis, has been associated rarely with glucocorticoid administration and with trauma or surgery involving the spinal cord. Gastric ulceration may occur concurrently. The pathogenesis of the colonic lesions developing in these circumstances is unclear. Ulcerative enterocolitis, with lesions apparently centered mainly on lymphoid tissue, as well as gastric ulcer, has been produced experimentally by administration of the analgesic drug indomethacin to dogs. Necrotizing colitis, ulceration, and perforation may occur rarely in dogs in uremia. The mechanism is uncertain, but colonic damage may be the effect of high concentrations of ammonia evolved by urease-producing colonic flora from urea diffusing into the gut from the blood. In canine intestinal hemorrhage syndrome, possibly associated with clostridial overgrowth in the gut, the colon may be involved or at least contain hemorrhagic content.

Trichuris vulpis, the whipworm of dogs, may cause mucosal colitis, which rarely evolves into a granulomatous transmural condition. Clinical trichuriasis is generally associated with a population of worms that extends from the usual site of infection in the cecum and proximal ascending colon into more distal parts of the large intestine. Rarely, trichuriasis may be complicated by infection with *Balantidium coli,* which possibly contributes to the development of mucosal erosion or ulceration. Ulcerative colitis in dogs is also caused rarely by *Entamoeba histolytica.* An ulcerative granulomatous transmural colitis is more common as one of the enteric manifestations of histoplasmosis. *Prototheca* also is a cause of distinctive but rare enterocolitis in dogs. Canine parvovirus causes colonic damage, but virtually never without lesions elsewhere. Canine coronavirus has also

been implicated as a cause of colonic as well as small intestinal lesions. The pathology of these conditions is discussed under Infectious and Parasitic Diseases of the Gastrointestinal Tract.

Spirochetes may be present in the canine colon, and although they are generally considered nonpathogenic, they are embedded in the microvillous border of surface epithelium and may be associated with mild mucosal colitis. *Campylobacter jejuni* is isolated from dogs with diarrhea, but its possible relationship to colitis in clinical cases is currently unclear. The association of giardiasis and colitis in dogs is considered to be fortuitous. The role of antigens gaining the mucosa is unknown. If they are significant, their identity, origin, and the factors predisposing to their entry are obscure. Colitis must be differentiated from ulcerating adenocarcinomas and infiltrative or ulcerative lymphosarcomas of the large intestine.

Most colitis in dogs is idiopathic and pathologically nonspecific; eosinophilic enterocolitis and histiocytic ulcerative colitis are the two distinctive patterns recognized microscopically.

Mild acute mucosal colitis, reflecting a grossly reddened, friable surface is characterized by congestion of superficial capillaries and venules, and proprial edema. Neutrophils are the most prominent inflammatory cells, and they are found mainly in the superficial lamina propria around vessels, and transmigrating or passing between surface epithelial cells into the lumen. The population of lymphocytes and plasma cells in the lamina propria may not differ subjectively from normal, but there is generally a moderate increase in mononuclear cells between glands. There is usually a reduced number of goblet cells on the surface and in glands, and surface epithelium may be basophilic, low columnar, or cuboidal (Fig. 1.16A,B). Hyperplasia of epithelium in glands is usually evident. Inflammatory cells, mainly neutrophils, may accumulate in a layer several cells deep along the mucosal side of the muscularis mucosae. The lesions in mild acute colitis in dogs often seem out of proportion to the severity of the clinical syndrome, which may be the result of irritation and tenesmus.

The spectrum of inflammation in colitis grades from acute toward an increasingly chronic infiltrate, which along with edema separates colonic glands and may accumulate deep in the mucosa between glands and muscularis mucosae (Fig. 1.16D). Neutrophils and eosinophils may be scattered in the propria and in glandular epithelium. Accumulation of granulocytes and necrotic debris in the lumen of glands forms so-called crypt abscesses. Greater severity of the lesion is reflected in attenuation and exfoliation of surface epithelium and the development of microerosions on the mucosal surface (Fig. 1.16C). Inflammatory cells, mainly neutrophils, and tissue fluid effuse into the lumen through defects in the epithelium. Persistent erosion or previous erosion in a healed mucosa is marked by the development of a thin, horizontally arrayed layer of connective tissue in the superficial lamina propria. With increasing chronicity in colitis of mild or moderate degree, there may be deposition of a collagenous stroma, throughout which inflammatory cells are interspersed, which separates glands abnormally throughout the mucosa. Downgrowth of glands into submucosal lymphoid follicles may occur in chronic colitis.

Severe erosion and ulceration is usually associated with local acute inflammation and with a heavy, mainly mononuclear-cell

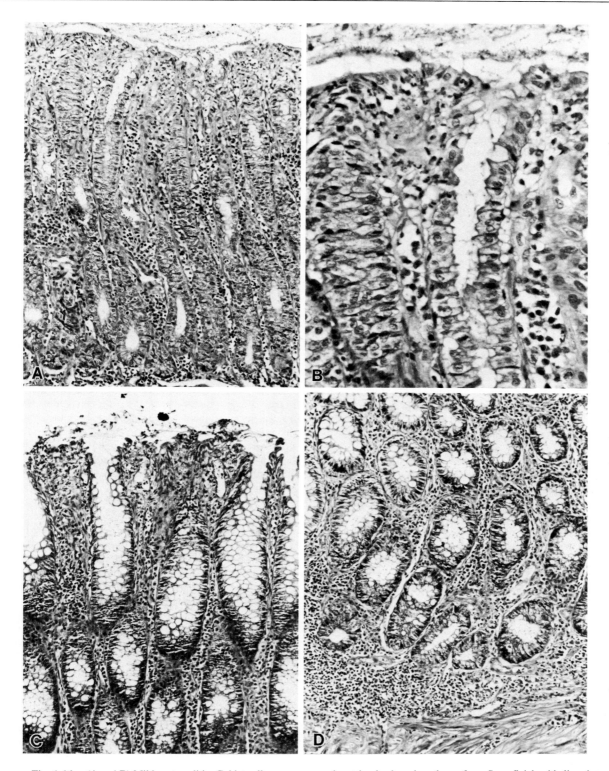

Fig. 1.16. (A and B) Mild acute colitis. Goblet cells are sparse or absent in glands and on the surface. Superficial epithelium is cuboidal and exfoliating in focal areas. Epithelium in glands is hyperplastic and crowded. The superficial lamina propria is edematous. (C and D) Chronic erosive colitis. Hypertrophic glands are lined by goblet cells. The mucosal surface has widespread erosion and effusion of tissue fluid and neutrophils. Edema of superficial lamina propria. Deeper in mucosa there is moderately increased population of mononuclear cells and increased fibrous stroma. Cells extend between base of glands and muscularis mucosae.

infiltrate in the lamina propria and, often, submucosa. The ulcerated areas extend usually no further than the muscularis mucosae and have a base of granulation tissue infiltrated heavily by neutrophils that effuse into the lumen of the bowel. The margin of surviving mucosa may overhang the ulcer. Crypt abscesses may be present in remaining mucosa, and all degrees of erosion and partial ulceration may be present. Idiopathic ulcerative colitis does not seem as severe as histiocytic ulcerative colitis of boxers and rarely comes to autopsy. Severely affected dogs may be cachectic, probably due in part to enteric loss of plasma protein. The mucosa in ulcerative colitis is usually deep red, swollen, folded, and granular due to edema and cellular infiltrates; the depressions may be punctate or up to several centimeters across, roughly round or oval, irregular or elongate. Their margins may be tattered or puckered. Colonic lymph nodes may be enlarged and edematous.

In canine colitis there is a broad, three-dimensional spectrum: in chronicity and density of the inflammatory infiltrate, in the distribution of the infiltrate within the wall of the bowel, and in the severity of the epithelial and mucosal change. Generally, milder lesions of superficial epithelium are associated with mild or moderate mucosal inflammation, which may be acute or chronic. In many cases of mild chronic mucosal colitis, the glands do not appear particularly hyperplastic; the mucosa may appear thin or atrophic. Severe erosion and ulceration are usually related to a more intense or heavy chronic inflammatory process, which may be limited to the mucosa, but which can extend into the submucosa. Truly granulomatous colitis is uncommon; when fully developed, perhaps as a component of a regional enteritis involving the ileocecocolic area, it is ulcerative and transmural.

Eosinophilic colitis forms part of the syndrome of eosinophilic gastroenteritis discussed previously. It conforms to the general description of the spectrum of lesions in idiopathic colitis, with the exception that eosinophils form a predominant part of the cellular infiltrate in the mucosa and superficial submucosa.

Histiocytic ulcerative colitis is a distinctive syndrome histologically, which has been recognized only in boxers and the related French bulldog. It is a chronic ulcerative colitis characterized by the presence of large numbers of macrophages, containing PAS-positive granules, in the deep mucosa and submucosa and in lymph nodes receiving drainage from the colon. Clinically, affected animals are usually under 2 years of age. This condition causes typical large bowel diarrhea, with mucus and blood; weight loss occurs, and chronic cases may become cachectic, probably due to protein loss into the gut.

Grossly, the colon of dogs with advanced disease is variably thickened, folded, and perhaps dilated and shortened, with some segmental or focal areas of scarring and stricture. Lesions on the mucosa may vary from patchy, punctate red ulcers to more extensive irregular, circular, or linear lesions that may coalesce, leaving only a few islands of persistent mucosa on a granulating colonic surface (Fig. 1.17A).

Early microscopic lesions are those of mild nonspecific inflammation. Microerosion of epithelium in the upper glands and on the surface is associated with local acute inflammation, migration of neutrophils into the epithelium, and effusion of neutrophils and tissue fluid into the lumen. Macrophages in these

areas may contain phagocytized necrotic debris and bacteria. In some areas the mucosa is thinned, and glands are relatively shortened, though lining epithelium appears hyperplastic. Macrophages with cytoplasmic vacuoles, which contain PAS-positive material, are mainly deep in the lamina propria and in the submucosa (Fig. 1.17B,C). Sometimes they may be relatively sparse in the mucosa, and may be missed in small biopsy specimens if the submucosa is not sampled. These same cells may be found about lymphatics in the muscularis and the serosa, and they may be numerous in subcapsular, cortical, and medullary sinuses in the draining lymph nodes. The cecum is often involved, to a lesser degree, with similar lesions. True granulomatous foci and giant cells are rarely encountered.

Ulceration seems to progress from the superficial epithelial erosion and destruction of the basement membrane seen in early lesions. Ulcers usually do not progress beyond the submucosa, and they are lined by granulation tissue. The bed of the ulcer is necrotic, and numerous neutrophils and erythrocytes may be passing into the lumen.

The cause of the condition is unknown, as is the origin of the material in the characteristic vacuoles in macrophages. Ultrastructural study suggests that these are digestion vacuoles, containing mainly remnants of phospholipid membranes. The material being digested may be phagocytosed cell debris and microorganisms picked up in the superficial lamina propria and carried in "constipated" macrophages to deeper structures. Certainly, bodies resembling microorganisms have been found in macrophages, and the involvement of chlamydiae, rickettsias, and mycoplasmas has been postulated. It seems that a defect in lysosomal function may exist in some boxer dogs that can lead to the accumulation of partially digested phospholipid membrane in macrophages, since similar histiocytes do not accumulate in ulcerative colitis in other breeds of dogs.

Colitis in Cats

Colitis in cats is rare. The most common cause is feline panleukopenia, in which over half the cases have colonic lesions. They are similar to, but rarely as severe or widespread as, the lesions found in the small intestine of all animals dying of the disease. The relative paucity and mildness of lesions in the colon is related to the lower rate of epithelial proliferation in comparison with the small intestine. The pathology of panleukopenia is considered under Infectious and Parasitic Diseases of the Gastrointestinal Tract.

Occasional cases of **mycotic colitis** are found in cats. These are associated with a hemorrhagic ulcerative colitis, in which focal or diffuse mucosal invasion by *Candida*, zygomycetes, or *Aspergillus* has occurred, sometimes causing microvascular thrombosis. These are mainly secondary to primary colonic damage and leukopenia caused by panleukopenia.

Necrotic colitis has also been described in cats, but very rarely. The condition is reported mainly in older animals, as a cause of chronic foul, and sometimes bloody, diarrhea. The colon and rectum are thickened, rough, and congested or hemorrhagic. The microscopic change is mucosal erosion or ulceration associated with severe damage to colonic glands (Fig. 1.17D). Crypt-lining cells are cuboidal or flattened, and necrotic debris may be in the lumen of glands. Some glands may be collapsed due to complete epithelial necrosis. The lesion resembles that of

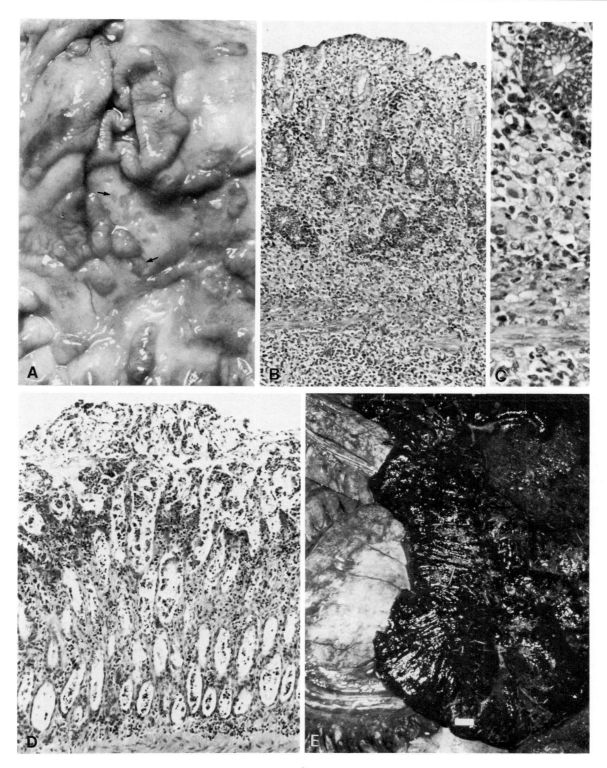

Fig. 1.17. (A–C) Histiocytic ulcerative colitis. Boxer dog. (A) Mucosa is thickened and edematous. There are numerous ulcers (arrows). (B) Accumulation of macrophages with extensive cytoplasm throughout mucosa, between base of glands and muscularis mucosae, and in submucosa. (C) Detail of macrophages in mucosa deep to crypts. (D) Necrotic colitis. Cat. Active necrosis on surface of mucosa. Glands are dilated, contain necrotic cellular debris, or are lined by extremely flattened epithelium. (Courtesy of J. S. Nimmo Wilkie.) (E) Acute colitis ("colitis X"). Horse. The mucosa is very congested and edematous.

panleukopenia but is generally more hemorrhagic and necrotic. The cause is unknown.

Ulcerative colitis, grossly and microscopically similar to idiopathic ulcerative colitis of the dog, occurs very rarely in cats. Granulomatous or pyogranulomatous foci in the subserosa or submucosa may cause regional enterocolitis, characterized by fibrosis and serosal nodularity of affected segments, usually without severe mucosal defects. Fibrinoid arteritis causing hemorrhage and edema in the colonic submucosa, and perhaps ischemic necrosis of the mucosa, is also reported. The granulomatous syndrome is attributed to feline infectious peritonitis, and there may be characteristic lesions in other organs.

Typhlocolitis in Horses

The diagnosis of acute colitis in horses resolves into the differentiation of peracute and acute salmonellosis from a similar condition, colitis X. Both of these must be differentiated from the sequelae of intestinal accidents and thromboembolism involving the large bowel.

Colitis X is a sporadic acute disease, usually but not always associated with profuse, foul-smelling, but rarely bloody, diarrhea. Some horses may die without having diarrhea. The remainder of the clinical syndrome is a reflection of the profound shock that occurs. At autopsy the animal is dehydrated, and there may be subcutaneous and serosal petechial hemorrhage. The blood is dark and clots poorly. Enteric lesions are virtually limited to the large bowel, which is distended with abnormally fluid content. The serosa of the cecum and large colon may appear cyanotic from congestion and hemorrhage in the mucosa (Fig. 1.17E) and perhaps submucosa. The deeper tissues of the intestinal wall are not themselves compromised, as is the case usually in volvulus and often in thromboembolic infarction. The mucosa and submucosa are commonly markedly edematous, and edema is often present at the mesenteric attachment of the gut and in the cecal and colic lymph nodes. The mucosa may appear brown and necrotic with focal fibrinohemorrhagic exudate on the surface. More commonly it is deeply congested with focal hemorrhage, but blood is rarely present to significant degree in the contents. Gross lesions in other organs are those consistent with circulatory or endotoxic shock.

The microscopic lesions in the large bowel include superficial or full-thickness necrosis of the mucosa, associated with dilatation and perhaps thrombosis of small mucosal and submucosal venules. There is hemorrhage and edema in the mucosa, and the submucosa is markedly edematous, with dilated lymphatics. Some neutrophils may be evident in the mucosa or submucosa, and fibrin may be effusing from the damaged mucosal surface in less advanced cases. Submucosal lymphoid follicles show evidence of recent severe lymphocytolysis. Congestion, microvascular thrombosis, and hemorrhage may be found in a variety of other organs, especially the adrenal cortex.

The pathogenesis of colitis X is uncertain and may be multifactorial. It seems likely that it, probably salmonellosis, and some even less well defined chronic diarrheas in horses are the result of dysbacteriosis of the large bowel. Animals developing these conditions frequently have a recent history of change in feed, hard training, shipment, surgery, antibiotic (especially tetracycline) therapy, or other intervention.

Proliferation of *Clostridium perfringens* type A has been associated with the development of signs consistent in some cases with colitis X. Increased protein in the ration may predispose to establishment of *C. perfringens,* which is apparently an uncommon inhabitant of the equine bowel. Toxin that is locally necrotizing may be the factor initiating mucosal damage, and perhaps observed changes in function of the liver and other organs are partly the result of absorbed toxin. Experimental infusion of extracts of *C. perfringens* type A exotoxin in ponies has marked systemic effects and causes severe edema and hemorrhage of the colonic mucosa and submucosa as well as sloughing of epithelium on the tips of villi in the small intestine. The proliferation of *C. perfringens* precedes the clinical episode, and the organism may not be numerous in the large bowel at death.

Endotoxin may also play a role, either by absorption through a mucosa already damaged by previous insult or by release of abnormal amounts following a change in the flora in the large intestine. Systemic effects of endotoxin may contribute to shock and to the microthrombosis and disseminated intravascular coagulation that sometimes occur.

The precedent for clostridial toxin- or endotoxin-mediated typhlocolitis following disruption of the gut flora lies in similar antibiotic-induced lesions in rabbits, guinea pigs, hamsters, and humans. Lincomycin-associated colitis resembling colitis X has been reported in horses. Tetracycline is excreted in the bile, and high concentrations in the gut may alter the flora in treated horses, permitting the intrusion of new inhabitants or proliferation of previously minor components.

Subacute and chronic diarrheas in horses may be associated with small intestinal malabsorption, but most involve the large intestine, with or without the small bowel. *Salmonella* typhlocolitis must be suspected in such cases. Salmonellosis in horses may have an extremely variable course and pathologic manifestations (see Infectious and Parasitic Diseases of the Gastrointestinal Tract). Suppurative ulcers involving lymphoid tissue in the typhlocolic mucosa, and cecal and colic lymphadenitis, characterize enteric infection with *Corynebacterium equi* in foals. Extensive mucosal involvement by larval cyathostomes and strongyles and, rarely, ulcerative typhlitis due to anoplocephalid tapeworms also may cause diarrhea and wasting; they are discussed with specific parasitisms. Chronic diarrhea and, possibly, cachexia may also result from persistent ulceration of the cecum or colon due to ischemic mucosal lesions. These may be the product of arterial thromboembolism and slow flow or, less likely, corrected strangulation with reflow. Phenylbutazone administration also has been associated with cecal and colonic ulceration and plasma protein loss.

The specific cause of extensive ulceration may be difficult to determine. Smaller chronic ulcers and widespread subacute erosion and ulceration are most likely the result of salmonellosis, rather than ischemia, and the agent should be sought by culture of the affected area, preferably by trituration of tissue and use of selective media.

Granulomatous and eosinophilic typhlocolitis in horses are extensions of the lesions considered previously with syndromes in the small bowel causing diarrhea and protein-losing enteropathy.

Chronic diarrhea occurs that does not appear to be related to morphologic lesions in the mucosa of the gut. Affected horses have a history of unformed cowpat-like feces, or overt diarrhea, which may persist for weeks, months, and occasionally, years with only periodic temporary remission. Examination of the feces may reveal none of the normal ciliate protozoan fauna, but often many flagellates, especially *Tritrichomonas,* are present. It seems likely that the large number of these flagellate protozoa, and the paucity of ciliates, reflect gross alterations in the micro-environment and flora in the large bowel. If these changes also cause altered fermentation of carbohydrate and, perhaps, reduced production and absorption of volatile fatty acids, the diarrhea, and gradual reduction in body condition that often occurs, might be explained. These horses will show transient response to therapeutic agents that affect anaerobic bacteria and protozoa, but they usually regress when medication is withdrawn. The response to implants of cecal or colonic content is variable and usually discouraging.

Typhlocolitis in Swine

The differential diagnosis of typholocolitis in swine revolves mainly around identifying swine dysentery, *Salmonella* enterocolitis, and the large bowel manifestations of the intestinal adenomatosis complex in weaned pigs. The latter condition is readily recognized by the consistent concurrent involvement of the terminal ileum by adenomatosis, with or without hemorrhage, or by necrotic ileitis. Mucosal thickening is reflected in the presence of the characteristic cerebriform folds of the serosal aspect of the bowel that is commonly seen. Lesions in the large bowel are present in a minority of cases and involve the cecum and proximal colon; they resemble the ileal lesions in being either adenomatous or necrotic.

Swine dysentery involves only the cecum and spiral colon. It is a catarrhal to mildly fibrinohemorrhagic erosive mucosal typhlocolitis. The colonic content is fluid and usually blood tinged. *Salmonella* enterocolitis, mainly due to *S. typhimurium,* is a fibrinous, erosive to focally ulcerative condition, mainly of the cecum and colon but perhaps involving the small intestine, especially terminal ileum. The content is fluid but usually not bloody. Mesenteric lymph nodes are prominent. Button ulcers or necrotic enteritis in the lower intestine may occur in chronic salmonellosis, in subacute to chronic forms of hog cholera, and perhaps in African swine fever.

Campylobacter associated with intestinal adenomatosis is readily identified in smears of affected mucosa stained with carbolfuchsin, and the large spirochetes causing swine dysentery may also be identified in mucosal scrapings at necropsy. Culture of affected tissues confirms these diagnoses and that of salmonellosis.

Escherichia coli may cause fibrinohemorrhagic enterocolitis in piglets about weaning, and intestinal adenomatosis may also occur in older suckling and in weanling piglets.

Fibrinohemorrhagic typhlitis is caused by heavy infestations with *Trichuris suis,* especially in weaned pigs with access to pastures and yards. Under similar circumstances, *Eimeria* infection rarely may cause ileotyphlocolitis.

Rectal stricture appears to be a product of ischemic proctitis, probably related in many cases to infection with *Salmonella typhimurium.*

Typhlocolitis in Ruminants

In cattle more than 2 or 3 months of age, diagnostic considerations in acute to subacute fibrinohemorrhagic typhlocolitis include salmonellosis, bovine virus diarrhea, rinderpest (in enzootic areas or populations at risk), coccidiosis, malignant catarrhal fever, and adenovirus infection. Lesions of the oral cavity and upper alimentary tract may be expected but are not necessarily present in bovine virus diarrhea, rinderpest, and malignant head catarrh; in the latter, lymphadenopathy and lesions of the trachea, bladder, parenchymatous organs, eye, and brain may also be present. Lesions affecting Peyer's patches in the small intestine strongly suggest bovine virus diarrhea or rinderpest. Coronavirus causes microscopic lesions in colonic crypts, as well as in small intestine, in young calves. Rarely, a mild fibrinous typhlocolitis is seen grossly. Salmonellosis affects all age groups from neonate to adult and may frequently involve both small and large intestine in catarrhal to fibrinohemorrhagic enteritis; mesenteric lymph nodes are usually enlarged. Coccidiosis may involve ileum and large intestine; it often can be diagnosed by mucosal scraping at autopsy. Adenovirus infection may cause severe hemorrhagic colitis, with few lesions elsewhere, as may malignant head catarrh on occasion. Arsenic, other heavy metals, and oak or acorn poisoning may also cause hemorrhagic typhlocolitis and dysentery. Rarely, trichuriasis causes a hemorrhagic mucosal typhlitis in calves.

Chronic fibrinous or ulcerative typhlocolitis may occur in salmonellosis, bovine virus diarrhea, and coccidiosis.

Granulomatous typhlocolitis associated with chronic diarrhea and wasting may occur in Johne's disease, concurrently with granulomatous ileitis and mesenteric lymphadenitis. The mucosa of the large bowel in these cases is thickened and rugose. Impressions of affected mucosa or ileocecal lymph node will contain acid-fast bacilli. Johne's disease in sheep and goats is associated usually with wasting but not diarrhea. The large bowel may be involved in a minority of cases; the ileum is consistently affected.

In sheep, hemorrhagic typhlocolitis may be present in animals with bluetongue; it is rarely the only lesion. Heavy-metal intoxication is the only other significant cause of hemorrhagic typhlocolitis and dysentery in older animals. Salmonellosis may cause fibrinohemorrhagic enteritis in lambs and pregnant ewes, and trichuriasis will occur rarely. Coccidiosis (*Eimeria* spp.) may be implicated in hemorrhagic ileotyphlocolitis in lambs and kids, though the small intestine is usually more commonly and severely involved; lesions of the large intestine are exceptional.

Hyperplastic and Neoplastic Diseases of the Intestine

Tumors of the intestine, either benign or malignant, are uncommon in domestic animals. Polyps are generally hyperplastic or regenerative rather than neoplastic. The exceptions are rectal polyps in dogs, which are usually adenomas or, less commonly, carcinomas. Highly malignant scirrhous adenocarcinomas occur in all species. The prevalence of this tumor in sheep is high in certain areas of the world.

Lymphosarcoma is the most common malignant tumor of

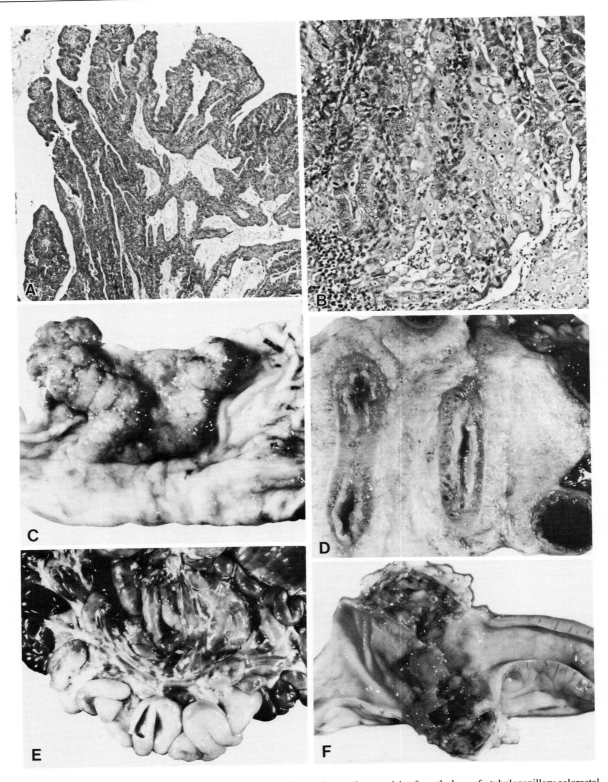

Fig. 1.18.   (**A**) Tubulopapillary colorectal polyp. Dog.   (**B**) Invasive carcinoma arising from the base of a tubulopapillary colorectal polyp in a dog.   (**C**) Rectal polyp. Dog.   (**D** and **E**) White areas of scirrhous intestinal adenocarcinoma invading colon (**D**) and ileum (**E**). Sheep.   (**F**) Annular ulcerating leiomyosarcoma. Cat.

mesenchymal origin in most animals; it is most prevalent in the cat. Lymphosarcoma may arise in the gut, although involvement of this area is more often part of multicentric disease (see the Hematopoietic System, Volume 3).

A hyperplastic condition of intestinal crypts in the ileum and colon in swine and some other species, called intestinal adenomatosis or proliferative ileitis, is described under *Campylobacter* Enteritis.

Colorectal Polyps in Dogs

These tumors are most common at the anal–rectal junction in middle-aged dogs. There is no apparent breed or sex predisposition. Prolapse of the polyp, rectal bleeding following defecation, chronic dyschezia, and diarrhea are the most common clinical signs associated with this tumor.

Macroscopically, the tumor is usually sessile or slightly pedunculated (Fig. 1.18C); it may be firm or friable and hemorrhagic. The mucosal surface is often ulcerated. It varies in size from one to several centimeters in diameter.

Microscopically, the polyp may have a predominantly tubular or papillary growth pattern (Fig. 1.18A). In well-oriented specimens the tubular pattern is characterized by branching crypts lined by usually well differentiated columnar to cuboidal epithelial cells. These are supported by the lamina propria. The papillary type consists of villus-like projections of proprial connective tissue covered by a single pseudostratified layer of columnar epithelial cells. There may be loss of nuclear polarity, and nucleoli are prominent in epithelium in both types of polyp. The number of mitotic figures varies from one tumor to another. The stalk of the tumor is highly vascular and is continuous with the lamina propria or submucosa of the rectum.

Some polyps are malignant (Fig. 1.18B). These are characterized by the presence of anaplastic epithelial cells *in situ* in the mucosa and, rarely, in the stalk of propria. There is little information on the biologic behavior of these tumors. Adequate surgical removal usually results in complete recovery. As in humans, the size of the tumor may be related to the prognosis. Polyps more than 1.0 cm in diameter tend to have a more anaplastic appearance and appear to recur more commonly. Some become invasive adenocarcinoma. Rectal polyps must be differentiated from rectal carcinoids, which they resemble grossly in dogs.

Polypoid Tumors in Other Species

Polypoid masses varying in diameter from one to several centimeters may be found at any level of the intestine in other species, especially cattle, They are usually an incidental finding except in those cases where they are large enough to cause partial obstruction. The tumors are raised, often pedunculated, gray to brown masses on the mucosal surface. They may occur in grape-like clusters. Miscroscopically, they resemble benign rectal polyps in the dog.

A high prevalence of intestinal adenomas and to a lesser extent adenocarcinomas in cattle has been reported in upland areas in Scotland and northern England. These tumors often coexist with papillomas and squamous-cell carcinomas of the upper alimentary tract (see Neoplasia of the Esophagus and Forestomachs). Three types of adenoma are recognized in the intestine of affected cattle in these endemic areas: a sessile plaque, an adenomatous polyp, and a more proliferative adenoma of the ampullae, where the bile and pancreatic ducts open into the duodenum.

Intestinal Adenocarcinoma

DOGS. Intestinal adenocarcinoma is uncommon in dogs. About 40% of all gastrointestinal carcinomas in dogs occur in the colon and rectum. The rest are equally divided between the stomach and small intestine, mainly duodenum. The average age of dogs with intestinal carcinomas is 8–9 years. Some investigators have reported a higher prevalence of intestinal carcinomas in male dogs, with a breed predisposition in boxers, collies, and German shepherds.

Macroscopically, the tumors appear as gray-white, firm, sometimes annular, stenotic areas that commonly affect the entire thickness of the intestinal wall (Fig. 1.19A). These tumors often do not ulcerate, and they usually do not project into the lumen of the gut. The papillary type of intestinal adenocarcinomas do form intraluminal masses, which tend to involve larger segments of the intestine, suggesting horizontal spread. There is dilation of the gut anterior to stenotic and obstructive tumors, and there may be hypertrophy of the intestinal muscularis proximal to such neoplasms.

On the basis of the microscopic appearance, intestinal carcinomas in dogs have been divided into four types, which may overlap. The **acinar type** is characterized by irregular glandular structures that obliterate the normal mucosa and infiltrate into submucosa and muscularis. The epithelial cells lining the acini are basophilic, cuboidal to columnar, and have small hyperchromatic nuclei in the basilar area of the cell. Amorphous eosinophilic material often fills the lumen of the glandular structures. Mucin is rarely found in this type of tumor. There is usually extensive necrosis, with marked inflammation and fibrosis in the gut wall of the affected areas. At the periphery of these tumors there may be hyperplasia of cryptal and villous epithelial cells.

In the **solid type** of intestinal carcinoma, the mucosa and gut wall are extensively infiltrated by nests and sheets of anaplastic epithelial cells. These have only a slight tendency to differentiate to acinar structures. The tumor cells have abundant amphophilic to basophilic cytoplasm and large vesicular nuclei with prominent nucleoli. There are some "signet-ring cells" and a few islets of mucin.

In the **mucinous type** of carcinoma, the anaplastic epithelial cells have pale eosinophilic cytoplasm. There are many "signet-ring cells." Large pools of extracellular mucin are evident in the stroma.

The **papillary type** consists of papilliferous projections into the lumen, covered by columnar, often highly anaplastic epithelial cells. The mitotic index tends to be high. There is goblet-cell hyperplasia of both crypts and villi. This type usually is only locally invasive.

With the exception of papillary adenocarcinomas, desmoplasia is is a prominent feature of these neoplasms, explaining their common tendency to cause stricture and obstruction of the intestine.

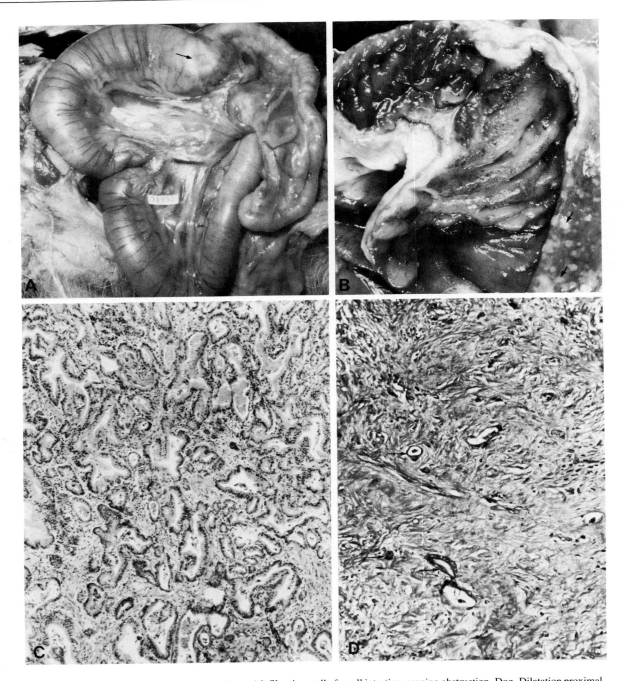

Fig. 1.19.   (**A**) Scirrhous adenocarcinoma (arrow) infiltrating wall of small intestine, causing obstruction. Dog. Dilatation proximal to obstruction and contraction of empty distal intestine.   (**B**) Intestinal carcinoma. Cow. There is annular thickening of intestine with carcinomatous serosal plaques (arrows).   (**C**) Well-differentiated intestinal adenocarcinoma. Cat.   (**D**) Intestinal adenocarcinoma. Sheep. Islands of neoplastic epithelium (arrows) scattered in extensive desmoplastic reaction.

All types, except possibly the papillary type, metastasize widely, mainly via the lymphatics to the regional nodes. Involvement of the small intestine leads to metastases mainly in the mesenteric lymph nodes, less commonly to other abdominal nodes, liver, spleen, and lungs. Colonic adenocarcinomas metastasize to colic, iliac, and other pelvic and abdominal nodes. Metastases may also occur in most abdominal organs and in the lungs. Implantation on serosal surfaces may result in obstruction of lymphatics, followed by ascites. In a few cases, malignant cells may migrate retrograde in the lymphatics of the abdomen and pelvic limbs, causing edema of the abdominal wall and legs.

CATS. Next to lymphosarcoma, intestinal adenocarcinoma is the most common intestinal tumor in cats. The prevalence of intestinal carcinomas is lower in cats than in dogs. They may be more common in Siamese cats compared to other breeds. As in dogs, male cats have been reported to have a higher prevalence of this tumor than females. The mean age of cats with intestinal carcinomas is 10 to 11 years with a range of 4 to 14 years.

The ileum is the most common site affected, followed by the jejunum. When the tumor is located at the ileocecal junction, both the large and small intestine are usually involved. Intestinal carcinomas in cats rarely arise in the large intestine. The clinical signs and gross appearance are similar to those in dogs.

With some minor variations, the morphologic types of intestinal carcinomas described for dogs also occur in cats (Fig. 1.19C). Osteochondroid metaplasia is a frequent feature of all types of adenocarcinoma in the cat. The rare carcinomas involving the large intestine have been mainly of the papillary type. They tend to be better differentiated and less scirrhous than carcinomas involving the small intestine.

The biologic behavior of intestinal carcinomas in cats is similar to that found in dogs.

SHEEP. Intestinal adenocarcinoma is relatively common in sheep in New Zealand, Iceland, Scotland, and southeastern Australia. The cause of the high prevalence of intestinal carcinomas in these areas is unknown but may be related to exposure to bracken fern. It occurs mainly in animals five years of age or older. Clinically, affected sheep lose weight and have distended abdomens.

The tumors are usually located in the middle or lower areas of the small intestine (Fig. 1.18E). They are dense, firm, white masses, $\frac{1}{2}$ to several centimeters long and up to 1.0 cm thick, which may form annular constrictive bands at the affected site. Cauliflower-like growths may be evident on the serosal surface. Polyps may protrude into the lumen, but ulceration of the mucosa is uncommon. The distal edge of the tumor is generally well demarcated. There is dilation of the intestine proximal to the lesion.

Metastasis occurs along the serosal lymphatics to the mesenteric lymph nodes. Implantations on serosal surfaces are common, and these appear as opaque to white plaques or diffusely thickened areas, which must be differentiated from mesothelioma. Obstruction of serosal lymphatics by tumor emboli may lead to ascites. Lung and liver metastases are rare.

Microscopically, the tumor is characterized by solid sheets or nests of highly anaplastic polyhedral, cuboidal, or columnar epithelial cells that may form irregular acinar structures. Mitotic figures and acinar differentiation are infrequent. The neoplastic cells infiltrate the submucosa and the muscularis through to the serosal surface, whence they spread via the lymphatics to the mesenteric lymph nodes. This is apparently followed by retrograde lymphogenous metastasis to the gut wall proximal to the primary tumor. These secondary tumors are particularly responsible for constriction of the gut lumen. The infiltrating tumor is always accompanied by a very scirrhous reaction (Figs. 1.18D and 1.19D). Sclerotic masses with anaplastic epithelial cells, which are located on the serosal surfaces of the abdominal organs, rarely infiltrate the parenchyma. Argentaffin cells may form part of some intestinal carcinomas, especially in lymph node metastases. Mineralization and osseous metaplasia may be evident in the stroma of some tumors.

OTHER SPECIES. Intestinal carcinomas generally are rare in cattle and swine (Fig. 1.19B), with the exception of those associated with bracken fern, papillomavirus, and upper alimentary cancer in cattle in certain parts of the United Kingdom, mentioned previously. They are usually an incidental finding at meat inspection. The location, morphology, and routes of metastasis are similar to those described for sheep, except that serosal lesions are less obvious. Liver and lung metastases may occur in cattle.

Carcinoid Tumors of the Intestine

Carcinoid tumors arise from endocrine or paracrine cells, which are located in the mucosal lining of a wide variety of organs, including the stomach and the intestine. These cells secrete vasoactive amines, which are responsible for the argentaffinic and argyrophilic tinctorial properties of the tumors. Functional derangements from excessive production of amines have not been reported in animals.

Carcinoid tumors of the gastrointestinal tract are rare in domestic animals. They have been reported mainly in aged dogs and occur rarely in the cat and cow. In dogs, carcinoids are mainly located in the duodenum, colon, and rectum. Clinically, they may cause intestinal obstruction and anemia due to hemorrhage from ulcers. Rectal carcinoids may protrude from the anus and resemble adenomatous polyps.

Macroscopically, carcinoids are usually lobulated, firm, dark red to cream-colored masses in the wall of the intestine. The tumor may result in submucosal or subserosal nodule formation. Microscopically, carcinoids have a distinct endocrine appearance. Round or oval to polyhedral cells have abundant finely granular eosinophilic or vacuolated cytoplasm and vesiculate nuclei with prominent nucleoli. They form nests, ribbons, rosettes, or diffuse sheets in the mucosa, submucosa, and muscularis. A fine, vascularized stroma divides the tumor masses. Amyloid may be present in intercellular and perivascular spaces. Multinucleate giant cells are occasionally seen.

Confirmation of the diagnosis requires special stains to reveal argentaffinic and argyrophilic properties. These histochemical reactions may be negative, especially in rectal carcinoids. They may also be lost during fixation in formalin. Electron microscopic examination helps to differentiate carcinoids from intestinal mast-cell tumors. Carcinoid tumor cells have dense, round to oval, membrane-bound secretory granules in the cytoplasm that vary in diameter from 75 to 300 nm. They have abundant rough endoplasmic reticulum, and the plasma membrane forms interdigitating processes. The ultrastructural characteristics of intestinal mast-cell tumors are described later. Carcinoid tumors are PAS-negative and do not show metachromasia with Giemsa stains.

Data on biologic behavior of intestinal carcinoids in dogs are limited. The few cases that have been reported were malignant. There may be extensive invasion of the gut wall and veins, with metastasis especially to the liver. In this respect their behavior is similar to intestinal carcinoids in humans.

Intestinal Mast-Cell Tumors

Intestinal mast-cell tumors are uncommon. They occur mainly in aged cats and, rarely, in dogs. They resemble carcinoid morphologically under the light microscope, and a definitive diagnosis requires histochemical and ultrastructural examination of tumor cells. They appear to be more common than intestinal carcinoid tumors in cats. Abnormal mast cells do not appear in circulation.

These tumors are mainly located in the small intestine, rarely in the colon. Affected areas in the gut are tan-colored, firm, thickened, and may be one to several centimeters in length. The overlying mucosa bulges into the gut lumen but rarely ulcerates. Nests, cords, and whorls of pleomorphic mast cells infiltrate the mucosa and adjacent areas of the gut wall. Cells in intestinal mast-cell tumors are unlike mast cells in mastocytomas involving the skin and other organs. The latter are round and have an intensely eosinophilic granular cytoplasm with distinct cytoplasmic borders and central oval nuclei. In contrast, cells in intestinal mastocytomas are polygonal to spindle-shaped. They have a finely granular or vacuolated cytoplasm with indistinct cytoplasmic borders and oval, hyperchromatic, eccentrically located nuclei. The degree of metachromatic staining varies considerably, and there is a marked variation in the number of eosinophils.

Ultrastructurally, the cells in most respects resemble typical degranulated mast cells. The cytoplasm contains many membrane-bound granules, which appear as singular or fused vesicles. Fine fibrillar material forms a loose network within these vesicles. A few tumor cells contains electron-dense fibrillar granules or intermediate forms. None of the tumor cells contains the crystalline, electron-dense granules present in normal mast cells and in mastocytomas in other sites.

Metastases occur most often in the mesenteric lymph nodes, followed by the liver, spleen, and rarely, the lungs. Ulceration of the gastrointestinal mucosa occurs commonly with visceral mast-cell tumors in cats and large cutaneous mastocytomas in dogs. Mucosal ulceration is not a feature of intestinal mast-cell tumors in the cat. This may be due to low levels of histamine in the cells in intestinal tumors.

Other Mesenchymal Intestinal Tumors

Leiomyomas and leiomyosarcomas (Fig. 1.18F) are probably more common than other types of mesenchymal tumors besides lymphosarcoma. These tumors occur most commonly in the small intestine, where they cause obstruction. They tend to be nodular rather than diffuse, and ulcerate and cavitate on the luminal surface. The histologic appearance is similar to smooth muscle tumors in other sites.

Infectious and Parasitic Diseases of the Gastrointestinal Tract

Viral Diseases

FOOT AND MOUTH DISEASE . Foot and mouth disease (aphthous fever) is a viral infection of ruminants and swine and of at least 30 species of wild animals. It is a problem of worldwide concern, being enzootic in large areas of Africa, Asia, Europe, and South America. In addition to these areas are others that are periodically visited by the virus and in whose susceptible populations the disease spreads rapidly. Some other areas, notably Japan, Australia, New Zealand, and North America, are currently free because of geographic isolation and quarantine restrictions. Foot and mouth disease is not notable for a high mortality rate, except in sucklings, but the morbidity rate is very high and in an affected population productivity is reduced substantially.

The virus of foot and mouth disease belongs to the Picornaviridae, in the genus *Aphthovirus* (*aphtha* = vesicles in the mouth). The virus is highly resistant under many circumstances but is inactivated by direct sunlight and moderate acidity. The acid production that accompanies rigor mortis in carcasses and meat inactivates the virus. The alteration in pH is not dependable, however, and the virus survives in offal, viscera, lymph nodes, and bone marrow for an indefinite period under refrigeration. It may survive on hay and other fomites for several weeks.

This resistance of the virus is of epidemiologic significance, especially where control policies involve slaughter rather than vaccination. But probably of much greater importance is the confirmation that many infected animals remain carriers. The carrier state has been observed in cattle, sheep, and African buffalo. Swine apparently become carriers, but less commonly than other species. Experimental transmission of virus from carrier swine to a susceptible animal, through contact, has never been accomplished. Virus recovered from carriers will infect susceptible animals by means of inoculation. Persistence of infection in convalescence has been extensively examined only in cattle, and the carrier state persists for up to 9 months. The virus is carried mainly in the pharynx and on the dorsal surface of the soft palate, but the host cells are unidentified and the carrier state exists even in animals with a significant level of serum neutralizing antibody.

Of equal importance to the persistence of the virus is its antigenic heterogeneity and instability. There are seven principal antigenic types, namely, the classical A, O, and C types, SAT-1, SAT-2, SAT-3, and Asia-1. These can be distinguished by serologic tests, although there are various degrees of overlap. In addition to being serologically different, these seven types are sufficiently different immunologically that infection with one type does not confer resistance to the other six. Within these seven major types there are antigenic subtypes, each different, to variable degrees, from the parent type. Generally, the subtypes cross-immunize to a useful degree, but exceptions do arise and become recognizable, especially when vaccination fails. Antigenic drift can also be demonstrated experimentally; new subtypes can be produced by passing the virus in immune or partially immune animals, or by growing the virus *in vitro* in the presence of immune serum. There are presently at least 60 distinct antigenic strains of the virus of natural origin and no reason to think that the possibility of recombination of subtypes is exhausted.

As well as differences and variability in antigenic characters, strains of the virus differ in virulence, and a given strain is probably able to vary in virulence although this is difficult to measure satisfactorily. Certainly, comparing different outbreaks, there is considerable variation in the severity of the disease produced in a given host species. Virulence also varies between species. Although the virus is pathogenic for all cloven-footed, domestic, and wild species, a given strain at any time is of different virulence for the different species. Some strains, for example, will infect pigs but not cattle, and others are pathogenic for cattle and not for pigs. A similar relationship pertains for sheep and goats, but in general, virus strains are intermediate between these extremes. There can be little doubt, however, that the adaptation to a host species does occur and that this adaptive relationship may establish a reservoir of infection.

In addition to the domestic hosts, humans can become infected, but not importantly, either clinically or epidemiologically. The hedgehog, coypu, and some marsupials are highly susceptible to infection and could be important in the transmission of the disease. Some laboratory animals are also susceptible, the white mouse in particular. Suckling mice inoculated intraperitoneally are susceptible enough to be used for detection of small amounts of virus. They consistently develop degeneration of skeletal musculature, and in ~50% there is myocardial degeneration and, in a variable percentage, pancreatic necrosis. Young adult guinea pigs can be infected by infection into the footpad. They regularly develop pancreatic necrosis, with some necrosis of skeletal and cardiac muscle. In terms of evolution and epithelial lesions, the disease in guinea pigs is similar to that in cattle.

The main portal of entry and primary site of viral multiplication is the mucosa of the upper respiratory tract, especially the pharynx. The ability of the virus to establish in this area is not affected by the presence of circulating antibodies. Primary multiplication is followed by a viremic stage of 4 or 5 days duration, after which the virus localizes, replicates, and produces characteristic vesicles in several different sites referred to later. The highest virus titers occur during the early stages of the disease. Virus persists in the sites of lesions for 3 to 8 days after the appearance of significant neutralizing titers in serum but seldom persists in lesions beyond the eleventh day of clinical illness. High titers of virus develop in all areas of skin, not necessarily related to lesions, and in several visceral tissues, including pancreas and hypophysis. Here they have been related to persistent aftereffects of natural and experimental infections.

The decline in virus titer follows within a week or so the development of neutralizing antibody. Ordinarily, antibody titers decline progressively and fairly rapidly. The duration of persistence of antibody is correlated with the initial titer. In general, animals are resistant to reinfection with homologous strains by natural exposure for about 2 to 4 years; susceptibility increases as the antibody titer declines.

The characteristic lesions of foot and mouth disease are seen only in those animals examined at the height of disease. Later, the lesions heal or are obscured by secondary bacterial infection. In cattle, there is appreciable loss of weight, and the buccal cavity contains much saliva. In the living animal, there is diffuse buccal hyperemia and mild catarrhal stomatitis, but the hyperemia disappears at death. Vesicles form on the inner aspects of the lips and cheeks, the gums, hard palate, dental pad, and especially on the sides and anterior portion of the dorsum of the tongue. Sometimes they form on the muzzle and exterior nares. The primary vesicles are small, but by coalescence they produce bullae that may be 5 to 6 cm across; these bullae rupture in 12 to 14 hr, leaving an intensely red, raw, and moist base to which shreds of epithelium may still adhere. A seropurulent exudate develops on the base of the erosion, and this coagulates to a scab, which in turn is replaced by regenerated epithelium in less than 2 weeks. Secondary infection may complicate this course.

Foot lesions occur in the majority of cases. There is inflammatory swelling of skin of the interdigital space, coronet, and heels a day or so before vesicles form. The swellings persist until the vesicles rupture and the resultant erosions heal; healing may be considerably delayed on the feet. Vesicles may also occur in the other sites but much less frequently. When the teats and udder are involved, there is severe swelling.

Fluorescent-antibody studies indicate that there is infection of individual cells in the stratum spinosum, adjacent to the papilla on mucosal surfaces, or in the follicular sheath in skin. The papilla serves as a bridge for transport of the virus from the vascular lamina propria to the avascular squamous epithelium. Immunofluorescence occurs in mononuclear cells of the lamina propria before there is evidence of virus in the epithelial cells. The infected epithelial cells progressively swell, develop eosinophilia of the cytoplasm, and undergo acantholysis. There is extensive spongiosis of the stratum spinosum, and this along with the necrosis of keratinocytes results in the formation of vesicles. Superficial lesions may be formed in the stratum corneum. These vesicles tend to rupture as soon as they develop, with leakage of vesicular fluid followed by desiccation. The cells in this type of lesion remain spherical and adhere to each other by proteinaceous material. The early microvesicles coalesce and become macroscopically visible, and these in turn may form bullae. The base of the vesicle is formed by the basal germinative layer of epithelium, which is not usually breached, and the underlying dermis or lamina propria, which is infiltrated by inflammatory cells and intensely hyperemic.

Additional to the vesiculate and erosive lesions, there may be catarrhal inflammation of the respiratory passages. In animals dying of the disease, there are petechial hemorrhages of the abomasum and intestine, with congestion and diapedesis into the lumen. The abomasal hemorrhages quickly develop to ulcers. Pulmonary edema, modest splenomegaly, and hydropericardium with petechiae on the cardiac serosa are nonspecific changes in this disease.

As indicated earlier, a malignant form of the disease without vesiculation does occur in young animals. In these, death is common and no doubt coupled with the myocarditis that develops. The myocardial lesion involves the ventricular musculature and the papillary muscle as poorly defined pale foci of varying size. It is characteristic enough to be referred to as the typical "tiger heart" on account of the striping and mottling. The myocarditis is acute, and hyaline degeneration and necrosis of muscle fibers is accompanied by an intense, principally lymphocytic, infiltrate. Similar lesions occur in skeletal muscle.

Prolonged convalescence or residual illness is frequently referred to in cattle but is difficult to evaluate. Residual bacterial infections are common complications, especially in the oral cavity and mammary glands, and on the feet. Additionally, syndromes of panting and hypertrichosis and disturbances of the regulation of body temperature, lactation, and fertility (including abortion) and of emaciation or obesity have been described. Such disturbances could be referable to disturbances of endocrine glands and of the hypothalamic–hypophyseal system, and nonspecific changes can be found in these locations. Clinical myocardial disease is frequent in convalescent cattle and is ascribed to myocardial degeneration with concurrent degeneration of the conduction system. Diabetes mellitus has been reported as a complication of the experimental and natural disease. The pancreatic islets may disappear almost completely, and the pancreas also shows acinar necrosis and regeneration, the latter evident as proliferation of tubular structures.

Foot and mouth disease is not well documented in sheep; they are, in general, less susceptible than cattle, and the infection runs a milder course, though there may be exceptions. The incubation period in sheep is commonly 3–8 days, with fever lasting ~4 days. Lesions may not develop. When they do, the dental pad is the preferred site in the oral cavity. Lingual lesions tend to occur on the posterior dorsal portion as underrunning necrotic erosions rather than vesicles. These are small and easily missed, and they heal within a few days. Lameness is prominent in acute outbreaks. Typical vesicles develop in the interdigital cleft and on the coronet and bulb of heel. They may occasionally involve all of the coronet and lead to eventual shedding of the hoof. Vesicles also occasionally occur on the teats, vulva, prepuce, and on the pillars of the rumen. The peracute form will occur in lambs.

In pigs there is also considerable variability in virulence of strains and acuteness of the disease. The incubation period is somewhat longer than in cattle and may extend for a week or more. Lesions occur in the usual sites, although more commonly on the feet than in the mouth. They may be present on the snout and behind its rim, and on the teats of lactating sows. Abortion and stillbirth of infected piglets has been recorded. The peracute form with high mortality occurs in young sucklings.

The lesions of foot and mouth disease must be differentiated from other viral vesicular diseases such as vesicular stomatitis, vesicular exanthema, and swine vesicular disease and in the latter stages from diseases producing erosive–ulcerative lesions of the oral cavity. Laboratory tests are essential to confirm or rule out a diagnosis of foot and mouth disease. Complement-fixation tests using vesicular fluid or epithelial cells from early lesions as antigen are the most commonly used procedures, because results may be available within 3 hr. False negative results are possible, and these should be followed up with fluorescent-antibody techniques, isolation attempts on tissue culture, and inoculation of susceptible animals.

VESICULAR STOMATITIS. Vesicular stomatitis is a specific viral disease occurring naturally among horses, cattle, and pigs, and it is transmissible experimentally to a number of laboratory animals, including guinea pigs and mice. The disease is important because it causes a loss in production, especially in dairy herds, and it must be differentiated from foot and mouth disease in cattle and pigs. Vesicular stomatitis is the only vesicular disease naturally occurring in horses. Sheep and goats do not appear to be susceptible to the disease. Several wildlife species, such as white-tailed deer, raccoons, and feral swine, are susceptible to vesicular stomatitis. In humans, the virus may cause an inapparent infection or a mild influenza-like condition.

Vesicular stomatitis is enzootic in Central and South America and occurs sporadically elsewhere in the Americas. It has a seasonal occurrence, outbreaks occurring in the warmer seasons and ceasing abruptly with the onset of cold weather. The seasonal nature of the disease suggests that it is transmitted by insects; however, insect transmission is not essential. It is not known how the virus spreads from one geographic area to another. The intact mucosa is resistant to infection, but abrasions in the susceptible site readily result in infection when contaminated with saliva or exudate from a lesion. Swine may become infected through ingestion.

The virus of vesicular stomatitis belongs to the Rhabdoviridae, genus *Vesiculovirus*. It contains single-stranded RNA, and the virion is large, rod-shaped, 80 × 120 nm, and it has an envelope. Apart from having a greater susceptibility to heat, being inactivated by pasteurization temperatures, it shares qualities of resistance with the aphthovirus. There are two serologically and immunologically distinct types of the virus. The more common and more virulent New Jersey strain has only one serotype, is restricted to vertebrate hosts, and extends farthest north into more temperate zones. The Indiana strain has three serotypes and occurs in vertebrate hosts but also in arthropods such as *Phlebotomus* flies, sand flies (*Culicoides*), and mosquitoes. The epidemiologic significance of this observation is unknown.

The lesions of vesicular stomatitis occur mainly on the oral mucosa; occasionally they do occur elsewhere, including the feet, and in swine, foot lesions are common. This is by no means a dependable feature, and outbreaks of the disease in cattle have been described in which the lesions were predominantly on the teats. The incubation period following exposure by abrasion is 24–48 hr, and there is a viremic phase that persists longer than the vesicular, but secondary lesions are rare. In cattle, intramuscular injections will not initiate the disease, a useful distinguishing feature from foot and mouth disease.

The lesions of vesicular stomatitis are indistinguishable from those of foot and mouth disease (Fig. 1.20A). Initially, in cattle, there is a raised, flattened, pale pink to blanched papule a few millimeters in diameter in or near the mouth. These papules rapidly become inflamed and hyperemic. In the course of a day or so, they develop into vesicles 2–3 cm in diameter and by coalescence may involve large areas. The shallow erosions that follow rupture of vesicles heal within 1 to 2 weeks unless secondary infections occur; in the mouth, the latter are expected.

The first microscopic changes are seen in the deeper layers of the stratum spinosum, where increasing prominence of the intercellular spaces and stretching of the desmosomes are ac-

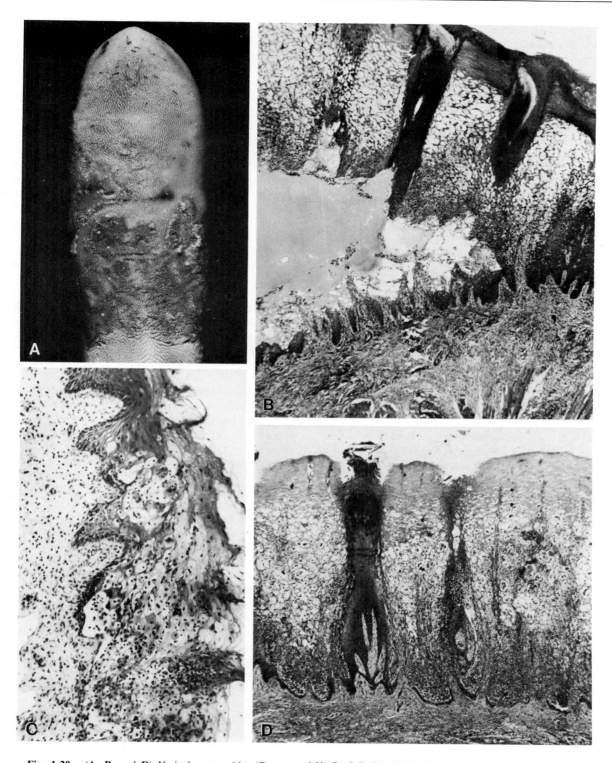

Fig. 1.20. (**A**, **B**, and **D**) Vesicular stomatitis. (Courtesy of H. R. Seibold and the *American Journal of Veterinary Research*.) (**A**) Erosion of vesicular lesions in tongue at 4 days postinoculation. (**B**) Edge of gross vesicle. (**C**) Margin of vesicle. Porcine vesicular exanthema. (**D**) Intraepithelial vesicle formation in vesicular stomatitis.

companied by a reduction in volume of the cell cytoplasm (Fig. 1.20B,D). This dissociation of cells proceeds to distinct intercellular edema (spongiosis), followed by further cytoplasmic retraction until the affected epithelial cells float freely in enlarging vacuoles, which in turn are loculated by strands of cytoplasmic debris. There is no hydropic degeneration of the epithelial cells, and the nuclei until now remain normal. With the onset of epithelial-cell necrosis there is a pleocellular inflammatory reaction in the mucosa and underlying lamina propria. Electron microscopic examination of epithelial cells adjacent to the vesicles confirms the intercellular edema and keratinocyte necrosis seen under the light microscope. Virions bud from the cytoplasmic membrane and are located in the dilated intercellular spaces. There is marked reduplication of desmosomes, and normal desmosomes are evident in the cytoplasm. These appear to be due to endocytosis of plasma membranes of adjacent damaged epithelial cells, and formation of desmosomes on invaginations of plasma membranes with subsequent migration into the cytoplasm of keratinocytes. The microvesicles coalesce to produce macroscopically visible ones. There are no inclusion bodies. The microscopic appearance of the lesions is not diagnostic.

The severity of vesicular stomatitis in swine approximates that of foot and mouth disease, but in other species it is much milder. Only ~30% of infected cattle develop vesicles. In light of its similarity to other vesicular diseases in cattle and swine, laboratory confirmation of vesicular stomatitis is essential.

VESICULAR EXANTHEMA.   Vesicular exanthema is an acute, febrile, viral disease of swine that is characterized by formation of vesicles on the mouth, skin, and feet. It was first diagnosed in southern California in the 1930s and eventually spread to most swine-producing states in the United States. The last reported outbreak of vesicular exanthema was in New Jersey in 1959.

The virus that causes vesicular exanthema belongs to the Caliciviridae, genus *Calicivirus*. It has a single-stranded RNA genome and has only one major polypeptide. It is about 35–40 nm in diameter, and characteristic cup-shaped structures (calyces) are evident in electron microscopic preparations. There are 13 immunologically distinct serotypes, which vary in virulence.

In 1973, a virus biophysically similar to vesicular exanthema virus was recovered from sea lions with vesicles on their flippers, off the coast of California near San Miguel Island. This virus, called San Miguel sea lion virus, produces lesions identical to those of vesicular exanthema when inoculated into swine. It has many distinct serotypes, which are considered to be another range of variants of swine vesicular exanthema virus. It is found in marine fish as well as sea lions and Pribilof fur seals.

Most outbreaks of vesicular exanthema have been associated with feeding of raw garbage containing pork waste. Therefore, the disease may be transmitted by direct contact and fomites. Spontaneous outbreaks of vesicular exanthema in swine due to San Miguel sea lion virus have not been documented, though undiagnosed vesicular disease of swine, associated with the feeding of marine products, has occurred in Tasmania and New Zealand.

After inoculation, there is an incubation period of about 18 to 72 hr, followed by fever and development of vesicles on the mouth, lips, tongue, on the mucosa of the oral cavity, and on the sole of the hoof, coronary band, and interdigital skin. Occasionally, they are present on the teats of nursing sows and on the skin of the metacarpus and metatarsus. Secondary infections of the feet are common, and the hooves may slough. Pregnant sows may abort. Without complications, affected pigs recover completely within about a week.

The vesicular lesions are indistinguishable from those of vesicular stomatitis, swine vesicular disease, and foot and mouth disease (Fig. 1.20C). Laboratory confirmation of clinical diagnosis should always be attempted. This is possible through inoculation of susceptible pigs and laboratory animals (e.g., hamsters). The virus does not grow in chick embryos but can be isolated in tissue cultures of swine origin.

SWINE VESICULAR DISEASE.   Swine vesicular disease is a highly contagious viral disease of pigs that is characterized by formation of vesicles around the coronary bands of the feet and to a lesser extent on the mouth, lips, and tongue.

The disease was first recognized in Italy in 1966, and it has since been reported from Hong Kong, the United Kingdom, Europe, and Asia. The economic importance of swine vesicular disease is related to losses in production and the fact that it is difficult to differentiate from other vesicular diseases in swine, including foot and mouth disease.

The cause of swine vesicular disease is a small RNA virus belonging to the Picornaviridae, genus *Enterovirus*. It is considered to be a porcine strain of human Coxsackie B5 enterovirus and occasionally infects humans, but not other domestic species. Swine vesicular disease virus is relatively resistant to environmental factors. Unlike foot and mouth disease virus, it is not inactivated at the low pH in muscle commonly associated with rigor mortis.

Most outbreaks of swine vesicular disease appear to originate by feeding raw garbage contaminated with pork products. Transmission within affected herds is by direct contact, especially during the early stages of the disease. The portal of entry is through damaged epithelium, and this is most likely to occur on the feet and to a lesser extent in the oral cavity. The tonsils and lower gastrointestinal tract may be routes of entry, but only when infective doses are high. Fluorescent studies and virus titer determinations have shown that swine vesicular disease virus has a strong affinity for the epithelial cells of the coronary band of the feet, tongue, snout, lips, lymphoid follicles of the tonsils, myocardial cells, and brain. Secretions and excretions have high viral titers for a period of 12 to 14 days. Feces may contain virus for up to 3 months, but titers are apparently not sufficiently high to transmit disease.

Clinically, vesicles are most common on the feet. Oral lesions occur only in ~10% of affected pigs. The foot lesions appear first at the junction between the heel and the coronary band. Initially, there is a 5.0-mm-wide, pale, swollen area that encircles the digit. A dark red to brown zone 2–3 mm wide surrounds the pale zone on both sides. In later stages a 1.0-cm-wide band of necrotic skin is located along the coronet. Well-demarcated areas of necrosis, resembling superficial abrasions, extend to the metacarpus, metatarsus, and interdigital cleft. Vesicles on the mouth, lips, and tongue occur in clusters, and they are small, ~2.0 mm in diameter, white, and opaque. They coalesce and rupture within 36 hr and may be covered by a pseudodiphtheritic membrane due to secondary bacterial infections.

The development of vesicles tends to follow a course similar to that reported for foot and mouth disease. The virus infects individual epithelial cells in the stratum spinosum, which leads to focal areas of keratinocyte degeneration and vesicle formation. Frequently, the necrosis involves the entire thickness of the epithelium, including the basal layer. There is an intense leukocytic reaction in the necrotic areas, which is mainly neutrophilic. Spongiosis is less prominent in swine vesicular disease, compared to vesicular stomatitis, although this depends to some extent on the location of the vesicle. Intra- and intercellular edema may be extensive in the snout lesions.

After 1 week there are indications of epithelial regeneration. These consist of an increase in mitotic figures, and long, flat epithelial cells at the periphery of the erosion. In contrast to lesions of foot and mouth disease, which tend to heal in an orderly fashion, in swine vesicular disease long cords of epithelial cells proliferate parallel and perpendicular to the skin surface. A moderate mononuclear-cell reaction and fibroplasia may be evident in the underlying dermis. Necrosis and inflammation involve the external root sheath of hair follicles and the subepithelial glands, especially of the mouth.

The early lesions in the tonsils are characterized by degeneration of the squamous epithelial cells, which are replaced by large droplets of foamy, basophilic, PAS-positive material. The tonsillar crypts are plugged with exudate. Similar changes are found in the inter- and intralobular collecting ducts of the salivary glands and pancreas. There is degeneration and hypertrophy of the renal pelvic epithelium. Foci of necrosis with a mild interstitial mononuclear-cell reaction may be found in the myocardium. There is necrosis and depletion of lymphocytes in most lymphoid tissues.

Nervous signs and lesions have been reported in field outbreaks and reproduced experimentally in swine vesicular disease. The characteristic lesions are those of a nonsuppurative meningoencephalitis involving most areas in the brain. Some reports indicate that the lesions are more severe in the brain stem. Nonviral, intranuclear, amphophilic inclusion bodies may be found in the amphicytes of the Gasserian and dorsal root ganglia.

The minor differences in the distribution and morphology of the lesions in swine vesicular disease, compared with the other vesicular diseases affecting swine, may be of some assistance in the differential diagnosis. However, further laboratory confirmation is necessary. If virus titers in infected tissues used as antigen are sufficiently high, the complement fixation test using vesicular fluid or scrapings from lesions may give results in 4 to 24 hr. Counterimmunoelectrophoresis appears to be the test of choice as a follow-up to a negative complement fixation test, since it is highly specific and produces rapid results. The virus may be isolated in cell cultures of swine origin.

BOVINE VIRUS DIARRHEA.　Virus diarrhea, as originally described in New York state in 1946, was an acute, highly contagious disease. The disease still occurs from time to time with these manifestations, but it also occurs sporadically. The fatal cases usually represent one or two severe infections in a group of animals otherwise subclinically affected.

Mucosal disease was described in 1953 in the United States as a disease with a morbidity rate of 2 to 50% and a mortality rate of ~100%. It was characterized by an initial febrile reaction, mucoid nasal discharge, anorexia, constant or intermittent watery diarrhea with feces often containing blood, rapid dehydration, and death. Erosions, ulcerations, and hemorrhages were always found in the alimentary canal.

Infection with bovine virus diarrhea virus results in a spectrum of signs that are compatible with both clinical syndromes: virus diarrhea and mucosal disease. The causative agent of bovine virus diarrhea is an RNA virus belonging to the Togaviridae, genus *Pestivirus*. It is antigenically related to hog cholera virus and the border disease virus. There is only one serotype of bovine virus diarrhea virus. Considerable variation in virulence is apparent among strains of the virus. Both cytopathic and noncytopathic strains may be isolated in tissue culture. Either may be virulent for cattle.

Transmission of the virus is still poorly understood; however, direct contact with clinically affected cattle or carriers and possibly with fomites is probably the main route. Aerosol transmission has been documented experimentally. A high prevalence is associated with the wide use of modified live virus vaccines.

After inoculation there is a viremia with a marked leukopenia. Fluorescent-antibody studies show that the virus infects a wide variety of tissues, including squamous epithelial cells of the upper alimentary tract and the interdigital area of the feet, glandular and cryptal epithelial cells of the lower alimentary tract, epithelial cells of the respiratory tract, and endothelial cells of submucosal vessels in the gut and several other organs. The virus has an affinity for lymphoid tissue, especially in the tonsils and Peyer's patches. Neurons, glomerular cells, and epithelial cells of renal convoluted tubules may be infected under certain conditions.

The virus may cross the placental barrier in pregnant animals. Depending on the stage of gestation, it may cause abortion, fetal mummification, or a wide spectrum of teratogenic lesions, including microencephaly, cerebellar hypoplasia and dysgenesis, hydranencephaly, hydrocephalus, and defective myelination of the spinal cord. Ocular lesions, such as microphthalmia, cataracts, retinal degeneration, atrophy and dysplasia, and optic neuritis, have all been associated with fetal infections by the virus (see the Nervous System, Volume 1). In addition, lesions of the alimentary tract similar to those seen in older animals may occur in fetuses and neonatal calves.

A condition in lambs, termed border disease, which is characterized by a hairy fleece, clonic rhythmic tremors, and unthriftiness, has been associated with prenatal infection by a togavirus that has a strong antigenic relationship to bovine virus diarrhea and hog cholera viruses. Affected animals are termed "hairy shakers" (see the Skin and Appendages, and the Nervous System, Volume 1).

All virulent strains of virus produce the same sort of experimental disease in susceptible calves. A slight fever with leukopenia at the third day is followed by a second phase of higher fever and more severe leukopenia at about the seventh day. At the end of this second, febrile phase oral hyperemia with some erosions may develop, and perhaps slight diarrhea. The severe fatal disease has seldom, if ever, been produced by experimental transmission.

These observations emphasize that the natural disease is usually very mild, or infection is commonly inapparent. It is also very widespread, as indicated by serologic surveys. Severe clinical or fatal cases are exceptional in spite of their apparent prevalence. When acute cases occur in a herd, it is usual that many other animals show the mild disease. The mildly affected may develop substantial levels of neutralizing antibody, while those severely affected tend not to. While deaths may occur within 1 or 2 days of illness and almost always within 2 weeks, some cases remain clinically affected for months. The failure of immunogenic response may be associated with immunotolerance or destruction of immunocompetent cells, which is reflected in lymphopenia. In addition to a lack of humoral antibody response, there is also depression of cell-mediated immunity, as indicated by a poor response of cultured peripheral lymphocytes to various mitogens. Animals with deficient humoral and cell-mediated immunity ultimately die. There may also be impairment of polymorphonuclear-cell function in cattle infected with bovine virus diarrhea virus, which may explain in part the observation that such cattle are susceptible to secondary bacterial infections.

Acute fulminant bovine virus diarrhea closely resembles rinderpest. The onset is febrile, with serous to mucoid nasal discharge. Discrete oral lesions are preceded by an acute catarrhal stomatitis and pharyngitis, the mucosae being hyperemic and pink and covered by a thin, gray film of catarrhal exudate. White necrotic foci 1–2 mm in size, surrounded by a margin of hyperemia, then appear on the muzzle and the buccal mucosa. These erode or ulcerate and expand irregularly; the margins remain fairly discrete, except for those on the soft palate and pharyngeal mucosa. There is severe diarrhea and tenesmus, with feces containing little or no blood or mucus. Animals may die quickly.

The more chronic cases also begin with fever and serous nasal discharge. The nasal discharge becomes more mucinous in a couple of days and dries on the muzzle, causing excoriation. The temperature returns to normal in 2 to 5 days, and then oral lesions and a watery diarrhea develop. These animals remain alert. The development of the oral lesions is like that found in acute cases; by the time chronic cases die, however, there is usually some evidence of healing. The watery diarrhea of the early phase gradually gives way to feces that are passed frequently, are scant in volume, and contain a large proportion of mucus flecked with blood. Late in the clinical course, there is lethargy, emaciation, ruminal stasis, and frequent attempts at defecation accompanied by severe tenesmus. Interdigital dermatitis affecting all four feet may be present in chronically affected animals. In these, the skin is dry and scurfy, especially over the neck, withers, and back, and that on the medial aspect of the thighs and forelegs and in the perineal region becomes moist and discolored a dirty yellow with encrustations.

The gross lesions vary considerably, especially in the acute disease, in which either upper alimentary or intestinal lesions may be absent, and less so in the chronic disease, in which a broader pathologic picture is often present, perhaps partially obscured by healing or evolution of lesions.

Erosions and shallow ulcers are present on the muzzle and nares of many affected cattle. The anterior edges of the lower lip and its cutaneous junction are similarly affected. A similar loss of epithelium from much of the oral cavity is common. Diffuse hyperemia of the mucosa may persist after death. The most conspicuous oral erosions are on the palate, on the tips of the buccal papillae and on the gingiva. Many, especially on the papillae and in the pharynx, are ulcers and expose a denuded, intensely hyperemic lamina propria. The tongue is not always affected. When present, lesions may be evident on all surfaces (Fig. 1.21A,B). Those on the smooth lateral surfaces are typically erosive and irregular, although in some early cases the degenerate epithelium may remain attached, to form flat, white plaques that may be scraped off. On the anterior half of the dorsum, the degenerate epithelium may accumulate and develop deep, irregular crevices and pits, or ulcerate to denude the greater portion of the surface.

In some cases the oral lesions are sharp, punched-out ulcers. These occur on the dental pad, palate, ventral and lateral surfaces of the tongue, the gums about the incisors, and the inside of the cheeks and pharynx. In some lesions of longer duration, the defect is filled in from the margin by thickened white proliferative epithelium.

Esophageal lesions are usually present. They are common in the upper third of the esophagus. In some acute cases, the lesions are shallow erosions rather than ulcers. The erosions are more or less linear but otherwise irregular, have a dirty brown base, and little or no reactive hyperemia (Fig. 1.21C). Shreds of adherent necrotic epithelium give the surface a rough, worn, tattered appearance in animals that have not been swallowing. In more advanced cases, discrete ulcerations occur. In many chronically affected animals, the ulcers begin to heal and appear as yellowish white, slightly elevated plaques of proliferative epithelium at the periphery of the mucosal defect.

Lesions are found in the rumenoreticulum and omasum, but not in the esophageal groove. The ruminal content in chronically affected animals with prolonged anorexia is usually scant and dry. The surface of the ingesta is frequently blackened, and the villi of the ruminal wall are thick, black, and dry. In most acute cases the ruminal content is usually liquid and putrid. The lesions on the wall of the rumen resemble those present elsewhere in the upper alimentary tract, and although they occur anywhere, they are best seen on the pillars and other smooth or nonvillous portions of the mucosa (Fig. 1.21E). The omasal lesions are most numerous along the edges of the leaves, sometimes causing a scalloped margin or perforation.

The morphogenesis of the lesions in the squamous mucosa of the upper alimentary tract begins with necrosis of the epithelium (Fig. 1.21D). Individual cells and groups of cells deep in the epithelium are eosinophilic and swollen, with pyknotic nuclei. These foci enlarge progressively and form areas of necrosis that extend to, and may involve, the basal layer. In the early stages there is little or no inflammation of the lamina propria, but leukocytes infiltrate the necrotic epithelium. These small necrotic foci are elevated above the surface and form the friable

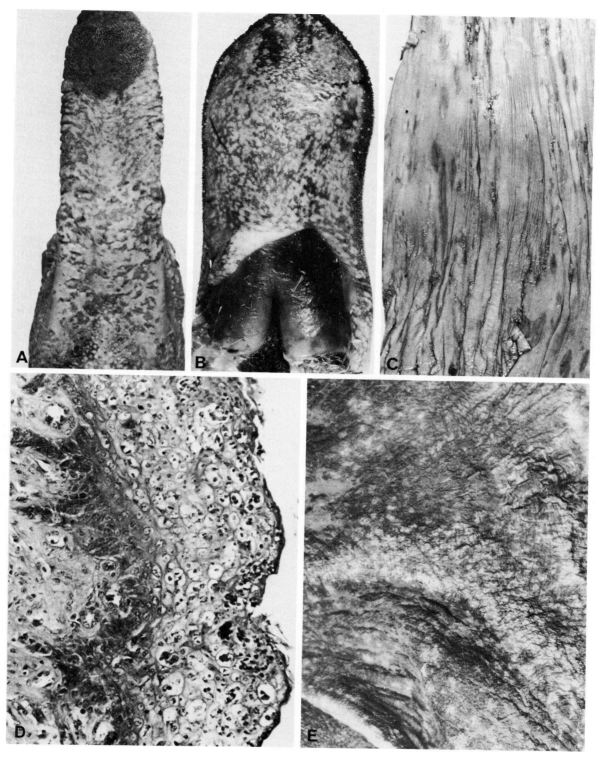

Fig. 1.21. Bovine virus diarrhea. (**A**) Dorsal and (**B**) ventral surface of tongue, showing multiple confluent ulcers. (**C**) Longitudinal erosions and ulcers on the esophagus. (**D**) Histologic appearance of esophageal lesion. (**E**) Focal and confluent lesions of dorsal sac of rumen.

plaques described earlier on the squamous mucosae. They enlarge progressively and by coalescence, and may form small cleavage vesicles along the proprial–epithelial junction (Fig. 1.23A). If the necrotic epithelium is abraded, erosions and ulcers develop.

The ulcerations of the squamous epithelium of the upper alimentary tract are accompanied by inflammation in the lamina propria, especially where this forms papillae (Fig. 1.23B). Capillaries are congested, the lymphatics are dilated, there is edema of the stroma, and a pleocellular inflammatory infiltrate is present. Focal hemorrhages may occur.

Changes are regularly present in the abomasum. The sides of the rugae bear what appear grossly to be ulcers, which may be punctate to 1.0 cm or more in diameter (Fig. 1.22A). They are lesions with raised margins and a distinct pale halo; there may also be some peripheral hemorrhage. The histologic changes in the glandular epithelium of the abomasum are characterized by epithelial necrosis, mainly in the depths of the glands. The necrotic cells fragment and slough and may cause dilation of affected glands. The mucosa is locally infiltrated by a variety of leukocytes and is edematous. In some affected foci, the glandular epithelium loses its differentiated appearance, becoming cuboidal, basophilic, and apparently mucus secretory. These glands too may be dilated with a small quantity of contained epithelial and leukocytic debris. In some abomasa, mucous metaplasia may be patchy but widespread and may reflect inflammation in the mucosa. There is some edema, hemorrhage, and modest leukocytic infiltration of the submucosa. Some necrotic foci in the abomasal glands appear to be associated with necrosis of adjacent mucosal lymphoid follicles.

The mucosa of the small intestine often appears normal over much of its length. There may be inspissated mucoid material in the lumen. In some cases the mucosa of the small intestine may have patchy or diffuse congestion. In rare cases, fibrin casts may be in the lumen of the small bowel. The wall is atonic but not dilated and may be greatly thickened by submucosal and subserosal edema, which may give a ground-glass appearance to the serosal surface.

In acute cases, it is usual to find coagulated blood and fibrin overlying and outlining Peyer's patches, the covering of which is eroded. This, when present, is a very distinctive lesion that is paralleled only in rinderpest. Severely affected Peyer's patches are often obvious through the serosa as red-black oval areas up to 10 to 12 cm long on the antimesenteric border of the gut (Fig. 1.22B). Less acutely affected Peyer's patches may be overlain by a diphtheritic membrane, while in milder or more chronic cases the patches may be depressed and covered by tenacious mucus. In chronic cases, exudate may not be evident over Peyer's patches, which become less obvious or sunken, resembling an ulcer. Mesenteric lymph nodes are usually not enlarged.

Lesions in the large bowel are highly variable. The mucosa may be congested, often in a "tiger stripe" pattern following the colonic folds. In acute cases there may be fibrinohemorrhagic typhlocolitis (Fig. 1.22D). In more chronic cases, fibrinous or fibronectrotic lesions and focal or extensive ulceration may be present at any level of the large bowel, but particularly in the cecum and rectum.

The characteristic lesion in the intestinal mucosa is destruction of the epithelial lining of the crypts of Lieberkühn. In the duodenum, a few glands only are affected, but more glands are affected more severely in the lower reaches of the small intestine and in the cecum and colon. Affected glands are dilated and filled with mucus, epithelial debris, and leukocytes. Remaining crypt-lining cells are attenuated in an attempt to cover the basement membrane. Reparative hyperplasia of crypt lining is rarely encountered. Crypt dropout may be evident microscopically. In the cecum and colon, extensive damage to crypts and attendant collapse of the lamina propria is the probable cause of ulceration seen grossly (Fig. 1.22E). Congestion of mucosal capillaries, and in acute or ulcerated cases, effusion of fibrin and neutrophils from the mucosal surface, may be evident.

The microscopic lesions of Peyer's patches are distinctive in bovine virus diarrhea, comparable lesions being caused only by rinderpest (Fig. 1.22C). In the acute phase of the disease, severe acute inflammation in the mucosa over Peyer's patches accompanies almost complete destruction of the underlying glands, collapse of the lamina propria, and lysis of the follicular lymphoid tissues. Later in the course of the disease, dilated crypts lined, at least in part, by cuboidal epithelium and filled with necrotic epithelial cells, mucus, and inflammatory cells appear to herniate into the submucosal space previously occupied by involuted lymphoid follicles. Peyer's patches should be sought assiduously at autopsy since their gross and microscopic appearance may provide useful evidence for diagnosis.

An important microscopic lesion, which may have been previously overlooked, is hyaline degeneration and fibrinoid necrosis of submucosal and mesenteric arterioles (Fig. 1.23C). A mild to moderate mononuclear inflammatory cell reaction is frequently present in the walls of the vessels and in perivascular areas. The vascular lesions are not limited to the intestine but may be present in a variety of other organs such as the heart, brain, and adrenal cortices, which may make it difficult to differentiate the disease from malignant catarrhal fever. The vascular lesions in bovine virus diarrhea are less consistently present and usually are milder.

In the acute disease, the lymph nodes of the head and neck are often enlarged and discolored reddish black by congestion and hemorrhage. Microscopically, the mesenteric lymph nodes show a diminished population of lymphocytes and necrosis of germinal centers. Similar lesions may be seen in the splenic lymphoid follicles, but they are not consistent and are difficult to interpret.

Coronitis may extend completely around the coronary band, with some separation of the skin–horn junction causing disturbance and overgrowth of the horn (Fig. 1.23D). Dermatitis may extend from the coronet up the back of the pastern. Milder dermatitis is generalized, with scurfiness especially from the ears to the withers. In sections of the skin of animals with virus diarrhea there are focal accumulations of necrotic epithelium, with intense hyperemia of the adjacent superficial dermis. The epithelial lesions are basically similar to those in the squamous mucosa of the upper alimentary tract (Fig. 1.23E). Necrosis often extends deeply to or through the basal layers; it results in minute erosions or ulcerations. These deeper lesions occur in the inner aspects of the legs and the perineum, and there is an exudation of serum in these areas. In chronically affected animals,

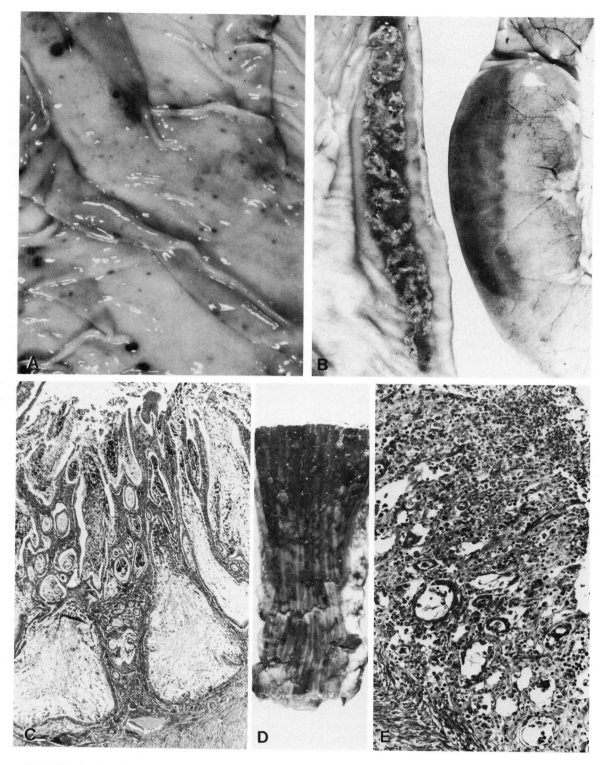

Fig. 1.22. Bovine virus diarrhea. (**A**) Hemorrhage and ulceration. Abomasum. (**B**) Fibrinohemorrhagic exudate over Peyer's patch in the ileum (left). Deep red Peyer's patch visible through serosa of small intestine (right). (**C**) Herniation of crypts of Lieberkühn into the submucosa, replacing necrotic lymphoid follicles in Peyer's patch. Mucus and inflammatory exudate is in the cystic glands and on the surface of the mucosa. (**D**) Fibrinohemorrhagic colitis. (**E**) Colon. Dilated and denuded glands, collapse of lamina propria, and pseudomembrane formation.

basal hyperplasia occurs in the skin. The overlying degenerate epithelium becomes disorderly and eventually is lifted off.

Some animals with chronic disease develop mycotic infections secondary to lesions in the forestomachs, abomasum, and Peyer's patches. The lesions are areas of hemorrhagic necrosis involving the mucosa, submucosa, and sometimes deeper layers of the wall. Fungal hyphae are found invading the stroma and causing thrombosis in venules.

Abortion in the acute febrile stage or in convalescence occurs in virus diarrhea. Enteric lesions of the disease may be observed in the fetus. Punctate hemorrhages with ulcers 1–3 mm in diameter may be profuse in the oral cavity, excepting the dorsum of the tongue, and in the esophagus, larynx, trachea, conjunctiva, and abomasum. The fetal lesions of squamous epithelium evolve in somewhat the same manner as those described above, with focal hemorrhages in the lamina propria and epithelial necrosis beginning in the basal layer.

More recently, a syndrome of inapparent persistent infection by the virus has been recognized. Virus is present in a variety of tissues and body fluids, but serum neutralizing antibodies are absent. These animals may be chronic shedders of virus and are an important source of infection for other animals. Although they do not show any evidence of infection clinically, they have microscopic lesions in the kidney and brain. The renal lesions consist of diffuse and focal thickening of the basement membranes of the glomerular tufts. There is an increase in mesangial cells. Fluorescent-antibody tests show antigen in glomeruli, epithelial cells of convoluted tubules, and endothelial cells in the interstitial blood vessels. The glomerular lesions are probably due to deposition of antigen–antibody complexes on the basement membrane.

Antigen is also present in the neurons, especially of the cerebral cortex. The neurons are pyknotic, and there is astrocytic and lymphocytic neuronal satellitosis. A few vessels are mildly cuffed by lymphocytes and have hypertrophic endothelial cells. The neuronal changes are probably due to direct action of the virus. Antigen is present in many other tissues that do not have microscopic lesions, such as vascular endothelial cells in many organs, mononuclear cells of the spleen, mesenteric and mediastinal lymph nodes, and cryptal epithelial cells. It has been suggested that the lack of serum neutralizing antibodies in these cattle is due to formation of antigen–antibody complexes in the kidney and other tissues.

Confirming a diagnosis of bovine virus diarrhea is often difficult. The wide variety in signs and lesions, coupled with inconsistent and often negative virologic and serologic results, can be a challenge to most diagnosticians. It is therefore important that clinical and pathologic findings should be supported by laboratory tests, including fluorescent-antibody techniques, and virus isolation. Spleen and Peyer's patch should be collected for these purposes. Serologic tests, preferably on acute and convalescent serum samples from several animals in a herd, should be carried out. Bovine virus diarrhea resembles rinderpest, thus it is important to confirm the diagnosis. Other diseases that must be differentiated include the vesicular diseases, malignant catarrhal fever, systemic infectious bovine rhinotracheitis, salmonellosis, and coccidiosis. The triad of erosive–ulcerative upper alimentary lesions, cryptal necrosis in large or small intestine, and lesions of Peyer's patches provides a presumptive diagnosis of bovine virus diarrhea on morphologic grounds, in areas where rinderpest does not occur.

RINDERPEST.   Otherwise known as "cattle plague," rinderpest is an acute, highly contagious disease of cattle characterized by erosive or hemorrhagic lesions of all mucous membranes. It is now enzootic in tropical Africa, the Middle East, and the Orient, to which places it is restricted by sanitary precautions. Unfortunately, the long and interesting history of its pandemic plunges across continents cannot be followed here.

The virus that causes rinderpest belongs to the Paramyxoviridae, genus *Morbillivirus*. It has a single-stranded RNA genome and is antigenically and morphologically closely related to the viruses causing canine distemper and human measles (rubeola). The three viruses have immunologically identical nucleocapsids and shared envelope antigens. The virus is highly fragile under ordinary environmental conditions; it is incapable of surviving more than a few hours outside the animal body under normal circumstances. The agent is readily adapted to the chorioallantoic membrane of the developing chick embryo and can be adapted to rabbits, although strains differ in the ease with which this is accomplished. Once adapted, the virus causes fever and characteristic grayish white, granular necrotic patches in the intestinal lymphoid tissue. Goats and sheep do respond, but inconsistently, to artificial inoculation, although their susceptibility to rinderpest in the field is unclear. Probably all cloven-hoofed animals are naturally susceptible to infection, but the expression of infection varies considerably.

The virus of rinderpest is antigenically uniform and, when suitably modified, is an effective vaccine. Control of the disease in endemic areas is impeded by difficulties inherent in systems of husbandry and in the coexistence of cattle with large populations of susceptible ungulate wildlife. The lability of the virus is such that the spread of infection from endemic areas is most likely to be by live animals with mild or subclinical disease.

The disease in cattle may be mild, especially in endemic areas, but probably will be acute or peracute in new foci. The different degrees of severity are in part due to real differences in virulence of strains, and largely due to differences in susceptibility of breeds or races of cattle. Such variations are well documented and apply also to modified vaccine strains, which although quite safe in some breeds of cattle cause high mortality in others.

The upper respiratory tract appears to be the main portal of entry in spontaneous cases of rinderpest. The virus localizes in the palatine tonsils and regional lymph nodes. This is followed after a 10- to 15-day incubation by a 2- to 3-day period of viremia that coincides with the fever seen clinically. In circulation, the virus is located mainly in lymphocytes. After the viremic stage, the virus replicates in all lymphoid tissues, the bone marrow, and the mucosa of the upper respiratory tract and the gastrointestinal tract. Nasal and oral secretions and the feces contain high titers of the virus. In general, excretion of virus ceases by about the ninth day of the clinical disease. Recovered animals do not appear to be carriers.

Fever and its attendant signs usher in the clinical syndrome

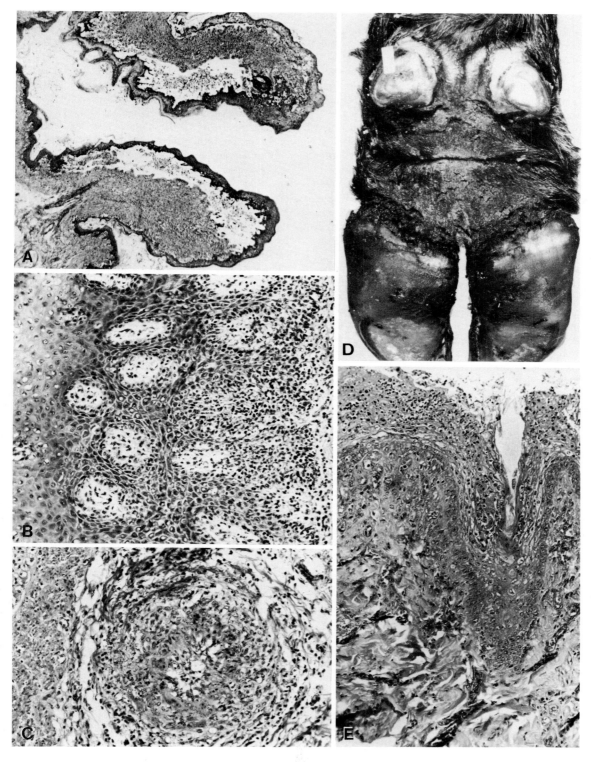

Fig. 1.23. Bovine virus diarrhea. (**A**) Cleavage vesicles in rumen papillae. (**B**) Early lesion. Edema of proprial papillae and acute focal inflammation of papilla and propria. There is necrosis of scattered cells deep in the epithelium. (**C**) Fibrinoid necrosis and mild periarteritis of a mesenteric arteriole. Colon. (**D**) Coronitis and erosive–ulcerative dermatitis of pastern. (**E**) Skin. Superficial epidermal necrosis extending into hair follicle. Hyperplasia of the stratum germinativum.

with early leukopenia. Fever reaches its maximum in ~3 days and falls with the onset of diarrhea. There is severe abdominal pain, tachypnea, occasional cough, severe dehydration and emaciation, and prostration. Death occurs in 6 to 12 days.

The gross morbid anatomic changes in rinderpest are characteristic but not pathognomic and are identical with bovine virus diarrhea. The lesions in the upper alimentary tract are necrotizing and erosive–ulcerative.

The virus of rinderpest has an affinity for the alimentary epithelium, which it gains hematogenously. Oral lesions are not invariably present. The oral lesions typically involve the inner side of the lower lips, the buccal papillae at the commissures, and the ventral surface of the free portion of the tongue. In severe cases, however, all mucous surfaces of the mouth may be involved, with the regular exception of the dorsal surface of the tongue. Esophageal erosions are usually mild and affect the anterior portion. The forestomachs rarely exhibit any lesions. When they do occur, the omasal leaves are involved.

The lesions of stratified squamous epithelium originate in the basal layer. A few and then many epithelial cells undergo necrosis, the nuclei become pyknotic and fragmented, and the cytoplasm coagulated and eosinophilic, but true vesicles do not develop. Multinucleate syncytia form in the epithelium (Fig. 1.24A–C). The necrotic foci produce, initially, white pinpoint papules. Natural movements cause the necrotic tissue to lift off and produce shallow erosions. This occurs so readily that erosions are usually the first lesions observed. Their margins are sharp, and the bases are reddened by the underlying congested capillaries. The initial minute erosions enlarge and coalesce to form extensive defects. Ulceration may supervene.

The abomasum is usually involved in this disease, its pyloric mucosa most consistently and severely. The lesions of the fundus are linear on the margins of the mucosal folds, and in the pylorus they are more rounded. The mucosa becomes necrotic and grayish in affected foci and then sloughs, leaving sharply marginated irregular erosions, the bases of which are intensely hyperemic and ooze blood. Ulcerations sometimes occur. There is usually a profuse submucosal edema that thickens the fundic plicae.

Lesions in the small intestine are less severe than those elsewhere but are of the same general character, streaks of congestion and erosion developing on the margins of mucosal folds. They are best developed in the upper duodenum and in the ileum. The ileocecal valve and surrounding cecal mucosa are congested and eroded. The linear lesions of the mucosal folds are well developed in the cecum and colon. Occasionally, the red foci are so numerous as to appear as diffuse hemorrhage, although they are, in reality, severely congested vessels of the lamina propria. The colon and rectum are more severely affected as a rule than the rest of the enteric mucosa.

The Peyer's patches and other gastrointestinal lymphoid follicles, especially at the cecocolic junction, become necrotic (Fig. 1.24D), and this may be extensive enough to cause necrosis of the overlying mucosa, leaving lesions resembling deep ulcers.

Microscopically, the cryptal epithelium in the small intestine may become necrotic, and syncytia may form in crypts. Associated villi may be somewhat atrophic. Small hemorrhages occur

from the intensely congested blood vessels. There is diffuse edema of the submucosa, but little leukocytic infiltration.

The rinderpest virus is tropic for lymphoid tissues. Necrosis of lymphocytes is extreme, but gross inspection, which reveals little abnormality except of nodes, is misleading. There is no hemorrhage or inflammation of lymph nodes. The necrosis begins in the germinal centers and proceeds until virtually all mature lymphocytes are lost in individual follicles, leaving only a reticular mesh (Fig. 1.24E). Multinucleate cells, similar to those in the mucosa, form in the lymph and hemolymph nodes. All or only some follicles may be involved, and there is often an increase of other leukocytes in the sinuses. Similar lesions occur in the spleen, tonsils, and as already noted, in the Peyer's patches.

Petechiae are common in the upper respiratory mucosae, and small erosions may develop on the larynx. Hemorrhages beneath the epicardium and endocardium are common but nonspecific, and there may be mild nonspecific myocardial degeneration. Mild erosive lesions develop in the mucosa of the bladder and vagina. Acute congestion and edema of the conjunctiva may be followed by purulent conjunctivitis and corneal ulceration. Skin lesions have been described, especially in buffalo, but are considered rare. A moist eczematous lesion of the udder, scrotum, inner aspect of thighs, neck, and flank may develop. Animals with such lesions usually die, but if recovery occurs, the dried scabs of exudate peel off, removing the superficial epithelium and hair.

The lesions of rinderpest can only provide a presumptive diagnosis. Confirmation of the diagnosis requires detection of antigen by immunodiffusion, using infected tissue such as lymph node; virus isolation and identification in bovine cell culture systems; and serologic tests such as virus neutralization and complement fixation. The virus may be isolated from unclotted blood, especially from the buffy coat, lymph nodes, and spleen, collected during the febrile and early erosive stages of the disease. Cellular syncytia and intranuclear and intracytoplasmic inclusion bodies occur in epithelial and lymphoid tissues and perhaps are found more easily in the tonsils than elsewhere. The presence of these may assist in differentiating rinderpest from bovine virus diarrhea on morphologic grounds.

PESTE DES PETITS RUMINANTS. *Peste des petits ruminants* (*kata,* stomatitis pneumoenteritis complex) is a disease of sheep and goats in west Africa that closely resembles rinderpest. The causative agent is closely related to rinderpest virus, with which it shares common antigenic determinants. The virus cross-reacts with rinderpest virus in the immunodiffusion and complement fixation tests. It does not infect cattle through contact; however, experimental infection stimulates antibody formation in cattle that is protective against challenge with rinderpest virus. Infection of sheep and goats with rinderpest virus will protect them against the *peste* virus. The clinical signs and lesions of the disease in sheep and goats are similar to those of rinderpest, except that the disease is more acute in onset, especially in goats, and follows a more rapid course.

MALIGNANT CATARRHAL FEVER. Malignant catarrhal fever (malignant head catarrh, *snotsiekte*) is of worldwide distribu-

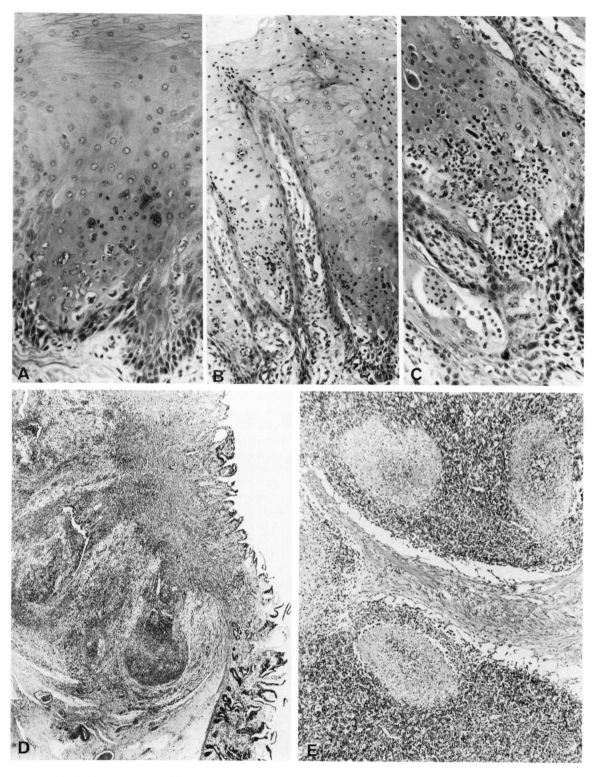

Fig. 1.24. Rinderpest. Ox. (AFIP 625840.) (**A**) Early stage of oral lesion, showing disorganization of epithelium above the basal layer and formation of syncytial cells. Tongue. (**B** and **C**) Slightly later stage, with beginning separation sparing basal cells. (**D**) Necrosis of Peyer's patch. Ileum. (**E**) Necrosis of germinal centers. Lymph node. (AFIP 623162.)

tion. It is generally sporadic in occurrence, although severe herd outbreaks have been reported in feedlot, dairy, and range cattle and zoo animals, mainly several species of deer, and bison. Other susceptible species of ungulates include banteng and greater kudu. Mortality usually reaches 100%, and although transmissible, it is apparently not contagious among cattle by direct contact. There are two forms of the disease: the African form, which occurs in cattle associated with wildebeest, and the sheep-associated form, which occurs in many other countries. The cause has only been determined for the African form of the disease. The cause of the sheep-associated form of malignant catarrhal fever has never been determined, in spite of numerous attempts. The diseases are clinically and morphologically very similar. Rabbits are susceptible to experimental inoculation with infective material from cattle affected with the African form of the disease. In these animals, lesions similar to those seen in cattle are produced.

The cause of the African, wildebeest-derived form of malignant catarrhal fever is an apparently cell-associated herpesvirus belonging to the alcelaphine herpes group. The cytopathic effect in calf thyroid monolayers is characterized by formation of intranuclear basophilic (Cowdry type A) inclusions and syncytia. Serial culture requires the transfer of cells because free virus is not present in the culture fluids. Freezing of infected tissues destroys most of the virus; however, infected tissue cell cultures can be stored at −70°C.

The cause of the sheep-associated form of malignant catarrhal fever is not known. A herpesvirus, morphologically and immunologically similar to that causing the African form, has been identified in cell cultures infected with material from an outbreak of malignant catarrhal fever in dairy cattle in Minnesota. Experimental inoculation of cattle with this virus failed to induce clinical disease. Cattle immunized with this agent survived a challenge with lethal doses of the virulent African strain. Several cell-associated polykaryon-forming viral agents, including a morbillivirus, have been recovered from cattle affected with malignant catarrhal fever in the United States. The significance of these isolates is not known. None of these isolates was related to the herpesvirus of the African form of malignant catarrhal fever.

The mode of natural transmission of malignant catarrhal fever is not known. Experimentally, the disease can be transmitted with large quantities of whole blood and lymphoid tissue, but not by cell-free filtrates. This indicates that the agent is cell associated, probably with lymphocytes. This virus is present in nasal secretions in wildebeest, and this may be important with regard to transmission to cattle, since steers have been infected experimentally via the respiratory route.

The incubation period of malignant catarrhal fever is 2–8 weeks but may on occasion be much longer than this. Initially, there is high fluctuating fever and depression. There is usually enlargement of the superficial lymph nodes, which may be readily visible. There is edema of the eyelids and conjunctivae and congestion of the nasal and buccal mucosae. There is copious lacrimation; nasal discharge dries on and excoriates the nasolabium and partially obstructs the nares. The conjunctivitis is accompanied by an increasing rim of opacity at the filtration angle, and later, the aqueous humor may become opaque. Cor-

neal edema and ulceration occur in some cases, but in those that die quickly the infiltration of the filtration angle may be all that is seen, and this is easily overlooked.

The clinical picture may be divided into four forms, namely, the peracute, the intestinal, the head and eye, and the mild. There is considerable overlap in the syndromes observed. The naturally acquired disease is usually fatal. In the peracute form, there is hyperthermia and hemorrhagic gastroenteritis. The clinical course is 1–3 days. The intestinal form is characterized by fever, diarrhea, diffuse exanthema, lacrimation, and enlargement of lymph nodes. The course is 4–9 days. The head and eye form is of slightly longer duration, and in addition to the above, there are nervous signs. This is the typical clinical syndrome. The mild form is an occasional experimental phenomenon and may be followed by recovery.

Gross morbid changes may not be present in animals that die of peracute malignant catarrhal fever, and in these the diagnosis must rest on the detection of the characteristic histologic changes and positive results of transmission experiments. With the sheep-associated disease, diagnosis is based usually on the microscopic findings. Bearing in mind the wide variation in the development and severity of lesions, the changes described below are what one hopes to see in any case.

The carcass is dehydrated and may be emaciated if the course has been prolonged. There is a mucopurulent conjunctivitis, which may glue the edematous eyelids together. The muzzle and nares are heavily encrusted and, if wiped, reveal irregular raw surfaces, although in some cases there may only be a slight serous discharge. Cutaneous lesions are common but often overlooked. There may be, acutely, a more or less generalized vesicular and papular exanthema, with sufficient exudation to wet and mat the hair and to form detachable crusts; in unpigmented skin there is obvious hyperemia. In due course, the crusts become 1.0 mm or more in thickness, and there is patchy loss of hair. Sometimes these cutaneous changes begin locally about the bases of the hooves and horns and on the loin and perineum and remain localized or become generalized.

The respiratory system may show minor or severe lesions (Fig. 1.26A). When the course is short, the nasal mucosa may show congestion and slight serous exudation only. Later, there is a copious discharge. The mucosa is then intensely hyperemic and edematous, and erosions of a few millimeters diameter are common. These are irregular in shape, with a hemorrhagic base. Occasionally, dirty brown pseudomembranes form, and if these are removed, raw surfaces remain. Lesions of severity similar to those on the septum and turbinates may develop in the sinuses. The pharyngeal and laryngeal mucosae are hyperemic and swollen and later develop multiple erosions or ulcerations and are often covered in part by grayish yellow pseudomembranes. The tracheobronchial mucosa is hyperemic and usually petechiated, but ulceration may occur, and in a small percentage of cases a pseudomembranous tracheobronchitis is present (Fig. 1.26B). The lungs are usually edematous and emphysematous, but in peracute cases they may appear perfectly healthy. A nonspecific bronchopneumonia may complicate chronic cases.

The alimentary mucosae may show no significant lesions in the peracute disease. Minor erosions are first observed on the lips adjacent to the mucocutaneous junction. Sometimes apparently normal epithelium on the surface of the tongue peels off in sheets (Fig. 1.25C). Later, erosive and ulcerative lesions may involve a large area of oral mucosa (Fig. 1.25A), occurring especially on all surfaces of the tongue, the tips of the buccal papillae, gingivae, both divisions of the palate, and the cheeks. In some areas, the cheesy or tattered necrotic epithelium may not be sloughed at the time of inspection. Esophageal erosions, similar to those that occur in the other diseases causing ulcerative stomatitis, occur in malignant catarrhal fever and, as in rinderpest, are most consistent in the anterior portion. Lesions of the same sort are revealed in the forestomachs by careful examination. The abomasal mucosa is hyperemic and edematous, diffusely or in patches, and sprinkled with petechiae. Hemorrhagic ulcerations may be present, especially on the margins of the plicae and along the greater curvature. The wall of the small intestine is firm and thickened by edema. Its serosa is dull, very finely granular, and often peppered with fine petechiae. Its content is mucoid or hemorrhagic. The mucosa is thickened and has few or many petechial hemorrhages and minor erosions. Similar lesions occur in the large intestine and rectum but are more obvious; there are lines of congestion along the longitudinal mucosal rugae, and severe ulceration and hemorrhage may be present. The contents of the large intestine are scant and may be dry and pasty or bloody.

Rather characteristic lesions may occur in the urinary system. Renal changes are not always present. They are infarcts or 2- to 4-mm foci of nonsuppurative interstitial nephritis (Figs. 1.25D and 1.27A). They may be numerous enough to produce a mottled appearance. These foci may form slight, rounded projections from the capsular surfaces. The pelvic and ureteral mucosa frequently have petechial and ecchymotic hemorrhages. Similar lesions are present on the mucosa of the urinary bladder, or there may be more severe hemorrhage associated with erosion and ulceration of the epithelium, and hematuria (Fig. 1.26F). Superficial lesions of the vagina, similar to those of the oral cavity and skin, occur.

The liver is slightly enlarged; close inspection will reveal, in some cases, a diffuse mottling with white foci that are periportal accumulations of mononuclear cells. There may be numerous small hemorrhages and a few erosions of the mucous membrane of the gallbladder.

Among the characteristic lesions of malignant catarrhal fever is enlargement of lymph nodes. All nodes may be involved, but some may appear grossly normal. Affected nodes may be many times the normal size, and some, including hemolymph nodes, which are usually too small to recognize, may become quite obvious. There is edema of the affected nodes, but on cross section it is apparent that much of the increase in size is due to lymphocytic hyperplasia. Some of the nodes are congested. The spleen is slightly enlarged, and the lymphoid follicles are prominent.

There is an excess of cerebrospinal fluid, which contains much protein and moderate numbers of mononuclear cells (Fig. 1.26C). The meninges are wet, and there is some cloudiness in the subarachnoid space of the sulci. There also may be scattered petechial hemorrhages in the meninges. These lesions are usually most concentrated in the cerebellar leptomeninges.

Gross changes usually are not visible in the heart and larger blood vessels. Polyarthritis, characterized by increased amounts of cloudy synovial fluid and red, swollen synovial membranes, has been reported in experimentally infected cattle.

Reliance must be placed on the histologic changes for the diagnosis of malignant catarrhal fever and its differentiation from similar diseases. The characteristic histologic changes are found in lymphoid tissues and in the adventitia and walls of arterioles and arteries in any organ, and these will be described before other lesions. The protean manifestations of this disease are due largely to the vascular lesions. They comprise fibrinoid necrotizing vasculitis and accumulation of mainly mononuclear cells in the adventitia (Figs. 1.25B,D, 1.26E, and 1.27B). These changes may be focal or segmental and may involve the full width of the wall or be confined more or less to one of the layers. When the intima is involved, there is often endothelial swelling and hyperplasia. Thrombi are difficult to demonstrate in damaged vessels. The media may be selectively affected, or perhaps the adventitia alone. The affected segments of vessel are replaced by a coagulum of homogeneous, eosinophilic material, in which nuclear remnants are seen. The altered nuclei are small, distorted, and fragmented. The perivascular accumulation of cells is particularly characteristic. They are mainly lymphoid cells with large, open nuclei and prominent nucleoli; occasionally, small lymphocytes and plasma cells may be present.

In some forms of the experimental disease, fibrinoid necrosis, endothelial-cell hyperplasia, and thrombosis are not prominent. Electron microscopic studies in these cases have shown that the endothelial reaction consists primarily of lymphocytes and macrophages rather than endothelial cells. The degree of the mononuclear-cell reaction in the vessel walls and the medial necrosis increase with progression of the disease.

These changes in the blood vessels strongly suggest malignant catarrhal fever; arteritis may be seen in bovine virus diarrhea, however, mainly in the submucosa in the lower alimentary tract. Fortunately for diagnostic purposes, arteritis is present in all cases of malignant catarrhal fever, whether peracute, acute, or mild with recovery, but it may be necessary to examine many sections to find it. The best organs to examine for vascular lesions are the brain and leptomeninges, carotid rete, kidney, liver, and adrenal capsule and medulla, and any area of skin or alimentary tract showing gross lesions.

Several hypotheses have been proposed to explain the pathogenesis of the vascular lesions, but none of these is well substantiated. Malignant catarrhal fever may be an immune-mediated disease, like other diseases that are characterized by vascular necrosis and vasculitis, such as equine viral arteritis of horses, Aleutian disease of mink, and periarteritis nodosa of humans. The vascular lesions of malignant catarrhal fever are similar to those seen in graft rejections. The long incubation period and prepatent viremic stage are also suggestive of an immune-mediated disease. The pathogenesis of the vascular lesions is discussed with the Cardiovascular System (Volume 3).

All lymphoid tissues show an active proliferation of lymphoblasts, which form extensive homogeneous populations of cells in the cortical and paracortical zone of the lymph node. There may be focal necrosis associated with arteritis in both cortex and medulla. The pathogenic mechanisms involved in the proliferation of lymphoid cells are poorly understood. Areas containing

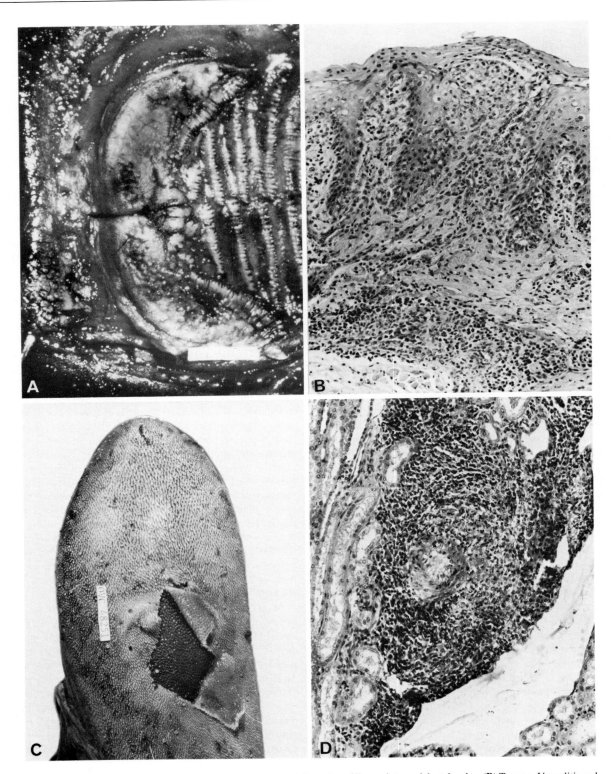

Fig. 1.25.   Malignant catarrhal fever. Ox.   **(A)** Erosion and ulceration of lips, palate, and dental pad.   **(B)** Tongue. Vasculitis and infiltration of lamina propria by lymphocytic cells, with developing ulcer over papilla.   **(C)** Separation of necrotic lingual epithelium from underlying propria.   **(D)** Extensive cuff of mononuclear cells, and fibrinoid necrosis in the wall of a small arteriole. Kidney.

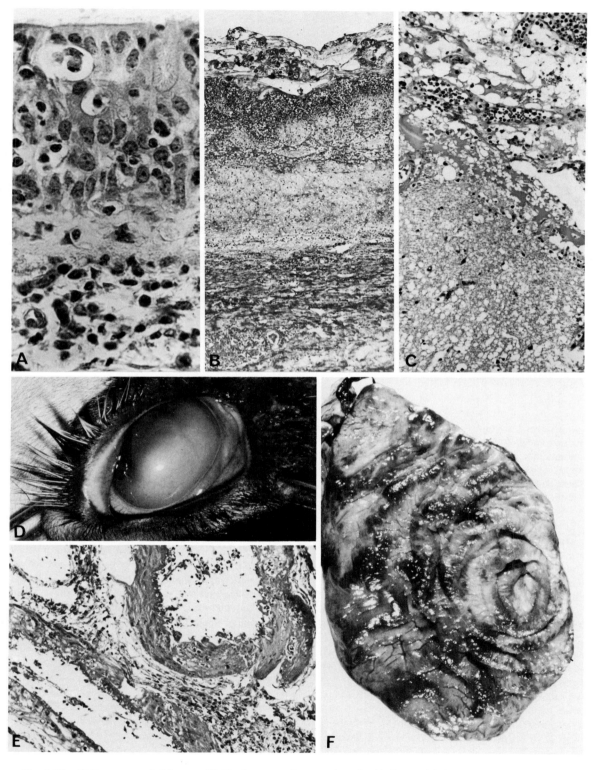

Fig. 1.26. Malignant catarrhal fever. (**A**) Nasal mucosa. Degeneration of epithelium and infiltration of lymphocytic cells in uncomplicated rhinitis. (**B**) Pseudomembranous tracheitis. (**C**) Meningeal exudate and vasculitis. (**D**) Edema of cornea. (**E**) Necrosis of arteries and periarterial reaction. Carotid rete. (**F**) Hemorrhages in mucosa of urinary bladder.

both B and T cells are obviously affected. Comparisons have been made to the lesions in lymphoid tissue in humans caused by the Epstein–Barr virus, another cell-associated herpesvirus.

Microscopic arteritis similar to that present in other organs occurs in the nervous system of many cases. Necrotizing arteritis, plasma exudation into the menginges or Virchow–Robin space, and the predominantly adventitial lymphocytic response are, in cattle, unique to malignant catarrhal fever and allow it to be differentiated from other nonsuppurative encephalitides (Fig. 1.26C). Degenerative changes in nervous parenchyma can be explained on the basis of the vascular changes.

The lesions in skin and squamous mucosae of the alimentary tract are histologically similar. The dermis or propria (and often the epithelium) is diffusely infiltrated with a mainly lymphocytic cell population. The dermis, especially its superficial portion, is edematous, and typical arteritis, involving small- and medium-sized vessels, is present. Epithelial changes are related to the presence of a diffuse mononuclear infiltrate and arteritis in the underlying dermis (Fig. 1.25B). Groups of cells become necrotic with swollen, strongly acidophilic cytoplasm; ultimately, the full thickness of epithelium in affected areas undergoes necrosis and erodes. Large areas of epithelium may thus be detached or lost, and there is not much acute leukocytic reaction in the exposed propria or dermis.

The severity of the lesions in the oral squamous mucosa is, in experimental cases at least, related to the degree of lymphoid-cell infiltration in the mucosa and underlying lamina propria rather than to the vascular thrombosis, which is minimal. The pathogenesis of the epithelial lesions has been compared to other lymphocyte-mediated reactions such as tuberculin, contact hypersensitivities, and graft rejection. The graft-rejection reaction, which is morphologically similar to malignant catarrhal fever in many respects, is purported to represent a model of B- and T-cell-mediated autoimmunity, and similar mechanisms may be involved in this disease. These lesions are all characterized by vasculitis, and perivascular mononuclear-cell reactions that extend into the epithelium.

These changes in the epithelium and its lamina propria account for the macroscopic lesions in the vagina, prepuce, bladder, and although there is often much less hemorrhage, oral cavity, nasal mucosa, esophagus, and forestomach. Although gross lesions are not present in the salivary glands, there are microscopic degenerative changes in the epithelium of the interlobular and excretory ducts, with multiple foci of parenchymal necrosis associated with arteritis.

The mottling of liver and the focal nephritis seen grossly is due to the accumulation of mononuclear cells in the portal triads of the liver (Fig. 1.27D) and in the cortices of the kidney. In the liver, these cuffs may be very large and invest the branches of the hepatic artery, which may undergo fibrinoid necrosis. Microscopic lesions are rather consistently present in the kidneys, even though gross lesions are not; they consist of vasculitis involving the smaller arteries and afferent arterioles (Fig. 1.25D). Extensive diffuse lymphocytic infiltrates disrupt the normal renal cortical architecture, and in some cases infarcts appear to be associated with vasculitis involving arcuate arteries.

The mucosa of the stomach and small and large intestine is also densely infiltrated focally and/or diffusely with large lymphocytes. Mucosal infiltrates and necrosis are associated with inflammation of arterioles in the underlying submucosa. In the abomasum, the glandular epithelium in affected areas becomes basophilic, cuboidal, or flattened mucous in type; eventually necrosis and focal ulceration occur. In the small intestine and large bowel, the lesion resembles ischemic damage. The superficial mucosa undergoes necrosis, and there is erosion and hemorrhage. Surviving crypts and glands are lined by flattened basophilic epithelium. In mucosa in which the epithelium is completely destroyed, the collapsed proprial stroma and mononuclear infiltrate are left resting on the muscularis mucosa (Fig. 1.27C). The full thickness of the intestinal wall is edematous, and there is often mesenteric arteritis.

The microscopic lesions in the joints are characterized by a marked, mainly lymphocytic reaction in the synovial membrane and underlying connective tissue, especially in the perivascular areas. Focal areas of necrosis and desquamation may be evident over regions that are heavily infiltrated by lymphocytes. Fibrinous exudate may cover the necrotic areas. Joint lesions have only been reported in experimental cases of malignant catarrhal fever, and a bovine syncytial virus was recovered from most of the affected joints. The significance of this agent in relation to the development of the arthritis is not known.

This completes a description of the histologic changes that are the basis of the gross lesions. These same changes may be found in any tissue, however, even in the absence of gross lesions. Rather constantly, there are vascular lesions of this sort in the neurohypophysis, but not the adenohypophysis, and in the adrenal glands. The adrenal changes are in the capsule and its vessels and trabeculae, and in the medullary vessels. There may be minor focal necrosis of the cortex in consequence, and more often there is disorganization of the medulla and a diffuse lymphocytic infiltrate.

Ophthalmitis occurs with some consistency, and its presence is a useful differential criterion from other ulcerative diseases of the alimentary tract. All portions of the globe may be affected. Rather consistently there is fibrinocellular exudation from hyperemic ciliary processes, and the accumulation of this exudate in the filtration angle is responsible for the rim of opacity observed clinically. Later and as a result of conjunctivitis and inflammation of the limbic vessels, the cornea is edematous and may be ulcerated and vascularized (Fig. 1.26D). There is a retinal vasculitis and, in some cases, hemorrhagic or inflammatory detachment of the retina in focal areas (Fig. 1.27B).

The differential diagnosis of malignant catarrhal fever in cattle should include other erosive–ulcerative diseases of the alimentary tract, including bovine virus diarrhea, rinderpest, bluetongue, and epizootic hemorrhagic disease in wildlife species. The African form of the disease may be confirmed by the isolation of the causative virus on bovine tissue cell cultures, especially thyroid. The diagnosis of the sheep-associated form is based on clinicopathologic findings and may be confirmed by reproduction of the disease following inoculation of whole blood into susceptible species.

BLUETONGUE AND RELATED DISEASES. **Bluetongue** is caused by a member of the genus *Orbivirus* (Reoviridae). There are more than 20 recognized serotypes of bluetongue virus dis-

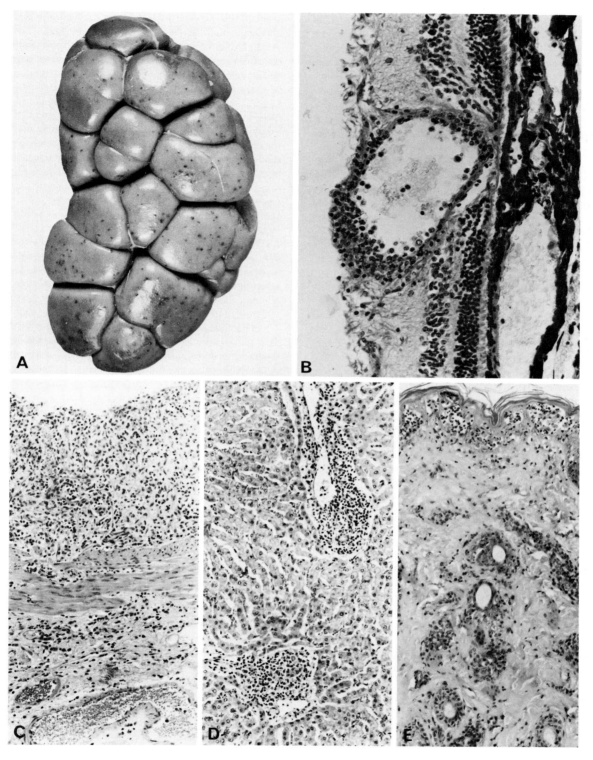

Fig. 1.27. Malignant catarrhal fever. (**A**) Focal nonsuppurative interstitial nephritis. (**B**) Vasculitis in retina. (**C**) Colitis with collapse of glands and edema of submucosa. (**D**) Accumulations of lymphocytic cells in portal triads. (**E**) Necrosis of epithelium. Skin.

tinguished by neutralization tests, though they may represent not so much distinct types as points in a spectrum of antigenicity brought about by recombination of the segmented orbivirus genome. Immunity to one serotype does not confer resistance against another and may cause "sensitization," with a more severe syndrome following infection by second type.

Epizootic hemorrhagic disease of deer is caused by a virus that represents another subgroup of *Orbivirus*. The virus causing **Ibaraki disease**, recognized in cattle in Japan, is closely related to, if not a variant of, epizootic hemorrhage disease virus; seropositive animals also have been found in Taiwan and Indonesia. Several other known orbiviruses are not associated with disease. Bluetongue, epizootic hemorrhagic disease, and related viruses are spread by *Culicoides*, known variously as midges, gnats, or sand flies. The virus multiplies by a factor of 10^3 to 10^4 in the *Culicoides* within 2 or 3 days of ingestion of the infected blood meal. Transovarian transmission of virus in *Culicoides* does not occur.

Bluetongue virus circulates in a broad belt across the tropics and warm temperate areas, with incursions or recrudescence during the *Culicoides* season, annually, or at irregular longer intervals, in cooler temperate areas. The condition is enzootic or seasonally epizootic in most of Africa, the Middle East, the eastern Mediterranean basin, the Indian subcontinent, the Caribbean, and the United States. A strain of bluetongue has been isolated from *Culicoides* in northern Australia, but spontaneous disease has not been recognized. It has made sporadic appearances in the Iberian peninsula, and seropositive cattle have been detected in Canada. Cattle, sheep, and goats are the susceptible domestic species wherever bluetongue occurs. Infection in cattle usually produces only inapparent infection or mild clinical disease. Goats, though susceptible to infection, rarely show signs; however, significant disease has occurred in goats in the Middle East and India. Sheep are the domestic species most highly susceptible to bluetongue, but there is considerable variation in expression of the disease, depending on the breed, age, and immune status of the sheep, the environmental circumstances under which they are held, and the strain of virus. In Africa, a wide variety of nondomestic ungulates and some small mammals may be inapparently infected; mortality has occurred in naturally or experimentally infected topi, cape buffalo, and kudu. In North America, wildlife species, particularly white-tailed deer, black-tailed or mule deer, elk (wapiti), bighorn sheep, and pronghorn antelope, are also infected. Bluetongue is responsible for significant mortality in all these species except elk, which usually develop mild or inapparent infection.

Epizootic hemorrhagic disease virus, or a closely related virus, has been isolated in Nigeria, but the natural vertebrate hosts there are not known. In North America, white-tailed deer, black-tailed or mule deer, pronghorn antelope, and elk are susceptible to infection. The white-tailed deer is extremely susceptible, and widespread epizootics have occurred among this species in the United States. A single outbreak has been recognized in Alberta, Canada. The rate of survival is much higher among black-tailed deer and pronghorn antelope, and elk are only very mildly affected. Clinical disease similar to that produced by bluetongue may occur in cattle, but sheep do not develop disease when infected with this virus. In Japan, the closely related virus

of Ibaraki disease also produces a clinical syndrome resembling bluetongue in cattle, but not in sheep.

The viruses of bluetongue and epizootic hemorrhagic disease circulate together in North America. Both viruses may be involved simultaneously in outbreaks of hemorrhagic disease in wild ruminants, and both have been isolated from *Culicoides* in a single locality at the same time. Cattle, among domestic animals, may play a major role as reservoir or overwintering host for bluetongue, since inapparent or latent infection may persist for a number of years, and recrudescence of viremia may be stimulated by the bites of *Culicoides*. Venereal transmission of bluetongue from an infected bull to the bred cow has been demonstrated, and infected progeny may result. Vertical transmission of bluetongue from dam to offspring also occurs in cattle, sheep, and elk. Immune tolerance may occur in prenatally infected calves.

The pathogenesis of bluetongue, epizootic hemorrhagic disease, and Ibaraki disease is fundamentally similar in all species in which disease is seen. Primary viral replication following insect bite probably occurs in regional lymph nodes and spleen. Viremia about 4–6 days after inoculation results in secondary infection of endothelium in arterioles, capillaries, and venules throughout the body, with microscopic lesions and fever beginning a day or so later, about a week after inoculation. Bluetongue virus in the blood appears to be closely associated with, or in, erythrocytes, and it may cocirculate with antibody. Endothelial damage caused by virus infection initiates local microvascular thrombosis and permeability. This is reflected microscopically by the presence of swollen endothelium, and fibrin and platelet thrombi in small vessels, with edema and hemorrhage in surrounding tissue. These lesions in turn mediate the full spectrum of gross findings. These are fundamentally ischemic necrosis of many tissues, edema due to vascular permeability, and hemorrhage resulting from vascular damage compounded, in severe cases, by consumption coagulopathy due to thrombocytopenia and depletion of soluble clotting factors.

Bluetongue in sheep is a highly variable disease; it may cause inapparent infection or an acute fulminant disease. Typically, leukopenia and pyrexia occur, even in mild infections, coincident with viremia. The degree and duration of fever do not correlate with the severity of the syndrome otherwise. In the early phase there is hyperemia of the oral and nasal mucosa, salivation, and nasal discharge within a day or two of the onset of fever. Hyperemia and edema of the eyelids and conjunctiva may occur, and edema of lips, ears, and the intermandibular area becomes apparent. Hyperemia may extend over the muzzle and the skin of much of the body, including the axillary and inguinal areas. Focal hemorrhage may be present on the lips and gums, and the tongue may become edematous and congested or cyanotic, giving the disease its name. Infarcted epithelium thickens and becomes excoriated, erosions and ulcerations develop along the margins of the tongue opposite the molars, and the mucosa of much of the tongue may slough. Excoriation and ulceration also occur on the buccal mucosa, the hard palate, and dental pad. Affected areas of skin may also become encrusted and excoriated with time, and a break in the wool can result in parts or much of the fleece being tender or cast. The coronet, bulbs, and interdigital areas of the foot may become hyperemic. Coronary swelling and streaky hemorrhages in the periople may be evident as a result of lesions in the underlying sensitive laminae. These hemorrhages may persist in the hoof as brown lines that move down the hoof as it grows. A defect parallel to the coronet may also be evident in the growing hoof in recovered cases.

Internally, in acute cases, there is subcutaneous and intermuscular edema, which may be serous or suffused with blood. Superficial lymph nodes are enlarged and juicy. Bruiselike gelatinous hemorrhages and contusions, which may be small and easily overlooked if not numerous, are often present in the subcutis and intermuscular fascial planes. Focal or multifocal pallid areas of streaky myodegeneration may be present throughout the carcass, perhaps partly obscured by petechial or ecchymotic hemorrhage. Resolving muscle lesions may be mineralized or fibrous.

Necrosis may be present deep in the papillary muscle of the left ventricle and perhaps elsewhere in the myocardium. The lesion that is perhaps most consistent and closest to pathognomonic for bluetongue is focal hemorrhage, petechial or up to 1.0 cm wide by 2 to 3 cm long, in the tunica media at the base of the pulmonary artery. These hemorrhages are visible from both the internal and adventitial surfaces and may be present in clinically mild cases with few other lesions. Petechial hemorrhage may also be present at the base of the aorta and in subendocardial and subepicardial locations over the heart.

There may also be edema and petechial or ecchymotic hemorrhage in the pharyngeal and laryngeal area. In severe cases the lungs may assume a purplish hue, with marked edematous separation of lobules. Animals with pharyngeal or esophageal myodegeneration may succumb to aspiration pneumonia.

Hyperemia, occasionally marked hemorrhage, or in advanced cases, ulceration of the mucosa may occur on rumen papillae, the pillars of the rumen, and the reticular plicae. In convalescent animals, stellate healing ulcers or scars on the wall of the forestomachs may be apparent. Petechial hemorrhage may be present in the abomasal mucosa, with congestion of the subserosa at the pylorus. The remainder of the intestinal mucosa may be congested, and occasionally there may be hemorrhage, particularly in the large bowel. Petechial hemorrhage of the mucosa of the gallbladder may also be seen.

The kidneys are commonly congested, and there may be petechial hemorrhage of the mucosa of the urinary bladder, urethra, and vulva or prepuce.

Acute lesions are characterized microscopically by microvascular thrombosis, and edema and hemorrhage, in affected sites recognized at autopsy. In squamous mucosa and skin, capillaries of the proprial and dermal papillae are involved, resulting in vacuolation and necrosis of overlying epithelium. There is a mild, local neutrophilic infiltrate acutely and a similarly mild mononuclear reaction in the dermis or propria in uncomplicated chronic lesions, which may granulate if widely or deeply ulcerated. Similar microvascular lesions are associated with necrosis and fragmentation of infarcted muscle. Muscle during the reparative phase follows the usual course of regeneration of fibers or fibrous replacement, depending on whether or not the sarcolemma retains its integrity.

In cattle, clinical bluetongue usually is apparent in only 5 to 10% of infected animals; mortality is low and often is attributed to secondary infection. Fever, loss of appetite, and leukopenia are usually seen after an incubation period of 6 to 8 days, and there may be a drop in milk production in dairy cattle. There is reddening of the epithelium of the mucous membranes, and of thin exposed skin, especially notable on the udder and teats. Edema of the lips and conjunctiva may be present. Salivation may become profuse, and as the disease progresses over the next several days, hyperemia and congestion of the mucosae become more intense. Ulcerations of the gingival, lingual, or buccal mucosa occur, most consistently on the dental pad. There may be necrosis of epithelium on the muzzle. Muscle stiffness is a feature of the disease in some animals. Laminitis, characterized by hyperemia and edema of the sensitive laminae at the coronet, may be apparent, and in some cases, hooves on affected feet may eventually slough. Sloughing or cracking of crusts of necrotic epithelium also may occur on affected parts of the skin, but the ulcerative or erosive defects heal readily. Viral antigen and thrombosis are present in small vessels in affected tissues during the acute phase.

The signs and lesions of Ibaraki disease are essentially similar to those of bluetongue in cattle, though perhaps a little more severe in some cases. As well as the signs and lesions described in cattle with bluetongue, there may be difficulty in swallowing in 20 to 30% of clinically affected animals, and the swollen tongue may protrude from the mouth. At autopsy, in addition to the lesions observable externally, there may be congestion, erosion, or ulceration of the mucosa of the abomasum, and less commonly, the esophagus and forestomachs. Ischemic necrosis and hemorrhage of the striated muscle in the tongue, pharynx, larynx, and esophagus causes the difficulty in swallowing seen clinically, and similar changes are seen in other skeletal muscles. Necrotizing aspiration pneumonia is a sequel to dysphagia in some animals.

The hemorrhagic diseases in bighorn sheep, pronghorn antelope, and white-tailed and black-tailed or mule deer in North America tend to resemble bluetongue in sheep. White-tailed deer may develop a particularly severe and fulminant acute hemorrhagic disease, with high mortality. Bluetongue in goats, though usually inapparent, can resemble bluetongue in sheep.

Bluetongue in sheep must be differentiated from foot and mouth disease, *peste des petits ruminants,* contagious ecthyma, and photosensitization in particular. In cattle, the condition must be differentiated from foot and mouth disease, vesicular stomatitis, bovine virus diarrhea, rinderpest, malignant head catarrh, and photosensitivity. In Japan, Ibaraki disease must in addition be differentiated, at least clinically, from ephemeral fever, and this would be the case in parts of Australia were the disease introduced into that continent.

In addition to the systemic disease described, abortion, perhaps unobserved, and birth of progeny with various congenital defects may follow bluetongue infection of pregnant sheep and cattle. In sheep, bluetongue infection of ewes early in gestation may result in hydranencephaly. Anomalous calves produced by bluetongue-infected cattle have excessive gingiva, an enlarged tongue, anomalous maxillae, dwarflike build, and rotations and contractures of the distal extremities. Hydranencephaly and arthrogryposis are also reported in calves infected *in utero* with bluetongue. Antibody may be sought in neonates that have not sucked, and attempts should be made to isolate virus, since some prenatally infected animals will have immune tolerance and persistent infection. The anomalies of the brain are considered further with the Nervous System (Volume 1).

BOVINE PAPULAR STOMATITIS. Papular stomatitis of cattle (infectious ulcerative stomatitis and esophagitis, proliferative stomatitis) has been known in Europe since at least the 1930s, and it occurs worldwide. It is generally an insignificant disease but needs to be differentiated from other, more serious diseases affecting the oral cavity and skin. It is caused by a DNA virus belonging to the Poxviridae, genus *Parapoxvirus*. The virus is closely related but not identical to the paravaccinia virus that causes pseudocowpox in cattle, and milker's nodules in humans. It is morphologically similar to, and shares at least one antigen with, the virus of contagious ecthyma (orf, contagious pustular dermatitis) of sheep and goats (see viral diseases of skin, in the Skin and Appendages, Volume 1).

Bovine papular stomatitis virus is host specific; it grows on tissue cultures and produces specific intracytoplasmic, acidophilic inclusions in infected epithelial cells. Neutralizing antibody is not readily demonstrated. Infection does not confer significant immunity, and successive crops of lesions and relapses can occur. The disease is more common in calves than in older animals, although the susceptibility of the latter may be increased by intercurrent debility or disease.

The papular lesions of this disease occur on the muzzle and in the anterior nares, on the gums, the buccal papillae, the dental pad, the inner aspect of the lips, the hard palate (Fig. 1.28A), the floor of the oral cavity behind the incisors, the ventral and lateral (not dorsal) surfaces of the tongue, and occasionally, in the esophagus (Fig. 1.28B) and forestomachs. The lesions may be few or many; they may be transient, or repeated crops of them may take a course of several months.

The initial lesions, which are likely to be detected on the muzzle or lips, are erythematous macules, about 2–15 mm in diameter. Shortly, the central portion becomes elevated as a low papule, although the elevation is not easy to see, and by the second day a grayish central zone of epithelial hyperplasia has developed on which there is superficial scaliness and necrosis. The lesions expand slowly to assume a "coin" shape, maintaining a hyperemic periphery and grayish center; the central necrotic area may slough to form a shallow craterous defect surrounded by a slightly raised red margin. The course of individual lesions is about a week.

Histologically, there is focal but intense hyperemia and edema in the papillae of the lamina propria, with the accumulation of a few mononuclear leukocytes. The epithelium is thickened, sometimes to twice its normal depth, by hyperplasia and ballooning degeneration in the deep layers (Fig. 1.28C). The cytoplasm of affected cells is clear, and the nucleus may be shrunken. A single round, dense, eosinophilic inclusion body lies in the vacuolate cytoplasm, especially in cells at the active margin of the lesion. In the central, more advanced part of the lesion, a mainly neutrophilic infiltrate into the superficial propria and epithelium is associated with erosion of the upper layers of necrotic cells. The basal layer survives and may be very flattened in eroded areas. Vesicles do not form.

Papular stomatitis is probably more common and widespread than reports indicate. Variation in the extent and gross appearance of the lesions is to be expected, depending on the usual host–parasite factors and the nature of superimposed infections. They may predispose to the development of necrotic stomatitis. The infection can be transmitted to humans to produce small papules, which may persist for several weeks on the skin, usually of the fingers or forearms.

Parapoxvirus particles may be demonstrated in negatively stained material from lesions examined under the electron microscope.

CONTAGIOUS ECTHYMA. Contagious ecthyma (orf, contagious pustular dermatitis) is a poxviral disease of sheep and goats that is characterized mainly by proliferative scabby lesions on the lips, face, and feet (see viral diseases of skin, in the Skin and Appendages, Volume 1). Lesions may extend into the oral cavity, involving the tongue, gingiva, dental pad, and palate. Involvement of the esophagus and forestomachs occurs but is very unusual. In general, the evolution of the lesions is similar to papular stomatitis of cattle, though they are more exudative and usually much more proliferative. In the upper alimentary tract they may consist of focal red, raised areas, which coalesce to form papules followed by pustules. The latter rupture, and on the muzzle and in the mouth they may become covered by a gray to brown scab, although scab formation may not occur in the mucosa of the upper alimentary tract.

INFECTIOUS BOVINE RHINOTRACHEITIS. Bovine herpesvirus type 1 has been associated with a wide range of clinicopathologic conditions in cattle. These include necrotizing rhinotracheitis, infectious pustular vaginitis and balanoposthitis, encephalitis, abortions, and latent infection (see appropriate chapters).

A systemic form of the disease may occur spontaneously in neonatal calves (in which it may be congenital, or acquired shortly after birth) and in feedlot cattle; it has been reproduced experimentally in young calves. Clinically affected animals have fever, leukocytosis, excessive salivation, nasal discharge, inspiratory dyspnea, depression, and often, diarrhea. The oral and nasal mucosae are hyperemic, and focal areas of necrosis, erosion, and ulceration, a few millimeters up to 3.0 cm in diameter, are located on the nares, dental pad, gums, buccal mucosa, palate, and caudal, ventral, and dorsal surfaces of the tongue. Characteristically, the lesions tend to be punctate with a slightly raised margin; the necrotic areas are covered by grayish white layer of fibrinonecrotic exudate, which leaves a raw, red base when removed.

The lesions may extend into the esophagus, usually only the upper third, and the forestomachs. In the esophagus, the erosions and ulcers may be irregular, circular, or linear and often have a punched-out appearance and a hyperemic border (Fig. 1.29A). The ruminal lesions, which are most commonly located in the dorsal and anterior ventral sacs, vary considerably. The earliest lesions consist of foci of necrosis and hemorrhage, a few millimeters in diameter. In some cases, the necrosis may involve

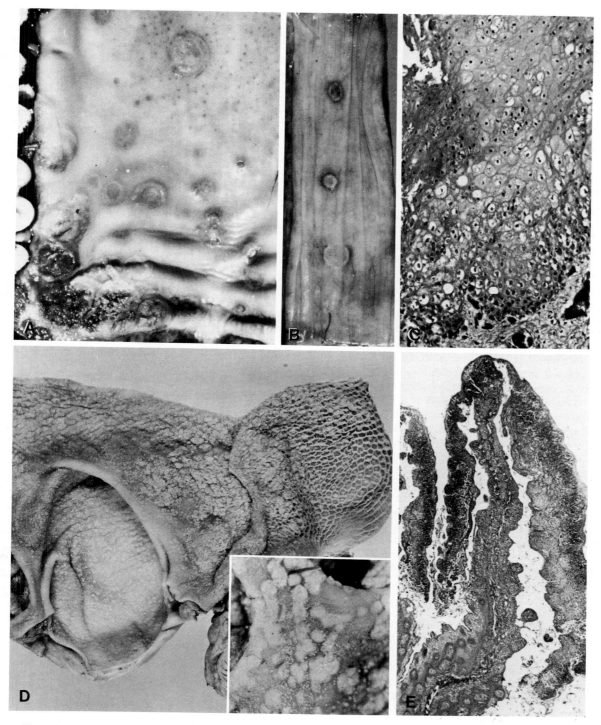

Fig. 1.28. (A–C) Bovine papular stomatitis. (A) Lesions at various stages of evolution in palate. (B) Lesions in esophagus. (C) Thickened epithelium at the margin of a lesion, with ballooning degeneration of cells in the deeper layers. (D and E) Infectious bovine rhinotracheitis. (D) Cheesy necrotic debris in rumen and reticulum. Calf. (Inset) Detail of rumen lesion. (E) Necrosis of omasal fold. Neonatal calf.

almost the entire surface of the ruminal mucosa, which becomes covered by a thick, dirty gray layer of exudate, resembling curdled milk, that adheres tightly to the wall (Fig. 1.28D). Similar lesions may be evident in the reticulum. Focal areas of necrosis result in the formation of holes, up to 1.5 cm in diameter, in the leaves of the omasum. In addition, these calves may have focal areas of necrosis in the abomasal mucosal folds, which may coalesce to form areas of necrosis 2–3 cm in diameter. The intestines are red and dilated, and the serosal surface may be covered by a thin layer of fibrinous exudate.

The enteric lesions may be accompanied by changes in the upper respiratory tract. When present, the respiratory lesions are similar to those described for older cattle, although they are milder and generally limited to the nasal mucosa, larynx, and upper third of the trachea (see the Respiratory System, this volume).

Gray to yellow necrotic foci 2–5 mm diameter may be evident macroscopically on the capsular and cut surfaces of the liver and the adrenal cortices, and in Peyer's patches.

Microscopically, the lesions in the squamous mucosa are characterized by focal areas of necrosis (Fig. 1.28E), erosion, and ulceration. A marked leukocytic reaction, predominantly neutrophilic, is evident in the basilar areas of the lesions, often extending from the underlying lamina propria. The epithelial cells at the periphery of the lesions are markedly swollen, and the cytoplasm is vacuolated. Severe necrosis may involve the entire papilla or mucosa more diffusely. Cowdry type A and B inclusions may be present in epithelial cells in the periphery of the lesion, although these are an inconsistent finding. They are more likely to be found if tissues are collected in the early stages of the disease and fixed in Bouin's fluid. The abomasal lesions consist of necrosis of glandular epithelial cells. Affected glands are dilated and filled with necrotic debris. Focal necrotic lesions involving crypts and lamina propria may be present in both the small intestine (Fig. 1.29B) and large bowel. Abomasal and intestinal lesions may predispose to the development of secondary mycosis, which is a common complication.

Foci of coagulation necrosis may occur in the liver, lymph nodes, Peyer's patches, spleen, and adrenal cortices. Typically, there is little inflammation associated with the necrosis. Herpes inclusions are inconsistently seen in cells at the periphery of the necrotic foci.

The lesions in the upper alimentary tract of cattle associated with bovine herpesvirus infection must be differentiated from those of calf diphtheria, bovine papular stomatitis, and bovine virus diarrhea. Bovine herpesvirus type 1 may be demonstrated in the lesions by means of electron microscopic examination-fluorescent-antibody technique, and tissue culture in a wide variety of systems. The ruminal lesions must be differentiated from those of bovine adenovirus infection and nonspecific rumenitis, described elsewhere in this chapter. The liver lesions may be confused with focal necrosis associated with septicemias, for example, listeriosis or salmonellosis (see Liver and Biliary System, this volume).

CAPRINE HERPESVIRUS.   A herpesvirus that shares some antigens with, but is immunologically distinct from, bovine herpesvirus-1 has been isolated from neonatal goat kids in California and Switzerland. The name caprine herpesvirus-1 has been suggested for this virus, which grows on embryonic bovine lung tissue cultures and causes severe systemic disease with erosions and ulcerations of the alimentary tract in neonatal goats. Adult goats may be latent carriers of the virus. Experimental infection of pregnant does causes abortion. The virus is nonpathogenic for calves and lambs.

The disease in neonatal kids is characterized by fever, conjunctivitis, ocular and nasal discharges, dyspnea, anorexia, abdominal pain, weakness, and death, usually within 1 to 4 days after onset of clinical signs. Affected kids have leukopenia and hypoproteinemia.

Macroscopic lesions are most obvious throughout the entire alimentary tract. Round or longitudinal erosions, which have a hyperemic border, are evident in the oral mucosa. These are particularly prominent on the gums around the incisor teeth and to a lesser extent in the pharynx and esophagus. Focal red areas of necrosis, which may be slightly elevated above the surrounding mucosa, occur in the rumen. In the abomasum, numerous longitudinal red erosions are located in the mucosa. The most severe lesions occur in the cecum and ascending colon, which are dilated, with a thickened wall, and contain focal to large areas of mucosal necrosis and ulceration, frequently covered by a pseudodiphtheritic membrane. The contents are yellow and mucoid. Hemorrhagic foci may be visible in the bladder mucosa.

Microscopically, the lesions in the upper alimentary tract are typical areas of necrosis and erosion of the squamous epithelial cells. The epithelial cells at the periphery of the necrotic areas are swollen and vacuolated, and these may contain herpes inclusions. There is marked inflammatory reaction in the underlying lamina propria. The abomasal lesions consist of acute foci of mucosal necrosis. Inclusions are particularly evident in this area. Lesions in the cecum and colon are more extensive and consist of large areas of mucosal ulceration and necrosis, which may involve the entire thickness of the wall. The submucosa is edematous and markedly infiltrated by inflammatory cells. The mesenteric nodes are edematous, and the germinal centers are depleted of lymphoid cells. Focal areas of necrosis with mild inflammatory cell reaction are evident in the bladder mucosa.

The alimentary lesions in goat kids in many respects resemble the lesions in calves infected with bovine herpesvirus type 1. Focal areas of necrosis in other organs, such as liver, spleen, and adrenal glands, which are often present in calves, are not reported in the goats.

OTHER HERPESVIRUSES.   **Canine herpesvirus** causes a systemic disease of neonatal puppies that is characterized by foci of necrosis and hemorrhage in a wide variety of organs, especially the lungs and renal cortices (see herpesvirus infections of the fetus and newborn, in the Female Genital System, Volume 3). Focal areas of necrosis may occur in the intestine as part of the systemic syndrome.

Feline viral rhinotracheitis virus (feline herpesvirus-1) causes alimentary tract lesions (see Erosive and Ulcerative Stomatitides). Viruses antigenically related to feline herpesvirus-1 have been isolated from dogs with diarrhea, but descriptions of lesions are not available.

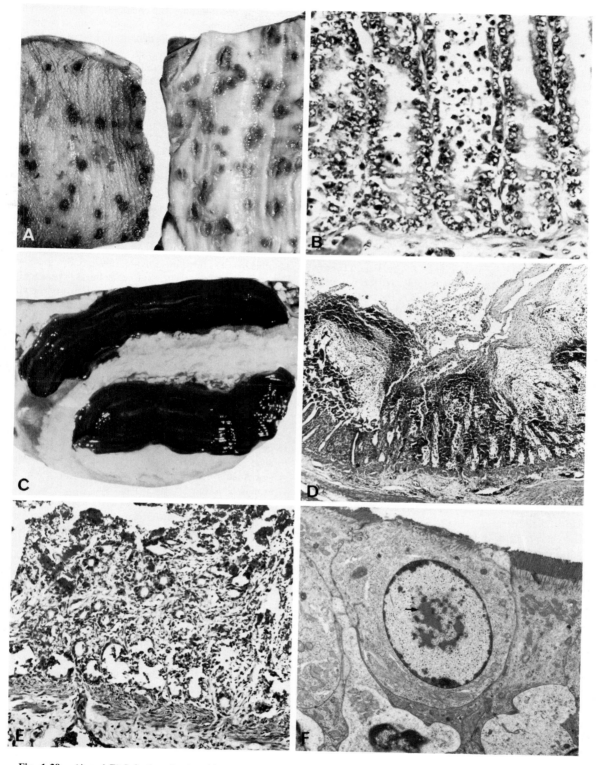

Fig. 1.29. (**A** and **B**) Infectious bovine rhinotracheitis. (**A**) Foci of necrosis on mucosa of esophagus and rumen. Neonatal calf. (**B**) Necrosis of epithelium in the crypts of Lieberkühn. Small intestine. Neonatal calf. (**C–E**) Bovine adenovirus infection. (**C**) Congested and hemorrhagic colon. (**D** and **E**) Infarctive necrosis and hemorrhage. Colon. (**F**) Porcine adenovirus infection. Adenovirus-infected cell in epithelium of dome over Peyer's patch. Note inclusion (arrow). (Courtesy of D. M. Hoover and S. E. Sanford.)

Adenovirus Enteritis

The adenoviruses that have been associated with enteric infections in humans, cattle, swine, horses, sheep, and dogs belong to the Adenoviridae, genus *Mastadenovirus*. *In vivo* and *in vitro* infection of cells results in the formation of both Cowdry type A and B inclusions. Adenoviruses are relatively heat resistant and can survive for several days at room temperature. Infected animals may remain carriers for weeks. Adenovirus infections in both humans and animals appear, in general, to be systemic, and disease seems to occur more commonly in immunologically compromised individuals. Certain strains have a tropism for the respiratory tract, others for the alimentary tract. Their enteric manifestations will be considered here.

BOVINE ADENOVIRUSES.   Serologic surveys indicate that adenovirus infections in cattle are worldwide in distribution. In many areas there is a high prevalence of antibodies, indicating that infection is common, but overt disease is sporadic. There are 10 different serotypes of bovine adenovirus, and this number is likely to increase. Infection has been mainly associated with keratoconjunctivitis and respiratory disease. Many strains have been isolated from normal cattle. Serotypes 3, 4, 5, 7, and 8 have all been associated with a pneumoenteritis complex. Experimental infection with most strains usually produces only a mild respiratory infection, and Koch's postulates have not been fulfilled for the enteric form of the disease. It appears that after an initial viremic stage, the virus localizes in the endothelial cells of vessels in a variety of organs, resulting in thrombosis with subsequent focal areas of ischemic necrosis.

Clinically, enteric infections with bovine adenovirus occur sporadically in 1- to 8-week-old calves and in feedlot animals. Affected animals have fever and diarrhea, which may contain blood. They are dehydrated, and the mucous membranes of the muzzle and mouth are congested. Dry encrusted exudate may cover the muzzle, and there may be serous to mucopurulent ocular and nasal discharges.

The macroscopic lesions may be present in the forestomachs, abomasum, and intestine. Those in the forestomachs are characterized by irregular, raised, red to gray necrotic areas 2–4 mm in diameter on the mucosa of both the dorsal and ventral sacs of the rumen. In some cases the areas of necrosis coalesce to give rise to a diffuse necrotizing rumenitis. Ulcers up to 1.5 cm in diameter may be located on the ruminal pillars, and these may be visible through the serosa. Similar lesions may be evident in the omasum. The abomasal mucosal folds are edematous and congested, with focal necrosis and ulceration in the mucosa, which, like those in the forestomachs, may be visible on the serosal surface.

The intestinal lesions vary from slight dilation and distention with excessive fluid to severe multifocal or diffuse fibrinohemorrhagic enteritis. The Peyer's patches are often necrotic and may be covered by a pseudodiphtheritic membrane. In feedlot cattle, the lesions may be most prominent in the colon. The mucosa is dark red, and there is marked edema of the mesocolon. The mesenteric lymph nodes are enlarged and edematous.

Microscopically, large, basophilic to amphophilic inclusions completely or partially fill the nuclei of endothelium in the vessels of the lamina propria and submucosa of the rumen, abomasum, and intestine. The endothelial cells are swollen and necrotic, and some veins and lymphatics contain thrombi. Foci of ischemic necrosis are evident in the overlying mucosa, and in more advanced lesions, the necrosis extends across the muscularis mucosae. Fibrinocellular exudate often covers the mucosal surface. There is usually marked submucosal edema, congestion, and fibrinous exudation. Foci of necrosis are evident in the lymphoid follicles of the Peyer's patches, which are also depleted of lymphocytes. Intestinal crypts are dilated, lined by flat epithelial cells, and usually contain necrotic debris.

Typical inclusions may also be found in endothelial cells of vessels and sinusoids of the adrenal glands, mesenteric lymph nodes, liver, spleen, glomeruli, and interstitial capillaries in the kidney and in the mucosa of the urinary bladder. Ultrastructurally, adenovirus particles are located in large numbers in the nuclei of endothelial cells.

Confirmation of enteric bovine adenovirus infection depends on the demonstration of the typical intranuclear inclusions in endothelial cells, the ultrastructural presence of virus particles, and isolation of the virus in tissue cell cultures. The latter is often difficult because different serotypes and strains of the virus require specific tissue cell cultures, and several blind passages may be required before cytopathic changes are evident.

Enteritis due to bovine adenovirus must be differentiated from bovine virus diarrhea, malignant catarrhal fever, the enteric form of infectious bovine rhinotracheitis, salmonellosis, coccidiosis, and enteric mycotic infections.

PORCINE ADENOVIRUS.   There are five different serotypes of adenoviruses in swine, which, according to serologic surveys, are all common. Serotype 4 appears to be the most widely distributed strain of the virus in Europe and North America. Asymptomatic infections are most common in swine, and the virus may be isolated from normal pigs.

The importance of adenoviruses as a cause of enteric disease in the field remains controversial. In Belgium, serotype 3 has been associated with diarrhea, occasional vomiting, dehydration, and reduced growth rate in 2- to 3-week-old pigs. Experimental oronasal infection of hysterotomy-derived, colostrum-deprived pigs with this same serotype produces diarrhea, after an incubation period of about 3 to 4 days. Diarrhea has also been produced experimentally with serotype 4 and other strains of the virus. Other lesions produced with serotype 4 are interstitial pneumonia, nonsuppurative meningoencephalitis, and focal interstitial nephritis. In general, however, these lesions do not appear to cause clinical disease.

The macroscopic lesions in the intestine consist of excessive yellow, watery contents and moderate enlargement of the mesenteric lymph nodes.

In contrast to the situation in calves, where the inclusions are located in the nuclei of endothelial cells, in pigs the inclusions are in enterocytes in the distal jejunum and ileum. Initially the inclusions are amphophilic to basophilic and fill the entire nucleus, and the nuclear membrane is thickened. In later stages of the infection, the inclusions are smaller and are surrounded by a halo. The infected nuclei are enlarged, round, and displaced to the apical portion of the cell. The inclusions are mainly located in cells on the sides of the villi, which may be short and blunt.

They are often seen in epithelium, and occasionally, in associated lymphocytes, on the dome over Peyer's patches. They may persist for up to 15 days postinfection. There may be a moderate mononuclear-cell reaction in the lamina propria. Inclusions are also found in the squamous epithelial cells of the tonsils.

Ultrastructurally, infected nuclei of enterocytes are round and swollen and contain numerous typical adenovirus particles (Fig. 1.29F). Affected enterocytes are cuboidal, and the apical portion protrudes slightly into the lumen. The cell membrane and microvilli are irregular, and the terminal web is absent. The rough endoplasmic reticulum shows local distension, with formation of large multivesicular bodies. Eventually, there is complete loss of microvilli, and the cell membrane ruptures with release of cell contents and virus particles into the gut lumen.

The presence of inclusions in enterocytes must be interpreted with caution. A survey in Canada revealed that 4.4% of 5-day- to 24-week-old pigs had adenovirus inclusions in enterocytes, mainly in the ileum. More than 50% of the pigs had diarrhea; however, other enteropathogenic organisms were found in most of these animals. Enteric adenovirus infection may be an incidental infection, and more research is needed to determine the prevalence and significance of adenovirus infection in swine.

The infection must be differentiated from other diseases that may cause villus atrophy, including rotavirus, coronavirus, and coccidiosis.

EQUINE ADENOVIRUS.   Equine adenovirus serotype 1 has a worldwide distribution. Subclinical infections are common. Clinical disease occurs mainly as an upper respiratory infection in foals less than 3 months of age. The infection is particularly important in Arabian foals with combined immunodeficiency, in which intestinal involvement is common. The virus is capable of replication in the intestinal epithelium and produces duodenal villus atrophy after experimental infection.

There is a single case report of an unidentified alimentary tract adenovirus infection in an Arabian foal that did not have lesions of combined immunodeficiency. The foal had diarrhea and progressive weight loss over a 2-month period. The macroscopic lesions consisted of ulcers in the distal esophagus and nonglandular mucosa of the stomach. The intestine contained soft to semifluid ingesta.

Histologically, there was necrosis and ulceration of the esophageal and gastric squamous mucosa. Typical adenoviral inclusions were found at all levels of the small intestine. These were most commonly located in the villous epithelial cells, less often in the crypts, and only occasionally in the submucosal glands. There was focal to diffuse villus atrophy through the small intestine.

ADENOVIRUSES IN OTHER SPECIES.   **Ovine adenovirus** type 1 has been recovered, in France, from feces of diarrheic lambs that also had coccidiosis. Serotype 4 replicates and persists in the alimentary tract of sheep, but there is no information on the pathogenesis and lesions associated with the virus in this site.

Diarrhea has been reported in dogs with **infectious canine hepatitis**. The virus has a particular tropism for hepatocytes and endothelial cells. The serosal hemorrhages in the gastrointestinal tract and possibly the diarrhea may be related to the

vascular damage in the serosa and mucosa, respectively (see the Liver and Biliary System, this volume).

Enteric Coronavirus Infection

Coronaviruses cause disease affecting a number of organ systems in a variety of species, many of which are outside our scope. Among domestic mammals, they cause mainly enteric infections; the major exceptions are feline infectious peritonitis and hemagglutinating encephalomyelitis virus of swine.

Coronavirus is the only genus in the Coronaviridae. These viruses have a single-stranded RNA genome. They are pleomorphic or roughly spherical and vary in size from about 70 to 200 nm in diameter, averaging approximately 100 to 130 nm. There is a phospholipid-bearing envelope probably derived in part from host cell membrane. They gain their name from the characteristic "corona" of petal- or droplet-shaped radial surface projections (peplomeres) visible under the electron microscope in negatively stained preparations. Some coronaviruses hemagglutinate. The coronaviruses infecting each species of host appear to be distinctive; some species are infected by more than one type of coronavirus. There are antigenic relationships among some viruses from various hosts, and experimental cross-infection will occur between some host species, generally without pathologic consequences.

Virus replication in the intestinal epithelium by coronaviruses is similar in all the species studied. Coronavirus infects and replicates in the apical cytoplasm of absorptive enterocytes on the tips and sides of intestinal villi. Virions are probably taken up by the apical border of the cell, perhaps by endocytosis or fusion with the plasmalemma. Replication and maturation appear to involve budding of virions from the cytosol through the membrane and into the lumen of vacuoles or cisternae in the smooth endoplasmic reticulum, where they accumulate. Virions are found in tubules of the Golgi apparatus. They may exit via that route from infected cells, by exocytosis at the apical cell membrane, or on the lateral cell surface, since virus particles are often seen lined up between microvilli or in the lateral intercellular space between infected cells. Coronaviruses will also infect some mesenchymal cells in villi and, probably, mesenteric lymph node.

By about 12 to 20 hr after infection, mitochondria in virus-infected cells swell, cisternae of smooth and rough endoplasmic reticulum dilate, the cytoplasm of infected cells loses its electron density, and cells lose their columnar profile. The terminal web is fragmented; microvilli swell and become irregular, perhaps in association with blebbing of the apical membrane. Damaged epithelium may lyse *in situ,* releasing virus retained in cytoplasmic vacuoles, or it may exfoliate into the lumen. Profuse diarrhea usually begins about the time that early cytologic changes become apparent, but before there is extensive epithelial exfoliation.

Exfoliation of damaged epithelium may be massive over a relatively short period of time, leading to the development of villus atrophy, the severity of which largely reflects the degree of initial viral damage. Villi may appear fused along their sides or tips, and during the exfoliative phase some villi with denuded tips may be present. The enterocytes present on villi shortly after the initial exfoliative episode are mainly poorly differentiated, low columnar, cuboidal, or squamous cells, with stubby irregular microvilli. Within 2 or 3 days, villi begin to regenerate and the epithelium becomes progressively more columnar, though still lacking a well-developed brush border and its complement of enzymes. Defective fat absorption is reflected in the accumulation of lipid droplets in the cytoplasm of enterocytes on villi. This is particularly marked over the period of about 2 to 5 days after experimental inoculation. With progressive epithelial regeneration from the crypts, the villus fusion, which may be the result of adhesion of temporarily denuded lamina propria of adjacent villi, regresses. Separation begins along the basal margins of the adhesions and progresses toward the tips of the villi. There may be focal acute inflammation in the lamina propria of temporarily denuded villi, and a mild mononuclear infiltrate in the stroma of collapsed villi. Though several cycles of virus replication may occur, poorly differentiated enterocytes appear relatively refractory to infection, and the virus titer falls, presumably as local immune mechanisms also come into play. Hyperplasia of epithelium in crypts usually results in eventual resolution of the villus atrophy, restoring normal function.

The diarrhea that occurs is a result of electrolyte and nutrient malabsorption, with some contribution by secretion from cells in crypts, and probably by poorly differentiated surface epithelium in the reparative phase. Mechanisms of diarrhea in villus atrophy have been discussed under Pathophysiology of Enteric Disease. Remission of signs occurs within about 4 to 6 days as regeneration of villi occurs, providing the animal survives the dehydration, electrolyte depletion, and acidosis brought about by diarrhea.

SWINE. Three coronaviruses cause gastrointestinal signs in swine. Hemagglutinating encephalomyelitis virus causes vomiting and wasting disease in suckling piglets; this is a condition mediated mainly by infection of the central and peripheral nervous system (see the Nervous System, Volume 1). **Transmissible gastroenteritis** virus and **coronavirus 777** (porcine epizootic diarrhea virus) both cause syndromes of acute diarrheal disease in all age groups, and chronic diarrhea and runting in weaned pigs. In some areas, coronaviruses, especially transmissible gastroenteritis, are the major cause of diarrhea in neonatal swine.

Transmissible gastroenteritis may affect swine of any age, causing vomition, severe diarrhea, and in piglets, high mortality. The disease is recognized throughout most of the world, including the United Kingdom, Europe, all of North America, Central and South America, and the Far East. Australia and New Zealand seem to be free.

The epizootiology of transmissible gastroenteritis depends on the overall immune status of the herd and of the various age groups within the herd. Introduction of virus into a naive herd results in a rapid spread of disease with high morbidity affecting all age groups. Sows and older pigs will show transient inappetence, possibly diarrhea, and perhaps vomition. Signs may be more severe in sows exposed to high virus challenge from infected baby pigs. Agalactia may occur in recently farrowed sows. Suckling piglets develop severe diarrhea, and mortality may approach 100% in piglets less than 10 to 14 days old. Older pigs usually develop less severe signs and have lower mortality. In herds with enzootic infection, high piglet mortality may occur in the offspring of recently introduced naive sows, and diarrhea

with lower mortality may occur in piglets more than about 2 to 3 weeks of age as milk intake and concomitant lactogenic immunity wane. Infected pigs in the late suckling or weanling age group may runt. Transmissible gastroenteritis is more prevalent in the winter months, perhaps because the virus is not resistant to summer environmental conditions of warmth and sunlight. Baby pigs that are chilled also seem less able to survive the effects of infection.

The severity of disease in baby pigs is related partly to their inability to withstand dehydration, due to their small size. Probably as significant is the differentiation, and low rate of turnover, of epithelium in the neonate. Villi in piglets under ~5 days of age are very tall, about 700–1200 μm long, with a villus:crypt ratio of about 7:1 to 9:1. The surface epithelium is mature and has an extensive vesicular network in the apical cytoplasm associated with uptake of macromolecules and colostrum during the first day or two after birth. Crypts are short and relatively inactive. The population of epithelium susceptible to infection on each villus is therefore large, and the capacity to regenerate new enterocytes is small. By ~3 weeks of age, villi are about 400–700 μm long, and crypts are longer and their epithelium is actively proliferative, so that the villus:crypt ratio is of the order of 3:1 or 4:1. Virus production by infected enterocytes in older pigs seems less efficient, and replacement of cells lost to infection is more rapid, contributing to the relative resistance seen in swine more than 2 to 3 weeks of age.

Pigs infected with transmissible gastroenteritis often continue to suck, and at necropsy the stomach may contain a milk curd. The small bowel is flaccid and contains yellow frothy fluid with flecks of undigested milk. Chyle is not usually evident in mesenteric lymphatics since there is fat malabsorption. The content of the large intestine is usually yellow, and watery to creamy in consistency. The carcass is dehydrated, and there is usually evidence of diarrhea at the perineum. Yellow granular deposits may be evident in the renal medulla and pelvis. These are urates precipitated as the result of dehydration (see the Urinary System, this volume).

The microscopic lesions are those of villus atrophy (Fig. 1.30A–C), the severity of which is a function of the age of the pig and the stage of the disease. The lesions are most severe about the time of the onset of diarrhea in young piglets. In later phases or in older pigs there may be subtotal to moderate atrophy, and the mucosa may be lined by cuboidal to low columnar epithelium, with irregular nuclear polarity and an indistinct brush border. Severe atrophy is readily recognized at necropsy of neonatal piglets, by examination of the mucosa under a dissecting microscope. Lesions are most common in the middle and lower small intestine, and villi in the duodenum are usually tall and cylindric. Lesions may be patchy, and several areas of lower small intestine must be examined before atrophy is considered not to be present. In animals beyond the neonatal age group, atrophy may not be so severe and readily recognized under the dissecting microscope, and the contrast with the normally shorter villi in the duodenum of older pigs is not as marked. Histologic assessment of the gut is essential.

Confirmation of a diagnosis of transmissible gastroenteritis is dependent on the demonstration of specific antigen in epithelium in frozen sections of lower small intestine by immunofluores-

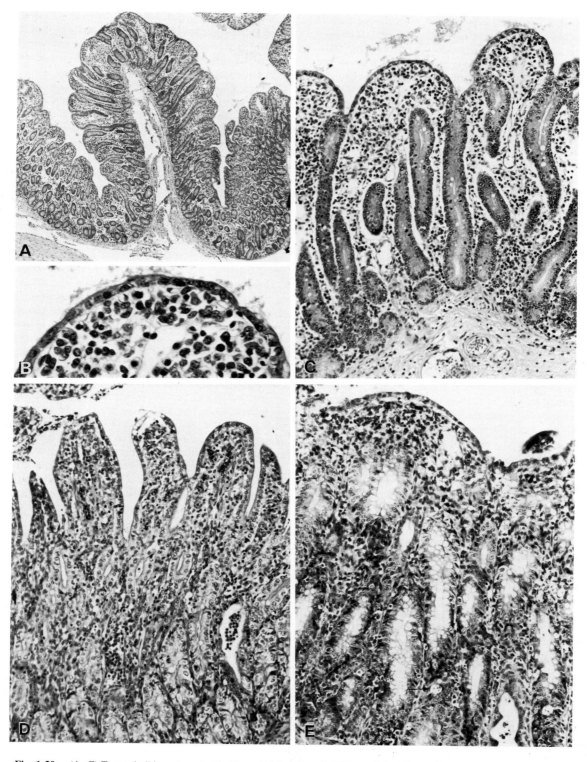

Fig. 1.30. (A–C) Transmissible gastroenteritis. Pig. (A) Atrophy of villi in small intestine. (B) Detail of (C). Enterocytes on surface of atrophic villus. (C) Atrophy of villi, with hypertrophy of crypts of Lieberkühn. Surface epithelium is cuboidal or flattened. (D and E) Bovine coronavirus infection. (Courtesy of M. Morin). (D) Blunt, fused villi with cuboidal surface epithelium. Small intestine. (E) Attenuation of surface epithelium and necrosis of gland epithelium (arrow). Colon.

cence or immunoperoxidase techniques. Coronavirus may be found by direct examination of negatively stained ileal or colonic content under the electron microscope. Immunoagglutination of virus in the content may improve the efficiency of this technique and allows differentiation from CV777. Isolation of virus in tissue culture on appropriate cell lines, especially swine testis, may be accomplished, but other methods of diagnosis are faster. To make a diagnosis it is essential to examine material taken from freshly killed piglets in the very early stages of clinical disease, before viral antigen is dissipated.

The differential diagnosis of diarrhea in suckling and weanling pigs includes, in piglets less than 5 days of age, transmissible gastroenteritis and enterotoxic *E. coli* diarrhea as the main candidates, with CV777 and clostridial enterotoxemia a possibility. Piglets 5 days of age to weaning may have transmissible gastroenteritis, CV777, rotavirus, adenovirus, *Isospora, Strongyloides,* or enteropathic *E. coli* infection.

Coronavirus 777 is reported mainly from England and Europe. It appears to cause disease that is essentially similar to transmissible gastroenteritis in epidemiology, pathogenesis, and pathology but may be milder.

CATTLE. Coronavirus infection is a common cause of diarrhea in neonatal beef and dairy calves, either alone or in combination with other agents, particularly rotavirus and *Cryptosporidium.* The virus is capable of infecting absorptive epithelium in the full length of the small intestine, and in the large bowel. Viral antigen is also found in macrophages in the lamina propria of villi and in mesenteric lymph nodes. In field infections, microscopic lesions are most consistently found in the lower small intestine and colon. Calves with coronavirus infection usually develop mild depression but continue to drink milk despite developing profuse diarrhea. With progressive dehydration, acidosis, and hyperkalemia, the animals become weak and lethargic, death ensuing as a result of hypovolemia, hypoglycemia, and potassium cardiotoxicosis. Diarrhea in survivors resolves in 5 or 6 days.

At autopsy, affected animals have the nonspecific lesions of undifferentiated neonatal calf diarrhea. Rarely, mild fibrinonecrotic typhlocolitis is recognized at necropsy in calves with coronavirus infection. Mesenteric lymph nodes may be somewhat enlarged and wet.

The microscopic lesions of coronavirus infection in calves vary with the severity and duration of the infection; villus atrophy in combination with colitis is typical (Fig. 1.30D,E). In the small intestine, villus atrophy is rarely as severe as that seen in neonatal swine. Rather, villi are moderately shortened or have subtotal atrophy, with a villus:crypt ratio of about 1:1 or 2:1. Villi are stumpy, club-shaped or pointed at the tips, and villus fusion may be common. In the early phase of the clinical disease, villi are often pointed and covered by cuboidal to squamous epithelium. Exfoliation of epithelium and microerosion may be evident. Later, the epithelium is cuboidal to low columnar and basophilic, with irregular nuclear polarity and an indistinct brush border. Cryptal epithelium is hyperplastic. The lamina propria may contain a moderate infiltrate of mainly mononuclear inflammatory cells, some of which may have pyknotic or karyorrhectic nuclei. In the early stages of infection, necrosis of

cells in mesenteric lymph nodes is associated with viral replication. Peyer's patches in animals examined after 4 or 5 days of clinical illness often appear involuted and are dominated by histiocytic cells. Whether this is the result of viral activity or the effect of endogenous glucocorticoids is unclear.

In the colon during the early phase of infection, surface epithelium may be exfoliating, flattened and squamous, or eroded in patchy areas, and some colonic glands lined by flattened epithelium will contain exfoliated cells and necrotic debris. A moderate mixed inflammatory reaction is present in the lamina propria, and neutrophils may be in damaged glands or effusing into the lumen through superficial microerosions. Later in infection, some dilated, debris-filled colonic glands will remain, but other glands will be lined by hyperplastic epithelium, and the surface epithelium will be restored to a cuboidal or low columnar cell type. Goblet cells are usually relatively uncommon. Colonic lesions may be recognizable in tissues from animals submitted dead, though postmortem change has obscured changes in the small intestine.

Live calves in the early stages of clinical disease are the best subjects for confirmation of an etiologic diagnosis. In calves becoming ill at less than 4 or 5 days of age, enterotoxic *E. coli* is the main alternative diagnosis. Rotavirus, *Cryptosporidium,* and combined infections must be considered in calves 5–15 days of age. Infectious bovine rhinotracheitis, salmonellosis, and bovine virus diarrhea must also be considered. Both salmonellosis and bovine virus diarrhea may be associated with depletion of Peyer's patches and colitis, which can be confused with that of coronavirus infection; neither is common in the strictly neonatal age group (less than 7 to 14 days of age). Demonstration of coronavirus antigen in frozen sections from the lower small intestine, in combination with direct electron microscopy or immunoelectron microscopy of content from the ileum or colon, will confirm the diagnosis. Hemadsorption–elution hemagglutination assay and enzyme-linked immunosorbent assay (ELISA) techniques have also been developed for demonstration of bovine coronavirus in intestinal contents or feces. Preferably, more than one animal should be examined to establish the cause of a herd problem. Isolation of the virus in cell culture can be accomplished in several systems but is not a practical means of rapid diagnosis.

In addition to its implication in neonatal diarrhea in calves, coronavirus has been associated with a diarrheal syndrome in older cattle in New Zealand, Japan, and France compatible with "winter dysentery." Mortality is low or nonexistent. Since it has been demonstrated in feces in the absence of other known pathogens, it has been considered causally associated with outbreaks of diarrhea. That coronavirus does cause colitis in calves makes it a plausible cause of transient colitis and diarrhea in older animals. Whether it is the agent (or one among others) responsible for winter dysentery is not known.

DOGS. A coronavirus was first associated with diarrhea in military dogs in Germany, and subsequent reports have emerged of coronavirus in normal canine feces, or associated with diarrhea, in Australia, North America, and Belgium. Although dogs of all age groups appear to be susceptible to infection by coronavirus, the condition is probably most important as a transient, generally nonfatal diarrhea in puppies. Coronaviruses were at first associated with the pandemic of diarrhea in dogs in 1978, which was subsequent demonstrated to be due to canine parvovirus-2. Coronavirus is probably widely prevalent in the dog population, but a cause of diarrhea in only a minority of animals. Very few animals with lesions consistent with coronavirus infection are submitted to biopsy or come to autopsy.

Viral replication is reported to occur in the enterocytes of the small intestine, and in experimental infections in neonatal puppies, the lesions resemble the villus atrophy associated with coronavirus infection in other species. Diarrhea began as early as 1 day after inoculation, and in most animals by 4 days. Onset of signs coincided with the development of moderate villus atrophy and fusion. Enterocytes on villi became cuboidal, contained lipid vacuoles, and had an indistinct brush border. Lesions were most consistent and severe in the ileum. Resolution of villus atrophy within 7 to 10 days was associated with remission of signs.

Colonic infection by canine coronavirus was not demonstrated by immunofluorescence in experimental animals, though mild colonic lesions were described, including loss of sulfomucins from goblet cells and some epithelial shedding. In the only available report of lesions due to spontaneous canine coronavirus infection, however, colonic infection and lesions were demonstrated. There was watery content in the lumen of the small and large intestine, and in the cecum and colon fibrin mixed with some blood was evident. Mesenteric lymph nodes were enlarged and edematous. Villus atrophy in the jejunum was inconsistent, but there was necrotic debris in many glands in the cecum and colon. Virus-infected cells were exfoliating into the lumen.

It seems, therefore, that canine coronavirus must be differentiated from common causes of small bowel diarrhea in the young dog, especially parvovirus infection, rotavirus infection, and coccidiosis, and from other forms of acute mucosal colitis. Demonstration of coronavirus particles in intestinal content or feces in association with villus atrophy and/or acute mucosal colitis, and preferably, demonstration of virus-infected cells under the electron microscope, would confirm an etiologic diagnosis in dogs.

OTHER SPECIES. Our understanding of the enteric implications of the coronavirus infections of **cats** is still confused. Feline infectious peritonitis is caused by a coronavirus that cross-reacts serologically with the virus of transmissible gastroenteritis in swine. Equivocal lesions, including mild villus atrophy, have been described in cats with feline infectious peritonitis, but intestinal lesions are not a feature of the disease. A morphologically similar, but probably different coronavirus, that also cross-reacts serologically with feline infectious peritonitis virus has been associated with diarrhea in cats. A third coronavirus, with distinctive peplomere morphology, has been described in the feces of clinically normal cats.

Coronaviruses have been recovered from the feces of **sheep** with transient diarrhea, and they have been associated with severe villus atrophy in several spontaneous outbreaks of diarrhea. No experimental confirmation of the pathogenicity of coronavirus in sheep is available.

Coronavirus infection may also be associated with diarrhea in **foals**, but again, experimental confirmation of pathogenicity is lacking.

Rotavirus Infection

Members of the genus *Rotavirus,* in the Reoviridae, infect the gastrointestinal tract of a very wide range of mammals and birds. In the earlier literature they are frequently referred to as reovirus-like. The ability to infect cells, and serologic specificity of individual types of rotaviruses, are conferred by elements of the outer capsid layer. Some strains of rotaviruses isolated from one species can be transmitted successfully to other species, sometimes producing significant lesions and disease in experimental infections. The factors influencing viral host specificity and virulence and their epizootiologic connotations are unclear. The viruses are probably generally host specific, however, with little significant zoonotic potential.

Rotaviruses infect the absorptive enterocytes and occasionally goblet cells on the tips and sides of the distal half or two-thirds of villi in the small intestine. Virus production and the pathogenesis of infection are similar in all species studied. The mode of entry of rotaviruses into the cell is unclear; presumably it is across the apical cell membrane or by endocytosis at the base of microvilli. Granular "viroplasm" containing incomplete virions is seen in the apical cytoplasm of infected cells, and virions acquire their complete capsid after budding into dilated cisternae of rough endoplasmic reticulum, where they accumulate. Elongate tubular structures are found in the nuclei and rough endoplasmic reticulum of some infected cells. Virus-infected cells are most prevalent 18–24 hr after experimental infection, and they tend to diminish in number rapidly, so that by 3 or 4 days after infection few cells containing viral antigen are present. Infected enterocytes lose cytoplasmic electron density, and mitochondria swell, as does the cell generally. Microvilli become irregular and somewhat stunted, and there may be some blebbing of membranes. Infected cells exfoliate into the intestinal lumen, and virus is probably released by lysis of damaged epithelium prior to or after exfoliation.

The pathogenesis of rotavirus infection resembles that of coronavirus. Exfoliation of infected epithelium over a relatively short period of time results in villus atrophy. The mucosal surface is covered by cuboidal, poorly differentiated epithelium that has an ill-defined microvillous border and may contain lipid droplets in the cytoplasm. Diarrhea is mediated probably by electrolyte and nutrient malabsorption, perhaps exacerbated by the effect of cryptal secretion. It begins about the time of early viral cytopathology, 20–24 hr after infection, and may persist for a variable period, from a few hours to a week or more. Regeneration of the mucosa by epithelium emerging from crypts, and differentiating on reformed villi, is associated with remission of signs in animals surviving the effects of diarrhea.

Rotaviruses are widespread, if not ubiquitous, among populations of most species, and they are relatively resistant to the external environment. Protection against infection in neonates is apparently conferred largely by the presence of lactogenic immunity. Probably, many individuals in a population undergo inapparent infection. Disease is seen in the various species when viral contamination of the environment is heavy, perhaps as a result of intensive husbandry practices, and lactogenic immunity is waning or absent. Though rotavirus infection is usually associated with younger age groups, naive older animals may become infected, sometimes with the development of diarrhea.

CATTLE.   Rotavirus infection is implicated mainly in diarrhea of neonatal beef and dairy calves, both suckled and artifically reared, though there are reports of its association with diarrhea in adult cattle. Diarrhea may be produced in calves by rotavirus infection alone, but the condition is usually considered to be relatively mild or transient in comparison with that induced by enterotoxic *E. coli* or coronavirus. Combinations of agents including rotavirus are frequently involved in outbreaks of diarrhea in neonatal calves. Rotavirus may be implicated in animals developing signs at any time over the period up to about 2 to 3 weeks of age, and it is more commonly encountered in animals more than 4 or 5 days of age.

The gross lesions of rotaviral infection are the nonspecific findings of undifferentiated neonatal diarrhea in calves. Microscopic lesions in the small intestine cannot be differentiated from those of coronavirus infection. They may vary somewhat, depending on the severity of the initial viral damage and the stage of evolution of the sequelae. Blunt, club-shaped villi, mild or moderate villus atrophy, and perhaps villus fusion may be present (Fig. 1.31B,C). Villi are covered by low columnar, cuboidal, or flattened surface epithelium with a poorly defined brush border. There is usually a moderate proprial infiltrate of mononuclear cells and eosinophils or neutrophils, and hypertrophic crypts may be evident. The distribution of lesions may vary between animals and perhaps with time after infection within an individual animal, since the onset of maximal viral damage may not occur synchronously throughout the full length of the intestine. Lesions and viral antigen always should be sought in the distal small intestine, and preferably at several sites along its length. Rotavirus does not cause gross or microscopic lesions in the colon, in contrast to coronavirus.

SWINE.   Rotavirus infection is widespread and enzootic in most swine herds, and subclinical infection of piglets is common. It assumes particular importance as a cause of diarrhea in pigs with reduced lactogenic immunity, either as a result of removal of piglets from the sow at an early age or following normal weaning practice. High environmental levels of virus may result in disease in piglets suckling the sow, but in these circumstances the signs are usually relatively mild. Rotavirus may be an important cause of "3-week," "white," or postweaning scours in piglets 2 to 7 or 8 weeks of age. The signs may resemble those of transmissible gastroenteritis, although rotavirus infection is considered to be less severe. Vomition is less commonly encountered than with transmissible gastroenteritis, but depression, diarrhea, and dehydration are usual. The character of the feces varies with the diet. Steatorrhea occurs in white scours of suckling piglets. Rotavirus infection in swine may be associated with other causes of diarrhea, including *E. coli,* coccidiosis, adenovirus infection, and *Strongyloides.*

The gross and microscopic lesions and pathogenesis of rotavirus infection in pigs resemble those of transmissible gastroenteritis (Fig. 1.31A).

OTHER SPECIES.   Rotavirus may cause diarrhea in neonatal **lambs** and has proved a useful model for the demonstration of the importance of lactogenic immunity in preventing the disease. Rotavirus may cause diarrhea in neonatal lambs alone or in combination with enterotoxic *E. coli* and *Cryptosporidium.* The pathogenesis and lesions of rotavirus infection in lambs are like those caused in other species, with the exception that viral infection of the colon may occur.

In **foals** less than 3 or 4 months of age, diarrhea may be associated with rotavirus infections. Limited experimental work indicates that rotavirus alone or in combination with enterotoxic *E. coli* is capable of inducing diarrhea in foals. The natural and experimental disease resembles that seen in other species, with significant viral infection limited to enterocytes in the small intestine, where villus atrophy occurs.

Diarrhea, occasionally fatal, may be caused by rotavirus infection in young **puppies**, especially those less than 1 or 2 weeks of age. Little information is available on the pathology of the disease in naturally or experimentally infected animals, but it is presumably like that in other species.

Rotavirus infection should be sought in cases of diarrhea in young animals of any species, and it should be particularly suspected in animals with villus atrophy in the small intestine.

Parvoviral Enteritis

Members of the genus *Parvovirus* infect a variety of species of laboratory and domestic animals. Syndromes associated with parvovirus infection include disease in cats, dogs, and mink, dominated clinically by enteritis; diarrhea in neonatal calves; and reproductive wastage in swine.

The bovine parvovirus is immunologically distinct. The parvoviruses infecting cats, mink, and dogs are antigenically related, though subtle antigenic differences do exist among them. On the basis of DNA restriction enzyme analysis, feline panleukopenia virus and mink enteritis virus are very closely related to each other and somewhat less related to canine parvovirus-2, the agent causing parvovirus enteritis in dogs. The latter virus is antigenically distinct from canine parvovirus-1, or minute virus of canids, which causes little or no disease. Feline panleukopenia virus, mink enteritis virus, and canine parvovirus-2 are each biologically distinct, varying somewhat in their hemagglutination characteristics, *in vitro* host-cell ranges, infectivity, and virulence in experimentally inoculated hosts. Feline panleukopenia virus and canine parvovirus-2 will infect the heterologous host when inoculated parenterally, apparently without producing significant disease.

Though parvoviruses may infect cells at any phase of the cell cycle, replication is dependent on cellular mechanisms functional only during nucleoprotein synthesis prior to mitosis. Hence the effects of parvovirus infection are greatest in tissues with a high mitotic rate; these include a variety of tissues during organogenesis in the fetus and neonate. In older animals, the proliferative elements of the enteric epithelium, hematopoietic, and lymphoid tissue are particularly susceptible. At the time of virus assembly, large basophilic or amphophilic Feulgen-positive intranuclear inclusions may be found in infected cells, especially in Bouin's-fixed tissues. Parvovirus may be demonstrated in these inclusions by electron microscopy. The chromatin in inclusion-bearing nuclei is usually clumped at the nu-

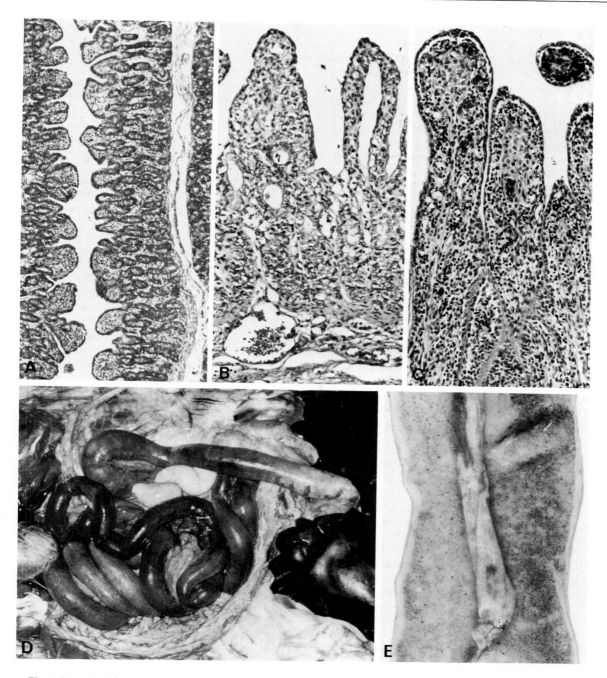

Fig. 1.31. **(A)** Porcine rotavirus infection. Atrophy of villi. Small intestine of 3-week-old piglet. **(B and C)** Bovine rotavirus infection. **(B)** Stumpy villi with severely attenuated surface epithelium. **(C)** Club-shaped villi with cuboidal or flattened epithelium. (Courtesy of M. Morin.) **(D)** Canine parvovirus infection. Segmental subserosal hemorrhage and mild fibrinous exudation on intestinal serosa. **(E)** Feline panleukopenia. Petechiae and fibrin cast on mucosal surface of small intestine.

clear membrane. Inclusions are most prevalent late in the incubation period, prior to extensive exfoliation or lysis of infected cells. Hence they are not commonly encountered in animals submitted for autopsy after a period of clinical illness culminating in death. Large nucleoli, seen in proliferative cells encountered in the intestine of parvovirus-infected animals, should not be confused with intranuclear inclusions.

The pathogenesis of feline panleukopenia and of canine parvovirus-2 infection is not firmly established but is probably sufficiently similar for them to be considered together here, followed by separate discussions of the specific diseases. Oronasal exposure results in uptake of virus by epithelium over Peyer's patches and, possibly, tonsils. Infection of draining lymphoid tissue is indicated by isolation of virus from mesenteric lymph nodes 2 days after experimental inoculation. Release of virus into lymph and dissemination of infected lymphoblasts from these sites may result in infection of other central and peripheral lymphoid tissues, including thymus, spleen, lymph nodes, and Peyer's patches, detected 3 or 4 days after infection. Lysis of infected lymphocytes in these tissues releases virus, reinforcing cell-free viremia. Viremia is terminated when neutralizing antibody appears in circulation about 5–7 days after infection. Moderate pyrexia occurs at about this time, perhaps associated with pyrogens released from lysing lymphocytes or with the formation of antigen–antibody complexes.

Infection of the gastrointestinal epithelium is a secondary event. It follows primary viral replication in lymphoid tissue and the resulting dissemination of virus by circulating lymphocytes and cell-free viremia. Peyer's patches are consistently infected at all levels of the intestine, and epithelium in crypts of Lieberkühn over or adjacent to Peyer's patches usually becomes infected a day or so later. Infection of gastrointestinal epithelium at other sites in the gut is less consistent. It may be the result of virus free in circulation or carried by infected lymphocytes homing to the mucosa. Maximal infection of cryptal epithelium occurs during the period about 5–9 days after infection. In experimental studies it tends to be heaviest in the duodenum and cranial jejunum early, but in the ileum later during the course of infection.

The occurrence and severity of enteric signs is determined by the extent of damage to epithelium in intestinal crypts. This seems to be a function of two main factors. The first is the availability of virus, which is influenced by the rate of proliferation of lymphocytes and, therefore, their susceptibility to virus replication and lysis. The second factor influencing the degree of epithelial damage is the rate of proliferation in the progenitor compartment in crypts of Lieberkühn. If many cells are entering mitosis, large numbers will support virus replication and subsequently lyse. Destruction of cells in the crypts of Leiberkühn, if severe enough, ultimately results in focal or widespread villus atrophy and, perhaps, mucosal erosion or ulceration. The recognition, evolution, and sequelae of radiomimetic insult to the intestine, such as that caused by parvovirus, have been described under Epithelial Renewal in Health and Disease.

Regeneration of cryptal epithelium and partial or complete restoration of mucosal architecture will occur if undamaged stem cells persist in most affected crypts and the animal survives the acute phase of clinical illness. In some survivors, focal villus atrophy is associated with local "drop out" of crypts completely destroyed by infection. Rarely, in animals recovering from acute disease, chronic malabsorption and protein-losing enteropathy are associated with persistent areas of ulceration caused by more extensive loss of crypts and collapse of the mucosa.

The relatively low rate of replication of intestinal epithelium in germ-free cats explains failure to produce significant intestinal lesions and clinical panleukopenia in experimentally infected animals. In spontaneous cases, the lower prevalence of parvoviral lesions in the colon and stomach, in comparison with the small intestine, reflects the relatively lower rate of epithelial proliferation in those tissues. The consistency of epithelial lesions in the mucosa over Peyer's patches probably results from high local concentrations of virus derived from infected lympho-

cytes in the dome and follicle. Possibly this is coupled with local stimulation of epithelial turnover by lymphokines released by T lymphocytes in the vicinity. Variations in the rate of epithelial proliferation related to age, starvation, and refeeding or concomitant parasitic, bacterial, or viral infections may also influence the susceptibility of crypt epithelium to infection and therefore affect the extent and severity of intestinal lesions and signs. It is difficult to duplicate fatal parvovirus infection experimentally, and work is required to define further the host factors influencing the severity of disease.

Diarrhea in parvovirus infections is mainly the result of reduced functional absorptive surface in the small intestine. Effusion of tissue fluids and blood from a mucosa at least focally denuded of epithelium probably also contributes to diarrhea. Dehydration and electrolyte depletion are the result of reduced fluid intake, enteric malabsorption, effusion of tissue fluid, and in some animals, vomition. Hypoproteinemia is common, and anemia may occur in severely affected animals; both are exacerbated by rehydration. Anemia reflects hemorrhage into the gut.

Proliferating cells in the bone marrow are also infected during viremia. Lysis of many infected cells is reflected in hypocellularity of the marrow caused by depletion of myeloid and erythroid elements, particularly the former. Megakaryocytes also may be lost, but they seem the least sensitive cell population in the marrow. Reduction in the number of neutrophils in circulation ensues quickly in severely affected animals. This is due to failure of recruitment from the marrow, and peripheral consumption, especially in the intestine. Transient neutropenia, of about 2 or 3 days duration, occurs consistently in cats, and less commonly in dogs. In surviving animals, regeneration of depleted myeloid elements from remaining stem cells results in restoration of the circulating population of granulocytes within a few days. Neutrophilic leukocytosis with left shift may occur during recovery.

Lymphopenia, relative or absolute, results consistently from viral lymphocytolysis in all infected lymphoid tissue. Relative lymphopenia is more consistently observed in dogs than neutropenia. When lymphopenia and neutropenia occur together, the combined leukopenia may be profound in both dogs and cats. In dogs surviving the lymphopenic phase, numbers of circulating lymphocytes return to normal within 2 to 5 days as regenerative hyperplasia occurs in lymphoid tissue throughout the body. Lymphocyte number increases rapidly, sometimes producing lymphocytosis in recovering dogs. However, there is evidence of at least transient immunosuppression in gnotobiotic pups subclinically infected with canine parvovirus-2. Transient depression of T-cell response to mitogens occurs in cats a week after experimental infection with feline panleukopenia virus, but immunosuppression by this agent appears to be of little practical significance.

Most infected cats and dogs do not develop clinical disease. When it occurs, signs usually begin during the late viremic phase, about 5–7 days after infection. Severe involvement of the gut is the major cause of mortality. Shedding of infective virus in feces begins about 3–5 days after infection, when Peyer's patches and cryptal epithelium first become infected. Virus shedding persists until coproantibody appears to neutralize virus entering the gut, about 6–9 days after infection. Virus-infected cells still may be detected in crypts and Peyer's patches at this time, and virus complexed with antibody may be found in feces or intestinal content by direct electron microscopy. Attempts to isolate virus from tissues or feces after several days of clinical disease or at death, however, are often thwarted by the fact that virus is neutralized by antibody present in tissue fluids. Persistent or sporadic shedding of virus by recovered animals may be the result of virus replication in cells entering mitosis days or weeks after they were infected during the viremic phase.

Infection of the fetus during late prenatal life by feline panleukopenia virus causes anomalies of the central nervous system, mainly hypoplasia of the cerebellum. Although reproductive success may be depressed in kennels infected with canine parvovirus-2, parvovirus infection has not been conclusively associated with fetal or congenital disease in dogs. Rarely, however, a syndrome of generalized infection may occur in neonatal dogs. Infection of proliferating cardiac myocytes in young puppies with canine parvovirus-2 results in a nonsuppurative myocarditis and sequelae of acute or chronic heart failure. Similar syndromes have not been associated with spontaneous feline panleukopenia infection.

PANLEUKOPENIA. The virus of panleukopenia (infectious feline enteritis) infects all members of the Felidae, as well as mink, raccoons, and some other members of the Procyonidae. Panleukopenia virus is ubiquitous in environments frequented by cats, and infection is common, though generally subclinical. The disease usually occurs in young animals exposed after decay of passively acquired maternal antibody, but it may occur in naive cats of any age. Clinical signs of several days duration, including pyrexia, depression, inappetence, vomition, diarrhea, dehydration, and perhaps anemia, may be evident in the history. Many cases, however, particularly poorly observed animals or those prone to wander, may present as "sudden death." The pathogenesis of panleukopenia has been considered above, with that of canine parvovirus-2 infection in dogs. Lesions of central nervous system in kittens are considered in the Nervous System (Volume 1).

At autopsy, external evidence of diarrhea may be present, the eyes may be sunken, and the skin is usually inelastic, with a tacky subcutis reflecting dehydration. Rehydrated animals may have edema, hydrothorax, and ascites due to hypoproteinemia. There is pallor of mucous membranes, fat, and internal tissues in anemic animals. Gross lesions of internal organs most consistently involve the thymus and the intestine. The thymus is markedly involuted and reduced in mass in young animals. Enteric lesions may be subtle and easily overlooked in some cases. Hence it is mandatory that intestine be examined microscopically despite the apparent absence of gross change.

The intestinal serosa may appear dry and nonreflective, with an opaque, ground-glass appearance. Uncommonly in cats there may be petechiae or more extensive hemorrhage in the subserosa or muscularis of the intestinal wall. The small bowel may be segmentally dilated and can acquire a hoselike turgidity in places, perhaps due to submucosal edema. However, turgidity is difficult to assess in the intestine of the cat. The content is usually foul smelling, scant, watery, and yellowish gray at all levels of the intestine. The mucosa may be glistening gray or

pink, with petechiae, perhaps covered by fine strands of fibrin (Fig. 1.31E). Patchy diphtheritic lesions may be present, especially over Peyer's patches in the ileum. Flecks of fibrin, and sometimes casts, may be in the content in the lumen. Formed feces are not evident in the colon. Lymph nodes may be prominent at the root of the mesentery. Gross lesions elsewhere in the carcass are usually restricted to pulmonary congestion and edema in some animals, and pale gelatinous marrow in normally active hematopoietic sites.

Microscopic changes are consistently found in fatal cases in the intestinal tract and are usual in lymphoid organs and bone marrow. The intestinal lesions vary with the severity and duration of disease. Their interpretation may be obscured by autolysis. Lesions may be patchy, and several levels of gut should be examined, preferably including ileum and, if possible, Peyer's patch. During the late incubation period and early phase of clinical disease, there is infection of crypt-lining epithelium. Intranuclear inclusions may be found, and there is exfoliation of damaged epithelium into the lumen of crypts. Crypts appear dilated and are lined by cuboidal or more severely attenuated epithelium. The lamina propria between crypts contains numerous neutrophils and eosinophils at this time, and some emigrate into the lumen of crypts, where they join the epithelial debris.

Subsequently, severely damaged crypts may be lined by extremely flattened cells and by scattered large, bizarre cells with swollen nuclei and prominent nucleoi (Fig. 1.32C). Enterocytes covering villi are not affected, but as they progress off the villus, they are replaced by a few cuboidal, squamous or bizarre epithelial cells, so that villi in affected areas undergo progressive collapse. If cryptal damage is severe and widespread, the mucosa becomes thin and eroded or ulcerated, with effusion of tissue fluids, fibrin, and erythrocytes. Inflammatory cells are usually sparse in the gut of such animals, and superficial masses of bacteria may be present, occasionally accompanied by locally invasive fungal hyphae or pseudohyphae. In less severely affected animals with disease of longer duration, corresponding to about 8 to 10 days after infection, scattered focal drop out of crypts, or focal mucosal collapse and erosion or ulceration, may be evident. Remaining crypts recovering from milder viral damage show regenerative epithelial hyperplasia (Fig. 1.32D) in these animals. Mucosal lesions are often most marked in the vicinity of Peyer's patches.

Lesions in the colon generally resemble those found in the small bowel, though they are frequently less severe or more patchy in distribution. When sought, colonic lesions are found in about half of fatal cases of panleukopenia. Gastric lesions resulting from damage to mitotic epithelium are relatively uncommon in cats. They are recognized by flattening of basophilic cells lining the narrowed isthmus of gastric fundic glands, with some reduction in number of parietal cells in the upper portion of the neck of glands.

Lesions of lymphoid organs during the early phase of the disease consist of lymphocytolysis in follicles and paracortical tissue in lymph nodes, in the thymic cortex and splenic white pulp, and in gut-associated lymphoid tissue. Infected cells rarely may contain inclusion bodies. Lymphocytes are markedly depleted in affected tissue, and large histiocytes are prominent, often containing the fragmented remnants of nuclear debris.

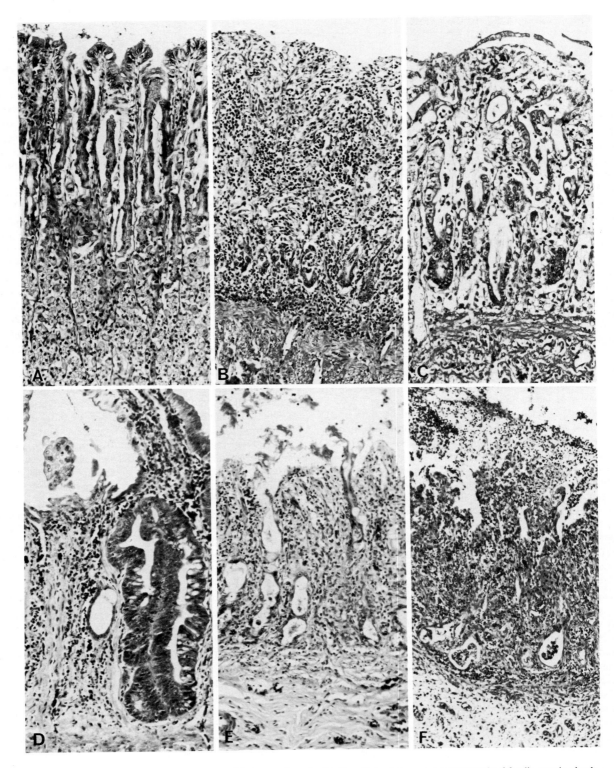

Fig. 1.32. (A–D) Parvovirus infections. (A) Attenuation of epithelium lining isthmus and upper neck of fundic gastric glands. Dog. (B) Loss of crypts of Lieberkühn and collapse of proprial stroma in small intestine. Remnants of crypt-lining epithelium persist deep in lamina propria. Dog. (C) Severe atrophy of villi associated with damage to crypts of Lieberkühn. Cat. Attenuation of surface epithelium and depletion of proprial inflammatory infiltrate. (D) Loss of crypts and collapse of proprial stroma. Gland is lined by hyperplastic epithelium. Mink virus enteritis. (E) Small intestinal mucosa following cyclophosphamide. Radiomimetic lesion, with attenuation of crypt-lining cells, and atrophy of villi. (F) Small intestine, sequel to transient ischemia 2 days previously. Ulcerated mucosa and dilated crypts lined by attenuated epithelium and containing necrotic debris. Inflammatory cells and fibrin exude from the mucosa, which is devoid of villi.

Follicular hyalinosis, the presence of amorphous eosinophilic material in the center of depleted follicles, may be seen. Erythrophagocytosis by sinus histiocytes may be seen in lymph nodes, especially those draining the gut. Severely depleted Peyer's patches may be difficult to recognize microscopically. Later in the course of clinical disease, corresponding to the period beyond about 7 or 8 days after infection, prominent regenerative lymphoid hyperplasia may be found.

In severely affected animals at the nadir of the leukopenia, virtually all proliferating elements in the bone marrow may be depleted. The extremely hypocellular, moderately congested marrow is populated only by scattered stem cells. Milder lesions affect mainly the neutrophil series, generally sparing megakaryocytes and the committed erythroid elements. During the later phases of the disease, marked hyperplasia of stem cells and, eventually, of amplifier populations in the various cell lines is evident.

In the liver, dissociation and rounding up of hepatocytes, and perhaps some periacinar atrophy and congestion, may be evident. This is probably associated with dehydration and anemia. Pancreatic acinar atrophy is also usual, reflecting inappetence. The lung may be congested and edematous. In leukopenic animals, few white cells are seen in circulation in any organ.

A diagnosis of feline panleukopenia may be made on the basis of the characteristic microscopic intestinal lesions, in association with evidence of involution or regenerative hyperplasia of lymphoid and hematopoietic tissues. Inclusions may be sought in these tissues but are usually present in significant numbers only during the late incubation and early clinical period. Application of fluorescent-antibody or immunoperoxidase techniques may identify viral antigen in tissue as late as 8 to 10 days after infection.

CANINE PARVOVIRUS-2 INFECTION. Canine parvovirus-2 infection presumably resulted by mutation of the virus of feline panleukopenia. It appeared spontaneously and virtually simultaneously in populations of dogs on several continents in 1978 and rapidly spread worldwide. Retrospective observation of antibody to this virus in the canine population suggests that it was circulating unnoticed in western Europe in late 1976 and 1977. In addition to domestic dogs, several species of wild canids, including coyotes, bush dogs, crab-eating foxes, raccoon dogs, and maned wolves, are susceptible to infection.

Enteric disease due to this virus was epizootic for several years in naive populations of dogs, affecting animals of all ages. As the prevalence of antibody due to natural infection and vaccination increased in the dog population, the problem subsided to one of an enzootic disease. It now affects those animals with reduced levels of passively acquired maternal immunity, or scattered naive individuals. During the epizootic period, nonsuppurative viral myocarditis due to canine parvovirus-2 was prevalent in the juvenile offspring of naive bitches unable to protect pups with maternal antibody. This syndrome has declined in frequency as the prevalence of antibody has increased in the reproductive population. Enteric and myocardial disease rarely occur together in the same individual or cohort of animals. Occasional cases of generalized parvovirus infection are reported in susceptible neonates. Necrosis and inclusion bodies are found in organs such as kidney, liver, lung, heart, gut, and vascular endothelium. They are presumably related to mitotic activity during organogenesis.

Dogs with typical disease due to canine parvovirus-2 become anorectic and lethargic and may vomit and develop diarrhea, perhaps in association with transient moderate pyrexia. Relative or absolute lymphopenia or leukopenia of 1 or 2 days duration may occur. Diarrhea may be mucoid or liquid, sometimes bloody, and is malodorous. After a period of 2 or 3 days, dogs either succumb to the effects of dehydration, hypoproteinemia, and anemia or begin to recover.

Gross findings at autopsy of fatal cases are those of dehydration, accompanied by enteric lesions characteristic of the disease. There is often segmental or widespread subserosal hemorrhage, often extending into the muscularis and submucosa of the intestine. The serosa frequently appears granular due to superficial fibrinous effusion (Fig. 1.31D). Peyer's patches may be evident from the serosal and mucosal aspects as deep red oval areas several centimeters long. The intestinal contents may be mucoid or fluid; sometimes they look like tomato soup due to hemorrhage. The mucosa is usually deeply congested and glistening or covered by a patchy fibrinous exudate. Severe enteric lesions may be widespread or segmental, and their distribution is irregular; thus tissues from several levels of the small intestine should be selected for microscopic examination. Gross changes are less common in the colon. The stomach may have a congested mucosa and contain scant bloody or bile-stained fluid. Mesenteric lymph nodes may be enlarged, congested, and wet, or reduced in size. Thymic atrophy is consistently present in young animals, and the organ may be so reduced in size as to be difficult to find. The lungs often appear congested and have a rubbery texture.

The microscopic lesions in stomach, small intestine (Fig. 1.32A,B), colon, lymphoid tissue, and bone marrow due to canine parvovirus-2 infection do not differ significantly from those described above in cats with panleukopenia. Gastric lesions are perhaps more frequently encountered in dogs with parvovirus infection. Small intestinal lesions are invariably severe in fatal cases. The colon is involved in a minority of animals. Pulmonary lesions such as alveolar septal thickening by mononuclear cells, congestion, and effusion of edema fluid and fibrin into the lumina of alveoli may be related in part to terminal Gram-negative sepsis. However, interstitial pneumonitis is commonly found and may be a function of uncomplicated viral infection. Periacinar atrophy and congestion in the liver are attributable to anemia, hypovolemia, and shock, and prominent Kupffer cells probably reflect endotoxemia.

The diagnosis of parvoviral enteritis in dogs follows the principles described for that of panleukopenia in cats. The disease must be differentiated from canine coronavirus infection, which appears to be very rarely fatal, and from canine intestinal hemorrhage syndrome, shock gut, intoxication with heavy metals or warfarin, infectious canine hepatitis, and other causes of hemorrhagic diathesis. Involution of gut-associated lymphoid tissue caused by parvovirus must be differentiated from that due to canine distemper.

BOVINE PARVOVIRUS INFECTION. The antigenically distinct bovine parvoviruses have been recognized since at least the 1960s and apparently occur widely in cattle populations. Bovine parvovirus is nondefective and replicates independently. Isolations have been made from the feces of normal and recently diarrheic calves as well as from conjunctiva, and from an aborted fetus. The role of bovine parvovirus infection as a significant pathogen is unclear. It is rarely diagnosed as a cause of death and unless sought specifically by culture or direct electron microscopy, would be missed as a cause of clinical diarrhea. Its significance may be greatest in neonatal calves and animals exposed while passive maternal antibody levels are waning.

The pathogenesis of infection with bovine parvovirus is not well defined. Viral antigen has been identified by immunofluorescence in the nuclei of epithelium in intestinal crypts and in cells in thymus, lymph nodes, adrenal glands, and heart muscle, suggesting similarities to the pathogenesis of feline panleukopenia and canine parvovirus-2. The pathology of natural or experimental infections has not been described. Intravenous inoculation of bovine parvovirus into young calves causes severe watery diarrhea and prostration. Milder diarrhea occurs in calves infected orally. The severity of the disease may be potentiated by concurrent infection with other enteric pathogens.

Bacterial Diseases

Escherichia coli

Escherichia coli infections in animals and humans cause disease by at least five different general mechanisms. The first is **enterotoxic colibacillosis**: secretory small bowel diarrhea stimulated by enterotoxins produced by *E. coli* colonizing the muscoa of the small intestine. This condition is an important cause of diarrhea in neonatal animals. The second mechanism involves **enterocyte-adherent** *E. coli* strains, which colonize the surface of epithelial cells, do not produce recognized enterotoxin, but are associated with villus atrophy. They currently are not known to occur in domestic animals. **Enterotoxemic colibacillosis** is represented by **edema disease** of swine. In this condition a toxin produced by specific strains of *E. coli* colonizing the small intestine is absorbed and has its pathogenic effect on tissues other than the gut. Postweaning *E. coli* enteritis is also caused by the same strains, presumably by different means. **Enteroinvasive** *E. coli* strains induce disease by a fourth mechanism. They have the capacity to invade the epithelium of the intestine and cause acute exudative enteritis, often endotoxemia, and perhaps terminal septicemia. Enteroinvasive colibacillosis is apparently rare in domestic animals. **Septicemic colibacillosis** is the final, and common, manifestation of disease caused by this organism. The intestine is not necessarily the portal of entry, and there may not be alimentary disease. The signs of *E. coli* septicemia are referable mainly to bacteremia, endotoxemia, and the effect of bacterial localization in a variety of tissue spaces throughout the body.

ENTEROTOXIC COLIBACILLOSIS. Enterotoxic colibacillosis is one of the major causes of diarrhea in neonatal pigs, calves, and lambs. It is also a significant cause of diarrhea in humans. Consequently, considerable information is available on the pathogenesis and prophylaxis of this condition.

Two major attributes confer virulence on certain diarrheagenic strains of *E. coli*. These are the ability to colonize the

intestine and the capacity to produce toxins that stimulate secretion of electrolyte and water by the intestinal mucosa. Colonization and enterotoxin production must occur together for disease to occur. The diarrhea produced by enterotoxic *E. coli* is accompanied by minor microscopic evidence of inflammation and by little or no architectural change in the mucosa. As a result, overt enteritis usually is not evident at autopsy, and the disease is part of the syndrome of undifferentiated diarrhea of neonatal animals.

Intestinal colonization results from the capacity of certain strains of *E. coli* to adhere to the surface of enterocytes on villi in the small intestine (Fig. 1.33A) and to proliferate there. By adhering to the mucosal surface, they are able to resist the normal peristaltic clearance mechanisms. Large numbers of organisms, of the order of 10^7 or more per gram of mucosa, or 20 to 30 per enterocyte, line the surface of villi. The ability to attach to enterocytes is conferred on most adhesive strains of *E. coli* by pili- (= fimbriae) fibrillar proteinaceous appendages that protrude from the surface of the bacterial cell; they bind with receptors on the surface of the cell (Fig. 1.33B). The cell receptors have not been clearly defined; carbohydrate moieties in mucosal glycolipids are probably involved. The pilar adhesins are distinct from type 1 fimbriae present on many strains of *E. coli*. Type 1 fimbriae do not confer recognized virulence characteristics on the organism.

A number of different pilar adhesins, which promote colonization, have been recognized on *E. coli* infecting domestic animals. **Adhesin K88** occurs in at least three combinations of four antigenic subunit variants, K88ab, ac, and ad, on *E. coli* infecting piglets. Five phenotypes of swine are recognized with resistance or susceptibility to enterocyte adhesion by the different K88 antigenic variants. **Adhesin 987P** is found on some strains of *E. coli* infecting piglets, as is F-41. **Adhesin K99** is also found on some strains infecting swine and is the only adhesin known to promote *E. coli* colonization in calves and lambs. Enterotoxic strains of *E. coli* lacking K88, K99, and 987P, but adherent to porcine enterocytes, are also recognized. Bacteria possessing K88 colonize the entire small bowel, while those with K99 or 987P adhere mainly in the jejunum and ileum.

Genetic control of pilus production is invested in plasmid DNA, with the exception of 987P, information for which appears to be encoded in chromosomal DNA. Combinations of more than one type of pilus adhesin occur on a single strain, exceptionally. Susceptibility to bacterial pilus adhesins appears to be somewhat age related; the ability of adhesin-bearing *E. coli* to colonize the small intestine is greatest in animals only a few days old. Stimulation of maternal immunity to appropriate pilus antigens causes antibody secretion in the milk, which agglutinates adhesins and prevents colonization of the gut of suckling animals.

Enterotoxin production is of two types, heat labile (LT) or heat stable (ST), both coded by plasmid DNA. In strains of *E. coli* causing diarrhea in animals, adhesin and enterotoxin production are generally controlled by separate plasmids. However, certain combinations of adhesin and toxin tend to occur together.

Heat-labile enterotoxin resembles cholera toxin in its structure and mechanism of action. It is a large molecular weight, antigenic protein, comprised of A and B subunits. The B sub-

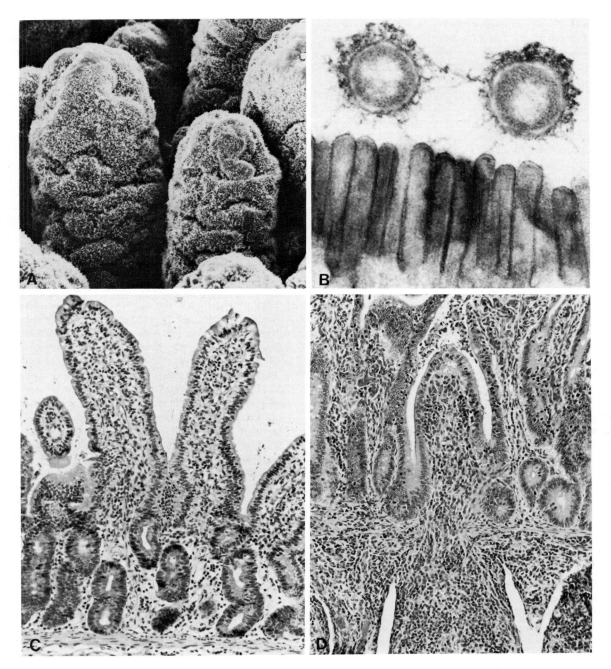

Fig. 1.33. (**A**) Scanning electron micrograph. *Escherichia coli* adherent to the surface of villi. Small intestine. Calf. (**B**) Transmission electron micrograph. Fimbriate *E. coli* adherent to microvilli. Small intestine. Calf. (**C**) Enterotoxic colibacillosis. Calf. Mild neutrophil infiltrate in lamina propria and between bases of villi. Atrophy of villi not evident, surface epithelium normal. (**A–C** courtesy of J. J. Hadad and C. L. Gyles.) (**D**) Enterotoxic colibacillosis. Calf. Neutrophil effusion into lumen over dome of Peyer's patch. (Courtesy of J. E. C. Bellamy.)

units bind to oligosaccharide moieties of ganglioside GM_1 in the apical cell membrane. The toxin complex then undergoes dissociation and the A subunit enters the cell, where it stimulates the adenyl cyclase system. Via mediation of cAMP it causes secretion of chloride, with sodium and water following, from the crypts. Cotransport of sodium chloride and associated water

absorption by enterocytes on villi is probably shut down at the same time, though other mechanisms of sodium and water absorption are not impaired.

Heat-stable enterotoxin is a poorly antigenic, low molecular weight polypeptide, which occurs in several forms with differing physical and functional characteristics. These are reflected by variations in host and age-group susceptibility to the toxin. The mechanism of action of the heat-stable toxin is not clearly understood. It may act by reducing chloride absorption and perhaps by causing cellular secretion of electrolyte and water, associated with accumulation of intracellular cGMP. This is probably mediated by stimulation of a transmembrane flux of calcium ions by toxin, with intracellular generation of prostaglandins that active guanylate cyclase. The rate of intestinal transit may also be reduced by ST-enhancing proliferation of *E. coli* and perhaps promoting absorption of toxin. The effect is rapid in onset and requires persistence of toxin, in contrast to that of the heat-labile toxin, which has a latent period after exposure and is relatively irreversible.

Enterotoxic colibacillosis in **pigs** is among the commonest causes of diarrhea in animals from a few hours old to about a week of age. At autopsy it cannot be separated readily from the other common causes of undifferentiated neonatal diarrhea without laboratory assistance. Generally there is dehydration, usually with evidence of diarrhea, or a history of its occurrence in the herd. Other than the presence of characteristic fluid content in the flaccid small and large bowel, perhaps with clotted milk still in the stomach, the internal findings are unremarkable. In order to establish the cause, one or more piglets early in clinical disease should be killed and examined. Tissue sections from several levels of the small bowel should be fixed rapidly. Bacterial cultures of intestinal content should be made. Intestinal content for electron microscopy, and mucosal smears or frozen tissue for fluorescent-antibody tests, should be reserved to incriminate or eliminate the intestinal viruses.

In contrast to the viruses and *Isospora,* enterotoxic *E. coli* does not consistently cause significant villus atrophy (Fig. 1.34A). Small clumps or a continuous layer of bacteria may be found on the surface of enterocytes on villi in mucosal sections (Fig. 1.34B). Neutrophils may be present in the proprial core of villi and transmigrating the epithelium into the lumen. Inflammation is not marked, however, and epithelial lesions and erosion generally are not seen in well-fixed tissue in enterotoxic colibacillosis. Rare cases of villus atrophy associated with *E. coli* infection do occur in neonatal swine. These are considered under Enteroinvasive Colibacillosis.

In **calves,** enterotoxic colibacillosis accounts for a significant proportion of cases of undifferentiated neonatal diarrhea; depending on the locality and circumstances, up to 20 to 30% of cases may be due to *E. coli.* The infections typically occur within the first 2 or 3 days of life, probably due to the resistance of enterocytes in older calves to K99 adhesion. In that age group they cause profuse yellow diarrhea and severe dehydration, with a high mortality in untreated animals. Enteric colibacillosis must be differentiated from the other major causes of undifferentiated diarrhea in neonatal animals; coronavirus, rotavirus, and *Cryptosporidium.* Enterotoxic *E. coli* is often found in combination with coronavirus or rotavirus infection. Experimental evidence suggests that prior or concomitant infection with rotavirus may permit or promote establishment by enterotoxic *E. coli* in calves older than 2 days. Combined infection may enhance the severity of disease in calves less than, and in some cases more than 2 days of age.

The gross findings in calves with enterotoxic colibacillosis are the nonspecific appearances of diarrhea and dehydration. The infection is differentiated in tissue sections from the other infectious causes of this syndrome in calves by the absence of severe villus atrophy and by the presence of bacteria on the surfaces of villi in the distal small intestine. As in piglets, application of a variety of presumptive or specific tests for the presence of enterotoxic *E. coli* in the intestine confirms the diagnosis.

Enterotoxic *E. coli* is not considered to induce diarrhea by villus atrophy and malabsorption, in contrast to the significant viruses and *Cryptosporidium,.* In the jejunum and ileum of calves, however, where bacterial colonization of the surface of enterocytes is heavy, stumpiness, lateral corrugation and contraction, or moderate atrophy of villi may be present. It is sometimes associated with villus fusion later in the course of the disease and as a result may resemble viral lesions. Cells on the surface of villi may be cuboidal, and subepithelial capillaries may be dilated. Transmigration of neutrophils from the lamina propria to the lumen is present in colonized areas of gut, especially in the vicinity of the domes over Peyer's patches (Fig. 1.33D). Colonization of the mucosa precedes the development of atrophy, which seems to occur prior to the onset of diarrhea. Atrophy of villi is related to degeneration and exfoliation of individual epithelial cells or small groups of enterocytes from the surface of villi, but the cause of the cell loss is unclear.

Enterotoxic colibacillosis should be suspected in neonatal calves having large numbers of Gram-negative rods in smears of ileal scrapings. Though enterotoxic *E. coli* may be isolated from mesenteric lymph nodes or other parenchymatous tissues at autopsy, systemic invasion is not a significant component of the disease. Enterotoxic colibacillosis must be differentiated from enteric colibacillosis in calves that appears to be due to enteroinvasive strains, and from septicemic colibacillosis.

Enterotoxic colibacillosis in **lambs** is a significant problem in some areas. The serotypes involved and pathogenesis and diagnosis of the condition are similar to those in calves. Strains of *E. coli* have been associated with diarrhea in neonates of other species, but their enterotoxigenicity and other attributes of virulence have not been adequately described.

EDEMA DISEASE OF SWINE AND POSTWEANING *ESCHERICHIA COLI* ENTERITIS.   Edema disease (gut edema) is a distinct syndrome in pigs characterized by sudden death, or the development of nervous signs, associated with enteric colonization by certain serotypes of usually hemolytic *Escherichia coli.* The disease occurs most commonly in pigs within a few weeks after weaning, or after other change in feeding or management. It often occurs in association with outbreaks of postweaning *E. coli* enteritis. Rare reports exist of edema disease in suckling and mature animals. The disease may be sporadic or occur as an outbreak, usually affecting the best animals in a group, and mortality often approaches 100% of affected animals. Edema disease and postweaning *E. coli* enteritis have apparently declined in prevalence in many parts of North America, perhaps with the use of concentrate rations based largely on soybeans and corn, rather than other grains.

Although the etiopathogenesis of edema disease is still incompletely understood, a soluble factor ("edema disease princi-

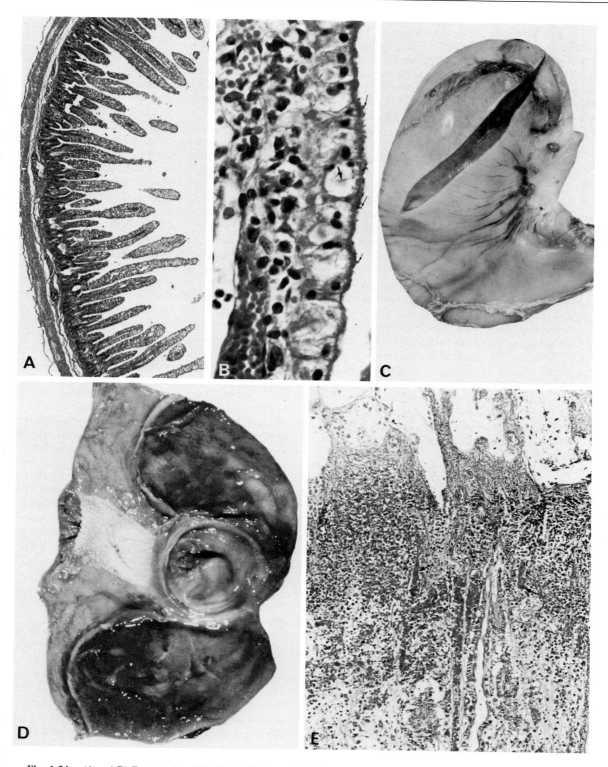

Fig. 1.34. (**A** and **B**) Enterotoxic colibacillosis. Piglet. (**A**) Villi are tall, and crypts short, as expected in a 2- to 3-day-old animal. (**B**) Bacteria are present on surface of enterocytes (arrows). Cytoplasmic vacuoles containing eosinophilic spicules (arrow) are normal in the ileal mucosa of young piglets. (**C**) Edema of stomach wall. Edema disease. Pig. (**D**) Postweaning colibacillosis in a pig. Deep red areas of venous infarction in the gastric mucosa. (**E**) Postweaning colibacillosis in a pig. Thrombosis of venules (arrows) and necrosis of the superficial gastric mucosa in venous infarction.

ple'' or ''E. coli neurotoxin'') released in the gut by some serotypes of E. coli (mainly O138, O139, O141) is implicated. The factors predisposing to enteric colonization and adhesion by these strains are unknown. Weaning, changes in ration, or accompanying alterations in the enteric microenvironment may favor proliferation of some strains of E. coli. The E. coli stick to the microvillus border of enterocytes on villi in the small intestine, presumably by the medium of some sort of ''adhesin'' or perhaps by mechanisms analogous to the enterocyte-adhesive strains in other species. They do not possess the K88, K99, or 987P pilus antigens, and pili are not obviously involved in adhesion.

The edema disease principle is not related to ''O'' or ''K'' antigens, nor to the hemolytic trait displayed by most, but not all, strains of E. coli causing the disease. It is heat labile but is distinguishable from both heat-labile and heat-stable enterotoxins responsible for the secretory diarrhea caused by some strains of E. coli. Some strains of E. coli that cause edema disease also produce secretory enterotoxin. Diarrhea is not a usual concomitant of edema disease in individual animals. However, some other animals in the group may develop typical E. coli ''postweaning'' diarrhea, described subsequently. Gross or microscopic lesions in the intestinal mucosa do not occur in edema disease, which appears to be classical enterotoxemia, the active principle being absorbed from the gut and acting at a distant site.

The edema disease principle can be neutralized by antitoxin prepared against crude toxin extracts. It shows specific titratable cytotoxicity for Vero cells grown in vitro and also may be assayed by intravenous injection in mice. It appears to be analogous to Shigella neurotoxin, which has been recognized for many years, and perhaps to certain ''verotoxins'' or ''neurotoxins'' produced by serotypes of E. coli of human origin.

The mechanism of action of the edema disease principle is uncertain. Its effect seems to be on the walls of small arteries and arterioles throughout the body. Lesions at this level of the vascular tree are sometimes seen in animals dying acutely and showing typical postmortem lesions of edema. They are more consistently encountered in survivors or in pigs with a subacute clinical course in which nervous signs are prominent but in which gross edema at autopsy is not. The angiopathy, in its early stages, is recognized by swelling of endothelial cells and pyknosis and karyorrhexis of smooth muscle nuclei, often accompanied by fibrinoid degeneration or hyaline change, in the tunica media. Proliferative mesenchymal elements are found in the tunica media and tunica adventitia in more advanced cases. Inflammation is not at any stage a prominent component of the angiopathy, nor of the associated edema in most sites, however, and thrombosis of vessels is rarely encountered. Edema is probably due to vessel damage during the early stages of the angiopathy, and perhaps to associated hypertension. The lesions are distinct from those that might be expected with the alternative hypotheses advanced to explain the pathogenesis of edema disease, either endotoxemia or a hypersensitivity to soluble factors released by E. coli.

Swine with edema disease may die without premonitory signs. Others may have anorexia or, more characteristically, show nervous signs, usually of less than a day's duration. An unsteady, staggering gait, knuckling, ataxia, prostration and tremors, convulsions, and paddling occur. A hoarse squeal attributed to laryngeal edema, and dyspnea, may also be noted clinically.

At autopsy, lesions in acute deaths may be subtle or absent. Typically, edema is variably present in one or more sites. It may be mild, however, and must be carefully sought, especially by ''slipping'' the suspected area over subjacent tissue. Subcutaneous edema may be present in the frontal area and over the snout, in the eyelids, and in the submandibular, ventral abdominal, and inguinal areas. Internally, there may be some hydropericardium and serous pleural and peritoneal effusion, perhaps accompanied by mild or moderate pulmonary edema. More commonly, the serous surfaces merely appear glistening and wet. Edema of the mesocolon, of the submucosa of the cardiac glandular area of the stomach over the greater curvature, and of mesenteric lymph nodes is most consistently found. The gastric submucosal edema should be sought by gently cutting through the muscularis to the submucosa. The edema fluid is clear and slightly gelatinous (Fig. 1.34C). It is rarely blood tinged, and overt hemorrhage is never present in uncomplicated edema disease. The stomach is often full of feed, but the small intestine is relatively empty and the mucosa grossly normal. The colon may contain somewhat inspissated feces.

In swine dying after a more prolonged clinical course, gross edema often is not present, though enlargement of mesenteric lymph nodes is present in a large proportion of cases. A few pigs may show usually bilaterally symmetric foci of yellowish malacia in the brain stem at various levels, from basal ganglia to medulla.

Edema in the sites of predilection mentioned above is the main microscopic lesion in swine dying acutely. It is generally devoid of much protein and contains few erythrocytes and inflammatory cells. A proportion of animals will also have meningeal edema and distended Virchow–Robin spaces in the brain. Vascular lesions may not be well developed in pigs dying suddenly. When present, they usually consist of mycocyte necrosis, edema, and hyalin degeneration in the tunica media. Angiopathy is more consistently found in cases of longer standing. Affected vessels may be found in any tissue in the carcass. Brain edema and focal encephalomalacia in the brain stem are associated with the presence of lesions in cerebral vessels; necrosis may be a sequel to edema and ischemia. The entity known as swine cerebrospinal angiopathy is probably a manifestation of edema disease.

A diagnosis of edema disease is based on nervous signs or sudden death in growing pigs, in association with typical gross and microscopic lesions, when they are present. In acute cases, heavy growth of hemolytic E. coli of one of the three common serotypes associated with edema disease is usual on culture of the small and large bowel. In animals with more chronic signs, these strains may have been superseded by others as the dominant E. coli populating the intestine. Tests for production of the edema disease principle by cultured bacteria, or for its presence in gut content, may become routine as techniques for in vitro assay are developed.

The disease must be differentiated from enteritis and endotoxemia due to E. coli in postweaning pigs, from mulberry-heart disease in animals dying suddenly, and from salt poisoning, Salmonella meningoencephalitis, and other infectious encephalitides in animals with nervous signs.

Postweaning *E. coli* **enteritis** (coliform "gastroenteritis" of weaned pigs) typically occurs during the first week or two following weaning or after some other change in feed or management. It is usually associated with hemolytic *E. coli* of the same three serotypes primarily implicated in edema disease, as well as serotype O149. The two diseases often occur in the same population of pigs, though usually affecting different animals. Typically, postweaning colibacillosis is a disease of high morbidity and variable mortality, with loss of condition in pigs suffering prolonged illness. Diarrhea is usually yellow and fluid and stains the perineum. Deaths that occur may or may not follow a prior episode of diarrhea and often appear to be related to endotoxemia.

In fatal cases, there may be bluish red discoloration of the skin and evidence of dehydration. Deep red gastric venous infarcts are present in almost all cases (Fig. 1.34D,E). The small intestine is flaccid. The mucosa may be normal in color and the content creamy. In other animals, the mucosa of the distal small intestine will be congested and the contents watery and perhaps blood stained or brown with flecks of yellow mucus (Fig. 1.35A). Cecal and colonic lesions are usually mild, but there may be some congestion and fibrinous exudate in the proximal large bowel. Mesenteric lymph nodes may be somewhat enlarged, congested, and juicy. Other organs are usually unremarkable grossly.

The pathogenesis of postweaning *E. coli* enteritis is poorly understood, and the microscopic pathology is not well described. In swine with diarrhea, *E. coli* is attached to the surface of villi by means not necessarily related to known adhesins. Atrophy of villi does not seem to be evident, and diarrhea is presumed to be enterotoxin mediated. Mortality in animals with prolonged diarrhea and few gross intestinal lesions may be ascribed to dehydration. In animals dying of more acute disease, there is local microvascular thrombosis in sections of congested mucosa, and the gross and microscopic lesions are suggestive of endotoxemia (Figs. 1.34E and 1.35B). Hemolytic *E. coli* of the implicated strains are consistently isolated in virtually pure culture from the lower small intestine and colon. They are present in the spleen and liver in only a minority of cases, however, suggesting terminal bacteremia but not usually septicemia.

The factors predisposing to the massive colonization of hemolytic *E. coli* are unclear. Loss of lactogenic immunity, a favorable environment for proliferation of bacterial strains with specific nutrient requirements, and promotion of epithelial colonization by the effects of antecedent rotavirus infection have been variously implicated.

A diagnosis of postweaning colibacillosis is suggested by the gross lesions in animals dying acutely or subacutely, and it is confirmed by culture and serotyping of associated strains of *E. coli*. The fatal disease must be differentiated from edema disease, intestinal adenomatosis complex, salmonellosis, and swine dysentery. Postweaning diarrhea due to uncomplicated rotavirus infection or transmissible gastroenteritis is usually nonfatal.

ENTEROINVASIVE COLIBACILLOSIS. Strains of *E. coli* are recognized, infecting humans and certain other species, that have the capacity to invade surface enterocytes of the small and large intestine. In this sense they resemble *Shigella* in primates, and *Salmonella*. The enteroinvasiveness of *Shigella* and some strains of *E. coli* appears to be correlated with the presence of a high molecular weight plasmid. Multiplication of the organism within cells results in local erosion and ulceration, associated with acute inflammation in the mucosa. Although in shigellosis septicemia does not usually occur, bacteria may be present in inflamed mesenteric lymph nodes or liver in some enteroinvasive *E. coli* infections in laboratory animals.

Among domestic animals, enteroinvasive colibacillosis has been confirmed experimentally only in neonatal swine, using a strain of O101 *E. coli*. Spontaneous enteritis, which appears to be due to enteroinvasive *E. coli*, is occasionally encountered in piglets up to weaning and in calves less than 2 weeks of age. Diarrhea in experimentally infected piglets is described as gray-yellow, watery, and containing small clots. The gross findings may not be remarkable, or the intestine may appear congested in comparison with that in most diarrheic piglets. In spontaneous cases suspected of being due to enteroinvasive *E. coli*, the gastric fundus may be congested also, and this correlates with the presence of venous infarction visible microscopically. Experimental enteroinvasive colibacillosis in piglets causes villus atrophy comparable in severity to that induced by the common viruses of neonates. Enterocytes appear cuboidal or flattened, and some are seen lysing. The lamina propria is edematous and capillaries are congested and infiltrated by neutrophils and other inflammatory cells. In spontaneous cases, thrombi may be evident in proprial capillaries and submucosal lymphatics. Neutrophils and tissue fluid effuse into the lumen between villi through epithelial discontinuities. Similar microthrombosis, proprial inflammation, enterocyte destruction, and effusion may be found in the cecum and colon. Intracellular organisms of strain O101 were demonstrated by immunoperoxidase staining in the experimental study but are not generally recognized in spontaneous cases suspected to be due to enteroinvasive *E. coli*. Edema and neutrophil accumulation in sinusoids of mesenteric lymph nodes are present. Experimental enteroinvasive colibacillosis in piglets has been associated with malabsorption and protein loss into the gut, presumably due to villus atrophy and effusive enteritis, respectively.

In calves, lesions suspected to be due to enteroinvasive *E. coli* grossly resemble mild salmonellosis. The mucosa of the lower small intestine, cecum, and spiral colon is congested and may be covered by a fine fibrinous exudate. The content is fluid and may appear blood tinged. Mesenteric lymph nodes are enlarged and wet. The microscopic lesions resemble those described above in pigs.

SEPTICEMIC COLIBACILLOSIS. Generalized systemic infection with *E. coli* occurs commonly in **calves** and less commonly or sporadically in young animals of the other domestic species. Predisposition to infection is a prerequisite for *E. coli* septicemia caused by a variety of strains. This usually results from reduced transfer or absorption of maternal immunoglobulin from colostrum, or intercurrent disease or debilitation. But certain strains of *E. coli*, especially O78:K80 and O2:K1, are particularly associated with septicemia in calves and lambs and may possess characteristics that enhance their ability to invade and proliferate systemically.

Among factors conferring virulence on these strains are plas-

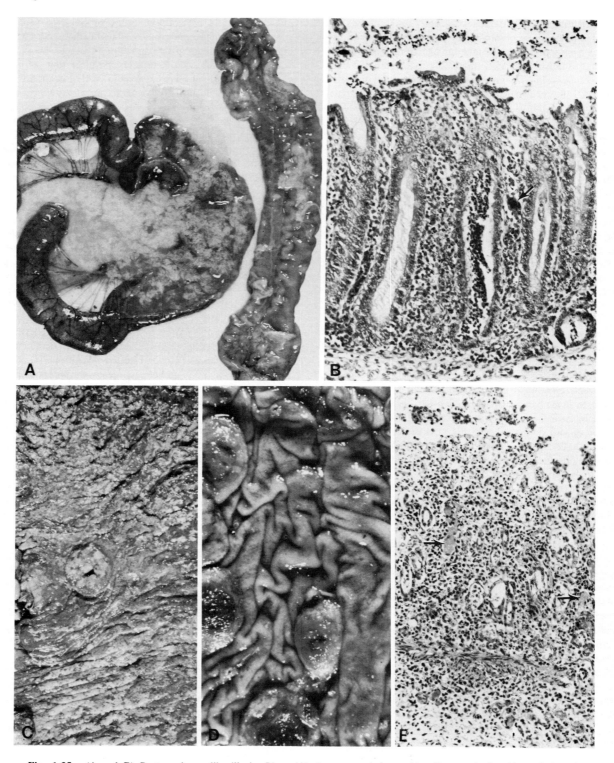

Fig. 1.35. (**A** and **B**) Postweaning colibacillosis. Pig. (**A**) Acute catarrhal enteritis. Congested, flaccid small intestine. (**B**) Erosion and effusion from colonic surface, and accumulation of neutrophils in glands, associated with thrombosis of some venules in the lamina propria (arrows). (**C–E**) Equine salmonellosis. (**C**) Focal and coalescent ulceration and diphtheresis involving ileocecal valve and cecal mucosa. (**D**) Nodular ulcerative lesions in colon. Chronic salmonellosis. (**E**) Superficial necrosis and effusion from colonic mucosa. Foal. *Salmonella typhimurium.* Several thrombosed vessels are in the propria (arrows).

mids coding for colicin V (Col V) and for the production of a specific toxin and surface antigen (Vir). Colicin V enhances the ability of the organism to resist host defense mechanisms, possibly by interfering with phagocytosis or complement activation. The Vir plasmid causes production of a toxin lethal in chicks and presumably active in other hosts. Hemolysin seems to promote virulence of some invasive strains of *E. coli* in experimental situations.

The portal of entry of *E. coli* causing septicemia is unclear and probably varies somewhat. The navel in the neonate, the upper respiratory tract, possibly the tonsil, and the intestine are likely sites. The nasopharyngeal route appears to be particularly important. Enteritis is not a necessary, or even common, concomitant of colisepticemia in animals. Invasive strains given to animals with adequate levels of immunoglobulin are usually limited to colonization of the intestine and local carriage to the mesenteric lymph nodes.

The lesions associated with colisepticemia in young animals of any species, especially calves, lambs, and foals, may vary from subtle to obvious. Mortality in hypogammaglobulinemic neonates may occur acutely with little in the way of abnormal gross findings. These may be limited to mildly congested or blue-red, slightly rubbery lungs and a firm spleen, perhaps with evidence of omphalitis. Microscopic changes in the lungs include thickening of alveolar septa by mononuclear cells and neutrophils, and effusion of lightly fibrinous exudate and a few neutrophils into alveoli. There may be a corona of neutrophils around white pulp in the spleen, and neutrophils may be present in abnormal numbers in circulation in many organs, including lung and hepatic sinusoids. Kupffer cells also may be prominent in sinusoids in the liver. Fibrin thrombi may be evident in pulmonary capillaries, glomeruli, and hepatic sinusoids. Some calves will develop acute interstitial nephritis with foci of neutrophil accumulation, which with time evolves into "white-spotted kidney" in surviving animals.

More severe acute cases will show evidence of serosal hemorrhage, including petechiae or ecchymoses on the epicardium and endocardium and perhaps parietal and visceral pleura. There may be slight serosanguinous pericardial fluid. The lungs may be deep red-blue and rubbery and fail to collapse. Interlobular septa may be slightly separated by edema, and froth or fluid may be present in the major airways. Meningeal vessels may be congested, and the meninges wet. The abomasum or stomach may have focal superficial ulcers or more extensive deep red areas of venous infarction. There may be evidence of diarrhea and dehydration, with congestion of the small intestine. Microscopic lesions resemble those previously described, with more severe congestion, thrombosis, and edema in lungs and, perhaps, other tissues. In cases not examined by some time after death, clumps of small bacilli may be seen in vessels throughout the body. The vascular permeability, thrombosis, and hemorrhage reflect endotoxemia.

Subacute cases may develop localized infection, often multiple, on serous surfaces, in the joints, meninges, and rarely, anterior chamber of the eye. Fibrinous peritonitis, pleuritis and pericarditis, and fibrinopurulent arthritis and meningitis are commonly found, alone or in variable combinations. Affected animals may have a history of lameness ascribable to arthritis,

nervous signs due to meningitis, or general debilitation. Microscopic examination reveals the lesions already described in animals with active systemic disease, with the addition of extensive congestion and edema of inflamed serous surfaces, associated with an acute inflammatory exudate.

In **lambs**, congestion and edema of the mucosa of turbinates and sinuses, perhaps with mucopurulent to hemorrhagic sinusitis, have been described. Fibrinous polyserositis and arthritis are sporadic manifestations of *E. coli* septicemia in **swine** and must be differentiated from the more significant *Haemophilus, Mycoplasma,* and *Streptococcus* infections causing these lesions. Colisepticemia is a sporadic cause of mortality in litters of young **puppies**.

Diagnosis of *E. coli* septicemia is based on the isolation of *E. coli* in large numbers from more than one parenchymatous organ or other internal site other than mesenteric lymph node (preferably liver, spleen, lung, or kidney) or from a site of serosal localization, in conjunction with compatible gross and/or microscopic lesions.

Salmonellosis

The genus *Salmonella* is named for D. E. Salmon, who was the first to describe one species, *S. choleraesuis,* in detail, although diseases in humans caused by members of this genus had been described earlier. Each antigenically distinct type is accorded species status and assigned a specific name. This usually designates the locality in which the specific type was first isolated and identified. Some 2000 or more serotypes have been defined, including members of the *arizona* group. All known types are pathogenic, or potentially so, for humans or animals or both. For the most part, however, salmonellosis is caused by a few types that are somewhat host specific, like *S. abortusovis,* and a few which are not host specific, like *S. typhimurium.* Salmonellosis is one of the most serious zoonotic diseases. Phage typing is indicated when there is evidence of transmission from animals to humans. This technique should also be used when the offending serotype is found in feed, or other epidemiologic tracing is necessary.

Knowledge of the pathogenesis of salmonellosis has not advanced in parallel with our more purely bacteriologic knowledge, so that much that is important about the disease remains vague. Probably, salmonellosis in animals (here excepting birds and humans) should be regarded as many diseases by reason of the variety of animal species that are susceptible, the variety of bacterial species that are pathogenic, and the poorly defined variety of circumstances in which host and pathogen interact to produce the disease. However, there are some general features of salmonellosis that may be noted here.

The more common "stress" factors that have been associated with salmonellosis in most species of domestic animals include transportation, starvation, changes in ration, overcrowding, age, pregnancy, parturition, exertion, anesthesia, surgery, intercurrent disease, and oral treatment with antibiotics and anthelmintics. A few of these factors will be considered in more detail.

There is clearly an age susceptibility to clinical disease and somewhat also to infection. Adult animals are less likely to suffer generalized or septicemic infections than are the young. When adults become infected, they are more likely to cast it off or become symptomless carriers for indefinite periods. The greater susceptibility of young animals is only partially explained by their failure to obtain specific antibody in colostrum; there is no sound explanation of why young animals are more susceptible than adults. The containment of many young animals in limited areas is conducive to high degrees of contamination of the local environment and to rapid spread of the infection. The concentration of animals is also of importance in adults, particularly horses and sheep. In these species, outbreaks are more common when the animals are closely confined. Often coupled with close confinement are the rigors attending it, especially during long travel with irregular and inadequate feeding and watering. Less tangible environmental effects are suggested by the seasonal occurrence of salmonellosis in pigs and horses.

There are many examples of enhancement of susceptibility to salmonellosis by intercurrent disease. The best known association is that between the virus of hog cholera and *Salmonella choleraesuis,* an association so close as to have caused early pathologists to disregard the bacterium as a primary pathogen. Salmonellosis sometimes complicates viral disease of carnivores and has also been observed in cattle infected with the viruses of foot and mouth disease and bovine virus diarrhea.

The disease in adult cattle is usually sporadic, and there are often noninfectious predisposing diseases such as parturient paresis, ketosis, mastitis, and parasitic infestations. The stress of anesthesia and surgery may account for the serious outbreaks of salmonellosis that occur in hospitalized animals at veterinary schools. The significance of antibiotic treatment in relation to salmonellosis is discussed under Typhlocolitis in Horses.

The pathogenesis of salmonellosis in domestic animals is poorly understood. The main route of transmission is undoubtedly by ingestion. Most of the more basic information on the pathogenesis has been obtained through experimental infection in laboratory animals. Although the data obtained from these experiments are valuable, they may not be completely applicable to domestic animals. There are obvious differences in susceptibility of animal species to particular serotypes of *Salmonella.* Some strains of *S. typhimurium* may cause a subclinical infection in mice but prove to be highly fatal for calves.

There are three basic requirements which must be met before infection with *Salmonella* induces disease. The bacteria have to be present in sufficient numbers; generally a minimal infective dose of 10^7 to 10^9 organisms is needed to infect large domestic animals. The strain must also colonize and invade enterocytes to produce enteritis; noninvasive strains of *Salmonella* are nonpathogenic. The ability to cause intestinal secretion is a property of some invasive strains.

Some *Salmonella* species have the ability to adhere to the brush border, but the mechanism by which this occurs is not understood. Adherence of *S. typhimurium* to the ileal mucosa of germ-free or specific-pathogen-free mice is not associated with O or H antigens or pili. In chicks, colonization and adherence of *Salmonella* occur more readily throughout the gastrointestinal tract in the absence of the normal microflora.

In experimental infections of guinea pigs, *Salmonella* invades the enterocytes, especially those in the ileum, and within 12 hr large numbers of organisms are present in the lumen, on the surface of the brush border, and in enterocytes. There is an

increase in the number of neutrophils in the gut lumen and within intercellular spaces, and some of these contain bacteria. Bacteria are also located in the lamina propria, mainly in macrophages. Degeneration of microvilli characterized by loss of filamentous cores is associated with close adherence of bacteria. Other degenerative changes consist of elongation, budding, and fusion of microvilli and loss of the terminal web. The organisms usually appear to invade the cells through the brush border; however, they may also enter the mucosa through the intercellular junctional complex. The bacteria are located in the cytoplasm within membrane-bound vacuoles, which may also contain remnants of microvilli and cytoplasmic debris. The *Salmonella* bacteria remain largely intact during their transcellular migration. Many bacteria are often present in a single enterocyte during the early stages of infection, but cellular damage is mild and transient. After 24 hr, most of the bacteria are located in macrophages in the lamina propria. Many organisms are evident in the lumina of crypts, but invasion of cryptal epithelial cells evidently does not take place.

In addition to causing obvious morphologic changes in the gut mucosa, some strains of invasive *Salmonella* are associated with fluid exsorption into the gut lumen. The secretion of fluid is probably toxin mediated. The significance of heat-labile or heat-stable enterotoxins, the effects of which are described under Enterotoxic Colibacillosis, is not defined for enteric salmonellosis. The cAMP system may play a role in secretion of fluids into the gut lumen, but the mechanism involved is poorly understood. *Salmonella* infection stimulates adenyl cyclase activity in the rabbit ileum, but the level of stimulation is considerably less than that produced by cholera toxins. Enterocolitis associated with salmonellosis may result in increased synthesis and secretion of prostaglandins, which in turn stimulate mucosal adenyl cyclase activity, causing abnormalities in fluid, sodium, and chloride transport.

As a result of the fluid exsorption that occurs, mainly in the lower small intestine, a large volume of fluid reaches the colon. Diarrhea is at least in part due to the inability of the damaged colon to absorb this fluid.

A cytotoxin similar to the cytotoxin or ''neurotoxin'' produced by *Shigella dysenteriae* has been associated with several serotypes of *Salmonella.* This toxin causes extensive detachment of intact Vero cells in tissue culture. The cytolytic activity is probably due to inhibition of protein synthesis rather than being a direct effect of the toxic factor on membrane integrity. The degeneration and necrosis of enterocytes in salmonellosis may be associated in part with such cytotoxin.

Vascular degeneration and thrombosis of mucosal vessels are common features of *Salmonella* enteritis. The vascular lesions may be due to action of large amounts of endotoxins absorbed through the damaged mucosa or released locally. The effects of cytotoxin on the endothelial cells also may be involved in the pathogenesis of these lesions.

Once the *Salmonella* organisms have crossed the mucosa, they may enter the blood stream via the lymphatics, perhaps carried in macrophages, and cause septicemia or transient bacteremia. Or they may remain indefinitely in the gut-associated lymphoid tissues and mesenteric lymph nodes. Increased susceptibility to salmonellosis in animals with intercurrent disease or subjected to stress may be related to relaxation of cell-mediated immunity to the organism. Septicemia may be of variable duration and severity, but as a rule, it is rapidly fatal in young animals. If, however, there is transient bacteremia, the organisms are removed by the fixed macrophages, especially of the spleen, liver, and bone marrow. They may continue to proliferate in such extravascular locations and cause another bacteremic phase that may be fatal as a septicemia or result in secondary localization.

The carrier state is of particular importance to the epidemiology of the disease. Swine especially may carry the organism in the intestine and excrete it in the feces. Whether *Salmonella* can maintain itself in the intestine is not clear; to some extent, at least, the fecal flora is likely to depend on intermittent seeding from the gallbladder or from macrophages in the lamina propria and gut-associated lymphoid tissue. The duration of the carrier state may be prolonged, or animals may rid themselves of the infection. The carrier state is an unstable one, for it appears that if the carrier is subjected to some stress or debilitating disease, it may succumb to disease; this often seems to be the case in adult cattle. The carrier animal is a potential threat to any other animal it contacts, either directly or through the medium of its excreta, or through by-products such as bone meal.

HORSES. The most common serotype in horses in most areas is *Salmonella typhimurium,* and its prevalence is increasing. Other serotypes are usually associated with sporadic outbreaks of disease. The high prevalence of salmonellosis in veterinary teaching hospitals has been mentioned. Many are carriers when they are admitted, and when they are stressed, diarrhea follows. Salmonellosis in horses may be manifested clinically as peracute, acute, chronic forms and as an asymptomatic carrier state.

The septicemic form occurs most commonly in foals 1–6 months of age. These animals are usually with their dams at pasture, and predisposing factors are unclear. The infection in foals tends to be fatal. Affected animals are lethargic and develop severe diarrhea, often with characteristic green color, which may contain casts and blood. They are febrile and waste rapidly, to die in 2 or 3 days. Some survive for a week or more, and these may develop signs of pneumonia, osteitis, polyarthritis, and meningoencephalitis.

The primarily enteric forms of the disease are more likely to occur in older horses. Most of the predisposing factors mentioned earlier apply to horses. Salmonellosis is an occupational hazard of horses since many are exposed to long periods of transport and exertion due to overwork or excessive training.

Clinically, the acute disease is characterized by diarrhea and fever for a period of 1 to 3 weeks, followed by recovery. The chronic form persists for weeks or months. Affected horses pass soft, unformed manure that resembles cow feces. They lose their appetite, with subsequent progressive loss of weight and condition. In later stages, they become dehydrated and emaciated. The carrier state is somewhat controversial. Some investigators were unable to confirm long-term carriers in horses; others were able to recover *Salmonella* from feces of recovered animals for months. Reinfection may complicate attempts to determine whether an animal is a carrier.

The gross lesions are those of enteritis and/or septicemia; the former are most consistently found at autopsy. As a rule, the longer the course, the lower in the intestine one finds the most severe lesions. Acute septicemic cases show small hemorrhages on the serous membranes, especially the pericardium and peritoneum, and enlargement of the spleen. In others, petechiae are present on the valvular endocardium, vesical mucosa, renal and adrenal cortices, and meninges, but none of these is consistent. The splenic enlargement is most marked in peracute cases, and the organ is dark and pulpy. Hepatic lipidosis seems to be common, but this may be related more to inanition than to the infection. The visceral lymph nodes are always enlarged, juicy, and often hemorrhagic.

The main lesions are in the stomach and intestines. In peracute cases, there is intense hyperemia of the gastric mucosa, probably venous infarction, with some edema and scattered hemorrhage. The small intestine may be congested with a mucous or hemorrhagic exudate. In acute cases, there is diffuse and intense hemorrhagic inflammation of the cecum and colon, overshadowing any lesions in the upper intestine and leading rapidly to superficial necrosis of the mucosa and a grayish red pseudomembrane (Fig. 1.35C). In chronic salmonellosis, enteric lesions may be few or subtle. Some animals have extensive or patchy fibrinous or ulcerative lesions of the cecum and colon. In others, raised circumscribed lesions about 2–3 cm in diameter may be evident, with a gelatinous submucosa and ulcerated mucosa. Some such lesions are more fibrinous and resemble button ulcers (Fig. 1.35D).

Histologic alterations of significance are usually limited to the intestine. In septicemic animals, however, there is sometimes focal Kupffer-cell hyperplasia in the liver, acute ileocecocolic lymphadenitis, and inflammation in sites of localization. Depending on the duration of the enteritis there may be hemorrhage, necrosis, or diphtheresis, but the infiltrating leukocytes are largely mononuclear. The superficial coagulation necrosis of the mucosa may extend over large areas. A layer of fibrinocellular exudate may cover the necrotic mucosa. Fibrin thrombi are frequently present in the capillaries of the lamina propria (Fig. 1.35E). There is usually marked congestion of submucosal vessels, which is accompanied by considerable edema.

Salmonellosis must be differentiated from septicemia due to *Actinobacillus equuli* in foals and colitis X and ischemic lesions of the large bowel in older horses. The differential diagnosis of typhlocolitis has been discussed previously. For some unknown reason, *Salmonella* is often difficult to isolate from horses that have typical signs and lesions of the disease. The tissues of choice for isolation are the mesenteric and ileocolic lymph nodes and gut, which should be ground up and inoculated into enrichment media. Repeated fecal cultures are necessary to identify carrier animals. It has been suggested that five consecutive negative cultures are required to rule out the carrier state.

CATTLE. There are differences between salmonellosis in young and adult cattle. The serotypes usually incriminated are *Salmonella typhimurium, S. enteritidis,* and *S. dublin,* the latter having often in the past been classified as *S. enteritidis.* These serotypes are of worldwide distribution. *Salmonella dublin* is not common in North America east of the Rockies, and wherever it is found it tends to show some specific adaptation to cattle and to occur in epizootics, whereas the other infections are more often sporadic. *Salmonella muenster* has become enzootic in cattle in Ontario and appears to be spreading to other eastern Canadian provinces and the northeastern United States. The behavior of this serotype is similar to that of *S. dublin*. Whatever the infecting serotype, the manifestations of infection in individual animals are the same.

It is unusual to find salmonellosis in calves less than 1 week of age, in contrast to colibacillosis, which usually affects very young animals. In calves, salmonellosis is a febrile disease typified by dejection, dehydration, and usually diarrhea. Diarrhea is not always present, but when it is, the feces are pulpy, yellow or grayish, and have a very unpleasant odor. In older calves there is often blood and mucus in the feces. In less acute cases there may be delayed evidence of localization in the lung and synovial structures. Morbidity and mortality may be considerable, especially in calves that are confined, such as in vealer operations. Experimental infections in calves indicate that survival is inversely related to the numbers of *Salmonella* in the inoculum and directly to the age of the calves.

The general appearance at autopsy of a calf with salmonellosis may be the same as one with colibacillosis. However, enlargement of mesenteric lymph nodes and gross enteric lesions are generally observed in salmonellosis. There are moderately severe gastrointestinal inflammation, acute swelling, and hemorrhage of the visceral lymph nodes, and some petechiation of serous membranes. The gastroenteritis may be catarrhal, but sometimes it is hemorrhagic or more commonly causes exudation of yellowish fibrin (Fig. 1.37A,B). The mucosa overlying the lymphoid tissues may become necrotic and slough. In animals with fibrinous enteritis, the bowel wall is somewhat turgid and the serosa may have a ground-glass appearance. There is often a diffuse, but perhaps mild, fibrinous peritonitis.

The intestinal lesions are usually most severe in the ileum, especially during the early stages of the disease. With time the jejunum and colon become involved, but the duodenum remains relatively normal. The regional distribution of the lesions may, at least in part, be related to differences in the level of bacterial colonization of the mucosa. Twelve hours after oral infection of calves with *Salmonella typhimurium,* the numbers of bacteria are generally lower in the abomasum and duodenum than in the lower intestinal tract, where they are relatively constant from the jejunum through to the rectum.

The early microscopic lesions in the small intestine consist of a thin layer of fibrinocellular exudate on the surface of short and blunt villi (Fig. 1.36B). This is followed by extensive necrosis and ulceration of the mucosa, with fibrin and neutrophils exuding from the ulcerated areas into the lumen (Fig. 1.36C,D). The lamina propria may be moderately infiltrated by mononuclear inflammatory cells. Fibrin thrombi are often evident in proprial capillaries. There is also marked submucosal edema, and the centers of lymphoid follicles in the Peyer's patches are necrotic. The mucosal damage is usually too extensive to be explained solely on the basis of ischemia due to microvascular thrombosis. Similar erosion, ulceration, and fibrinous effusion occur in the proximal large bowel.

Scanning electron microscopy of small intestine shows large numbers of bacteria on a tattered mucosal surface. Clusters of enterocytes slough off short and blunt villi (Fig. 1.36A). Strands

of fibrin emerge from the mucosal defects and cover the mucosa. Ultrastructurally, the lesions are similar to those described above for guinea pigs, except that there is more damage to epithelium in calves experimentally infected with *Salmonella typhimurium.*

Characteristic changes usually occur in the liver and spleen but may be absent in peracute septicemic cases. There is often fibrinous inflammation in the gallbladder. In acute cases, the spleen is enlarged and pulpy as a result of congestion, but this is soon replaced by acute splenitis, present as miliary, tiny foci of necrosis or as reactive nodules. The liver is often pale and beset with many minute foci of necrosis, which may require microscopy for detection. They are referred to as "paratyphoid nodules," although all transitional stages from foci of simple nonspecific necrosis to reactive granulomas occur. Typically there are few neutrophils, and whether the nodules are necrotic or reactive depends on their duration. The initial change is focal coagulation necrosis. About the margins, the macrophages accumulate and form small histiocytic granulomas, which expand and displace the surrounding parenchymal cords. In the spleen, macrophage reaction is sometimes diffuse. "Paratyphoid" granulomas may also be found microscopically in the kidney, lymph nodes, and bone marrow. In calves with acute septicemia, interstitial thickening of pulmonary alveolar septa by mononuclear cells and edema is usually found. There may be thrombosis of septal capillaries, and some effusion of edema fluid and macrophages into alveolar spaces.

In chronic salmonellosis, there is almost always an anterior bronchopneumonia, usually with adhesions and small abscesses, and purulent exudation in synovial cavities. The organism is recoverable in pure culture from such affected joints and tendon sheaths but may be mixed with *Corynebacterium* and *Pasteurella* in the lungs.

Salmonellosis in adult cattle may occur in outbreaks as it does in calves, but more often it is sporadic. The source of infection is usually the carrier animal. Other sources, such as feed containing protein of animal origin or bone meal, should be considered when the disease is caused by an uncommon serotype. Abortions are common with *Salmonella dublin* and *S. muenster* but may occur with any serotype. In some herds this may be the only clinical evidence of infection, although other animals often excrete the offending serotype in the feces. The morbid changes in adults correspond to those in calves, except that there is more pleural hemorrhage and the enteritis may be more hemorrhagic and fibrinous. The histologic changes seen in the liver and other organs are the same as those seen in calves with salmonellosis.

SHEEP.   As well as abortion caused by *Salmonella abortus-ovis*, abortion and neonatal death may attend infection of pregnant ewes by any species of *Salmonella*. Otherwise it is not a common disease in sheep, but outbreaks are always severe and may cause very heavy losses. Predisposing influences are necessary, and these are usually provided by circumstances that enforce congregation. Deprivation of food and water for 2 or 3 days may be sufficient and, coupled with fatigue, is the usual predisposing factor when sheep are transported or confined in holding yards. Deaths usually continue for a week to 10 days after debilitating circumstances have been remedied.

The serotypes usually found in sheep are *Salmonella ty-*

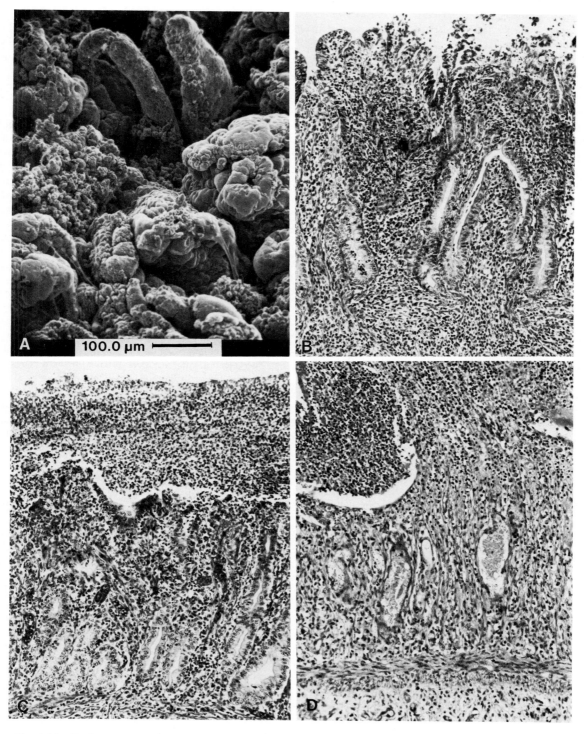

Fig. 1.36. Bovine salmonellosis. **(A)** Scanning electron micrograph. Ileum. Calf 12 hr postinoculation with *Salmonella typhimurium*. Villi are atrophic, and rounded cells are exfoliated from surface. **(B)** Atrophy of villi, exfoliation of surface epithelium, and effusion of neutrophils in ileum 12 hr after inoculation with *S. typhimurium*. **(C)** Atrophy of villi, erosion, and effusion of neutrophils and fibrin into lumen. Some thrombosis of proprial vessels. Thirty-six hours after inoculation with *S. typhimurium*. (A–C courtesy of R. C. Clarke and C. L. Gyles.) **(D)** Eroded ileal mucosa, largely devoid of crypts of Lieberkühn. Fibrin and neutrophils in lumen.

phimurium, S. arizona, and *S. enteritidis. Salmonella dublin* is increasing in prevalence in Great Britain and the midwestern states of the United States. They produce the same sort of disease, which closely resembles that seen in cattle both clinically and at autopsy. The major findings are fibrinohemorrhagic enteritis and septicemia.

SWINE. Many serotypes of *Salmonella* have been isolated from swine, and with poultry they form the most important reservoir of the organism. The bacteria are carried in the intestine but also in the regional lymph nodes of the alimentary tract so that carrier animals may not excrete the organism in the feces.

Salmonellosis occurs in feeder pigs, usually those 2–4 months of age. It is very uncommon in sucklings and adult swine.

Three syndromes are associated with *Salmonella* infections in swine. **Septicemic salmonellosis** is usually associated with *S. choleraesuis* var. *kunzendorf,* although enteric lesions may be present with this serotype. Sporadic infections with *S. dublin* have also been associated with septicemia in nursing pigs. *Salmonella typhimurium* most commonly causes **acute** or **chronic enterocolitis,** including a necrotizing proctitis that may lead to rectal structure. *Salmonella typhisuis* infection is characterized by **caseous tonsillitis** and **lymphadenitis** as well as ulcerative enterocolitis. Detailed consideration of the three syndromes just outlined is warranted because salmonellosis is one of the most important diseases of swine.

Salmonella choleraesuis was once thought to be the cause of hog cholera because gross lesions of the two diseases are similar. Hog cholera may be complicated by *S. choleraesuis.* It has been estimated that the bacterium may be recovered from 10 to 50% of hog cholera infections. Other predisposing factors mentioned earlier generally also apply to salmonellosis in swine.

The major clinical manifestations of *Salmonella choleraesuis* infection are septicemia and enteritis; they usually occur separately. Septicemia is more common. It is probable that the pathogenesis of the infection follows the system given for *Salmonella* in general. The bacteremic phase may develop into a fatal septicemia, or the organism may localize in the intestine, causing enteritis that is not necessarily chronic or even clinically manifest.

Salmonellosis that is clinically septicemic is usually fatal. Death may occur quickly without observed illness, or after a course of a week or more. There is a high fever; characteristic but not pathognomonic blue discoloration of the skin, especially of the tail, snout, and ears; posterior weakness; dyspnea, which often leads to misdiagnosis of primary pneumonia; and sometimes terminal convusions. Pigs recover from this phase may have dry gangrene of the ears and tail, posterior paralysis, blindness, and diphtheritic enteritis. The chronic or enteric form may develop from the acute but is usually insidious from the onset. It is characterized by loose yellow feces containing flakes of fibrin, progressive emaciation and debility, and eventual death. Some recover but fail to thrive, often partly owing to chronic bronchopneumonia.

At autopsy there is a bluish or purplish discoloration of the skin, which may be very intense about the head and ears. There may be superficial necrosis of the ears. The internal lesions are typically hemorrhagic; the hemorrhages are petechial. The lymph nodes are almost invariably hemorrhagic but not much enlarged unless the course is prolonged. The visceral nodes are more frequently and obviously involved than the peripheral ones, with the exception of those of the throat, which are consistently hemorrhagic. The mesenteric lymph nodes are greatly enlarged; they may be speckled with parenchymal hemorrhages, or the extravasations may be in the peripheral sinus.

There may be hemorrhages, petechial or as small discrete blebs, on the laryngeal mucosa (Fig. 1.37D). The lungs do not collapse because there is frothy fluid in the respiratory passages. They may be pale blue or purple. Beneath the visceral pleura there are small dark foci of hemorrhage. The lungs are wet, and there is fluid in the interlobular tissue. The changes are best appreciated in the posterior lobes, because the anterior lobes are often the seat of acute lobular pneumonia. These pulmonary changes account for the respiratory signs observed clinically. The pneumonia is interstitial because of the influence of the organism on the alveolar vessels. The lobar anteroventral pneumonia may be due to ascending *Salmonella* alveolitis and bronchiolitis. Occasionally, the injury to the alveolar septa by *Salmonella* results in copious outpouring of fibrin and extensive fibrinous pneumonia of the posterior lobes. The cardiac serosae often bear petechiae, and in some more virulent infections there is fibrinohemorrhagic pericarditis with scant fluid exudation.

The spleen is enlarged, deep blue, with sharp edges. There may be petechiae on the capsule, but the small marginal infarcts of hog cholera or the larger ones of porcine erysipelas are not present. The enlargement of the spleen and absence of infarcts distinguish salmonellosis from hog cholera. In acute erysipelas, the spleen is enlarged but the sectioned surface is the same blue color as the capsular surface and is firm and rubbery. These points are made as generalizations and are not totally reliable. Other causes of splenomegaly must be differentiated.

The liver is usually congested, and focal hemorrhages may be visible in the capsule. In some cases the hemorrhages are very large, involving up to half of the central area in a lobule. They may be scattered at random throughout the liver or grouped, often at the edge of a lobe. Occasionally, almost every lobule is affected, and the lesions may resemble those of hepatosis dietetica. In some, there are tiny yellow foci of necrosis, the "paratyphoid nodules" described above for calves (Fig. 1.37C).

Pinpoint hemorrhages are consistently present in the renal cortex. There may be only a few in each kidney, or they may be so numerous as to cause the "turkey egg" appearance. The kidneys may be of normal color, or the cortices may be pale and the medulla intensely congested as in other septicemias. In some, there are petechiae in the pelvic and ureteral epithelium. In almost all cases, hemorrhages are present beneath the epithelium of the bladder.

The stomach shows the intense red-black color of the severe congestion and infarction common to endotoxemia in postweaned pigs. If the animal survives a week or more, the superficial layers of the affected gastric epithelium slough. There may be no lesions in the intestine. There may be a catarrhal enteritis, or more frequently, the enteritis is hemorrhagic, increasing in severity lower in the tract and terminating in a hemorrhagic ileitis. The mucosae of the colon and cecum may be normal, but

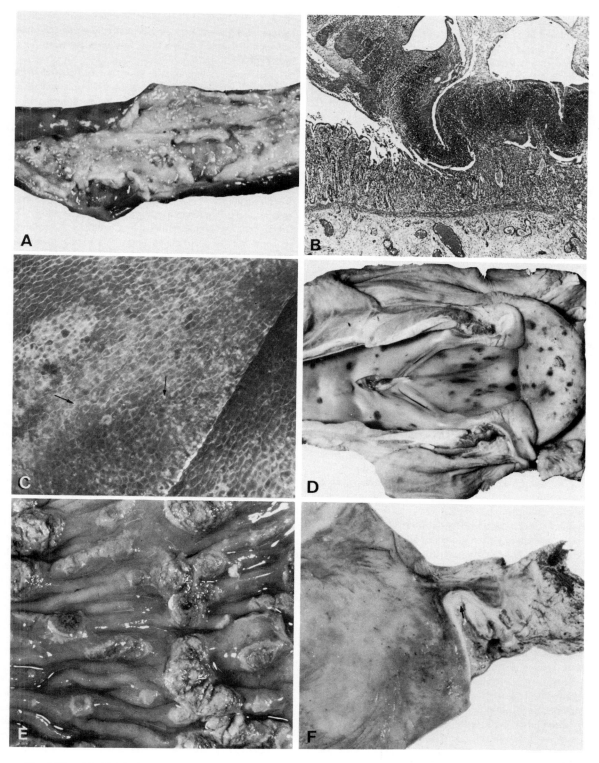

Fig. 1.37. (A) Diphtheritic enteritis. *Salmonella enteritidis*. Calf. (B) Bovine salmonellosis. Diphtheritic membrane on the surface of the ileum. Exudate arises from eroded mucosa, in which crypts of Lieberkühn are sparse or absent. (C–F) Porcine salmonellosis. (C) Paratyphoid nodules (arrows) in liver. *Salmonella* septicemia. (D) Laryngeal hemorrhages. (E) Ulcers in colon. (F) Rectal stricture. Opened colon is massively dilated anterior to stricture in rectum (arrow).

if the course if prolonged, there is hyperemia or fibrinohemorrhagic inflammation.

Petechial hemorrhages may occur in the meninges and brain, but there is no sign of gross inflammation. Localization sometimes occurs in synovial membranes, producing polysynovitis and sometimes polyarthritis. It is more usual to have an increase in the volume of fluid with red, velvety hypertrophy of the synovial villi.

The gross features that have been described are a composite, and they are usually not all present in any one case. The splenic, gastric, renal, and lymphatic lesions are most consistent.

The development of the experimental intestinal lesions in salmonellosis has been well described. The morphogenesis and microscopic appearance of the enteritis resemble those described in calves. The result may be diffuse diphtheritic enteritis in the cecum and colon and, occasionally, ileum, or focal "button ulcers." Focal ulcers in salmonellosis may occur at points where the bacteria have breached the epithelium, or they may be centered on Peyer's patches and solitary lymphoid follicles. Button ulcers that occur along the cecum and colon are to be distinguished from nonspecific ulcers that occasionally occur on and about the ileocecal valve. Necrotic enteritis due to secondary invasion of the eroded ileum and large bowel by pathogenic anaerobes and *Balantidium coli* may also supervene. Porcine adenomatosis is probably a more important forerunner of necrotic enteritis.

The histologic changes that occur in internal organs in acute disease are mainly associated with endothelial damage due to endotoxin and focal localization of bacteria. The discoloration of the skin is initially due to intense dilation, congestion, and thrombosis of capillaries and venules in the dermal papilla. There is activation and necrosis of the endothelial cells in affected vessels. The renal lesions vary but affect principally the glomeruli. In some there is diffuse glomerulitis, and this is associated with mild nephrosis and hyaline casts. In others the glomerulitis is exudative and hemorrhagic, and in these a great many capillary loops contain hyaline thrombi. The hemorrhages seen grossly come mainly from glomeruli and the wide venules of the outer cortex, although some are from intertubular capillaries; this is always the case in the medulla. Embolic bacterial colonies are occasionally seen in the glomerular and intertubular capillaries. Fibrin thrombi may also be found in the afferent arterioles and interlobular arteries.

It has been suggested that the pathogenesis of the renal vascular lesions can be explained on the basis of a generalized Shwartzman reaction. However, disseminated intravascular coagulation initiated by endotoxemia may be all that is necessary to cause these and other vascular lesions in septicemia due to Gram-negative bacteria.

The microscopic pulmonary lesions similarly are characterized by thrombosis and vasculitis and a largely mononuclear cellular response in alveolar septa. There is a flooding of the alveoli by edema fluid and moderate numbers of alveolar macrophages. This is the usual histologic picture; the extremes are an acute fibrinous inflammation or only a few scattered parenchymal hemorrhages.

In the spleen there are some scattered hemorrhages, but the overall histologic impression is of increased histiocytes with a scattering of neutrophils. The follicles are small and rather inactive. Very small foci of necrosis, containing many bacteria, are scattered in the sections or are relatively numerous, and these develop a reactive macrophage response and form the typical paratyphoid nodules.

Meningoencephalomyelitis occurs in a proportion of cases of septicemic salmonellosis. The lesion is fundamentally a vasculitis. There may be petechiae in the meninges, but microscopically, there is an infiltration of large mononuclear cells in the pia–arachnoid and concentrated about the veins. There is also sludging of these cells and polymorphs, including eosinophils, in the veins. Similar lesions may occur at any level in the brain. In some cases the walls of many veins are necrotic, and there may be a mononuclear-cell reaction in the walls and surrounding neuropil. Only a few neutrophils and eosinophils form part of the inflammatory cell reaction in these areas. The parenchymal lesions consist of a disseminated focal granulomatous encephalitis. Areas of malacia may be associated with the granulomas. Microabscesses form in those few cases in which bacterial emboli are detectable. Glial nodules are typical of the healed phase. These lesions occur in the spinal cord as well.

Salmonella typhimurium infection in swine produces a syndrome that differs from *S. choleraesuis* in a number of ways. Clinically, the disease occurs in feeder pigs and is characterized by fever, inanition, and yellow, watery diarrhea, which may contain blood and mucus, especially in the later stages. The diarrhea may be chronic and intermittent. There is a high morbidity but low mortality. Most pigs recover but may remain carriers for variable periods of time.

The pathogenesis and morphology of the enteric lesions are similar to those described for *Salmonella choleraesuis* enteritis. The lesions with *S. typhimurium* infection are mainly confined to the colon (Fig. 1.37E), cecum, and rectum, however, with rare involvement of the distal small intestine.

Rectal stricture is thought to be a sequel in most cases to ulcerative proctitis of ischemic origin caused by *Salmonella typhimurium*. It is characterized clinically by marked progressive distension of the abdomen, loss of appetite, emaciation, and soft feces. At autopsy, there is marked dilatation of the colon, which is caused by narrowing of the rectum, 1–10 cm anterior to the anus (Fig. 1.37F). The stricture is usually less than 1.0 cm in diameter and varies in length from 0.5 to 20 cm. There is marked fibrous thickening of the rectal wall, which may contain microabscesses. The dilatation of the colon, anterior to the stricture, may consist of a well-demarcated, widened area several centimeters long and wide. The colonic mucosa in this area is usually ulcerated and may be covered by fibrinous exudate. In some cases, there is more gradual dilatation of the entire colon, with ulceration of the mucosa just anterior to the stricture. The mucosa is always excessively corrugated; this is mainly the result of marked thickening of the internal muscularis. Localized chronic peritonitis is often associated with the dilated segments of the colon.

Microscopically, the strictures are the result of marked fibrosis of the gut wall, with almost complete obliteration of the normal structures. The mucosa is generally completely absent. The luminal surface is covered by debris, fibrin, and neutrophils. A few veins in the wall contain well-organized thrombi. The colonic lesions are those of a mild to severe necrotizing ulcerative colitis, described earlier.

The stricture is located in an area of rectum that has a relatively poor blood supply, namely, the junction of the circulatory fields of the caudal mesenteric and pudendal arteries. Ulcerative proctitis is consistently found in swine with typhlocolitis due to *Salmonella typhimurium* infection. Granulation of such lesions probably leads to cicatrization and stricture. The location, the persistent nature of this lesion in some pigs, and its limited capacity to heal are probably related to the restricted blood supply of the affected area. The lesions in the colon and cecum, with greater collateral blood supply, heal more rapidly, usually without further complications. At the time of autopsy, *S. typhimurium* may not be isolated due to loss of the carrier state. Alternatively, rectal stricture in some cases may result from ischemia due to noninfectious causes, such as rectal prolapse.

Salmonella typhisuis infection is an uncommon condition in pigs, with a limited geographic distribution. The disease is called paratyphoid in Europe. It is a progressive disease of 2- to 4-month-old pigs that is clinically characterized by intermittent diarrhea, emaciation, and frequently, massive enlargement of the neck region. The lesions are those of circular or button-like to confluent ulceration of the mucosa of the ileum, cecum, and colon. Other typical findings are caseous palatine tonsillitis and cervical lymphadenitis, parotid sialoadenitis, and caseous lymphadenitis of the mesenteric lymph nodes.

The differential diagnosis of septicemic salmonellosis includes other septicemias that occur in feeder swine, such as peracute erysipelas, *Haemophilus*, and *Steptococcus* infections. It is important to differentiate *Salmonella choleraesuis* infection from hog cholera and African swine fever.

The enteric forms of salmonellosis must be differentiated from other enteritides in postweaning swine, particularly postweaning *E. coli* enteritis, swine dysentery, and *Campylobacter* enteritis.

CARNIVORES. *Salmonella* may often be recovered from dogs. However, primary disease rarely, if ever, occurs. Salmonellosis is most commonly secondary to canine distemper and may cause bronchopneumonia, acute gastroenteritis, splenic swelling, serosal hemorrhages, and foci of necrosis in the liver and other organs. There is also enlargement of the mesenteric lymph nodes. Salmonellosis has also been reported in dogs with lymphosarcoma, shortly after the initiation of chemotherapy. The immunosuppressive effect of the treatment probably predisposes to the development of disease.

Various serotypes have been isolated from cats, and most of these appear to cause subclinical infections. Salmonellosis may be a problem in catteries and hospitals, however, affecting animals subjected to the usual stressful conditions mentioned earlier. *Salmonella typhimurium* is most commonly associated with such outbreaks. The disease is characterized by gastroenteritis and septicemia.

Because of their close association with humans, especially children and the aged, dogs and cats, which are carriers, may be a source of zoonotic infection.

Yersiniosis

Yersinia enterocolitica causes sporadic cases of mucoid enterocolitis in young dogs and produces ulcerative ileocolitis in humans. The significance of the organism in human disease has finally been recognized. Strains of *Y. enterocolitica* from dogs, and from pigs, which are regarded as reservoirs of infection, cause disease in humans. Outbreaks of disease in pigs and goats due to *Y. enterocolitica* have been recorded. In goats, sudden deaths sometimes preceded by diarrhea occur; the diarrhea is associated with acute catarrhal enteritis. Kids are particularly susceptible. Certain strains of *Y. enterocolitica* are enterotoxigenic and/or invasive. Invasion occurs via the lymphoid tissue of the ileum and cecum.

Yersinia (Pasteurella) pseudotuberculosis infection may cause enteritis and diarrhea in animals. The organism is carried in the alimentary tract of rats, mice, and birds. Following oral infection, a local lesion in the intestine may be produced. In some animals, systemic spread, with multifocal hepatic necrosis and splenitis, occurs. Captive wild ruminants commonly show enteric lesions as well as visceral lesions, and this combination is seen occasionally in sheep. In dogs and cats, signs of enteritis occur, but lesions have not been described. *Yersinia pseudotuberculosis* occasionally can be isolated from small green abscesses in the mesenteric lymph nodes of asymptomatic dogs and cats. The organism also causes pneumonia and septicemia in foals and sporadic abortions in ruminants.

Campylobacter Enteritis

Enteritis in animals and humans associated with *Campylobacter*, or *Campylobacter*-like organisms, appears in two forms. The first is characterized by adenomatous proliferation of epithelium in the crypts of Lieberkühn in the small intestine (especially ileum) and in mucosal glands in large bowel. Bacteria that have been confirmed as *Campylobacter* or that resemble *Campylobacter* morphologically are found within proliferating epithelial cells. Conditions that fall into this category include ileal hyperplasia or proliferative ileitis in hamsters, typhlitis in rabbits, duodenal hyperplasia in guinea pigs, intestinal adenomatosis affecting the cecum and colon in blue foxes, proliferative colitis in ferrets, intestinal adenomatosis in horses, and a cluster of syndromes in swine grouped under the name intestinal adenomatosis complex. Terminal ileitis or regional enteritis in lambs has not been firmly associated with intracellular *Campylobacter*-like organisms. The second group of conditions comprises enteritis and mucosal colitis associated with apparently noninvasive *C. jejuni* and perhaps *C. coli*. Diarrhea in humans, dogs, and cattle is associated with *C. jejuni*. The causal role of *C. jejuni* and *C. coli* in spontaneous enteritis in sheep, cats, and swine is less clearly established.

The intestinal adenomatosis complex of swine, the most significant expression of *Campylobacter*-associated proliferative enteritis, and the syndromes associated with *C. jejuni* and *C. coli*, will be considered more fully.

INTESTINAL ADENOMATOSIS COMPLEX OF SWINE. This group of conditions is associated with intracellular proliferation of *Campylobacter* spp. in the mucosal glands of the ileum and proximal large bowel of swine. Its components have been variously recognized in the past as intestinal adenoma of swine, adenomatous intestinal hyperplasia, terminal regional ileitis, regional ileitis, terminal ileitis, proliferative ileitis, and as part of hemorrhagic bowel syndrome, necrotic enteritis, and ileal muscular hypertrophy.

The agent associated most commonly with the intestinal adenomatosis complex is *Campylobacter sputorum* var. *mucosalis*, which has been isolated from the mucosal lesion and from the oral cavity of swine in affected herds. It has proved difficult consistently to reproduce the disease, or its essential lesions, even using crude inocula comprised of infected intestinal mucosa. Cultures of the organism may inconsistenly produce disease in Caesarian-derived, colostrum-deprived, but not germ-free pigs. A second species, *C. hyointestinalis*, has been recovered commonly, alone or in association with *C. sputorum* var. *mucosalis*, from lesions in naturally infected swine. Immunofluorescence suggests that *C. hyointestinalis* is more numerous and widespread in cells in hypertrophic crypts, while *C. sputorum* var. *mucosalis* is limited to more superficial foci in affected tissue. The etiologic significance of each of these agents and their possible interactions with each other and the rest of the enteric flora remain to be clarified.

A number of clinicopathologic syndromes comprise the intestinal adenomatosis complex in swine. They may be found concurrently in a single herd and are manifestations of different phases of the interaction between the host and the invasive *Campylobacter*. The fundamental lesion is porcine intestinal adenomatosis—proliferation of *Campylobacter*-infected epithelial cells in crypts and glands and associated mucosal alterations (Fig. 1.38A). Necrotic enteritis, regional ileitis, and proliferative hemorrhagic enteropathy are the other defined components of the complex. Each syndrome will be discussed in turn.

Porcine intestinal adenomatosis and its sequelae, necrotic enteritis or regional ileitis, occur most commonly in postweaning feeder pigs. Piglets as young as 3 weeks of age, however, as well as adults, may have lesions of adenomatosis. Intestinal adenomatosis is associated with a syndrome that may vary from subtle subclinical disease with a mild decrease in growth rate to diarrhea and unthriftiness. Animals with extensive lesions, developing necrotic enteritis, or regional ileitis may show anorexia, intermittent or persistent diarrhea, and severe weight loss. Death may follow a period of diarrhea and progressive cachexia, or it may occur occasionally as a result of perforation of an ulcerated intestine in regional ileitis.

In adenomatosis, infection of cells lining mucosal glands may occur initially in the vicinity of Peyer's patches and mucosal lymphoid aggregates in the ileocecal colic region. In some experimental studies, lesions were first seen there, and in mildly affected spontaneous cases, lesions sometimes seem associated with these structures preferentially. *Campylobacter* invades epithelium in crypts and glands, where the bacteria lie free in the apical cytoplasm and replicate. Goblet cells disappear from affected glands, and infected epithelium is transformed to a population of highly mitotic cells. These form a crowded, pseudostratified columnar epithelium, with basophilic cytoplasm. Nuclei may be open and vesiculate with prominent nucleoli, or laterally compressed. Glands become elongate, dilated, and branching, causing thickening of the mucosa. Isolated plaques of affected mucosa may project above adjacent unaffected tissue. The derivation of the term adenomatosis to describe such a change is obvious. Hypertrophic glands sometimes protrude into lymphoid tissue in the submucosa.

Enterocyte migration from crypt to lumen appears to decline, and villi undergo progressive atrophy so that they may be entirely absent in well-established lesions. Adenomatous areas merge sharply with adjacent normal mucosa. Masses of *Campylobacter* are readily recognized in silver-stained tissue sections as curved rods, sometimes seagull- or W-shaped, infecting especially the apical cytoplasm of cells in adenomatous glands (Fig. 1.38B). *Campylobacter* also has been identified ultrastructurally in degenerate cells and macrophages in the lamina propria. However, proprial and submucosal inflammation in areas of uncomplicated adenomatosis is not marked.

How *Campylobacter* induces such lesions is unknown. The lesion may be the result of cell-mediated immune reactions stimulating, by lymphokine, crypt-cell hyperplasia. Proliferation of the bacteria appears to be largely intracellular, and the effect of continual mitosis of cells in crypts may be to increase the population of cells able to support bacterial growth and replication.

In animals with the relatively mild syndrome of uncomplicated intestinal adenomatosis, lesions are always found in the terminal portion of the ileum, extending proximally from the ileocecal–colic orifice for usually less than a meter. In a proportion of cases they involve the cecum and proximal third of the spiral colon. Lesions of the cecum and colon do not occur without ileal involvement. In mild cases, which are likely to be subclinical, only a few ridge- or plaquelike thickened areas project above the remainder of the mucosa. However, more typical widespread lesions cause the thickened mucosa to form irregular longitudinal or transverse folds or ridges. The surface may be intact, but commonly, small foci of fibrin exudation or necrosis may be evident (Fig. 1.38F).

Thickening of the adenomatous mucosa, and perhaps some edema of the submucosa, is reflected in accentuation of the normal reticular pattern on the serosa of the ileum (Fig. 1.38D). This results in a ''cerebral'' or gyrate pattern of projections and depressions on the serosal aspect of the intestine, which is readily recognized and virtually pathognomonic for this condition. Mucosal lesions in the large intestine often form thickened plaquelike or almost polypoid masses, which may be confluent in some areas. Serosal folds may be evident on extensively affected large intestine. The ileocolic lymph nodes are enlarged and hyperplastic. Occasionally, microscopic foci of adenomatous epithelium may be found in submucosal lymphatics or the regional lymph node.

Coagulation necrosis of adenomatous mucosa occurs commonly. **Necrotic enteritis** may be partly the result of pathogenic anaerobic large bowel flora, colonizing the affected terminal ileum. There may be effusion of fibrin from superficial lesions, and a pseudodiphtheritic membrane or luminal fibrin cast may be present. Caseous yellow-brown or blood-tinged necrotic mucosa may be found focally or widely in the distal ileum and proximal large intestine. The cerebral pattern of serosal folding is evident in such cases (Fig. 1.39B). Necrotic enteritis may be a sequel to other enterocolitides in swine, but adenomatosis is probably the most common primary lesion.

Microscopically, coagulation necrosis of the mucosa may be focal and superficial, with local effusion of neutrophils and fibrin into the lumen and an acute inflammatory infiltrate at the margin of the necrotic tissue. Frequently, necrosis extends to

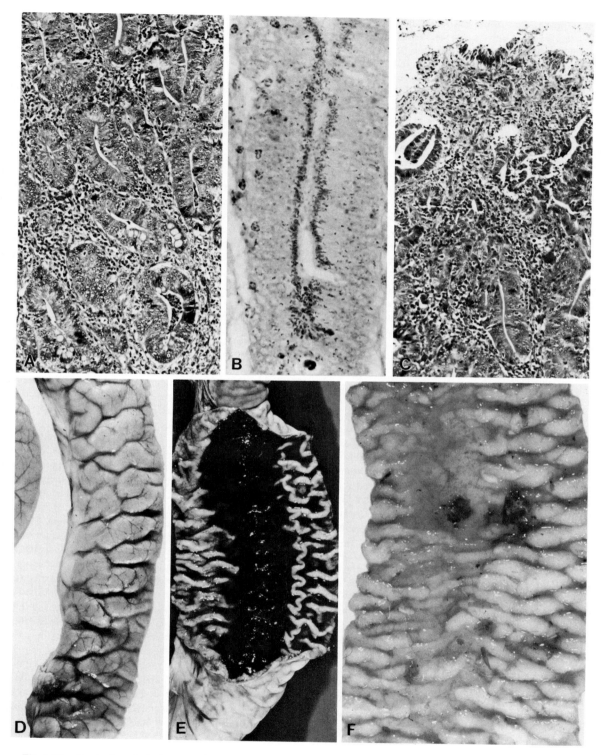

Fig. 1.38. Porcine intestinal adenomatosis complex. (**A**) Adenomatous change in glands in lamina propria. (**B**) Masses of silver-stained *Campylobacter* in cytoplasm of hyperplastic epithelium lining intestinal glands. (**C**) Proliferative hemorrhagic enteropathy. Superficial necrosis of mucosa associated with thrombosis of small vessels, hemorrhage, and effusion of fibrin and neutrophils. (**D**) Exaggerated reticular pattern of folds on serosal aspect of the ileum. (**E**) Proliferative hemorrhagic enteropathy. Hemorrhage and blood clot in terminal ileum. Nodular folded mucosa. (**F**) Raised nodular or ridgelike areas of thickened mucosa in the ileum, resulting from hypertrophy of glands.

involve most the thickness of the mucosa, sometimes penetrating to the submucosa. A few islands of viable adenomatous crypts or glands may be left deep among the necrotic debris. Tissue in the upper ileum at the proximal margin of the zone of mucosal necrosis should be examined for adenomatosis, since in severe cases of necrotic enteritis, no remnants of abnormal mucosa may persist elsewhere. Masses of bacteria, presumably fecal anaerobes, are found superficially in the necrotic tissue. With time, granulation tissue develops in ulcerated areas.

Regional ileitis is the term applied to contracted tubular distal ileum, which may have an ulcerated mucosa, perhaps with a few raised foci of surviving proliferative mucosa. Granulation of ulcerated gut may result in progressive stricture of the lumen. More characteristically, there is hypertrophy of the external muscle layer. Idiopathic ileal muscular hypertrophy also occurs in swine, apparently independent of antecedent adenomatosis. Granulomatous regional ileitis and mesenteric lymphadenitis in swine, nontuberculous and distinct from adenomatosis, has been described from Finland.

Proliferative hemorrhagic enteropathy is the fourth syndrome in the intestinal adenomatosis complex. It is a distinctive clinical entity, characterized by acute or subacute intestinal hemorrhage and anemia. Animals may exsanguinate so quickly as to die without passing blood. Others pass dark, tarry feces for several days. This syndrome is more common in young adults rather than growing pigs. It is usually sporadic or of relatively low morbidity, but up to half the clinically recognized cases may die.

Animals dead of proliferative hemorrhagic enteropathy are pale. The typical cerebral pattern is evident on the external surface of the distal ileum, which is thickened and turgid (Fig. 1.39A). Fluid blood, or a loose or firm fibrin and blood clot, may be present in the ileum (Fig. 1.38E), and the contents of the cecum and colon may contain dark, bloody digesta and feces. The mucosa of the affected ileum usually resembles that in uncomplicated adenomatosis, and overt points of hemorrhage or ulceration are rarely appreciated grossly. Rather, the animals appear to suffer widespread diapedesis from the mucosa. In tissue section there is extensive degeneration and necrosis of adenomatous epithelium (Fig. 1.38C). An acute inflammatory infiltrate is present in the upper lamina propria, small vessels are thrombosed, and heavy effusion of neutrophils onto the mucosal surface and into lumina of glands is evident. Fibrin and hemorrhage emanating from superficial mucosal vessels are in the intestinal lumen. More extensive coagulation necrosis of the mucosa is associated occasionally with the hemorrhagic syndrome. It has been suggested that proliferative hemorrhagic enteropathy is the result of a hypersensitivity reaction to release of normally occult intracellular bacterial antigen from its intracellular location, by degeneration or phagocytosis of infected epithelium.

The diagnosis of proliferative hemorrhagic enteropathy at autopsy is based on the presence in the distal ileum of gross lesions characteristic of adenomatosis, in association with massive hemorrhage from the lower small intestine. The condition must be differentiated from hemorrhagic ulceration of the pars esophagea, mesenteric torsion, and acute swine dysentery as well as from less common causes of gastrointestinal bleeding in swine. Less hemorrhagic manifestations of the adenomatosis complex must be differentiated from acute or chronic salmonellosis.

The diagnosis of components of the intestinal adenomatosis complex is confirmed by finding *Campylobacter*. They may be seen in smears of mucosal scrapings stained by the modified Koster's acid-fast method or with specific immunofluorescent techniques. Their intracellular location and association with typical adenomatous lesions is demonstrated in silver-stained tissue sections.

ENTERITIS ASSOCIATED WITH OTHER *CAMPYLOBACTER* SPECIES. *Campylobacter jejuni* and *C. coli* have been recognized recently as common causes of diarrhea in humans. *Campylobacter* enteritis rivals salmonellosis in significance in this regard in many areas. Like salmonellosis, *Campylobacter* infection may be zoonotic. Many human infections appear to be acquired by drinking raw milk or come from other animal foodstuffs, especially poultry products. Chickens are common asymptomatic shedders of *C. jejuni*. Some human cases have been associated with diarrhea in family pets, particularly puppies.

Despite the fact that it can be isolated from nondiarrheic animals, *Campylobacter jejuni* has been associated with diarrhea characterized by the presence of blood and mucus in some dogs. It has also been isolated from dogs with parvoviral enteritis and other viral infections; it is not known if concurrent infection with these agents is synergistic. The role of *Campylobacter* as a significant primary pathogen in dogs is not proven. Mild enteritis and colitis have been described in naturally infected dogs, while in experimentally infected gnotobiotic dogs, lesions are limited to mild mucosal colitis.

Campylobacter jejuni, *C. fetus* subsp. *fetus*, and *C. fecalis* have been isolated from the feces of normal cattle and from diarrheic calves and cattle, many of them suffering from disease due to other agents. Experimental inoculation of these agents has resulted in passage of dark, fluid feces with mucus and flecks of blood. The intestine was described as thickened and patchily reddened, especially in the ileum, cecum, and colon. Mild enteritis with stunting of villi and some accumulation of neutrophils in crypts was described in sections of the small intestine. There was hyperplasia of lymphoid tissue in Peyer's patches and mesenteric lymph nodes. *Campylobacter jejuni* and perhaps other species are thought to be primary agents causing diarrhea in cattle, but further work is needed to define their significance. For many years *Campylobacter (Vibrio) coli* was proposed as the cause of "winter dysentery," a clinical entity in cattle, the etiology of which has not been determined.

Campylobacter jejuni, in addition to causing a significant proportion of "vibrionic" abortions, is isolated from the intestine of sheep with diarrhea, but its causal association is unproven. The same agent also has been isolated from the feces of a number of scouring foals, but the significance of the infection is unclear. *Campylobacter jejuni* is also isolated commonly from cats, but not usually in association with diarrhea.

Campylobacter coli is the species commonly isolated from the intestine of swine. As "*Vibrio coli*" it was long associated with swine dysentery but did not induce enteritis in experimentally inoculated gnotobiotic pigs. More recent reports of diarrhea in conventional swine inoculated orally with *C. coli* need confirmation.

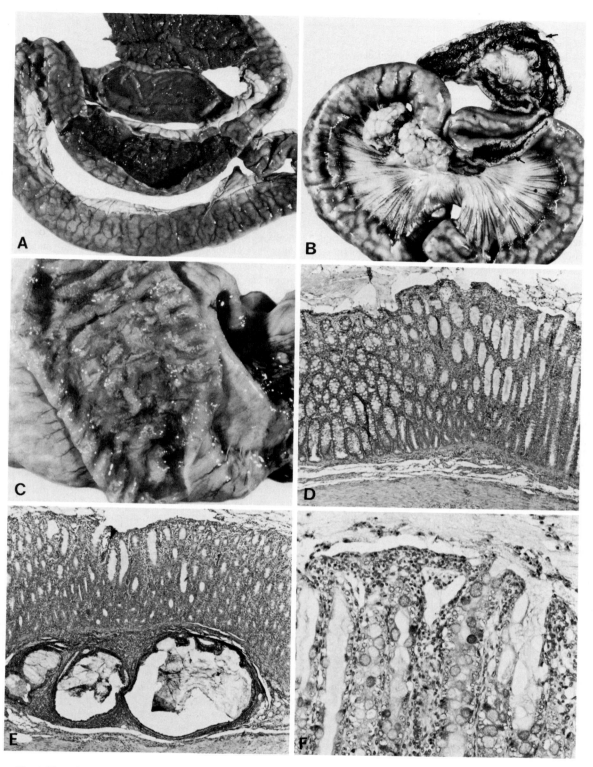

Fig. 1.39. (**A** and **B**) Porcine intestinal adenomatosis complex. (**A**) Folded necrotic mucosa, and fibrinohemorrhagic exudate in terminal ileum. (**B**) Necrotic enteritis. Thick ileal wall (arrows), enlarged lymph nodes, and opaque mesentery. (**C–F**) Swine dysentery. (**C**) Patchy fibrinocatarrhal exudate on the colonic mucosa. (**D**) Hyperplastic glands with few goblet cells adjacent to mucosa with normal density of goblet cells. Mucus in large amounts on mucosal surface. (**E**) Hyperplastic glandular lining virtually devoid of goblet cells; "colitis cystica profunda," or herniation of mucous glands into submucosal lymphoid tissue. (**F**) Flattened and exfoliating epithelium on mucosal surface, and edema of superficial lamina propria. Mucus in glands and on surface, mixed with neutrophils and exfoliated epithelium.

SWINE DYSENTERY. Swine dysentery is a highly infectious disease mainly of weaned pigs that is characterized by diarrhea, with mucus, blood, or fibrin in the feces. The disease has been reported from a number of countries and probably occurs wherever swine are raised. It has been recognized for nearly half a century, and as long ago as 1924 was known to be experimentally transmissible by dosing young pigs with colonic contents from affected swine. *Campylobacter coli* (formerly *Vibrio coli*) was thought to be the etiologic agent of swine dysentery for many years, but *Treponema hyodysenteriae* is now considered to be the causative agent. It is a Gram-negative, anaerobic but oxygen-tolerant spirochete, 6–8.5 μm long and 0.5 μm in diameter. It produces strong β-hemolysis on blood agar plates. The organism is motile, moving in serpentine fashion; it is loosely coiled and has 7–13 axial filaments. Swine dysentery can be reproduced by feeding pure cultures of *T. hyodysenteriae* to specific pathogen-free and conventionally reared swine. Experimental reproduction of the disease in gnotobiotic pigs requires the presence of anaerobic bacteria indigenous to the normal colon, along with *T. hyodysenteriae*. There is apparently a synergistic action between the spirochete and the other anaerobes, mainly *Bacteroides* and fusiforms. These probably provide a suitable microenvironment for the *Treponema* to proliferate. *Treponema hyodysenteriae* is also pathogenic for guinea pigs and mice. Oral inoculation causes colitis in both species.

Other *Treponema* organisms occur in the colon of normal pigs. These spirochetes are approximately half the size of *T. hyodysenteriae*, are nonhemolytic or only weakly so, and differ in other biochemical reactions. It has been suggested that these spirochetes be called *T. innocens*. Their role in spontaneous disease is controversial, since they have been associated with diarrhea that resembled a mild form of swine dysentery. It appears that at least some strains of *T. innocens* are mildly pathogenic for swine.

The pathogenesis of swine dysentery is still incompletely understood. *Treponema hyodysenteriae* invades the epithelial cells of the superficial mucosa of the colon. Although there is no evidence to suggest that invasion is essential for epithelial necrosis to occur, lesions in the mucosa are associated with the presence of large numbers of spirochetes and other anaerobic bacteria. Only the spirochetes invade the epithelial cells. It has been suggested that liberation of large amounts of toxins by *T. hyodysenteriae* and possibly other anaerobes results in the superficial necrosis of the mucosa. *Treponema* usually does not invade beyond the mucosal epithelial cells. The morphologic lesion is mucosal colitis characterized by hypersecretion of mucus, and superficial erosion with hyperplasia of cells in colonic glands. Thrombosis of capillaries and venules in the superficial areas of the mucosa in the colon and the gastric fundic mucosa (venous infarction) is probably due to absorption of endotoxins released by Gram-negative bacteria.

The diarrhea in swine dysentery is due to failure of absorption of fluids and electrolytes in the colon. This presumably results from damage to the superficial colonic epithelium. The normal colon of the pig has a tremendous absorptive capacity. Interference with this absorption results in severe diarrhea and dehydration. There is no evidence of active fluid secretion associated with bacterial enterotoxins. Fluid and electrolyte transport are normal in the small intestine. Thus the pathogenesis of diar-

rhea associated with swine dysentery differs from that seen with enterotoxigenic *E. coli* and *Salmonella* spp. Prostaglandins released during the inflammation do not appear to be implicated in the development of diarrhea, as they are in salmonellosis.

Histories usually recount the introduction of pigs, presumably carriers, into a herd some days, weeks, or even months before the disease breaks out. Once established in a herd, the infection tends to remain enzootic, and although treatment can effect a rapid clinical amelioration, it is not curative, and relapses at greater or lesser intervals are the rule. Apparently infection is not followed by a substantial immunity, although individual pigs are resistant to challenge with *Treponema hyodysenteriae* after recovery. The morbidity may reach 90% and mortality 30%. Many of the factors predisposing to salmonellosis also apply to swine dysentery. Pigs fed diets deficient in vitamin E and selenium develop more severe signs and lesions of swine dysentery.

The disease occurs in pigs of all ages more than about 2 to 3 weeks old, but particularly in pigs 8 to 14 weeks of age. Once initiated, it spreads rapidly by pen contact. The disease is initially febrile, but with the onset of diarrhea, fever tends to subside. The initial diarrheic feces are thin, semisolid, and without blood or mucus; it is usually only after 1 or 2 days of diarrhea that blood and mucus appear in the feces. Some pigs die peracutely without showing diarrhea and many that show diarrhea do not have dysentery but pass feces composed almost wholly of mucus.

Pigs that die of swine dysentery are usually gaunt with a contracted abdomen, the eyes are sunken, and there may be bluish discoloration of the abdominal skin. Incidental lesions may include pericardial serous effusion and intense congestion and infarction of the stomach. The intestinal lesions, especially in young pigs dying acutely, can be easily overlooked because the mucosal colitis may be mild, patchy, and often more catarrhal than fibrinous.

In typical cases, dehydration gives to the serosa a semiopaque, ground-glass appearance, and the wall of the cecum and colon is thickened. The colonic content in these cases is usually scant and of a porridge-like, dirty gray to reddish brown and greasy appearance. The mucosa, with patchy foci of light fibrin exudation, has the velvety thickening of catarrhal secretion (Fig. 1.39C). The most severe lesions approach those of salmonellosis in extent and severity of fibrinous effusion. The production of mucus in swine dysentery becomes copious in many chronic cases, and there is a remarkable goblet-cell metaplasia. It is common to find foul-smelling straw and bedding in the stomach and colon of such cases, evidence of pica.

The earliest microscopic lesions are characterized by expulsion of mucus from the basilar portions of the crypts (Fig. 1.39D). There are discrete areas of necrosis and erosion in the superficial mucosa. Thin layers of fibrinocellular exudate cover the eroded areas. In more advanced cases, the areas of necrosis become more diffuse but remain superficial, and exudation is more copious (Fig. 1.39F). There may be minor bleeding from small vessels in eroded mucosa. Fibrin thrombi are evident in the capillaries and venules of the superficial lamina propria. There is usually some edema of the lamina propria, submucosa, and serosa. Many crypts are dilated and contain necrotic debris; others show marked goblet-cell hyperplasia. In response to the increased turnover of epithelial cells associated with the superficial necrosis, there is hyperplasia of cells deeper in the glands. The crypts are elongated, lined by proliferative basophilic epithelial cells that have large nuclei, and have few differentiated goblet cells (Fig. 1.39E).

Large numbers of spirochetes are easily demonstrated using Warthin–Starry silver stain or similar stains. They are mainly located in the areas of superficial erosion and in the lumen of crypts.

Ultrastructurally, large numbers of spirochetes are located on the surface and within the cytoplasm of epithelial cells. Fewer organisms are present in the intercellular spaces between superficial epithelial cells, in the lumen of crypts, and occasionally in the lamina propria. Degenerative changes in the epithelial cells are characterized by loss of microvilli, clumping of nuclear chromatin, and swelling of the mitochondria and the rough endoplasmic reticulum.

The diagnosis of swine dysentery is usually based on the characteristic clinical signs and gross and microscopic lesions, since it is difficult to isolate the causative agent under practical conditions. Selective media are required to isolate *Treponema hyodysenteriae*. Colonic contents may be examined by phase contrast or dark field microscopy. Large numbers of the characteristic motile spirochetes are present in affected cases. Fluorescent-antibody and special stains such as crystal violet, Victoria 4-R, and modified acid fast are all used to demonstrate the spirochetes in mucosal smears. However, culture is required conclusively to differentiate *T. hyodysenteriae* from other spirochetes such as *T. innocens*.

The differential diagnosis of swine dysentery from salmonellosis, especially that due to *Salmonella typhimurium*, intestinal adenomatosis complex, and trichurosis, is discussed under Typhlocolitis in Swine.

Diseases Associated with Enteric Clostridial Infections

Most of the important enteric clostridial diseases occur in herbivores and are caused by one or other of the five toxigenic types of *Clostridium perfringens*. Occasionally, other members of the genus are associated with enteric disease, examples being *C. sordellii* and *C. botulinum* in cattle and *C. strasburgense* in dogs.

There are five types of *Clostridium perfringens*, designated A–E, which are differentiated on the basis of their production of the four major antigenic lethal exotoxins. A strain formerly classified as type F is now regarded as a subtype of type C. The major exotoxins are alpha (α), beta (β), epsilon (ϵ), and iota (ι); the relationships between the five types and the four toxins are tabulated here:

Toxin	α	β	ϵ	ι
Type A	++	−	−	−
B	+	++	+	−
C	+	++	−	−
D	+	−	++	−
E	+	−	−	++

++, Significant toxin; +, small amount, −, none produced.

Eight minor toxins (antigens) are produced by *Clostridium perfringens*, and it is suggested that some of these may be useful in identification of types and in division of types A, B, and C into varieties.

The α toxin is a lecithinase that acts on cell membranes, producing hemolysis or necrosis of cells. The chemical nature of the β toxin is not clear. It is common to those strains (B and C) that cause enteritis and is necrotizing, trypsin labile, and appears to have a paralyzing effect on the intestine. The ϵ toxin is produced as an inactive prototoxin that is activated by enzymatic digestion. In culture, the appropriate enzymes [the minor toxins kappa (κ) and lambda (λ)] may be produced by the organism. In the intestine, trypsin is an effective activator. The prototoxin is produced only during periods of growth. The ι toxin also is elaborated as a prototoxin and activated by proteolytic enzymes either in culture (λ toxin) or in the intestine. The κ toxin is a collagenase, and λ a nonspecific proteinase. Other minor toxins include mu (μ), a hyaluronidase, and delta (δ), a hemolysin. The enterotoxin produced by certain strains is discussed below.

There is not always a clear distinction between the different types of *Clostridium perfringens*. Some strains lose their ability to produce one or more of their toxins when stored or cultured, and this complicates the identifications of isolates and the assessment of their significance in disease outbreaks.

Clostridial diseases of the intestine often are called enterotoxemias. Disease produced by *Clostridium perfringens* type D, whose ϵ exotoxin is elaborated in the intestine but exerts its important effects on distant organs such as brain and kidney, is an enterotoxemia. The hemolytic disease attributed to type A is also an enterotoxemia, but in general the other types produce local intestinal lesions. The production of an enterotoxin, distinct from the classical exotoxins, by some types of *C. perfringens* is potentially confusing. This enterotoxin is elaborated only by sporulating cells and is released on lysis of the cells. It is almost exclusively a product of type A strains but is identified occasionally from type C and very rarely from type D strains. The enterotoxin is not involved in the pathogenesis of enterotoxemia ("pulpy-kidney disease") caused by the latter strains. It is significant in food poisoning by type A strains in humans.

CLOSTRIDIUM PERFRINGENS TYPE A. *Clostridium perfringens* type A is the most common of the five types and is the only one associated with the microflora of both soil and intestinal tract. Its major toxin is the α toxin and it also produces the enterotoxin. Some type A strains may produce either very small amounts or no α toxin. Strains yielding large quantities of this toxin are rare.

Clostridium perfringens type A is one of several clostridia that produce gas gangrene in humans and animals. The production of gas gangrene in wound and puerperal infections probably is a composite effect of the major and minor toxins elaborated by the organism. The necrotizing and hemolytic activity of the α toxin is assisted by the collagenase and hyaluronidase, which disrupt connective tissues and permit the infection to spread. Other wound contaminants, not necessarily clostridial, also can be important in lesion development.

The significance of type A strains in enteric diseases other than food poisoning in humans and necrotic enteritis of chickens is not clear. Their postulated causative association with equine colitis X is discussed elsewhere. A very rare disease of calves and lambs characterized by acute intravascular hemolysis is also associated with type A infections. Affected animals may be found dead or moribund, and jaundice and hemoglobinuria may be evident clinically. At autopsy, icterus, anemia, and other changes of severe acute intravascular hemolysis are prominent. Severe diarrhea may occur in calves, but enteric lesions are likely to be obscured by rapid autolysis. This hemolytic disease must be distinguished from other causes of acute intravascular hemolysis such as leptospirosis, bacillary hemoglobinuria caused by *Clostridium novyi* type D (*haemolyticum*), and chronic copper poisoning. Presumably the hemolytic effect of this toxin is responsible for the intravascular hemolysis. Given that type A strains are commonly found in the intestines of ruminants, and that α toxin given intravenously is destroyed rapidly, it is apparent that there must be complex pathogenetic requirements for the development of this disease. The pathogenesis may be somewhat analogous to that of enterotoxemia caused by type D, which is discussed below.

CLOSTRIDIUM PERFRINGENS TYPE B.   *Clostridium perfringens* type B is reported from Europe, South Africa, and the Middle East, but not from North America and Australasia. It causes "lamb dysentery," usually in lambs up to about 10 to 14 days of age, dysentery in calves of approximately the same age, and dysentery in foals within the first few days of life.

In **lambs**, death may occur without premonitory signs, but there is usually abdominal pain, especially when forced to rise, and passage of semifluid dark feces mixed or coated with blood. The abdomen is often tympanitic. A more chronic form in older lambs, which among other diseases is known as "pine" in England, is characterized by unthriftiness and depression, reluctance to suckle, and a peculiar stretching when the animal rises; such cases are reputed to respond well to specific antiserum. Proof of the nature of their illness is lacking, although epidemiologically it does appear to be a chronic form of this disease.

Typical lesions are usually present, although in exceptional peracute cases they may be indistinct. The first impression on opening the abdominal cavity is that there is intestinal strangulation, an occasional accident in young lambs. The characteristic lesion is an extensive hemorrhagic enteritis. Discrete and then confluent ulcerations develop if the course is long enough. In peracute cases, there may be only a few small patches of necrosis. The peritoneal cavity often contains a small amount of serous or bloodstained fluid.

In cases with more severe and deeply penetrating mucosal ulcerations, there may be an overlying peritonitis with red fibrin strands on the local mesentery and intestinal adhesions. The ulcers are usually visible through the serosa as purplish areas, and they may be limited to the small intestine or also involve the large intestine. On the mucosal surface, they are irregular but well defined by a sharp margin and rim of intense hyperemia, and they contain a yellow necrotic deposit; they may coalesce to form extensive areas of necrosis. Usually the intestinal contents are bloodstained and may appear to be composed of pure blood, but in lambs that live for 3 or 4 days, there may be little or no staining with blood. In acute cases, the abomasal mucosa may be intensely congested. The mesenteric lymph nodes are edematous or intensely congested. Histologically, the wall of the intes-

tine is suffused with blood, and the areas of necrosis extend deeply into the mucous membrane and may penetrate the muscularis mucosa to the muscle layers and peritoneum. In the necrotic tissue, there are large numbers of typical bacilli, but the cellular inflammatory response is slight.

The lesions in other organs are those of severe toxemia. The liver is usually pale and friable but may be congested. The spleen is normal or slightly enlarged and pulpy, owing to congestion and dissolution of its delicate reticulum. The kidneys may be enlarged, edematous, pale, and soft from toxic degeneration. The pericardial sac contains abundant clear gelatinous fluid, the myocardium is pale and soft, and hemorrhages beneath the serous membranes of the heart are almost constant. The lungs are often slightly congested and very edematous.

In areas in which this disease occurs, the diagnosis can be made with reasonable certainty on the basis of the history and the presence of the typical macroscopic lesions. Confirmation depends on finding large numbers of clostridia in the necrotic tissue of the ulcers and on the detection of toxins in the intestinal contents of fresh cadavers. The organism may be isolated only from the intestine of fresh cadavers.

The disease in **calves** caused by type B *Clostridium perfringens* closely resembles that in lambs, usually affecting sucklings less than 10 days of age, with a course of 2 to 4 days characterized by prostration and dysentery. Older calves up to 10 weeks of age sometimes are affected. It appears that calves are more likely to recover, albeit slowly, than lambs. The intestinal lesion is an acute hemorrhagic enteritis with extensive mucosal necrosis and patchy diphtheritic membrane formation, especially in the ileum.

In **foals** also there is hemorrhagic enteritis with severe diarrhea. Suckling foals of 2 days to, rarely, some weeks of age are affected. The course of the illness is 1 or 2 days. The intestine is intensely hyperemic, with a number of dark foci up to 1.0 cm in diameter that may develop into ulcerations. The contents of the intestine are bloodstained. The disease is apparently rare in foals but should be differentiated bacteriologically from infection with *Actinobacillus equuli*, and from salmonellosis, which more typically involves the large bowel.

CLOSTRIDIUM PERFRINGENS TYPE C.   *Clostridium perfringens* type C has a worldwide distribution and causes disease in adult sheep and goats, feeder cattle, and lambs, calves, foals, and baby pigs. The prevalence of disease varies widely between countries, and between regions and species within countries. There appear to be several varieties within type C that possibly are associated with different diseases.

In **adult sheep**, *Clostridium perfringens* type C causes "struck," a disease of pastured animals that has a mortality rate of 5 to 15% in some areas. The disease in adult goats probably is similar in most respects to that in sheep. Death usually occurs suddenly with terminal convulsive episodes, but some animals, with infections not so peracute, stand in a straining position that probably indicates acute abdominal pain. In adult sheep there is no diarrhea or convulsions.

At autopsy, the peritoneal cavity contains up to 3 liters of clear, pale yellow fluid that clots on exposure to air and that becomes stained with hemoglobin if autopsy is delayed. The peritoneal vessels, especially of the omentum, small intestine, and urinary bladder, are intensely congested, and multiple subperitoneal hemorrhages may be present. The small intestine is intensely hyperemic, either in patches or along most of its length, and in the zones of hyperemia there may be ulcers that vary in size, in diameter from 2 to 3 mm and in length from 6 to 12 cm. Ulcers usually are present, mostly in the jejunum, and are surrounded by a zone of hyperemia with deep red base, although in some the necrotic material is dark green and adherent. The large intestine is normal. The primary intestinal lesion is superficial mucosal necrosis, which advances more deeply into a developing leukocytic reaction, congestion, and hemorrhage. The organisms do not invade the healthy mucosa but appear in tissue already necrotic, apparently invading from the lumen of the bowel.

Lesions in other organs are those of severe toxemia and include copious pleural and pericardial transudate of gelatinous fluid and hemorrhages beneath the serous membranes of the heart. There is congestion and sometimes gross hemorrhage of the zona reticularis of the adrenal.

The causative organism is usually distributed in all organs, and this accounts for the very different appearance when autopsy is delayed for some hours. In such instances, there is extensive bloodstained gelatinous fluid in the intermuscular septa and subcutis, and fluid in the serous cavities is stained. The muscles are soft, stained pink to black with blood, and emphysematous. Because of this change, "struck" may be confused with blackleg if postmortem examination is delayed.

The disease in **feedlot cattle** is similar to "struck." Animals are found either dead or moribund, and congestion and hemorrhage of the gastrointestinal tract are prominent. The jejunal and ileal content is bloody with fibrin clots and necrotic debris. Excessive straw-colored pleural and pericardial fluid and petechiation of epicardium and endocardium are present. Autolysis and postmortem bloat occur rapidly, and differentiation from ruminal tympany and other clostridial diseases is necessary.

The diseases caused by type C in **calves**, **lambs**, and **foals** are very similar and will be discussed together. Affected animals are young sucklings, which contract the disease within the first few days of life, often within the first 12 hr if they have been confined. Foals and most clinically affected lambs die, but in calves, subacute cases may occur in which there is diarrhea and unthriftiness.

Often, affected animals are found dead. Sick lambs may shiver, show abdominal pain, abdominal distension, dysentery, and prostration and die in 12 hr or less. Sick calves show abdominal pain, some show diarrhea of sudden onset, and death is preceded by spasmodic convulsions.

Similar lesions occur at autopsy in all species but may be less severe in lambs. In lambs, the intestinal changes vary from catarrhal to acute hemorrhagic enteritis with mucosal necrosis, which, like lamb dysentery, suggests strangulation. The most prominent changes occur in the jejunum and ileum, the lumen of which may contain free blood, which forms a clotted cast in fresh cadavers; sometimes there is merely acute hyperemia of a segment of jejunum with edema of the wall, a scant creamy intestinal content, and a few small ulcerations of the mucosa.

The peritoneal cavity contains a small quantity of serous, bloodstained fluid, and the local mesentery and peritoneum are often mildly inflamed, hyperemic, and bear red strands of fibrin. The mesenteric nodes are enlarged, wet, and congested. There is usually an excess of pericardial fluid, and pulmonary interstitial edema. Ecchymoses on the serous membranes are nearly constant, and in a few cadavers all tissues, but especially the meninges and brain, are liberally sprinkled with small hemorrhages; these are sites of bacterial embolism, a massive terminal bacteremia by *Clostridium perfringens* occurring in such cases.

Other lesions are those of toxemia, and the histologic changes are the same as those of lamb dysentery; indeed, there is no reliable distinction between the two diseases except for the geography of their occurrence and the results of toxin analyses, which must be performed both on the intestinal contents and the cultured organism since only the β toxin may be detectable in the intestinal contents.

Clostridium prefringens type C causes hemorrhagic enteritis of **suckling piglets** in many parts of the world. The disease occurs as epizootics in affected herds and regions and may then remain enzootic. Whole litters are affected, usually within the first week of life and often within the first 24 hr; the clinical course is ~1 day. Rarely, epizootics occur in 2- to 4-week-old pigs and in weaned pigs. Affected animals pass bloodstained feces in the terminal stages, and there is marked hyperemia of the anus just prior to death. The predominant lesions occur in the small intestine, especially the jejunum, but the cecum and spiral colon often are involved, and occasionally lesions are confined to the large intestine. Lesions are similar in all areas and in acute cases consist of intestinal and mesenteric hyperemia, extensive necrosis of the intestinal mucosa, and staining of the contents (Fig. 1.41A). There may be emphysema of the intestinal wall, which becomes fragile. Mesenteric lymph nodes are red, and sanguinous peritoneal and pleural fluid is present. Fibrinous intestinal adhesions may develop.

Microscopically, the necrotic process extends deeply and sometimes penetrates the muscularis mucosa. Numerous typical bacilli inhabit the necrotic tissue and line up along the margin of involved villi. Older pigs may not show intestinal hemorrhage but do show mucosal necrosis and peritoneal and pericardial effusion.

Infection is acquired from the sow's feces, and lesions begin in the jejunum with adhesion to and necrosis of epithelium on the villus tips. The cells are sloughed, and extension of the necrotizing process then is nonselective and involves all the structures of the villi as it extends toward the crypt. The disease is not reproducible with toxins of *Clostridium perfringens* type C but requires viable organisms with the ability to attach to the enterocytes.

CLOSTRIDIUM PREFRINGENS TYPE D. Enterotoxemia ("pulpy-kidney disease," "braxy-like disease," "overeating disease") through the toxins of *Clostridium perfringens* type D is an important disease of sheep and goats, with a worldwide distribution. It occurs occasionally in calves. Focal symmetric encephalomalacia of sheep is caused by the epsilon toxin of type D.

In most lambs and calves with type D enterotoxemia, the

course is peracute and the animal is found dead. Lambs and calves may die in a few minutes in convulsions, and calves often bawl as from severe pain. Animals that survive longer may show excessive salivation, rapid breathing, hyperesthesia, straining, opisthotonus, and terminal coma or convulsions. In adult sheep, in which the clinical course may be 2 days, diarrhea with the passage of dark, semifluid feces is common. In sheep, subacute cases may occur and be followed by recovery. In some such cases, neurologic signs may develop. These include blindness, ataxia, head pressing, and posterior paresis, and the lesions of focal symmetric encephalomalacia are present in the brains of such cases. On other occasions these lesions are not preceded by signs of enterotoxemia. In goats, signs of enterotoxemia similar to those in sheep and lambs may be seen, but chronic enterotoxemia characterized by abdominal distension and pain, depression, and dark green diarrhea may persist for several days to weeks. Focal symmetric encephalomalacia does not occur in goats.

In **lambs** dead of acute enterotoxemia, the carcass usually is well nourished. In those with a course of 1 or 2 days, often there is evidence of a dark scour about the buttocks. Putrefactive changes occur rapidly. In some rapidly fatal cases there are no lesions. Often there is excessive straw-colored pericardial fluid that clots on exposure to air, congestion and edema of the lungs that may be severe enough to produce froth in all the respiratory passages, and hemorrhage beneath the endocardium of the left ventricle. There may be hemorrhages beneath other serous membranes (Fig. 1.40A), such as the epicardium, and blotchy hemorrhages beneath the parietal peritoneum are characteristic. Sometimes the liver is congested and the spleen enlarged and pulpy. There is no gastrointestinal inflammation visible at autopsy, although there is a mild microscopic enteritis. Short lengths of the small intestine are distended with gas and are pink from hyperemia. The intestinal content is creamy in cases of rapid death, but in those that live for some hours, the contents, especially the lower intestine, are more fluid and dark green.

In experimental cases and natural cases examined immediately after death there are no specific renal lesions. The kidneys often are congested, and postmortem degeneration leads within a few hours to the intertubular "hemorrhages" characteristic of the disease (Fig. 1.40D). Similarly, autolysis that is unusually rapid is responsible for the "pulpy kidney" of enterotoxemia. Both of these "lesions" can be useful diagnostic aids.

In **adult sheep**, the lesions are the same as those in lambs but are more constant and more developed, with the exception of renal autolytic changes, which occur less rapidly and rarely progress to the stage of "pulpiness."

Brain lesions occur in lambs with enterotoxemia that is not immediately fatal, and these are sufficiently constant to be of diagnostic significance. They develop in two patterns; each is bilaterally symmetric. The commonest pattern involves the basal ganglia, internal capsule, dorsolateral thalamus, and substantia nigra; there are some minor variations of the pattern, but the lesions always are of the same type and are symmetric (Fig. 1.40B). The second pattern affects the white matter of the frontal gyri, sparing only the communicating U fibers. The lesion begins with edema and the leakage of plasma and then red cells from the venules and capillaries in the affected area. The altered

permeability of the vessels is diffuse throughout the brain, sparing only heavily myelinated tracts such as the optic tracts and corpus callosum. This is well demonstrated by vital staining with trypan blue. The least change visible by light microscopy is the accumulation of protein droplets around small venules. Electron microscopically severe damage to vascular endothelium is apparent, and there is swelling of protoplasmic astrocytes. The foot processes around blood vessels and the processes around neurons are most severely swollen. Edema and hemorrhage lead to malacia in the affected areas.

In goats with chronic enterotoxemia, enterocolitis occurs and is characterized by atrophy of villi and mucosal ulceration. Specific systemic signs do not develop.

Lesions in **calves** dying of enterotoxemia caused by *Clostridium perfringens* type D closely resemble those in lambs. Affected calves are usually 1–3 months of age. Splenic swelling is more common in calves than in lambs, and rapid autolysis of the kidney is not a prominent finding. Subcapsular congestion and hemorrhage occur (Fig. 1.40C), however, and sometimes a blackish clot of blood up to 1.0 cm thick forms a rather even cast for the kidney.

The histologic changes in enterotoxemia include, in addition to the brain lesions described above, mild degeneration and necrosis of the epithelium of the proximal convoluted tubules with edema, congestion and interstitial hemorrhage in the renal cortex, and congestion of the medulla (these are autolytic changes but are useful diagnostically); superficial desquamation in the intestine with congestion, and numerous typical bacilli in the contents; congestion and hemorrhage of the spleen with disruption of reticulum; subepicardial hemorrhage and degeneration in the Purkinje network; and proteinaceous edema fluid in the lungs. All of these changes are secondary to endothelial damage produced by the ε toxin. The nature of the clinical syndrome, including the severity and extent of the nervous disorder, probably depends on the amount and rate of absorption of this toxin.

Significant biochemical abnormalities that occur in enterotoxemia include hemoconcentration and hyperglycemia. Hemoconcentration is secondary to loss of fluid into tissues and cavities through injured vascular endothelium. The increase in blood glucose is due to rapid mobilization of hepatic glycogen, possibly stimulated by hepatocyte-bound ε toxin. The blood glucose may reach 400 mg % and spills into the urine, providing the basis of very good circumstantial evidence for diagnosis of the disease. The absence of glucosuria after some hours postmortem is of no significance, as early postmortem growth of bacteria in the urine destroys the glucose. Glucosuria may occur in calves and presumably in kids but does not occur in starved animals with depleted glycogen stores.

CLOSTRIDIUM PERFRINGENS TYPE E. *Clostridium perfringens* type E causes a rare disease that occurs in calves and rabbits. Calves die acutely and have a congested ulcerated abomasum and hemorrhagic enteritis, which occurs segmentally along the small intestine. Mesenteric nodes are enlarged and red, and pericardial effusion and serosal hemorrhages may be present.

Hemorrhagic canine gastroenteritis (canine gastrointestinal hemorrhage syndrome) occurs sporadically in associa-

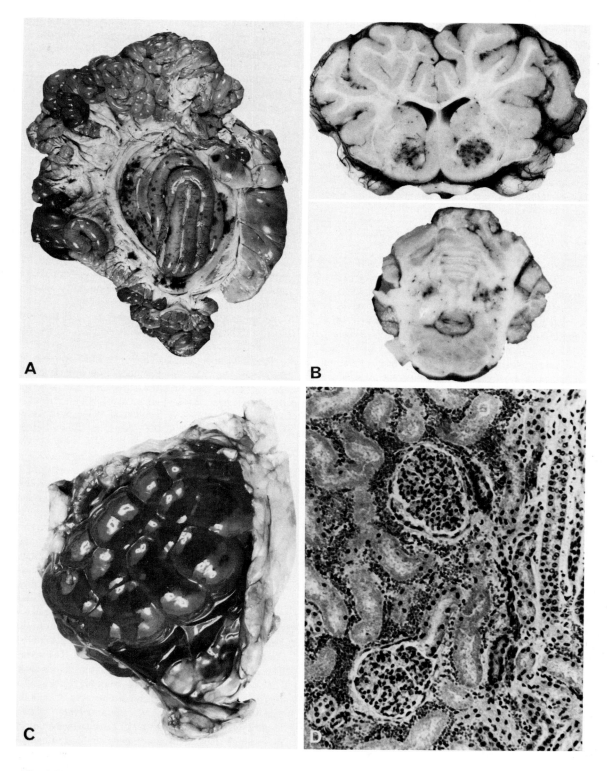

Fig. 1.40. *Clostridium perfringens* type D enterotoxemia. (**A**) Peritoneal hemorrhages. Sheep. (**B**) Focal symmetric encephalomalacia. Sheep. Hemorrhages and softening in internal capsules and cerebellar white matter. (**C**) Renal cortical hemorrhage. Calf. (**D**) Nephrosis and intertubular hemorrhage. Sheep.

tion with *Clostridium perfringens*. Usually a peracute hemorrhagic gastroenteritis develops, and the specific *C. perfringens* type is not identified; recurrent diarrhea associated with a type A strain has also been recorded. Dogs with the peracute disease often are found dead, lying in a pool of bloody excreta. Sometimes hemorrhage from the anus is noted prior to death. Autopsy reveals hemorrhagic enteritis and colitis, and sometimes superficial gastritis is present. Colonic lesions tend to be more severe. Microscopically, there is hemorrhagic necrosis of the intestinal mucosa, with accumulation of necrotic cells in crypts. Numerous clostridia may line the necrotic intestinal structures or be distributed through the detritus. The condition must be differentiated from canine parvoviral enteritis, canine hepatitis, shock gut, and warfarin toxicity or other coagulopathy.

Pathogenesis and Diagnosis of Clostridial Enteric Infections

The pathogenesis of some of the enteric clostridial disease is extraordinarily circuitous. More is known of the pathogenesis of enterotoxemia caused by *Clostridium perfringens* type D than of the others, and this can be exemplary: disease due to types A and E may develop in the same way, but types B and C usually affect the newborn and probably have a more simple pathogenesis. In all of the diseases, the organism multiplies rapidly in the intestine and disease results from the activity of the bacterial exotoxins. (The contribution of enterotoxin from type A strains to enteric diseases of animals probably is minimal.) Many animals harbor the specific clostridial organisms in their alimentary canal for greater or lesser periods but in small and harmless numbers. Under certain circumstances they grow profusely and produce toxins in overwhelming concentration.

Enterotoxemia of pastured lambs occurs mainly in the spring, when pastures are abundant and lush, and usually the best lambs are affected. It is possible that intestinal hypomotility may be a primary factor that allows clostridia to proliferate in the small intestine instead of being carried by peristalsis to the colon. Whether it is the level of nutrients or other factors in ingested pasture that predispose to the development of enterotoxemia is unclear. "Pulpy kidney" is not solely a disease of green, lush pastures; it also occurs on pastures of little but coarse fibrous grass, and in sheep fed pelleted feeds. In these circumstances the relationship to diet is obscure.

Lambs fed large amounts of grain or concentrate are highly susceptible, thus the synonym "overeating disease." The manner in which overeating leads to clostridial enterotoxemia is complex. Cultures of *Clostridium perfringens* type D given orally are largely destroyed in the rumen and abomasum. The few organisms that reach the intestine proliferate rapidly and produce toxin, but when the numbers are no longer reinforced by escapees from the stomachs, they are rapidly cleared from the intestine by peristalsis. If the cultures are administered into the duodenum, the concentrations of organisms and toxin in the intestine become much larger than after oral dosing but not large enough to cause anything but diarrhea. The disease can be reproduced successfully if the diet of the sheep is suddenly changed to grain or concentrate before administering the culture.

The critical factor is almost certainly the presence of starch in the small intestine, providing a suitable substrate for these saccharolytic bacteria, and they proliferate to immense numbers perhaps more than 1×10^9 organisms per gram of intestinal contents, and produce correspondingly large amounts of toxin. When the rumen is provided suddenly with excessive quantities of food, or food of a different type, there is a delay before the ruminal flora can adapt; in this period, undigested or partially digested food may escape into the intestine, and if starch is there, as it is with overeating on grain, *Clostridium perfringens* type D is likely to take advantage of it.

It appears that the concentration of toxin must be maintained at high levels for several hours on end if it is to cause intoxication rather than just diarrhea. The outcome depends not only on the concentration of toxin in the intestine but also on the length of time it is maintained, the size of the sheep, and whether there is circulating antitoxin. Some sheep possess ϵ antitoxin, attesting to previous nonfatal intoxication, and they are highly resistant to the disease. Even with high intestinal concentrations of toxin, only small amounts reach the blood stream. A high concentration of ϵ toxin facilitates its own absorption from the intestine, probably in part by increasing the permeability of the mucosa. Necrosis of epithelium and moderate atrophy of villi is evident in some animals with type D enterotoxemia, and it is reasonable to assume that epithelial damage must precede the facilitated absorption.

Probably the disease develops in the same way in the calf as in the sheep. The virtual confinement of the disease to calves that are overfed suggests that this is the case. The acute disease in goats likely has a similar pathogenesis, but the chronic disease, with lesions confined to the intestine, appears to be caused by local effects of type D toxins. This form of the disease has not been investigated in detail.

The pathogenesis of disease produced by type A bacteria is obscure. In lambs it occurs under circumstances similar to type D enterotoxemia. Nothing is known of the permeability of the ruminant intestine to α toxin, but the syndrome described in both lambs and calves is consistent with the action of a hemolytic toxin in the circulation.

The diseases caused in young animals by *Clostridium perfringens* types B and C are principally diseases of the intestine, and this suggests that the pathogenesis is more direct. This is particularly true of type C hemorrhagic enteritis in pigs.

Cultures of type B or C given orally produce disease much more consistently than type D. Types B and C possess the β toxin, which is probably responsible for the severe intestinal lesion, and it is possible that these types need not attain the high concentration in the intestine that type D must to initiate illness. The β toxin is trypsin labile, and circumstances such as low enzyme levels in young animals, very high levels of toxin, or trypsin inhibitors could be important. Although both "lamb dysentery" and "hemorrhagic enterotoxemia" occur in pastured animals, they are most serious in confined animals. Under these circumstances, disease spreads rapidly among the susceptible age group, as would be expected of any virulent infection.

Often the most vigorous and presumably the best nourished lambs and calves succumb, and on occasion there may be a nutritional predisposition to these diseases. "Pig bel," a necrotizing jejunitis of humans in New Guinea that probably is caused by the β toxin, has been causally related to consumption of heat-stable trypsin inhibitors in sweet potatoes. Naturally occurring protease inhibitors in soybeans appear to have a similar effect in guinea pigs.

"Struck" in adult sheep, caused by type C, is prevalent when the grass is short in late winter or early spring. It is also a disease of the best conditioned sheep, but the place of nutritional factors in its pathogenesis, and in the pathogenesis of disease caused by type C in feedlot cattle, has not been examined.

The diagnosis of outbreaks of enteric diseases caused by clostridia usually is not difficult. A history of sudden deaths in appropriate environmental circumstances, age groups, etc. should provoke a suspicion. Gross lesions in one or more reasonably fresh carcasses are often characteristic enough to provide a working diagnosis. Glucosuria may be demonstrable in type D enterotoxemia, but its absence does not preclude the disease. Confirmation of type D enterotoxemia can be based on microscopic brain lesions, but in this and other suspected clostridial diseases, bacteriologic proof should be sought. Examinations should be made as soon after death as is possible. Very autolyzed carcasses generally are unsuitable as the toxin is rapidly destroyed postmortem and the intestinal flora very quickly becomes mixed.

The contents of the small intestine should be examined for toxin; in adult sheep that have shown diarrhea, it is well to examine the contents of cecum and colon if toxin is not found in the small intestine. One drop of chloroform per 10 ml of content should be added to preserve the toxin. There is no critical concentration of toxin diagnostic for pulpy-kidney disease or other enteric clostridial diseases. The presence of toxin in conjunction with typical lesions is considered significant. The absence of demonstrable toxin does not preclude a presumptive diagnosis if other characteristic findings are evident.

Negative results on a toxin analysis made more than 4 hr after death do not eliminate clostridial disease as the cause of death. Gram-stained smears should be made from various levels of the intestine or from discrete mucosal lesions. The smears should reveal large numbers of bacilli with the morphology of *Clostridium perfringens*. In pulpy-kidney disease, and the other clostridial enteritides, the bacteria are present in smears in pure, or virtually pure, population.

ENTEROCOLITIS OF FOALS CAUSED BY *CORYNEBACTERIUM EQUI*. *Corynebacterium equi*, thought formerly to be primarily a soil-associated organism, is now believed to be part of the normal intestinal flora of horses. The organism usually is associated with pyogranulomatous pneumonia of foals (see the Respiratory System, this volume). About half the pneumonic foals also have ulcerative colitis. In some foals intestinal lesions occur alone.

The development of intestinal lesions appears to be dose related in that reproduction of the disease requires repeated oral infection. In natural disease, continual exposure to bacteria in swallowed respiratory exudate probably is an important source of infection in those animals with pneumonia.

Gross lesions may occur throughout the small and large intestines but usually are most severe in the cecum, large colon, and related lymph nodes. Mucosal lesions consist of irregular ulcers up to 1 to 2 cm in diameter, often covered by purulent or necrotic

debris (Fig. 1.41D). Edema of the wall of the gut may be severe. Lymph nodes often are massively enlarged by edema and by caseous or purulent foci that may destroy the structure of the node (Fig. 1.41C). Occasionally, massively enlarged abscessed lymph nodes are found without evidence of concurrent enteritis.

Microscopically, infection seems to occur by penetration of the specialized epithelium over intestinal lymphoid follicles. An initial neutrophilic response occurs, and erosions of the epithelium develop. Macrophages and a few neutrophils accumulate in the lamina propria. The macrophages contain *Corynebacterium equi* but do not destroy them. Later, multinuclear giant cells form, deep ulcers develop, and necrosis of lymphoid follicles occurs. Lymphangitis and pyogranulomatous mesenteric lymphadenitis characterize the chronic enteric disease.

Mycobacterial Enteritis

Various *Mycobacterium* species may cause enteric disease in animals. *Mycobacterium avium* has been incriminated as a cause of colonic ulceration and of granulomatous enteritis in horses; *M. intracellulare* has been isolated from granulomas in mesenteric lymph nodes of pigs in various countries, but enteric lesions have not been described; the primary complex of *M. bovis* may include an enteric lesion (see tuberculosis, in the Respiratory System, this volume). All of these infections are of minor importance compared to that caused by *M. paratuberculosis* in ruminants.

JOHNE'S DISEASE. Johne's disease (paratuberculosis) is a specific infectious disease of ruminants caused by *Mycobacterium paratuberculosis*. Infections by *M. paratuberculosis* can be produced in pigs and horses, but gross lesions are modest or absent. Typical histologic lesions may develop, but are mild. The disease can be transmitted to mice, hamsters, rats, and rabbits.

There are several strains of *Myobacterium paratuberculosis*, differing in cultural characteristics and in pathogenicity for different species. A pigmented strain that produces an intensely orange pigment in tissues and in cultures sometimes is isolated from sheep and occasionally from cattle. Each strain can infect and produce disease in cattle, sheep, and goats.

The epidemiology and pathogenesis of Johne's disease are best understood in cattle. It is assumed that the disease develops in sheep and goats in a similar way. Young animals are more susceptible than the old to experimental infection. Adults may become infected but are less likely to develop the disease and often recover from the infection. The critical age determining susceptibility to an infection that will ultimately produce clinical disease is not known. For many calves it is probably ~6 months. This age-dependent resistance is reflected in the ability of the macrophages of resistant animals to restrict intracellular growth of bacteria, but not to lyse them.

Although the major lesions of Johne's disease usually are confined to the ileum, colon, and draining lymph nodes, the infection is generalized; organisms may be excreted in milk, semen, and urine, and intrauterine infections occur. Bovine fetuses may be infected as early as 2 months of gestation. The excretion of the organism in milk and the fact of intrauterine infection have important implications for the epidemiology of

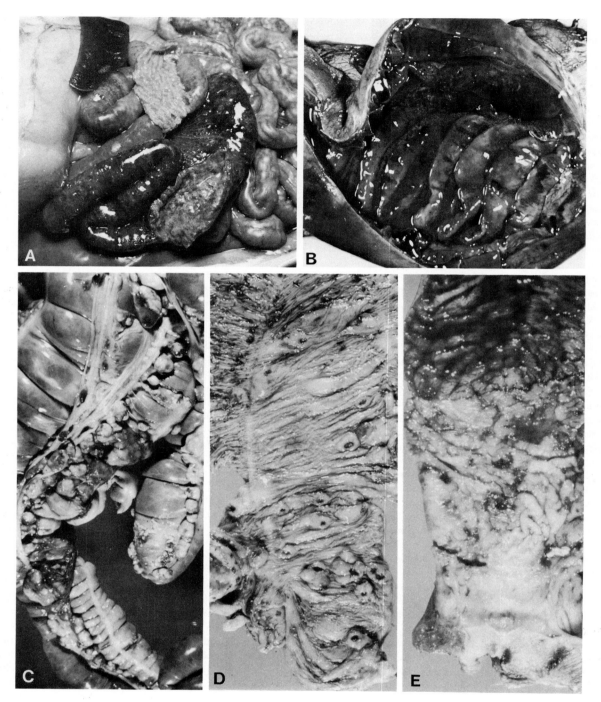

Fig. 1.41. (**A**) Necrotizing enteritis. *Clostridium perfringens* type C. Piglet. (**B**) Braxy-like clostridial abomasitis (*C. septicum*). Calf. (**A** and **B** courtesy of M. Bergeland.) (**C**) *Corynebacterium equi* infection. Foal. Enlarged suppurative cecal and colic lymph nodes. (**D**) *Corynebacterium equi* infection. Foal. Craterous ulcerated lesions on colonic mucosa. (**E**) Ulcerative colitis. Dog. Histoplasmosis.

the disease. A prevalence of 50% has been reported for intrauterine infection when the dam is clinically diseased.

Intrauterine infection can occur when the dam is clinically normal. In both clinical and nonclinical cases of the disease, the organism can be cultured from a variety of parenchymatous organs and widely distributed lymph nodes and has also been found in the gonads of both sexes. In fulminating infections, there is a bacteremia, and it is in these unusual cases that the organism is excreted in the milk. Excretion of the organism in the milk of ewes has not been demonstrated, but congenital and uterine infections have.

The incubation period of Johne's disease is protracted and irregular. Following oral infection, *Mycobacterium paratuberculosis* enters the lymphatic system through the tonsils (and probably the intestinal mucosa) and spreads through the body. It localizes mainly in the small intestine, and in the first 2 to 3 months after infection the organisms multiply there. Depending on their resistance, some animals clear themselves of infection while others become carriers. In the latter, bacteria persist in the mucosa and draining lymph nodes. Some carriers may be infected for life without showing signs of disease. This tolerance to infection may result from compromised immunologic reactivity at the time of infection. Fetal infection may fall into this category. When there is a breakdown of tolerance, hypersensitivity and cell-mediated immunity develop, the mucosal lesions progress, and clinical disease occurs. Shifts between levels of tolerance and hypersensitivity probably are responsible for the clinical exacerbations that are characteristic of the disease.

The diarrhea of Johne's disease has a complex pathogenesis. It is related to the moderate villus atrophy that develops, probably as a result of the immune response in the lamina propria. In addition, there is leakage of plasma proteins, amino acid malabsorption, and increased gut motility with decreased intestinal transit time.

Exacerbations of clinical disease often are associated with parturition, a low nutritional plane, heavy milk yield, and intercurrent disease. A change of environment often leads to clinical disease. Often this can be attributed to differences in the lime content and pH of the soil; soils high in lime tend to inhibit clinical breakdowns, and transfer from alkaline to acid soils often precipitates clinical disease within a few weeks.

The typical manifestation of Johne's disease is profuse diarrhea passed effortlessly. Emaciation is progressive and ultimately fatal, but the appetite is retained, and animals remain bright until the terminal stages. Clinically affected animals are usually 2 years of age or older, and Channel Island breeds and beef shorthorn cattle appear to be unusually susceptible.

Johne's disease in sheep and goats is comparable to that in cattle, occurring in adults and characterized by chronic wasting. The feces are soft, but there is usually no diarrhea, except intermittently in the terminal stages.

There is no correlation between the severity of the clinical syndrome and the severity of the lesions. Many animals allowed to die have gross and microscopic lesions so slight that they would be easily missed unless looked for specifically, and in some of these even detailed gross inspection is unrewarding; on the other hand, severe lesions can be found in animals that appear healthy. In goats and sheep, gross changes usually are minimal.

Advanced cases of Johne's disease are emaciated with gelatinous atrophy of fat depots, intermandibular edema, and serous effusion in the body cavities, more voluminous in sheep and goats than in cattle. Specific gross lesions occur in the intestine and regional nodes. The mesenteric nodes, particularly the ileocecal, are always enlarged, sometimes remarkably so, pale so that there is little corticomedullary distinction, and edematous, especially in the medulla. Lymphangitis of some degree is constant, and the lymphatic vessels can often be traced as thickened cords from the intestine through the mesentery to the mesenteric nodes. Often, lymphangitis is the only recognizable gross change and is specific enough to justify a diagnosis of Johne's disease. In sheep and goats, the lymphatics may be knotted as well as corded, the knots being focal granulomatous accumulations of epithelioid cells and lymphocytes. Sometimes lymphangitis is not recognizably grossly. The intestinal serosa has a slight granular and diffusely opaque appearance because of subserosal edema and cellularity (Fig. 1.42A).

The specific intestinal lesions may occur from the duodenum to the rectum, but in many animals both of these regions are unaffected. Lesions are usually best developed in the lower jejunum and ileum (Fig. 1.42B). Reference is frequently made to enlargement of the ileocecal valve, and to this vicinity as the earliest and most consistently affected, but specific changes of, and immediately adjacent to, the valve are so inconsistent as to deserve deemphasis. The classical intestinal change is diffuse hypertrophy, with the mucosa folded into thick, tranverse rugae, like the convolutions of the cerebral cortex.

When well developed, the mucosal folds cannot be smoothed out by stretching, and they fissure if the intestinal wall is bent sharply. These mucosal changes are partly due to thickenings of the mucosa itself, but largely they are due to abundant accumulations of epithelioid cells in the submucosa. The crests of the folds are often slightly reddened by congestion, and the mucosal surface is velvety, but there is no excess of mucus except in occasional sheep and goats. The minimal recognizable gross change is a very slight fleshy or velvety thickening of the mucosa.

In sheep and goats, enteric lesions are usually mild, resembling the minimal lesions of cattle. Occasionally the bowel is quite remarkably thickened and contains nodules of caseation and calcification. Necrosis occurs rarely in the lesions in cattle, but there is almost never any caseation or calcification. This is a distinguishing feature from intestinal tuberculosis of cattle. Other distinguishing features are the diffuseness of the lesion and the absence of ulceration in Johne's disease. The lesion in cattle is characterized by the virtual absence of necrosis, the absence of inflammatory hyperemia, and the absence of reactionary fibrosis. Orange pigmentation of the mucosa and lymph nodes may be seen in sheep infected with the pigmented strain of the organism.

When gross lesions are well developed, histologic changes are obvious and very characteristic, but in those bovine cases in which gross changes are minimal or absent, the microscopic changes in the mucosa are more indefinite; this is probably true

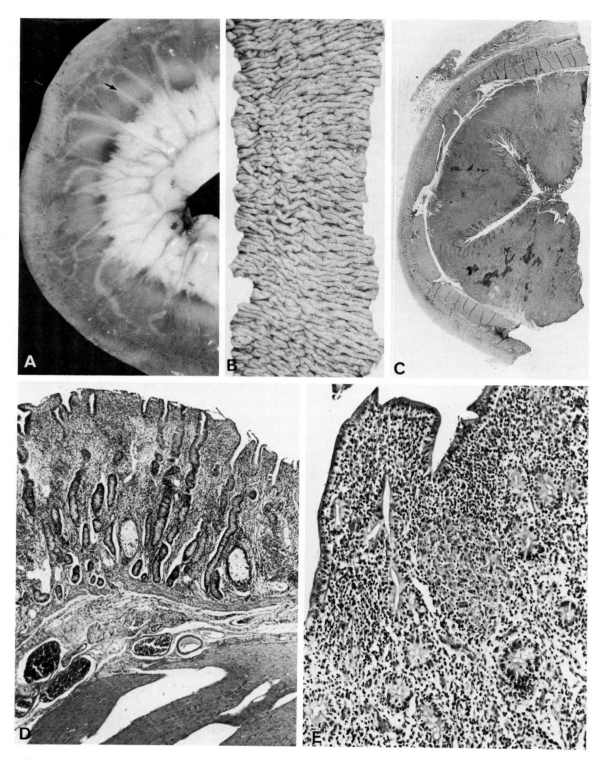

Fig. 1.42. Johne's disease. (**A**) Serosal edema and lymphangitis (arrow). Sheep. (**B**) Thickened mucosal folds. Jejunum. Cow. (**C**) Hemisection of ileum, showing diffuse infiltration of cells and small (dark) areas of necrosis. (**D**) Blunt atrophic ileal villi and hyperplastic, and occasionally cystic, crypts. Edema of the lamina propria, submucosa, and muscularis. A heavy inflammatory infiltrate is in the lamina propria. Cow. (**E**) Macrophages in hypercellular lamina propria.

too of very early lesions. In these, the lamina propria is diffusely but loosely infiltrated with lymphocytes and plasma cells and a large number of eosinophils. There may be very few epithelioid cells (Fig. 1.42E), and the most characteristic change is usually a loose infiltration of lymphocytes and plasma cells in the submucosa and in association with the submucosal and mesenteric lymphatics. As the epithelioid cells increase in number, the other cells are proportionately reduced. In single sections of bowel, the epithelioid cells may infiltrate diffusely from the onset, especially when the outer layers of the mucous membranes are involved, or the infiltrations may be predominantly nodular, either in the tips or the bases of the villi.

The cell accumulations tend to be progressive, and they gradually compress and obliterate the crypts, although some glands persist for a while as cystic remnants containing cellular detritus (Fig. 1.42D). The infiltrating cells congregate in the submucosa, and when gross thickening of the intestine occurs, it is largely due to this submucosal infiltration of typical epithelioid cells. Almost invariably there are lymphocytes in the cellular masses, both as a diffuse distribution of isolated cells and as microscopic foci. Giant cells may be present. Foci of necrosis occur within the cell masses, but in cattle, caseation and calcification are extremely rare (Fig. 1.42C).

A significant proportion of sheep and goats develop foci of tubercle-like caseation with some calcification in the mucosa, the submucosa, on the peritoneal surface of the bowel, in the lymphatics, and in the lymph nodes; some are recognizable grossly as whitish foci, 1–4 mm in diameter, and there is modest surrounding fibrosis. These lesions in sheep are the only suggestion that affected animals may develop resistance or hypersensitivity comparable to that seen in tuberculosis. It is usual for the organism to be demonstrable in vast numbers both intracellularly and extracellularly in the lesions when appropriately stained by acid-fast techniques. When there are few organisms, they are best demonstrated by fluorescent staining; this technique is applicable to tissue but not to feces, as these exhibit autofluorescence. The pigmented strains of the organism are invariably present in large numbers in sheep, but in those infected with nonpigmented strains and showing evidence of tubercle formation, the organisms may be too few to be demonstrated except by culture.

Lymphangitis is one of the most consistent changes. Initially the lymphatics are surrounded by lymphocytes and plasma cells, and many contain plugs of epithelioid cells in the lumen. These changes are progressive, and small mononuclear cells are replaced by large ones; epithelioid granulomas form in the wall and project into the lumen. These nodules frequently show some necrosis.

Specific lesions similar to those in the intestine occur also in the lymph nodes. In the early stages, the subcapsular sinus is infiltrated loosely with epithelioid cells. The infiltrations are progressive, forming follicular or diffuse areas of epithelioid and giant cells, which may ultimately replace much of the cortex. When tubercles form in the intestine of sheep and goats, they form in lymph nodes, too, and may be large enough to replace much of the node.

Of the other organs and tissues in which the bacilli may be found, lesions have been described only in the liver, tonsils, and lymph nodes. These lesions are of characteristic type. They are common in the liver and consist of foci of epithelioid cells and lymphocytes in the triads and indiscriminately in the lobules. These lesions contain bacilli, which can be readily demonstrated.

Antemortem diagnosis of Johne's disease and infection with *Mycobacterium paratuberculosis* is difficult. Various immunologic tests are more or less useful, depending on the immune status of the host and the stage of the disease. Textbooks of medicine and the Bibliography should be consulted for details.

Biopsy of the ileocecal lymph node appears to be a useful diagnostic test, much more so than rectal biopsy, since rectal infection often is absent. The examination of feces for organisms is a useful diagnostic aid in clinical cases; it is too cumbersome and too often negative for use as a screening procedure on preclinical cases. In fecal smear examinations, individual acid-fast organisms are ignored (they are probably incidental saprophytes) and significance is given only to clumps of two or more organisms of typical size. It may be validly objected that such organisms may be merely ingested ones being passed in the feces even when they are certainly *Mycobacterium paratuberculosis*, but nevertheless, reliance can be placed on positive smears when the animals are typically diseased and other causes of chronic diarrhea have been eliminated by appropriate means. A negative fecal smear should not be given any significance. The slow growth of the organism in culture and the variable requirements for growth of different strains limits this examination to the experimental rather than the diagnostic procedure.

Enteritis Due to Chlamydia psittaci

Chlamydiae are obligate intracellular parasites. There are two species, *Chlyamydia trachomatis*, which infects humans, and *C. psittaci,* which infects animals and humans. *Chlamydia psittaci* is divisible into two types: type 1 is associated with abortion, pneumonia, or enteric disease; type 2 with polyarthritis, encephalitis, or conjunctivitis. The nonenteric diseases are discussed in the appropriate chapters.

The intestinal tract is the natural habitat for chlamydiae. Most infections probably are inapparent, but the intestine may be an important portal of entry in the development of systemic infections leading to arthritis, encephalitis, pneumonia, and abortion in ruminants. Enteritis may accompany or presage these diseases, and occasionally chlamydiae cause severe enteric disease in calves.

Following oral infection, chlamydiae infect mainly the enterocytes on the tips of ileal villi. These cells are in the G_1 phase of the cell cycle; cells in this phase are required by chlamydiae as a site for multiplication. Chlamydiae also infect other cells, including goblet cells, enterochromaffin cells, and macrophages. Macrophages may transport chlamydiae systemically prior to destruction by the organisms they carry.

Chlamydiae are adsorbed on the brush border of enterocytes and enter the cell by pinocytosis. Following multiplication of organisms in the supranuclear region, the cells degenerate. Chlamydiae are released into the gut lumen and into the lamina propria, where they infect endothelial cells of lacteals, are released, and become systemic.

Gastrointestinal disease caused by chlamydiae usually is a problem of calves less than 10 days old but may affect older calves and may produce recurrent diarrhea. Watery diarrhea, dehydration, and death are often accompanied by lesions, though not necessarily signs, of arthritis. Gross lesions may occur in the abomasum and throughout the intestinal tract but are most consistent and severe in the terminal ileum. Mucosal edema, congestion, and petechiae, sometimes with ulceration, are usually observed. Serosal hemorrhages and focal peritonitis may occur. Histologically, chlamydial inclusions may be demonstrable with Giemsa stain in the supranuclear region of the enterocytes. Central lacteals and capillaries are dilated, and neutrophils and monocytes infiltrate the lamina propria. Occasionally, granulomatous inflammation occurs in the intestinal submucosa and extends into the mesentery and to the serosa to produce the peritonitis observed grossly. Crypts in the small and large intestine may be dilated, lined by flattened epithelium, and contain inflammatory exudate.

Mycotic Diseases of the Gastrointestinal Tract

Mycotic invasion of the wall of the gastrointestinal tract is a common sequel to many diseases and lesions affecting the mucosa. Although it is generally agreed that one or more of lowered host resistance, disruption of the normal flora, or a local lesion is required for establishment of mycotic disease in the gut, it is possible that spores are carried across the mucosa in macrophages.

Organisms usually associated with alimentary tract mycoses are zygomycetes of the genera *Absidia*, *Mucor*, and *Rhizopus*, and the phaeohyphomycete *Aspergillus*. *Candida* may also invade the wall of the alimentary canal (see below). Zygomycoses are characterized in their invasive mycelial form by infrequent septation and broad, coarse hyphae. *Aspergillus* has a filamentous tissue form with relatively numerous septa.

Lesions occur anywhere in the gastrointestinal tract, including the forestomachs of ruminants. Clinical signs may be related specifically to the location of lesions (vomition, bloody diarrhea) or be nonspecific (malaise, weight loss) or absent. Three types of lesion are produced: hemorrhagic and infarctive, caseating, and granulomatous. Hemorrhagic and infarctive lesions are illustrated by mycotic rumenitis following grain overload in ruminants (Fig. 1.8A,B). They often complicate Peyer's patch necrosis in cattle with bovine virus diarrhea and are seen along the tips of the abomasal folds in calves in the later stages of bacterial gastroenteritis. The fungi have a propensity to invade mucosal and submucosal veins, producing thrombosis and necrosis. Usually there is full-thickness necrosis of the gut wall, which is edematous and blue-black due to venous stasis (Fig. 1.11A–C). Often there is a relatively mild inflammatory response to the fungi. Spread to the liver and other organs via portal and systemic circulations is common (Fig. 1.8D). Mycotic ileitis and colitis in cats occasionally may be a sequel to panleukopenia. Intestinal lesions caused by the fungi (usually *Aspergillus*) may be hemorrhagic and necrotizing with a prominent cellular response but sometimes are small, localized, and difficult to find. In the latter cases, lesions of panleukopenia in the intestine and multifocal mycotic emboli in the lung suggest

the pathogenesis. The lung appears to be the favored site of dissemination in cats. Mycotic enteritis with dissemination is a rare sequel to canine parvovirus enteritis.

The gastrointestinal tract is probably a common portal of entry for many sporadic, disseminated zygomycoses in animals. The presence of fungal hyphae in mesenteric lymph node granulomas of many clinically normal cattle indicates that contrary to general impressions, invasion by these agents across the intestinal mucosa does not lead invariably to systemic disease. It seems likely that the ability of the fungus to cause thrombosis and necrosis determines whether generalization occurs. In the absence of infarctive lesions, fungi may produce a localized granulomatous lesion in specialized lymphoid tissue of the Peyer's patch or may be carried to the regional lymph node while the mucosal lesion heals. In the lymph nodes, a granulomatous response with giant cells that contain hyphal fragments often develops; asteroid bodies may form around *Aspergillus*. Usually the granulomatous lesions produce no or moderate enlargement of lymph nodes, but sometimes a massive, caseating lymphadenitis with adhesions to adjacent structures results.

CANDIDIASIS.   *Candida* species are normal inhabitants of the alimentary tract of animals, existing as budding yeasts in association with mucosal surfaces. When there are changes in the mucosae, particularly squamous mucosae, or in the mucosal flora, the yeasts may become invasive, and branching, filamentous pseudohyphae largely replace the yeast forms. In order of prevalence, the species producing candidiasis in animals are *C. albicans*, *C. slooffii*, and *C. parapsilosis*.

Changes in the mucosal flora usually result from antibiotic therapy, which reduces the numbers of bacteria and allows proliferation of *Candida*. Antibiotics may also inhibit antibody synthesis and phagocyte activity and may directly injure the mucosa, but these effects probably are of minor significance. Treatment with anticancer and antiinflammatory agents may also predispose to candidiasis.

Pseudohypha formation is favored by carbohydrates such as sucrose or polysaccharides, which are less readily fermentable than glucose. Glucose is necessary for keratolysis by the fungus. An endotoxin released during reproduction and death of *Candida* organisms probably causes local irritation and damage and permits deeper penetration into squamous epithelium.

Candida occasionally is an opportunistic invader of mucosal lesions anywhere in the alimentary tract, but other fungi are more likely to take advantage of this kind of lesion, particularly in older animals. Candidiasis is mainly a disease of keratinized epithelium in young animals, especially pigs, calves, and foals. Accumulation of keratin due to anorexia probably contributes to the extensiveness of lesions in all species by increasing the substrate available to the fungus.

In **pigs**, *Candida* often invades the parakeratotic material that accumulates in the gastric squamous mucosa. Apparently these infections are innocuous. "Thrush" is candidiasis of the oral cavity; it is seen occasionally in young pigs, especially those raised on artificial diets, or in pigs with intercurrent disease. Lesions may be confined to the tongue, hard palate, or pharynx but often involve the esophagus and gastric squamous mucosa as well. Rarely, the glandular stomach is involved. Grossly, the lesions are yellow-white, smooth or wrinkled plaques, more or less covering the mucosa. Histologically, the epithelium is spongy and contains abundant pseudohyphae and, particularly with *C. albicans* infections, pockets of neutrophils and bacteria beneath the cornified layer. There is congestion of vessels, and a few inflammatory cells are present under the epithelium. Desquamation of the epithelium may produce small ulcers.

In **calves**, candidiasis occurs following prolonged antibiotic therapy and in association with rumen putrefaction. Lesions are seen most often in the ventral sac of the rumen but may involve the omasum and reticulum and occasionally the abomasum. Grossly, the lesions resemble those of thrush in pigs, but the keratinaceous layer tends to be thicker, less diffuse, and light gray. In the omasum, the leaves may be stuck together by the mass of fungus-riddled keratin. Disseminated candidiasis occurs more often in calves than in pigs, probably because of the relatively prolonged survival of calves with alimentary lesions. Candidiasis in calves must be differentiated from alimentary herpesvirus infections.

Gastroesophageal candidiasis in **foals** involves the squamous epithelium and is associated with ulceration adjacent to the margo plicatus. Colic and anorexia are seen and are probably related to the development of the ulcers, which may perforate, causing peritonitis.

In tissues, the presence of blastospores mixed with pseudohyphae or hyphae permits a provisional identification of *Candida.*

INTESTINAL HISTOPLASMOSIS. *Histoplasma capsulatum* is a soil organism of worldwide distribution. The disease histoplasmosis is endemic in certain areas for example, the Mississippi and Ohio River Valleys of the United States. In is important in humans and dogs and occurs sporadically in other species. Infection usually occurs via inhalation of spores, and if lesions occur, usually they are confined to the lungs. Dissemination with hepatic, splenic, and sometimes gastrointestinal lesions develops in some dogs and probably requires a degree of host immunoincompetence. Infection can be produced by ingestion, and possibly the rare examples of disease confined to the gastrointestinal tract develop in this manner. Intestinal infection by ingestion of infected sputum also is possible.

Disseminated histoplasmosis is a disease predominantly of young dogs, which usually present with weight loss, generalized lymphadenopathy, and often, diarrhea with blood, and tenesmus. Intestinal histoplasmosis has been reported as part of a disseminated disease of cats and as an isolated lesion in a horse.

At postmortem there may be hemorrhagic enteritis involving the small and large intestine, or granulomatous thickening of the mucosa and intestinal wall with ulceration (Fig. 1.41E), or no apparent lesions. Mesenteric lymph nodes often are markedly enlarged. Histologically, lesions may occur in the stomach and small or large intestine. The nonulcerated areas of the mucosa contain focal to diffuse infiltrations of macrophages laden with *Histoplasma capsulatum* organisms within cytoplasmic vacuoles. The mucosa may be grossly thickened by the infiltrate, causing necrosis and ulceration. The cellular reaction may extend through the muscularis to the serosa. Macrophages filled with organisms are particularly prominent in the lymphoid tissue

of the gut and the mesenteric nodes. Microscopic diagnosis of gastrointestinal histoplasmosis is not difficult, but grossly the disease must be distinguished from intestinal lymphoma and, in the colon, from colitis of other types. Histoplasmosis is discussed in detail with the Hematopoietic System (Volume 3).

Protothecal Enterocolitis

Prototheca species are colorless algae closely related to the blue-green alga *Chlorella*. They are ubiquitous in raw and treated sewage and in water and are found in feces, plant sap, and slime flux of trees.

Lesions caused by *Prototheca* include cutaneous infections of cats (see the Skin and Appendages, Volume 1) and humans, mastitis in cows, and disseminated infections in dogs. The intestine and the eye (see the Eye and Ear, Volume 1) are the most commonly involved sites in prototheciosis of dogs.

Clinically, chronic, intractable, bloody diarrhea or passage of bloodstained feces are frequent presenting signs. Hemorrhagic and ulcerative colitis is a prominent enteric lesion, but changes may develop also in the small intestine. Mesenteric lymph nodes may be enlarged. Characteristic of prototheciosis is the mild host response to infection; usually only a few lymphocytes and monocytes are present. In early lesions, the organisms are scattered in the lamina propria, but later they fill the lamina propria and often are packed in cords between the connective tissue of the submucosa. Lacteals are distended, while the lymphatics proximal to them and the sinuses of draining lymph nodes are filled with organisms.

Factors predisposing to the development of intestinal protothecosis are poorly understood. Skin infections are thought to result from traumatic inoculation, and it is possible that in the alimentary tract, *Prototheca* is an opportunistic invader of existing mucosal lesions. The chronicity of the disease and the mild host response are inconsistent with a virulent infection. Two species, *P. zopfii* and *P. wickerhamii,* cause disease in animals; infections with both may occur in the same animal.

Prototheca in sections somewhat resembles cryptococcal organisms. They range from 5-mm spheres to 9×12 μm ovoids and are positive with PAS and silver stains. The presence of endosporulation with formation of 2 to 20 sporangiospores within a single sporangium characterizes *Prototheca* and *Chlorella*. *Chlorella* contains PAS-positive cytoplasmic starch granules that are PAS-negative following diastase digestion; *Prototheca* does not contain these granules. Differentiation of the genera by a fluorescent-antibody test using formalin-fixed material is also possible.

Clinically, and grossly at postmortem, protothecal enterocolitis must be distinguished from histiocytic ulcerative colitis of boxer dogs, histoplasmosis, and intestinal lymphoma.

Gastrointestinal Helminthosis

The diagnosis of disease due to gastrointestinal helminths must be made with knowledge of their pathogenic potential and the mechanisms by which it is expressed. Parasites are much more common than the diseases they cause, and *helminthiasis,* the state of infection, must be differentiated clearly from *helminthosis,* the state of disease.

Gastrointestinal helminths fall into five categories, according to pathogenesis of disease. The first group resides free in the lumen of the intestine, competing with the host for nutrients in the gut content. They are of generally low pathogenicity, except for rare overwhelming infections, and are not likely to cause lethal infection, except by obstruction. These worms, present in sufficient numbers, may cause subclinical disease, such as inefficient growth, or clinical disease in the form of ill thrift. The ascarids, small stronglyes (cyathostomes), and tapeworms such as *Moniezia* and *Taenia* fall into this group, as may *Physaloptera,* in the stomach of carnivores.

A second group of helminths, all nematodes, causes disease exclusively or primarily by causing blood loss. These worms feed on the mucosa, causing bleeding, or actively suck blood. Anemia, hypoproteinemia, and their sequelae cause production loss, clinical disease, and death. *Haemonchus* in the abomasum, and in the intestine the hookworms of carnivores and ruminants, the large strongyles of horses, and *Oesophagostomum radiatum* in cattle are the main examples.

The third group, composed of nematodes and some flukes, in heavy infestations causes mainly protein-losing gastroenteropathy, usually associated with inappetence and diarrhea. In the abomasum, *Ostertagia* and *Trichostrongylus axei* cause mucous metaplasia and hyperplasia of gastric glands, achlorhydria, and diarrhea. In the intestine, several species cause villus atrophy. This may cause malabsorption of nutrients, electrolytes, and water. But probably more important is the associated loss of endogenous protein into the gut. *Cooperia* and *Nematodirus* live in the lumen, coiled among villi, against which they brace. Longitudinal cuticular ridges (the synlophe) may aid them in holding position among villi, resisting peristalsis. The members of the genera *Strongyloides* and *Trichostrongylus* are buried, at least partly, in tunnels within, but not normally beneath, the epithelium about the base of villi (Fig. 1.45A,B). Flukes, especially larval paramphistomes in sheep and cattle, attach by their suckers to the mucosa.

The villus atrophy that occurs in these infections may be largely immune mediated. Crypts become hypertrophic, and cells on the mucosal surface in animals with subtotal or total villus atrophy are often attenuated. There may be transient "leaks" of tissue fluid and inflammatory cells through the epithelium, and microerosion of the mucosa occurs in severe cases. Physical damage to the mucosa due to feeding activity of the nematodes is unlikely; however, in fluke infestations this may be superimposed. Disease due to these agents is marked by diarrhea and weight loss, the latter probably mainly the result of the interaction of inappetence and enteric protein loss.

In infection of the cecum and colon by *Trichuris,* the worms reside partly in tunnels in the epithelium on the mucosal surface. Mucosal typhlocolitis results, which may be in part related to the immunoinflammatory response to the worms. In heavy infestations, erosion results in loss of absorptive function and effusion of tissue fluids, or in severe cases, hemorrhagic exudate. More subtle alteration in colonic function, perhaps again immune mediated, is caused by *Oesophagostomum columbianum* in sheep. Mucus hypersecretion and diarrhea occur.

The fourth group causes physical trauma to the intestinal wall by burrowing into or inciting inflammatory foci in the submucosa or deeper layers. In the stomach, various species of spirurids embed in the mucosa or establish in cystic spaces in the submucosa. In the intestine, Acanthocephala cause local ulceration by their thorny holdfast organ; larval stages of equine cyathostomes, and *Oesophagostomum,* become encapsulated in the submucosa. Protein loss may occur from ulcerated areas or when larvae emerge from the submucosa. The potential exists for perforation of the stomach or bowel, or for complications due to sepsis of submucosal nodules. Adhesion of inflamed serosal surfaces associated with nodules or perforations may impair motility.

Finally, some intestinal helminths, among them a few in the categories above, have effects at sites distant from the gut. This is usually the result of migrating larval stages of the worm, either in definitive or intermediate hosts. Larval *Habronema,* ascarids, hookworms, and equine strongyles may cause lesions in a variety of extraintestinal sites in the definitive host. Larval ascarids and taeniid cestodes may cause lesions or signs due to migration in nonenteric locations in accidental or intermediate hosts.

A diagnosis of helminthosis should be reserved for cases where, ideally, three criteria are met: the helminth is present, and in numbers consistent with disease; the lesions (if any) typically caused by the agent are identified; and there is a syndrome compatible with the pathogenic mechanisms known to be associated with the worm. A presumptive diagnosis only can be made if the syndrome, and preferably lesions, are present, but worms are not. This is appropriate only if treatment is very recent, and the condition of the animal is such that it would have been virtually moribund prior to therapy, since response to treatment is usually rapid.

In many cases, it may be necessary and reasonable to base the diagnosis only on the presence of an adequate number of worms, associated with an appropriate syndrome, since autolysis may preclude critical examination of intestinal tissues. This is also appropriate for the establishment of a rapid presumptive diagnosis at autopsy. However, quantitation of the worm burden is highly desirable. To this end, appropriate samples of gastric and intestinal content and mucosa should be collected, and estimates made of the number of worms they contain, using standard parasitologic techniques. Many species of nematodes are difficult to see and impossible to enumerate with the naked eye. Others, such as hookworms, though usually visible, may be so sparsely distributed that they are overlooked or dismissed. An accurate estimate of their number might indicate that they were present in numbers sufficient to represent a significant burden.

It is not acceptable to diagnose helminthosis only on the basis of the presence of worms, without evidence of an appropriate disease state. Nor it is an acceptable diagnosis when a syndrome such as wasting and diarrhea, or anemia, is recognized without identifying the presence of worms or their characteristic lesions.

Parasitic Diseases of the Abomasum and Stomach

OSTERTAGOSIS. Ostertagosis is probably the most important parasitism in grazing sheep and cattle in temperate climatic zones throughout the world. It causes subclinical loss in production, and clinical disease characterized by diarrhea, wasting, and in many cases, death. *Ostertagia ostertagi, O. lyrata,* and *O. leptospicularis* infect cattle; the first species is most important. Sheep and goats are infected by *O. circumcincta,* which is most significant, and by *O. trifurcata.* Some cross-infection by these species occurs between sheep and cattle but is of minor significance. Related genera, including *Marshallagia, Teladorsagia,* and *Camelostrongylus,* may infect sheep and goats; their development and behavior resemble those of *Ostertagia.*

The life cycle is direct. Third-stage larvae exsheath in the rumen and enter glands in the abomasum, where they undergo two molts. Normally, early fifth-stage larvae emerge to mature on the mucosal surface, beginning between the eighth and twelfth days after infection in *Ostertagia circumcincta* infections in sheep, and about 17–21 days after *O. ostertagi* infection in cattle. A proportion of larvae ingested may persist in glands in a hypobiotic state at the early fourth stage, however, only to resume development and emerge at a future time, perhaps many months hence. The prepatent period is ~3 weeks.

During the course of larval development, the normal architecture of the gastric mucosa is altered by interstitial inflammation, and mucous metaplasia and hyperplasia of the epithelium lining glands. In sheep infected with *Ostertagia circumcincta,* mucous metaplasia and hyperplasia occur in infected and surrounding glands early in infection, reaching a peak about the time of emergence of larvae onto the mucosal surface. In cattle with *O. ostertagi* (Fig. 1.43D), only glands infected with larvae undergo significant mucous change until about the time larvae leave the glands for the surface of the mucosa (Fig. 1.43E). Mucous change then becomes more widespread, involving uninfected glands in the vicinity of those that contained larvae.

In both species, affected glands are lined by mucous neck cells, which proliferate, displacing parietal cells. Glands elongate, and the affected areas of mucosa thicken. In developing lesions the gland lining is cuboidal or low columnar, and mitotic figures are frequent. In infected glands the lining in many cases is flattened adjacent to worms (Fig. 1.43F) but is composed of tall columnar mucous cells elsewhere in the gland. The undifferentiated mucous cells lining uninfected glands also eventually differentiate into tall columnar mucous cells. If infection is not heavy, lesions are limited to a radius of a few millimeters around infected or previously infected glands. These form raised, nodular pale areas in the mucosa, often with a slightly depressed center. Confluence of these lesions in heavily infected animals leads to the development of widespread areas of irregularly thickened mucosa with a convoluted surface pattern, likened to Morocco leather. With time, severely affected mucosa may be comprised almost totally of somewhat dilated, elongate glands lined by columnar mucous cells. With loss of the worm burden, through treatment or natural attrition, the mucosa gradually returns to normal.

Mucous metaplasia and hyperplasia are accompanied by a mixed population of inflammatory cells in the lamina propria. As has been speculated earlier, under Gastritis, the epithelial lesion itself may be immune mediated. Infiltrates of lymphocytes are present between glands deep in infected mucosa within a few days after infection of sheep with *Ostertagia,* and lymphoid follicles with germinal centers evolve in these sites. Lymphocytes, plasma cells, eosinophils, and a few neutrophils are present between glands in the infected abomasum. There may be edema of the lamina propria associated with permeability of proprial vessels, which in experimental *Camelostrongylus* infection occurs as early as 4 days after infection. Globule leukocytes are common in the lining of infected glands. A few eosinophils, neutrophils, and effete epithelial cells may be seen in the lumen of glands.

Mucosal lesions lead to achlorhydria, elevation of plasma pepsinogen levels, and loss of plasma protein. Widespread replacement of parietal cells by mucous neck cells results in progressive and massive decline in hydrogen-ion secretion. In severe cases, the abomasal content has a pH of up to 7 or more, and a high sodium-ion concentration. The pathogenic significance of associated failure to hydrolyze protein in the abomasum, and of increased numbers of bacteria in content, is unclear. Mucous metaplasia and achlorhydria in ovine ostertagosis occur in the face of substantially increased gastrin secretion, which is not stimulated simply by failure of antral acidification. The permeability of the mucosa is also increased, which is reflected in back diffusion of pepsinogen from the lumen of glands to the propria, and ultimately to the circulation. Intercellular junctions between poorly differentiated mucous neck cells are permeable also to plasma protein in tissue fluids, emanating from the leaky small vessels in the inflamed lamina propria. Significant loss of protein occurs into the lumen of the abomasum.

The cardinal signs of ostertagosis in sheep and cattle are loss of appetite, diarrhea, and wasting. The cause of reduced appetite is unclear. Diarrhea is associated with marked elevation in abomasal pH, but the mechanism by which it occurs is also obscure. Plasma protein loss into the gastrointestinal tract, in combination with reduced feed intake, seems largely responsible for the weight loss and hypoproteinemia that occur in clinical ostertagiosis, and for loss in productive efficiency that occurs in subclinical disease. The interaction of protein-losing gastroenteropathy and nutrition has been discussed previously.

Clinical ostertagosis occurs under two sets of circumstances. The first, type I disease, is seen in lambs or calves at pasture during or shortly following a period of high availability of infective larvae. It is due to the direct development, from ingested larvae, of large numbers of adult worms over a relatively short period of time. In contrast, type II disease is due to the synchronous maturation and emergence of large numbers of hypobiotic larvae from the mucosa, and it occurs when intake of larvae is likely low or nonexistent. It may occur in yearlings during the winter in the northern hemisphere, or during the dry summer period in Mediterranean climates. Heifers about the time of parturition may succumb, and this syndrome is also occasionally seen in animals experiencing environmental stress of any type.

Type I and II ostertagosis do not differ fundamentally in the signs or lesions they present. Animals will have a history of depression, inappetence, and diarrhea, and weight loss consistent with the severity and duration of the other signs. There may be edema of subcutaneous tissues and mesenteries, and accumulation of fluid in the body cavities. The carcass may be wasted, and the liver is often atrophic and the gallbladder dilated as a result of inanition. The content of the abomasum is fluid. It may be slightly foul smelling, in contrast to the normal sharply

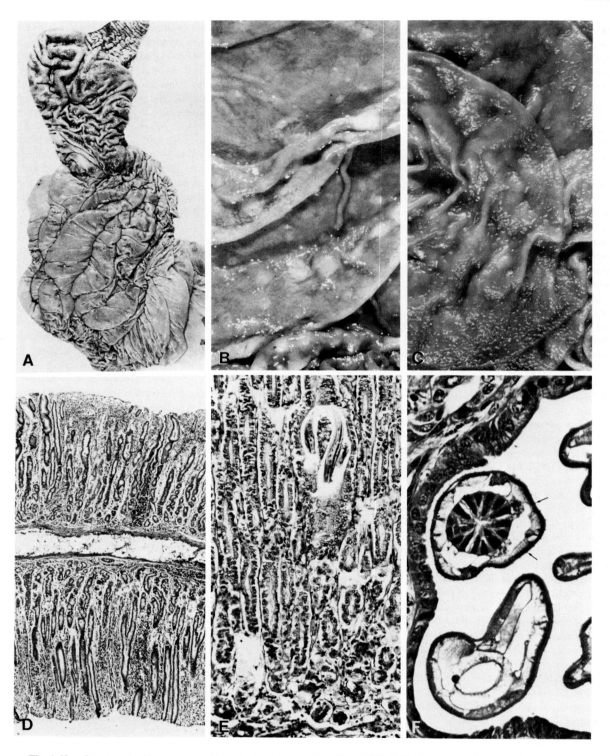

Fig. 1.43. Ostertagosis. Abomasum. (**A**) Acute edematous gastritis. Ox. (**B**) Individual nodules and some confluent lesions are present. Sheep. (**C**) Confluent thickening of hyperplastic glandular mucosa. Sheep. (**D**) Mucous metaplasia and hyperplasia thickening fundic mucosa on an abomasal fold. Moderate inflammatory infiltrate in propria between glands. Ox. (**E**) Mucous metaplasia and hyperplasia deep in fundic mucosa. Larva in section in gland. Ox. (**F**) *Ostertagia* in a dilated gland lined by cuboidal, mucous neck cells. The longitudinal cuticular ridges are visible as fine projections on the nematode in cross section (arrows).

acidic odor of abomasal content. The rugae often have substantial submucosal edema (Fig. 1.43A). The mucosa will have widespread individual or confluent thickened pale mucosal nodules (Fig. 1.43B,C) or will show diffuse thickening and corrugation over much of the gastric lining. Both fundic and pyloric areas are involved. The mucosa may be reddened and perhaps focally eroded, with a superficial light fibrinous exudate in occasional cases.

The diagnosis is indicated at autopsy by an abnormally elevated abomasal pH (>4.5), in association with typical gross lesions on the mucosa. The adult worms are brown and threadlike, up to 1.5 cm long but very difficult to see on the mucosa with the unaided eye. Abomasal contents and washings should be quantitatively examined for the presence of emergent or adult *Ostertagia* and other nematodes. The mucosa, or a known portion of it, should be digested to permit recovery and quantitation of preemergent stages. Significant worm burdens in sheep are in the range 10,000 to 50,000 or more. In cattle, more than 40,000 to 50,000 adult worms may be present, and in outbreaks of type II disease, hundreds of thousands of hypobiotic larvae are often detected in the abomasal mucosa. Typically, there is widespread mucous metaplasia and hyperplasia in dilated glands in sections of abomasum. *Ostertagia* is recognized, in glands, or on the mucosal surface, in sections by the presence of prominent longitudinal cuticular ridges that project from the surface of worms cut transversely (Fig. 1.43F). In some cases, the worm burden may have been lost through attrition or treatment, and the diagnosis must be presumptive, based on the characteristic mucosal lesions.

Ostertagosis must be differentiated in sheep from other gastrointestinal helminthoses (except haemonchosis) and from chronic coccidiosis. In cattle, gastrointestinal helminthosis, chronic bovine virus diarrhea, chronic salmonellosis, and in older animals, Johne's disease, must be considered.

HAEMONCHOSIS. Haemonchosis may be a common and severe disease in parts of the world where it occurs. *Haemonchus contortus* infects mainly sheep and goats, while *H. placei* occurs mainly in cattle. Though *H. contortus* and *H. placei* will infect the heterologous host, the host–parasite relationship appears to be less well adapted, and the species do appear to be genetically distinct. *Mecistocirrus digitatus* causes disease very similar to haemonchosis in cattle and sheep in Southeast Asia and Central America. *Haemonchus* species require a period of minimum warmth and moisture for larval development on pasture. As a result, they tend to be most important in tropical or warm temperate climates with hot, wet summers. By exploitation of hypobiosis or retardation of larvae, populations of *H. contortus* are able to persist in the abomasum of the host through periods of climatic adversity, such as excessive cold or dryness. Disease can be expected in animals, especially females, experiencing the synchronous "spring rise" or periparturient development and maturation of previously hypobiotic larvae, and in young animals heavily stocked at pasture during periods of optimal larval development and availability. Resistance to reinfection occurs much more reliably in calves infected with *H. placei* than in sheep infected with *H. contortus*.

Haemonchus, commonly called the large stomach worm or barberpole worm, is ~2.0 cm long. Females give the species its common name by their red color, against with the white ovaries and uterus stand out. The male is a little shorter and a uniform deep red. These worms are equipped with a buccal tooth or lancet, and fourth-stage and adult worms suck blood. Ingested third-stage larvae enter glands in the abomasum, where they molt to the fourth stage and persist as hypobiotic larvae, or from which they emerge as late fourth-stage larvae to continue development in the lumen. The prepatent period of *H. contortus* in sheep is about 15 days, and for *H. placei* in cattle about 26–28 days.

Haemonchosis may present as peracute or acute disease, resulting from the maturation or intake of large numbers of larvae. It may cause more insidious chronic disease if worm burdens are low or moderate. The pathogenicity of *Haemonchus* infection, whatever its manifestation, is the result of anemia and hypoproteinemia caused by bloodsucking activity. Large numbers of *Haemonchus* administered to sheep cause changes resembling those occurring in ostertagosis, including achlorhydria, increased plasma pepsinogen, and some architectural alterations in the abomasal glands. These appear to be experimental phenomena, however, and do not contribute to the spontaneous disease.

Individual *Haemonchus* worms in sheep cause the loss of ~0.05 ml of blood per day. Of the order of a tenth to a quarter of the erythrocyte volume may be lost per day by heavily infected lambs; the plasma loss is concomitant, several hundreds of milliliters. The potential for the rapid development of profound anemia and hypoproteinemia in heavily infected animals is obvious. Such animals succumb quickly, some even before the maturation of the worm burden. Less severely affected animals may be able to withstand the anemia and hypoproteinemia for a period of time. They compensate by expanding erythropoiesis two- or threefold and increasing hepatic synthesis of plasma protein. They are unable adequately to compensate for the enteric iron loss, however, despite intestinal reabsorption of a proportion of the excess and they ultimately succumb some weeks later to iron-loss anemia, when iron reserves are depleted. Low-level infections may contribute to subclinical loss of production or ill thrift through chronic enteric protein and iron loss.

The clinical syndrome may vary somewhat. Some animals are found dead, without the owner's observing illness. Others lack exercise tolerance, fall when driven, or are reluctant to stand or move, so weak are they from anemia. Sometimes edema of dependent portions, especially the submandibular area or head in grazing animals, is observed. In primary haemonchosis, there is no diarrhea; this sign may be present if intercurrent infection with large numbers of other gastrointestinal helminths occurs.

The postmortem appearance of animals with haemonchosis is dominated by the extreme pallor of anemia, apparent on the conjunctiva and throughout the internal tissues. The liver is pale, friable, and perhaps somewhat fatty. There is usually edema of subcutaneous tissues and mesenteries, with hydrothorax, hydropericardium, and ascites, reflecting the severe hypoproteinemia. In animals with more chronic disease, perhaps complicated by a low plane of nutrition, there may be depletion of fat depots and atrophy of muscle mass. The abomasal content is usually fluid and dark red-brown, due to the presence of blood (Fig. 1.44D). The abomasal rugae may be edematous due to hypoproteinemia, and focal areas of hemorrhage are evident over the surface. In animals not decomposing, the worms will be evident to the naked eye: if alive, writhing on the mucosal surface; if dead, less obvious and free in the content. The mucosa should be washed and the washings combined with content for determination of the worm burden.

In clinically affected sheep and goats, usually about 1000–12,000 worms are found. The severity of the disease is partly a function of the number of worms, and to some extent, the size of the animal. In lambs, 2000–3000 worms is a heavy burden, while in adult sheep and goats, 8000–10,000 are associated with fatal infection. Burdens of less than 500 to 1000 *Haemonchus* worms are unlikely to cause death in animals on a good plane of nutrition but may contribute to inefficiency in production or cause ill thrift and perhaps mortality if the quality of feed declines.

A high egg count is usually found on fecal flotation since *Haemonchus* is a prolific egg layer. In peracute prepatent infections, however, no eggs will be present. In recently treated animals, no worms may be present, and the diagnosis may have to be presumptive. On the other hand, animals returned to contaminated pasture may succumb to reinfection within 2 to 3 weeks of treatment. A diagnosis of haemonchosis in one or two animals from a group indicates the necessity of treatment and a move to clean pasture for the remainder of the flock or herd.

Other causes of acute anemic syndromes in sheep and goats, from which haemonchosis should be differentiated, include *Bunostomum* infection, acute fascioliasis, coccidiosis, and eperythrozoonosis. Chronic copper poisoning is more marked by icterus than anemia, though hemolytic anemia occurs. In cattle, sucking lice, infections with *Bunostomum, Oesophagostomum radiatum,* coccidiosis, and hemolytic anemias due to babesiosis, anaplasmosis, leptospirosis, and bacillary hemoglobinuria must be considered. At some stage, all of the hemolytic anemias cause hemoglobinuria, and icterus is often present. Neither occurs in haemonchosis.

TRICHOSTRONGYLUS AXEI INFECTION.   *Trichostrongylus axei* infects the abomasum of cattle, sheep, and goats, and the stomach of horses. It has a direct life cycle, third-stage infective larvae entering tunnels in the epithelium of the foveolae and isthmus of gastric glands in fundic and pyloric areas. The worms live throughout their life at least partly embedded in intraepithelial tunnels at about this level of the mucosa. They molt to the fourth stage about a week after being ingested and to the fifth stage by ~2 weeks after infection. The prepatent period is ~3 weeks in calves and sheep and ~25 days in horses.

Infections with *Trichostrongylus axei* are usually part of a mixed gastrointestinal helminthosis. In all hosts, however, this species alone is capable of inducing disease if present in sufficient numbers. After a period of several weeks, mucous metaplasia and hyperplasia are seen in glands in infected areas of the mucosa. Mucous neck cells replace parietal and peptic cells, and the glands increase markedly in depth and appear slightly dilated. This change is associated with an infiltrate of eosinophils and lymphocytes, especially in the superficial lamina propria. In

severely affected animals, flattening of surface epithelium with desquamation, or erosion of the mucosa, develops, accompanied by effusion of neutrophils, eosinophils, and tissue fluid. The inflammatory reaction in the propria is most intense in the vicinity of erosions, and no specific reaction is associated with worms in epithelial tunnels. Fibroplasia may occur in the superficial propria in eroded areas.

In light infestations there may be no changes visible in the abomasum, other than congestion of the mucosa. The gross lesions present in heavy *Trichostrongylus axei* infections reflect the hypertrophy of glands and superficial erosion. Circular or irregular, raised white plaques of thickened infected mucosa stand out against the background of more normal tissue. The surface of the mucosa generally is covered by a heavy layer of mucus. Erosions or shallow ulcers may be present, especially on the tips of abomasal folds. In severe infections the entire mucosa appears edematous and congested.

Infection in horses is uncommon and is related usually to sharing pasture with sheep or cattle. In chronically infected horses, white raised plaques (Fig. 1.44B) or nodular areas of mucosa are present, covered by tenacious mucus and surrounded by a zone of congestion. Mucosal lesions may be confluent in heavily infected animals, and erosions and superficial ulceration may be encountered. Infection may extend into the proximal duodenum, where polypoid masses of hypertrophic glandular mucosa are occasionally observed.

Achlorhydria develops in heavily infected sheep and cattle, associated with diarrhea particularly in the latter species. Dehydration may prove severe in scouring calves. Plasma pepsinogen levels increase, and hypoproteinemia and wasting occur. This suggests that the mucous metaplasia in the glands is associated with increased permeability and that plasma protein loss occurs into the gastrointestinal tract.

Though *Trichostrongylus axei* is not common as a primary cause of disease in any species, it should be sought at autopsy of animals with signs of wasting and perhaps diarrhea. The typical gross lesions in the stomach are distinctive in horses. They must be differentiated from those due to *Ostertagia*, with which animals may be intercurrently infected, in ruminants. The worms are very fine, and gastric washes or digestion are required to recover them quantitatively. The distinctive intraepithelial location of *T. axei* in section differentiates it from other nematodes inhabiting the abomasum of ruminants and the stomach of horses.

GASTRIC PARASITISM IN HORSES.   The commonest parasites of the equine stomach are larvae of the botflies of the genus *Gasterophilus*. Though they are not helminths, it is convenient to consider them here. There are six species of the genus, the common ones being *G. intestinalis, G. nasalis,* and *G. haemorrhoidalis,* and the uncommon ones *G. pecorum, G. nigricornis,* and *G. inermis*. The ova are deposited on the ends of the coat hairs. The larvae of *G. inermis* and *G. haemorrhoidalis* are able to penetrate the cheeks of horses, but those of *G. intestinalis* and *G. pecorum* must be licked to stimulate hatching and to convey the larvae to the mouth. The first-stage larvae penetrate the oral mucosa and migrate down the alimentary canal.

Gasterophilus intestinalis usually wanders about in the super-

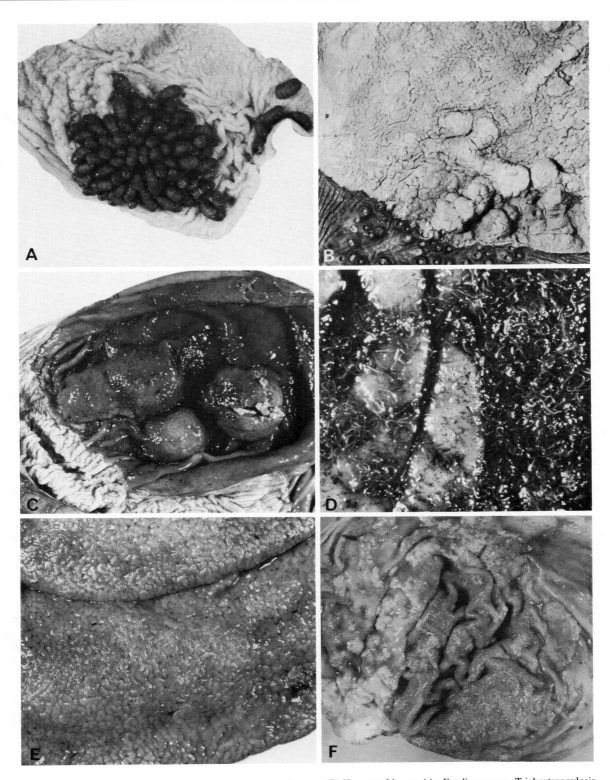

Fig. 1.44. (A) *Gasterophilus* larvae on gastric mucosa. Horse. (B) Hypertrophic gastritis. Fundic mucosa. Trichostrongylosis. Horse. (Courtesy of N. O. Christensen and the *Skandinavisk Veterinartidskrift*.) (C) Nodules containing *Draschia megastoma* in the submucosa of glandular mucosa, near margo plicatus. Purulent content in sectioned nodule. (D) *Haemonchus contortus* in acid/hematin-tinged abomasal content. Sheep. (E) Hyostrongylosis. Abnormally rugose mucosa. Pig. (F) Hyostrongylosis. Pig. Hypertrophic catarrhal gastritis.

ficial tissues of the tongue or gums for 3 to 4 weeks before molting and moving on. This is the most common species, and in the stomach it attaches itself to the squamous mucosa of the cardia to complete its subsequent molts. The larvae of *G. nasalis* first invade the gums, then pass to the stomach and settle on the pyloric mucosa and in the duodenum. Members of any of these species may occasionally be found attached to the pharynx and esophagus, but except for *G. pecorum,* which congregates in the pharynx and causes pharyngitis, these preliminary migrations are uneventful for the host. In the summer following the deposition of the ova, the larvae leave the stomach and pass out in the feces to pupate. Those of *G. pecorum* and *G. haemorrhoidalis* may attach themselves for a short while to the wall of the rectum.

It is generally assumed that the larvae of *Gasterophilus* have little effect on their host. They may, however, produce significant gastric lesions. Infestations by bots usually involve scores or occasionally hundreds, scattered or more commonly grouped together in rosette-like colonies (Fig. 1.44A). The larvae fasten themselves to the mucosa by the chitinous oral hooks, and they bore into the mucosa. They apparently subsist on blood, exudate, and detritus and produce focal erosions and ulcerations at the point of contact. These defects in the cardia are surrounded by a narrow rim of hyperplastic squamous epithelium. Usually the number of epithelial defects exceeds the number of larvae, suggesting that they move about on the mucosa. Undoubtedly many are removed mechanically, and often some are found free in the ingesta. Severe infestations produce a dense, pockmarked appearance with chronic inflammatory thickening. Ulcers may occur in the glandular mucosa, and a large proportion of the pyloric mucosa may be lost. Healing occurs when the larvae migrate, but may be complicated by secondary bacterial infection. Histologically, the ulcers penetrate the submucosa, which is chronically inflamed. The deep layers of eroded epithelium and the epithelial margins of ulcers in the squamous mucosa become hyperplastic and develop rete pegs. Other exceptional untoward sequelae include subserosal abscessation, or perforation with hemorrhage or peritonitis, and inflammatory stricture of the pylorus.

The spirurid nematodes *Draschia megastoma, Habronema majus* (formerly *microstoma*), and *H. muscae* are also parasitic in the stomachs of horses. The adult worms are 1–2 cm in length. The latter two species lie on the mucosal surface and are probably pathogenetically insignificant except possibly for a few erosions and mild gastritis. *Draschia megastoma* burrows into the submucosa to produce large, tumor-like nodules (Fig. 1.44C). *Habronema majus* mainly uses *Stomoxys calcitrans* as its intermediate host, and the other two species use various muscid flies. The *Habronema* larvae in the feces are swallowed by maggots of the appropriate intermediate host and persist through pupation and maturation of the fly. They leave the host fly via the proboscis when it eats. Horses may also be infected when they swallow parasitized flies. Larvae deposited on or in cutaneous wounds invade them and provoke an intense local reaction that becomes granulomatous and densely infiltrated with eosinophils (see the Skin and Appendages, Volume 1).

The only one of concern in the stomach is *Draschia megastoma,* which burrows into the submucosa of the fundus, usually within a few centimeters of the margo plicatus. Within the sub-

mucosa, the worms provoke a surrounding granulomatous reaction, which contains them in a central core of necrotic and cellular detritus. Eosinophils are present in large numbers. The granulomas cause the overlying mucosa to bulge into the gastric lumen. Except for a small fistulous communication through which the ova pass, the epithelium is not defective, even though the protrusions may be 5.0 cm or so in diameter. The nodules generally produce no clinical disturbance though they have been considered to lead rarely to abscessation or perforation when secondarily infected with pyogenic bacteria.

Trichostrongylus axei in horses has been considered in the previous section.

GASTRIC PARASITISM IN SWINE.   Gastric parasitism is not of great clinical or pathologic importance in swine and is rare in pigs reared in modern total-confinement systems. *Ascaris suum,* normally inhabiting the small intestine, may migrate or reflux to the stomach after death. *Hyostrongylus rubidus* is probably the most significant parasite of the stomach of swine, while the various spirurids are more common in pigs allowed to forage. *Ollulanus tricuspis* has been reported to occur in pigs. It is more commonly encountered in cats and is discussed under Gastric Parasitism in Dogs and Cats.

Hyostrongylus rubidus is a trichostrongylid nematode with a typical life cycle. Third-stage larvae enter glands in the stomach, especially in the fundic region, where they develop and molt twice. Preadult and adult worms emerge onto the gastric mucosa about 18–20 days after ingestion. The lesions produced by *Hyostrongylus* resemble those caused by *Ostertagia* in ruminants. During the course of larval development, there is mucous metaplasia and hyperplasia of the lining of infected and neigboring glands, and dilation of infected glands. The lamina propria in infected mucosa is edematous and infiltrated by lymphocytes, plasma cells, and eosinophils, and lymphoid follicles develop deep in the mucosa. Neutrophils and eosinophils may transmigrate the epithelium into dilated glands, the lining of which may become quite attenuated. Effusion of neutrophils and fibrin may occur through transient gaps, or more extensive erosions, in the surface of the mucosa. Larval nematodes are found in the gastric glands in sections, while adults are mainly on the surface of the mucosa.

During the course of development of the worms, the mucous metaplasia and hyperplasia cause the formation of pale nodules in the vicinity of infected glands (Fig. 1.44F). In heavy infections these may become confluent, causing the development of an irregularly thickened convoluted mucosa (Fig. 1.44E), most notable in the fundic area and along the lesser curvature. Adult worms are fine, red, and threadlike in the gastric mucus; they are difficult to see with the naked eye. Mucosal nodularity is most apparent during larval development and perhaps persists around glands containing inhibited larvae. In established heavy infections, the mucosa is not so thickened. It is pinkish brown, corrugated, and covered with excess mucus. There may be focal or diffusely eroded areas with pale fibrin evident on the surface, and occasionally ulceration of the glandular mucosa has been associated with hyostrongylosis.

Experimental infections of moderate degree do not produce obvious clinical signs or loss of production. Plasma protein loss has been documented in *Hyostrongylus* infections, however, following heavy doses of larvae. Inappetence, diarrhea, and reduced weight gains also occur in these circumstances. In the field, hyostrongylosis is associated mainly with the "thin-sow syndrome." It seems probable that hyostrongylosis may interact with nutritional and metabolic factors in contributing to this syndrome. Hyostrongylosis is confirmed by total worm count on the gastric mucosa and digests, in association with compatible gross and microscopic lesions in the stomach.

Spirurid nematodes parasitizing the porcine stomach include *Physocephalus sexalatus*, *Ascarops strongylina*, *A. dentata*, and *Simondsia paradoxa*. *Physocephalus* and *Ascarops* utilize dung beetles as intermediate hosts; the intermediate host of *Simondsia* is not known. *Ascarops* and *Physocephalus* are common in swine with access to grazing in many parts of the world. Large numbers of worms are required to cause disease. Worms in affected pigs may be free in the lumen or partly embedded in the mucosa, which may be congested and edematous, or eroded and ulcerated with a fibrinous exudate on the surface. *Simondsia* is found in swine in Europe and Asia. The posterior portion of the female worms is globular and embedded in palpable nodules up to 6 to 8 mm in diameter in the gastric mucosa. *Gnathostoma hispidum* may cause lesions in the liver, and submucosal nodules in the gastric wall of pigs, similar to those produced by *G. spinigerum* in carnivores.

GASTRIC PARASITISM IN DOGS AND CATS. Parasites are relatively uncommonly encountered in the stomach of dogs and cats at autopsy, and most are incidental findings or postmortem migrants from the intestine to the stomach.

Gnathostoma spinigerum occurs in the stomach of dogs and cats and a variety of nondomestic carnivores. It is more common in areas with warm climates. The life cycle of this spirurid nematode involves *Cyclops* as an aquatic invertebrate intermediate host, and a variety of fish, amphibians, or reptiles as second intermediate hosts. Third-stage larvae may also persist in the tissues of a variety of mammalian transport hosts. The life cycle dictates that infected animals have the opportunity to forage and scavenge. Ingested third-stage larvae may migrate in the liver, leaving tracks of necrotic debris, which eventually heal by fibrosis. In heavy infections, lesions associated with larval migration may be found elsewhere in the abdominal and pleural cavities.

Adults are found in groups of up to 10 in nodules in the gastric submucosa. Nodules are up to ~5.0 cm in diameter, and open into the gastric lumen. Portions of nematodes may protrude through this opening. The worms lie in a pool of blood-tinged purulent exudate in the lumen of the nodule, the wall of which is comprised of granulation tissue and reactive fibrous stroma. A mixed inflammatory infiltrate is in the wall of the nodules, and focal granulomas may center on nematode ova trapped in the connective tissue. Infection with *Gnathostoma* has been considered significant. Illness and death may be associated with disturbance of motility, chronic vomition, and occasional rupture of verminous nodules onto the gastric serosa, leading to peritonitis.

A number of species of *Physaloptera*, including *P. praeputialis* (cat), *P. rara* (dogs and wild Canidae and Felidae), and *P. canis* (dog), are found in the stomach of dogs and cats. These nematodes utilize arthropod intermediate hosts, and probably some vertebrate transport hosts. The adult worms, which may be mistaken for small ascarids, are found in the stomach, where they may be free in the lumen. More commonly they are attached as individuals or in small clusters to the gastric mucosa. Ulcers may be formed, and the anterior end of the worm may be embedded in the submucosa. A hyaline, PAS-positive material surrounds the anterior end of some worms, perhaps anchoring them in the tissue. These nematodes are not highly pathogenic, though heavy burdens may have the potential to cause significant gastric damage and protein loss into the lumen.

Cylicospirura felineus and members of the genus *Cyathospirura* may be found in the stomach of domestic and wild felids. *Cylicospirura* is usually found in the submucosal nodules, similar to those formed by *Gnathostoma*, while *Cyathospirura* is usually found free in the lumen, or sometimes associated with *Cylicospirura* in gastric nodules. The pathogenicity of these species is poorly defined, but is likely low.

Ollulanus tricuspis is a small trichostrongyle, ~1.0 mm long, which inhabits the stomach of cats and swine. It is viviparous, and third stage larvae developing in the uterus of the female are transmitted in vomitus. As a result, infection is usually not detected by usual coprologic examination, and infection with this species may go unnoticed. In some parts of the world it is common, particularly in cat colonies and cats that roam. Clinical signs and gross lesions due to *O. tricuspis* are uncommon.

The worms lie beneath the mucus on the surface of the stomach, or partly in gastric glands. Infection is associated with the presence of increased numbers of lymphoid follicles deep in the gastric mucosa, increased interstitial connective tissue in the mucosa, and elevated numbers of globule leukocytes in the gastric epithelium. Heavy infection results in mucous metaplasia and hyperplasia of gastric glands, causing the surface of the stomach to be thrown into thickened, convoluted folds. Gastric glands are separated by the heavy, reactive fibrous stroma in the mucosa. *Ollulanus* is characterized in section by the numerous longitudinal cuticular ridges recognized as projections on the surface of sectioned worms.

Capillaria putorii has also been reported from the stomach of cats. It is probably an uncommonly recognized inhabitant of the intestine, found in the stomach due to intestinal reflux at or after death. It is likely of little significance in either site.

Ascarids, hookworms, and tapeworms normally found in the small intestine may also be found as postmortem artifacts in the stomach.

Intestinal Nematode Infection

STRONGYLOIDES INFECTION. *Strongyloides* species parasitize all species of domestic animals considered here. Ruminants are infected by *S. papillosus*, horses by *S. westeri*, swine mainly by *S. ransomi*, dogs by *S. stercoralis*, and cats by *S. cati*, perhaps *S. stercoralis*, and *S. tumefaciens* in the colon. The parasitic worms are parthenogenetic females, which produce larvae capable of direct infection of the host, or of development into a free-living generation of males and females. The offspring of this generation then adopt a parasitic existence.

Infection by third-stage larvae takes place by skin penetration, or to a lesser extent by ingestion and probably subsequent penetration of the gastrointestinal mucosa. Larvae attain the bloodstream, and in young animals they break out into pulmonary alveoli. They migrate to the large airways, whence they are carried up the mucociliary escalator to be swallowed, and established in the small intestine. Alternatively, prenatal, or much more importantly, transmammary, infection occurs. Infective early fourth-stage larvae are mobilized from muscle or adipose tissue in the periparturient female. They may cross the placenta shortly before birth or are shed in the milk for several weeks after parturition. No somatic migration is required prior to establishment of these larvae in the gut of the new host.

The suckling young may develop patent infections within 1 or 2 weeks of birth. The prepatent period is short, and development of free-living larvae or the free-living generation is rapid. If sanitation is poor, and large numbers of larvae derived from parasitic or free-living generations of the worm are in the substrate, infection through the skin may be considerable. Dermatitis of contact surfaces may be associated with skin penetration (see the Skin and Appendages, Volume 1). Heavy intestinal infections may be a significant cause of morbidity and mortality in neonatal or suckling animals under appropriate epizootiologic circumstances.

Typically infecting the anterior small intestine of all species, *Strongyloides* larvae establish in tunnels in the epithelium about the base of villi, and they persist in that location (Fig. 1.45A). Adult worms are small, only 2–6 mm long, depending on species. In sufficient numbers, they cause the development of villus atrophy, associated with a mixed but mainly mononuclear inflammatory cell infiltrate into the lamina propria. Cryptal epithelium is hyperplastic. Villi are stumpy, or there is subtotal villus atrophy. Surface epithelium is usually low columnar to cuboidal, with an indistinct brush border. It may be squamous or, in some cases, eroded. In such circumstances, local effusion of neutrophils and tissue fluid into the lumen is seen. The nematodes are usually seen in tunnels in the surface epithelium, not beneath the basal lamina. In animals with severe atrophy, they may be in crypts of Lieberkühn. Embryonated or larvating ova may be retained in epithelial tunnels and help to distinguish this nematode in tissue section from *Trichostrongylus* in hosts in which both species occur.

Strongyloides ransomi is responsible for diarrhea in suckling piglets in some parts of the world. Minor local hemorrhage occurs as larvae migrate through the lungs and thickening of alveolar septa, associated with scattered aggregates of lymphocytes and plasma cells is reported. In the duodenum, villus atrophy is associated with local malabsorption of amino acids and with protein loss into the gut. In heavy infections, amino acid malabsorption is not compensated for by increased absorption in more distal intestine. Diarrhea occurs, presumably the result of malabsorption. Debilitation is the product of anorexia, protein loss into the gut, and nutrient malabsorption. Plasma gastrin levels are elevated in this infection, but the pathogenetic significance of this is obscure. This disease must be considered in enzootic areas and differentiated from the other causes of undifferentiated diarrhea in suckling piglets more than 6 to 10 days of age. Specific gross lesions other than those associated with diarrhea may be absent. Moderate to severe clinical disease in 3-month-old pigs is associated with 20,000 to 70,000 worms, most in the anterior 30 to 40% of the small intestine. Worms are evident in mucosal scrapings at autopsy.

Strongyloides westeri commonly infects foals. It is associated with diarrhea, occasionally fatal, in some animals less than 4 to 5 months of age. It is claimed that skin lesions by larval penetration may permit entry of *Corynebacterium equi*, which causes lymphadenitis. Millions of infective larvae are necessary to cause fatal infections experimentally. The gross findings at necropsy do not indicate the etiology, which may be suggested by finding worms in gut scrapings, and confirmed by their association with atrophic villi in tissue section.

In suckling ruminants, or young animals artifically reared, *Strongyloides papillosus* may cause diarrhea and, in occasional overwhelming infection, death. The pathology, and presumably the pathogenesis of *S. papillosus* infection, are typical of the genus.

Strongyloides stercoralis infections are most commonly fatal in puppies up to 2 to 3 months old, often from kennel environments. Affected dogs are wasted and dehydrated with evidence of diarrhea, perhaps blood tinged, but the intestine may only be congested or unremarkable at autopsy. Severe villus atrophy and heavy mononuclear interstitial infiltrates are evident in the duodenum of affected dogs. Occasionally, larvae may be present in granulomas in the lamina propria and submucosa. This suggests the possibility of autoinfection, or penetration and systemic migration by larvae originating in the gut. This may occur in *S. stercoralis* infections in humans and primates but is not confirmed in dogs.

Strongyloides tumefaciens in cats has been associated rarely with chronic diarrhea. It differs from the other species discussed above, however, being associated with the formation in the colon of submucosal nodules of proliferative glands infected by *Strongyloides*. It is uncertain whether this is a specific lesion induced by infection, or merely herniation of infected colonic glands into space left by involution of a submucosal lymphoid follicle.

TRICHOSTRONGYLOSIS.   Members of the genus *Trichostrongylus* parasitize the anterior small intestine of ruminants the world over. They cause significant subclinical inefficiency in production, or clinical disease characterized by diarrhea, ill thrift, and in some cases, death. The most important species infecting sheep and goats are probably *T. colubriformis*, *T. vitrinus*, and *T. rugatus*; others include *T. longispicularis*, *T. falculatus*, *T. capricola*, and *T. probolurus*. *Trichostrongylus colubriformis* and *T. longispicularis* also parasitize cattle. Though some *T. axei* may be found in the duodenum of cattle and sheep, this species is primarily parasitic in the abomasum and has been considered earlier with parasites of that organ.

Trichostrongylosis is most important in zones with a cool wet climate at some time of the year, but without extreme winters. It is an extremely important problem in many sheep-grazing areas of New Zealand, Australia, South Africa, South America, and the United Kingdom in particular. Though gastrointestinal helminthosis is usually a mixed infection, *Trichostrongylus* often dominates and appears to be a significant pathogen in its own right.

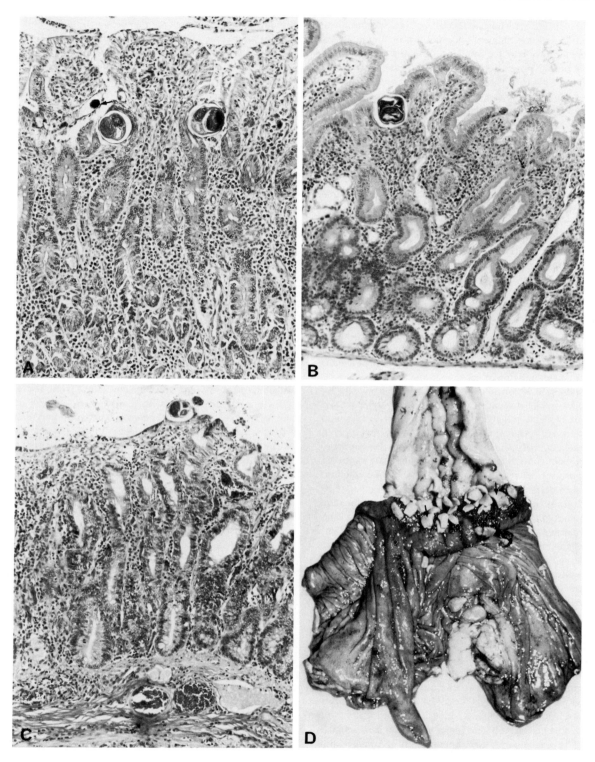

Fig. 1.45. (**A**) *Strongyloides westeri* in tunnels at base of a moderately atrophic villus. Intestine of foal with diarrhea. An ovum is in a tunnel on an adjacent villus (arrow). (**B**) Subtotal villus atrophy. *Trichostrongylus colubriformis*. Intestine. Sheep. Exfoliation of enterocytes, focal effusion of tissue fluid, dilated crypts, and mononuclear cells in lamina propria. (**C**) Severe villus atrophy in intestinal trichostrongylosis. Sheep. Surface epithelium is attenuated or eroded, and crypts are hyperplastic. Nematode in tunnel in surface epithelium. (**D**) *Anoplocephala perfoliata* (arrows) at ileocecal junction. Horse. Local ulceration and hemorrhage.

The life cycle is direct. Ingested third-stage larvae exsheath in the acid abomasal environment and establish preferentially in the proximal 5 to 6 m of the small intestine in sheep. A small proportion of the population settles in the abomasal antral mucosa near the pylorus. The larvae in the intestine enter tunnels above the basal lamina, between enterocytes, mainly at the base of villi, and they persist throughout their life at least partially embedded in the epithelium. Usually, infecting larvae all develop, over about 2 weeks, into adult worms, with a prepatent period of about 16 to 18 days. Hypobiosis appears to be relatively uncommon among members of the genus *Trichostrongylus*, and the circumstances by which it is stimulated are unclear. When it occurs, larvae are retarded in development at the parasitic third stage.

Experimental infections of all *Trichostrongylus* species studied indicate that the pathology and pathogenesis of disease caused by them is similar (Fig. 1.45B,C). Villus atrophy occurs in areas of intestine populated heavily by the worms, and the severity of the lesion within individual animals is correlated with the local density of the worms. The mechanism by which the atrophy occurs has not been investigated. In experimental infections, however, hyperplasia of cryptal epithelium seems to precede the onset of villus atrophy. It may be that the lesion is induced by cell-mediated immune mechanisms that stimulate proliferation by the epithelial proliferative compartment and interfere with differentiation of cells emerging from crypts.

The established lesion is characterized microscopically by villus atrophy, which may vary considerably in severity, in association with elongate, dilated, often straight crypts, containing many mitotic cells. Goblet cells may be numerous in crypts in some infected animals. In animals with subtotal villus atrophy, the surface epithelium may vary from tall columnar, relatively normal-appearing cells, to more domed or cuboidal epithelium lacking a well-defined brush border. Ultrastructurally, such epithelium appears poorly differentiated, containing numerous polyribosomes in the cytoplasm, and with stumpy, sparse, and irregularly oriented microvilli. The levels of brush-border enzymes, notably alkaline phosphatase, peptidases, and maltase, are diminished in affected areas of intestine. In animals with subtotal villus atrophy, exfoliating, rounded enterocytes are seen, as are focal and probably transient "leaks" of neutrophils and tissue fluids through the epithelial surface. In animals with more severe atrophy, the surface epithelium is flattened between the openings of crypts, and erosions of the mucosa may be evident, from which inflammatory cells and tissue fluid effuse.

The lamina propria in the affected area of intestine is populated by a moderately heavy mixed inflammatory cell population. Lymphocytes and plasma cells are prominent between crypts, with an admixture of eosinophils. Globule leukocytes may be present in the epithelium of crypts and occasionally villi, but this is often not marked in severely affected mucosa. In the superficial lamina propria, neutrophils often accumulate beneath the epithelium, and in areas of erosion or previous erosion, there may be a thin, transversely oriented layer of connective tissue. No specific attraction of inflammatory cells is evident to worms in tunnels in the surface epithelium. Abnormal permeability of the endothelium of capillaries and venules in heavily infected mucosa has been demonstrated, and edema of the lamina propria may be evident in these areas.

The disease is marked clinically by depression, inappetence that may be mild or profound, diarrhea, and wasting. The cause of the inappetence is unclear. It is suggested that it may be related to abormalities in levels of some gastrointestinal hormones, and it can be associated with concurrent gastric hyposecretion of acid and apparent atrophy of fundic parietal cell mass. The pathogenesis of the diarrhea is also uncertain. It too is associated with the period when inappetence and gastric dysfunction occur. Though local malabsorption of nutrients, and presumably electrolyte and water, occurs in the duodenum, it seems unlikely that the absorptive capacity of the remaining small intestine and large bowel would be overwhelmed.

Weight loss or reduced productive efficiency is not related to nutrient malabsorption, since net absorption of nutrients over the length of the small intestine does not seem to be severely affected. Rather, the interaction of reduced feed consumption with increased loss of endogenous nitrogen into the gut seems to be responsible. There is considerable effusion of plasma protein into the intestine of infected animals, and this, coupled with exfoliation of epithelium, which appears to be turning over at an increased rate, is the source of protein loss. The pathogenesis of protein-losing gastroenteropathy has been discussed earlier. In trichostrongylosis, compensation for increased catabolism of plasma protein and mucosal epithelial protein is at the expense of anabolic processes elsewhere in the body. Wool and muscle growth are hindered in subclinical disease. In severely affected animals, breaks in the wool, muscle wasting, reduced skeletal growth, and osteoporosis are related to reduced deposition, or catabolism, of somatic and cutaneous protein, associated probably with functional hyperadrenalcorticism. In addition, reduced mineralization of bone may be attributable to reduced intestinal absorption of calcium and phosphorus (see osteoporosis, in Bones and Joints, Volume 1). The pathogenesis of trichostrongylosis in calves and goats is similar to that in sheep.

Animals succumbing to trichostrongylosis are usually cachectic and dehydrated. Dark green, scoured feces will be on the skin or wool of the escutcheon or breech. There may be serous atrophy of internal fat depots, and marked atrophy of skeletal muscle. The subcutis is tacky. There may be edema of the mesentery and perhaps serous effusion into the body cavities, associated with hypoproteinemia, if dehydration is not severe. Mesenteric lymph nodes are enlarged and juicy. The content of the abomasum is abnormally fluid, and its pH may be greater than 4. The intestines are flaccid, and the small bowel contains thin, fluid, green content, which in the duodenum may appear somewhat mucoid. The large intestine may contain similar fluid or pasty green feces. These are usually foul smelling, probably due to products of bacterial action on protein.

The mucosa of the duodenum in the freshly killed animal may be glistening and pink, but in spontaneous mortalities with superimposed postmortem change, it will be unremarkable. Examination of the duodenal mucosa of freshly dead animals using a hand lens or dissecting microscope will reveal patchy or diffuse atrophy of villi, and fine white or translucent, threadlike worms, about 5–8 mm long, entwined on the mucosal surface. The proximal third of the small intestine (about 5–7 m) contains the bulk of the population of *Trichostrongylus*. A worm count on the small bowel usually reveals 15,000–80,000 *Trichostrongylus* in severe clinical infections. Subclinical or mild disease may be associated with fewer worms. The diagnosis is based on recovery of substantial populations of *Trichostrongylus* in association with the clinicopathologic syndrome and villus atrophy described above. Mixed infections with other genera are common, and the additive effects of populations of several species of worms should be considered.

NEMATODIRUS AND COOPERIA INFECTION.   *Nematodirus* species infect the anterior third of the small intestine of ruminants. The most important species are *N. helvetianus,* which infects cattle; *N. spathiger* and *N. filicollis,* which infect sheep, goats, and cattle; and *N. battus,* which is a parasite mainly of sheep.

The life cycle is direct. However, the hatch of infective larvae of *Nematodirus battus* and *N. filicollis* from the egg is delayed. Eggs of *N. battus* deposited on the ground in one year hatch the next spring, following a period of conditioning by cold over winter. The epizootiologic pattern is that of infection of a susceptible lamb crop during one year by larvae produced by the previous year's lambs. Under these conditions, with high availability of infective larvae, parasitic enteritis dominated by *Nematodirus* may occur. The larvae of *N. spathiger* and *N. helvetianus* are not delayed in hatching, and their epizootiologic pattern resembles that of *Trichostrongylus* in grazing animals. They often form part of a mixed population of worms in parasitic gastroenteritis in grazing lambs and calves. The disease may occur in yarded calves as well as animals at pasture.

Third-stage larvae enter the deeper layers of the mucosa, perhaps penetrating into crypts. Larvae emerge at the fourth or fifth stage to take up residence coiled among the villi, with their posterior ends protruding toward the lumen. They normally do not penetrate the epithelium.

The presence of large numbers of *Nematodirus* is associated with the development of villus atrophy, which is usually moderate in comparison with that induced by *Strongyloides* or *Trichostrongylus*. The villi are compressed by the pressure of entwined nematodes, and the impression of the longitudinal cuticular ridges is present on the surface of enterocytes adjacent to the worms. Local erosions may occur at such sites. Villi are stumpy, bifurcate, perhaps fused; or ridgelike surface alterations may replace the normal villous structures. Crypts may appear elongate and dilated. The surface epithelium may be domed, with loss of the prominent brush border, and irregular nuclear polarity. Ultrastructurally, such cells appear poorly differentiated and have irregular, defined microvilli. Biochemical studies reveal reduction in levels of mucosal alkaline phosphatase and disaccharidases, which correlate with the severity of diarrhea in affected sheep. If villus atrophy is severe, the ability of the worms to maintain their position may be compromised. They may enter crypts with their anterior end, move to more normal mucosa lower in the small bowel, or perhaps be lost from the gut.

The pathogenesis of the villus atrophy has not been determined, but it may be related to the development of immune responses to the presence of nematodes in the lumen. A moderate mixed inflammatory response with substantial numbers of lymphocytes, plasma cells, and eosinophils is evident in the lamina propria. The presence of such an infiltrate, and moderate shortening of villi associated with poorly differentiated surface enterocytes, is consistent with the postulated induction of villus atrophy by cell-mediated immune activity in the lamina propria.

Lambs and calves with nematodirosis develop severe dark green diarrhea, which stains the escutcheon or the breech of lambs. Affected animals may become inappetent, scour and waste for several weeks before recovering, or may die acutely. Disease is presumably mainly related to malabsorption and loss of appetite. Protein loss into the gut apparently has not been investigated. At necropsy, other than the changes associated with dehydration and perhaps cachexia, findings are limited to fluid mucoid content in the upper small intestine, and soft or fluid feces in the colon. The mucosa of the duodenum is usually unremarkable or perhaps hyperemic with excess mucus on the surface. Worm counts will reveal tangled, cottony masses of elongate, lightly coiled nematodes in heavy *Nematodirus* infections. Clinical disease is associated with populations of about 10,000 to 50,000 or more *Nematodirus* worms.

Cooperia infect the upper small intestine of ruminants. The important species include *C. curticei,* mainly in sheep and goats, and *C. pectinata, C. punctata,* and *C. oncophora,* mainly in cattle. Though both sheep and cattle may suffer from mixed burdens of helminths containing or dominated by populations of *Cooperia,* this genus seems to be most significant in cattle, especially in cool temperate regions. *Cooperia oncophora* appears to be less pathogenic for cattle than *C. pectinata* or *C. punctata.*

Cooperia has a typical trichostrongylid life cycle, but larvae do have the capacity to undergo hypobiosis to carry the population through periods of regular climatic adversity. The normal prepatent period is about 16–20 days. Like *Nematodirus,* *Cooperia* does not tunnel in the epithelium, but rather the worms brace or coil themselves among villi to maintain their place in the intestine. In sections, the compression of epithelium adjacent to the worms, and the impressions left on enterocytes by the longitudinal cuticular ridges, are apparent. In light infections, the worms are concentrated in the anterior third of the small intestine. Heavier infections, perhaps because they are associated with villus atrophy and therefore loss of the substrate against which to brace, are more evenly distributed down the intestine.

Heavy burdens of *Cooperia* in calves, in excess of 70,000 to 80,000 nematodes, may be associated with reduced weight gain, or weight loss and diarrhea. The associated atrophy of villi is concomitant with reductions in the brush-border enzymes. The syndrome is typical of intestinal helminthosis, and the diagnosis is confirmed by finding large numbers of the fine, coiled *Cooperia* in the small intestine.

HOOKWORM INFECTION.   Members of the Ancylostomatidae infect dogs, cats, ruminants, and swine. Hookworms of the genus *Globocephalus* appear to be of little significance in swine. In dogs, *Ancylostoma caninum, A. braziliense,* and *A. ceylanicum* occur. The former is most common in tropical, subtropical, and warm temperate zones of Africa, Australia, Asia, and North America, where adequate humidity for larval development occurs. *Ancylostoma braziliense* occurs in dogs and cats in the tropics and subtropics, while *A. ceylanicum* is found in both species in Sri Lanka and Southeast Asia. *Uncinaria stenocephala* occurs in dogs in cool temperate regions of Europe and North America. *Ancylostoma tubaeformae* occurs only in the cat.

Members of the genus *Ancylostoma* are capable of infecting the host by four routes: orally, with direct development to adult worms in the intestine; by skin penetration, resulting in movement through the bloodstream to the lungs, and thence via the trachea to the pharynx and gut; by the lactogenic transmission of third-stage larvae mobilized from dormancy in the skeletal muscle of parturient bitches; and in occasional instances, by prenatal transplacental transmission of mobilized larvae in pregnant bitches. The latter route of transmission does not apparently occur in *A. braziliense* infection. Some larvae of *A. caninum* may become arrested at the third stage in the intestine, to resume development at a later time.

Ancylostoma species all usually inhabit the small intestine, where they move about the surface, several times a day attaching to feed, then moving on. They penetrate deeply into the mucosa, sometimes to, or through, the muscularis mucosa, taking a plug of tissue into the large buccal capsule. Tissue is lacerated by the prominent teeth, and anticoagulant is released permitting persistent blood flow. Bloodsucking activity begins when larvae enter the adult stage, in *A. caninum* ~8 days after infection. Blood loss is maximal while worms are attaining maturity, between 12 and 16 days after infection, and then again during the peak period of egg production, after ~$3\frac{1}{2}$ weeks of infection. The prepatent period for *A. caninum* is ~15 days.

Ancylostomosis is the result of persistent blood loss, resulting in anemia and hypoproteinemia. There is considerable variation in the bloodsucking activity, and therefore the pathogenicity, of the members of the genus. *Ancylostoma caninum* consumes in the range of 0.01 to 0.2 ml of blood per worm per day. The amount of blood lost per worm is least in heavier infections. Pups several months old with populations of the order of 300 to 400 worms may lose 10 to 30% of their blood volume per day, depending on body weight. *Ancylostoma ceylanicum* also causes anemia, but *A. braziliense* seems to cause insignificant blood loss. *Ancylostoma tubaeformae* in cats is a significant bloodsucker. Experimentally, ~200 worms may cause anemia, weight loss, and mortality in 1.5-kg cats. The anemia in ancylostomosis is at first normochromic and normocytic. If adequate iron reserves and hematopoietic capacity are mustered, the animal may be able to equilibrate the rate of red cell production with the increased rate of loss, stabilizing the mass of the reduced circulating red cell population. Small size, poor iron reserves, and the low level of iron in bitch's milk make suckling pups with ancylostomosis susceptible to rapid development of the microcytic hypochromic anemia characteristic of iron deficiency.

Acute fatal ancylostomosis occurs most commonly in pups only 2–3 weeks of age, infected via the bitch's milk. Heavy infections acquired by this route may result in death from anemia and hypoproteinemia within a few days of the initiation of bloodsucking activity, and before eggs are present in the feces. Ane-

mia may also lead to mortality of pups after a course of longer duration. Percutaneous infection results in disease in older dogs held in runs or kennels under conditions of moisture and temperature conducive to larval development on the ground. Dermatitis due to larval penetration may be observed between the toes or on ventral contact surfaces of the body. The condition is usually typified by anemia, lack of exercise tolerance, weakness, and emaciation. Feces may be diarrheic, dark red or black, and often mucoid. Though diarrhea may occur, and there is some evidence for mild malabsorption and subtle atrophy of the intestinal mucosa, the major effect of ancylostomosis is due to increased loss of erythrocytes, iron, and plasma protein.

Animals dying of ancylostomosis are characteristically extremely pale. There is often glistening edema of subcutaneous tissues and mesenteries, and serous effusion into body cavities, attributable to hypoproteinemia. In chronic infections, cachexia may be evident. If recent exposure to heavy percutaneous infection has occurred, there may be dermatitis and numerous focal hemorrhages scattered in the pulmonary parenchyma, reflecting disruption of vessels by larvae breaking out into alveoli. The liver has the blotchy pallor of anemia. The intestinal content throughout the entire length is mucoid and deep red, from the erythrocytes voided into it by the worms. The latter are visible, about 1.0–1.5 cm long, translucent, gray or red (depending on when they last consumed blood), and dispersed over the mucosa, sometimes into the large intestine. They are often attached to the mucosa, and pinpoint, red sites of recent feeding activity may be scattered over the intestinal surface. Relatively few *Ancylostoma caninum* worms are required to cause death. In a young pup, as few as 20 to 50 may be present in fatal infections, and they may be sufficiently sparsely scattered as to be overlooked if not sought. In older animals with chronic or more acute fatal disease, 300 to 400, or less commonly, several thousands of worms, may be present.

Uncinaria stenocephala infects mainly by the oral route; percutaneous infection is not efficient, though dermatitis may result; and prenatal and lactogenic transmission appear not to occur. This species sucks little blood and is much less pathogenic than *Ancylostoma caninum*. Heavy infections with this species, however, arising usually in contaminated communal kennel environments, may cause clinical disease and, occasionally, mortality in pups. Nonspecific lethargy, inappetence, and ill thrift are signs of infection, perhaps with diarrhea; anemia does not occur. Disease is associated with burdens of a thousand or more worms, each about 5–10 mm long, in the small intestine. Worms may be particularly distributed in the distal small bowel in heavy infections and are often embedded in the mucosa in freshly dead animals. The intestinal mucosa appears thickened, and focal hemorrhages at sites of attachment may be scattered over it.

The presence of large numbers of worms is associated with moderate atrophy and thickening of villi. The surface epithelium is irregular. Focal aggregates of mononuclear cells and some neutrophils are in the vicinity of the anterior ends of worms embedded deep in the mucosa, a plug of tissue within their buccal cavity. It seems that disease due to *Uncinaria stenocephala* may be related to villus atrophy, perhaps with malabsorption and protein loss into the gut, since hypoproteinemia, but not anemia, may be evident. A similar syndrome may be associated with heavy infections of *Ancylostoma braziliense,* in which hypoproteinemia also occurs.

The **hookworms** of **ruminants** include, in cattle, *Bunostomum phlebotomum,* and in India and Indonesia, *Agriostomum vryburgi;* in sheep, *B. trigonocephalum,* and in India and Southeast Asia and Africa, *Gaigeria pachyscelis.* The life cycle of these nematodes is typical of hookworms. *Bunostomum* third-stage larvae infect by the oral or percutaneous routes, while *Gaigeria* infects only across the skin. Eggs and larval stages on the ground are extremely susceptible to desiccation, and hookworm disease in ruminants is most common in tropical or subtropical areas during wet seasons. However, stabled animals in cooler temperate areas may suffer disease resulting from larvae invading the skin from contaminated bedding. Following skin penetration, the usual pattern is seen, with migration of larvae to the lungs, where they molt to the fourth stage, subsequently passing up the trachea to the digestive tract. Larvae taken in by ingestion spend some time in the deep mucosa of the intestine before emerging to mature in the lumen of the small intestine. The prepatent period of *Bunostomum* is long, about 7–8 weeks. *Gaigeria* larvae migrate via the lungs, and worms begin to lay eggs ~10 weeks after infection.

Both *Bunostomum* and *Gaigeria* cause hemorrhagic anemia and hypoproteinemia, especially in animals under a year of age. These species often occur with mixed gastrointestinal helminth burdens, and their effects are at least additive to those of the other worms. They may be primary pathogens. Several hundred *Bunostomum* worms may cause signs in lambs, and a few hundred to a few thousand are found in clinical or fatal infections in calves. As few as 20 to 30 *Gaigeria* worms will cause anemia and hypoproteinemia in lambs, though several times that number may be more usual in fatal cases. The size of the animal, the status of its iron reserves, and the plane of nutrition, especially the level of protein, likely influence the pathogencity of these species.

At autopsy, the lesions expected in anemia and hypoproteinemia are evident. *Bunostomum* are found often in the lower half of the small intestine, while *Gaigeria* tends to be concentrated high in the duodenum. Blood spots and bite marks may be evident on the mucosa in the infected areas of intestine, but hemorrhage may be occult. The relatively low numbers of worms associated with disease, and their peculiar distribution, dictate that the entire gut be examined and flushed and a careful search be made for these species in suspect cases. Haemonchosis may occur concurrently or should be eliminated as a diagnosis, as should fascioliasis, and in cattle, *Oesophagostomum radiatum* infection.

TRICHURIS INFECTION. *Trichuris* species, the whipworms, are so called because of their long, thin anterior end and shorter, stouter posterior portion. They inhabit the cecum and, occasionally, the colon of all the domestic animals considered here, except the horse. The host–parasite relationships include, in dogs, *T. vulpis;* in cats, *T. campanula* and *T. serrata;* in swine, *T. suis;* in sheep and goats, *T. ovis, T. globulosa,* and *T. skrjabini;* in cattle, *T. discolor* and, less commonly, *T. ovis* and *T. globulosa.*

The life cycle is direct. Larvated ova are resistant to climatic insult and persist in contaminated environments for several years. Ingestion of larvated eggs leads to release of third-stage larvae, which enter the mucosa of the anterior small intestine for up to 7 to 10 days before returning to the lumen and passing on to the cecum, where they establish their adult existence. The prepatent period varies from about 6 to 7 weeks in the case of *T. suis* to 11 to 12 weeks for *T. vulpis.* In rare instances, disease may occur during the prepatent period, in which case ova will not be in the feces.

In all species the anterior ends of the worms are embedded at least partially in tunnels within the surface epithelium (Fig. 1.50E), but not normally breaching the basal lamina. Light infections apparently cause little morphologic alteration in the mucosa, and no disease. While *Trichuris* worms are reputed to ingest blood, disease associated with them is not related to this activity. Moderate infection of *T. vulpis* in dogs, at least, is associated with a mild mucosal colitis. There is a moderate mixed inflammatory infiltrate in the lamina propria between glands. Superficial vessels are congested, and scattered neutrophils may be present in the lamina propria beneath the surface epithelium. There is at least focal loss of goblet cells on the surface. These are replaced by low columnar or cuboidal cells, some of which may be exfoliating. Focal erosion may also be evident, and effusion of a few neutrophils and tissue fluid is evident through "leaks" or erosions on the surface. Goblet cells may be sparser than normal in glands in affected areas, which often appear longer than usual, and are lined by hyperplastic epithelium.

Heavy infection with *Trichuris* is associated with severe and often hemorrhagic typhilitis or typhlocolitis in all species. In the dog, large populations of worms overflow their normal habitat and infect the mucosa of the ascending, and often more distal, colon, sometimes extending to the rectum. The signs are chronic diarrhea or dysentery, perhaps with some weight loss. The blood and foul odor of the feces is related to hemorrhage and effusion of tissue fluid from the eroded mucosal surface. The mucosa is thickened, red, and edematous. The colonic content is fluid or porridge-like, and brown, tinged pink or red. Masses or tangled worms are visible on the mucosa (Fig. 1.50D). Microscopically, the mucosa is widely eroded or mildly ulcerated, and effusion of inflammatory exudate and blood is evident. Glandular epithelium is hyperplastic. Occasionally, *T. vulpis* infection may be associated with local or regional transmural lesions, with granulomatous foci and fibroplasia in deeper layers of the mucosa. Sometimes ova or worms are in these aberrant locations. Other transmural lesions may be the result of bacteria entering through mucosa damaged by *Trichuris. Balantidium* infection has been reported as a rare complication of *Trichuris* infection, in dogs with access to swine yards.

Trichuris suis infection in swine, if heavy enough, may cause mucohemorrhagic typhlocolitis associated with anorexia, diarrhea or dysentery, dehydration, ill thrift, and in some cases, death. The disease is most common in animals exposed to dirt yards contaminated with infective *Trichuris* ova. The lesion is one of mucosal colitis, resembling that described in the dog. There is thickening of the mucosa, with ultimate mucus hypersecretion from hypertrophic glands, coupled with erosion of, and effusion from, the mucosal surface. Lesions are more severe in swine with conventional gut flora than in those reared germ free or free of known enteric pathogens. Some contribution of the normal anaerobe flora to the development of lesions more severe than mild catarrhal colitis is apparent.

The large bowel in swine with *Trichuris* is thickened and congested, possibly with focal hemorrhages. The surface is glistening with mucus, perhaps with some fibrin exudation. The appearance may resemble that found in swine dysentery. Since the microscopic lesions are similar, this is logical. However, closer examination at autopsy will reveal the presence of the nematodes over the mucosa. Usually the thicker posterior ends of the worms are noted. They may resemble at first glance *Oesophagostomum,* and only on more careful observation is the elongate, threadlike anterior end seen.

The signs of the disease appear to be referable to loss of colonic absorptive function, and probably partly to effusion of protein into the lumen. Though erythrocyte loss does occur, it is a minor component of the pathogenesis.

Trichurosis in sheep and cattle resembles that described in swine. The disease usually occurs in animals concentrated in areas contaminated by ova. Hence it may occur in stabled or yarded calves or cattle. Outbreaks in sheep may be associated with hand feeding or congregation of animals at watering points. Affected animals develop chronic diarrhea with brown feces or dysentery and loss of condition. At autopsy the lesions are those of cachexia and hypoproteinemia, associated with a mucohemorrhagic typhlitis or typhlocolitis.

A diagnosis of trichurosis in all species is usually readily made at autopsy. The worms have a characteristic morphology and are usually easily seen on the inflamed mucosal surface. In section, the thin anterior end of the nematodes, embedded in tunnels in the surface epithelium, contains the stichosome esophagus typical of members of the Trichuroidea. The ova may be seen in the body of worms, in the gut lumen, or occasionally in tissue. They are barrel-shaped, have a thick wall, and plugs at both poles of the egg. *Capillaria* worms and ova may be similar in tissue section but are not expected in the cecum and colon of domestic animals.

OESOPHAGOSTOMUM AND *CHABERTIA* INFECTION. Members of the genus *Oesophagostomum* infect sheep, cattle, and swine. Their pathogenic effects are related to the formation of inflammatory nodules in the wall of the intestine incited by histotropic stages, and to ill thrift and diarrhea induced by adult populations in the lumen of the colon.

In sheep, two species, *Oesophagostomum columbianum* and *O. venulosum,* are probably most significant; the former is considerably more pathogenic and is particularly important in warm temperate to tropical areas. Third-stage *O. columbianum* larvae penetrate deep into the lamina propria, or sometimes to the submucosa, mainly in the small intestine, where they normally spend a week or so. They molt, emerge, and mature in the colon. However, a proportion of fourth-stage larvae enter a second histotropic phase in nodules in the colonic submucosa. Adult worms in the colon may be pathogenic for lambs. Burdens of only a few hundred *O. columbianum* worms are associated with anorexia, mucoid feces or diarrhea, and ill thrift, associated

perhaps with hypoproteinemia. The effects of infection may be exacerbated by intercurrent malnutrition.

At autopsy of animals with clinical oesophagostomosis, the carcass is emaciated, the mesenteric lymph nodes are enlarged, and the colonic mucosa is thickened, congested, and covered by a layer of mucus in which the worms are scattered. There is hyperplasia of goblet cells, and the lamina propria contains a heavy mixed inflammatory infiltrate with eosinophils and many immune-active cells. Globule leukocytes are in epithelium of glands. Nodules caused by histotropic fourth-stage larvae, mainly in the large intestine, are 0.5–3 cm in diameter and comprise a central caseous or mineralized core surrounded by a thin, fibrous, encapsulating stroma. Microscopically, the nematode or its remnants are present among a mass of necrotic debris in which eosinophils are prominent. Giant cells and macrophages may surround the necrotic material. Similar nodules may be found in liver, lungs, mesentery, and mesenteric lymph nodes. Those in the deeper layers of the gut project from the serosal surface, hence the name "pimply gut." They may cause adhesion to adjacent loops of gut or to other organs, and rarely may incite intussusception or peritonitis. In most cases, however, nodules are incidental findings at autopsy. They are probably the response to histotropic fourth-stage larvae in hosts sensitized by third-stage larvae, or the result of prior infection. The nodules caused by the histotropic third stage consist of small concentrations of suppurative exudate, which resolve as minor foci of granulomatous inflammation after the evacuation of the larvae. *Oesophagostomum venulosum* is a much less significant parasite. It seldom causes significant nodule formation; when it does, the nodules are small and mainly in the cecum and colon. Adult worm burdens are usually not considered particularly pathogenic.

In cattle, two species, *Oesophagostomum radiatum* and *O. venulosum* occur, the former being the significant parasite. The life cycle is similar to that of *O. columbianum.* The disease caused by *O. radiatum* is characterized by loss of appetite, reduced productive efficiency, anemia, hypoproteinemia, and diarrhea. Anemia results from hemorrhage at sites of larval emergence, and from mucosal erosions and discontinuities in the gland lining, associated with maturing and adult populations of worms. Blood loss is exacerbated by impaired coagulation, probably the result of consumption of clotting factors, the iniating mechanism for which is unclear. Considerable exudation of tissue fluids and plasma protein from colonic lesions, in addition to that due to hemorrhage, contributes to the hypoproteinemia and gastrointestinal protein loss. Reduced growth, or loss in condition, is mainly the product of the interaction between protein effusion into the gut and inappetence. Diarrhea presumably results in part from loss of colonic absorptive capacity.

Oesophagostomosis may be fatal in calves. Animals may be pale from anemia, and edematous from hypoproteinemia. Cases of some duration will be cachectic. Colonic lymph nodes are enlarged. The mucosa of the colon is grossly thickened and folded by edema and increased mixed inflammatory cell infiltrates, including many immune-active cells, in the lamina propria. Colonic submucosal lymphoid follicles are large and active. Effusion of tissue fluid and blood cells may be evident through small leaks between cells, or from erosions in glands or on the surface. Pathogenic burdens in calves are in the range of about 1000 to 10,000 *Oesophagastomum radiatum* worms. Although repeated exposure to infective larvae may result in the accumulation of large numbers of fourth-stage worms in nodules, formation of nodules has little pathogenic significance in cattle.

In swine, *Oesophagostomum dentatum, O. quadrispinulatum,* and several other species occur in the large intestine; the two mentioned are most widespread. The life cycle is typical of the genus. Third-stage larvae enter the wall of the cecum and colon, where they encyst and molt to the fourth stage, emerging about a week later to mature in the lumen. The larvae initially lie about the level of the base of the mucosa. They incite a reaction causing local loss of the muscularis mucosae, so that the nodule formed involves both mucosa and submucosa, and the larvae ultimately reside in the submucosa. The nodules are grossly about 1–20 mm in diameter, umbilicate, and may contain yellow or black, cheesy exudate in the center. An eosinophilic "cyst" wall surrounds the third-stage larva. Nearby lymphatics may undergo thrombosis. Once the larvae molt and begin to move to the lumen, an intense influx of eosinophils and neutrophils occurs into the nodules, and a focus of necrotic debris and fibrin lies over the evacuated nodule. Mucosal and submucosal edema cause thickening of the wall of the large bowel and contraction of the cecum. Gross and microscopic lesions resolve over the ensuing weeks as most larvae leave the mucosa.

Oesophagostomosis in swine is a mild, usually subclinical disease. Occasional diarrhea, depression in weight gain, and inefficiency of feed conversion may occur, especially during the period of emergence of larvae and maturation of worms in the lumen of the large intestine. Burdens of about 3000 to 20,000 adult worms are associated with subclinical disease experimentally. The nematodes are about 1–2 cm long, white, and present in mucus on the surface of the gut or in luminal content. Occasionally, infection with *Oesophagostomum,* particularly mucosal damage precipitated by larval encystment, may predispose to necrotic enteritis in association with anaerobic flora and perhaps *Balantidium.* Massive repeated challenge will cause severe typhlocolitis, but this seems to be purely an experimental phenomenon. Mortality should rarely, if ever, be ascribed to esophagostomosis in pigs.

Chabertia ovina, a robust worm about 1–2 cm long, inhabits the colon of sheep, goats, and cattle. It is particularly a problem in cooler climatic zones, mainly in sheep. The life cycle resembles that of *Oesophagostomum,* third-stage larvae encysting in the wall of the small intestine, then emerging to mature in the cecum and colon. Disease in sheep is associated with the presence of mature worms in the colon. Feces are soft, mucoid, and perhaps blood flecked, and ill thrift may occur. The adults penetrate to the muscularis mucosae and take a plug of mucosa into the buccal capsule; minor hemorrhage may be related to physical trauma to the mucosa. More significant is loss of plasma protein from the mucosa, associated with numerous focal sites of trauma, and widespread areas of mononuclear infiltration in the mucosa and submucosa. There is also hyperplasia of goblet cells. Grossly, the lesions are characterized by edema of all layers of the wall of infected parts of the colon, and enlargement of colonic lymph nodes. Worms are generally concentrated in

the proximal portion of the spiral colon, and the area they inhabit may have numerous hemorrhagic foci corresponding to sites of former attachment. Pathogenic burdens may be as few as 150 worms, and the species must be sought in its usual site of predilection or be missed.

EQUINE STRONGYLOSIS. Members of the Strongylidae are abundant and common nematode parasites of the cecum and colon in horses, usually present as mixed infections. The subfamily Strongylinae are the large strongyles, including the important genus *Strongylus* and the less significant genera *Triodontophorus, Oesophagodontus,* and *Craterostomum.* Members of this group are plug feeders or bloodsuckers, and *Strongylus* species undergo extensive extraintestinal migrations. The subfamily Cyathostominae, or small strongyles, includes eight genera of nematodes, among several of which the species of the superseded genus *Trichonema* have now been dispersed. Adults of this group feed mainly on intestinal contents and are of little pathogenic significance. However, emergence of histotropic larval stages from the gut wall may cause disease.

Strongylus vulgaris is common and the most significant nematode parasitic in horses. Larval forms cause endoarteritis in the mesenteric circulation, resulting in colic and thromboembolic infarction of the large bowel, while the adults cause anemia and ill thrift. Infective third-stage larvae, ingested from pasture, penetrate the mucosa of the small and large intestine and molt to the fourth stage. They enter the lumina of small arterioles, up which they migrate, on or under the intima, to reach the cranial mesenteric artery within 3 weeks. Three or four months later, after molting in that location to the fifth stage, the immature adults return down the mesenteric arteries to the wall of the cecum or colon, where they encapsulate in the subserosa, forming nodules about 5–8 mm in diameter. Returning larvae in nodules are surrounded by necrotic debris, neutrophils, some eosinophils, and perhaps some macrophages, and the adjacent arteriole may be thrombosed. They eventually break into the lumen of the large bowel, especially cecum and right ventral colon, where they mature in another month or two, about 6–7 months after infection. Some larvae may become trapped and encapsulated in arterioles in the mesentery on their way back to the gut and remain there to eventually die.

Endoarteritis associated with migration and establishment of larvae in the cranial mesenteric artery and its branches is discussed with the Cardiovascular System (Volume 3), as are the consequences of aberrant migration in the aorta, coronary artery, brachiocephalic trunk, and spermatic and renal arteries. Lesions of the cranial mesenteric artery and of the cecal and colic arteries may lead to colic as a result of reduced perfusion or thromboembolism, or perhaps due to impingement on autonomic ganglia in the vicinity of the arterial root at the aorta. The recognition and diagnosis of infarctive lesions of the equine bowel, and their sequelae, have been discussed with ischemia and infarction of the intestine. Though many older horses are infected with adult worms, or have arterial lesions, the complications of colic and infarction caused by this parasite are most common in young horses. An acute syndrome, characterized by pyrexia, anorexia, depression and weight loss, diarrhea or constipation, colic, and infarction of intestine, occurs in foals infected with large numbers of larvae, but not often in animals previously exposed to infection.

Strongylus edentatus is also common and has a life cycle characterized by extensive larval migration. Third-stage larvae enter the intestinal wall and pass in the portal system to the liver, where they incite inflammatory foci. Here they molt to the fourth stage, and ~30 days after infection, begin migrating through the hepatic parenchyma. The foci of inflammatory reaction in the liver are probably related to antigens released by migrating and trapped larvae. They consist of a core of necrotic eosinophils, with a surrounding fibrous capsule, a mixture of neutrophils, eosinophils, and mononuclear cells, or recent necrotic foci or tracks infiltrated by neutrophils and a few eosinophils.

By 8 to 10 weeks after infection, larvae are migrating from the liver via the hepatic ligaments. Hemorrhagic tracks may be produced in the hepatic parenchyma. Parenchymal scars and tags of fibrous tissue on the hepatic capsule, especially the diaphragmatic surface, commonly found at autopsy, are the legacy of migrating *Strongylus edentatus*. Those migrating in the hepatorenal ligament enter the retroperitoneal tissue of the flank, where they are frequently encountered, often associated with local hemorrhage. Larvae in aberrant locations in the omentum, hepatic ligaments, and diaphragm may become encapsulated in eosinophilic granulomas and destroyed. Omental adhesions may also be a sequel to aberrant larval migration. In the flank, larvae persist for several months, molting to the fifth stage before returning from the right flank via the cecal ligament to the cecum and origin of the colon. There they form nodules and hemorrhagic foci in the wall of the gut, eventually perforating to the lumen, where they mature and begin to lay eggs about 10–12 months after infection. Lesions associated with the larval migration of *S. edentatus* are usually incidental findings at autopsy.

Strongylus equinus is relatively less prevalent and abundant than the other two members of the genus. Exsheathed third-stage larvae penetrate to the deeper layers of the wall of the cecum and colon, molt to the fourth stage, and produce hemorrhagic subserosal nodules before moving to the liver through the peritoneal cavity. They migrate in the hepatic parenchyma for 6 to 7 weeks, then leave the liver, probably via the hepatic ligaments, to the pancreas and peritoneal cavity, where they molt to the fifth stage ~4 months after infection. They regain the lumen of the cecum, and to a lesser extent, the colon, by an unknown route, probably by direct penetration from the peritoneal cavity or pancreas. Eggs appear in the feces of the horse about 8–9 months after infection. Larval migration by this species causes lesions in the bowel wall and hepatic parenchyma similar to those produced by *S. edentatus*.

Hemomelasma ilei is the term applied to slightly elevated subserosal hemorrhagic plaques, up to 1 to 2 by 3 to 4 cm in size, found usually along the antimesenteric border of the distal small intestine or, rarely, on the large bowel. They are associated with trauma by migrating larvae of *Strongylus edentatus* in particular but may be caused by larvae of any species of *Strongylus*. These lesions are composed of edema, hemorrhage, and a mixed population of leukocytes, with macrophages ingesting erythrocytes prominent in evolving lesions. Occasionally a fragment of nematode or cuticle, or a migration track, may be found in section. With time these lesions resolve to yellow, brown, or tan

fibrotic plaques, as red cells engulfed by macrophages are destroyed and the products of hemoglobin breakdown reduced to iron and bile pigments and removed from the site, which scars. The presence of hemomelasma ilei is sometimes associated with clinical, but nonfatal, colic. The lesion is not uncommon as an incidental finding, however, and probably is a rare cause of clinical signs.

The other genera in the Strongylinae, *Triodontophorus*, *Oesophagodontus*, and *Craterostomum*, have life cycles that probably involve local migration of developing larvae into the deeper layers of the mucosa or the submucosa in the large intestine. Here they form small nodules before emerging to mature in the lumen of the cecum and colon. Larval members of these genera may contribute to the syndrome associated with emergence of larval cyathostomes, described below.

Adults of all species in the Strongylinae are plug feeders and bloodsuckers. In sufficient numbers they may cause ill thrift, and perhaps anemia, as the result of active hematophagia and blood loss from recent sites of feeding activity. Increased albumin catabolism causing accelerated turnover of the plasma pool, and reduced red cell survival, have been demonstrated in horses infested with relatively low numbers (<100) of *Strongylus vulgaris*. *Triodontophorus tenuicollis*, the most important species of that genus, tends to attach to the mucosa in clusters, usually in the right dorsal colon, causing local congestion and ulceration. *Triodontophorus* may be associated with significant blood loss.

The small strongyles, or cyathostomes, are essentially nonpathogenic as adults, despite the fact that tens or hundreds of thousands may be in the content of the large bowel and may browse on the mucosal surface to some extent. The larval stages migrate into the deep mucosa or submucosa of the large bowel to molt and develop before emerging to the lumen to molt again and mature. In the mucosa they are surrounded by a fibrous capsule, and there may be a moderate mixed inflammatory reaction containing eosinophils in the mucosa and adjacent submucosa. A similar but more intense reaction is seen around larvae in the submucosa. Emergence of larvae causes rupture of the muscularis mucosae and intense local eosinophilia and edema, followed by infiltration of neutrophils and macrophages. The larvae of some species may undergo hypobiosis or retarded development, persisting in the mucosa, only to mature sporadically, or perhaps more synchronously, as the adult population in the lumen turns over or is lost.

Mucosal nodules are up to only a few millimeters in diameter, slightly raised, red or blackish, and maybe umbilicate. Incision reveals a small, translucent, gray or red larval nematode. In heavy infections, the mucosa of the cecum and colon may be diffusely pocked by such nodules, which may attain a density of up to 60 per square centimeter.

Disease attributable to larval cyathostomes usually occurs in heavily infected horses at the time of turnover of the adult population and is due to emergence of large numbers of hypobiotic larvae over a short period. This occurs in the late winter, spring, and early summer in northern temperate climates. It is a disease of horses over a year of age. Little resistance is apparent to repeated infection. Animals develop a syndrome characterized by diarrhea, ill thrift or cachexia, and hypoalbuminemia, perhaps with passage of immature cyathostomes in the feces. In animals dying or killed at this time, numerous nodules, containing immature cyathostomes or recently ruptured, are present in the mucosa of the cecum and colon. The mucosa and submucosa are edematous, and the mucosa congested. If mucosal damage is severe, there may be a fibrinous exudate on the eroded or ulcerated surface. Many recently emerged fourth-stage or early fifth-stage larvae may be in the luminal content. The cecal and colic lymph nodes may be enlarged and wet, and the mesentery of the large bowel edematous. Diarrhea and wasting are presumably due to reduced absorptive function, and loss of protein is associated with the damage to the colonic mucosa caused by emerging larvae.

ASCARID INFECTION.   Members of the Ascaridae are common and important parasites of swine, horses, dogs, cats, and to a lesser extent, cattle. They do not occur normally in sheep and goats. Their importance is related to incidental and sometimes significant lesions caused by larvae during migration in the tissues of definitive and accidental hosts, and to the effects of adult worms in the small intestine of the definitive host.

Ascaris suum is a large parasite, females measuring up to 40 cm long, usually found in the upper half of the small intestine of swine. The life cycle is direct. Infective larvae, present in the resistant egg, are released in the intestine and penetrate the mucosa to be carried in the portal blood to the liver. They then pass to the lungs in the blood and break out of capillaries into alveoli. Third-stage larvae may be found in liver and lung 3–5 days after infection. Larvae move up the respiratory tree to the pharynx, where they are swallowed, arriving in the intestine about a week after infection. Worms mature in the intestine and begin to lay eggs ~2 months after infection. Small doses of eggs more commonly give rise to patent infections than large doses. This probably results from excessive loss of migrating larvae due to resistance incited by the antigenic mass of the heavier infections.

Larval migration induces lesions in the liver and lungs (Fig. 1.46). Infections heavy enough to cause clinical signs are rare in swine reared under conditions of good hygiene and husbandry. However, respiratory signs characterized by dyspnea (commonly termed "thumps") may occur in piglets if large numbers of larvae migrate through the lungs. Gross lesions in pigs, associated with pulmonary migration of ascarids, are limited largely to numerous focal hemorrhages scattered over and through the pulmonary parenchyma. There may be some edema, congestion, and failure of the lung to collapse at autopsy, due to bronchiolar constriction and alveolar emphysema.

Microscopically, there is an eosinophilic bronchiolitis. Bronchioles are surrounded by macrophages and eosinophils, and the bronchiolar mucosa is thrown into small folds, the epithelium frequently disorganized or perhaps eroded. The bronchiolar wall is infiltrated by eosinophils, which are also present, with necrotic debris, in the lumen. The architecture of small airways may be obscured or obliterated by the reaction, the outlines of some bronchioles recognizable only by the persistent smooth muscle of the wall. Interstitial infiltrates of eosinophils and macrophages are most dense about bronchioles, but diffuse out into surrounding parenchyma, thickening alveolar septa and diminishing the size of alveoli. Small branches of the pulmonary artery are also cuffed by eosinophils, lymphocytes, and macrophages, and eosinophils may be seen transmigrating the wall of vessels.

Larvae are usually readily found in section. They may be present in alveoli, alveolar ducts, bronchioles, or bronchi, perhaps surrounded by eosinophils. In more chronic cases, larvae in tissue are in eosinophilic granulomas. The worms may be dead in cases of some standing and are recognized only as an eosinophilic remnant or some bits of cuticle. Like all larval ascarids of mammals, *Ascaris suum* in the lungs have lateral alae visible in section.

Lesions in the liver due to migrating *Ascaris suum*, though not causing clinical disease, do result in considerable economic loss from condemnation at meat inspection. At first exposure to larvae, the lesions are related to mechanical damage caused by the worms, subsequent repair, and hypersensitivity reactions to excretory and secretory products of the larvae. Initially, hemorrhagic tracks are present near portal areas and throughout lobules. They are visible through the capsule as pinpoint red areas, perhaps slightly depressed and surrounded by a narrow pale zone. Erythrocytes, and within a few days, neutrophils and eosinophils, fill the space left in the parenchyma by the larva. These lesions collapse and heal by fibrosis, causing scarring, which involves most intensely the adjacent portal tracts. Fibrosis extends diffusely through more distant tracts, however, emphasizing lobular outlines. There is a heavy eosinophil infiltrate in fibrotic septa, which becomes most obvious beginning about 10–14 days after infection. In sensitized pigs, fewer larval tracks and hemorrhages occur, but a heavy infiltrate of eosinophils is found in portal tracts within a few days of infection, followed several weeks later by the formation of lymphocyte aggregates and follicles. Granulomatous foci containing giant cells, macrophages, and eosinophils may center on the remnants of larvae trapped and destroyed in the liver.

The inflammatory infiltrates in livers of animals exposed to larval ascarids may become severe and diffuse, and this is reflected in the gross appearance of the liver, which has extensive "milk spots" and prominent definition of lobules. The liver is firm, and heavy scars may become confluent, obliterating some lobules and extending out to exaggerate interlobular septa throughout the liver. Where pigs are raised intensively, it is now rare to encounter extreme fibrosis of the liver associated with ascarid migration.

The pathogenicity of adult ascarids in the intestine is poorly defined. Heavy infections may obstruct the gut, being visible as ropelike masses through the intestinal wall. Ascarids may occasionally pass to the stomach and be vomited or migrate up the pancreatic or bile ducts. Sometimes biliary obstruction and icterus, or purulent cholangitis, may ensue. Rarely, intestinal perforation occurs. Relatively subtle morphologic changes are induced in the intestine by *Ascaris* infection in swine. These include substantial hypertrophy of the muscularis externa and elongation of the crypts of Lieberkühn, though height of villi is not significantly reduced. Hypertrophy and exhaustion of the goblet-cell population and increased prorial infiltrates of eosinophils and mast cells are also observed in infected intestine. The presence of about 80 to 100 worms in 3-month-old

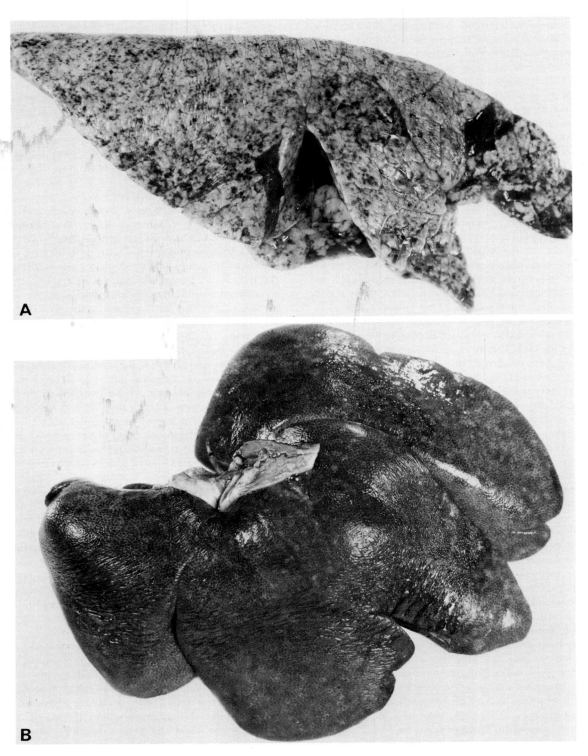

Fig. 1.46. (**A**) *Ascaris suum*. Lung. Pig.   (**B**) Interstitial hepatitis caused by larvae of *Ascaris suum*. Pig.

swine fed low-protein rations may depress feed intake and the efficiency of feed conversion. *Ascaris lumbricoides* in humans interferes with carbohydrate, fat, and protein absorption, and *A. suum* probably has a similar influence. The effects of infection seem to be most apparent in animals on diets marginal in energy and in quantity and quality of protein.

Ascaris suum also infects animals other than swine. In sheep, and occasionally cattle, immature ascarids may be found in the intestine. Eosinophilic granulomas and interstitial hepatitis and fibrosis with heavy eosinophil infiltrates may occur in the livers of sheep-grazing areas contaminated by ascarid ova. Larval ascarids may be found in section. In calves exposed to yards contaminated by pig feces containing *Ascaris* eggs, severe acute interstitial pneumonia may occur. Respiratory signs typified by dyspnea, tachypnea, coughing, and increased expiratory effort are usually first seen about 7–10 days after exposure when large numbers of larvae are present in the lungs. Deaths may ensue over the following few days, and the lungs are moderately consolidated, light pink to deep red, with alveolar and interstitial emphysema and interlobular edema. Microscopically, there is thickening of alveolar septa, and effusion of fibrin, proteinaceous edema fluid, and macrophages into alveoli. Hemorrhage into alveoli may also occur. Larvae are present in alveoli and bronchioles and provoke acute bronchiolitis. Neutrophils are found around larvae in bronchioles; eosinophils may be present but are not prominent in animals dying acutely. In addition to being usually readily observed in tissue sections, larvae may be recovered from the airways by washing with saline, or from minced lung in saline or digestion fluid by use of a Baermann apparatus. Tens of thousands to millions of larvae may be present in the lungs of fatal cases.

Parascaris equorum is the ascarid of horses. It is widespread and common in young horses; it may contribute to ill thrift and occasionally causes death. *Parascaris equorum* is a large nematode, females being up to $\frac{1}{2}$ m long. The life cycle resembles that of *Ascaris suum*. Similarly, hepatic and pulmonary lesions are associated with larval migration, and coughing may occur at the time larvae are in the lungs if infections are heavy. The prepatent period is about 10–15 weeks. The lesions in the lungs of foals with migrating *Parascaris* larvae, ~2 weeks after infection, are like those described in swine with *Ascaris*. Animals with resolving pulmonary lesions develop subpleural nodular accumulations of lymphocytes up to 1.0 cm in diameter, and there may be lymphocytic cuffing of pulmonary vessels.

It is possible to establish heavy infections of *Parascaris equorum* in the intestines of foals a few months old, but not in yearlings, where larvae appear to be killed during hepatopulmonary migration. In heavily infected foals, however, many worms are lost from the intestine prior to patency, suggesting the possibility of an effect of crowding on the population of growing worms. A heavy burden of ascarids in the intestine may reduce weight gains in growing foals. Inappetence occurs, but increased plasma protein catabolism or loss into the gut does not. Reduced weight gain and hypoalbuminemia may be due to decreased protein intake. Ascarid infection may reduce rate of intestinal transit. Heavy burdens can be associated with obstruction, intussusception, or rarely, perforation of the intestine.

The ascarids of small animals are *Toxascaris leonina,* infecting both cats and dogs, and *Toxocara canis* and *T. cati*, infecting the dog and cat, respectively. All occur in the small intestine, mainly in young animals. *Toxascaris leonina* has a life cycle that may be direct but can involve an intermediate host. In the definitive host, larvae ingested in infective ova enter the wall of the gut, where they remain for several weeks, molting to the fourth stage and emerging to the intestinal lumen to molt again and mature. The prepatent period is about 10–11 weeks. In the intermediate host, such as the mouse, third-stage larvae are found encapsulated in granulomas in many tissues but mainly the wall of the intestine, there they may be visible as pale foci 1–2 mm in diameter. They are infective to the definitive host if the intermediate is eaten.

Toxocara canis has a complex life cycle. Puppies may be infected by ingestion of larvated ova, in which case they follow the pathway of hepatopulmonary movement in the bloodstream, and tracheal migration to the pharynx and gut, though some larvae reach other tissues in the circulation. In older dogs, most larvae ingested in eggs are disseminated in the circulation to various tissues, where they encyst still in the second stage rather than undergoing development and a tracheal migration. In the pregnant bitch, these larvae are mobilized, crossing the placenta to infect the fetus in the 7 to 10 days before parturition. In the fetus, they molt in the liver and pass to the lungs as third-stage larvae, where they are present at birth. Transmammary transmission of mobilized second-stage larvae also occurs, infecting the neonate via the colostrum. In addition, paratenic hosts may be infected by ingestion of larvated eggs. In a wide variety of species, second-stage larvae are disseminated hematogenously to many organs, where they settle mainly in muscle. In some abnormal hosts, including humans, a syndrome termed visceral larva migrans has been described, characterized by eosinophilia, general malaise, and perhaps signs related to granulomatous reactions to larvae in the eye, liver, lungs, and brain. Larvae in paratenic hosts eaten by dogs develop in the gut of the definitive host.

Toxocara cati may infect cats directly from the larvated egg, via paratenic hosts, or in kittens, by the transmammary route from the postparturient queen. Prenatal infection apparently does not occur. Second-stage larvae hatching from eggs migrate via the liver, lungs, and trachea, while those taken in from milk or prey do not. Following tracheal migration or ingestion in milk or prey, larvae molt to the third stage in the gastric wall, while fourth-stage larvae are found in the gastric contents and the wall and lumen of the small intestine. *Toxocara cati* may also be a cause of visceral larva migrans in humans.

Heavy infections of ascarids in puppies and kittens, usually those reared in unhygienic communal environments, may result in ill thrift or occasionally death. The most significant effects are those caused in the stomach and intestine by maturing *Toxocara canis* in young puppies infected prenatally or in the bitch's milk. The animals may develop weakness, lethargy, and vomition, which is occasionally fatal. At autopsy, the animal appears poorly grown for its age, potbellied, and cachectic, and masses of maturing worms are present in the intestine and perhaps stomach. Sometimes up to 20% of the body weight of young puppies may be accounted for by the worm burden. *Toxocara cati* may be associated with clinical disease but usually not death, in kittens up to several months of age. Pathogenic effects are rarely attributed to *Toxascaris leonina*. Mature *Toxocara cati* are up to ~10 cm long, *T. canis* up to ~18 cm long. In freshly dead animals they are often coiled like a spiraled spring. They may maintain their place in the intestine by bracing against the gut wall in this way. The mechanism by which adults of these ascarids in the intestinal lumen impair growth has not been investigated. Ascarids occasionally enter the bile or pancreatic ducts, and many perforate those structures or the intestine.

Focal hemorrhages may be found in the lungs of puppies with migrating *Toxocana canis* larvae. Larval *T. canis* is occasionally found in or associated with granulomas in the tissues of pups and older dogs, though a clinical syndrome comparable to visceral larva migrans occurs only very rarely, if at all, in the dog. Inflammatory foci are most commonly seen grossly in the kidney, as white, elevated spots 1–2 mm in diameter in the cortex beneath the capsule. They may be encountered in section in any organ and are composed of a small focus of macrophages, lymphocytes, and plasma cells, perhaps with a few eosinophils, and possibly containing a larva. Larvae may be destroyed in such foci, which heal by scarring. Considering the large numbers of larvae that must move through the tissues of dogs, and in many cases be sequestered there, relatively few are encountered incidentally, free or encapsulated in granulomas. Occasionally, granulomas incited by *T. canis* larvae may be found in the eye on ophthalmoscopic examination. There are rare reports of encapsulated *T. canis* larvae associated with eosinophilic gastroenteritis in German shepherd dogs, and a somewhat similar syndrome has been produced experimentally by superinfection with large numbers of *T. canis*.

Larval *Toxocara cati* developing in the mucosa of the stomach and intestine may provoke a mild granulomatous response comprising lymphocytes and a few macrophages about the coiled larva. Larvae free of such a response are also found in the mucosa and submucosa.

Toxocara (Neoascaris) vitulorum infects the small intestine of young calves of domestic Bovidae, mainly in the tropics and subtropics, and it is significant especially in water buffalo. The life cycle involves transmammary transmission of third-stage larvae mobilized from the tissues of the dam. The larvae apparently do not migrate through the lungs of the calf. Patency occurs within about a month of birth, but worms are expelled within a short time, and after a few months, none are present. Signs of infection include foul diarrhea and ill thrift, and perhaps colic suggestive of impaction. Heavily infected calves may die in an emaciated state, with burdens of up to 400 to 500 worms as much as 30 cm long in the intestine. Occasionally, migration up the bile duct and perforation of the gut may occur.

PROBSTMAYRIA AND OXYURIS. *Probstmayria vivipara*, the small pinworm of horses, is viviparous, and as a result, massive proliferation of the population can occur endogenously. The worms are small, ~3.0 mm long, and may be present in the millions on the mucosa and in the content of the cecum and right ventral colon. Despite the large number that may be present, they do not appear to be pathogenic.

Oxyuris equi, the large pinworm of horses, also is relatively nonpathogenic. The fourth-stage larvae in the dorsal colon do have a large buccal capsule and feed on plugs of mucosa; in massive numbers they may be of significance. The adults probably live in the content. The male is ~1.0 cm long, but the female may be 4–15 cm, with a narrow tail comprising up to 75% the body length. They lay eggs on the perianal area, and their main significance is the irritation this activity causes.

Cestode Infection

Adult tapeworms inhabit the gastrointestinal tract or the ducts of the liver and pancreas, where they are generally of minor pathologic significance. They are flattened, segmented colonies of sequentially maturing hermaphroditic reproductive units, or proglottids, forming an elongate strobila a few millimeters to many meters long. The Eucestoda are attached to the host by a specialized holdfast organ (scolex), which usually has four suckers, and perhaps a rostellum, sometimes armed with hooks. The Cotyloda may have elongate muscular grooves (bothridia) on the scolex. Cestodes lack an alimentary tract and absorb nutrients through the specialized absorptive surface or tegument of the proglottids. Any effects they have on the host are related to competition for nutrients in the lumen of the intestine or result from tissue damage caused by scolices of species that embed themselves deeply in the mucosa or submucosa.

Carnivores may be infected by tapeworms that use as intermediate hosts certain prey species. Metacestodes, or larvae, of members of the Taeniidae use as intermediate hosts some species of domestic animals and, accidentally, humans. They may cause disease, result in economic loss due to condemnation of tissues or organs at meat inspection, or have zoonotic significance.

Adult cestodes in tissue section are flattened, with internal organs in a loose, parenchymatous matrix, often containing calcareous corpuscles in the outer region and lacking tubular digestive structures. They are segmented, and the scolex may be encountered at the anterior end, attached to the intestine.

In ruminants, the more common and widely distributed intestinal tapeworms are *Moniezia expansa*, *M. benedini*, and *Thysaniezia (Helictometra) giardi*. *Stilesia globipuncta* is found in the small intestine of sheep and goats in Europe, Asia, and Africa, while *S. hepatica* occurs in the bile ducts of ruminants in Africa and Asia. *Thysanosoma actinioides* occurs in the small intestine and pancreatic and bile ducts of ruminants in North and South America. *Avitellina* species occur in the small intestines of sheep and other ruminants in parts of Europe and Asia. The intermediate hosts of these tapeworms are oribatid mites or psocids (book lice).

Heavy infestations of the small intestine by *Moniezia*, *Thysaniezia*, and *Avitellina* may be associated with diarrhea and ill thrift in young lambs and calves. Concomitant gastrointestinal nematode parasitism may well be present and of greater significance.

The solex of *Stilesia globipuncta* may be embedded in mucosal nodules 6–10 mm in diameter in the upper small intestine, with the threadlike strobila streaming into the lumen. There is a chronic inflammatory reaction around the scolex, which is deep in the mucosa, plugs of tissue being grasped by the suckers. Glands in the vicinity are hyperplastic, causing the nodules. The presence of up to a hundred of these nodules has been associated with wasting, edema, and in some animals, diarrhea. Enteric protein loss perhaps occurs from the sites of attachment in the nodules.

Stilesia hepatica and *Thysanosoma actinioides* may cause mild fibrosis and ectasia of the bile ducts. Worms are often concentrated in the segmented, saclike dilations in the duct. These worms cause economic loss through condemnation of infected livers at meat inspection, and in areas where infection is common, this cost may be very significant.

In horses, the cestodes found are *Anoplocephala perfoliata*, which colonizes the proximal cecum, especially at the ileocecal junction, and *A. magna* and *Paranoplocephala mamillana* in the small intestine and occasionally the stomach. The latter worm is small, less than 5.0 cm in length, and is rarely associated with disease or lesions. *Anoplocephala magna* tends to live in the lower small intestine, where it can attain a length of up to 80 cm and a width of 2.5 cm. All use oribatid mites as intermediate hosts. Heavy infections have been associated with erosive or ulcerative enteritis, and rarely with intestinal perforation. *Anoplocephala perfoliata* is more commonly associated with lesions, and occasionally with mortality. In areas of concentrated mucosal attachment by clusters of this stumpy species, especially at the ileocecal orifice, erosion and ulceration of the mucosa occur (Fig. 1.45D). The depressed surface is often covered by a fibrinous exudate, perhaps with some hemorrhage, or there may be a local verrucous granulating mass projecting into the lumen. Chronic lesions of this sort may be associated with unthriftiness. Partial obstruction of the ileocecal orifice may occur rarely, but no relationship is established between infection with *A. perfoliata* and the development of ileal muscular hypertrophy. Ileocecal and cecal–cecal intussusception, and occasionally, perforation of the intestine, have also been associated with infection by this tapeworm.

Dogs may be parasitized by *Diphyllobothrium latum*, as may be humans, cats, occasionally swine, and many other fish-eating mammals. The adults can be large, attaining lengths of up to 12 to 15 m in humans, though those in animals tend to be shorter. The worm is ~2.0 cm across, and marked centrally by the dark uterus and eggs. Ova passed in feces are operculate, and the hatched coracidium is ingested by a copepod, where it develops into a procercoid stage. This in turn develops into a wormlike plerocercoid in the body cavity of various predatory fish. Plerocercoids develop into the adult worm in the intestine of piscivorous mammals. Macrocytic hypochromic anemia associated with vitamin B_{12} deficiency, probably induced by competitive absorption from the gut by the worm, has been reported in some infected people. Infection by *D. latum* is rarely, if ever, associated with clinical disease in animals.

Spirometra species are, like *Diphyllobothrium*, members of the class Cotyloda, and their life cycle is similar. The taxonomy of the genus is difficult, but among recognized species are *S. mansonoides*, infecting dogs, cats, and raccoons in North and South America, *S. mansoni* in dogs and cats in eastern Asia and South America, and *S. erinacei*, found in cats and dogs in Australia and the Far East. Prospective hosts must have the opportunity for predation, since they are infected by the plerocercoid or "sparganum" found in the body cavity of the second inter-

mediate host, usually an amphibian or reptile, or in another transport host. Spargana can also occur in carnivores, swine, or even humans if the procercoid in the first intermediate host, *Cyclops*, is ingested, usually while drinking. Spargana are white, ribbon-like, but otherwise structureless worms up to several centimeters long. They may be found free or encysted in a thin, noninflammatory fibrous capsule in the peritoneal cavity and intermuscular or subcutaneous tissue. A chronic inflammatory reaction may occur about dead spargana. The adult worms are nonpathogenic. Plerocercoids are of significance in humans, where they migrate mainly in the subcutaneous tissues.

Mesocestoides occasionally infects dogs, as well as other mammals and some birds, in North America, Europe, Asia, and Africa. These members of the Eucestoda have a life cycle involving an insect or mite, and a vertebrate as intermediate hosts. In the latter, infective tetrathyridia, about 1–2 cm long, flat, narrow, and bearing an invaginated scolex with four suckers, are found in body cavities, liver and lung. Tetrathyridia have the capacity for asexual multiplication, and massive infections of intermediate hosts such as amphibians and reptiles may result. In definitive hosts, *Mesocestoides* adults may also replicate asexually, and heavy intestinal infections may occur as a result of this or of the consumption of larger numbers of tetrathyridia in an intermediate host. Animals infected with intestinal *Mesocestoides* may develop diarrhea. Tetrathyridia in the abdominal cavity of dogs and cats may cause peritoneal effusion and adhesions.

Dipyllidium caninum occurs in the dog, cat, fox, and occasionally, children. It is ubiquitous. The narrow worms, up to $\frac{1}{2}$ m long, have distinctive cucumber-seed-like segments and are often encountered incidentally in the small intestine at autopsy. They are of no pathologic significance. Cysticercoids develop in fleas and perhaps in the dog louse *Trichodectes canis*. Infection in the normal definitive hosts, or in accidental ones such as humans, is by ingestion of fleas containing cysticercoids.

Tapeworms of the genus *Taenia* are the most important in domestic animals, not because of the effects of the adult worm in the carnivorous definitive host, but rather because of the metacestodes or larval forms. Taeniid metacestodes assume four basic forms. Single oncospheres hatch in the upper small intestine, penetrate the epithelium, and are carried in the portal blood to the liver. Some migrate in the liver, eventually to enter the peritoneal cavity. Others persist to develop in the liver, while still other metacestodes pass on to the heart, lungs, and systemic circulation, establishing in muscle or a variety of other sites and tissues. The **cysticercus** is a fluid-filled, thin-walled, but muscular cyst, into which the scolex and neck of a single larval tapeworm are invaginated. The **strobilicercus** is a modification on this theme; late in larval development the scolex evaginates and becomes connected to the terminal bladder by a segmented strobila, so that it resembles a tapeworm, several centimeters long. The **coenurus** is a single or loculated fluid-filled cyst, on the inner wall of which up to several hundred nodular invaginated scolices are present in clusters. Each scolex is capable of developing into a single adult cestode in the intestine of the definitive host. The **hydatid cyst** is a uni- or multilocular structure, on the inner germinal membrane of which develop brood capsules. Within the brood capsules, invaginated protoscolices form. Brood capsules may float free in the cyst fluid, where they are termed "hydatid sand." Internal daughter cysts can develop. Release of brood capsules or protoscolices into tissues, as a result of rupture of the hydatid cyst, may lead to development of new cysts. The alveolar hydatid cyst proliferates by budding externally.

Taenia taeniaeformis infects the intestine of domestic cats and some wild felids, and the strobilicercus, *Cysticercus fasciolaris,* is found in the liver of small rodents. The adults are up to 60 cm long, have no neck, and posterior segments are somewhat bell-shaped, so this species is readily differentiated from the other cestodes found in the feline small intestine. Usually only a few worms are present in the cat, and they are of little consequence.

Taenia pisiformis is common in the small intestine in dogs and some wild canids that prey on rabbits and hares. *Cysticercus pisiformis* migrates in the liver of the intermediate host, causing hemorrhagic tracks that are infiltrated by a mixed inflammatory reaction and ultimately heal by scarring. The pea-size cysticerci encyst in a thin, noninflammatory fibrous capsule on the mesentery or omentum or on the ligaments of the bladder. Occasionally cysticerci persist beneath the hepatic capsule. Burdens of up to 20 to 30 worms, sometimes more, may be present in the intestine of the dog.

Taenia hydatigena infects the dog, and the metacestode, *Cysticercus tenuicollis,* the long-necked bladder worm, or false hydatid, is found in the peritoneal cavity of sheep, cattle, swine, and occasionally, other species. Immature cysticerci in the liver migrate through the parenchyma for several weeks as they develop, before emerging to encyst on the peritoneum anywhere in the abdominal cavity. The immature cysticerci are less than a centimeter long, ovoid, and translucent. They cause tortuous hemorrhagic tracks similar to those produced by immature liver flukes, and if large numbers are present, they may cause a syndrome of depression and icterus identical to acute fascioliasis. Heavily infected livers, with 4000 or 5000 actively migrating cysticerci, are mottled due to the subcapsular and parenchymal hemorrhagic foci and tracks. Cysticerci up to 6 to 8 mm long may be present beneath or breaching the capsule by ~3 weeks after infection. In severe cases, hemorrhage into the abdominal cavity may occur, but this is uncommon. Hepatic necrosis due to migrating cysticerci may predispose to germination of clostridial spores and the development of black disease or bacillary hemoglobinuria, though these are more often complications of fascioliasis. Cysterci trapped in the liver may persist in a fibrous capsule or be destroyed in a cystic eosinophilic granuloma, which may mineralize; this is common on the diaphragmatic surface, where the falciform ligament is attached. Usually the intensity of infection is low, and a few, but occasionally scores of cysticerci, delicate, translucent, fluctuant, fluid-filled cysts up to 5.0 cm or more in diameter, are contained in individual thin, noninflammatory fibrous capsules scattered on the peritoneal serosa. A single invaginated scolex on a long neck is present in each cysticercus. When a cyst degenerates, it is destroyed by a granulomatous reaction, and the fibrotic mass may mineralize.

Taenia ovis infects the intestine of the dog, while the metacestode, *Cysticercus ovis,* is in the muscle of sheep, where is causes cysticercosis, or "sheep measles." Cysticercosis of muscle caused by *C. ovis, C. bovis* in cattle, and *C. cellulosae* in swine is considered with disease of muscle (in Muscles and Tendons, Volume 1). The adult stages of the latter two cysticerci, *T. saginata* and *T. solium,* respectively, occur in the small intestine of humans.

Taenia serialis infects dogs and foxes throughout the world. The larval coenurus is found in the subcutaneous and intermuscular connective tissue of lagomorphs. Usually, large numbers of tapeworms are found in individual infected dogs, presumably due to the development of many individuals from the numerous scolices in one or more coenuri.

Taenia multiceps occurs in the intestine of dogs and wild canids, but the metacestode, *Coenurus cerebralis,* develops in the brain and spinal cord of sheep and other ungulates, and rarely, humans. In the goat, coenuri may also occur in other organs, beneath the skin and intramuscularly. The migration of small metacestodes in the central nervous system may cause tortuous red or yellowish gray tracks in the brain due to traumatic hemorrhage and malacia, and nervous signs or death may occur at this stage. More commonly, signs of central nervous disease, termed "sturdy" or "gid," do not develop until coenuri, up to 4 to 5 cm in diameter, have developed more fully, 4–8 months after infection. Cysts may be present at any level and depth in the brain and spinal cord and projecting into the cerebral ventricles, but they are most common near the surface of the parietal cortex in the cerebrum. They cause increased intracranial pressure, hydrocephalus, necrosis of adjacent brain, and sometimes lysis, perhaps extending to perforation, of the overlying cranial bone. Coenuri developing in the spinal cord may cause paresis.

Cysticerci and coenuri are recognized in tissue sections as generally cystic structures with an eosinophilic outer layer or tegument, which may appear fibrillar or almost ciliate on the outermost surface. Beneath the tegumental cells a less cellular area, which may contain calcareous corpuscles, gives way to a light, weblike, lightly cellular matrix, and the central, open, fluid-filled portion of the cyst. No internal organs are seen. Muscular inverted scolices, with suckers and (in all but *Cysticercus bovis*) hooks on the rostellum, may be encountered in favorable sections, extending into the center of the metacestode. Immature migrating metacestodes lack organized scolices. The reader is referred to other sources for details on the taxonomy and specific identification of adult and larval taeniid tapeworms.

Echinococcus tapeworms occur in the small intestine of a number of species of carnivores, predominantly canids. In enzootic areas the distinctive metacestodes, or hydatid cysts, are commonly found in normal or accidental intermediate hosts. Humans may become infected with the metacestode, and echinococcosis or hydatidosis is a significant public health problem where carnivores carrying *Echinococcus* come in close contact with people.

The taxonomy of the genus is complex and in dispute. There appear to be four species, of which at least some have strains or biotypes that may be recognized on the basis of biochemical characteristics, biologic behavior, and ecology. These strains seem to be based on adaptations to prey–predator relationships among definitive and intermediate hosts, which are relatively isolated geographically and ecologically. Since *Echinococcus* species may be self-fertilizing, they have a high potential for forming double recessives. The large number of genetically identical worms that may result from asexual reproduction by the cystic metacestode developing from a single oncosphere gives the genus a high capacity for establishment of mutant populations. These adaptive advantages may predispose to the development of strains. The species recognized are *E. granulosus, E. multilocularis, E. oligarthus,* and *E. vogeli*. The latter two involve sylvatic cycles in South America, with felids and canids as definitive hosts, respectively, and rodents as intermediate hosts. The other two species may use domestic animals as definitive hosts and will be considered further here.

Echinococcus granulosus uses the dog and some other canids as the definitive host. The most widespread strain uses a sheep–dog cycle and has been disseminated wherever there is pastoral husbandry of sheep. It is significant as a potential zoonosis in many parts of Eurasia and the Mediterranean region, some parts of the United Kingdom, North and South America, continental Australia, and Africa. Eradication has been accomplished, or virtually so, in Iceland, New Zealand, and Tasmania. Other strains affecting domestic animals use horse–, cattle–, camel–, pig–, buffalo–, goat–, and human–dog cycles. Sylvatic cycles include, in North America, moose–wolf; in Argentina, hare–fox; in Sri Lanka, deer–jackal; and in Australia, macropod–dingo. Typically, cysts that develop in the intermediate host to which the strain is adapted are fertile, and a high proportion contains brood capsules and protoscolices. Oncospheres infecting other hosts either may not establish or, more commonly, develop into sterile cysts that do not produce protoscolices. Thus knowledge of the local cycles of *E. granulosus* permits interpretation and prediction of the patterns of fertility and sterility of cysts found in the various potential intermediate hosts.

In the small intestine of the definitive host, protoscolices evaginate and establish between villi and in the crypts of Lieberkühn. The scolex distends the crypt, and the epithelium is gripped by the suckers and occasionally eroded. The worms that develop are short, usually less than 6 to 7 mm long. They commonly have only three or four proglottids, the caudal gravid one making up almost half the length of the worm. Burdens of *Echinococcus granulosus* are often heavy, no doubt due to the large numbers of protoscolices ingested at a meal containing one or more hydatid cysts. The heavily infected intestine is carpeted by the tiny white, blunt projections, partially obscured between the villi; the lesion may resemble lymphangiectasia. Enteric signs are not normally encountered in dogs with intestinal hydatid tapeworms.

Penetration of oncospheres released from eggs in the intestine of the intermediate host takes them into the subepithelial capillaries, or perhaps the lacteal. The majority probably migrate via the liver, some carrying on to the lungs and general circulation. Those gaining the lacteal may bypass the liver, however, entering the vena cava with the lymph, and are either filtered out in the pulmonary circulation or disseminated. Hydatid cysts occur most commonly in the liver and lung, with some species varia-

tion in the relative prevalence in these organs. In sheep, they may be more common in lungs, while in cattle and horses, the liver is the usual site of establishment. Less commonly, the brain, heart, and bone may be sites of development of hydatid cysts.

Hydatid cysts are usually spherical, turgid, and fluid filled. They commonly measure 5–10 cm in diameter in domestic animals; rarely, cysts in animals may be larger, but in humans, hydatid cysts can become huge. On the other hand, some fertile cysts in horse livers may be as small as 2 to 3 mm across. The lining of fertile cysts is studded with small, granular brood capsules, and hydatid sand is in the fluid. The lining of sterile cysts is smooth. Though the potential exists for development of internal daughter cysts, and rare exogenous budding by herniated cysts, most hydatid cysts in domestic animals are unilocular. They may be irregular or distorted in shape, however, due to the variable resistance of parenchyma and portal tracts or bronchi and the differing profiles of bone or other resistant tissues. A single cyst or up to several hundred may be present, displacing tissue in infected organs. Disease is rarely attributed to hydatidosis in animals, even in those heavily infected.

Immature hydatid cysts are surrounded by an infiltrate of mixed inflammatory cells including giant cells and eosinophils. As they develop, a layer of granulation tissue, which may contain round cells and eosinophils, invests the cysts, and this evolves so that the inner portion of the fibrous capsule is composed of mature collagenous connective tissue, which is relatively acellular. Within this, and in close apposition, is the lamellar hyaline outer layer of the hydatid cyst wall, which with time may become hundreds of micrometers thick. The cyst is lined by the thin, cellular germinal layer, from which the brood capsules form on fine pedicles.

Hydatid cysts frequently degenerate. The inner structures collapse, and the mass becomes caseous and may mineralize. Degenerate hydatid cysts may resemble tuberculous lesions or squamous-cell carcinoma but for the fact that they can often be shelled out of the fibrous capsule. In section, among necrotic debris, macrophages and giant cells, remnants of the lamellar outer membrane, and perhaps the rostellar hooklets of degenerate protoscolices may be recognized, confirming the origin of the lesion.

Echinococcus multilocularis has a holarctic distribution, the adults occurring mainly in foxes, and the metacestodes in small rodents, especially voles and lemmings. Dogs and cats may also become infected with the worms in enzootic areas. Though the parasite is principally arctic, the cycle is found in the northern prairie area of North America as far south as Iowa, and in parts of central and western Europe. The mature cestodes in the intestine are similar to, but smaller than, *E. granulosus*. In the intermediate host, the metacestode infects mainly the liver, forming a cystic structure with internal brood capsules and protoscolices; but it is capable of external budding. As a result, racemose proliferative masses of metacestodes infiltrate infected livers. They may metastasize via the bloodstream to the lungs or bone, or implant in the peritoneal cavity. The inflammatory reaction to alveolar hydatids is composed of macrophages, perhaps giant cells, lymphocytes, and plasma cells in an encapsulating fibrous stroma. The metacestodes are rarely found in domestic animals but they infect humans exposed to the eggs shed by infected carnivores.

Intestinal Fluke Infection

Trematode infections of the intestine of domestic animals are, on the whole, uncommon. Dogs and cats in many parts of the world may be infected with *Alaria*, the second intermediate hosts for which are frogs or other amphibians. *Heterophyes heterophyes*, *Metagonimus yokagawi*, and *Echinochasmus perfoliatus* may infect dogs and cats fed fish containing metacercariae. The former two occur in the Mediterranean area and the Far East; the latter in Eurasia. *Cryptocotyle*, most commonly parasitic in piscivorous birds, may also be found in dogs, cats, and mink fed infected marine fish. Enteritis is attributed to *Alaria*, *Echinochasmus*, and *Cryptocotyle*. The effects are related to attachment of flukes to the mucosa by suckers, and perhaps to local irritation, erosion, and ulceration, which large numbers of them may induce. The production of excessive intestinal mucus, and hemorrhagic enteritis, have been associated with intestinal fluke infection in small animals. The flukes involved are small, less than 4 to 5 mm long, and must be sought carefully at autopsy.

Nanophyetus salmincola occurs in the small intestine of dogs and cats, and a wide variety of fish-eating wild mammals, birds, and people in the northwestern United States and eastern Siberia. Its distribution is determined by that of the snails that are the first intermediate hosts. The second intermediate hosts are various fish, especially Salmonidae. The adult flukes inhibit the small intestine, where they penetrate and attach to the mucosa. Large numbers may cause mucoid or hemorrhagic enteritis. *Nanophyetus salmincola*, however, transmits the distinct rickettsia of Elokomin fluke fever and salmon-poisoning disease. The former is caused by a distinct rickettsia and affects a wide range of carnivores, while salmon-poisoning disease may be caused by *Neorickettsia helminthoeca* alone or possibly in combination with the agent of Elokomin fluke fever. *Neorickettsia helminthoeca* causes disease only in Canidae. Both diseases are reported only in North America.

Salmon poisoning disease has an incubation period of about 5 to 7 days and is characterized clinically by pyrexia, anorexia, depression, weakness, and weight loss. There may be serous nasal discharge and mucopurulent conjunctivitis. Diarrhea with tenesmus develops; feces are scant, yellowish, and mucoid or watery, perhaps with some blood. The condition usually is fatal, only 5–10% of infected dogs recovering. These dogs are immune to reinfection. At autopsy, lesions are most consistently found in the lymphoid tissues. There is generalized enlargement of lymph nodes, especially in the abdominal cavity. Involved nodes are edematous, and on cut surface they have a yellowish hue with prominent cortical follicles. Enlarged tonsils are everted from their fossae. The thymus is often increased in size in young dogs, and the spleen may be swollen and congested. Prominent splenic lymphoid tissue has been reported in foxes but is not obvious in dogs. Intestinal lymphoid tissue stands out prominently. Peyer's patches and other intestinal lymphoid aggregates are elevated above the mucosal surface, and there may

be petechial hemorrhages on the mucosa. Lymphoid tissue near the ileocecalcolic valve may ulcerate and bleed. Ileocolic intussusception occurs in many cases. The liver of foxes becomes friable and may rupture, causing hemorrhage into the peritoneal cavity. Focal hemorrhages may be seen in the mucosa of the bladder, and subpleural hemorrhages up to 2.0 cm in diameter usually occur.

The microscopic changes in lymph nodes include depletion of lymphocytes, focal necrosis with neutrophilic infiltrates, and an increase in the number of histiocytes in the cortex and medulla. Similar changes may occur in the thymus, and splenic follicles may undergo necrosis. Elementary bodies of *Neorickettsia* may be demonstrated by use of Giemsa or Macchiavello stains in the cytoplasm of macrophages in lymphoid tissue and in other visceral organs. In the small intestine, the flukes may be present embedded deep in the mucosa, though usually little reaction to them is present.

Lesions of the central nervous system occur in the great majority of cases. Leptomeninges may be somewhat opaque, but the lesions are best recognized microscopically. They are composed of macrophage accumulations in the leptomeninges and Virchow–Robin spaces, and focal gliosis in the parenchyma. Meningeal reaction is perhaps most consistent over the cerebellum and is composed of mild or moderate perivascular or more diffuse accumulations of histiocytes. Similar cells may cuff small- and medium-sized vessels throughout the parenchyma. Focal gliosis is relatively sparsely distributed but seems most common in the brain stem. Elementary bodies are also demonstrable in macrophages in the central nervous system, and the diagnosis is usually made on the basis of this finding in macrophages in lymphoid tissue and/or brain. The organisms can be isolated and grown on primary canine monocyte cultures and in several other cell culture systems, but this is not a routine procedure.

Paramphistome infections in **ruminants** may cause significant intestinal disease. Adults of the genera *Paramphistomum*, *Cotylophoron*, *Calicophoron*, *Ceylonocotyle*, *Gastrothylax*, *Fischoederius*, and *Carmyerius* occur in the forestomachs of ruminants, including sheep or cattle, or both, in various areas around the world. Infection is most common in warm temperate to tropical areas. In the rumen, the reddish, pear-shaped adult flukes, with their characteristic anterior and posterior suckers, are considered innocuous, though some papillae may become atrophic and slough. Metacercariae encysted on herbage give rise to immature flukes, which inhabit the duodenum, where massive infections may cause severe enteritis. In cattle, water buffalo, and bison, the species incriminated in disease include *P. cervi*, *P. microbothrium*, *P. explanatum*, *Calicophoron calicophorum*, and various species of *Cotylophoron*, *Gastrothylax*, and *Fischoederius*. In sheep and goats, *P. microbothrium*, *P. ichikawai*, *P. cervi*, *P. explanatum*, *G. crumenifer*, *Cotylophoron cotylophorum*, and *F. cobboldi* have been associated with disease. The species involved vary with the host and geographic area. After about 3 to 5 weeks in the small intestine, the worms normally migrate forward, through the abomasum, to establish and mature in the reticulorumen. If massive infection occurs, however, growth in the small intestine is retarded, and flukes may persist for months in the duodenum, prolonging the course of disease.

Calves and lambs with intestinal paramphistomosis are depressed and inappetent. Fetid diarrhea usually develops within several weeks of infection and may contain immature flukes. Soiling of the perineum and escutcheon, and tenesmus, may be severe. Hypoproteinemia is reflected in submandibular edema in some animals, and anemia has been reported to occur occasionally. Sheep may die within 5 to 10 days, and cattle and water buffalo after a course of 2 to 3 weeks of disease. Morbidity and mortality can be substantial, and survivors may suffer considerable loss in condition. The carcass may be in good or cachectic condition, depending on the duration of the disease, and there may be edema of subcutaneous tissues, abomasal folds, and mesentery and fluid in the body cavities, due to hypoproteinemia. The gallbladder is frequently distended with bile, associated with inappetence. The mesenteric lymph nodes are enlarged and edematous. The anterior small intestine appears congested externally, and immature paramphistomes, deeply penetrating the intestinal wall, may be visible through the serosa. Occasionally they will perforate the gut and be found free in the abdominal cavity. The mucosal surface of the duodenum is edematous, thickened, corrugated, and covered with mucus. Many immature pink or brown paramphistomes, a few millimeters long, are scattered over the surface and embedded in the mucosa. Some are free in clusters in the lumen, and the digesta, which is thin and mucoid, may appear somewhat blood tinged. Most larval paramphistomes are in the first 3 m of small intestine. In advanced infections, some may be present migrating forward on the abomasal mucosa, or already in the forestomachs.

In section, small larval paramphistomes are found deep in the lamina propria, occasionally in the submucosa, or perhaps in Brunner's glands. Larger immature forms are attached to the surface of the mucosa by a plug of tissue taken into the acetabulum. There is atrophy of villi, elongation of crypts, and possibly erosion or ulceration of the mucosa in heavily infected areas. A mixed inflammatory infiltrate is in the lamina propria, but often, little specific reaction is present to flukes in tissue, the lesions are somewhat reminiscent of those in severe trichostrongylosis but for the difference in appearance of the offending helminths. Protein loss into the gut, coupled with loss of appetite, seems to be the most important pathophysiologic consequence. The pathogenesis of the diarrhea is unclear.

The other fluke occurring in the intestine of ruminants is *Skjrabinotrema ovis*, associated with catarrhal enteritis in sheep in Eurasia.

In swine, the paramphistomes *Gastrodiscoides* and *Gastrodiscus* may be found in the colon, where they are of little significance. *Fasciolopsis buski* may also infect the small intestine of swine as well as humans. It is of little importance in pigs other than as a reservoir for human infection.

In horses in Africa and India, the paramphistomes *Gastrodiscus aegyptiacus* and *Pseudodiscus colinsi* occur in the large bowel. Larvae of the former species have been associated with severe colitis in horses, but they are generally nonpathogenic.

Intestinal schistosomiasis, due mainly to *Schistosoma* in ruminants, and *Heterobilharzia* in dogs, may cause protein-losing enteropathy, associated perhaps with granulomatous enteritis in response to deposition of ova in mucosal venules (see the Cardiovascular System, Volume 3).

Flukes in tissue section are generally somewhat flattened or globose, with a loose mesenchymal parenchyma in which the internal structures are suspended. The cuticle is eosinophilic and may be spiny. Muscular oral and acetabular suckers, and pharynx, may be encountered in sections. Ceca are usually present, and elements of the male and female reproductive systems in these typically hemaphroditic adult worms (excepting the schistosomes) may be seen. The uterus may contain ova with a tan-yellow or brown shell, perhaps with an operculum, and ova are often seen in the intestinal lumen or in tissue. The developing miracidium may be present in ova. Schistosomes are recognized by their intravascular location and sexual dimorphism, the leaf-like male perhaps enveloping the slender cylindrical female within the gynocophoric canal in section.

Acanthocephalan Infection

The Acanthocephala are a phylum of parasitic animals, apparently related to the Nematoda, that have an elongate, saclike body, no internal alimentary canal, and use as the holdfast a spiny protrusible proboscis. The life cycle typically involves obligate development in an intermediate host, usually an arthropod, and perhaps the utilization of a paratenic host to facilitate transmission. The Acanthocephala of concern in domestic animals are in the genera *Macracanthorynchus* and *Oncicola*.

Macracanthorynchus hirudinaceus is the thorny-headed worm of swine, infecting the small intestine. The life cycle involves dung beetles or other Scarabaeidae, and foraging or rooting swine are prone to infection. Males are ~10 cm long, and the females up to 30 to 40 cm long, slightly pink, curved, and tapering posteriorly. The proboscis has about six rows of hooks and is used to penetrate deeply the intestinal wall. It incites a local granulomatous nodule called a "strawberry mark," with a purulent focus about the embedded proboscis. The proboscis may penetrate the muscularis, and the nodules, up to a centimeter or more in diameter, may be visible on the serosal surface of the gut as gray or yellow suppurative foci, surrounded by a halo of hyperemic tissue. They occasionally perforate, causing peritonitis. As the parasites move about in the gut, abandoned sites of attachment granulate, forming a firm, fibrous nodule, which may persist for some time in the wall of the gut. Severely infected pigs may suffer ill thrift and perhaps anemia, probably related partly to the potential for plasma protein loss and hemorrhage from numerous focal ulcerative lesions. *Macracanthorynchus catalinum* and *M. ingens* are smaller but similar thorny-headed worms that inhibit the intestine of a variety of wild carnivores, and occasionally the dog.

Oncicola canis occurs in the small intestine of wild carnivores, and occasionally the dog and cat. Intermediate hosts are presumably arthropods, with insectivorous vertebrates acting as paratenic hosts. Up to several hundred worms, 0.5–1.5 cm long and dark gray, may infest the small intestine; infections usually are light. The proboscis is embedded to the subserosal level, and a focal nodular lesion develops about it. Associated disease, or complications such as perforation, are apparently rare.

Protozoal Enteritis

Coccidiosis

The coccidia are members of the protozoan phylum Apicomplexa, intracellular parasites characterized at some stage of the life cycle by a typical "apical complex" of organelles at one end of the organism. Members of the suborder Eimeriina, which we shall consider together here, all have a similar basic life cycle. It begins with infection of a cell, usually in the intestinal mucosa, by a sporozoite released from a sporocyst in the lumen of the gut. One or more stages of asexual division, termed schizogony or merogony, follow, and the merozoites produced infect other cells. Separate sexual stages or gamonts subsequently develop into nonmotile macrogametes and motile male forms or microgametes. A nonmotile zygote produced by union of micro- and macrogametes forms an oocyst. Sporogony, or production of sporocysts containing infectious sporozoites within the oocyst, may occur in the host, or more commonly after the resistant oocysts are passed in feces. Members of the genus *Eimeria* are homoxenous, sexual and asexual development taking place in a single host. *Isospora* may be homo- or heteroxenous (*Cystoisospora*), with asexual stages occurring in an intermediate host. The members of the genera *Toxoplasma*, *Sarcocystis*, *Hammondia*, *Besnoitia*, and *Frenkelia* are all heteroxenous. The heteroxenous genera exploit natural prey–predator relationships. Sexual development takes place in the intestinal mucosa of a predator. At least one generation of asexual replication, often several, occurs in the tissues of one or more species of prey.

In the domestic animals we are considering, asexual and sexual development of *Eimeria* is limited normally to the intestinal mucosa and may involve stages within the lamina propria or epithelium. In the definitive host, asexual and sexual development of the *Isospora* species parasitic in domestic animals is also usually limited to the intestinal mucosa. In the heteroxenous *Isospora*, *Toxoplasma*, *Sarcocystis*, *Hammondia*, *Besnoitia*, and *Frenkelia*, asexual stages in the intermediate hosts may be found in a variety of tissues. Depending on the parasite and the stage of development, the range of tissues infected may be wide or narrow. As examples, *Toxoplasma* may infect phagocytic and parenchymal cells in many organs in the intermediate host, while *Sarcocystis* typically infects endothelium and, finally, myocytes.

The endogenous stages of coccidia are all intracellular, except, temporarily, the merozoite and microgamete. Mature developmental stages are usually readily recognized; immature forms may not be easily identifiable. Trophozoites, small, undifferentiated, rounded, basophilic forms with a single nucleus, within a parasitophorous vacuole in the host cell, are found in three stages of the life cycle: following invasion by the infective sporozoite, prior to merogony; following invasion by a merozoite, prior to a subsequent generation of merogony; following invasion by a merozoite, prior to differentiation into a recognizable gamont. Developing meronts or schizonts are multinucle-

ate. Merogony may occur by a variety of mechanisms that may or may not involve apparent "budding" of merozoites from the periphery of the meront or from infoldings of it. A single residual body, surrounded by slightly curved, fusiform, or banana-shaped, uninucleate merozoites, or many spherical clusters of merozoites with a central residuum, may be present. The location of a schizont, and the number of merozoites it contains, vary with the species and the generation of schizogony. A very few, or up to tens or hundreds of thousands of merozoites, may be released from a single schizont.

Microgamonts mature in two steps. The first involves enlargement of the gamont and proliferation of nuclei. During the second phase, the microgametes differentiate about the periphery of the gamont, which may become deeply folded or fissured by invaginations. Immature microgametocytes during these stages may resemble developing schizonts. However, fully differentiated microgametes differ from merozoites in being small, densely basophilic, comma-shaped, with two or three flagella. They may be present in swirling masses, perhaps with some residual bodies, in mature microgametocytes. Macrogametes, the female stage, have a large nucleus with a prominent nucleolus and with time usually enlarge to contain refractile eosinophilic "plastic granules" or wall-forming bodies, which give rise to the layers of the oocyst wall. Mature macrogametes typically have prominent wall-forming bodies and contain clear or PAS-positive amylopectin granules and a large nucleus and nucleolus.

Fertilization by the microgamete leads to development of the zygote and subsequent formation of the oocyst wall. The oocyst wall is composed of one or two clear or eosinophilic, refractile membranes in most species of coccidia, but the outer wall of some species can be very thick and densely amphophilic. The contained sporont is spherical, with nucleus and nucleolus, and amylopectin granules in the cytoplasm. Sporulation usually occurs outside the host, but in *Sarcocystis* and *Frenkelia*, it occurs in the tissue of the definitive host. Sporozoites are enclosed within sporocysts, which in turn are contained by the oocyst wall. Oocysts of most coccidia, or sporocysts of *Sarcocystis* and *Frenkelia*, are passed in the feces.

Coccidia are typically highly host, organ, and tissue specific. Species of coccidia rarely occur in more than one genus of host. Similar coccidia occurring in related genera of hosts, when tested, usually prove incapable of cross-infection. The coccidia of sheep and goats exemplify this, and our concepts of the species infecting these hosts have been modified considerably as a result. The epizootiologic connotations of high host specificity are obvious. Within a host, infections are commonly organ or site and tissue specific, so that a given life-cycle stage of a species of coccidium typically infects a certain type of cell at a particular level of the intestine or other target site. Asexual and sexual stages may have different site and tissue specificites. The location of the endogenous stages, and their morphology, may give a strong indication of the species of coccidium infecting the animal.

The economic cost of coccidiosis in cattle, sheep, and pigs is considerable, in terms of mortality, morbidity, subclinical disease, and the cost of prevention and treatment. It is even more so in chickens. In dogs and cats, coccidiosis is a minor problem, and in horses, coccidia probably do not cause disease. The development of coccidiosis is a function of the innate virulence of the organism, the size and viability of the inoculum, and the susceptibility of the host. Some species of coccidia are much more commonly associated with disease than others. Species virulence reflects a number of factors. Among these are the location and type of cell infected by various stages of the organism, the function of infected cells, and the degree of host reaction stimulated by infection. The biotic potential of the organism within the host (i.e., the degree of asexual replication) coupled with the size of inoculum determines to some extent the number of cells infected by subsequent asexual and sexual generations of the coccidium. Provided the later generations are pathogenic, a high biotic potential increases the virulence of the organism.

The effects of infection on the host cell are several and vary somewhat with the infecting species. Infected cells may be functionally compromised. They may hypertrophy; nuclei may enlarge or a considerable amount of cytoplasm may be displaced; and the outer membrane of infected cells may be modified highly, perhaps to facilitate metabolic exchange. The intercellular relationships may be affected. The rate of movement of infected epithelial cells up villi appears to be altered in some cases, and epithelial cells infected by some species seem more resistant to autolysis. At least in chickens, and perhaps in mammals, epithelial cells infected by coccidia may migrate into the lamina propria. The release of merozoites and oocysts is cytolytic, and if this is synchronous and widespread, as may occur in heavy infections, considerable loss of function may be expected. This may result in villus atrophy if many surface epithelial cells are lost, as in piglets infected by *Isospora suis*. On the other hand, massive coccidial infection and cytolysis in the intestinal crypts and glands may have a radiomimetic effect; erosion and ulceration of the colon is a sequel to severe cryptal damage in bovine coccidiosis.

Immunoinflammatory reactions may be incited by coccidial infection. In experimental systems, resistance to coccidial infection is thymus dependent and is largely mediated by functions of T cells other than as helper cells for immunoglobulin production. It seems to be directed mainly against asexual stages in the life cycle. Villus atrophy may also be related to cell-mediated immune reactions. In chickens infected with *Eimeria acervulina*, atrophy of villi is preceded by a hyperproliferative state in the crypts of Lieberkühn, characteristic of atrophy associated with cell-mediated immunity. In *E. neischultzi*–infected rats, the development of villus atrophy is also associated with competent cell-mediated immune mechanisms. Villus atrophy associated with chronic coccidiosis in sheep and goats perhaps has a similar pathogenesis.

In mammals, acute inflammatory reactions in intestinal coccidiosis are most commonly associated with heavy infection and destruction of cells by the sexual stages and oocysts, rather than in response to asexual stages. This contrasts with *Eimeria necatrix* infection in chickens, where acute hemorrhage occurs around schizonts in the lamina propria. In toxoplasmosis, necrosis and focal acute or chronic inflammatory reactions may be incited by actively replicating asexual stages in many organs. A syndrome characterized by hemorrhage occurs in some species infected with asexual stages of *Sarcocystis*, about the time that merogony occurs in vascular endothelium. This may be mediated in part by endothelial damage and by activation and consumption of clotting factors.

The effects of intestinal coccidiosis in mammals vary with the host–parasite system. They mainly relate to malabsorption induced by villus atrophy, or to anemia, hypoproteinemia, and dehydration due to exudative enteritis and colitis caused by epithelial erosion and ulceration. Many species of coccidia appear to have little pathogenic effect under normal circumstances. This may reflect relative insulation from host defense mechanisms due to their largely intraepithelial location or it may be associated with a relatively low biotic potential. However, even some species of coccidia developing in cells in the lamina propria, in large numbers, seem innocuous.

Coccidiosis is typically a disease of intensively managed animals. It is especially important in susceptible young animals exposed to a high level of infection. This is predisposed by high contamination rates associated with crowding, yarding, or high stocking rates on pasture. A damp substrate promotes oocyst sporulation and survival, and practices such as feeding on the ground, or the natural propensity of young animals to nibble or perhaps indulge in coprophagy, may promote infection. Although infections may not proceed to patency, chronic ingestion of oocysts may cause an intestinal immune response, villus atrophy, and perhaps ill thrift in some situations. Immune reactions may only halt development of, but not kill, endogenous asexual stages. Epizootiologic evidence suggests that under some circumstances there may be relaxation of resistance and resumption of development of the organisms, ultimately expressed in disease. This seems the likely explanation for outbreaks of bovine coccidiosis occurring during midwinter in freezing climates, or in postparturient stabled dairy cattle.

The members of the genera *Eimeria* and *Isospora,* and coccidiosis caused by them in the various species, will be considered further here. Cryptosporidiosis and the heteroxenous cyst-forming organisms, including *Toxoplasma* and *Sarcocystis,* will be considered subsequently.

CATTLE. About 13 species of *Eimeria* parasitize cattle; of these, *E. zuernii* and *E. bovis* are potentially highly pathogenic, while several others, notably *E. ellipsoidalis* and *E. auburnensis,* may cause diarrhea, but probably not death. Coccidial infection is common and usually comprises a mixture of species. Disease occurs mainly in calves or weaned feeder cattle under about a year of age, if one or both of the potentially pathogenic species produce heavy infection. It may occur in animals at range, concentrated at waterholes, but is most common in animals in feedlots or yards, where the level of sanitation is not high. The stress of shipping, cold weather, or intercurrent disease may be associated with outbreaks, which can occur in midwinter, when oocyst transmission is expected to be poor. Morbidity may be high, but mortality is usually low. The disease is characterized by diarrhea, which may progress to dysentery with mucus, and tenesmus, perhaps causing rectal prolapse. Animals dehydrate and become hyponatremic and perhaps anemic. The duration of severe disease is about 3–10 days, after which most cases recover, since infection is essentially self-limiting. Some animals develop concurrent nervous signs, including tremors, nystagmus, opisthotonus, and convulsions, and many of these die within a few days.

The signs in bovine coccidiosis due to *Eimeria zuernii* and *E. bovis* occur when the epithelium in the glands of the cecum and colon is infected by second-generation schizonts and gametocytes. In heavily infected animals, disease, and perhaps death, can occur before many oocysts are passed in the feces. The life cycles of both agents are similar, two schizogonous generations preceding gametogony. The first-generation schizont of *E. bovis* infects hypertrophic endothelial cells in lacteals on the upper part of villi in the lower small intestine, several meters proximal to the ileocecal valve. These schizonts may be large, up to ~300 μm in diameter, and are visible to the naked eye as pinpoint white nodular foci in the mucosa. They contain tens of thousands of merozoites but are invested by only a narrow rim of mononuclear inflammatory cells, unless they degenerate, when a marked local mixed reaction develops, including neutrophils and macrophages. Merozoites released from these schizonts about 14–18 days after infection enter cells deep in cecal and colonic glands. In heavy infections, crypts of Lieberkühn in the terminal ileum may also be infected. Here they produce small, second-generation schizonts, which in turn release merozoites, infecting other cells in the gland. Gametogony may begin as early as 15 days after infection, and oocyst production peaks about 19–21 days after infection.

The first generation schizonts of *Eimeria zuernii* may be about the same size as those of *E. bovis*. They are most common in the terminal meter of the ileum, however, and are located in the lamina propria below the crypt–villus junction, often deep near the muscularis mucosae rather than in the endothelium of the lacteal. Hence, they are not so readily visible grossly as those of *E. bovis*. The second-generation schizonts and gamonts of *E. zuernii* also occur in glands of the cecum and colon, but not the terminal ileum. The merozoites tend to be somewhat longer (up to 15 μm) and the schizonts more numerous and of greater diameter (~14 μm) than those of *E. bovis*. The timing of the development of *E. zuernii* infection is similar to that of *E. bovis*.

Animals dying of coccidiosis have fecal staining of the hindquarters, and may be somewhat cachectic and anemic. The gross lesions in severe cases are those of fibrinohemorrhagic typhlocolitis, which may extend to the rectum; if *Eimeria bovis* is involved, the terminal ileum may be affected (Fig. 1.47A), and perhaps a few schizonts will be visible in ileal villi. The contents of the large bowel are usually abnormally fluid and may vary from brown to black to overtly bloody, possibly with flecks of mucus or fibrin. The mucosa is edematous, with exaggerated longitudinal and perhaps transverse folds, which may be congested in a "tiger stripe" pattern, or more diffusely petechiated. Submucosal edema is also marked. Fibrin strands or a patchy diphtheritic membrane may be present on the mucosa (Fig. 1.47B), and fibrin casts can form. In milder cases, lesions are limited to congestion and edema of the mucosa.

In animals dying at the peak of infection, virtually all cells lining cecal and colonic glands in many areas are infected by small schizonts, gamonts, or developing oocysts. Cells infected by *Eimeria bovis* tend to dissociate and project into the lumen of the gland. Where infected epithelium remains more or less intact, the surface does not erode, and effusion of exudate is not apparent. As cells are disrupted and oocysts are released into the lumen of glands, however, the remaining glandular epithelium becomes extremely attenuated, or the gland collapses (Fig. 1.47C,E). Concurrently, the surface epithelium becomes squamous, or the mucosa is eroded, and effusion of fibrin, neutrophils, and some hemorrhage occurs from dilated, congested superficial vessels. Oocysts released into the lumen of the colon may be seen in the exudate (Fig. 1.47D). At the same time, the mucosa begins to collapse, and the lamina propria is infiltrated by neutrophils, eosinophils, lymphocytes, macrophages, and plasma cells. Oocysts trapped in denuded glands in the collapsed mucosa may be surrounded by small giant cells.

If destruction is widespread, and the animal survives sufficiently long, the mucosa may ulcerate to the level of the muscularis mucosae and begin to granulate. In areas where the lesion is patchy, glands that have been relatively spared may become lined with hyperplastic epithelium, making an attempt to regenerate the mucosa. Flattened epithelial cells spread from these glands across the denuded surface, beneath the diphtheritic exudate. A few crenated oocysts in small giant cells in the stromal remnants of the mucosa may be all the evidence of coccidiosis found in lesions in animals surviving for 7 to 10 days.

Malabsorption due to mucosal damage in the cecum and colon, and inflammatory effusion and hemorrhage, explain the enteric signs of coccidiosis. The nervous signs in bovine coccidiosis are not associated with recognized lesions in the brain, and their cause remains unknown.

The gross lesions of coccidiosis in cattle must be differentiated from those in salmonellosis, bovine virus diarrhea, rinderpest, malignant catarrhal fever, and bovine adenovirus infection, all of which may cause typhlocolitis. Coccidiosis can often be simply confirmed at autopsy by finding developing stages in mucosal scrapings. Oocysts of *Eimeria bovis* are ovoid, smooth, and about 28 × 21 μm; those of *E. zuernii* are subspherical to ovoid, smooth, and about 18 × 15 μm.

While other coccidia are unlikely to be the primary cause of diarrhea or death in cattle, several have distinctive endogenous stages that may be recognized in tissue section. *Eimeria auburnensis* has a giant first-generation schizont that may be confused with those of *E. bovis* and *E. zuernii*. They are present, however, usually 6–12 m cranial to the ileocecal valve, and form in the epithelium deep in crypts of Lieberkühn, though this may not be apparent due to plane of section or migration into the lamina propria. Second-generation schizonts and gamonts of *E. auburnensis* develop in the lamina propria in the ileum, small schizonts in villi, and gamonts in the deeper lamina propria. Microgametocytes may be several hundred micrometers across. Oocysts are about 38 × 23 μm. The other bovine coccidium with gamonts apparently developing in the lamina propria is *E. bukidnonensis*. Oocysts of this species are large, about 48 × 35 μm and thick walled, with a micropyle, and have been found in the lamina propria. *Eimeria alabamensis* develops in vacuoles within the nucleus of epithelial cells in small intestine and, in heavy infections, the large bowel. Both schizonts and gamonts may be found together within the same nucleus. Gamonts of *E. kosti* have been described in the epithelium deep in the abomasal glands. None of these organisms is considered particularly pathogenic.

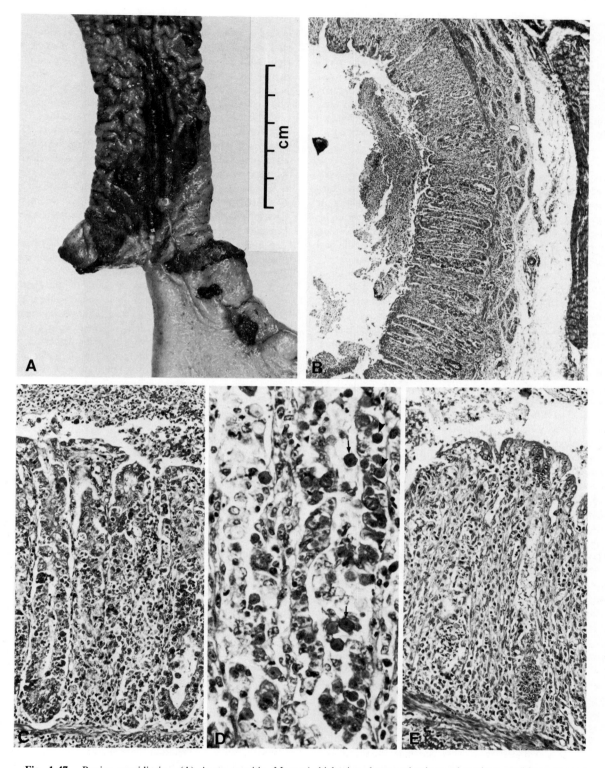

Fig. 1.47. Bovine coccidiosis. (**A**) Acute enteritis. Mucosal thickening, large and minute ulcerations, and hemorrhages. (**B**) Damaged colonic glands and inflammatory exudate. (**C**) Heavy infection and destruction of colonic glands by gamonts. Exudate covers mucosa. (**D**) Destruction of colonic glands by developing gamonts (arrowheads). Oocysts are in the lumen of some glands (arrows). (**E**) Destruction of colonic glands. Only a few glands remain in the mucosa.

Eimeria bareillyi is associated with clinical coccidiosis in water buffalo calves. The serosal vessels in the distal half of the small intestine are congested, and the lumen of the lower small bowel contains creamy or yellow fluid content in which some mucus, fibrin, or blood may be present. Focal to coalescent pale raised plaques or polypoid masses may be present on the mucosa, or the surface may appear granular and necrotic, with petechial hemorrhages. The gross changes are caused by hypertrophy of crypts and villi, upon which virtually every cell is infected with developing gamonts or oocysts.

SHEEP AND GOATS. Coccidial infection is virtually universal in sheep and goats, and coccidiosis can be a significant problem in the young of both species. Consideration of the etiology of coccidiosis in these species is complicated by the morphologic similarity of the coccidia infecting sheep and goats. Former assumptions on the potential for cross-infection of coccidia between sheep and goats, and of the species found in each host, have been revised considerably as new taxonomic and biologic information has come to light.

At present, about a dozen species of coccidia each are found in sheep and goats. Of these, seven (*Eimeria crandallis, E. faurei, E. granulosa, E. intricata, E. pallida, E. parva,* and *E. punctata*) are recognized in both sheep and goats, and among these further taxonomic revision is expected. *Eimeria ninakohlyakimovae, E. arloingi, E. christenseni, E. caprovina,* and *E. caprina* occur in goats; *E. ahsata, E. ovinoidalis* (formerly *E. ninakohlyakimovae*), *E. ovina* (formerly *E. arloingi* "A"), *E. weybridgensis* (formerly *E. arloingi* "B"), and *E. marsica* are found in sheep. In addition, giant schizonts of unknown coccidia, termed *Globidium gilruthi,* are seen incidentally as pinpoint white foci in the abomasum of sheep and goats. The taxonomic confusion has been carried over into descriptions of the natural or experimental disease, since many infections were of mixed species, resulted from inocula of poorly defined species of coccidia, or occurred under circumstances where the oocysts associated were not described. While the taxonomic picture has changed, the syndromes associated with coccidiosis in sheep and goats have not.

Coccidiosis in these species is a disease of young animals. Under conditions of intensive pastoral husbandry or confinement, lambs and kids are exposed to oocysts of many species of coccidia within the first few days of life. Oocyst production peaks fairly rapidly between 20 and 90 days of age, sometimes at levels of millions of oocysts per gram of feces. It then gradually drops off, but usually persists for the rest of the animal's life. A degree of protection against subsequent challenge with oocysts of a species of coccidium is conferred by previous infection with that species. Coccidiosis seems to occur mainly in susceptible animals, those with relatively limited experience of infection, exposed to conditions where infection pressure is relatively high. Hence the disease may occur in lambs and kids held in sheds or yards with the ewes or does. Under these circumstances, animals as young a 3 weeks of age may develop signs and perhaps die. Weaned lambs, presumably exposed to only light infections while at range, are also prone to coccidiosis when brought into feedlots. In young, suckled animals and those in feedlots, exposed to large numbers of oocysts, signs may occur before oocysts are passed. Suckling lambs, about 5–8 weeks old, reared at pasture at relatively heavy stocking rates, may also develop signs and occasionally die. Under these conditions, the disease needs to be differentiated from gastrointestinal helminthosis, which may be concurrent.

Outbreaks of coccidiosis in confined lambs and kids are usually acute and characterized by moderate morbidity and low mortality; there is green or yellow, watery diarrhea, occasionally with blood or mucus. Yarded and grazing animals may also suffer weight loss or subclinical ill thrift. Signs are usually associated with infection by species developing in the lower small intestine and perhaps large bowel, including *Eimeria ovinoidalis, E. ahsata,* and *E. ovina* in lambs, and their analogs in goats, *E. ninakohlyakimovae, E. christenseni,* and *E. arloingi.* Infections are usually mixed, and gross and microscopic lesions may be expected to reflect this.

Eimeria ovinoidalis in sheep and *E. ninakohlyakimovae* in goats presumably have similar endogenous development. In the sheep, giant schizonts up to 300 μm in diameter develop in cells deep in the lamina propria, in the terminal ileum. They release merozoites that enter epithelium in the glands of the cecum and colon, and perhaps distal ileum. There small, second-generation schizonts evolve, and other cells in glands in the same area subsequently become infected by the gametocytes. These species are considered highly pathogenic, and *E. ovinoidalis* is a species often encountered in association with disease in feedlot lambs. Lesions other than those related to diarrhea, dehydration, and hypoproteinemia are limited to the terminal ileum, and especially the cecum and proximal colon, and are associated with second-generation schizogony and gametogony. Affected areas of gut are edematous and thickened, and there may be focal or more diffuse congestion and hemorrhage in the mucosa. Heavily infected animals may have bloodstained feces. Occasionally, pinpoint white foci, the giant schizonts, may be seen in the mucosa of the ileum. In sections, schizonts and gamonts are in many or most cells lining glands in affected areas. Neutrophils and macrophages may accumulate in response to merozoites released from ruptured giant schizonts, but the most significant microscopic lesions are those in the cecum and colon, which resemble those in cattle due to *E. bovis* and *E. zuernii.*

Eimeria christenseni and *E. arloingi* in goats and *E. ahsata* and *E. ovina* in sheep are also associated with serious disease. They seem to have somewhat similar developmental cycles and lesions, though interpretation of the literature is clouded by confusion among these species. Many cases of coccidiosis in lambs attributed to *E. arloingi* (*E. ovina*) may have in fact been due to *E. ahsata,* since the unsporulated oocysts, though of differing sizes, can be confused.

Eimeria christenseni has a developmental cycle that involves giant schizonts up to nearly 300 μm across in the endothelium of the lacteal in villi in the middle small intestine. The more mature of these may detach and appear to lie free in the lacteal, dilating the villi. Second-generation schizogony, and gametogony, occur in epithelial cells lining the crypts and villi, mainly in the small intestine 4–6 m below the abomasum, but in heavy infections, also in terminal small bowel. Gamonts are usually below the host-cell nucleus, though this is variable, and multiple infections of host cells are common. In heavy infections, every cell in a number of contiguous crypt–villus units may be infected. Though there may be an acute local reaction around ruptured primary schizonts, clinical disease is associated with the subsequent stages of development, diarrhea occurring during the late prepatent and patent periods. Affected intestine may be congested and edematous. Numerous pale white or yellow foci from a few millimeters up to a centimeter in diameter, often visible from the serosa, are present as slightly raised plaques on the mucosa of the small bowel. These foci are areas of intense infection of cryptal and villus epithelium by gamonts and developing oocysts. There may be some hemorrhage into the intestine, but the feces are rarely bloody.

Eimeria arloingi undergoes a development similar to that of *E. christenseni* (Fig. 1.48C,D) and causes similar gross and microscopic lesions in goats, with minor differences. First-generation schizonts are most numerous in the lacteals of villi in the lower jejunum, gamonts are mainly above the host-cell nucleus, and the associated, grossly visible plaques in the mucosa (Fig. 1.48A,B) may tend to be more distal in the small intestine, and occasionally involve the large bowel; *E. ahsata* and *E. ovina* in sheep are similar.

Nodular polypoid structures, sometimes pedunculate and about 0.3–1.5 cm in diameter, are encountered in the small intestinal mucosa of sheep and goats, usually as an incidental finding. These masses are composed of hypertrophic crypt–villus units, in which virtually every epithelial cell is infected by mainly gametocytic stages of coccidia. Adjacent mucosa appears normal and is uninfected. The term ''pseudoadenomatous'' has been used to describe these polypoid lesions and the plaques discussed above in coccidia-infected sheep and goats. The infected epithelial cells also appear somewhat hypertrophic, with eosinophilic cytoplasm, and often these coccidia-infected cells do not slough rapidly postmortem, in contrast to their uninfected fellows. This may aid a histologic diagnosis in otherwise autolytic gut in clinical cases. Why nodular masses of infected cells apparently persist in chronically infected animals without clinical disease is unclear.

Large schizonts are often encountered incidentally in submucosal lymphatics or in the subcortical or medullary sinusoids of mesenteric lymph nodes in sheep and goats. Sometimes they may be visible grossly in these locations as pinpoint white foci. Occasionally, coccidial gametocytes or oocysts may also develop in the mesenteric lymph nodes, where they may invoke a mild granulomatous reaction. These stages probably result from establishment of sporozoites or primary merozoites swept from the lacteal into the lymphatic drainage early in infection. Development in such locales is to be regarded as not uncommon, but aberrant, and likely dead-end. The species involved appear mainly to be those considered above, with a giant primary schizont developing in the lacteal.

Ill thrift and diarrhea in suckling or weanling lambs 5–6 weeks old, heavily stocked on pasture, may also be due to coccidiosis. In the United Kingdom, *Eimeria crandallis*, which develops largely in the ileum, and *E. ovinoidalis* are associated mainly with this syndrome. *Eimeria weybridgensis* (*E. arloingi* ''B''), which infects most of the length of the small intestine, may contribute also. Under some circumstances, several of these species cause villus atrophy in infected areas of intestine.

Villi may be stumpy or absent, and crypts are straight, hypertrophic, and contain proliferative epithelium. Asexual or, more commonly, sexual stages of coccidia are present in epithelium on the surface of the mucosa. Such lesions, if widespread, may cause malabsorption or perhaps be associated with protein-losing enteropathy. It is unclear whether atrophy of villi is the result of excess loss of epithelium directly due to the effects of coccidial infection or is mediated by an immune response. In addition to villus atrophy, which may cause subclinical disease, perhaps diarrhea but rarely death, mortality may be associated with the presence of a grossly congested or edematous thickened intestine or segment thereof.

Oocyst numbers are usually high in feces, but this is neither constant in, nor necessarily indicative of, coccidiosis. Mucosal scrapings or tissue sections of mucosa containing large numbers of asexual and gametogenous coccidial forms, in association with diarrhea, and perhaps some hemorrhage into the intestine, support the diagnosis in the absence of other syndromes such as gastrointestinal helminthosis. Bacterial enteritis, particularly clostridial enterotoxemia and septicemic pasteurellosis, and in young lambs and kids, viral diarrhea or cryptosporidiosis, must be differentiated. In light of the large number of relatively innocuous species of coccidia infecting sheep and goats, and the uncertainty of the lesions associated with some, sporulation and positive identification of oocysts in mucosal scrapings or feces is desirable.

HORSES. The only coccidium of horses reported with any frequency is *Eimeria leuckarti,* which is found in horses and donkeys the world over. In one survey of foals in the United States, it was found in nearly 60%. It may also occur in older animals. Its reputation for pathogenicity rests largely on the distinctive large gamonts found by pathologists in the lamina propria of the small intestine in animals dead of obscure enteric disease. Implication of *E. leuckarti* in the disease process is rarely, if ever, convincing, however, and it is encountered incidentally in the intestine of horses dead of other clearly defined conditions. Furthermore, heavy experimental inoculations, producing many gamonts in the gut and heavy oocyst passage, have failed to elicit clinical signs.

The stages present in the lamina propria of villi are giant microgametocytes and macrogametes, developing in markedly hypertrophic host cells, probably of mesenchymal origin (Fig. 1.48E). The microgametocytes are up to ~250 μm in diameter, and when mature they contain swirling masses of microgametes. Immature microgametocytes very much resemble some of the giant schizonts of other species of coccidia and have frequently been referred to as such; this stimulated the application of the term *Globidium* to the organism. Schizonts containing merozoites have never been recognized in this organism, however, nor in several similar species of coccidia developing in the lamina propria in other hosts. The macrogametes have distinctive large eosinophilic or PAS-positive granules, which may be individual or confluent. The host cells are markedly hypertrophic with a fibrillar periphery, and the enlarged nucleus forms a crescent along one side of the parasitophorous vacuole. There is no inflammatory response to the gamonts, and only a mild reaction to degenerate stages in the lamina propria.

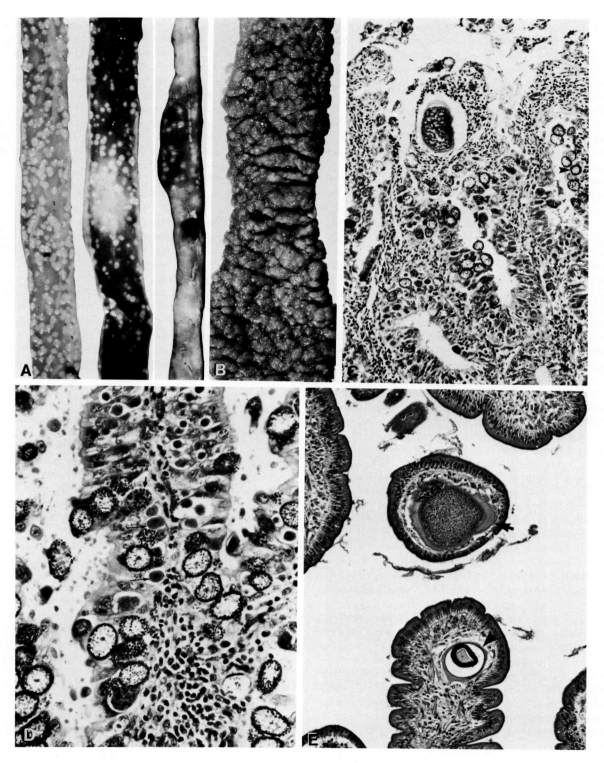

Fig. 1.48 Coccidiosis. **(A–D)** Goat. **(A)** White nodules on mucosa are visible from serosa (right). Hemorrhage in lumen. *Eimeria arloingi.* (Courtesy of P. A. Taylor.) **(B)** Chronic coccidiosis, showing mucosal hypertrophy. **(C)** *Eimeria arloingi.* Ileum. Large schizont in lacteal and gamonts (arrow) and developing occysts (arrowhead) in epithelium of crypts and villi. **(D)** *Eimeria arloingi.* Goat. Undifferentiated gamonts (long arrow), macrogametocytes (short arrow), and microgametocytes infect epithelial cells. **(E)** Microgametocyte (arrow) and developing oocyst (arrowhead) of *E. leuckarti* in lamina propria. Horse.

SWINE.   At least 8 to 10 species of *Eimeria* are thought to occur in swine, as does a single species of *Isospora*. The latter, *I. suis,* is the most important, causing porcine neonatal coccidiosis, a disease of piglets from about 5 or 6 days to about 2 to 3 weeks of age. This disease is recognized in the United States, Canada, the United Kingdom, and western Europe; it also occurs in Australia, and probably wherever swine are reared intensively. The condition is most severe in herds where continuous farrowing and total confinement are practiced, and some laboratories report a prevalence of 10 to 50% among scouring baby pigs.

Porcine neonatal coccidiosis has a high morbidity, and usually a low but variable mortality. It causes yellow, watery diarrhea, dehydration, loss of condition, and death, or at least temporary check in growth. Some animals may runt severely. Illness usually begins at about 7 to 10 days of age. Piglets continue to nurse but may vomit clotted milk. At autopsy, many piglets have the typical appearance of undifferentiated neonatal diarrhea, with no specific gross findings in the gastrointestinal tract other than fluid yellow content. The intestine in animals with coccidiosis may look turgid rather than flaccid, however, and in a minority of animals, a fibrinous or fibrinonecrotic exudate is present in the lower portion of the small intestine. Occasionally, casts will form.

Isospora suis replicates in the epithelium on the distal third of villi, mainly in the jejunum and ileum, though infected cells may be found in the duodenum and colon in a few animals. Piglets usually become infected within the first day or two of life, perhaps by coprophagy of the sow's feces. Merogony occurs in two phases in vacuoles in the cytoplasm of the host cell. Infection of host cells is maximal 4 or 5 days after infection, and by 5 days, gametogony is evident. The onset of lesions and clinical signs corresponds with this period of heavy infection of cells. Villi may become markedly atrophic (Fig. 1.49A). The surface epithelium that remains is cuboidal to squamous, and infected epithelial cells may be seen undergoing lysis. Erosions may develop at the tips of villi (Fig. 1.49B). In the remnant of the villus, neutrophil infiltration, a moderate increase in round cells, and an eosinophilic proteinaceous material, perhaps collagen, may be present in the lamina propria. Effusion of neutrophils and fibrin from the eroded tips of villi contributes to the fibrinonecrotic membrane seen in some animals, and ulceration can occur. Gram-positive cocci are often present in the exudate. In animals surviving for a few days, the cryptal epithelium may be markedly hyperplastic.

The severity of the lesions is a function of the size of the inoculum and the age of the pigs. Heavier inocula, within limits, produce more cellular damage and villus atrophy; fibrinonecrotic enteritis indicates ingestion of a large dose of oocysts. Severe lesions may not be associated with heavy shedding of oocysts, however, since relatively few gamonts are able to develop in the reduced population of epithelial cells remaining on villi. The severity of lesions and signs is much greater in piglets a few days old in comparison with those 2 weeks of age. This relates partly to the lower rate of replication of epithelium in the crypts of young piglets, and therefore, the development of more severe villus atrophy. The smaller size of young piglets also makes them more susceptible to dehydration. Animals previously exposed to *Isospora suis* have relatively strong resistance to challenge.

A diagnosis of coccidiosis must be considered in scouring piglets of the appropriate age group and is suggested strongly by the presence of fibrinonecrotic enteritis in the distal small bowel. Atrophy of villi may be recognized at autopsy using a hand lens or stereomicroscope, or in tissue section. Asexual or sexual stages may be found in smears of mucosal scrapings. The distinctive binucleate type 1 meronts and pairs of large (12–18 μm in smears, 8–13 μm in sections) type 1 merozoites may be found in jejunal mucosa in the early phase of diarrheal disease. Multinucleate type 2 meronts and numerous small type 2 merozoites are the predominant stage during the clinical phase of disease. In section, these form clusters of 2 to 16 organisms like bunches of bananas, perhaps with a small residual body, in the parasitophorous vacuole.

Macro- and microgamonts are present in moderate numbers by the fifth day of infection, and a few oocysts may also be seen. Microgametocytes are about 9–16 μm in diameter and are multinucleate while developing. Oocysts in tissue sections are oval, about 15 × 12 μm, while those in smears are about 18 × 16 μm. Coccidial stages may be difficult to find in animals that have been ill for several days. Oocysts may not be found in feces, either because the infection is not yet patent, the patent period has passed, or the lesions are very severe, reducing the number of oocysts produced.

Coccidiosis may occur concurrently with the other infectious and parasitic diseases causing diarrhea in neonatal pigs, and it also must be differentiated from them. If coccidia are found in atrophic mucosa, even associated with other agents, they should be considered potentially significant. Enterotoxic colibacillosis usually affects a younger age group, though some piglets with coccidiosis may also have adherent *Escherichia coli*. Rotavirus and coronavirus also cause villus atrophy and are the main conditions to differentiate from coccidiosis in animals with atrophic villi. When they occur together with coccidiosis, they may have additive effects.

Coccidiosis in older swine is due to several *Eimeria* species and is uncommon. It typically occurs in animals with access to yards or pasture contaminated with oocysts. Weaners and growing pigs are affected. The species considered potentially pathogenic include *E. debliecki, E. scabra,* and *E. spinosa*. Rare massive infections of some other species may also cause disease. Coccidiosis in swine due to *Eimeria* is usually sporadic or affects a few pigs in a group. Typically it causes diarrhea of a few days durations, loss of appetite, and perhaps transient ill thrift, or in severe cases, emaciation. Occasionally animals die.

Lesions are usually limited to the lower small intestine, which may be congested or hemorrhagic, though overt blood is rarely found in the feces. Large numbers of schizonts, gamonts, and developing oocysts are in epithelial cells on villi and sometimes in crypts. Atrophy of villi or erosion and local hemorrhage may be evident, the lamina propria is edematous, and desquamated epithelium and oocysts are in the lumen of the gut. Rarely, heavily infected animals may have lesions in the large intestine. The species involved are diagnosed on the basis of the morphology of oocysts in feces or mucosal scrapings.

Coccidial gamonts and oocysts of a species resembling

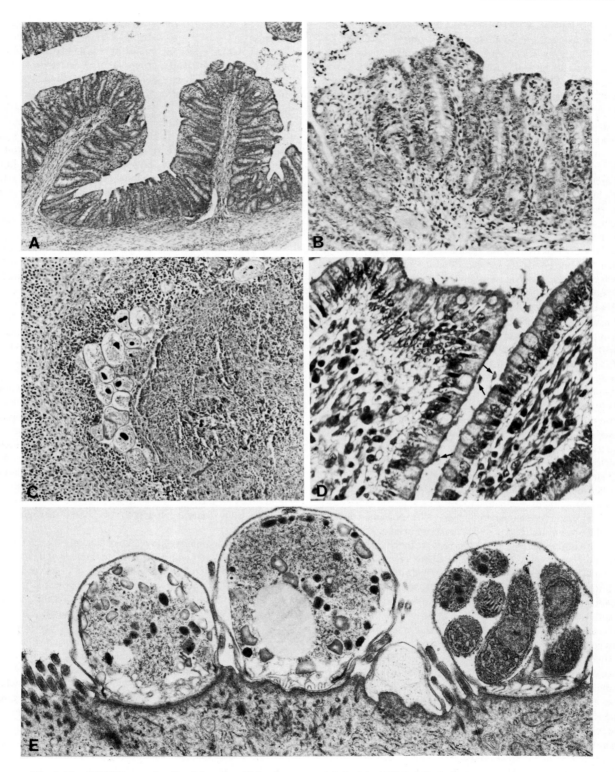

Fig. 1.49. **(A)** Villus atrophy. Small intestine. Piglet. *Isospora suis* infection. **(B)** Detail of **(A)**. Surface epithelium is severely attenuated, and there is some erosion and effusion at tips of villi. **(C)** *Balantidium coli* in ulcerated colon of pig with intestinal adenomatosis and necrotic enteritis. **(D)** *Giardia lamblia* (arrows) applied to brush border of enterocytes on villi. Cat. **(E)** Cryptosporidia attached to apex of enterocytes in small intestine. Two macrogametes, and a schizont containing merozoites. (Courtesy of S. Tzipori.)

Eimeria debliecki have been found infecting epithelium on the papilliform mucosa of cystic bile ducts in porcine liver. This is probably an aberrant site of development.

DOGS AND CATS.   Although several species of *Eimeria* have been reported from dogs and cats, their status as genuine parasites of these hosts is in doubt. The significant coccidia of dogs and cats are members of the genus *Isospora*, considered here, and *Toxoplasma, Sarcocystis, Hammondia,* and *Besnoitia,* dealt with subsequently.

Isospora is characterized by oocysts that are passed unsporulated in feces, and that when sporulated have two sporocysts, each with four sporozoites. Some species are apparently homoxenous, others heteroxenous. Following ingestion of sporulated oocysts, transport hosts, usually prey species such as mice and other small rodents, but sometimes other hosts, are infected by large sporozoite-like "hypnozoites" in phagocytic cells in lymph nodes and other tissues. These, when ingested by the predator, resume development in the intestine and lead to asexual and sexual development in the definitive host. Heteroxenous passage is not obligatory, and sporulated oocysts are also directly infective to the definitive host.

Coccidiosis in the dog and cat is largely a clinical entity, usually nonfatal. The lesions of coccidiosis in small animals are poorly defined, and care must be taken not to ascribe disease to these organisms simply on the basis of the presence of endogenous stages in the mucosa of animals dead of enteric disease. Rotavirus and coronavirus might be expected to produce similar signs. Some genuine cases of fatal coccidiosis do occur, however, though few are recorded in the literature. Affected animals are young and usually from environments such as pet shops, animal shelters, or kennels, where standards of sanitation may not be high. There is a history of diarrhea of several days duration, and the animal is dehydrated. Other than mild hyperemia of the mucosa and excessively fluid content of the small intestine and colon, gross lesions in the gut may not be evident. Microscopically, there may be moderate atrophy of villi, with attenuation of surface enterocytes, and perhaps effusion of acute inflammatory exudate from the tips of some eroded villi. Asexual and sexual stages of coccidia will be evident in moderate to large numbers in the epithelium or lamina propria of villi. In some cases the large bowel may be infected, with exfoliation of surface epithelium and the accumulation of necrotic debris in some dilated glands.

In dogs, four species of *Isospora* have been recognized, and the endogenous stages of these must be differentiated from those of *Hammondia* and *Sarcocystis*. Meronts of *I. canis* develop in the subepithelial lamina propria of the villi in the distal small intestine and, to a lesser extent, in large bowel. Gamonts occur beneath and within the epithelium of the ileum and large intestine, and the oocyst is the largest among *Isospora* of dogs, being about 38 × 30 μm. Endogenous stages of *I. burrowsi* occur in epithelial cells and in the lamina propria of the tips of villi in the distal two-thirds of the small intestine. *Isospora neorivolta* develops mainly in proprial cells beneath the epithelium in the tips of villi in the distal half of the small intestine, and rarely in the cecum and colon. Occasional stages may be in the epithelium.

Isospora ohioensis develops exclusively in epithelial cells, mainly in the distal portions of villi along the length of the small bowel, especially in the ileum, and occasionally in the large bowel. The oocysts of *I. burrowsi, I. ohioensis,* and *I. neorivolta* are similar. Original literature should be consulted for details that permit differentiation of these species in tissue. *Isospora canis* and *I. ohioensis* are known to be heteroxenous.

In cats, two heteroxenous *Isospora* species occur. Meronts and gamonts of *I. felis* develop in epithelium of villi in the small intestine, and occasionally in epithelium in the large bowel. The oocyst is large, about 43 × 33 μm. *Isospora rivolta* also develops in epithelium on villi and in crypts and glands in the small and large intestine. Oocysts are ovoid, about 25 × 23 μm.

TOXOPLASMA, SARCOCYSTIS, BESNOITIA, HAMMONDIA, AND FRENKELIA.   These heteroxenous members of the Apicomplexa utilize carnivores as definitive hosts and have one or more generations of merogony in the tissues of various species of prey. *Frenkelia,* as far as is known, utilizes only raptorial birds as definitive hosts, and small rodents as intermediate hosts. It will not be considered further.

Toxoplasma gondii uses members of the Felidae as definitive hosts. The organism is optionally heteroxenous; cats may be infected directly by ingestion of oocysts, or probably most commonly by ingestion of asexual stages developing in the tissues of prey species. These intermediate hosts are infected by oocysts shed in the feces of cats, or perhaps by a variety of other routes considered below. Five stages of asexual development have been recognized in the intestinal epithelium of cats infected with tissue cysts from intermediate hosts. The gametocytes also develop in epithelium on villi, especially in the ileum. In heavy infections, exfoliation of infected epithelium from villi is associated with the development of villus atrophy, and occasional spontaneous cases of diarrhea in kittens seem to be caused by *Toxoplasma*-induced atrophy of villi and malabsorption.

In intermediate hosts, and in cats, extraintestinal asexual development occurs in a variety of organs and tissues. Rapidly dividing forms (tachyzoites) may proliferate in many sites for an indefinite number of generations and are the stage associated with acute toxoplasmosis in cats and other species. Eventually, tachyzoites enter host cells, induce the formation of a cyst wall, and divide slowly by endodyogeny, forming bradyzoites.

Toxoplasma gondii is unique among the protozoa in its ability to parasitize a wide range of hosts and tissues. It is one of the most ubiquitous of organisms; experimentally, essentially all homeothermic animals can be infected, and natural infections have been shown to occur in nonhuman primates, rodents, insectivores, herbivores, and carnivores, including domestic species and humans. Serologic surveys indicate that infection is widespread in most species of domestic animals; except for abortions in sheep and goats, however, overt disease is sporadic.

Transmission may occur by a number of different routes. The shedding of oocysts in the feces of cats and wild Felidae has been mentioned earlier. Transplacental infection occurs commonly in sheep and goats and sporadically in swine and humans. Carnivorous animals and humans may become infected by ingesting cysts containing bradyzoites in tissues of infected animals. Prolonged excretion of *Toxoplasma gondii* in the semen of goats and rams has been observed experimentally. The importance of venereal transmission, under field conditions, is unknown and warrants further investigation.

Tachyzoites have been demonstrated in milk from experimentally infected goats. However, the chance of the organisms being in the milk of spontaneously infected goats is very small. Apparently, large numbers of infecting oocysts are required for tachyzoites to be excreted in the milk. Consumption of raw goat milk has been associated with human cases of toxoplasmosis. Milk is, however, not considered to be an important source of toxoplasma for humans because tachyzoites are destroyed by gastric juices and pasteurization. *Toxoplasma* has also been isolated from the milk of lactating sows, and in this species it may be a source of infection to neonatal piglets.

Systemic toxoplasmosis occurs most commonly in young animals, especially neonates. In the latter age group the infection may be acquired pre- or postnatally. After ingestion, *Toxoplasma* organisms penetrate the intestinal mucosa. In cats, the enterointestinal cycle and systemic infection occur almost simultaneously. In other animals the tachyzoites are the first stage of infection, after the bradyzoite is released from the cysts in the intestine.

Dissemination of *Toxoplasma* occurs in lymphocytes, macrophages, granulocytes, and as free forms in plasma. From the intestine the organism may follow two routes. It may spread via the lymphocytes to the regional nodes and from there via the thoracic duct to the lungs; or it may pass in the portal circulation to the liver and from there to the lungs. Further dissemination from the lungs occurs to a wide variety of organs. Entry to the host cell may be the result of both phagocytosis and active penetration. The ability of *Toxoplasma* to survive in the intracellular environment is apparently due to failure of fusion of lysosomal membranes with membranes of the parasitophorous vacuole. The reasons for this failure of phagocytic degradation of *Toxoplasma* are still poorly understood. Cell-to-cell transmission may occur within infected organs.

Necrosis is a feature in organs heavily infected with tachyzoites, and this appears to be directly related to the rapid replication of the organism. There is no evidence that *Toxoplasma gondii* produces a toxin. The outcome of infection is determined by a number of factors, including the number and strain of *Toxoplasma* in the infecting dose, and the species, age, and immune status of the host. Lesions in visceral organs are usually evident within 1 to 2 weeks after oral infection. Variable numbers of tachyzoites are usually found in the vicinity of the necrotic areas. Specific immunity develops within a few days after infection. This reduces the severity of infection but usually does not terminate it. Immune animals develop a chronic or dormant form of *Toxoplasma* infection characterized by the formation of cysts, containing bradyzoites, which are mainly located in the brain, skeletal muscle, and myocardium. The formation of cysts is accompanied by the disappearance of tachyzoites from the circulation and visceral organs. Cyst formation may take place as early as 1 to 2 weeks after infection, and they may persist for months, possibly years. Intracellular encystment protects the bradyzoites from both cellular and humoral immune mechanisms. Inflammation is usually not associated with cysts.

When the level of immunity drops below a critical level, for example, due to treatment with immunosuppressive drugs, intercurrent disease, or other factors that depress immunity, a chronic infection may become reactivated. The cysts rupture and cause a severe inflammation that is mainly hypersensitive in character. Apparently, released bradyzoites rarely infect other cells.

The clinical signs of toxoplasmosis vary considerably, depending on the organs affected. The most consistent signs that have been reported are fever, lethargy, anorexia, ocular and nasal discharges, and respiratory distress. Neurologic signs include incoordination, circling, tremors, opisthotonus, convulsions, and paresis. Paresis is often associated with radiculitis and myositis. In dogs, toxoplasmosis may coexist with canine distemper and signs are, in any case, not sufficiently distinctive to allow ready differentiation. Immunosuppression by intercurrent distemper may activate latent *Toxoplasma* infection.

Systemic toxoplasmosis has been reported in most species of domestic animals. Pulmonary lesions are probably most consistently found, followed by central nervous system lesions. The lesions in the various organs are morphologically similar in most species, varying mainly in degree.

Macroscopic lesions in the lung vary from irregular, gray foci of necrosis on the pleural surface to a hemorrhagic pneumonia with confluent involvement of the ventral portions. Careful examination of the liver usually reveals either areas of focal necrosis or irregular mottling and edema of the gallbladder. The spleen is enlarged, as are lymph nodes, which are wet and freqently red. Pleural, pericardial, and peritoneal effusions occur irregularly. Pale areas may be evident in the myocardium and skeletal muscle. Occasionally, the pancreas is the most severely affected organ, in which case an acute hemorrhagic reaction may involve the entire organ. Yellow, small, superficial intestinal ulcers with a hyperemic border have been reported in piglets. Large pale areas of necrosis may be present in the renal cortices, mainly in goats and kittens. Chronic granulomatous toxoplasmosis may involve the intestine in older cats and produce annular areas of thickening. The mucosa overlying the granulomas may be ulcerated.

Microscopically, the early pulmonary lesions are characterized by diffuse interstitial pneumonia, and the alveolar septa are thickened due to a predominantly mononuclear inflammatory cell reaction with a few neutrophils and eosinophils. Large numbers of macrophages and fibrinous exudate fill the alveoli. Foci of necrosis involving the alveolar septa, bronchiolar epithelial cells, and blood vessels are scattered throughout the lobules. These lesions are soon followed by regenerative changes characterized by hyperplasia and hypertrophy of alveolar lining cells, mainly type II pneumocytes: so-called epithelialization of alveoli. In some areas this may be so marked as to give the affected areas an adenomatous appearance. Tachyzoites are usually evident in variable numbers in alveolar macrophages and may also be found in bronchiolar epithelial cells and the walls of blood vessels.

In the liver, irregular foci of coagulation necrosis are scattered at random throughout the lobules. There is usually little evidence of inflammation associated with the necrotic areas. Variable numbers of tachyzoites may be present in hepatocytes and Kupffer cells, usually at the periphery of the lesions. A moderate lymphocytic reaction may be found in periportal areas and around central veins in cats. In this species, tachyzoites have also been observed in bile duct epithelial cells. If the pancreas is involved, there is extensive peripancreatic fat necrosis, with areas of coagulation necrosis in parenchyma. Numerous tachyzoites are usually evident in both ductal and acinar cells.

Lesions in lymph nodes are often associated with infection in the corresponding organ. They are characterized by irregular areas of coagulation necrosis, mainly in the cortex. A moderate inflammatory reaction may be evident at the periphery of the necrotic areas. There may be necrosis and depletion of lymphocytes in the follicles. In more chronic cases, the changes are those of nonspecific hyperplasia of lymphoid cells in cortical and paracortical areas, with a large macrophage population in the medullary sinusoids. Tachyzoites may be seen in phagocytic cells in sinusoids. Similar lesions may occur in the spleen. Necrotic areas are mainly located in the red pulp in this organ.

In the heart and skeletal muscle, foci of necrosis and mononuclear-cell inflammation may be part of toxoplasmosis. There is often some difficulty in distinguishing between tachyzoites and mineralization of mitochondria in myocytes, but at some distance from areas of acute reaction, inert cysts can usually be identified in healthy fibers.

The development of brain lesions is inconsistent. In the most fulminating cases, cerebral lesions may be relatively inconspicuous. They consist of a nonsuppurative meningoencephalitis with multifocal areas of necrosis and often malacia. There is swelling of endothelial cells, necrosis of vessel walls, and vasculitis. There may be marked perivascular edema and hyperplasia of perithelial cells. Tachyzoites and occasionally cysts may be found in vessel walls and in necrotic areas in both gray and white matter at all levels of the brain. If survival is prolonged, residual cerebral lesions consist of microglial nodules along with more extensive hyperplasia of perithelial cells and perivascular fibrosis, which tends to make the vessels very obvious. At this stage, tachyzoites are rare, and cysts 30 μm in diameter with a wall of amorphous acidophilic material ~1 μm thick, located in areas away from the lesions, may be the only form seen. Spinal cord lesions resemble those seen in the brain.

The placental and fetal lesions associated with *Toxoplasma* infection are described with the Female Genital System (Volume 3), and ocular lesions with the Eye and Ear (Volume 1).

The finding of tachyzoites and/or cysts in association with areas of coagulation necrosis in one or more organs is highly suggestive of toxoplasmosis. With the exception of the dormant cysts, which may be found in brain, the accidental discovery of *Toxoplasma* in routine sections is rare. The inference from this is that in spite of the ubiquity of the infection, when *Toxoplasma* is found in sections in association with lesions, it is probably significant. The encephalitic form of toxoplasmosis in pigs must be differentiated from pansystemic viral infections with brain lesions, such as pseudorabies, hog cholera, African swine fever, and viral encephalitides. These diseases are discussed elsewhere. In sheep and horses, lesions of the central nervous system due to *Toxoplasma*-like organisms must be differentiated from those due to *Sarcocystis,* which tend to be associated with vessels. The lung lesions in cats with toxoplasmosis resemble those of feline calicivirus infection (see the Respiratory System, this volume).

Serologic tests such as the Sabin–Feldman dye test and the indirect hemagglutination test are of limited value in the diagnosis of disease associated with *Toxoplasma gondii* infection. The fluorescent-antibody technique is available for application to infected tissues. Intraperitoneal inoculation of infected tissue into mice may be needed to differentiate toxoplasmosis from other protozoan infections, such as *Sarcocystis.*

Hammondia species are obligatorily heteroxenous organisms, with the cat (*H. hammondi*) and dog (*H. heydorni*) as definitive hosts. They are also known as *Toxoplasma hammondi* and *Isospora bahiensis,* respectively. *Toxoplasma*-like oocysts are shed in the feces of the definitive host and are infectious to intermediate hosts, normally prey species. There, bradyzoites develop in cysts in striated muscle. Disease is not associated with infection of intermediate hosts; diarrhea may occur in heavily infected dogs.

Sarcocystis is obligatorily heteroxenous. Sexual stages occur in the subepithelial lamina propria at the tips of villi in the small intestine of carnivores, and oocysts sporulate in tissue, producing two sporocysts within a thin oocyst wall. Sporocysts containing four sporozoites shed in feces are infective to intermediate hosts, in which several generations of schizogony occur in vascular endothelium, and a final cyst containing merozoites (bradyzoites) is formed in myocytes and, occasionally, other cells. Ingestion of tissue cysts containing bradyzoites initiates gametogony in the definitive host. There is apparently no resistance to the development of gamonts, and no disease is associated with them in the definitive host. Many species of *Sarcocystis* are recognized, based on prey–predator cycles. Gametogony of a given species usually occurs in only one species of carnivore. The number of vertebrates capable of acting as intermediate hosts may be narrow or wide, depending on the species of *Sarcocystis.*

Sarcocystis cysts in ovine muscle may be grossly visible, causing losses at meat inspection. It is unclear whether *Sarcocystis* is involved in the etiology of eosinophilic myositis in cattle. *Sarcocystis* infection in cattle, sheep, goats, and swine may cause chronic ill thrift or an acute fatal disease characterized by anemia and widespread hemorrhage. Both syndromes are initiated during the endothelial phase of the infection. Abortion occurs during this phase of infection in some species. Abortion associated with the acute disease in pregnant animals is the result of the systemic illness, and the fetus usually is not infected. In cattle, however, some abortions, seen in otherwise clinically normal animals, are associated with schizonts of *Sarcocystis* in the vascular endothelium of the fetus, especially in the brain, and with nonsuppurative encephalitis. Encephalitis is occasionally associated with *Sarcocystis* infection in sheep, and in horses, *Sarcocystis* is the cause of protozoal myeloencephalitis.

Besnoitia is also obligatorily heteroxenous. Some stages of merogony, and gametogony, occur in the intestine of the definitive host, cats, where they are not known to be pathogenic. Oocysts are shed unsporulated. When sporulated, they are *Isospora*-like, and so-called large forms of *I. bigemina* are probably *Besnoitia* spp. Meronts in the intermediate host develop in mesenchymal cells, probably fibroblasts, which become massively hypertrophic, forming cysts containing many clusters of merozoites (bradyzoites) in the host-cell cytoplasm. Among domestic animals, cysts of *B. besnoiti* may assume some significance in the skin of cattle (see the Skin and Appendages, Volume 1).

CRYPTOSPORIDIOSIS. *Cryptosporidium* is a small apicomplexan protozoan parasite found on the surface of epithelium in the gastrointestinal (Fig. 1.49E) and respiratory tracts of mammals, birds, reptiles, and fish. Respiratory infection seems most significant in birds. Disease in mammals is enteric. *Cryptosporidium* has a typical coccidian life cycle, with merogony, gametogony, and sporogony occurring in the brush border of infected epithelial cells. The organisms are within a vacuole formed by apposition of two unit membranes of the host cell, probably caused by inversion of a microvillus by the infecting sporozoite or merozoite. A specialized ''feeder'' organelle is often present at the attachment zone in the base of the vacuole, between the infecting organism and the cytoplasm of the host cell. Developmental stages are small, in most cases about 2–6 μm in diameter. Undifferentiated meronts and gamonts are recognized as small basophilic trophozoites. Mature schizonts contain small, falciform merozoites. Macrogamonts are ~5 μm in diameter and contain small granules. Oocysts in tissue sections often are collapsed into a crescent shape. The various stages may be recognized in wax- or plastic-embedded sections under the light microscope but are best studied with the electron microscope. Oocysts may be demonstrated by fecal flotation or in fecal smears stained with Giemsa, by a modified Ziehl–Neelsen technique, or with auramine O and examined with fluorescent light.

The number of generations of schizogony and the significance of possible autoinfection by oocysts sporulated in the intestine of the host are unclear. The massive number of organisms that may be present in clinically affected animals suggests that extensive proliferation may take place within the host following ingestion of oocysts.

Although most coccidia are considered host specific, *Cryptosporidium* is not. Experimental cross-infection using cryptosporidia recovered from humans and a variety of mammals has been accomplished, with other species of mammals, and sometimes birds, susceptible to infection. Some strain variations may exist, however, reflected in the relative host susceptibility and site of proliferation. Cryptosporidiosis is a zoonosis, some human cases being associated with exposure to infected animals.

The pathogenicity of cryptosporidia was not recognized for a long time, and the mechanism by which disease is induced is unclear. In some hosts, infection appears always to be asymptomatic. However, neonatal ruminants seem particularly susceptible to disease induced by cryptosporidia. Diarrhea, anorexia, and depression in calves occur usually between about 1 and 3 or 4 weeks of age, and in lambs about 5–14 days old. Cryptosporidiosis is incriminated sporadically as a cause of diarrhea in other species, including piglets and cats. In humans, immunosuppression may be contributory to the development of cryptosporidiosis, and heavy infections have occurred in Arabian foals with combined immunodeficiency. However, severe immunodeficiency does not appear to be a necessary concomitant of infection. Cryptosporidia frequently occur concurrently with enterotoxic *E. coli,* rotavirus, or coronavirus infection in neo-

natal ruminants, but it is clear from experimental work that *Cryptosporidium* can be a primary pathogen.

In all species, intestinal cryptosporidiosis is associated with villus atrophy of varying severity, with blunting and some fusion of villi and hypertrophy of crypts of Lieberkühn (Fig. 1.50A,C). Surface epithelium is usually cuboidal, rounded, or low columnar, and sometimes exfoliating or forming irregular projections at tips of villi. Large numbers of cryptosporidia are usually visible in the microvillus border of cells on the villi (Fig. 1.50B) and not in crypts of Lieberkühn, although occasionally the reverse is true. Organisms are most heavily distributed in the distal half of the small intestine, especially in the ileum. They may occur in the cecum and colon, however, where they infect cells on the surface and occasionally in glands. In heavily infected large bowel, some attenuation of surface epithelium and dilation of crypts with necrotic debris may be evident. Mild proprial infiltrates of neutrophils and mixed mononuclear cells are present in both small and large intestine.

Diarrhea in cryptosporidiosis may be related to malabsorption associated with villus atrophy, and perhaps to the occupation of a large proportion of the surface area of absorptive cells in the distal small bowel by cryptosporidia. Mucosal lactase activity in infected calves is significantly reduced, even at uninfected or lightly infected sites in the anterior small intestine. This suggests that the effects on mucosal digestion and absorption are not solely related to physical alteration of villi or microvilli and associated loss of functional surface area.

Cryptosporidiosis is most significant in calves, as a cause of undifferentiated neonatal diarrhea, in which it must be differentiated particularly from coronavirus and rotavirus infection. Frequently it is concurrent with other agents causing this syndrome. A similar situation occurs in lambs, though disease does not appear to be as common or well recognized in that species. It is a sporadic or minor cause of fatal diarrhea in other species, usually but not always occurring in the neonatal age group. Though cryptosporidiosis can be induced experimentally in piglets, it is a relatively rare cause of spontaneous disease in them. The pathologic diagnosis is based on the presence of large numbers of cryptosporidia in sections of freshly fixed lower small intestine. Examination of smears of ileal mucosa stained with Giemsa may allow a more rapid answer or permit a diagnosis on tissue from an animal dead for some hours. In neonatal animals, other infectious causes of diarrhea should be sought at the same time.

Other Protozoa

AMOEBIASIS. *Entamoeba histolytica* is the cause of amoebiasis in humans, nonhuman primates, and occasionally in other species, including dogs and cattle; cats are susceptible to experimental infection. Among domestic animals, spontaneous amoebiasis occurs with any frequency only in dogs. Even then, it is uncommon or rare in most areas. Infection in dogs appears to have a low prevalence, and most cases are sporadic, probably acquired by exposure to cysts in feces from infected people. Dogs tend not to pass encysted amoebae; hence it has been suggested that they present little public health hazard and are unlikely to support spread from dog to dog. Under some circumstances, however, cysts may be shed, and fecal material contain-

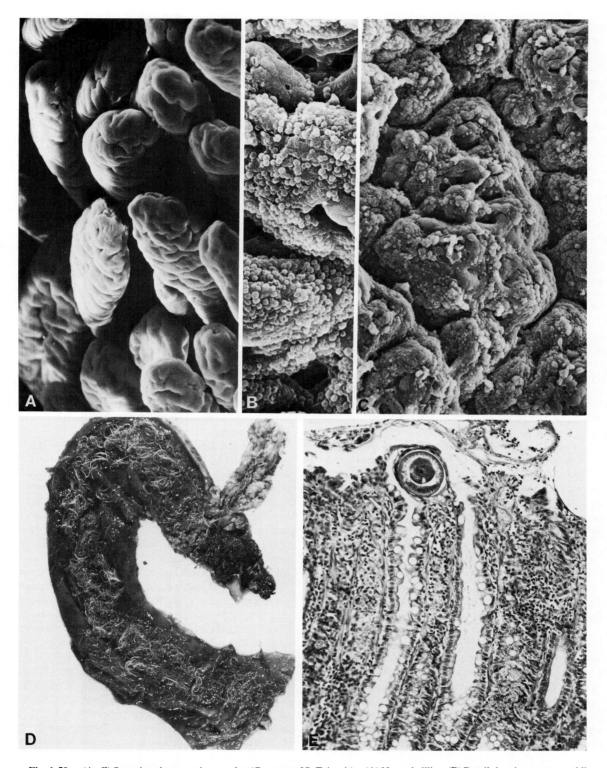

Fig. 1.50. (**A–C**) Scanning electron micrographs. (Courtesy of S. Tzipori.) (**A**) Normal villi. (**B**) Detail showing cryptosporidia (arrows). (**C**) Villus atrophy associated with cryptosporidiosis. Cryptosporidia are visible as minute spheres on the mucosal surface. (**D**) *Trichuris vulpis* typhlocolitis. Dog. (**E**) Mild erosive colitis. *Trichuris vulpis*. Dog. Anterior end of nematode is in tunnel in surface epithelium. There is exfoliation of epithelium, and effusion of neutrophils and fibrin from the surface.

ing motile trophozoites has been used to transmit infection orally to dogs.

Amoebae usually are nonpathogenic inhabitants of the lumen of the large bowel, but sometimes they cause colitis. The diet and immune status of the host and virulence attributes of various strains of the organism seem to influence pathogenicity. Large forms of *Entamoeba histolytica* are potentially invasive, and pathogenic strains are erythrophagocytic. Amoebiasis in dogs is associated with diarrheic or mucoid feces, perhaps with some blood, or with dysentery. Erosive mucosal colitis or ulcerative colitis occurs in dogs with amoebiasis, and disease seems more common or severe in animals with concomitant *Trichuris* or *Ancylostoma* infection.

Early lesions in human amoebiasis seem to be a diffuse acute mucosal colitis, with focal erosions or ulcerations. Amoebae, though scarce, may be found in mucus on the colonic surface but are most numerous in the fibrinocellular exudate over erosions or superficial ulcers. Ulcers advance as an area of necrosis and predominantly neutrophilic infiltrate, causing loss of glands, and extend for the full depth of the mucosa. Established ulcerative amoebic colitis classically has a flask-shaped ulcer, the narrow neck through the mucosa, and the broad base in the submucosa. There amoebae, and necrosis, expand laterally, apparently less constrained by the architecture of the tissue. The ragged mucosal margin of the ulcer overhangs the excavation in the submucosa. The muscularis is rarely invaded. Amoebae may attain the deeper tissue via mucosal blood vessels or lymphatics. A mixed inflammatory reaction is present about the periphery of areas of necrosis. Amoebae may be present, commonly in small clusters, in necrotic debris or in adjacent viable tissue, often not involved in an inflammatory reaction. Amoebae in tissue, often surrounded by a clear halo, may be spherical or irregular, with extended pseudopodia, and are about 6 to 40 or 50 μm in diameter. The nucleus has a central dense karyosome and peripheral chromatin clumps. The cytoplasm may appear foamy, can contain remnants of erythrocytes in phagolysosomes, and contains glycogen, which makes the cytoplasm PAS-positive. The lesions of established amoebiasis in the colon of dogs resemble those in humans, as may the early lesions.

Although dissemination of amoebae, with localization in other organs, especially liver, lung, and brain, is a relatively common complication in humans, it seems rare in dogs. One such case occurred in an animal with canine distemper.

GIARDIA AND OTHER FLAGELLATES. *Giardia* species are flagellate protozoa that inhibit the small intestine of a wide range of vertebrates. The taxonomy of the genus is confused. In the past, species status has been conferred on *Giardia* found in various hosts. Now it appears that a relatively small number of species exists, however, each with a relatively wide host range. *Giardia* infection is common in humans and is associated with disease in a proportion of them. *Giardia* from people are infective for a wide range of mammals, and there is circumstantial evidence that giardiasis in humans may be zoonotic in some cases. *Giardia* occurs in dogs, cats, cattle, sheep, and horses and has been associated with disease, with varying degrees of credibility, in each of these hosts.

Giardia trophozoites are pyriform in outline, about 10 to 20

μm long by 5 to 15 μm wide and 2 to 4 μm thick, and convex on the dorsal surface. The concave ventral surface is modified by the presence of an adhesive disk, which functions in attachment. Nutrient absorption seems to occur through the dorsal surface. A pair of nuclei, two axonemes, two medial bodies, and four pairs of flagella are present. The organisms apply their ventral aspect to the microvillous surface of enterocytes (Fig. 1.49D), usually between villi, in folds on the villous surface, or occasionally in crypts of Lieberkühn. *Giardia* has been demonstrated in the mucosa, but this is an unusual and probably aberrant location. Relatively resistant oval cysts are passed in the feces, and transmission is by the fecal–oral route.

The significance of *Giardia* as a pathogen in humans and other species has been controversial, since asymptomatic infection is the rule. There now seems little doubt that under some circumstances *Giardia* may cause disease. How the host–parasite relationship is modified to cause disease, and the pathogenesis of disease, are still unclear. In young dogs and cats, in which the disease is most important, though still uncommon, the main sign is intermittent or chronic diarrhea, which may persist for several months. The stool is soft, pale, mucoid, and greasy. Though appetite is not usually impaired, there may be a reduced growth rate or weight loss, suggesting malabsorption. A poor hair coat is attributed to deficiency of fat-soluble vitamins. Gastrointestinal dysfunction has not been extensively documented in animals. Some people with *Giardia* infection have malabsorption of *d*-xylose and vitamin B_{12}, and steatorrhea and hypocarotinemia. Excess fecal fat has been found in infected cats, but *d*-xylose malabsorption was not demonstrated in one dog with giardiasis.

Several mechanisms have been proposed to explain these findings. Although villous atrophy may occur in human patients with giardiasis, this usually occurs mainly in a subgroup of patients with hypogammaglobulinemia. Marked histologic abnormality is not found in many cases of giardiasis in humans, and this seems also to be true for dogs and cats. In experimental murine giardiasis, infection is associated with hypertrophy of crypts and increased production of cells, combined with an increased rate of movement of enterocytes along villi. Intraepithelial lymphocytes are common in infected intestine, and altered epithelial kinetics may be related to cell-mediated immune reactions in the mucosa. Atrophy of villi has been associated with restoration of cell-mediated immune competence in *Giardia*-infected athymic mice, suggesting that immune phenomena may be involved in the pathogenesis of giardiasis.

Selective deficiencies in some brush-border enzymes occur in people with giardiasis. Possibly these are related to altered villus transit times or to the direct effects of *Giardia* on microvilli, which may be deformed adjacent to adherent organisms. *Giardia* may also inhibit the activity of pancreatic lipase, causing fat malabsorption. Bacterial overgrowth of the small intestine may occur with *Giardia* infection, however, and associated bile salt deconjugation could explain steatorrhea in giardiasis. Possibly, *Giardia* is capable of deconjugating bile salts.

Giardiasis is usually diagnosed clinically on the basis of typical cysts in fecal flotations, or trophozoites in intestinal aspirates or fecal smears, coupled with remission of clinical signs following therapy and an inability to identify other potential causes of the signs. A diagnosis is sometimes based on findings in biopsies of small intestine, or at autopsy. In dogs and cats, morphologic changes in the mucosa are not well defined. The mucosa may appear normal, but there may be equivocal blunting of villi, perhaps associated with a moderate infiltrate of mononuclear cells into the core of the villus, or a heavy population of intraepithelial lymphocytes. *Giardia* should be sought in animals with malabsorption syndromes. They lie between villi and are usually evident as crescent shapes, applied by their concave surface to the brush border of epithelial cells. In favorable sections through the level of the nuclei, they may appear to have a pair of "eyes." Trophozoites oriented along the plane of section may look as they do in smears, the paired nuclei giving the organism a facelike appearance. An abnormal number of bacteria, suggestive of overgrowth, may be present in the mucus and content in the vicinity, in symptomatic animals. A diagnosis of giardiasis should always be reserved for those cases in which no other explanation for the syndrome can be identified. Giardiasis has been associated with mucosal colitis in dogs, but the association is probably coincidental.

Among animals other than dogs and cats, *Giardia* seems most convincingly to be associated with enteric signs in cattle. However, the significance of infection in that and other species is very poorly defined.

Trichomonas, or similar flagellates, are sometimes encountered in the feces of horses, dogs, cats, and cattle with diarrhea, but there is no established causal association between the organisms and disease. The association of trichomonads with diarrhea in horses is discussed briefly with typhlocolitis in horses.

BALANTIDIUM. *Balantidium* is a large, oval protozoan about 50–60 μm or more long, with a macronucleus and micronucleus and covered by many cilia arrayed in rows along its surface. *Balantidium coli* occurs in the large bowel of swine, humans, and nonhuman primates. It is very common in pigs, and many infected people live in close contact with swine. It has also been reported from several dogs with access to swine yards, as a complication of trichurosis.

Balantidium is normally present as a commensal in the lumen of the cecum and colon but is capable of opportunistic invasion of tissues injured by other diseases. Its capacity to invade may be related to production of hyaluronidase. In swine, where the organisms are most commonly encountered by veterinary pathologists (Fig. 1.49C), *Balantidium* may be found at the leading edge of the necrotizing or ulcerative lesions of the large intestine that develop secondarily to intestinal adenomatosis, swine dysentery, or perhaps salmonellosis. Likely, *Balantidium* interacts with the anaerobic colonic flora in perpetuating and advancing the necrotizing lesions that are themselves complications of the primary bacterial infection. *Balantidium* is recognized in tissue by large size, ovoid shape, the dense, curved or kidney-shaped macronucleus, and the presence of cilia (which may be accentuated by silver stains) on the surface.

ACKNOWLEDGMENTS

We wish to acknowledge the helpful criticism of portions of the manuscript by Drs. J. E. C. Bellamy, R. C. Clarke, C. L. Gyles, F. D. Horney, J. F. Prescott, and J. Thorsen.

BIBLIOGRAPHY

Congenital Oral Defects

Crowell, W. A., Stephenson, C., and Gosser, H. S. Epitheliogenesis imperfecta in a foal. *J Am Vet Med Assoc* **168:** 56–58, 1976.

Dennis, S. M. Perinatal lamb mortality in Western Australia. 7. Congenital defects. *Aust Vet J* **51:** 80–82, 1975.

Dennis, S. M., and Leipold, H. W. Agnathia in sheep: external observations. *Am J Vet Res* **33:** 339–347, 1972.

Donald, H. P., and Wierer, G. Observations on mandibular prognathism. *Vet Rec* **66:** 479–483, 1954.

Done, J. T. Facial deformity in pigs. *Vet Annu* **17:**96–102, 1977.

Edmonds, L., Crenshaw, D., and Selby, L. A. Micrognathia and cerebellar hypoplasia in an Aberdeen Angus herd. *J. Hered* **64:** 62–64, 1973.

Evans, H. E., and Sack, W. O. Prenatal development of domestic and laboratory mammals: growth curves, external features and selected references. *Anat Histol Embryol* **2:** 11–45, 1973.

Haynes, P. F., and Qualls, C. W., Jr. Cleft soft palate, nasal septal deviation, and epiglottic entrapment in a thoroughbred filly. *J Am Vet Med Assoc* **179:** 910–913, 1981.

Hewitt, M. P., Mills, J. H. L., and Hunter, B. Case report: epitheliogenesis imperfecta in a black Labrador puppy. *Can Vet J* **16:** 371–374, 1975.

Huston, R., Saperstein, G., and Leipold, H. W. Congenital defects in foals. *J Equine Med Surg* **1:** 146–161, 1977.

Hutt, F. B., and De Lahunta, A. A lethal glossopharyngeal defect in the dog. *J Hered* **62:** 291–293, 1971.

Johnson, J. H., Hull, B. L., and Dorn, A. S. The mouth. *In* "Veterinary Gastroenterology," N. V. Anderson (ed.), pp. 337–372. Philadelphia, Lea & Febiger, 1980.

Karbe, E. Lateral neck cysts in the dog. *Am J Vet Res* **26:** 112, 1965.

Leipold, H. W., and Schalles, R. Genetic defects in cattle: transmission and control. *VM SAC* **72:** 80–85, 1977.

Logue, D. N., Breeze, R. G., and Harvey, M. J. A. Arthrogryposis-palatoschisis and a 1/29 translocation in a Charolais herd. *Vet Rec* **100:** 509–510, 1977.

Mulvihill, J. J. Congenital and genetic disease in domestic animals. *Science* **176:** 132–137, 1972.

Oksanen, A. Congenital defects in Finnish calves. *Nord Vet Med* **24:** 156–161, 1972.

Saperstein, G., Harris, S., and Leipold, H. W. Congenital defects in domestic cats. *Feline Pract* **6:** 18–43, 1976.

Saperstein, G., Leipold, H. W., and Dennis, S. M. Congenital defects of sheep. *J Am Vet Med Assoc* **167:** 314–322, 1975.

Selby, L. A., Hopps, H. C., and Edmonds, L. D. Comparative aspects of congenital malformations in man and swine. *J Am Vet Med Assoc* **159:** 1485–1490, 1971.

Swartz, H. A., Vogt, D. W., and Kintner, L. D. Chromosome evaluation of Angus calves with unilateral congenital cleft lip and jaw (cheilognathoschisis). *Am J Vet Res* **43:** 729–731, 1982.

Diseases of Teeth and Dental Tissues

Al-Talabani, N. G., and Smith, C. J. Experimental dentigerous cysts and enamel hypoplasia: their possible significance in explaining the pathogenesis of human dentigerous cysts. *J Oral Pathol* **9:** 82–91, 1980.

Baker, G. J. Some aspects of equine dental decay. *Equine Vet J* **6:** 127–130, 1974.

Barnicoat, C. R. Wear in sheep's teeth. *NZ J Sci Technol [A]* **38:** 583–632, 1957.

Bell, A. F. Dental disease in the dog. *J Small Anim Pract* **6**: 421–428, 1965.

Drieux, H. *et al.* Hypotrichose congénitale avec anodontie, acérie et macroglossie chez le veau. *Recl Med. Vet.* **126**: 385–399, 1950.

Dubielzig, R. R., Higgins, R. J., and Krakowka, S. Lesions of the enamel organ of developing dog teeth following experimental inoculation of gnotobiotic puppies with canine distemper virus. *Vet Pathol* **18**: 684–689, 1981.

Dyson, D. A., and Spence, J. A. A cystic jaw lesion in sheep. *Vet Rec* **105**: 467–468, 1979.

Franklin, M. C. The influence of diet on dental development in the sheep. *Bull CSIRO (Aust)* **252**: 34, 1950.

Harris, M., and Toller, P. The pathogenesis of dental cysts. *Br Med Bull* **31**: 159–163, 1975.

McGhee, J. R., and Michalek, S. M. Immunobiology of dental caries: microbial aspects and local immunity. *Annu Rev Microbiol* **35**: 595–638, 1981.

Page, R. C., and Schroeder, H. E. Spontaneous chronic periodontitis in adult dogs. A clinical and histopathological survey. *J Periodontol* **52**: 60–73, 1981.

Page, R. C., and Schroeder, H. E. ''Periodontitis in Man and Other Animals. A Comparative Review.'' Basel, Karger, 1982.

Schneck, G. W. A case of enamel pearls in a dog. *Vet Rec* **92**: 115–117, 1973.

Schneck, G. W., and Osborn, J. W. Neck lesions in the teeth of cats. *Vet Rec* **99**: 100, 1976.

Schwartz, R. R., and Massler, M. Tooth accumulated materials: a review and classification. *J Periodontol.-Periodontics* **40**: 31/407–37/413, 1969.

Spence, J. A. *et al.* Broken mouth (premature incisor loss) in sheep: the pathogenesis of periodontal disease. *J Comp Pathol* **90**: 275–292, 1980.

Thesleff, I., and Hurmerinta, K. Tissue interactions in tooth development. *Differentiation* **18**: 75–88, 1981.

Weinreb, M. W., and Sharav, Y. Tooth development in sheep. *Am J Vet Res* **25**: 891–908, 1964.

Miscellaneous Stomatitides

Andrews, J. J. Ulcerative glossitis and stomatitis associated with exudative epidermitis in suckling swine. *Vet Pathol* **16**: 432–437, 1979.

Arnbjerg, A. *Pasteurella multocida* from canine and feline teeth, with a case report of *Glossitis calcinosa* in a dog caused by *P. multocida*. *Nord Vet Med* **30**: 324–332, 1978.

Baker, G. J., Breeze, R. G., and Dawson, C. O. Oral dermatophilosis in a cat: a case report. *J Small Anim Pract* **13**: 649–653, 1972.

Crandell, R. A. Feline viral rhinotracheitis (FVR). *Adv Vet Sci Comp Med* **17**: 201–224, 1973.

Evermann, J. F., Bryan, G. M., and McKiernan, A. J. Isolation of a calicivirus from a case of canine glossitis. *Canine Pract* **8**: 36–39, 1981.

Gaskell, R. M., and Gruffydd-Jones, T. J. Intractible feline stomatitis. *Vet Annu* **17**: 195–199, 1977.

Gillespie, J. H., and Scott, F. W. Feline viral infections. *Adv Vet Sci Comp Med* **17**: 163–200, 1973.

Gupta, P. P., and Tisha, B. P. Oral dermatophilosis associated with actinomycosis in cattle. *Zentralbl Veterinaermed [B]* **25**: 211–215, 1978.

Hoover, E. A., and Kahn, D. E. Lesions produced by feline picornaviruses of different virulence in pathogen-free cats. *Vet Pathol* **10**: 307–322, 1973.

Hume, W. J., and Potten, C. S. Advances in epithelial kinetics—an oral view. *J Oral Pathol* **8**: 3–22, 1979.

Johnson, R. P., and Povey, R. C. Effect of diet on oral lesions of feline calicivirus infection. *Vet Rec* **110**: 106–107, 1982.

Kaplan, M. L., and Jeffcoat, M. K. Acute necrotizing ulcerative gingivitis. *Canine Pract* **5**: 35–38, 1978.

Kharole, M. U. *et al.* Oral streptothricosis in cow calves and a buffalo calf. *Indian J Anim Sci* **45**: 119–122, 1975.

Mebus, C. A., Underdahl, N. R., and Twiehaus, M. J. Exudative epidermitis. *Pathol Vet* **5**: 146–163, 1968.

Nesbitt, G. H., and Schmitz, J. A. Contact dermatitis in the dog: a review of 35 cases. *J Am Anim Hosp Assoc* **13**: 155–163, 1977.

Neufeld, J. L., Burton, L., and Jeffery, K. R. Eosinophilic granuloma in a cat. Recovery of virus particles. *Vet Pathol* **17**: 97–99, 1980.

Parker, W. M. Autoimmune skin diseases in the dog. *Can Vet J* **22**: 302–304, 1982.

Potter, A. Eosinophilic granuloma of Siberian huskies. *J Am Anim Hosp Assoc* **16**: 595–600, 1980.

Povey, R. C. A review of feline viral rhinotracheitis (feline herpesvirus 1 infection). *Comp Immunol Microbiol Infect Dis* **2**: 373–387, 1979.

Povey, R. C., and Hale, C. J. Experimental infections with feline caliciviruses (picornaviruses) in specific pathogen–free kittens. *J Comp Pathol* **84**: 245–256, 1974.

Scott, D. W. *et al.* The comparative pathology of non-viral bullous skin diseases in domestic animals. *Vet Pathol* **17**: 257–281, 1980.

Zinter, D. E., and Migaki, G. *Gongylonema pulchrum* in tongues of slaughtered pigs. *J Am Vet Med Assoc* **157**: 301–303, 1970.

Deep Stomatitides

Coyle-Dennis, J. E., and Lauerman, L. H. Biological and biochemical characteristics of *Fusobacterium necrophorum* leukocidin. *Am J Vet Res* **39**: 1790–1793, 1978.

Davis, C. L., and Stiles, G. W. Actinobacillosis in rams. *J Am Vet Med Assoc* **95**: 754–756, 1939.

Hayston, J. T. Actinobacillosis in sheep. *Aust Vet J* **24**: 64–66, 1948.

Jensen, R. *et al.* Laryngeal diphtheria and papillomatosis in feedlot cattle. *Vet Pathol* **18**: 143–150, 1981.

Johnston, K. G. Nasal actinobacillosis in a sheep. *Aust Vet J* **30**: 105–106, 1954.

Langworth, B. F. *Fusobacterium necrophorum:* its characteristics and role as an animal pathogen. *Bacteriol Rev* **41**: 373–390, 1977.

M'Fadyean, J. Actinomycosis and actinobacillosis. *J Comp Pathol* **45**: 93–105, 1932.

Newsom, I. E., and Cross, F. Some complications of sore mouth in lambs. *J Am Vet Med Assoc* **78**: 539–544, 1931.

Nimmo-Wilkie, J. S., and Radostits, O. Fusobacteremia in a calf with necrotic stomatitis, enteritis and granulocytopenia. *Can Vet J* **22**: 166–170, 1981.

Till, D. H., and Palmer, F. P. A review of actinobacillosis with a study of the causal organism. *Vet Rec* **72**: 527–533, 1960.

Salivary Gland (Excluding Tumors)

Chandler, E. A. Mumps in the dog. *Vet Rec* **96**: 365–366, 1975.

Crump, M. H. Slaframine (slobber factor) toxicosis. *J Am Vet Med Assoc* **163**: 1300–1302, 1973.

Glen, J. B. Canine salivary mucoceles: results of sialographic examination and surgical treatment of 50 cases. *J Small Anim Pract* **13**: 515, 1972.

Hagler, W. M., and Behlow, R. F. Salivary syndrome in horses: identification of slaframine in red clover hay. *Appl Environ Microbiol* **42**: 1067–1073, 1981.

Harrison, J. D., and Garrett, J. R. An ultrastructural and histochemical study of a naturally occurring salivary mucocele in a cat. *J Comp Pathol* **85**: 411–416, 1975.

Harvey, C. E. Parotid salivary duct rupture and fistula in the dog and cat. *J Small Anim Pract* **18**: 163–168, 1977.

Harvey, H. J. Pharyngeal mucoceles in dogs. *J Am Vet Med Assoc* **178**: 1282–1283, 1981.

Karbe, E., and Nielson, S. W. Canine ranulas, salivary mucoceles and branchial cysts. *J Small Anim Pract* **7**: 625–630, 1966.

Kelly, D. F. *et al.* Histology of salivary gland infarction in the dog. *Vet Pathol* **16**: 438–443, 1979.

Mitten, R. W., Fleming, C., and Gooey, P. D. Concurrent parotiditis (mumps) in a child and a dog. *Aust Vet J* **58**: 39, 1982.

Schmidt, G. M., and Betts, C. W. Zygomatic salivary mucoceles in the dog. *J Am Vet Med Assoc* **172**: 940–942, 1978.

Smith, D. F., and Gunson, D. E. Branchial cyst in a heifer. *J Am Vet Med Assoc* **171**: 64–66, 1977.

Spreull, J. S. A., and Head, K. W. Cervical salivary cysts in the dog. *J Small Anim Pract* **8**: 17–35, 1967.

Neoplastic and Like Lesions of the Oral Cavity and Salivary Gland

Borthwick, R., Else, R. W., and Head, K. W. Neoplasia and allied conditions of the canine oropharynx. *Vet Annu* **22**: 248–269, 1982.

Brodey, R. S. The biological behaviour of canine oral and pharyngeal neoplasms. *J Small Anim Pract* **11**: 45–53, 1970.

Brodey, R. S. Alimentary tract neoplasms in the cat: a clinicopathologic survey of 46 cases. *Am J Vet Res* **27**: 74–80, 1966.

Dee, J. F., Mickley, J., and O'Quinn, J. L. Canine lingual myoblastoma. *J Am Anim Hosp Assoc* **8**: 303–306, 1972.

Dodd, D. C. Mastocytoma of the tongue of a calf. *Pathol Vet* **1**:69–72, 1964.

Dorn, C. R., and Priester, W. A. Epidemiologic analysis of oral and pharyngeal cancer in dogs, cats, horses and cattle. *J Am Vet Med Assoc* **169**: 1202–1206, 1976.

Dubielzig, R. R. Proliferative dental and gingival diseases of dogs and cats. *J Am Anim Hosp Assoc* **18**: 577–584, 1982.

Dubielzig, R. R., Adams, W. M., and Brodey, R. S. Inductive fibro-ameloblastoma, an unusual dental tumor of young cats. *J Am Vet Med Assoc* **174**: 720–722, 1979.

Dubielzig, R. R., Goldschmidt, M. H., and Brodey, R. S. The nomenclature of periodontal epulides in dogs. *Vet Pathol* **16**: 209–214, 1979.

Dubielzig, R. R., and Thrall, D. E. Ameloblastoma and keratinizing ameloblastoma in dogs. *Vet Pathol* **19**: 596–607, 1982.

Dyrendahl, S., and Henricson, B. Hereditary hyperplastic gingivitis in silver foxes. *Acta Vet Scand* **1**: 121–139, 1960.

Eversole, L. R. Histogenic classification of salivary tumors. *Arch Pathol* **92**: 433–443, 1971.

Giles, R. C., Montgomery, C. A., and Izen, L. Canine lingual granular cell myoblastoma: a case report. *Am J Vet Res* **35**: 1357–1359, 1974.

Gorlin, R. J., Meskin, L. H., and Brodey, R. Odontogenic tumors in man and animals: pathologic classification and clinical behavior—a review. *Ann NY Acad Sci* **108**:722–771, 1963.

Harvey, H. J. *et al.* Prognostic criteria for dogs with oral melanoma. *J Am Vet Med Assoc* **178**: 580–582, 1981.

Hayden, D. W., and Nielsen, S. W. Canine alimentary neoplasia. *Zentralbl Veterinaermed* [A] **20**: 1–22, 1973.

Head, K. W. Tumors of the upper alimentary tract. *Bull WHO* **53**: 145–166, 1976.

Henson, W. R. Carcinoma of the tongue in a horse. *J Am Vet Med Assoc* **94**: 124, 1939.

Jarrett, W. F. H. *et al.* High incidence area of cattle cancer with a possible interaction between an environmental carcinogen and a papilloma virus. *Nature* **274**: 215–217, 1978.

Karbe, E., and Schiefer, B. Primary salivary gland tumours in carnivores. *Can Vet J* **8**: 212–214, 1967.

Koestner, A., and Buerger, L. Primary neoplasms of the salivary glands in animals compared to similar tumors in man. *Pathol Vet* **2**: 201–226, 1965.

Ladds, P. W., and Webster, D. R. Pharyngeal rhabdomyosarcoma in a dog. *Vet Pathol* **8**: 256–259, 1971.

McClelland, R. B. Melanosis and melanomas in dogs. *J Am Vet Med Assoc* **98**: 504–507, 1941.

Olafson, P. Oral tumors of small animals. *Cornell Vet* **29**: 222–237, 1939.

Patnaik, A. K. *et al.* Extracutaneous mast-cell tumor in the dog. *Vet Pathol* **19**: 608–615, 1982.

Patnaik, A. K., Hurvitz, A. I., and Johnson, G. F. Canine gastrointestinal neoplasms. *Vet Pathol* **14**: 547–555, 1977.

Pirie, H. M. Unusual occurrence of squamous carcinoma of the upper alimentary tract in cattle in Britain. *Res Vet Sci* **15**: 135–138, 1973.

Roberts, M. C., Groenendyk, S., and Kelly, W. R. Ameloblastic odontoma in a foal. *Equine Vet J* **10**:91–93, 1978.

Sobel, H. J., Schwartz, R., and Marquet, E. Light- and electron-microscopy study of the origin of granular-cell myoblastoma. *J Pathol* **109**: 101–111, 1973.

Spradbrow, P. B. Papillomaviruses, papillomas and carcinomas. *In* "Advances in Veterinary Virology," T. G. Hungerford (ed.), Proc. No. 60, pp. 15–20. University of Sydney Postgraduate Committee in Veterinary Science, Sydney, Australia, 1982.

Stackhouse, L. L., Moore, J. J., and Hylton, W. E. Salivary gland adenocarcinoma in a mare. *J Am Vet Med Assoc* **172**: 271–273, 1978.

Todoroff, R. J., and Brodey, R. S. Oral and pharyngeal neoplasia in the dog: a retrospective survey of 361 cases. *J Am Vet Med Assoc* **175**: 567–571, 1979.

Wells, G. A. H., and Robinson, M. Mixed tumour of salivary gland showing histological evidence of malignancy in a cat. *J Comp Pathol* **85**: 77–85, 1975.

Werner, R. E., Jr. Canine oral neoplasia: a review of 19 cases. *J Am Anim Hosp Assoc* **17**: 67–69, 1981.

Withers, F. Squamous-celled carcinoma of the tonsil in the dog. *J Pathol Bacteriol* **49**: 429–432, 1939.

Esophagus

Alexander, J. W. *et al.* Hiatal hernia in the dog: a case report and review of the literature. *J Am Anim Hosp Assoc* **11**: 793–797, 1975.

Bailey, W. S. *Spirocerca lupi:* a continuing inquiry. *J Parasitol* **58**: 3–22, 1972.

Barber, S. M., McLaughlin, B. G., and Fretz, P. B. Esophageal ectasia in a quarterhorse colt. *Can Vet J* **24**: 46–49, 1983.

Bishop, L. M. *et al.* Megaloesophagus and associated gastric heterotopia in the cat. *Vet Pathol* **16**: 444–449, 1979.

Brodey, R. S. *et al. Spirocerca lupi* infection in dogs in Kenya. *Vet Parasitol* **3**: 49–59, 1977.

Caywood, D. D., and Feeney, D. A. Acquired esophagobronchial fistula in a dog. *J Am Anim Hosp Assoc* **18**: 590–594, 1982.

Chhabra, R. C., and Singh, K. S. Life-history of *Spirocerca lupi:* route of migration of histiotropic juveniles in dog. *Indian J Anim Sci* **42**: 540–541, 1972.

Clifford, D. H. Myenteric ganglial cells of the esophagus in cats with achalasia of the esophagus. *Am J Vet Res* **34**: 1333–1336, 1973.

Collins, G. H., Atkinson, E., and Charleston, W. A. G. Studies on *Sarcocystis* species III: the macrocystic species of sheep. *NZ Vet J* **27**: 204–206, 1979.

Cox, V. S. *et al.* Hereditary esophageal dysfunction in the miniature schnauzer dog. *Am J Vet Res* **41**: 326–330, 1980.

Diamant, N., Szczepanski, M., and Mui, H. Idiopathic megaesophagus in the dog: reasons for spontaneous improvement and a possible method of medical therapy. *Can Vet J* **15:** 66–71, 1974.

Dodman, N. H., and Baker, G. J. Tracheo-oesophageal fistula as a complication of an oesophageal foreign body in the dog—a case report. *J Small Anim Pract* **19:** 291–296, 1978.

Duncan, I. D., and Griffiths, I. R. Canine giant axonal neuropathy: some aspects of its clinical, pathological and comparative features. *J Small Anim Pract* **22:** 491–501, 1981.

Ellison, G. W. Vascular ring anomalies in the dog and cat. *Compend Contin Educ Pract Vet* **2:** 693–706, 1980.

Gaskell, C. J., Gibbs, C., and Pearson, H. Sliding hiatus hernia with reflux esophagitis in two dogs. *J Small Anim Pract* **15:** 503–509, 1974.

Keane, D. P., Horney, F. D., and Ogilvie, T. H. Congenital esophago-tracheal fistula as the cause of bloat in a calf. *Can Vet J* **24:** 57–59, 1983.

Kornegay, J. N. *et al.* Polymyositis in dogs. *J Am Vet Med Assoc* **176:** 431–438, 1980.

Munday, B. L. Cats as definitive hosts for *Sarcocystis* of sheep. *NZ Vet J* **26:** 166, 1978.

Murray, M. Incidence and pathology of *Spirocerca lupi* in Kenya. *J Comp Pathol* **78:** 401–405, 1968.

Pearson, H. *et al.* Pyloric and oesophageal dysfunction in the cat. *J Small Anim Pract* **15:** 487–501, 1974.

Pearson, H. *et al.* Reflux esophagitis and stricture formation after anaesthesia: a review of seven cases in dogs and cats. *J Small Anim Pract* **19:** 507–519, 1978.

Pearson, H., Gibbs, C., and Kelly, D. F. Oesophageal diverticulum formation in the dog. *J Small Anim Pract* **19:** 341–355, 1978.

Pope, C. E. Pathophysiology and diagnosis of reflux esophagitis. *Gastroenterology* **70:** 445–454, 1976.

Scott, E. A. *et al.* Intramural esophageal cyst in a horse. *J Am Vet Med Assoc* **171:** 652–654, 1977.

Slocombe, R. F., Todhunter, R. J., and Stick, J. A. Quantitative ultrastructural anatomy of esophagus in different regions in the horse: effects of alternate methods of tissue processing. *Am J Vet Res* **43:** 1137–1142, 1982.

Stephens, L. C., Gleiser, C. A., and Jordine, J. H. Primary pulmonary fibrosarcoma associated with *Spirocerca lupi* infection in a dog with hypertrophic pulmonary osteoarthropathy. *J Am Vet Med Assoc* **182:** 496–498, 1983.

Strombeck, D. R. Pathophysiology of esophageal motility disorders in the dog and cat. *Vet Clin North Am* **8:** 229–244, 1978.

Wilkinson, T. Chronic papillomatous oesophagitis in a young cat. *Vet Rec* **87:** 355–356, 1970.

Woods, C. B. *et al.* Esophageal deviation in four English bulldogs. *J Am Vet Med Assoc* **172:** 934–940, 1978.

Forestomachs

Ahrens, F. A. Histamine, lactic acid and hypertonicity as factors in the development of rumenitis in cattle. *Am J Vet Res* **28:** 1335–1342, 1967.

Allison, M. J. *et al.* Grain overload in cattle and sheep: changes in microbial populations in the caecum and rumen. *Am J Vet Res* **36:** 181–185, 1975.

Bartley, E. E. *et al.* Ammonia toxicity in cattle. I. Rumen and blood changes associated with toxicity and treatment methods. *J Anim Sci* **43:** 835–841, 1976.

Boray, J. C. The pathogenesis of ovine intestinal paramphistomosis due to *Paramphistomum ichikawai. In* "The Pathology of Parasitic Disease," S. M. Gaafar (ed.), pp. 209–216. Lafayette, Indiana, Purdue Univ. Press, 1971.

Brent, B. E. Relationship of acidosis to other feedlot ailments. *J Anim Sci* **43:** 930–935, 1976.

Bryant, M. P. Bacterial species of the rumen. *Bacteriol Rev* **23:** 125–153, 1959.

Clarke, R. T. J., and Reid, C. S. W. Foamy bloat of cattle: a review. *J Dairy Sci* **57:** 753–785, 1974.

Davidovich, A. *et al.* Ammonia toxicity in cattle. III. Absorption of ammonia gas from the rumen and passage of urea and ammonia from the rumen to the duodenum. *J Anim Sci* **46:** 551–558, 1977.

Dougherty, R. W. *et al.* Physiologic studies of experimentally grain-engorged cattle and sheep. *Am J Vet Res* **36:** 833–835, 1975.

Dunlop, R. H. Pathogenesis of ruminant lactic acidosis. *Adv Vet Sci Comp Med* **16:** 259, 1972.

Elam, C. J. Acidosis in feedlot cattle: practical observations. *J Anim Sci* **43:** 898–901, 1976.

Ellicott, D. H., and Jones, A. Right-sided rumen in a Friesian heifer. *Vet Rec* **99:** 318–319, 1976.

Fell, B. F. *et al.* The role of ingested animal hairs and plant spicules in the pathogenesis of rumenitis. *Res Vet Sci* **13:** 30–36, 1972.

Greene, H. J. *et al.* Effects of polyethylene roughage substitute on the rumen of fattening steers. *Can Vet J* **15:** 191–197, 1974.

Howarth, R. E. A review of bloat in cattle. *Can Vet J* **16:** 281–294, 1975.

Huber, T. L. Lactic acidosis and renal function in sheep. *J Anim Sci* **29:** 612–615, 1969.

Huber, T. L. Physiological effects of acidosis on feedlot cattle. *J Anim Sci* **43:** 902–909, 1976.

Hungate, R. E. *et al.* Microbiological and physiological changes associated with acute indigestion in sheep. *Cornell Vet* **42:** 432, 1952.

Irwin, L. N. *et al.* Amine production by sheep with glucose-induced lactic acidosis. *J Anim Sci* **35:** 267, 1972.

Jensen, R. *et al.* The rumenitis–liver abscess complex in beef cattle. *Am J Vet Res* **15:** 202–216, 1954.

Jensen, R., Connell, W. E., and Deem, A. W. Rumenitis and its relation to rate of change of ration and the proportion of concentrate in the ration of cattle. *Am J Vet Res* **15:** 425–428, 1954.

Kay, M., Fell, B. F., and Boyne, R. The relationship between the acidity of the rumen contents and rumenitis, in calves fed on barley. *Res Vet Sci* **10:** 181–187, 1969.

Kennedy, P. M., and Milligan, L. P. The degradation and utilization of endogenous urea in the gastrointestinal tract of ruminants: a review. *Can J Anim Sci* **60:** 205–221, 1980.

Landsverk, T. Indigestion in young calves. IV. Lesions of ruminal papillae in young calves fed barley and barley plus hay. *Acta Vet Scand* **19:** 377–391, 1978.

Leek, B. F. Reticulo-ruminal function and dysfunction. *Vet Rec* **84:** 238–243, 1969.

Lindsay, D. B. The significance of carbohydrate in ruminant metabolism. *Vet Rev Annot* **5:** 103–128, 1959.

McGavin, M. D., and Morrill, J. L. Scanning electron microscopy of ruminal papillae in calves fed various amounts and forms of roughage. *Am J Vet Res* **37:** 497–508, 1976.

Maeide, Y. Observations on the ruminal fluids of clinically healthy cows, especially on the changes of the characters by storage. *Jpn J Vet Res* **17:** 85, 1969.

Mills, J. H. L., and Christian, R. G. Lesions of bovine ruminal tympany. *J Am Vet Med Assoc* **157:** 947–952, 1970.

Morrow, L. L. *et al.* Laminitis in lambs injected with lactic acid. *Am J Vet Res* **34:** 1305–1307, 1973.

Mullen, P. A. Overfeeding in cattle: clinical, biochemical and therapeutic aspects. *Vet Rec* **98:** 439–443, 1976.

Osborne, A. D. Hairballs in veal calves. *Vet Rec* **99:** 239, 1976.

Roberts, D. S. Toxic, allergenic and immunogenic factors of *Fusiformis necrophorus. J Comp Pathol* **80:** 247–257, 1970.

Rowland, A. G. Diet and rumenitis. *Vet Annu* **12:** 15–20, 1973.

Rowland, A. C., Wieser, M. F., and Preston, T. R. The rumen pathology of intensively managed beef cattle. *Anim Prod* **11:** 499–504, 1969.

Slyter, L. L. Influence of acidosis on rumen function. *J Anim Sci* **43:** 910–929, 1976.

Suber, R. L. *et al.* Blood and ruminal fluid profiles in carbohydrate-foundered cattle. *Am J Vet Res* **40:** 1005–1008, 1979.

Svendsen, P. The effect of volatile fatty acids and lactic acid on rumen motility in sheep. *Nord Vet Med* **25:** 226–231, 1973.

Telle, P. P., and Preston, R. L. Ovine lactic acidosis: intraruminal and systemic. *J Anim Sci* **33:** 698–705, 1971.

Vestweber, J. G. E., and Leipold, H. W. Experimentally induced ovine ruminal acidosis: pathologic changes. *Am J Vet Res* **35:** 1537–1540, 1974.

Vestweber, J. G. E., Leipold, H. W., and Smith, J. E. Ovine ruminal acidosis: clinical studies. *Am J Vet Res* **35:** 1587–1590, 1974.

Warner, E. D. The organogenesis and early histogenesis of the bovine stomach. *Am J Anat* **102:** 33–64, 1958.

Papillomatosis and Neoplasia of the Esophagus and Forestomachs

Bailey, W. S. *Spirocerca* associated esophageal sarcomas. *J Am Vet Med Assoc* **175:** 148–150, 1979.

Camp, M. S. *et al.* A new papillomavirus associated with alimentary cancer in cattle. *Nature* **286:** 180–182, 1980.

Carb, A. V., and Goodman, D. G. Oesophageal carcinoma in the dog. *J Small Anim Pract* **14:** 91–99, 1973.

Georgsson, G. Carcinoma of the reticulum of a sheep. *Vet Pathol* **10:** 530–533, 1973.

Jarrett, W. F. H. *et al.* High incidence of cattle cancer with a possible interaction between an environmental carcinogen and a papillomavirus. *Nature* **274:** 215–217, 1978.

Jarrett, W. F. H. *et al.* Virus-induced papillomas of the alimentary tract of cattle. *Int J Cancer* **22:** 323–328, 1978.

Plowright, W., Linsell, C. A., and Peers, F. G. A focus of rumenal cancer in Kenyan cattle. *Br J Cancer* **25:** 72–80, 1971.

Spradbrow, P. B. Papillomaviruses, papillomas and carcinomas. In "Advances in Veterinary Virology," T. G. Hungerford (ed.), Proc. No. *60*, pp. 15–20. University of Sydney Postgraduate Committee in Veterinary Science, Sydney, Australia, 1982.

Normal Gastric Form and Function

Anderson, W. D., and Anderson, B. G. Comparative anatomy. *In* "Veterinary Gastroenterology," N. V. Anderson (ed.), pp. 127–171, Philadelphia, Lea & Febiger, 1980.

Argenzio, R. A., Southworth, M., and C. E. Stevens. Sites of organic acid production and absorption in the equine gastrointestinal tract. *Am J Physiol* **226:** 1043–1050, 1974.

Becker, M., and Ruoff, H.-J. Inhibition by prostaglandin E_2, somatostatin and secretin of histamine-sensitive adenylcyclase in human gastric mucosa. *Digestion* **23:** 194–200, 1982.

Cranwell, P. D., and Hansky, J. Serum gastrin in newborn, suckling and weaned pigs. *Res Vet Sci* **29:** 85–88, 1980.

Eastwood, G. L. Gastrointestinal epithelial renewal. *Gastroenterology* **72:** 962–975, 1977.

Hansky, J., McNaughtan, J., and Nairn, R. C. Distribution of G cells in the canine gastrointestinal tract. *Aust J Exp Biol Med Sci* **50:** 391–394, 1972.

Hargis, A. M., Prieur, D. J., and Gaillard, E. T. Chlamydial infection of the gastric mucosa in twelve cats. *Vet Pathol* **20:** 170–178, 1983.

Johnson, L. R. (ed.) "Physiology of the Gastrointestinal Tract." New York, Raven Press, 1981. [See chapters by A. Allen (pp. 617–639), G. Flemstrom (603–616), D. Fromm (733–748), M. I. Grossman (659–672), P. H. Guth and K. W. Ballard (709–731), and S. Ito (517–550)]

Lipkin, M. Proliferation and differentiation of gastrointestinal cells in normal and disease states. *In* "Physiology of the Gastrointestinal Tract," L. R. Johnson (ed.), pp. 145–168, New York, Raven Press, 1981.

McLeay, L. M., and Titchen, D. A. Gastric, antral and fundic pouch secretion in sheep. *J Physiol (Lond)* **248:** 595–612, 1975.

Murray, M. The fine structure of bovine gastric epithelia. *Res Vet Sci* **11:** 411–416, 1970.

Sommerville, R. I. The histology of the ovine abomasum and the relation of the globule leukocyte to nematode infestations. *Aust Vet J* **32:** 237–240, 1956.

Strombeck, D. R. Gastric structure and function. *In* "Small Animal Gastroenterology," pp. 78–97. Davis, California, Stonegate Press, 1979.

Weber, A. F., Hasa, O., and Sautter, J. H. Some observations concerning the presence of spirilla in the fundic glands of dogs and cats. *Am J Vet Res* **19:** 677–680, 1958.

Willems, G. Control of cell proliferation and differentiation in the normal stomach. *Rend Gastro-Enterol* **5:** 196–203, 1973.

Willems, G., Vansteenkiste, Y., and Smets, P. Cell proliferation in the mucosa of Heidenhain pouches after feeding in dogs. *Dig Dis* **17:** 671–674, 1972.

Pyloric Stenosis

Barth, A. D., Barber, S. M., and McKenzie, N. T. Pyloric stenosis in a foal. *Can Vet J* **21:** 234–236, 1980.

Happe, R. P., Van Der Gaag, I., and Wolvekamp, W. T. C. Pyloric stenosis caused by hypertrophic gastritis in three dogs. *J Small Anim Pract* **22:** 7–17, 1981.

Pearson, H. Pyloric stenosis in the dog. *Vet Rec* **105:** 393–394, 1979.

Pearson, H. *et al.* Pyloric and oesophageal dysfunction in the cat. *J Small Anim Pract* **15:** 487–501, 1974.

Twaddle, A. A. Congenital pyloric stenosis in two kittens corrected by pyloroplasty. *NZ Vet J* **19:** 26–27, 1971.

Gastric Dilation, Displacement, and Impaction

Barclay, W. P. *et al.* Primary gastric impaction in the horse. *J Am Vet Med Assoc* **181:** 682–683, 1982.

Bolton, J. R. *et al.* Normal abomasal electromyography and emptying in sheep and the effects of intra-abomasal volatile fatty acid infusion. *Am J Vet Res* **37:** 1387–1392, 1976.

Breukink, H. J., and de Ruyter, T. Abomasal displacement in cattle: influence of concentrates in the ration on fatty acid concentrations in ruminal, abomasal and duodenal contents. *Am J Vet Res* **37:** 1181–1184, 1976.

Caywood, D. *et al.* Gastric gas analysis in the canine gastric dilatation–volvulus syndrome. *J Am Anim Hosp Assoc* **13:** 459–462, 1977.

Coppock, C. E. Displaced abomasum in dairy cattle: etiological factors. *J Dairy Sci* **57:** 926–933, 1974.

Habel, R. E., and Smith, D. F. Volvulus of the bovine abomasum and omasum. *J Am Vet Med Assoc* **179:** 447–455, 1981.

Muir, W. W. Gastric dilatation–volvulus in the dog, with emphasis on cardiac arrhythmias. *J Am Vet Med Assoc* **180:** 739–742, 1982.

Muir, W. W. Acid–base and electrolyte disturbances in dogs with gastric dilatation–volvulus. *J Am Vet Med Assoc* **181:** 229–231, 1982.

Muir, W. W., and Weisbrode, S. E. Myocardial ischemia in dogs with gastric dilatation–volvulus. *J Am Vet Med Assoc* **181:** 363–366, 1982.

Neal, P. A., and Edwards, G. B. Vagus indigestion in cattle. *Vet Rec* **82:** 396–402, 1968.

Osborne, A. D. Hairballs in veal calves. *Vet Rec* **99:** 239, 1976.

Poulsen, J. S. D. Aetiology and pathogenesis of abomasal displacement in dairy cattle. *Nord Vet Med* **28:** 299–303, 1976.

Smith, D. F. Right sided torsion of the abomasum in dairy cows: classification of severity and evaluation of outcome. *J Am Vet Med Assoc* **173:** 108–111, 1978.

Svendsen, P. Abomasal displacement in cattle. *Nord Vet Med* **22:** 571–577, 1970.

Van Kruiningen, H. J., Gregoire, K., and Meuten, D. J. Acute gastric dilatation: A review of comparative aspects, by species, and a study in dogs and monkeys. *J Am Anim Hosp Assoc* **10:** 294–324, 1974.

Wingfield, W. E., Betts, C. W., and Rawlings, C. A. Pathophysiology associated with gastric dilatation–volvulus in the dog. *J Am Anim Hosp Assoc* **12:** 136–142, 1976.

Circulatory Disturbances, Response to Insult, and Gastritis

Barker, I. K., and Titchen, D. A. Gastric dysfunction in sheep infected with *Trichostrongylus colubriformis*, a nematode inhabiting the small intestine. *Int J Parasitol* **12:** 345–356, 1982.

Barsanti, J. A., Attleberger, M. H., and Henderson, R. A. Phycomycosis in a dog. *J Am Vet Med Assoc* **167:** 293–297, 1975.

Cheville, N. F. Uremic gastropathy in the dog. *Vet Pathol* **16:** 292–309, 1979.

Eustis, S. L., and Bergeland, M, E. Suppurative abomasitis associated with *Clostridium septicum* infection. *J Am Vet Med Assoc* **178:** 732–734, 1981.

Hansen, O. H. *et al.* Relationship between gastric acid secretion, histopathology and cell proliferation kinetics in human gastric mucosa. *Gastroenterology* **73:** 453–456, 1977.

Hargis, A. M. *et al.* Chronic fibrosing gastritis associated with *Ollulanus tricuspis* in a cat. *Vet Pathol* **19:** 320–323, 1982.

Hayden, D. W., and Fleischman, R. W. Schirrhous eosinophilic gastritis in dogs with gastric arteritis. *Vet Pathol* **14:** 441–448, 1977.

Isaacson, P. Immunoperoxidase study of the secretory immunoglobulin system and lysozyme in normal and diseased gastric mucosa. *Gut* **23:** 578–588, 1982.

Jeffries, G. N. Gastritis. *In* "Gastrointestinal Disease," M. H. Sleisenger and J. S. Fordtran (eds.), 2nd ed., pp. 733–743. Philadelphia, Saunders, 1978.

Kelly, D. G. *et al.* Giant hypertrophic gastropathy (Menetrier's disease): pharmacologic effects on protein leakage and mucosal ultrastructure. *Gastroenterology* **83:** 581–589, 1982.

Kipnis, R. M. Focal cystic hypertrophic gastropathy in a dog. *J Am Vet Med Assoc* **173:** 182–184, 1978.

Krohn, K. J. E., and Finlayson, N. D. C. Interrelations of humoral and cellular immune responses in experimental canine gastritis. *Clin Exp Immunol* **14:** 237–245, 1973.

Lev, R., Siegel, H. I., and Glass, G. B. J. Effects of salicylates on the canine stomach: a morphological and histochemical study. *Gastroenterology* **62:** 970–980, 1972.

McLeod, C. G., Langlinais, P. C., and Brown, J. C. Ulcerative histiocytic gastritis and amyloidosis in a dog. *Vet Pathol* **18:** 117–120, 1981.

Murray, M., Jennings, F. W., and Armour, J. Bovine ostertagiasis: structure, function and mode of differentiation of the bovine gastric mucosa and kinetics of the worm loss. *Res Vet Sci* **11:** 417–427, 1970.

Neitzke, J. P., and Schiefer, B. Incidence of mycotic gastritis in calves up to 30 days of age. *Can Vet J* **15:** 139–144, 1974.

Osborne, A. D., and Wilson, M. R. Mycotic gastritis in a dog. *Vet Rec* **85:** 487–489, 1969.

Smith, J. M. B. Mycoses of the alimentary tract of animals. *NZ Vet J* **16:** 89–100, 1968.

Strickland, R. G., and Mackay, I. R. A reappraisal of the nature and significance of chronic atrophic gastritis. *Am J Dig Dis* **18:** 426–440, 1973.

Strombeck, D. R. Acute gastritis. *In* "Small Animal Gastroenterology," pp. 98–109. Davis, California, Stonegate Press, 1979.

Strombeck, D. R. Chronic gastritis, gastric retention and gastric neoplasms. *In* "Small Animal Gastroenterology," pp. 110–124. Davis, California, Stonegate Press, 1979.

Strombeck, D. R., Doe, M., and Jang, S. Maldigestion and malabsorption in a dog with chronic gastritis. *J Am Vet Med Assoc* **179:** 801–805, 1981.

Van Der Gaag, I., Happe, R. P., and Wolvekamp, W. T. C. A boxer dog with chronic hypertrophic gastritis resembling Menetrier's disease in man. *Vet Pathol* **13:** 172–185, 1976.

Van Kruiningen, H. J. Giant hypertrophic gastritis of Basenji dogs. *Vet Pathol* **14:** 19–28, 1977.

Gastroduodenal Ulceration

Adair, H. M. Epithelial repair in chronic gastric ulcers. *Br J Exp Pathol* **59:** 229–236, 1978.

Ader, P. Penetrating gastric ulceration in a dog. *J Am Vet Med Assoc* **175:** 710–713, 1979.

Carrig, C. B., and Seawright, A. A. Mastocytosis with gastrointestinal ulceration in a dog. *Aust Vet J* **44:** 503–507, 1968.

Dobson, K. J., Davies, R. L., and Cargill, C. F. Ulceration of the pars oesophagia in pigs. *Aust Vet J* **54:** 601–602, 1978.

Dodd, D. C. Hyostrongylosis and gastric ulceration in the pig. *NZ Vet J* **8:** 100–103, 1960.

Else, R. W., and Head, K. W. Some pathological conditions of the canine stomach. *Vet Annu* **20:** 66–81, 1980.

Ewing, G. O. Indomethacin-associated gastrointestinal hemorrhage in a dog. *J Am Vet Med Assoc* **161:** 1665–1668, 1972.

Fatimah, I., Butler, D. G., and Physick-Sheard, P. W. Perforated duodenal ulcer in a cow. *Can Vet J* **23:** 173–175, 1982.

Gross, T. L., and Mayhew, I. G. Gastroesophageal ulceration and candidiasis in foals. *J Am Vet Med Assoc* **182:** 1370–1373, 1983.

Hani, H., and Indermuhle, N. A. Esophagogastric ulcers in swine infected with *Ascaris suum*. *Vet Pathol* **16:** 617–618, 1979.

Happe, R. P. *et al.* Zollinger–Ellison syndrome in three dogs. *Vet Pathol* **17:** 177–186, 1980.

Happe, R. P., and van den Brom, W. E. Duodenogastric reflux in the dog, a clinicopathological study. *Res Vet Sci* **33:** 280–286, 1982.

Hemmingsen, I. Erosiones et ulcera abomasi bovis. *Nord Vet Med* **18:** 354–365, 1966.

Howard, E. B. *et al.* Mastocytoma and gastroduodenal ulceration. *Pathol Vet* **6:** 146–158, 1969.

Jensen, R. *et al.* Fatal abomasal ulcers in yearling feedlot cattle. *J Am Vet Med Assoc* **169:** 524–526, 1976.

Jones, B. R., Nicholls, M. R., and Badman, R. Peptic ulceration in a dog associated with an islet cell carcinoma of the pancreas and an elevated plasma gastrin level. *J Small Anim Pract* **17:** 593–598, 1976.

Kadel, W. L., Kelley, D. C., and Coles, E. H. Survey of yeastlike fungi and tissue changes in esophagogastric region of stomachs of swine. *Am J Vet Res* **30:** 401–408, 1969.

Kowalczyk, T. *et al.* Gastric ulcers in swine under modern intensified husbandry. *VM SAC* **66:** 1185–1196, 1971.

Lev, R., Siegel, H. I., and Glass, G. B. J. Effects of salicylates on the canine stomach: a morphological and histochemical study. *Gastroenterology* **62:** 970–980, 1972.

MacKay, R. J. *et al.* Effects of large doses of phenylbutazone administration to horses. *Am J Vet Res* **44:** 774–780, 1983.

Maxwell, C. W. *et al.* Effect of dietary particle size on lesion development and on the contents of various regions of the swine stomach. *J Anim Sci* **30:** 911–922, 1970.

Maxwell, C. V. *et al.* Use of tritiated water to assess, *in vivo*, the effect of dietary particle size on the mixing of stomach contents in swine. *J Anim Sci* **34:** 212–216, 1972.

Moore, R. W., and Withrow, S. J. Gastrointestinal hemorrhage and pancreatitis associated with intervertebral disk disease in the dog. *J Am Vet Med Assoc* **180:** 1443–1447, 1982.

Murray, M. *et al.* Peptic ulceration in the dog. a clinicopathological study. *Vet Rec* **91:** 441–447, 1972.

O'Brien, J. J. Gastric ulcers. *In* "Diseases of Swine," A. D. Leman *et al.* (eds.), 5th ed., pp. 632–646. Ames, Iowa State Univ. Press, 1981.

Phillips, B. M. Aspirin-induced gastrointestinal microbleeding in dogs. *Toxicol Appl Pharmacol* **24:** 182–189, 1973.

Pocock, E. F. *et al.* Dietary factors affecting the development of esophagogastric ulcer in swine. *J Anim Sci* **29:** 591–597, 1969.

Rebhun, W. C., Dill, S. G., and Power, H. T. Gastric ulcers in foals. *J Am Vet Med Assoc* **180:** 404–407, 1982.

Robert, A. Prostaglandins and the gastrointestinal tract. *In* "Physiology of the Gastrointestinal Tract," L. R. Johnson (ed.), pp. 1407–1434. New York, Raven Press, 1982.

Rooney, J. R. Gastric ulceration in foals. *Pathol Vet* **1:** 497–503, 1964.

Roudebush, P., and Morse, G. E. Naproxen toxicosis in a dog. *J Am Vet Med Assoc* **179:** 805–806, 1981.

Seawright, A. A., and Grono, L. R. Malignant mast cell tumor in a cat with perforating duodenal ulcer. *J Pathol Bacteriol* **87:** 107–111, 1964.

Sorjonen, D. C. *et al.* Effects of dexamethasone and surgical hypotension on the stomach of dogs: clinical, endoscopic and pathologic evaluations. *Am J Vet Res* **44:** 1233–1237, 1983.

Straus, E., Johnson, G. F., and Yalow, R. S. Canine Zollinger–Ellison syndrome. *Gastroenterology* **72:** 380–381, 1977.

Swerczek, T. W. Toxicoinfectious botulism in foals and adult horses. *J Am Vet Med Assoc* **176:** 217–220, 1980.

Tannock, G. W., and Smith, J. M. B. The microflora of the pig stomach and its possible relationship to ulceration of the pars oesophagea. *J Comp Pathol* **80:** 359–367, 1970.

Zamora, C. S. *et al.* Effects of prednisone on gastric secretion and development of stomach lesions in swine. *Am J Vet Res* **36:** 33–39, 1975.

Gastric Neoplasms

Chapman, W. L., and Smith, J. A. Abomasal adenocarcinoma in a cow. *J Am Vet Med Assoc* **181:** 493–494, 1982.

Conroy, J. D. Multiple gastric adenomatous polyps in a dog. *J Comp Pathol* **79:** 465–467, 1969.

Cotchin, E. Some tumors of dogs and cats of comparative veterinary and human interest. *Vet Rec* **71:** 1040–1050, 1959.

Grundmann, E., and Schlake, W. Histological classification of gastric cancer from initial to advanced stages. *Pathol Res Pract* **173:** 260–274, 1982.

Happe, R. P. *et al.* Multiple polyps of the gastric mucosa in two dogs. *J Small Anim Pract* **18:** 179–189, 1977.

Hayden, D. W., and Nielsen, S. W. Canine alimentary neoplasia. *Zentralbl Veterinaermed [A]* **20:** 1–22, 1973.

Head, K. W. Tumors of the lower alimentary tract. *Bull WHO* **53:** 167–186, 1976.

Lingeman, C. H., Garner, F. M., and Taylor, D. O. N. Spontaneous gastric adenocarcinomas of dogs: a review. *JNCI* **47:** 137–153, 1971.

Meagher, D. M. *et al.* Squamous cell carcinoma of the equine stomach. *J Am Vet Med Assoc* **164:** 81–84, 1974.

Meuten, D. J. *et al.* Gastric carcinoma with pseudohyperparathyroidism in a horse. *Cornell Vet* **68:** 179–195, 1978.

Murray, M. *et al.* Primary gastric neoplasia in the dog: a clinicopathological study. *Vet Rec* **81:** 474–479, 1972.

Patnaik, A. K., Hurvitz, A. I., and Johnson, G. F. Canine gastrointestinal neoplasms. *Vet Pathol* **14:** 547–555, 1977.

Patnaik, A. K., Hurvitz, A. I., and Johnson, G. F. Canine gastric adenocarcinoma. *Vet Pathol* **15:** 600–607, 1978.

Patnaik, A. K., and Lieberman, P. H. Gastric squamous cell carcinoma in a dog. *Vet Pathol* **17:** 250–253, 1980.

Sautter, J. H., and Hanlon, G. F. Gastric neoplasms in the dog: a report of 20 cases. *J Am Vet Med Assoc* **166:** 691–696, 1975.

Tennant, B. *et al.* Six cases of squamous cell carcinoma of the stomach of the horse. *Equine Vet J* **14:** 238–243, 1982.

Turk, M. A. M., Gallina, A. M., and Russell, T. S. Nonhematopoietic gastrointestinal neoplasia in cats: a retrospective study of 44 cases. *Vet Pathol* **18:** 614–620, 1981.

Wester, P. W., Franken, P., and Hani, H. J. Squamous cell carcinoma of the equine stomach. *Vet Q.* **2:** 95–103, 1980.

Normal Intestinal Morphology, Immune Events, and Microflora

Allen, W. D., and Porter, P. The relative distribution of IgM and IgA cells in intestinal mucosa and lymphoid tissues of the young unweaned pig and their significance in ontogenesis of secretory immunity. *Immunology* **24:** 493–501, 1973.

Anderson, J. C. The response of gut-associated lymphoid tissue in gnotobiotic piglets to the presence of bacterial antigen in the alimentary tract. *J Anat* **124:** 555–562, 1977.

Argenzio, R. A. Functions of the equine large intestine and their interrelationship in disease. *Cornell Vet* **65:** 303–330, 1975.

Atkins, A. M., and Schofield, G. C. Lymphoglandular complexes in the large intestine of the dog. *J Anat* **113:** 169–178, 1972.

Aumaitre, A., and Corring, T. Development of digestive enzymes in the piglet from birth to 8 weeks. II. Intestine and intestinal disaccharidases. *Nutr Metab* **22:** 244–255, 1978.

Banks, K. L. Host defence in the newborn animal. *J Am Vet Med Assoc* **181:** 1053–1056, 1982.

Banta, C. A. *et al.* Sites of organic acid production and patterns of digesta movement in the gastrointestinal tract of dogs. *J Nutr* **109:** 1592–1600, 1979.

Befus, A. D., and Bienenstock, J. Immunity to infectious agents in the gastrointestinal tract. *J Am Vet Med Assoc* **181:** 1066–1068, 1982.

Befus, A. D., and Bienenstock, J. Factors involved in symbiosis and host resistance at the mucosa–parasite interface. *Prog Allergy* **31:** 76–177, 1982.

Bellamy, J. E. C., Latshaw, W. K., and Nielsen, N. O. The vascular architecture of the porcine small intestine. *Can J Comp Med* **37:** 56–62, 1973.

Bienenstock, J. *et al.* Mast cell heterogeneity: derivation and function, with emphasis on the intestine. *J Allergy Clin Immunol* **70:** 407–412, 1982.

Bienenstock, J., and Befus, A. D. Mucosal immunology. *Immunology* **41:** 249–270, 1980.

Bronson, R. T. Ultrastructure of macrophages and karyolytic bodies in small intestinal villi of macaque monkeys and baboons. *Vet Pathol* **18:** 727–737, 1981.

Canfield, P. J., Bennett, A. M., and Watson, A. D. J. Large intestinal biopsies from normal dogs. *Res Vet Sci* **28:** 6–9, 1980.

Chu, R. M. *et al.* Lymphoid tissues of the small intestine of swine from birth to one month of age. *Am J Vet Res* **40:** 1713–1719, 1979.

Chu, R. M. Glock, R. D., and Ross, R. F. Gut-associated lymphoid tissues of young swine with emphasis on dome epithelium of aggregated lymph nodules (Peyer's patches) of the small intestine. *Am J Vet Res* **40**: 1720–1728, 1979.

Clamp, J. R. The role of mucus secretions in the protection of the gastrointestinal mucosa. *In* "The Mucosal Immune System," F. J. Bourne (ed.), pp. 389–397. The Hague, Martinus Nijhoff, 1981.

Eastwood, G. L. Gastrointestinal epithelial renewal. *Gastroenterology* **72**: 962–975, 1977.

Gardner, J. D., Brown, M. S., and Laster, L. The columnar epithelial cell of the small intestine: digestion and transport. *N Engl J Med* **283**: 1196–1202, 1264–1271, and 1317–1324, 1970.

Granger, D. N., and Barrowman, J. A. Microcirculation of the alimentary tract. II. Pathophysiology of edema. *Gastroenterology* **84**: 1035–1049, 1983.

Gregory, M. W. The globule leukocyte and parasitic infection—a brief history. *Vet Bull* **49**: 821–827, 1979.

Hall, J. G. The physiology of intestinal immunity. *In* "The Ruminant Immune System," J. E. Butler (ed.), pp. 623–632. New York, Plenum, 1981.

Hart, I. R. The distribution of immunoglobulin-containing cells in canine small intestine. *Res Vet Sci* **27**:269–274, 1979.

Hintz, H. F. Digestive physiology of the horse. *J S Afr Vet Assoc* **46**: 13–16, 1975.

Hoskins, J. D., Henk, W. G., and Abdelbaki, Y. Z. Scanning electron microscopic study of the small intestine of dogs from birth to 337 days of age. *Am J Vet Res* **43**: 1715–1720, 1982.

Husband, A. J. Ontogeny of the gut-associated immune system. *In* "The Ruminant Immune System," J. E. Butler (ed.), pp. 633–647. New York, Plenum, 1981.

Inokuchi, H., Fujimoto, S., and Kawai, K. Cellular kinetics of gastrointestinal mucosa, with special reference to gut endocrine cells *Arch Histol Jpn* **46**: 137–157, 1983.

Jeffcott, L. B. Passive immunity and its transfer with special reference to the horse. *Biol Rev* **47**: 439–464, 1972.

LeFevre, M. E., Hammer, R., and Joel, D. D. Macrophages of the mammalian small intestine. A review. *J Reticuloendothel Soc* **26**: 553–573, 1979.

Lyscom, N., and Brueton, M. J. Intraepithelial, lamina propria and Peyer's patch lymphocytes of the rat small intestine: isolation and characterization in terms of immunoglobulin markers and receptors for monoclonal antibodies. *Immunology* **45**: 775–783, 1982.

MacDonald, T. T., Bashore, M., and Carter, P. B. Nonspecific resistance to infection expressed within the Peyer's patches of the small intestine. *Infect Immun* **37**: 390–392, 1982.

McGuire, T. C. *et al.* Failure of colostral immunoglobulin transfer in calves dying from infectious disease. *J Am Vet Med Assoc* **169**: 713–718, 1976.

McGuire, T. C. *et al.* Failure of colostral immunoglobulin transfer as an explanation for most infections and deaths of neonatal foals. *J Am Vet Med Assoc* **170**: 1302–1304, 1977.

Madara, J. L. Cup cells: structure and distribution of a unique class of epithelial cells in guinea pig, rabbit and monkey small intestine. *Gastroenterology* **83**: 981–984, 1982.

Mebus, C. A., Newman, L. E., and Stair, E. L. Scanning electron, light and transmission electron microscopy of intestine of gnotobiotic calf. *Am J Vet Res* **36**: 985–993, 1975.

Miller, H. R. P., Huntley, J. F., and Dawson, A. M. Mucus secreton in the gut, its relationship to the immune response in *Nippostrongylus*-infected rats. *In* "The Mucosal Immune System," F. J. Bourne (ed.), pp. 402–430. The Hague, Martinus Nijhoff, 1981.

Moon, H. W. Epithelial cell migration in the alimentary mucosa of the suckling pig. *Proc Soc Exp Biol Med* **137**: 151–154, 1971.

Moon, H. W. Vacuolated villous epithelium of the small intestine of young pigs. *Vet Pathol* **9**: 3–21, 1972.

Moon, H. W., and Joel, D. D. Epithelial cell migration in the small intestine of sheep and calves. *Am J Vet Res* **36**: 187–189, 1975.

Moon, H. W., Kohler, E. M., and Whipp, S. C. Vacuolation: a function of cell age in porcine ileal absorptive cells. *Lab Invest* **28**: 23–28, 1973.

Murata, H., and Namioka, S. The duration of colostral immunoglobulin uptake by the epithelium of the small intestine of neonatal piglets. *J Comp Pathol* **87**: 431–439, 1977.

Newby, T. J., and Bourne, F. J. The nature of the local immune system of the bovine small intestine. *Immunology* **31**: 475–480, 1976.

Ogra, P. L. Mucosal immunity and macromolecular absorption. *Nutr Res* **2**: 367–369, 1982.

Porter, P., Noakes, D. E., and Allen, W. D. Intestinal secretion of immunoglobulins in the preruminant calf. *Immunology* **23**: 299–312, 1972.

Pout, D. The mucosal surface patterns of the small intestine of grazing lambs. *Br Vet J* **126**: 357–363, 1970.

Reid, L., and Clamp, J. R. The biochemical and histochemical nomenclature of mucus. *Br Med Bull* **34**: 5–8, 1978.

Roberts, M. C. Carbohydrate, digestion and absorption in the equine small intestine. *J S Afr Vet Assoc* **46**: 19–27, 1975.

Roberts, M. C., and Hill, F. W. G. The mucosa of the small intestine of the horse: a microscopical study of specimens obtained through a small intestinal fistula. *Equine Vet J* **6**: 74–80, 1974.

Ruitenberg, E. J., and Elgersma, A. Response of intestinal globule leucocytes in the mouse during a *Trichinella spiralis* infection and its independence of intestinal mast cells. *Br J Exp Pathol* **60**: 246–251, 1979.

Sawyer, M. *et al.* Passive transfer of colostral immunoglobulins from ewe to lamb and its influence on neonatal lamb mortality. *J Am Vet Med Assoc* **171**: 1255–1259, 1977.

Smith, M. W., and Jarvis, L. G. Growth and cell replacement in the newborn pig intestine. *Proc R Soc Lond* **[B]** **203**: 69–89, 1978.

Spiro, H. M. Visceral viewpoints: the rough and the smooth—some reflections on diet therapy. *N Engl J Med* **293**: 83–85, 1975.

Staley, T. E., Jones, E. W., and Corley, L. D. Fine structures of duodenal absorptive cells in the newborn pig before and after feeding of colostrum. *Am J Vet Res* **30**: 567–581, 1969.

Strobel, S., Miller, H. R. P., and Ferguson, A. Human intestinal mucosal mast cells: evaluation of fixation and staining techniques. *J Clin Pathol* **34**: 851–858, 1981.

Thomas, J., and Anderson, N. V. Interepithelial lymphocytes in the small intestinal mucosa of conventionally reared dogs. *Am J Vet Res* **43**: 200–203, 1982.

Thrall, D. E., and Leininger, J. R. Irregular intestinal mucosal margination in the dog: normal or abnormal *J Small Anim Pract* **17**: 305–312, 1976.

Torres-Medina, A. Morphologic characteristics of the epithelial surface of aggregated lymphoid follicles (Peyer's patches) in the small intestine of newborn gnotobiotic calves and pigs. *Am J Vet Res* **42**: 232–236, 1981.

Ulyatt, M. J. *et al.* Structure and function of the large intestine of ruminants. *In* "Digestion and Metabolism in the Ruminant," I. W. Macdonald and A. C. I. Warner (eds.), pp. 119–133. Armidale NSW, University of New England, 1975.

Ward, G. E., and Nelson, D. I. Effects of dietary milk fat (whole milk) and propionic acid on intestinal coliforms and lactobacilli in calves. *Am J Vet Res* **43**: 1165–1167, 1982.

Welsh, M. J. *et al.* Crypts are the site of intestinal fluid and electrolyte secretion. *Science* **218**: 1219–1221, 1982.

Willard, M. D. *et al.* Number and distribution of IgM cells and IgA cells in colonic tissue of conditioned sex- and breed-related dogs. *Am J Vet Res* **43**: 688–692, 1982.

Willard, M. D., and Leid, R. W. Nonuniform horizontal and vertical distributions of immunoglobulin A cells in canine intestines. *Am J Vet Res* **42**: 1573–1580, 1981.

Intestinal Anomalies

Barth, A. D., Barber, S. M., and McKenzie, N. T. Pyloric stenosis in a foal. *Can Vet J* **21:** 234–236, 1980.

Carr, P. M. An apparently inherited inguinal hernia in the Merino ram. *Aust Vet J* **48:** 126–127, 1972.

Clark, W. T., Cox, J. E., and Birtles, M. J. Atresia of the small intestine in lambs and calves. *NZ Vet J* **26:** 120–122, 1978.

Cork, L. C., Munnel, J. F., and Lorenz, M. D. The pathology of feline G$_{M2}$ gangliosidosis. *Am J Pathol* **90:** 723–734, 1978.

Dennis, S. M., and Leipold, H. W. Atresia ani in sheep. *Vet Rec* **91:** 219–222, 1972.

Doughri, A. M., Altera, K. P., and Kainer, R. A. Some developmental aspects of the bovine fetal gut. *Zentralbl Veterinaermed [A]* **19:** 417–434, 1972.

Estes, R., and Lyall, W. Congenital atresia of the colon: a review and report of four cases in the horse. *J Equine Med Surg* **3:** 495–498, 1979.

Feron, V. J., and Mullink, J. W. M. A. Mucosal cysts in the gastrointestinal tract of beagle dogs. *Lab Anim* **5:** 193–201, 1971.

Gonzalez-Licea, A., Carranza-Portocarrero, A., and Escobedo, M. Duodenal gangliosidosis in a cat: ultrastructural study. *Am J Vet Res* **39:** 1342–1347, 1978.

Grant, B. D., and Tennant, B. Volvulus associated with Meckel's diverticulum in the horse. *J Am Vet Med Assoc* **162:** 550–551, 1973.

Hayes, H. M., Jr. Congenital umbilical and inguinal hernias in cattle, horses, swine, dogs and cats: risk by breed and sex among hospital patients. *Am J Vet Res* **35:** 839–842, 1974.

Hoffsis, G. F., and Bruner, R. R., Jr. Atresia coli in a twin calf. *J Am Vet Med Assoc* **171:** 433–434, 1977.

Hultgren, B. D. Ileocolonic aganglionosis in white progeny of overo spotted horses. *J Am Vet Med Assoc* **180:** 289–292, 1982.

Huston, R., Saperstein, G., and Leipold, H. W. Congenital defects in foals. *J Equine Med Surg* **1:** 146–161, 1977.

Ladds, P. W., and Anderson, N. V. Atresia ilei in a pup. *J Am Vet Med Assoc* **158:** 2071–2072, 1971.

Leipold; H. W. *et al.* Intestinal atresia in calves. *VM SAC* **71:** 1037–1039, 1976.

Leipold, H. W., and Dennis, S. M. Atresia jejuni in a lamb. *Vet Rec* **93:** 644–645, 1973.

Leipold, H. W., and Saperstein, G. Rectal and vaginal constriction in Jersey cattle. *J Am Vet Med Assoc* **166:** 231–232, 1975.

Lenghaus, C., and White, W. E. Intestinal atresia in calves. *Aust Vet J* **49:** 587–588, 1973.

McAfee, L. T., and McAfee, J. T. Atresia ani in a dog. *VM SAC* **71:** 624–627, 1976.

Nihleen, B., and Eriksson, K. A hereditary lethal defect in calves—atresia ilei. *Nord Vet Med* **10:** 113–127, 1958.

Norrish, J. G., and Rennie, J. C. Observations on the inheritance of atresia ani in swine. *J Hered* **59:** 186–187, 1968.

Osborne, J. C., Davis, J. W., and Farley, H. Hirschsprung's disease: a review and report of the entity in a Virginia swine herd. *Vet Med* **63:** 451–453, 1968.

Osborne, J. C., and Legates, J. E. Six cases of bovine intestinal anomaly. *J Am Vet Med Assoc* **142:** 1104, 1963.

Rawlings, C. A., and Capps, W. F., Jr. Rectovaginal fistula and imperforate anus in a dog. *J Am Vet Med Assoc* **159:** 320–326, 1971.

Smart, M. E., Fletch, S. M., and Black, F. Congenital absence of jejunum and ileum in two neonatal Alaskan malamute pups. *Can Vet J* **19:** 22–23, 1978.

Steenhaut, M. *et al.* Intestinal malformations in calves and their surgical correction. *Vet Rec* **98:** 131–133, 1976.

Van Der Gaag, I., and Tibboel, D. Intestinal atresia and stenosis in animals: a report of 34 cases. *Vet Pathol* **17:** 565–574, 1980.

Vonderfecht, S. L., Trommershausen Bowling, A., and Cohen, M. Congenital intestinal aganglionosis in white foals. *Vet Pathol* **20:** 65–70, 1983.

Miscellaneous Intestinal Diseases, Displacements, and Obstruction

Arrick, R. H., and Kleine, L. J. Intestinal pseudoobstruction in a dog. *J Am Vet Med Assoc* **172:** 1201–1205, 1978.

Barlow, R. M. Neuropathological observations in grass sickness of horses. *J Comp Pathol* **79:** 407–411, 1969.

Blue, M. G., and Wittkopp, R. W. Clinical and structural features of equine enteroliths. *J Am Vet Med Assoc* **179:** 79–82, 1981.

Boles, C. L., and Kohn, C. W. Fibrous foreign body impaction colic in young horses. *J Am Vet Med Assoc* **171:** 193–195, 1977.

Bundza, A., Lowden, J. A., and Charlton, K. M. Niemann–Pick disease in a poodle dog. *Vet Pathol* **16:** 530–538, 1979.

Cordes, D. O., and Dewes, H. F. Diverticulosis and muscular hypertrophy of the small intestine of horses, pigs and sheep. *NZ Vet J* **19:** 108–111, 1971.

Cordes, D. O., and Mosher, A. H. Brown pigmentation (lipofuscinosis) of intestinal muscularis. *J Pathol Bacteriol* **92:** 197–206, 1966.

Ducharme, N. G., Smith, D. F., and Koch, D. B. Small intestinal obstruction caused by a persistent round ligament of the liver in a cow. *J Am Vet Med Assoc* **180:** 1234–1236, 1982.

Gilmour, J. S., Brown, R., and Johnson, P. A negative serological relationship between cases of grass sickness in Scotland and *Clostridium perfringens* type A enterotoxin. *Equine Vet J* **13:** 56–58, 1981.

Gilmour, J. S., and Mould, D. L. Experimental studies of neurotoxic activity in blood fractions from acute cases of grass sickness. *Res Vet Sci* **22:** 1–4, 1977.

Hackett, R. P. Nonstrangulated colonic displacement in horses. *J Am Vet Med Assoc* **182:** 235–240, 1983.

Hammond, P. B. *et al.* Experimental intestinal obstruction in calves. *J Comp Pathol* **74:** 210–222, 1964.

Hayes, K. C., Neilsen, S. W., and Rousseau, J. E., Jr. Vitamin E deficiency and fat stress in the dog. *J Nutr* **99:** 196–209, 1969.

Hodson, N. *et al.* Grass sickness of horses: changes in the regulatory peptide system of the bowel. *Vet Rec* **110:** 276, 1982.

Howell, J. McC., Baker, J. R., and Ritchie, H. E. Observations on the coeliaco–mesenteric ganglia of horses with and without grass sickness. *Br Vet J* **130:** 265–270, 1974.

Meyer, R. C., and Simon, J. Intestinal emphysema (pneumatosis cystoides intestinalis) in a gnotobiotic pig. *Can J Comp Med* **41:** 302–305, 1977.

Moon, H. W. Vacuolated villous epithelium of the small intestine of young pigs. *Vet Pathol* **9:** 3–21, 1972.

Ochoa, R., and de Velandia, S. Equine grass sickness: serologic evidence of association with *Clostridium perfringens* type A enterotoxin. *Am J Vet Res* **39:** 1049–1051, 1978.

Sellers, A. F. *et al.* The reservoir function of the equine cecum and ventral large colon—its relation to chronic non-surgical obstructive disease with colic. *Cornell Vet* **72:** 233–241, 1982.

Sellers, A. F. *et al.* Retropulsion–propulsion in equine large colon. *Am J Vet Res* **43:** 390–396, 1982.

Smith, B. H., and Welter, L. J. Pneumatosis intestinalis. *Am J Clin Pathol* **48:** 455–465, 1967.

Speirs, V. C., Hilbert, B. J., and Blood, D. C. Dorsal displacement of the left ventral and dorsal colon in two horses. *Aust Vet J* **55:** 542–544, 1979.

Strombeck, D. R. Obstruction of the intestinal tract. *In* "Small Animal Gastroenterology," pp. 291–300. Davis, California, Stonegate Press, 1979.

Svendsen, P., and Kristensen, B. Cecal dilatation in cattle. An experimental study of the etiology. *Nord Vet Med* **22:** 578–583, 1970.

Tate, L. P., and Donawick, W. J. Recurrent abdominal distress caused by enteroliths in a horse. *J Am Vet Med Assoc* **172:** 830–832, 1978.

Van Kruiningen, H. J. *et al.* A granulomatous colitis of dogs with histologic resemblance to Whipple's disease. *Pathol Vet* **2:** 521–544, 1965.

Wimberley, H. C., Andrews, E. J., and Haschek, W. M. Diaphragmatic hernias in the horse: a review of the literature and an analysis of six additional cases. *J Am Vet Med Assoc* **170:** 1404–1407, 1977.

Intestinal Ischemia and Infarction

Anderson, G. A. *et al.* Fatal acorn poisoning in a horse: pathologic findings and diagnostic considerations. *J Am Vet Med Assoc* **182:** 1105–1110, 1983.

Angus, K.W., Coop, R. L., and Mapes, C. J. Pathological changes or postmortem changes in parasitic infections: the influence of slaughter methods on intestinal histopathology. *Int J Parasitol* **2:** 485–486, 1972.

Bennett, D. G. Predisposition to abdominal crisis in the horse. *J Am Vet Med Assoc* **161:** 1189–1194, 1972.

Bounous, G. Menard, D., and de Medicis, E. Role of pancreatic proteases in the pathogenesis of ischemic enteropathy. *Gastroenterology* **73:** 102–108, 1977.

Cawthorne, R. J. G., Taylor, S. M., and Purcell, D. A. Pathological changes in parasitic infections of the intestine of calves and lambs: a technique for avoiding post-mortem artefacts. *Int J Parasitol* **3:** 447–449, 1973.

Chiu, C.-J. *et al.* Intestinal mucosal lesion in low-flow states. I. A morphological hemodynamic, and metabolic reappraisal. *Arch Surg* **101:** 478–483, 1970.

Fell, B. F. Cell shedding in the epithelium of the intestinal mucosa: fact and artefact. *J Pathol Bacteriol* **81:** 251–254, 1961.

Gay, C. C., and Speirs, V. C. Parasitic arteritis and its consequences in horses. *Aust Vet J* **54:** 600–601, 1978.

Granger, D. N. *et al.* Intestinal blood flow. *Gastroenterology* **78:** 837–863, 1980.

Gunson, D. E., and Rooney, J. R. Anaphylactoid purpura in a horse. *Vet Pathol* **14:** 325–331, 1977.

Haglund, U. *et al.* Mucosal lesions in the human small intestine in shock. *Gut* **16:** 979–984, 1975.

Lanciault, G., and Jacobson, E. D. The gastrointestinal circulation. *Gastroenterology* **71:** 851–873, 1976.

Menge, H., and Robinson, J. W. L. Early phase of jejunal regeneration after short term ischemia in the rat. *Lab Invest* **40:** 25–30, 1979.

Meyers, K. *et al.* Circulating endotoxin-like substance(s) and altered hemostasis in horses with gastrointestinal disorders: an interim report. *Am J Vet Res* **43:** 2233–2238, 1982.

Moore, J. N. *et al.* Effect of intraluminal oxygen in intestinal strangulation obstruction in ponies. *Am J Vet Res* **41:** 1615–1620, 1980.

Moore, J. N. *et al.* Endotoxemia following experimental intestinal strangulation obstruction in ponies. *Can J Comp Med* **45:** 330–332, 1981.

Nelson, A. W., and Adams, O. R. Intestinal infarction in the horse: acute colic arterial occlusion. *Am J Vet Res* **27:** 707–710, 1966.

Nelson, A. W., Collier, J. R., and Griner, L. A. Acute surgical colonic infarction in the horse. *Am J Vet Res* **29:** 315–327, 1968.

Pearson, G. R., and Logan, E. F. The rate of development of postmortem artefact in the small intestine of neonatal calves. *Br J Exp Pathol* **59:** 178–182, 1978.

Penning, P. D., and Treacher, T. T. Intestinal haemorrhage syndrome in artificially-reared lambs. *Vet Rec* **88:** 613–615, 1971.

Robinson, J. W. L. *et al.* Functional and morphological response of the dog colon to ischaemia. *Gut* **13:** 775–783, 1972.

Rooney, J. R. Volvulus, strangulation and intussusception in the horse. *Cornell Vet* **55:** 644–653, 1965.

Rowland, A. C., and Lawson, G. H. K. Intestinal haemorrhage syndrome in the pig. *Vet Rec* **93:** 402–404, 1973.

Slone, D. E. *et al.* Noniatrogenic rectal tears in three horses. *J Am Vet Med Assoc* **180:** 750–751, 1982.

Smart, M. E. *et al.* Intussusception in a Charolais bull. *Can Vet J* **18:** 244–246, 1977.

Speirs, V. C., Hilbert, B. J., and Blood, D. C. Dorsal displacement of the left ventral and dorsal colon in two horses. *Aust Vet J* **55:** 542–544, 1979.

Tepperman, B. L., and Jacobson, E. D. Mesenteric circulation. *In* "Physiology of the Gastrointestinal Tract," L. R. Johnson (ed.), pp. 1317–1336. New York, Raven Press, 1981.

Thorpe, E., and Thomlinson, J. R. Autolysis and postmortem bacteriological changes in the alimentary tract of the pig. *J Pathol Bacteriol* **93:** 601–610, 1967.

Todd, J. N. *et al.* Intestinal haemorrhage and volvulus in whey fed pigs. *Vet Rec* **100:** 11–12, 1977.

Tulleners, E. P. Surgical correction of volvulus of the root of the mesentery in calves. *J Am Vet Med Assoc* **179:** 998–999, 1981.

Wagner, R., Gabbert, H., and Hohn, P. Ischemia and post-ischemic regeneration of the small intestinal mucosa. *Virchows Arch B [Cell Pathol]* **31:** 259–276, 1979.

White, N. A. Intestinal infarction associated with mesenteric vascular thrombotic disease in the horse. *J Am Vet Med Assoc* **178:** 259–262, 1981.

White, N. A., Moore, J. N., and Trim, C. M. Mucosal alterations in experimentally induced small intestinal strangulation obstruction in ponies. *Am J Vet Res* **41:** 193–198, 1980.

Whitehead, R. The pathology of intestinal ischaemia. *Clin Gastroenterology* **1:** 613–637, 1972.

Wilson, G. P., and Burt, J. K. Intussusception in the dog and cat: a review of 45 cases. *J Am Vet Med Assoc* **164:** 515–518, 1974.

Yale, C. E., and Balish, E. The importance of clostridia in experimental intestinal strangulation. *Gastroenterology* **71:** 793–796, 1976.

Epithelial Renewal in Health and Disease

Angus, K. W., Coop, R. L., and Sykes, A. R. The rate of recovery of intestinal morphology following anthelintic treatment of parasitised sheep. *Res Vet Sci* **26:** 120–122, 1979.

Barker, I. K., and Ford, G. E. Development and distribution of atrophic enteritis in the small intestine of rabbits infected with *Trichostrongylus retortaeformis*. *J Comp Pathol* **85:** 427–435, 1975.

Barratt, M. E. J., Strachan, P. J., and Porter, P. Antibody mechanisms implicated in digestive disturbances following ingestion of soya protein in calves and piglets. *Clin Exp Immunol* **31:** 305–312, 1978.

Batt, R. M., and Scott, J. Response of the small intestinal mucosa to oral glucocorticoids. *Scand J Gastroenterol* **17:** Suppl 74, 75–88, 1982.

Bloom, S. R., and Polak, J. M. The hormonal pattern of intestinal adaptation. A major role for enteroglucagon. *Scand J Gastroenterol* **17:** Suppl 74, 93–103, 1982.

Castro, G. A. Immunological regulation of epithelial function. *Am J Physiol* **243:** G321–G329, 1982.

Dowling, R. H. Small bowel adaptation and its regulation. *Scand J Gastroenterol* **17:** Suppl 74, 53–74, 1982.

Ferguson, A., and Jarrett, E. E. E. Hypersensitivity reactions in the small intestine. I. Thymus dependence of experimental partial villous atrophy. *Gut* **16:** 114–117, 1975.

Fernando, M. A., and McCraw, B. M. Changes in the generation cycle of duodenal crypt cells in chickens infected with *Eimeria acervulina*. *Z Parasitenkd* **52:** 213–218, 1977.

Johnson, L. R. Regulation of gastrointestinal growth. *In* "Physiology of the Gastrointestinal Tract," L. R. Johnson (ed.), pp. 169–196. New York, Raven Press, 1981.

Kent, T. H., and Moon, H. W. The comparative pathogenesis of some enteric diseases. *Vet Pathol* **10**: 414–469, 1973.

Kilshaw, P. J., and Slade, H. Villus atrophy and crypt elongation in the small intestine of preruminant calves fed with heated soyabean flour or wheat gluten. *Res Vet Sci* **33**: 305–308, 1982.

Lipkin, M. Proliferation and differentiation of gastrointestinal cells in normal and disease states. *In* "Physiology of the Gastrointestinal Tract," L. R. Johnson (ed.), pp. 145–168. New York, Raven Press, 1981.

MacDonald, T. T., and Ferguson, A. Hypersensitivity reactions in the small intestine. III. The effects of allograft rejection and of graft-versus-host disease on epithelial cell kinetics. *Cell Tissue Kinet* **10**: 301–312, 1977.

Manson-Smith, D. F., Bruce, R. G., and Parrott, D. M. V. Villous atrophy and expulsion of intestinal *Trichinella spiralis* are mediated by T cells. *Cell Immunol* **47**: 285–292, 1979.

Mouwen, J. M. V. M. White scours in piglets. II. Scanning electron microscopy of the mucosa of the small intestine. *Vet Pathol* **8**: 401–413, 1971.

Rijke, R. P. C. *et al.* The effect of ischemic villus cell damage on crypt cell proliferation in the small intestine. Evidence for a feedback control mechanism. *Gastroenterology* **71**: 786–792, 1976.

Symons, L. E. A. Kinetics of the epithelial cells and morphology of villi and crypts in the jejunum of the rat infected by the nematode *Nippostrongylus brasiliensis*. *Gastroenterology* **49**: 158–168, 1965.

Watson, A. J., Appleton, D. R., and Wright, N. A. Adaptive cell-proliferative changes in the small-intestinal mucosa in coeliac disease. *Scand J Gastroenterol* **17**: Suppl 74, 115–127, 1982.

Weser, E., Vandeventer, A., and Tawil, T. Non-hormonal regulation of intestinal adaptation. *Scand J Gastroenterol* **17**: Suppl 74, 105–113, 1982.

Williamson, R. C. N. Intestinal adaptation. *N Engl J Med* **298**: 1393–1402, 1444–1450, 1978.

Williamson, R. C. N. Intestinal adaptation: factors that influence morphology. *Scand J Gastroenterol* **17**: Suppl 74, 21–29, 1982.

Wright, N. A. The experimental analysis of changes in proliferative and morphological status in studies on the intestine. *Scand J Gastroenterol* **17**: Suppl 74, 3–10, 1982.

Malabsorption and Diarrhea

Argenzio, R. A. Physiology of diarrhea—large intestine. *J Am Vet Med Assoc* **173**: 667–672, 1978.

Argenzio, R. A., and Whipp, S. C. Effect of *Escherichia coli* heat-stable enterotoxin, cholera toxin and theophylline on ion transport in porcine colon. *J Physiol (Lond)* **320**: 469–487, 1981.

Banwell, J. G. *et al.* Phytohemagglutinin derived from red kidney bean (*Phaseolus vulgaris*): a cause for intestinal malabsorption associated with bacterial overgrowth in the rat. *Gastroenterology* **84**: 506–515, 1983.

Batt, R. M. The molecular basis of malabsorption. *J Small Anim Pract* **21**: 555–569, 1980.

Batt, R. M., Bush, B. M., and Peters, T. J. Biochemical changes in the jejunal mucosa of dogs with naturally occurring exocrine pancreatic insufficiency. *Gut* **20**: 709–715, 1979.

Bolton, J. R. *et al.* Normal and abnormal xylose absorption in the horse. *Cornell Vet* **66**: 183–197, 1976.

Butler, D. G. *et al.* Transmissible gastroenteritis: mechanisms responsible for diarrhea in an acute viral enteritis in pigs. *J Clin Invest* **53**: 1335–1342, 1974.

Bywater, R. J., and Logan, E. F. The site and characteristics of intestinal water and electrolyte loss in *Escherichia coli*–induced diarrhea in calves. *J Comp Pathol* **84**: 599–610, 1974.

Duffy, P. A., Granger, D. N., and Taylor, A. E. Intestinal secretion induced by volume expansion in the dog. *Gastroenterology* **75**: 413–418, 1978.

Gardner, J. D. Pathogenesis of secretory diarrhea. *In* "Secretory Diarrhea," M. Field, J. S. Fordtran, and S. G. Schultz (eds.), pp. 153–158. Bethesda, Maryland, Am. Physiol. Soc., 1980.

Giannella, R. A. *et al.* Pathogenesis of *Salmonella*-mediated intestinal fluid secretion. *Gastroenterology* **69**: 1238–1245, 1975.

Gray, G. M. Carbohydrate digestion and absorption. *N Engl J Med* **292**: 1225–1230, 1975.

Hoenig, M. Intestinal malabsorption attributed to bacterial overgrowth in a dog. *J Am Vet Med Assoc* **176**: 533–535, 1980.

Isaacs, P. E. T., and Kim, Y. S. The contaminated small bowel syndrome. *Am J Med* **67**: 1049–1057, 1979.

Joy, C. L., and Patterson, J. M. Short bowel syndrome following surgical correction of a double intussusception in a dog. *Can Vet J* **19**: 254–259, 1978.

Kertzner, B. *et al.* Transmissible gastroenteritis: sodium transport and the intestinal epithelium during the course of viral enteritis. *Gastroenterology* **72**: 457–461, 1977.

King, C. E., and Toskes, P. P. Small intestine bacterial overgrowth. *Gastroenterology* **76**: 1035–1055, 1979.

Moon, H. W. Mechanisms in the pathogenesis of diarrhea: a review. *J Am Vet Med Assoc* **172**: 443–448, 1978.

Rachmilewitz, D. Prostaglandins and diarrhea. *Dig Dis Sci* **25**: 897–899, 1980.

Riley, J. W., and Glickman, R. M. Fat malabsorption—advances in our understanding. *Am J Med* **67**: 980–988, 1979.

Rogers, W. A. *et al.* Simultaneous evaluation of pancreatic exocrine function and intestinal absorptive function in dogs with chronic diarrhea. *J Am Vet Med Assoc* **177**: 1128–1131, 1980.

Sleisenger, M. H., and Kim, Y. S. Protein digestion and absorption. *N Engl J Med* **300**: 659–663, 1979.

Strombeck, D. R., Doe, M., and Jang, S. Maldigestion and malabsorption in a dog with chronic gastritis. *J Am Vet Med Assoc* **179**: 801–805, 1981.

Sykes, A. R., Coop, R. L., and Angus, K. W. Experimental production of osteoporosis in growing lambs by continuous dosing with *Trichostrongylus colubriformis* larvae. *J Comp Pathol* **85**: 549–559, 1975.

Tate, L. P. *et al.* Effects of extensive resection of the small intestine of the pony. *Am J Vet Res* **44**: 1187–1191, 1983.

Tennant, B., Harrold, D., and Reina-Guerra, M. Physiologic and metabolic factors in the pathogenesis of neonatal enteric infections in calves. *J Am Vet Med Assoc* **161**: 993–1007, 1972.

Weser, E., Fletcher, J. T., and Urban, E. Short bowel syndrome. *Gastroenterology* **77**: 572–579, 1979.

Whipp, S. C. Physiology of diarrhea—small intestines. *J Am Vet Med Assoc* **173**: 662–666, 1978.

Whitenack, D. L., Whitehair, C. K., and Miller, E. R. Influence of enteric infection on zinc utilization and clinical signs and lesions of zinc deficiency in young swine. *Am J Vet Res* **39**: 1447–1454, 1978.

Protein Metabolism in Enteric Disease and Syndromes Associated with Malabsorption and Protein-Losing Enteropathy

Bank, S. *et al.* The lymphatics of the intestinal mucosa. *Am J Dig Dis* **12**: 619–632, 1967.

Barker, I. K. Intestinal pathology associated with *Trichostrongylus colubriformis* infection in sheep: vascular permeability and ultrastructure of the mucosa. *Parasitology* **70**: 173–180, 1975.

Barton, C. L. *et al.* The diagnosis and clinicopathological features of canine protein-losing enteropathy. *J Am Anim Hosp Assoc* **14**: 85–91, 1978.

Bartsch, R. C., and Irvine-Smith, B. Eosinophilic gastroenteritis: report of a case in a dog. *J S Afr Vet Med Assoc* **43**: 263–265, 1972.

Batt, R. M., Bush, B. M., and Peters, T. J. Morphological and biochemical studies of a naturally occurring enteropathy in the dog resembling chronic tropical sprue in man. *Gastroenterology* **76**: 1096, 1979.

Breitschwerdt, E. B. *et al.* Serum proteins in healthy Basenjis and Basenjis with chronic diarrhea. *Am J Vet Res* **44**: 326–328, 1983.

Castro, G. A. Gastrointestinal function in the parasitized host. *Isot Radiat Parasitol 4 Proc Advis Group Meet 1979* pp. 143–153, 1981.

Cello, J. P. Eosinophilic gastroenteritis—a complex disease entity. *Am J Med* **67**: 1097–1104, 1979.

Cheville, N. F., Cutlip, R. C., and Moon, H. W. Microscopic pathology of the gray collie syndrome. *Pathol Vet* **7**: 225–245, 1970.

Coffman, J. R., and Hammond, L. S. Weight loss and the digestive system in the horse: a problem specific data base. *Vet Clin North Am: Large Anim Pract* **1**: 237–249, 1979.

Coop, R. L. Feed intake and utilization by the parasitized ruminant. *Isot Radiat Parasitol 4 Proc Advis Group Meet 1979* pp. 129–141, 1981.

Dargie, J. D. The pathophysiological effects of gastrointestinal and liver parasites in sheep. *In* "Digestive Physiology and Metabolism in ruminants," Y. Ruckebusch and P. Thivend (eds.), pp. 349–371. Lancaster, England, MTP Press, 1980.

DiBartola, S. P. *et al.* Regional enteritis in two dogs. *J Am Vet Med Assoc* **181**: 904–908, 1982.

Dietz, H.H., and Nielsen, K. Turnover of ^{131}I-labelled albumin in horses with gastrointestinal disease. *Nord Vet Med* **32**: 369–373, 1980.

Doe, W. F. An overview of intestinal immunity and malabsorption. *Am J Med* **67**: 1077–1084, 1979.

Finco, D. R. *et al.* Chronic enteric disease and hypoproteinemia in 9 dogs. *J Am Vet Med Assoc* **163**: 262–271, 1973.

Flesja, K., and Yri, T. Protein-losing enteropathy in the Lundehund. *J Small Anim Pract* **18**: 11–23, 1977.

Frank, B. W., and Kern, F. Intestinal and liver lymph and lymphatics. *Gastroenterology* **55**: 408–422, 1968.

Griffiths, G. L., Clark, W. T., and Mills, J. N. Lymphangiectasia in a dog. *Aust Vet J* **59**: 187–188, 1982.

Hart, I. R., and Kidder, D. E. The quantitative assessment of mucosa in canine small intestinal malabsorption. *Res Vet Sci* **25**: 163–167, 1978.

Hayden, D. W., and Fleischman, R. W. Scirrhous eosinophilic gastritis in dogs with gastric arteritis. *Vet Pathol* **14**: 441–448, 1977.

Hayden, D. W., and Van Kruiningen, H. J. Eosinophilic gastroenteritis in German shepherd dogs and its relationship to visceral larva migrans. *J Am Vet Med Assoc* **162**: 379–384, 1973.

Hayden, D. W., and Van Kruiningen, H. J. Lymphocytic–plasmacytic enteritis in German shepherd dogs. *J Am Anim Hosp Assoc* **18**: 89–96, 1982.

Hendrick, M. A spectrum of hypereosinophilic syndromes exemplified by six cats with eosinophilic enteritis. *Vet Pathol* **18**: 188–200, 1981.

Hill, F. W. G. Malabsorption syndrome in the dog: a study of thirty-eight cases. *J Small Anim Pract* **13**: 575–594, 1972.

Hill, F. W. G., and Kelly, D. F. Naturally occurring intestinal malabsorption in the dog. *Dig Dis* **19**: 649–665, 1974.

Landsverk, T., and Gamlem, H. Scanning electron microscopy of the Lundehund enteropathy. *J Ultrastruct Res* **69**: 153–154, 1979.

Malo, D., Gosselin, Y., and Papageorges, M. Enteropathie, avec perte de protéines, secondaire à une lymphangiectasie intestinale, chez trois chiens. *Can Vet J* **23**: 129–131, 1982.

Merritt, A. M. *et al.* Plasma clearance of [^{51}Cr]albumin into the intestinal tract of normal and chronically diarrheal horses. *Am. J Vet Res* **38**: 1769–1774, 1977.

Merritt, A. M., Cimprich, R. E., and Beech, J. Granulomatous enteritis in nine horses. *J Am Vet Med Assoc* **169**: 603–609, 1976.

Meuten, D. J. *et al.* Chronic enteritis associated with malabsorption and protein-losing enteropathy in the horse. *J Am Vet Med Assoc* **172**: 326–333, 1978.

Nielsen, K., and Andersen, S. Intestinal lymphagiectasia in cattle. *Nord Vet Med* **19**: 31–35, 1967.

Olson, N. C., and Zimmer, J. F. Protein-losing enteropathy secondary to intestinal lymphangiectasia in a dog. *J Am Vet Med Assoc* **173**: 271–274, 1978.

Pass, D. A., and Bolton, J. R. Chronic eosinophilic gastroenteritis in the horse. *Vet Pathol* **19**: 486–496, 1982.

Quigley, P. J., and Henry, K. Eosinophilic enteritis in the dog: a case report with a brief review of the literature. *J Comp Pathol* **91**: 387–392, 1981.

Randall, R. W., and Gibbs, H. C. Effects of clinical and subclinical gastrointestinal helminthiasis on digestion and energy metabolism in calves. *Am J Vet Res* **42**: 1730–1734, 1981.

Roberts, M. C., and Kelly, W. R. Granulomatous enteritis in a young standardbred mare. *Aust Vet J* **56**: 230–233, 1980.

Rothschild, M. A., Oratz, M., and Schreiber, S. S. Albumin metabolism. *Gastroenterology* **64**: 324–337, 1973.

Van Kruiningen, J. H. Giant hypertrophic gastritis of Basenji dogs. *Vet Pathol* **14**: 19–28, 1977.

Vardy, P. A., Lebenthal, E., and Shwachman, H. Intestinal lymphangiectasia: a reappraisal. *Pediatrics* **55**: 842–851, 1975.

Waldmann, T. A. Protein losing gastroenteropathies. *In* "Gastroenterology," H. L. Bockus (ed.), 3rd ed., Vol. 2, pp. 361–385. Philadelphia, Saunders, 1974.

Inflammation of the Large Intestine

Blaser, M. J., Parsons, R. B., and Wang, W.-L. L. Acute colitis caused by *Campylobacter fetus* ss. *jejuni. Gastroenterology* **78**: 448–453, 1980.

Bolton, G. R., and Brown, T. T. Mycotic colitis in a cat. *VM SAC* **67**: 978–981, 1972.

Bowe, P. S., Van Kruiningen, H. J., and Rosendal, S. Attempts to produce granulomatous colitis in boxer dogs with a mycoplasma. *Can J Comp Med* **46**: 430–433, 1982.

Damron, G. W. Gastrointestinal trichomonads in horses: occurrence and identification. *Am J Vet Res* **37**: 25–27, 1976.

Ewing, G. O. Feline ulcerative colitis: a case report. *J Am Anim Hosp Assoc* **8**: 64–65, 1972.

Ewing, G. O., and Gomez, J. A. Canine ulcerative colitis. *J Am Anim Hosp Assoc* **9**: 395–406, 1973.

Ferguson, H. W., Neill, S. D., and Pearson, G. R. Dysentery in pigs associated with cystic enlargement of submucosal glands in the large intestine. *Can J Comp Med* **44**: 109–114, 1980.

Gomez, J. A. *et al.* Canine histiocytic ulcerative colitis. An ultrastructural study of the early mucosal lesion. *Dig Dis* **22**: 485–496, 1977.

Greatorex, J. C. Diarrhea in horses associated with ulceration of the colon and caecum resulting from *S. vulgaris* larval migration. *Vet Rec* **97**: 221–225, 1975.

Hill, F. W. G., and Sullivan, N. D. Histiocytic ulcerative colitis in a boxer dog. *Aust Vet J* **54**: 447–449, 1978.

Kennedy, P. C., and Cello, R. M. Colitis of boxer dogs. *Gastroenterology* **51**: 926–931, 1966.

LeVeen, E. G. *et al.* Urease as a contributing factor in ulcerative lesions of the colon. *Am J Surg* **135**: 53–56, 1978.

McGavin, M. D., Gronwall, R. R., and Mia, A. S. Pathologic changes in experimental equine anaphylaxis. *J Am Vet Med Assoc* **160**: 1632–1636, 1972.

Manahan, F. F. Diarrhea in horses with particular reference to a chronic diarrhea syndrome. *Aust Vet J* **46**: 231–234, 1970.

Merritt, A. M., Bolton, J. R., and Cimprich, R. Differential diagnosis of diarrhoea in horses over six months of age. *J S Afr Vet Assoc* **46**: 73–76, 1975.

Moore, R. W., and Withrow, S. J. Gastrointestinal hemorrhage and pancreatitis associated with intervertebral disk disease in the dog. *J Am Vet Med Assoc* **180:** 1443–1447, 1982.

Nielsen, K., and Vibe-Petersen, G. Entero-colitis in the horse. A description of 46 cases. *Nord Vet Med* **31:** 376–384, 1979. [in Danish]

Nimmo-Wilkie, J. S. Necrotic colitis in two cats—description of the lesions. *Can Vet J* **23:** 197–199, 1982.

Ochoa, R., and Kern, S. R. The effects of *Clostridium perfringens* type A enterotoxin in Shetland ponies—clinical, morphologic and clinicopathologic changes. *Vet Pathol* **17:** 738–747, 1980.

Owen, R. Post stress diarrhoea in the horse. *Vet Rec* **96:** 267–270, 1975.

Patton, N. M., and Blankevoort, M. Colitis cystica profunda in pygmy goats. *J Comp Pathol* **86:** 371–375, 1976.

Prescott, J. R. *et al. Campylobacter jejuni* colitis in gnotobiotic dogs. *Can J Comp Med* **45:** 377–383, 1981.

Raisbeck, M. F., Holt, G. R., and Osweiler, G. D. Lincomycin-asociated colitis in horses. *J Am Vet Med Assoc* **179:** 362–363, 1981.

Rooney, J. R. *et al.* Exhaustion shock in the horse. *Cornell Vet* **56:** 220–235, 1965.

Russell, S. W., Gomez, J. A., and Trowbridge, J. O. Canine histiocytic ulcerative colitis. The early lesion and its progression to ulceration. *Lab Invest* **25:** 509–515, 1971.

Schiefer, H. B. Equine colitis X, still an enigma. *Can Vet J* **22:** 162–165, 1981.

Stewart, T. H. M. *et al.* Ulcerative enterocolitis in dogs induced by drugs. *J Pathol* **131:** 363–378, 1980.

Toombs, J. P. *et al.* Colonic perforation following neurosurgical procedures and corticosteroid therapy in four dogs. *J Am Vet Med Assoc* **177:** 68–72, 1980.

Turek, J. J., and Meyer, R. C. Studies on a canine intestinal spirochete: scanning electron microscopy of canine colonic mucosa. *Infect Immun* **20:** 853–855, 1978.

Umemura, T. *et al.* Histopathology of colitis X in the horse. *Jpn J Vet Sci* **44:** 717–724, 1982.

Van der Gaag, I. *et al.* Histiocytic ulcerative colitis in a French bulldog. *J Small Anim Pract* **19:** 283–290, 1978.

Van Kruiningen, H. J. The ultrastructure of macrophages in granulomatous colitis of boxer dogs. *Vet Pathol* **12:** 446–459, 1975.

Van Kruiningen, H. J., and Dobbins, W. O., III Feline histiocytic colitis. A case report with electron microscopy. *Vet Pathol* **16:** 215–222, 1979.

Van Kruiningen, H. J., Ryan, M. J., and Shindell, N. M. The classification of feline colitis. *J Comp Pathol* **93:** 275–294, 1983.

Vaughan, J. T. The acute colitis syndrome. Colitis X. *Vet Clin North Am* **3:** 301–313, 1973.

Watson, A. D. J. Giardiosis and colitis in a dog. *Aust Vet J* **56:** 444–447, 1980.

Wierup, M. Equine intestinal clostridiosis. *Acta Vet Scand [Suppl]* **62:** 1–182, 1977.

Wierup, M., and DiPietro, J. A. Bacteriologic examination of equine fecal flora as a diagnostic tool for equine intestinal clostridiosis. *Am J Vet Res* **42:** 2167–2169, 1981.

Tumors of the Intestinal Tract

Alroy, J. *et al.* Distinctive intestinal mast cell neoplasms of domestic cats. *Lab Invest* **33:** 159–167, 1975.

Brodey, R. A. Alimentary tract neoplasms in the cat: a clinicopathologic survey of 46 cases. *Am J Vet Res* **27:** 74–80, 1966.

Brodey, R. S., and Cohen, D. An epizootiologic and clinicopathologic study of 95 cases of gastrointestinal neoplasms in the dog. *Proc 101st Annu Meet Am Vet Med Assoc* pp. 167–179, 1964.

Carakostas, M. C. *et al.* Malignant foregut carcinoid tumor in a domestic cat. *Vet Pathol* **16:** 607–609, 1979.

Cotchin, E. Neoplasms in cats. *Proc R Soc Med* **45:** 671–674, 1952.

Cotchin, E. Some tumors of dogs and cats of comparative veterinary and human interest. *Vet Rec* **71:** 1040–1050, 1959.

Cotchin, E. A general survey of tumours in the horse. *Equine Vet J* **9:** 16–21, 1977.

Dodd, D. C. Adenocarcinoma of the small intestine of sheep. *NZ Vet J* **8:** 109–112, 1960.

Garner, F. M., and Lingeman, C. H. Mast-cell neoplasms of the domestic cat. *Pathol Vet* **7:** 517–530, 1970.

Georgsson, G., and Vigfusson, H. Carcinoma of the small intestine of sheep in Iceland. A pathological and epizootiological study. *Acta Vet Scand* **14:** 392–409, 1973.

Giles, R. C., Jr., Hildebrandt, P. K., and Montgomery, C. A., Jr. Carcinoid tumor in the small intestine of a dog. *Vet Pathol* **11:** 340–349, 1974.

Hayden, D. W., and Neilsen, S. W. Canine alimentary neoplasia. *Zentralbl Veterinaermed [A]* **20:** 1–22, 1973.

Head, K. W., and Else, R. W. Neoplasia and allied conditions of the canine and feline intestine. *Vet Annu* **21:** 190–208, 1981.

Kolaja, G. J., and Fairchild, D. G. Leiomyosarcoma of the duodenum in a dog. *J Am Vet Med Assoc* **163:** 275–276, 1973.

Lingeman, C. H., and Garner, F. M. Comparative study of intestinal adenocarcinomas of animals and man. *JNCI* **48:** 325–346, 1972.

Lingeman, C. H., Garner, F. M., and Taylor, D. O. N. Spontaneous adenocarcinomas of dogs: a review. *JNCI* **47:** 137–153, 1971.

McDonald, J. W., and Leaver, D. D. Adenocarcinoma of the small intestine of Merino sheep. *Aust Vet J* **41:** 269–271, 1965.

Olin, F. H., Lea, R. B., and Kim, C. Colonic adenoma in a cat. *J Am Vet Med Assoc* **153:** 53–56, 1968.

Palumbo, N. E., and Perri, S. F. Adenocarcinoma of the ileum in a cat. *J Am Vet Med Assoc* **164:** 607–608, 1974.

Patnaik, A. K., Hurvitz, A. I., and Johnson, G. F. Canine gastrointestinal neoplasms. *Vet Pathol* **14:** 547–555, 1977.

Patnaik, A. K., and Lieberman, P. H. Canine goblet-cell carcinoid. *Vet Pathol* **18:** 410–413, 1981.

Patnaik, A. K., Liu, S.-K., and Johnson, G. F., Feline intestinal adenocarcinoma. A clinicopathologic study of 22 cases. *Vet Pathol* **13:** 1–10, 1976.

Ross, A. D. Small intestinal carcinoma in sheep. *Aust Vet J* **56:** 25–28, 1980.

Ross, A. D., and Day, W. A. Intestinal polyps in a lamb. *NZ Vet J* **27:** 172–173, 1979.

Schaffer, E., and Schiefer, B. Incidence and types of canine rectal carcinomas. *J Small Anim Pract* **9:** 491–496, 1968.

Seiler, R. J. Colorectal polyps of the dog: a clinicopathologic study of 17 cases. *J Am Vet Med Assoc* **174:** 72–75, 1979.

Simpson, B. H., and Jolly, R. D. Carcinoma of the small intestine in sheep. *J Pathol* **112:** 83–92, 1974.

Sykes, G. P., and Cooper, B. J. Canine intestinal carcinoids. *Vet Pathol* **19:** 120–131, 1982.

Turk, M. A. M., Gallina, A. M., and Russell, T. S. Nonhematopoietic gastrointestinal neoplasia in cats: a retrospective study of 44 cases. *Vet Pathol* **18:** 614–620, 1981.

Vitovec, J. Carcinomas of the intestine in cattle and pigs. *Zentralbl Veterinaermed [A]* **24:** 413–421, 1977.

Diagnosis of Diarrhea in Neonatal Ruminants, Swine, and Foals

Acres, S. D., Saunders, J. R., and Radostits, O. M. Acute undifferentiated neonatal diarrhea of beef calves: the prevalence of enterotoxigenic *E. coli*, reo-like (rota) virus and other enteropathogens in cow-calf herds. *Can Vet J* **18:** 113–121, 1977.

Bergeland, M. E., and Henry, S. C. Infectious diarrheas of young pigs. *Vet Clin North Am: Large Anim Pract* **4**: 389–399, 1982.

Bohl, E. H. *et al.* Porcine pararotavirus: detection, differentiation from rotavirus, and pathogenesis in gnotobiotic pigs. *J Clin Microbiol* **15**: 312–319, 1982.

Bulgin, M. S. *et al.* Infectious agents associated with neonatal calf disease in southwestern Idaho and eastern Oregon. *J Am Vet Med Assoc* **180**: 1222–1226, 1982.

Cilli, V., and Castrucci, G. Viral diarrhea of young animals: a review. *Comp Immunol Microbiol Infect Dis* **4**: 229–242, 1981.

Dea, S., Roy, R. S., and Elazhary, M. A. S. Y. Virus-like particles, 45 to 65 nm, in intestinal contents of neonatal calves. *Can J Comp Med* **47**: 88–91, 1983.

Durham, P. J. K., and Johnson, R. H. Viral diarrhoea in young animals. *In* "Advances in Veterinary Virology," T. G. Hungerford (ed.), Proc. No. 60, pp. 211–222. University of Sydney Postgraduate Committee in Veterinary Science, Sydney, Australia, 1982.

Eugster, A. K., and Sneed, L. Viral intestinal infections of animals and man. *Comp Immunol Microbiol Infect Dis* **2**: 417–435, 1980.

Gibbs, E. P. J., Smale, C. J., and Voyle, C. A. Electron microscopy as an aid to the rapid diagnosis of virus diseases of veterinary importance. *Vet Rec* **106**: 451–458, 1980.

Marsolais, G. *et al.* Diagnosis of viral agents associated with neonatal calf diarrhea. *Can J Comp Med* **42**: 168–171, 1978.

Mebus, C. A., Rhodes, M. B., and Underdahl, N. R. Neonatal calf diarrhea caused by a virus that induces villous epithelial cell syncytia. *Am J Vet Res* **39**: 1223–1228, 1978.

Moon, H. W. *et al.* Pathogenic relationships of rotavirus, *Escherichia coli* and other agents in mixed infections in calves. *J Am Vet Med Assoc* **173**: 577–583, 1978.

Morin, M. *et al.* Neonatal diarrhea of pigs in Quebec: infectious causes of significant outbreaks. *Can J Comp Med* **47**: 11–17, 1983.

Morin, M., Lariviere, S., and Lallier, R. Pathological and microbiological observations made on spontaneous cases of acute neonatal calf diarrhea. *Can J Comp Med* **40**: 228–240, 1976.

Saif, L. J. *et al.* Rotavirus-like, calicivirus-like and 23-nm virus-like particles associated with diarrhea in young pigs. *J Clin Microbiol* **12**: 105–111, 1980.

Schwartz, W. L. Laboratory diagnosis of swine diseases. *Vet Clin North Am: Large Anim Pract* **4**: 201–223, 1982.

Snodgrass, D. R. Astroviruses in diarrhea of young animals and children. *In* "Comparative Diagnosis of Viral Diseases," E. Kurstak and C. Kurstak (eds.), Vol. 6, pp. 659–669. New York, Academic Press, 1981.

Storz, J. *et al.* Parvoviruses associated with diarrhea in calves. *J Am Vet Med Assoc* **173**: 624–627, 1978.

Svendsen, J. *et al.* Preweaning mortality in pigs. 4. Diseases of the gastrointestinal tract in pigs. *Nord Vet Med* **27**: 85–101, 1975.

Tzipori, S. The aetiology and diagnosis of calf diarrhoea. *Vet Rec* **108**: 510–514, 1981.

Tzipori, S. *et al.* Diarrhea in lambs: experimental infections with enterotoxigenic *Escherichia coli*, rotavirus, and *Cryptosporidium* sp. *Infect Immun* **33**: 401–406, 1981.

Woode, G. N., and Bridger, J. C. Isolation of small viruses resembling astroviruses and caliciviruses from acute enteritis of calves. *J Med Microbiol* **11**: 441–452, 1978.

Infectious Gastroenteritis in Dogs and Cats

Ducatelle, R. *et al.* Concurrent parvovirus and distemper virus infections in a dog. *Vet Rec* **108**: 310, 1980.

Evermann, J. F. *et al.* Diarrheal condition in dogs associated with viruses antigenically related to feline herpesvirus. *Cornell Vet* **72**: 285–291, 1982.

Hammond, M. M., and Timoney, P. J. An electron microscopic study of viruses associated with canine gastroenteritis. *Cornell Vet* **73**: 82–97, 1983.

Osterhaus, A. D. M. E. *et al.* Canine viral enteritis: prevalence of parvo-corona- and rotavirus infections in dogs in the Netherlands. *Vet Q* **2**: 181–236, 1980.

Williams, F. P. Astrovirus-like, coronavirus-like, and parvovirus-like particles detected in the diarrheal stools of beagle pups. *Arch Virol* **66**: 215–226, 1980.

Vesicular Diseases

Anderson, E. C. The pathogenesis of foot and mouth disease in the African buffalo (*Syncercus caffer*) and the role of this species in the epidemiology of the disease in Kenya. *J Comp Pathol* **89**: 541–549, 1979.

Anonymous. Foot and mouth disease in non-domestic animals. *Bull Epizoot Dis Afr* **11**: 143–146, 1963.

Baker, K. B. Swine vesicular disease. *Vet Annu* **22**: 135–139, 1982.

Barboni, E., Manocchio, I., and Asdrubali, G. Observations on diabetes mellitus associated with experimental foot and mouth disease in cattle. *Vet Ital* **17**: 362–368, 1966.

Blackwell, J. H., and Yilma, T. Localization of foot and mouth disease viral antigens in mammary gland of infected cows. *Am J Vet Res* **42**: 770–773, 1981.

Brooksby, J. B. Epizootiology of foot and mouth disease in developing countries. *World Anim Rev* **1**: 10–13, 1972.

Burrows, R. Studies on the carrier state of cattle exposed to foot and mouth disease virus. *J Hyg (Lond)* **64**: 81–90, 1966.

Burrows, R. *et al.* The pathogenesis of natural and simulated natural foot and mouth disease infection in cattle. *J Comp Pathol* **91**: 599–609, 1981.

Chow, T. L., Hansen, R. R., and McNutt, S. H. Pathology of vesicular stomatitis in cattle. *Proc Am Vet Med Assoc* pp. 119–124, 1951.

Chow, T. L., and McNutt, S. H. Pathological changes of experimental vesicular stomatitis of swine. *Am J Vet Res* **14**: 420–424, 1953.

Chu, R. M., Moore, D. M., and Conroy, J. D. Experimental swine vesicular disease: pathology and immunofluorescence studies. *Can J Comp Med* **43**: 29–38, 1979.

Crawford, A. B. Experimental vesicular exanthema of swine. *J Am Vet Med Assoc* **90**: 380–395, 1937.

Gailiunas, P., and Cottral, G. E. Presence and persistence of foot and mouth disease virus in bovine skin. *J Bacteriol* **91**: 2333–2338, 1966.

Geering, W. A. Foot and mouth disease in sheep. *Aust Vet J* **43**: 485–489, 1967.

Gibbs, E. P. J. (ed.) "Virus Diseases of Food Animals," Vol. 2 New York, Academic Press, 1981.

Henderson, W. M. Foot-and-mouth disease and related vesicular diseases. *Adv Vet Sci* **6**: 19–77, 1960.

Hyslop, N. St.G., and Fagg, R. H. Isolation of variants during passage of a strain of foot and mouth disease virus in partly immunized cattle. *J Hyg (Lond)* **63**: 357–368, 1965.

Leman, A. D. *et al.* (eds.) "Diseases of Swine," 5th ed. Ames, Iowa State Univ. Press, 1981.

Lenghaus, C. *et al.* Neuropathology of experimental swine vesicular disease in pigs. *Res Vet Sci* **21**: 19–27, 1976.

Lenghaus, C., and Mann, J. A. General pathology of experimental swine vesicular disease. *Vet Pathol* **13**: 186–196, 1976.

Mann, J. A., and Hutchings, G. H. Swine vesicular disease: pathways of infection. *J Hyg (Lond)* **84**: 355–363, 1980.

Mebus, C. A. Ulcerative diseases of animals with an infectious etiology. *J Oral Pathol* **7**: 365–371, 1978.

Mohanty, S. B., and Dutta, S. K. "Veterinary Virology," pp. 87–274. Philadelphia, Lea & Febiger, 1981.

Murray, M. D., and Snowdon, W. A. The role of wild animals in the spread of exotic diseases in Australia. *Aust Vet J* **52:** 547–554, 1976.

Platt, H. The localization of lesions in experimental foot-and-mouth disease. *Br J Exp Pathol* **41:** 150–159, 1960.

Proctor, S. J., and Sherman, K. C. Ultrastructural changes in bovine lingual epithelium with vesicular stomatitis virus. *Vet Pathol* **12:** 362–377, 1975.

Ribelin, W. The cytopathogenesis of vesicular stomatitis virus infection in cattle. *Am J Vet Res* **19:** 66–72, 1958.

Sawyer, J. C. Vesicular exanthema of swine and San Miguel sea lion virus. *J Am Vet Med Assoc* **169:** 707–709, 1976.

Scott, R. W., Cottral, G. E., and Gailiunas, P. Persistence of foot and mouth disease virus in external lesions and saliva of experimentally infected cattle. *Am J Vet Res* **27:** 1531–1536, 1966.

Siebold, H. R., and Sharp, J. B. A revised concept of the pathologic changes of the tongue in cattle with vesicular stomatitis. *Am J Vet Res* **21:** 35–51, 1960.

Smith, A. W., and Akers, T. G. Vesicular exanthema of swine. *J Am Vet Med Assoc* **169:** 700–703, 1976.

Sutmoller, P., McVicar, J. W., and Cottral, G. E. The epizootiological importance of foot and mouth disease carriers. I. Experimentally produced foot and mouth disease carriers in susceptible and immune cattle. *Arch Virus* **23:** 227–235, 1968.

Watson, W. A. Vesicular diseases: recent advances and concepts of control. *Can Vet J* **22:** 311–320, 1981.

Yilma, T. Morphogenesis of vesiculation in foot and mouth disease. *Am J Vet Res* **41:** 1537–1542, 1980.

Bovine Virus Diarrhea

Ames, T. R. *et al.* Border disease in a flock of Minnesota sheep. *J Am Vet Med Assoc* **180:** 619–621, 1982.

Badman, R. T. *et al.* Association of bovine viral diarrhoea virus infection to hydranencephaly and other central nervous system lesions in perinatal calves. *Aust Vet J* **57:** 306–307, 1981.

Baker, J. A. *et al.* Virus diarrhea in cattle. *Am J Vet Res* **15:** 525–531, 1954.

Bistner, S. I., Rubin, L. F., and Saunders, L. Z. The ocular lesions of bovine viral diarrhea–mucosal disease. *Pathol Vet* **7:** 275–286, 1970.

Bohac, J. G., and Yates, W. D. G. Concurrent bovine virus diarrhea and bovine papular stomatitis infection in a calf. *Can Vet J* **21:** 310–313, 1980.

Carbrey, E. A. *et al.* Natural infection of pigs with bovine viral diarrhea virus and its differential diagnosis from hog cholera. *J Am Vet Med Assoc* **169:** 1217–1219, 1976.

Coria, M. F., and McClurkin, A. W. Specific immune tolerance in an apparently healthy bull persistently infected with bovine viral diarrhea virus. *J Am Vet Med Assoc* **172:** 449–451, 1978.

Cutlip, R. C., McClurkin, A. W., and Coria, M. F. Lesions in clinically healthy cattle persistently infected with the virus of bovine viral diarrhea–glomerulonephritis and encephalitis. *Am J Vet Res* **41:** 1938–1941, 1980.

Done, J. T. *et al.* Bovine virus diarrhea–mucosal disease virus: pathogenicity for the fetal calf following maternal infection. *Vet Rec* **106:** 473–479, 1980.

French, E. L., and Snowdon, W. A. Mucosal disease in Australian cattle. *Aust Vet J* **40:** 99–105, 1964.

Inui, S., Narita, M., and Kumagai, T. Bovine virus diarrhea–mucosal disease. I. Pathological changes in natural and experimental cases. *Natl Inst Anim Health Q (Tokyo)* **18:** 109–117, 1978.

Johnson, D. W. Immunologic abnormalities in calves with chronic bovine virus diarrhea. *Am J Vet Res* **34:** 1139–1141, 1975.

Kahrs, R. F. Effects of bovine virus diarrhea on the developing fetus: a review. *J Am Vet Med Assoc* **163:** 877–878, 1973.

Kent, T. H., and Moon, H. W. The comparative pathology of some enteric diseases. *Vet Pathol* **10:** 414–469, 1973.

Lambert, G., Fernelius, A. L., and Cheville, N. F. Experimental bovine viral diarrhea in neonatal calves. *J Am Vet Med Assoc* **154:** 181–189, 1969.

Lambert, G., McClurkin, A. W., and Fernelius, A. L. Bovine viral diarrhea in the neonatal calf. *J Am Vet Med Assoc* **164:** 287–289, 1974.

Loken, T., Bjorkas, I., and Hyllseth, B. Border disease in goats in Norway. *Res Vet Sci* **33:** 130–131, 1982.

Meyling, A. Distribution of VD-virus by the fluorescent antibody technique in tissues of cattle affected with bovine viral diarrhea (mucosal disease). *Acta Vet Scand* **11:** 59–72, 1970.

Muscoplat, C. C., Johnson, D. W., and Stevens, J. B. Abnormalities of *in vitro* lymphocyte responses during bovine viral diarrhea virus infection. *Am J Vet Res* **34:** 753–755, 1973.

Niemi, S. M. *et al.* Border disease virus isolation from postpartum ewes. *Am J Vet Res* **43:** 86–88, 1982.

Parsonson, I. M. *et al.* The effects of bovine viral diarrhea–mucosal disease (BVD) virus on the ovine foetus. *Vet Microbiol* **4:** 279–292, 1979.

Peter, C. P. *et al.* Cytopathologic changes of lymphatic tissues of cattle with the bovine virus diarrhea–mucosal disease complex. *Am J Vet Res* **29:** 939–948, 1968.

Plant, J. W., Gard, G. P., and Acland, H. M. A mucosal disease virus infection of the pregnant ewe as a cause of a border disease–like condition. *Aust Vet J* **52:** 247–249, 1976.

Potts, B. J., Johnson, K. P., and Osburn, B. I. Border disease: tissue culture studies of the virus in sheep. *Am J Vet Res* **43:** 1460–1463, 1982.

Potts, B. J., Osburn, B. I., and Johnson, K. P. Border disease: experimental reproduction in sheep, using a virus replicated in tissue culture. *Am J Vet Res* **43:** 1464–1466, 1982.

Pritchard, W. R. *et al.* A transmissible disease affecting the mucosae of cattle. *J Am Vet Med Assoc* **128:** 1–5, 1956.

Reggiardo, C., and Kaeberle, M. L. Detection of bacteremia in cattle inoculated with bovine viral diarrhea virus. *Am J Vet Res* **42:** 218–221, 1981.

Roth, J. A., Kaeberle, M. L., and Griffith, R. W. Effects of bovine viral diarrhea virus infection on bovine polymorphonuclear leukocyte function. *Am J Vet Res* **42:** 244–250, 1981.

Steck, F. *et al.* Immune responsiveness in cattle fatally affected by bovine virus diarrhea–mucosal disease. *Zentralbl Veterinaermed* [B] **27:** 429–445, 1980.

Terlecki, S. Border disease: a viral teratogen of farm animals. *Vet Annu* **17:** 74–79, 1977.

Terlecki, S., Herbert, C. N., and Done, J. T. Morphology of experimental border disease of lambs. *Res Vet Sci* **15:** 310–317, 1973.

Tyler, D. E., and Ramsey, F. K. Comparative pathologic, immunologic and clinical responses produced by selected agents of the bovine mucosal disease–virus diarrhea complex. *Am J Vet Res* **26:** 903–913, 1965.

Ward, G. M. *et al.* A study of experimentally induced bovine viral diarrhea–mucosal disease in pregnant cows and their progeny. *Cornell Vet* **59:** 525–538, 1969.

Rinderpest and Peste des Petits Ruminants

Appel, M. J. G. *et al.* Morbillivirus diseases of animals and man. *In* "Comparative Diagnosis of Viral Diseases," E. Kurstak and C. Kurstak (eds.), Vol. 4, pp. 235–297. New York, Academic Press, 1981.

Bawa, H. S. Rinderpest in sheep and goats in Ajmermerwara. *Indian J Vet Sci* **10:** 103–112, 1940.

Hamdy, F. M. *et al.* Etiology of the stomatitis, pneumonenteritis complex in Nigerian dwarf goats. *Can J Comp Med* **40:** 276–284, 1980.

Joshi, R. C., Chaudhary, P. G., and Bansal, R. P. Occurrence of cutaneous eruptions in rinderpest outbreak among bovine. *Indian Vet J* **54:** 871–873, 1977.

Liess, B., and Plowright, W. Studies on the pathogenesis of rinderpest in experimental cattle. I. Correlation of clinical signs, viraemia and virus excretion by various routes. *J Hyg (Lond)* **62:** 81–100, 1964.

Maurer, F. D. *et al.* The pathology of rinderpest. *Proc 92nd Annu. Meet Am Vet Med Assoc* pp. 201–211, 1956.

Plowright, W. The role of game animals in the epizootiology of rinderpest and malignant catarrhal fever in East Africa. *Bull Epizoot Dis Afr* **11:** 149–162, 1963.

Plowright, W. Studies on the pathogenesis of rinderpest in experimental cattle. II. Proliferation of the virus in different tissues following intranasal infection. *J Hyg (Lond)* **62:** 257–281, 1964.

Plowright, W. Rinderpest. *Vet Rec* **77:** 1431–1438, 1965.

Rowland, A. C., Scott, G. R., and Hill, D. H. The pathology of an erosive stomatitis and enteritis in West African dwarf goats. *J Pathol* **98:** 83–87, 1969.

Scott, G. R. Rinderpest and peste des petits ruminants. *In* "Virus Diseases of Food Animals," E. P. Gibbs (ed.), Vol. 2, pp. 401–432. New York, Academic Press, 1981.

Scott, G. R., DeTray, D. E., and White, G. Rinderpest in pigs of European origin. *Am J Vet Res* **23:** 452–456, 1961.

Taylor, W. P. *et al.* Studies on the pathogenesis of rinderpest in experimental cattle. IV. Proliferation of the virus following contact infection. *J Hyg (Lond)* **63:** 497–506, 1965.

Malignant Catarrhal Fever

Boever, W. J., and Kurka, B. Malignant catarrhal fever in greater kudus. *J Am Vet Med Assoc* **165:** 817–819, 1974.

Castro, A. E. *et al.* Malignant catarrhal fever in an Indian gaur and greater kudu: experimental transmission, isolation, and identification of a herpesvirus. *Am J Vet Res* **43:** 5–11, 1982.

Castro, A. E., and Daley, G. G. Electron microscopic study of the African strain of malignant catarrhal fever virus in bovine cell cultures. *Am J Vet Res* **43:** 576–582, 1982.

Coulter, G. R., and Storz, J. Identification of a cell-associated morbillivirus from cattle affected with malignant catarrhal fever: antigenic differentiation and cytologic characterization. *Am J Vet Res* **40:** 1671–1677, 1979.

Hamdy, F. M. Etiology of malignant catarrhal fever outbreak in Minnesota. *Proc 82nd Annu Meet US Anim Health Assoc* pp. 248–267, 1978.

Kalunda, M. *et al.* Malignant catarrhal fever. III. Experimental infection of sheep, domestic rabbits and laboratory animals with malignant catarrhal fever virus. *Can J Comp Med* **45:** 310–314, 1981.

Kalunda, M., Dardiri, A. H., and Lee, K. M. Malignant catarrhal fever. I. Response of American cattle to malignant catarrhal fever virus isolated in Kenya. *Can J Comp Med* **45:** 70–76, 1981.

Liggitt, H. D. *et al.* Experimental transmision of malignant catarrhal fever in cattle: gross and histopathologic changes. *Am J Vet Res* **39:** 1249–1257, 1978.

Liggitt, H. D. *et al.* Synovitis and bovine syncytial virus isolation in experimentally induced malignant catarrhal fever. *J Comp Pathol* **90:** 519–533, 1980.

Liggitt, H. D., and De Martini, J. C. The pathomorphology of malignant catarrhal fever. I. Generalized lymphoid vasculitis. *Vet Pathol* **17:** 58–72, 1980.

Liggitt, H. D., and DeMartini, J. C. The pathomorphology of malignant catarrhal fever. II. Multisystemic epitheial lesions. *Vet Pathol* **17:** 73–83, 1980.

Orsborn, J. R. *et al.* Diagnostic features of malignant catarrhal fever outbreaks in the western United States. *Proc Am Assoc Vet Lab Diagn* **20:** 215–224, 1977.

Pierson, R. E. *et al.* An epizootic of malignant catarrhal fever in feedlot cattle. *J Am Vet Med Assoc* **163:** 349–350, 1973.

Pierson, R. E. *et al.* Clinical and clinicopathologic observations in induced malignant catarrhal fever of cattle. *J Am Vet Med Assoc* **173:** 833–837, 1978.

Plowright, W. Malignant catarrhal fever. *J Am Vet Med Assoc* **152:** 795–806, 1968.

Plowright, W. *et al.* Congenital infection of cattle with the herpesvirus causing malignant catarrhal fever. *Res Vet Sci* **13:** 37–45, 1972.

Plowright, W., Ferris, R. D., and Scott, G. R. Blue wildebeest and the aetiological agent of bovine malignant catarrhal fever. *Nature* **188:** 1167–1169, 1960.

Reid, H. W. *et al.* An outbreak of malignant catarrhal fever in red deer (*Cervus elephus*). *Vet Rec* **104:** 120–123, 1979.

Rossiter, P. B. Antibodies to malignant catarrhal fever virus in sheep sera. *J Comp Pathol* **91:** 303–311, 1981.

Rossiter, P. B. Immunoglobulin response of rabbits infected with malignant catarrhal fever virus. *Res Vet Sci* **33:** 120–122, 1982.

Ruth, G. R. *et al.* Malignant catarrhal fever in bison. *J Am Vet Med Assoc* **171:** 913–917, 1977.

Rweyemamu, M. M. *et al.* Malignant catarrhal fever virus in nasal secretions of wildebeest: a probable mechanism for virus transmission. *J Wildl Dis* **10:** 478–487, 1974.

Selman, I. E. *et al.* Transmission studies with bovine malignant catarrhal fever. *Vet Rec* **102:** 252–257, 1978.

Storz, J. *et al.* Virologic studies on cattle with naturally occurring and experimentally induced malignant catarrhal fever. *Am J Vet Res* **37:** 875–878, 1976.

Zimmer, M. A., McCoy, C. P., and Jensen, J. M. Comparative pathology of the African form of malignant catarrhal fever in captive Indian gaur and domestic cattle. *J Am Vet Med Assoc* **179:** 1130–1135, 1981.

Bluetongue and Related Diseases

Della-Porta, A. J. *et al.* Classification of the orbiviruses. Confusion in the use of terms bluetongue virus, bluetongue-like virus, bluetongue-related virus and the overall nomenclature. *Aust Vet J* **58:** 164–165, 1982.

Erasmus, B. J. Bluetongue in sheep and goats. *Aust Vet J* **51:** 165–170, 228–232, 1975.

Erasmus, B. J. The epizootiology of bluetongue: the African situation. *Aust Vet. J* **51:** 196–198 and 228–232, 1975.

Fletch, A. L., and Karstad, L. H. Studies on the Pathogenesis of experimental epizootic hemorrhagic disease of white-tailed deer. *Can J Comp Med* **35:** 224–229, 1971.

Hoff, G. L., and Trainer, D. O. Bluetongue and epizootic hemorrhagic disease viruses: their relationship to wildlife species. *Adv Vet Sci Comp Med* **22:** 111–132, 1978.

Hoff, G. L., and Trainer, D. O. Hemorrhagic diseases of wild ruminants. *In* "Infectious Diseases of Wild Mammals," J. W. Davis, L. H. Karstad, and D. O. Trainer (eds.), pp. 45–53. Ames, Iowa State Univ. Press, 1981.

Hourrigan, J. L., and Klingsporn, A. L. Bluetongue: the disease in cattle. *Aust Vet J* **51:** 170–174, 1975.

Hourrigan, J. L., and Klingsporn, A. L. Epizootiology of bluetongue: the situation in the United States of America. *Aust Vet J* **51:** 203–208, 1975.

House, J. A., Groocock, C. M., and Campbell, C. H. Antibodies to bluetongue viruses in animals imported into United States zoological gardens. *Can J Comp Med* **46:** 154–159, 1982.

Inaba, Y. Ibaraki disease and its relationship to bluetongue. *Aust Vet J* **51**: 178–185, 1975.

Karstad, L., and Trainer, D. O. Histopathology of experimental blue-tongue disease of white-tailed deer. *Can Vet J* **8**: 247–254, 1967.

Luedke, A. J. *et al.* Clinical and pathologic features of bluetongue in sheep. *Am J Vet Res* **25**: 963–970, 1964.

Luedke, A. J., Jochim, M. M., and Jones, R. H. Bluetongue in cattle: effects of *Culicoides variipennis*–transmitted bluetongue virus in pregnant heifers and their calves. *J Am Vet Med Assoc* **38**: 1687–1695, 1977.

Metcalf, H. E., and Luedke, A. J. Bluetongue and related diseases. *Bovine Pract* **15**: 188–193, 1980.

Omori, T. Ibaraki disease: a bovine epizootic disease resembling blue-tongue. *Natl Inst Anim Health Q* (*Tokyo*) **10**: Suppl 45–55, 1970.

Pini, A. A study on the pathogenesis of bluetongue: replication of the virus in the organs of infected sheep. *Onderstepoort J Vet Res* **43**: 159–164, 1976.

Sellers, R. F. Bluetongue and related diseases. *In* "Virus Diseases of Food Animals," E. P. J. Gibbs (ed.), Vol. 2, pp. 567–584. New York, Academic Press, 1981.

Stair, E. L., Robinson, R. M., and Jones, L. P. Spontaneous bluetongue in Texas white-tailed deer. *Pathol Vet* **5**: 164–173, 1968.

Stott, J. L., Lauerman, L. H., and Luedke, A. J. Bluetongue virus in pregnant elk and their calves. *Am J Vet Res* **43**: 423–428, 1982.

Thomas, A. D., and Neitz, W. O. Further observations on the pathology of bluetongue in sheep. *Onderstepoort J Vet Sci Anim Ind* **22**: 27–36, 1947.

Tsai, K., and Karstad, L. The pathogenesis of epizootic hemorrhagic disease of deer. *Am J Pathol* **70**: 379–392, 1973.

Uren, M. F., and Squire, K. R. E. The clinico-pathological effect of bluetongue virus serotype 20 in sheep. *Aust Vet J* **58**: 11–15, 1982.

Bovine Papular Stomatitis and Contagious Ecthyma

Carson, C. A., and Kerr, K. M. Bovine papular stomatitis with apparent transmission to man. *J Am Vet Med Assoc* **151**: 183–187, 1967.

Cheville, N. F., and Shey, D. J. Pseudocowpox in dairy cattle. *J Am Vet Med Assoc* **150**: 855–861, 1967.

Crandell, R. A., and Gosser, H. S. Ulcerative esophagitis associated with poxvirus infection in a calf. *J Am Vet Med Assoc* **165**: 282–283, 1974.

Griesemer, R. A., and Cole, C. R. Bovine papular stomatitis. III. Histo-pathology. *Am J Vet Res* **22**: 482–486, 1961.

Nagington, J., Lauder, I. M., and Smith, J. S. Bovine papular stom-atitis, pseudocowpox and milker's nodules. *Vet Rec* **81**: 306–313, 1967.

Robinson, A. J., and Balassu, T. C. Contagious pustular dermatitis (orf). *Vet Bull* **51**: 771–782, 1981.

Infectious Bovine Rhinotracheitis Virus and Other Herpesviruses Infections of the Alimentary Tract

Baker, J. A., McEntee, K., and Gillespie, J. H. Effects of infectious bovine rhinotracheitis–infectious pustular vulvovaginitis (IBR–IPV) virus on newborn calves. *Cornell Vet* **50**: 156–170, 1960.

Berrios, P. E., McKercher, D. G., and Knight, H. D. Pathogenicity of a caprine herpesvirus. *Am J Vet Res* **36**: 1763–1769, 1975.

Burkhardt, E., and Paulsen, J. Nachweis von Bovinem Herpesvirus 1 (IBR/IPV) bei Rindern mit Affektionen des Verdauungstraktes. *Berl Muench Tieraerztl Wochenschr* **91**: 480–486, 1978.

Ehrensperger, F., and Polenz, J. Infektiose Bovine Rhinotracheitis bei Kalbern. *Schweiz Arch Tierheilkd* **121**: 635–642, 1979.

Fernelius, A. L., and Ritchie, A. E. Mixed infections or contaminations of bovine viral diarrhea virus with infectious bovine rhinotracheitis virus. *Am J Vet Res* **27**: 241–248, 1966.

Kahrs, R. F. Infectious bovine rhinotracheitis: a review and update. *J Am Vet Med Assoc* **171**: 1055–1064, 1977.

Mettler, F. *et al.* Herpesvirus-infektion bei Zicklein in der Schweiz. *Schweiz Arch Tierheilkd* **121**: 655–662, 1979.

Miller, R. B., Smith, M. W., and Lawson, K. F. Some lesions observed in calves born to cows exposed to the virus of infectious bovine rhinotracheitis in the last trimester of gestation. *Can J Comp Med* **42**: 438–445, 1978.

Reed, D. E., Bicknell, E. J., and Bury, R. J. Systemic form of infectious bovine rhinotracheitis in young calves. *J Am Vet Med Assoc* **163**: 753–755, 1973.

Rogers, R. J. *et al.* Bovine herpesvirus-1–infection of the upper alimen-tary tract of cattle and its association with a severe mortality. *Aust Vet J* **54**: 562–565, 1978.

Saito, J. *et al.* A new herpesvirus isolate from goats: preliminary report. *Am J Vet Res* **35**: 847–848, 1974.

Adenovirus Enteritis

Bulmer, W. S., Tsai, K. S., and Little, P. B. Adenovirus infection in two calves. *J Am Vet Med Assoc* **166**: 233–238, 1975.

Corrier, D. E., Montgomery, D., and Scutchfield, W. L. Adenovirus in the intestinal epithelium of a foal with prolonged diarrhea. *Vet Pathol* **19**: 564–567, 1982.

Coussement, W. *et al.* Adenovirus enteritis in pigs. *Am J Vet Res* **42**: 1905–1911, 1981.

Derbyshire, J. B. Porcine adenovirus infections. *In* "Diseases of Swine," A. D. Leman *et al.* (eds.), 5th ed., pp. 261–264. Ames, Iowa State Univ. Press, 1981.

Ducatelle, R., Coussement, W., and Hoorens, J. Sequential patholog-ical study of experimental porcine adenovirus enteritis. *Vet Pathol* **19**: 179–189, 1982.

Gleeson, L. J., Studdert, M. J., and Sullivan, N. D. Pathogenicity and immunological studies of equine adenovirus in specific-pathogen-free foals. *Am J Vet Res* **39**: 1636–1642, 1978.

Horner, G. W., Hunter, R., and Thompson, E. J. Isolation and charac-terization of a new adenovirus serotype from a yearling heifer with systemic infection. *NZ Vet J* **28**: 165–167, 1982.

Mattson, D. E. Adenovirus infection in cattle. *J Am Vet Med Assoc* **163**: 894–896, 1973.

Mattson, D. E. Naturally occurring infection of calves with a bovine adenovirus. *Am J Vet Res* **34**: 623–629, 1973.

Reed, D. E., Wheeler, J. G., and Lupton, H. W. Isolation of bovine adenovirus type 7 from calves with pneumonia and enteritis. *Am J Vet Res* **39**: 1968–1971, 1978.

Sharp, J. M., Rushton, B., and Rimer, R. D. Experimental infection of specific pathogen–free lambs with ovine adenovirus type 4. *J Comp Pathol* **86**: 621–628, 1976.

Thompson, K. G., Thomson, G. W., and Henry, J. N. Alimentary tract manifestations of bovine adenovirus infections. *Can Vet J* **22**: 68–71, 1981.

Enteric Coronavirus Infections

Appel, M. *et al.* Canine viral enteritis. *Can Pract* **7**: 22–36, 1980.

Bass, E. P., and Sharpee, R. L. Coronavirus and gastroenteritis in foals. *Lancet* **2**: 822, 1975.

Binn, L. N. *et al.* Recovery and characacterization of a coronavirus from military dogs with diarrhea. *Proc 78th Annu Meet US Anim Health Assoc* pp. 359–366, 1974.

Chu, R. M., Glock, R. D., and Ross, R. F. Changes in gut-associated lymphoid tissues of the small intestine of eight-week-old pigs infected with transmissible gastroenteritis virus. *Am J Vet Res* **43:** 67–76, 1982.

Coussement, W. *et al.* Pathology of experimental CV777 coronavirus enteritis in piglets. I. Histological and histochemical study. *Vet Pathol* **19:** 46–56, 1982.

Dea, S., Roy, R. S., and Elazhary, M. A. S. Y. La diarrhée neonatale due au coronavirus de veau. Une revue de la littérature. *Can Vet J* **22:** 51–58, 1981.

Doughri, A. M., and Storz, J. Light and ultrastructural pathologic changes in intestinal coronavirus infection of newborn calves. *Zentralbl Veterinaermed [B]* **24:** 367–385, 1977.

Ducatelle, R. *et al. In vivo* morphogenesis of a new porcine enteric coronavirus, CV777. *Arch Virol* **68:** 35–44, 1981.

Ducatelle, R. *et al.* Pathology of experimental CV777 coronavirus enteritis in piglets. II. Electron microscopic study. *Vet Pathol* **19:** 57–66, 1982.

Espinasse, J. *et al.* Winter dysentery: a coronavirus-like agent in the faeces of beef and dairy cattle with diarrhea. *Vet Rec* **110:** 385, 1982.

Haelterman, E. O. On the pathogenesis of transmissible gastroenteritis of swine. *J Am Vet Med Assoc* **160:** 534–540, 1972.

Hayashi, T. *et al.* Enteritis due to feline infectious peritonitis virus. *Jpn J Vet Sci* **44:** 97–106, 1982.

Hooper, B. E., and Haelterman, E. O. Lesions of the gastrointestinal tract of pigs infected with transmissible gastroenteritis. *Can J Comp Med* **33:** 29–36, 1969.

Horvath, I., and Mocsari, E. Ultrastructural changes in the small intestinal epithelium of suckling pigs affected with a transmissible gastroenteritis (TGE) –like disease. *Arch Virol* **68:** 103–113, 1981.

Hoshino, Y., and Scott, F. W. Coronavirus-like particles in the feces of normal cats. *Arch Virol* **63:** 147–152, 1980.

Keenan, K. P. *et al.* Intestinal infection of neonatal dogs with canine coronavirus 1-71: studies by virologic, histologic, histochemical, and immunofluorescent techniques. *Am J Vet Res* **37:** 247–256, 1976.

Kerzner, B. *et al.* Transmissible gastroenteritis: sodium transport and the intestinal epithelium during the course of viral enteritis. *Gastroenterology* **72:** 457–461, 1977.

Langpap, T. J., Bergeland, M. E., and Reed, D. E. Coronaviral enteritis of young calves: virologic and pathologic findings in naturally occurring infections. *Am J Vet Res* **40:** 1476–1478, 1979.

Larson, D. J. *et al.* Mild transmissible gastroenteritis in pigs suckling vaccinated sows. *J Am Vet Med Assoc* **176:** 539–542, 1980.

Lewis, L. D., and Phillips, R. W. Pathophysiologic changes due to coronavirus-induced diarrhea in the calf. *J Am Vet Med Assoc* **173:** 636–642, 1978.

Mebus, C. A. Pathogenesis of coronaviral infection in calves. *J Am Vet Med Assoc* **173:** 631–632, 1978.

Mebus, C. A. *et al.* Pathology of neonatal calf diarrhea induced by a coronavirus-like agent. *Vet Pathol* **10:** 45–64, 1973.

Moon, H. W. *et al.* Age-dependent resistance to transmissible gastroenteritis of swine. III. Effects of epithelial cell kinetics on coronavirus production and on atrophy of intestinal villi. *Vet Pathol* **12:** 434–445, 1975.

Moon, H. W., Norman, J. O., and Lambert, G. Age dependent resistance to transmissible gastroenteritis of swine (TGE). I. Clinical signs and some mucosal dimensions in small intestine. *Can J Comp Med* **37:** 157–166, 1973.

Morin, M., Lariviere, S., and Lallier, R. Pathological and microbiological observations made on spontaneous cases of acute neonatal calf diarrhea. *Can J Comp Med* **40:** 228–240, 1976.

Morin, M., and Morehouse, L. G. Transmissible gastroenteritis in feeder pigs: observations on the jejunal epithelium of normal feeder pigs and feeder pigs infected with TGE virus. *Can J Comp Med* **38:** 227–235, 1974.

Olsoh, L. D. Induction of transmissible gastroenteritis in feeder swine. *Am J Vet Res* **32:** 411–417, 1971.

Olson, D. P., Waxler, G. L., and Roberts, A. W. Small intestinal lesions of transmissible gastroenteritis in gnotobiotic pigs: a scanning electron microscopic study. *Am J Vet Res* **34:** 1239–1245, 1973.

Pass, D. A. *et al.* Intestinal coronavirus-like particles in sheep with diarrhoea. *Vet Rec* **111:** 106–107, 1982.

Pedersen, N. C. *et al.* An enteric coronavirus infection of cats and its relationship to feline infectious peritonitis. *Am J Vet Res* **42:** 368–377, 1981.

Pospischil, A., Hess, R. G., and Bachmann, P. A. Light microscopy and ultrahistology of intestinal changes in pigs infected with epizootic diarrhoea virus (EVD): comparison with transmissible gastroenteritis (TGE) virus and porcine rotavirus infections. *Zentralbl Veterinaermed [B]* **28:** 564–577, 1981.

Reynolds, D. J., and Garwes, D. J. Virus isolation and serum antibody responses after infection of cats with transmissible gastroenteritis virus. *Arch Virol* **60:** 161–166, 1979.

Schnagl, R. D., and Holmes, I. H. Coronavirus-like particles in stools from dogs, from some country areas of Australia. *Vet Rec* **102:** 528–529, 1978.

Shepherd, R. W. *et al.* The mucosal lesion in viral enteritis. Extent and dynamics of the epithelial response to virus invasion in TGE in piglets. *Gastroenterology* **76:** 770–777, 1979.

Shimizu, M., and Shimizu, Y. Demonstration of cytotoxic lymphocytes to virus-infected target cells in pigs inoculated with transmissible gastroenteritis virus. *Am J Vet Res* **40:** 208–213, 1979.

Storz, J., Doughri, A. M., and Hajer, I. Coronaviral morphogenesis and ultrastructural changes in intestinal infections of calves. *J Am Vet Med Assoc* **173:** 633–635, 1978.

Takeuchi, A. *et al.* Electron microscope study of experimental enteric infection in neonatal dogs with a canine coronavirus. *Lab Invest* **34:** 539–549, 1976.

Takahashi, E. *et al.* Epizootic diarrhoea of adult cattle associated with a coronavirus-like agent. *Vet Microbiol* **5:** 151–154, 1980.

Thake, D. C. Jejunal epithelium in transmissible gastroenteritis of swine. An electron microscopic and histochemical study. *Am J Pathol* **53:** 149–168, 1968.

Thake, D. C., Moon, H. W., and Lambert, G. Epithelial cell dynamics in transmissible gastroenteritis of neonatal pigs. *Vet Pathol* **10:** 330–341, 1973.

Turgeon, D. C. *et al.* Coronavirus-like particles associated with diarrhea in baby pigs in Quebec. *Can Vet J* **22:** 100–101, 1981.

Tyrrell, D. A. J. *et al.* Coronaviridae: second report. *Intervirology* **10:** 321–328, 1978.

Tzipori, S. *et al.* Enteric coronavirus-like particles in sheep. *Aust Vet J* **54:** 320–321, 1978.

Vandenberghe, J. *et al.* Coronavirus infection in a litter of pups. *Vet Q* **2:** 136–141, 1980.

Wagner, J. E., Beamer, P. D., and Ristic, M. Electron microscopy of intestinal epithelial cells of piglets infected with a transmissible gastroenteritis virus. *Can J Comp Med* **37:** 177–188, 1973.

Woods, R. D., Cheville, N. F., and Gallagher, J. E. Lesions in the small intestine of newborn pigs inoculated with porcine, feline, and canine coronaviruses. *Am J Vet Res* **42:** 1163–1169, 1981.

Rotavirus Infection

Bohl, E. H. Rotaviral diarrhea in pigs: brief review. *J Am Vet Med Assoc* **174:** 613–615, 1979.

Bohl, E. H. *et al.* Rotavirus as a cause of diarrhea in pigs. *J Am Vet Med Assoc* **172:** 458–463, 1978.

Bridger, J. C. Rotavirus: the present situation in farm animals. *Vet Annu* **20:** 172–179, 1980.

Carpio, M., Bellamy, J. E. C., and Babiuk, L. A. Comparative virulence of different bovine rotavirus isolates. *Can J Comp Med* **45:** 38–42, 1981.

Conner, M. E., and Darlington, R. W. Rotavirus infection in foals. *Am J Vet Res* **41:** 1699–1703, 1980.

Crouch, C. F., and Woode, G. N. Serial studies of virus multiplication and intestinal damage in gnotobiotic piglets infected with rotavirus. *J Med Microbiol* **11:** 325–334, 1978.

Debouck, P., and Pansaert, M. Experimental infection of pigs with Belgian isolates of the porcine rotavirus. *Zentralbl Veterinaermed* [*B*] **26:** 517–526, 1979.

De Leeuw, P. W. *et al.* Rotavirus infections in calves in dairy herds. *Res Vet Sci* **29:** 135–141, 1980.

Eugster, A. K., and Sidwa, T. Rotaviruses in diarrheic feces of a dog. *VM SAC* **74:** 817–819, 1979.

Fahey, K. J. *et al.* IgG$_1$ antibody in milk protects lambs against rotavirus diarrhoea. *Vet Immunol Immunopathol* **2:** 27–33, 1981.

Fulton, R. W. *et al.* Isolation of a rotavirus from a newborn dog with diarrhea. *Am J Vet Res* **42:** 841–843, 1981.

Halpin, C. G., and Caple, I. W. Changes in intestinal structure and function of neonatal calves infected with reovirus-like agent and *Escherichia coli. Aust Vet J* **52:** 438–441, 1976.

Hoskins, Y. *et al.* Isolation and characterization of a canine rotavirus. *Arch Virol* **72:** 113–125, 1982.

Hoskins, Y., Baldwin, C. A., and Scott, F. W. Isolation and characterization of feline rotavirus. *J Gen Virol* **54:** 313–323, 1981.

Lecce, J. G., King, M. W., and Mock, R. Reovirus-like agent associated with fatal diarrhea in neonatal pigs. *Infect Immun* **14:** 816–825, 1976.

McAdaragh, J. P. *et al.* Pathogenesis of rotaviral enteritis in gnotobiotic pigs: A microscopic study. *Am J Vet Res* **41:** 1572–1581, 1980.

Mebus, C. A. *et al.* Pathology of neonatal calf diarrhea induced by a reolike virus. *Vet Pathol* **8:** 490–505, 1971.

Mebus, C. A. *et al.* Intestinal lesions induced in gnotobiotic calves by the virus of human infantile gastroenteritis. *Vet Pathol* **14:** 273–282, 1977.

Middleton, P. J. Pathogenesis of rotaviral infection. *J Am Vet Med Assoc* **173:** 544–546, 1978.

Moon, H. W. *et al.* Pathogenic relationships of rotavirus, *E. coli* and other agents in mixed infections in calves. *J Am Vet Med Assoc* **173:** 577–583, 1978.

Morin, M., Lariviere, S., and Lallier, R. Pathological and microbiological observations made on spontaneous cases of acute neonatal calf diarrhoea. *Can J Comp Med* **40:** 228–240, 1976.

Mouwen, J. M. V. M. *et al.* Some biochemical aspects of white scours in piglets. *Tijdschr Diergeneeskd* **97:** 65–90, 1972.

Narita, M., Fukusho, A., and Shimizu, Y. Electron microscopy of the intestine of gnotobiotic piglets infected with porcine rotavirus. *J Comp Pathol* **92:** 589–597, 1982.

Pearson, G. R., and McNulty, M. S. Pathological changes in the small intestine of neonatal pigs infected with a pig reovirus-like agent (rotavirus). *J Comp Pathol* **87:** 363–375, 1977.

Pearson, G. R., and McNulty, M. S. Ultrastructural changes in small intestinal epithelium of neonatal pigs infected with pig rotavirus. *Arch Virol* **59:** 127–136, 1979.

Rodger, S. M., Craven, J. A., and Williams, I. Demonstration of reovirus-like particles in intestinal contents of piglets with diarrhoea. *Aust Vet J* **51:** 536, 1975.

Scrutchfield, W. L. *et al.* Rotavirus infections in foals. *Proc Am Assoc Equine Pract* **25:** 217–223, 1979.

Snodgrass, D. R. *et al.* Small intestine morphology and epithelial cell kinetics in lamb rotavirus infection. *Gastroenterology* **76:** 477–481, 1979.

Snodgrass, D. R., Angus, K. W., and Gray, E. W. A rotavirus from kittens. *Vet Rec* **104:** 222–223, 1979.

Stair, E. L. *et al.* Neonatal calf diarrhea: electron microscopy of intestines infected with a reovirus-like agent. *Vet Pathol* **10:** 155–170, 1973.

Strickland, K. L. *et al.* Diarrhoea in foals associated with rotavirus. *Vet Rec* **111:** 421, 1982.

Studdert, M. J., Mason, R. W., and Patten, B. E. Rotavirus diarrhoea of foals. *Aust Vet J* **54:** 363–364, 1978.

Theil, K. W. *et al.* Pathogenesis of porcine rotaviral infection in experimentally inoculated gnotobiotic pigs. *Am J Vet Res* **39:** 213–220, 1978.

Torres-Medina, A., and Underdahl, N. R. Scanning electron microscopy of intestine of gnotobiotic piglets infected with porcine rotavirus. *Can J Comp Med* **44:** 403–411, 1980.

Tzipori, S. *et al.* Enteritis in foals induced by rotavirus and enterotoxigenic *Escherichia coli. Aust Vet J* **58:** 20–23, 1982.

Tzipori, S., and Williams, I. H. Diarrhoea in piglets inoculated with rotavirus. *Aust Vet J* **54:** 188–192, 1978.

Woode, G. N., and Bohl, E. H. Porcine rotavirus infection. *In* "Diseases of Swine," A. D. Leman *et al.* (eds.), 5th ed., pp. 310–322. Ames, Iowa State Univ. Press, 1981.

Woode, G. N., and Crouch, C. F. Naturally occurring and experimentally induced rotaviral infections of domestic and laboratory animals. *J Am Vet Med Assoc* **173:** 522–526, 1978.

Parvovirus Infection

Afshar, A. Canine parvovirus infections—a review. *Vet Bull* **51:** 605–612, 1981.

Azetaka, M. *et al.* Studies on canine parvovirus isolation, experimental infection and serologic survey. *Jpn J Vet Sci* **43:** 243–255, 1981.

Bachmann, P. A. *et al.* Parvoviridae: second report. *Intervirology* **11:** 248–254, 1979.

Boosinger, T. R. *et al.* Bone marrow alterations associated with canine parvoviral enteritis. *Vet Pathol* **19:** 558–561, 1982.

Carlson, J. H., and Scott, F. W. Feline panleukopenia. II. The relationship of intestinal mucosal cell proliferation rates to viral infection and development of lesions. *Vet Pathol* **14:** 173–181, 1977.

Carlson, J. H., Scott, F. W., and Duncan, J. R. Feline panleukopenia. I. Pathogenesis in germ-free and specific pathogen–free cats. *Vet Pathol* **14:** 79–88, 1977.

Carlson, J. H., Scott, F. W., and Duncan, J. R. Feline panleukopenia. III. Development of lesions in the lymphoid tissues. *Vet Pathol* **15:** 383–392, 1978.

Carman, P. S., and Povey, R. C. Successful experimental challenge with canine parvovirus-2. *Can J Comp Med* **46:** 33–38, 1982.

Carpenter, J. L. *et al.* Intestinal and cardiopulmonary forms of parvovirus infection in a litter of pups. *J Am Vet Med Assoc* **176:** 1269–1273, 1980.

Cockerell, G. L. Naturally occurring acquired immunodeficiency diseases of the dog and cat. *Vet Clin North Am* **8:** 613–628, 1978.

Cooper, B. J. *et al.* Canine viral enteritis. II. Morphologic lesions in naturally occurring parvovirus infection. *Cornell Vet* **69:** 134–144, 1979.

Csiza, C. K. *et al.* Feline viruses. XIV. Transplacental infections in spontaneous panleukopenia of cats. *Cornell Vet* **61:** 423–439, 1971.

Doi, K. *et al.* Histopathology of feline panleukopenia in domestic cats. *Natl Inst Anim Health Q (Tokyo)* **15:** 76–85, 1975.

Eugster, A. K., Bendele, R. A., and Jones, L. P. Parvovirus infection in dogs. *J Am Vet Med Assoc* **173:** 1340–1341, 1978.

Gillespie, J. H., and Scott, F. W. Feline viral infections. *Adv Vet Sci Comp Med* **17:** 163–200, 1973.

Gooding, G. E., and Robinson, W. F. Maternal antibody, vaccination and reproductive failure in dogs with parvovirus infection. *Aust Vet J* **59:** 170–174, 1982.

Hayes, M. A., Russell, R. G., and Babiuk, L. A. Sudden death in young dogs with myocarditis caused by parvovirus. *J Am Vet Med Assoc* **174:** 1197–1203, 1979.

Jacobs, R. M. *et al.* Clinicopathologic features of canine parvoviral enteritis. *J Am Anim Hosp Assoc* **16:** 809–814, 1980.

Jefferies, A. R., and Blakemore, W. F. Myocarditis and enteritis in puppies associated with parvovirus. *Vet Rec* **104:** 221, 1979.

Kahn, D. E. Pathogenesis of feline panleukopenia. *J Am Vet Med Assoc* **173:** 628–630, 1978.

Kilham, L., Margolis, G., and Colby, E. D. Cerebellar ataxia and its congenital transmission in cats by feline panleukopenia virus. *J Am Vet Med Assoc* **158:** 888–906, 1971.

Krakowka, S. *et al.* Canine parvovirus infection potentiates canine distemper encephalitis attributable to modified live-virus vaccine. *J Am Vet Med Assoc* **180:** 137–139, 1982.

Langheinrich, K. A., Nielsen, S. W. Histopathology of feline panleukopenia: a report of 65 cases. *J Am Vet Med Assoc* **158:** 863–872, 1971.

Larsen, S., Flagstad, A., and Aalback, B. Experimental feline panleukopenia in the conventional cat. *Vet Pathol* **13:** 216–240, 1976.

Lenghaus, C., and Studdert, M. J. Generalized parvovirus disease in neonatal pups. *J Am Vet Med Assoc* **181:** 41–45, 1982.

McAdaragh, J. P. *et al.* Experimental infection of conventional dogs with canine parvovirus. *Am J Vet Res* **43:** 693–696, 1982.

Meunier, P. C. *et al.* Canine parvovirus in a commercial kennel: epidemiologic and pathologic findings. *Cornell Vet* **71:** 96–110, 1981.

Nelson, D. T. *et al.* Lesions of spontaneous canine viral enteritis. *Vet Pathol* **16:** 680–686, 1979.

Osterhaus, A. D. M. E. *et al.* Canine viral enteritis: prevalence of parvo-, corona- and rotavirus infections in dogs in the Netherlands. *Vet Q* **2:** 181–190, 1980.

Osterhaus, A. D. M. E., van Steenis, G., and de Kreek, P. Isolation of a virus closely related to feline panleukopenia virus from dogs with diarrhea. *Zentralbl Veterinaermed [B]* **27:** 11–21, 1980.

Pollock, R. V. H. Experimental canine parvovirus infection in dogs. *Cornell Vet* **72:** 103–119, 1982.

Rice, J. B. *et al.* Comparison of systemic and local immunity in dogs with canine parvovirus gastroenteritis. *Infect Immun* **38:** 1003–1009, 1982.

Robinson, W. F., Huxtable, C. R., and Pass, D. A. Canine parvoviral myocarditis: a morphologic description of the natural disease. *Vet Pathol* **17:** 282–293, 1980.

Schultz, R. D., Mendel, H., and Scott, F. W. Effect of feline panleukopenia virus infection on development of humoral and cellular immunity. *Cornell Vet* **66:** 324–332, 1976.

Stokes, R. Intestinal mycosis in a cat. *Aust Vet J* **49:** 499–500, 1973.

Storz, J. *et al.* Parvovirus associated with diarrhea in calves. *J Am Vet Med Assoc* **173:** 624–627, 1978.

Tratschin, J. D. *et al.* Canine parvovirus: relationship to wild-type and vaccine strains of feline panleukopenia virus and mink enteritis virus. *J Gen Virol* **61:** 33–41, 1982.

Escherichia coli

Acosta-Martinez, F., Gyles, C. L., and Butler, D. G. *Escherichia coli* heat-stable enterotoxin in feces and intestines of calves with diarrhea. *Am J Vet Res* **41:** 1143–1149, 1980.

Acres, S. D., Forman, A. J., and Kapitany, R. A. Antigen-extinction profile in pregnant cows, using a K99-containing whole-cell bacterin to induce passive protection against enterotoxigenic colibacillosis of calves. *Am J Vet Res* **43:** 569–575, 1982.

Anderson, M. J., Whitehead, J. S., and Kim, Y. S. Interaction of *Escherichia coli* K88 antigen with porcine intestinal brush border membranes. *Infect Immun* **29:** 897–901, 1980.

Ansari, M. M., Renshaw, H. W., and Gates, N. L. Colibacillosis in neonatal lambs: onset of diarrheal disease and isolation and characterization of enterotoxigenic *Escherichia coli* from enteric and septicemic forms of the disease. *Am J Vet Res* **39:** 11–14, 1978.

Askaa, J., Jacobsen, K. B., and Sorensen, M. Neonatal infections in puppies caused by *Escherichia coli* serogroups 04 and 025. *Nord Vet Med* **30:** 486–488, 1978.

Awad-Masalmeh, M. *et al.* Pilus production, hemagglutination, and adhesion by porcine strains of enterotoxigenic *Escherichia coli* lacking K88, K99, and 987P antigens. *Infect Immun* **35:** 305–313, 1982.

Bellamy, J. E. C., and Acres, S. D. Enterotoxigenic colibacillosis in colostrum-fed calves: pathologic changes. *Am J Vet Res* **40:** 1391–1397, 1979.

Bijlsma, I. G. W. *et al.* Different pig phenotypes affect adherence of *Escherichia coli* to jejunal brush borders by K88ab, K88ac, or K88ad antigen. *Infect Immun* **37:** 891–894, 1982.

Boedeker, E. C. Enterocyte adherence of *Escherichia coli:* its relation to diarrheal disease. *Gastroenterology* **83:** 489–492, 1982.

Cantey, J. R., and Blake, R. K. Diarrhea due to *Escherichia coli* in the rabbit: a novel mechanism. *J Infect Dis* **135:** 454–462, 1977.

Duchet-Suchaux, M. *et al.* Experimental *Escherichia coli* diarrhoea in colostrum deprived lambs. *Ann Rech Vet* **13:** 259–266, 1982.

Field, M. Modes of action of enterotoxins from *Vibrio cholerae* and *Escherichia coli.* *Rev Infect Dis* **1:** 918–925, 1979.

Formal, S. B. *et al.* Invasive *Escherichia coli.* *J Am Vet Med Assoc* **173:** 596–598, 1978.

Frisk, C. S., Wagner, J. E., and Owens, D. R. Hamster (*Mesocricetus auratus*) enteritis caused by epithelial cell-invasive *Escherichia coli.* *Infect Immun* **31:** 1232–1238, 1981.

Gaastra, W., and de Graff, F. K. Host-specific fimbrial adhesions of noninvasive enterotoxigenic *Escherichia coli* strains. *Microbiol Rev* **46:** 129–161, 1982.

Gay, C. C. Problems of immunization in the control of *Escherichia coli* infection. *Ann NY Acad Sci* **176:** 336–349, 1971.

Goodman, M. L., Way, B. A., and Irwin, J. W. The inflammatory response to endotoxin. *J Pathol* **128:** 7–14, 1979.

Greenberg, R. N., and Guerrant, R. L. *E. coli* heat-stable enterotoxin. *Pharmacol Ther* **13:** 507–531, 1981.

Gyles, C. L. Comments on pathogenesis of neonatal enteric colibacillosis of pigs. *J Am Vet Med Assoc* **160:** 592–584, 1972.

Hadad, J. J., and Gyles, C. L. The role of K antigens of enteropathogenic *Escherichia coli* in colonization of the small intestine of calves. *Can J Comp Med* **46:** 21–26, 1982.

Hadad, J. J., and Gyles, C. L. Scanning and transmission electron microscopic study of the small intestine of colostrum-fed calves infected with selected strains of *Escherichia coli*. *Am J Vet Res* **43:** 41–49, 1982.

Harnett, N. M., and Gyles, C. L. Enterotoxigenicity of bovine and porcine *Escherichia coli* of 0 groups 8, 9, 20, 64, 101, and X46. *Am J Vet Res* **44:** 1210–1214, 1983.

Harris, J. R. *et al.* High-molecular-weight plasmid correlates with *Escherichia coli* enteroinvasiveness. *Infect Immun* **37:** 1295–1298, 1982.

Inman, L. R., and Cantey, J. R. Specific adherence of *Escherichia coli* (strain RDEC-1) to membranous (M) cells of the Peyer's patch in *Escherichia coli* diarrhea in the rabbit. *J Clin Invest* **71:** 1–8, 1983.

Isaacson, R. E., Moon, H. W., and Schneider, R. A. Distribution and virulence of *Escherichia coli* in the small intestines of calves with and without diarrhea. *Am J Vet Res* **39:** 1750–1755, 1978.

Isaacson, R. E., Nagy, B., and Moon, H. W. Colonization of porcine small intestine by *Escherichia coli:* colonization and adhesion factors of pig enteropathogens that lack K88. *J Infect Dis* **135:** 531–539, 1977.

Johnston, N. E., Estrella, R. A., and Oxender, W. D. Resistance of neonatal calves given colostrum diet to oral challenge with a septicemia-producing *Escherichia coli*. *Am J Vet Res* **38:** 1323–1326, 1977.

Kohler, E. M. Neonatal enteric colibacillosis of pigs and current research on immunization. *J Am Vet Med Assoc* **173:** 588–591, 1978.

Lariviere, S., Lallier, R., and Morin, M. Evaluation of various methods for the detection of enteropathogenic *Escherichia coli* in diarrheic calves. *Am J Vet Res* **40:** 130–134, 1979.

Larsen, J. L. Differences between enteropathogenic *Escherichia coli* strains isolated from neonatal *E. coli* diarrhoea (N.C.D.) and post weaning diarrhoea (P.W.D.) in pigs. *Nord Vet Med* **28:** 417–429, 1976.

Lecce, J. G. *et al.* Rotavirus and hemolytic enteropathogenic *Escherichia coli* in weanling diarrhea of pigs. *J Clin Microbiol* **16:** 715–723, 1982.

Lopez-Alvarez, J., and Gyles, C. L. Occurrence of vir plasmid among animal and human strains of invasive *Escherichia coli*. *Am J Vet Res* **41:** 769–774, 1980.

Lund, A., Fossum, K., and Liven, E. Serological, enterotoxin-producing and biochemical properties of *Escherichia coli* isolates from piglets with neonatal diarrhea in Norway. *Acta Vet Scand* **23:** 79–87, 1982.

Mason, R. W., and Corbould, A. Coliseptocaemia of lambs. *Aust Vet J* **57:** 458–460, 1981.

Moon, H. W. Protection against enteric colibacillosis in pigs suckling orally vaccinated dams: evidence of pili as protective antigens. *Am J Vet Res* **42:** 173–177, 1981.

Moon, H. W. *et al.* Pathogenic relationships of rotavirus, *Escherichia coli*, and other agents in mixed infections in calves. *J Am Vet Med Assoc* **173:** 577–583, 1978.

Moon, H. W., and McDonald, J. S. Antibody response of cows to *Escherichia coli* pilus antigen K99 after oral vaccination with live or dead bacteria. *Am J Vet Res* **44:** 493–496, 1983.

Moon, H. W., Whipp, S. C., and Skartvedt, S. M. Etiologic diagnosis of diarrheal diseases of calves: frequency and methods for detecting enterotoxin and K99 antigen production by *Escherichia coli*. *Am J Vet Res* **37:** 1025–1029, 1976.

Morin, M., Lariviere, S., and Lallier, R. Pathological and microbiological observations made on spontaneous cases of acute neonatal calf diarrhea. *Can J Comp Med* **40:** 228–240, 1976.

Pearson, G. R., and Logan, E. F. The pathogenesis of enteric colibacillosis in neonatal unsuckled calves. *Vet Rec* **105:** 159–164, 1979.

Pearson, G. R., and Logan, E. F. Ultrastructural changes in the small intestine of neonatal calves with enteric colibacillosis. *Vet Pathol* **19:** 190–201, 1982.

Pearson, G. R., Logan, E. F., and Brennan, G. P. Scanning electron microscopy of the small intestine of a normal unsuckled calf and a calf with enteric colibacillosis. *Vet Pathol* **15:** 400–406, 1978.

Pearson, G. R., McNulty, M. S., and Logan, E. F. Pathological changes in the small intestine of neonatal calves with enteric colibacillosis. *Vet Pathol* **15:** 92–101, 1978.

Prochazka, Z. *et al.* Protein loss in piglets infected with different enteropathogenic types of *Escherichia coli*. *Br Vet J* **138:** 295–304, 1982.

Raskova, H., and Raska, K. Enterotoxins from gram-negative bacteria relevant for veterinary medicine. *Vet Res Commun* **4:** 195–224, 1980.

Runnels, P. L., Moon, H. W., and Schneider, R. A. Development of resistance with host age to adhesion of K99+ *Escherichia coli* to isolated intestinal epithelial cells. *Infect Immun* **28:** 298–300, 1980.

Sack, R. B. Enterotoxigenic *Escherichia coli*: identification and characterization. *J Infect Dis* **142:** 279–286, 1980.

Schneider, R. A., and To, S. C. M. Enterotoxigenic *Escherichia coli* strains that express K88 and 987P pilus antigens. *Infect Immun* **36:** 417–418, 1982.

Sembrat, R. *et al.* Acute pulmonary failure in the conscious pony with *Escherichia coli* septicemia. *Am J Vet Res* **39:** 1147–1154, 1978.

Shaw, W. B. *Escherichia coli* in newborn lambs. *Br Vet J* **127:** 214–219, 1971.

Shimizu, M., and Terashima, T. Appearance of enterotoxigenic *Escherichia coli* in piglets with diarrhea in connection with feed changes. *Microbiol Immunol* **26:** 467–477, 1982.

Sivaswamy, G., and Gyles, C. L. Characterization of enterotoxigenic bovine *Escherichia coli*. *Can J Comp Med* **40:** 247–256, 1976.

Smith, C. J. *et al.* K99 antigen-positive enterotoxigenic *Escherichia coli* from piglets with diarrhea in Sweden. *J Clin Microbiol* **13:** 252–257, 1981.

Smith, H. W. Transmissible pathogenic characteristics of invasive strains of *Escherichia coli*. *J Am Vet Med Assoc* **173:** 601–607, 1978.

Smith, H. W., and Halls, S. The experimental infection of calves with bacteraemia-producing strains of *Escherichia coli*: the influence of colostrum. *J Med Microbiol* **1:** 61–78, 1968.

Smith, H. W., and Huggins, M. B. Experimental infection of calves, piglets and lambs with mixtures of invasive and enteropathogenic strains of *Escherichia coli*. *J Med Microbiol* **12:** 507–510, 1979.

Snodgrass, D. R., Chandler, D. S., and Makin, T. J. Inheritance of *Escherichia coli* K88 adhesion in pigs: identification of nonadhesive phenotypes in a commercial herd. *Vet Rec* **109:** 461–463, 1981.

Snodgrass, D. R., Smith, M. L., and Kraitil, F. L. Interaction of rotavirus and enterotoxigenic *Escherichia coli* in conventionally-reared dairy calves. *Vet Microbiol* **7:** 51–60, 1982.

Soderlind, O., and Mollby, R. Studies on *Escherichia coli* in pigs. V. Determination of enterotoxicity and frequency of 0 groups and K88 antigen in strains from 200 piglets with neonatal diarrhoea. *Zentralbl Veterinaermed [B]* **25:** 719–728, 1978.

Svendsen, J., and Larsen, J. L. Studies of the pathogenesis of enteric *E. coli* infections in weaned pigs. The significance of the milk of the dam in preventing the disease. *Nord Vet Med* **29:** 533–538, 1977.

Tzipori, S. R. *et al.* Clinical manifestations of diarrhea in calves infected with rotavirus and enterotoxigenic *Escherichia coli*. *J Clin Microbiol* **13:** 1011–1016, 1981.

Tzipori, S. *et al.* Diarrhea in lambs: experimental infections with enterotoxigenic *Escherichia coli*, rotavirus, and *Cryptosporidium* sp. *Infect Immun* **33:** 401–406, 1981.

Tzipori, S. *et al.* Experimental colibacillosis in gnotobiotic piglets exposed to 3 enterotoxigenic serotypes. *Aust Vet J* **59:** 93–96, 1982.

Tzipori, S. *et al.* Intestinal changes associated with rotavirus and enterotoxigenic *Escherichia coli* infection in calves. *Vet Microbiol* **8:** 35–43, 1983.

Welch, R. A. *et al.* Haemolysin contributes to virulence of extraintestinal *E. coli* infections. *Nature* **294:** 665–667, 1981.

Whipp, S. C., Moon, H. W., and Argenzio, R. A. Comparison of enterotoxic activities of heat-stable enterotoxins from class 1 and class 2 *Escherichia coli* of swine origin. *Infect Immun* **31:** 245–251, 1981.

Wilkie, I. W. Polyserositis and meningitis associated with *Escherichia coli* infection of piglets. *Can Vet J* **22:** 171–173, 1981.

Wray, C., and Thomlinson, J. R. Lesions and bacteriological findings in colibacillosis in calves. *Br Vet J* **130:** 189–199, 1974.

Salmonellosis

Arbuckle, A. B. R. Villous atrophy in pigs orally infected with *Salmonella cholerae-suis*. *Res Vet Sci* **18:** 322–324, 1975.

Barnes, D. M., and Bergeland, M. E. *Salmonella typhisuis* infection in Minnesota swine. *J Am Vet Med Assoc* **152:** 1766–1770, 1968.

Barron, N. S., and Scott, D. C. *S. dublin* infection in adult cattle. *Vet Rec* **61**: 35, 1949.

Brown, D. D., Ross, J. G., and Smith, A. F. G. Experimental infections of sheep with *Salmonella typhimurium*. *Res Vet Sci* **21**: 335–340, 1976.

Buckley, H. G., and Donnelly, W. J. C. *Salmonella dublin* infection in piglets. *Ir Vet J* **24**: 74–78, 1970.

Calvert, C. A., and Leifer, C. E. Salmonellosis in dogs with lymphosarcoma. *J Am Vet Med Assoc* **180**: 56–58, 1982.

Carter, M. E., Dewes, H. G., and Griffiths, O. V. Salmonellosis in foals. *NZ Vet J* **3**: 78–83, 1979.

Cook, W. R. Diarrhea in the horse associated with stress and tetracycline therapy. *Vet Rec* **93**: 15–17, 1973.

Dimock, W. W., Edwards, P. R., and Bruner, D. W. The occurrence of paratyphoid infection in horses following treatment for intestinal parasites. *Cornell Vet* **30**: 319–320, 1940.

Dorn, C. R. *et al.* Neutropenia and salmonellosis in hospitalized horses. *J Am Vet Med Assoc* **166**: 65–67, 1975.

Ehrensperger, F. *et al.* Megacolon in fattening pigs. *Schweiz Arch Tierheilkd* **120**: 477–483, 1978.

Eiklid, K., and Olsnes, S. Animal toxicity of *Shigella dysenteriae* cytotoxin: evidence that the neurotoxic, enterotoxic, and cytotoxic activities are due to one toxin. *J Immunol* **130**: 380–384, 1983.

Eugster, A. K., Whitford, H. W., and Mehr, L. E. Concurrent rotavirus and *Salmonella* infections in foals. *J Am Vet Med Assoc* **173**: 857–858, 1978.

Fisher, E. W., and Martinez, A. A. Studies of neonatal calf diarrhoea. III. Water balance studies in neonatal salmonellosis. *Br Vet J* **131**: 643–651, 1975.

Fromm, D. *et al.* Ion transport across isolated ileal mucosa invaded by *Salmonella*. *Gastroenterology* **66**: 215–225, 1974.

Furness, G., and Ferreira, I. The role of macrophages in natural immunity to Salmonellae. *J Infect Dis* **104**: 203–206, 1959.

Giannella, R. A. Pathogenesis of *Salmonella* mediated intestinal fluid secretion. *Gastroenterology* **69**: 1238–1245, 1975.

Giannella, R. A. Importance of the intestinal inflammatory reaction in *Salmonella*-mediated intestinal secretion. *Infect Immun* **23**: 140–145, 1979.

Gibbons, D. F. Equine salmonellosis: a review. *Vet Rec* **106**: 356–359, 1980.

Grady, G. F., and Keusch, G. T. Pathogenesis of bacterial diarrhoeas. *N Engl J Med* **285**: 831–841 and 891–900, 1971.

Hall, G. A. *et al.* Experimental oral *Salmonella dublin* infection in cattle: effects of concurrent infection with *Fasciola hepatica*. *J Comp Pathol* **90**: 227–233, 1981.

Hall, G. A., Jones, P. W., and Aitken, M. M. The pathogenesis of experimental intra-ruminal infections of cows with *Salmonella dublin*. *J Comp Pathol* **88**: 409–417, 1978.

Harp, J. A. *et al.* Role of *Salmonella arizonae* and other infective agents in enteric disease of lambs. *Am J Vet Res* **42**: 596–599, 1981.

Henning, M. W. Calf paratyphoid. I. A general discussion of the disease in relation to animals and man. *Onderstepoort J Vet Sci* **26**: 3–23, 1953.

Higgins, R. *et al. Salmonella choleraesuis* septicemia in a calf. *Can Vet J* **22**: 269, 1981.

Hohmann, A. W., Schmidt, G., and Rowley, D. Intestinal colonization and virulence of *Salmonella* in mice. *Infect Immun* **22**: 763–770, 1978.

Hunter, A. G. *et al.* An outbreak of *S. typhimurium* in sheep and its consequences. *Vet Rec* **98**: 126–130, 1976.

Johnston, K. G., and Jones, R. T. Salmonellosis in calves due to lactose fermenting *Salmonella typhimurium*. *Vet Rec* **98**: 276–278, 1975.

Ketaren, K. *et al.* Canine salmonellosis in a small animal hospital. *J Am Vet Med Assoc* **179**: 1017–1018, 1981.

Lawson, G. H. K., and Dow, C. The pathogenesis of oral *Salmonella cholerae-suis* infection in pigs. *J Comp Pathol* **75**: 75–81, 1965.

Lawson, G. H. K., and Dow, C. Experimental infection of pigs with smooth and rough strains of *Salmonella cholerae-suis*. *J Comp Pathol* **75**: 83–88, 1965.

Lawson, G. H. K., and Dow, C. Porcine salmonellosis: a study of the field disease. *J Comp Pathol* **76**: 363–371, 1966.

Meinershagen, W. A., Waldhalm, D. G., and Frank, F. W. *Salmonella dublin* as a cause of diarrhea and abortion in ewes. *Am J Vet Res* **31**: 1769–1771, 1970.

Merritt, A. M., Bolton, J. R., and Cimprich, R. Differential diagnosis of diarrhea in horses over six months of age. *J S Afr Vet Assoc* **46**: 73–76, 1975.

Morse, E. V. Canine salmonellosis. *J Am Vet Med Assoc* **167**: 817–820, 1975.

Morse, E. V. Salmonellosis in equidae. *Cornell Vet* **66**: 198, 1976.

Nordstoga, K. Porcine salmonellosis. I. Gross and microscopic changes in experimentally infected animals. *Acta Vet Scand* **11**: 361–369, 1970.

Norstoga, K., and Fjolstad, M. Porcine salmmonellosis. II. Production of the generalized Schwartzman reaction by intravenous injections of disintegrated cells of *Salmonella cholerae-suis*. *Acta Vet Scand* **11**: 370–379, 1970.

Nordstoga, K., and Fjolstad, M. Porcine salmonellosis. III. Production of fibrinous colitis by intravenous injections of a mixture of viable cells of *Salmonella cholerae-suis* and disintegrated cells of the same agent, or hemolytic *Escherichia coli*. *Acta Vet Scand* **11**: 380–389, 1970.

Owen, R. ap R. *et al.* Studies on experimental enteric salmonellosis in ponies. *Can J Comp Med* **43**: 247–254, 1979.

Owen, R. ap R., Fullerton, J. and Barnum, D. A. Effects of transportation, surgery, and antibiotic therapy in ponies infected with *Salmonella*. *Am J Vet Res* **44**: 46–50, 1983.

Petrie, L. *et al.* Salmonellosis in young calves due to *Salmonella enteritidis*. *Vet Rec* **101**: 398–402, 1977.

Richardson, A. Salmonellosis in cattle. *Vet Rec* **96**: 329–331, 1975.

Roberts, M. C., and O'Boyle, D. A. The prevalence and epizootiology of salmonellosis among groups of horses in south east Queensland. *Aust Vet J* **57**: 27–35, 1981.

Romane, W. M. *et al.* Systemic salmonellosis in foals. *Southwest Vet* **26**: 113–118, 1972.

Slavin, G. Experimental paratyphoid infection in pigs. *J Comp Pathol* **61**: 168–179, 1951.

Smith, B. P. *et al.* Equine salmonellosis: experimental production of four syndromes. *Am J Vet Res* **40**: 1072–1077, 1979.

Smith, B. P. *et al.* Bovine salmonellosis: experimental production and characterization of the disease in calves, using oral challenge with *Salmonella typhimurium*. *Am J Vet Res* **40**: 1510–1513, 1979.

Smith, B. P., Reina-Guerra, M., and Hardy, A. J. Prevalence and epizootiology of equine salmonellosis. *J Am Vet Med Assoc* **172**: 353–356, 1978.

Smith, H. W., and Halls, S. The simultaneous oral administration of *Salmonella dublin*, *S. typhimurium* and *S. choleraesuis* to calves and other animals. *J Med Microbiol* **1**: 203–209, 1968.

Takeuchi, A. Electron microscope studies of experimental *Salmonella* infection. I. Penetration into the intestinal epithelium by *Salmonella typhimurium*. *Am J Pathol* **50**: 109–136, 1967.

Timoney, J. F., Niebert, H. C., and Scott, F. W. Feline salmonellosis: a nosocomial outbreak and experimental studies. *Cornell Vet* **68**: 211–219, 1978.

Wenkoff, M. S. *Salmonella typhimurium* septicemia in foals. *Can Vet J* **14**: 284–287, 1973.

Wilcock, B. P. Experimental *Klebsiella* and *Salmonella* infection in neonatal swine. *Can J Comp Med* **43**: 200–206, 1979.

Wilcock, B. P., and Olander, H. J. The pathogenesis of porcine rectal stricture. II. Experimental salmonellosis and ischemic proctitis. *Vet Pathol* **14**: 43–55, 1977.

Wilcock, B. P., and Olander, H. J. Neurologic disease in naturally occurring *Salmonella choleraesuis* infection in pigs. *Vet Pathol* **14**: 113–120, 1977.

Wray, C., and Sojka, W. J. Experimental *Salmonella typhimurium* infection in calves. *Res Vet Sci* **25**: 139–143, 1978.

Wray, C., Sojka, W. J., and Bell, J. C. *Salmonella* infection in horses in England and Wales, 1973 to 1979. *Vet Rec* **109**: 398–401, 1981.

Yersiniosis

Christensen, S. G. *Yersinia enterocolitica* in Danish pigs. *J Appl Bacteriol* **48**: 377–382, 1980.

Kaneko, K., Hamada, S., and Katom E. Occurrence of *Yersinia enterocolitica* in dogs. *Jpn J Vet Sci* **39**: 407–414, 1977.

Mair, N. S. *et al. Pasteurella pseudotuberculosis* infection in the cat: Two cases. *Vet Rec* **81**: 461–462, 1967.

Obwolo, M. J. A review of yersiniosis (*Yersinia pseudotuberculosis* infection). *Vet Bull* **46**: 167–171, 1976.

Papageorges, M., Higgins, R., and Gosselin, Y. *Yersinia enterocolitica* enteritis in two dogs. *J Am Vet Med Assoc* **182**: 618–619, 1983.

Spearman, J. G., Hunt, P., and Nayar, P. S. G. *Yersinia pseudotuberculosis* infection in a cat. *Can Vet J* **20**: 361–364, 1979.

Campylobacter

Al-Mashat, R. R., and Taylor, D. J. *Campylobacter* spp. in enteric lesions in cattle. *Vet Rec* **107**: 31–34, 1980.

Al-Mashat, R. R., and Taylor, D. J. Production of diarrhoea and dysentery in experimental calves by feeding pure cultures of *Campylobacter fetus* subspecies *jejuni*. *Vet Rec* **107**: 459–464, 1980.

Al-Mashat, R. R., and Taylor, D. J. Production of enteritis in calves by the oral inoculation of pure cultures of *Campylobacter fecalis*. *Vet Rec* **109**: 97–101, 1981.

Atherton, J. G., and Ricketts, S. W. *Campylobacter* infection from foals. *Vet Rec* **107**: 264–265, 1980.

Blaser, M. J., and Reller, L. B. *Campylobacter* enteritis. *N Engl J Med* **305**: 1444–1452, 1981.

Campbell, S. G., and Cookingham, C. A. The enigma of winter dysentery. *Cornell Vet* **68**: 423–441, 1978.

Cross, R. F., Smith, C. K., and Parker, C. F. Terminal ileitis in lambs. *J Am Vet Med Assoc* **162**: 564–566, 1973.

Dodd, D. C. Adenomatous intestinal hyperplasia (proliferative ileitis) of swine. *Pathol Vet* **5**: 333–341, 1968.

Duhamel, G. E., and Wheeldon, E. B. Intestinal adenomatosis in a foal. *Vet Pathol* **19**: 447–450, 1982.

Elwell, M. R., Chapman, A. L., and Frenkel, J. K. Duodenal hyperplasia in a guinea pig. *Vet Pathol* **18**: 136–139, 1981.

Firehammer, B. D., and Myers, L. L. *Campylobacter fetus* subsp *jejuni*: its possible significance in enteric disease of calves and lambs. *Am J Vet Res* **42**: 918–922, 1981.

Fox, J. G. *et al.* Proliferative colitis in ferrets. *Am J Vet Res* **43**: 858–864, 1982.

Gebhart, C. J. *et al. Campylobacter hyointestinalis* (new species) isolated from swine with lesions of proliferative ileitis. *Am J Vet Res* **44**: 361–367, 1983.

Holt, P. E. *Campylobacter* infections in small animals. *Vet Annu* **23**: 168–172, 1983.

Jonsson, L., and Martinsson, K. Regional ileitis in pigs. Morphological and pathogenetical aspects. *Acta Vet Scand* **17**: 223–232, 1976.

Jopp, A., and Orr, M. B. Enteropathy and nephropathy associated with "winter scour" in hoggets. *NZ Vet J* **28**: 195, 1980.

Kurtz, H. J., and Chang, K. Demonstration of a new *Campylobacter* species in lesions of proliferative enteritis in swine. *Proc Int Pig Vet Soc Congr* p. 60, 1982.

Landsverk, T. Intestinal adenomatosis in a blue fox (*Alopex lagopus*). *Vet Pathol* **18**: 275–278, 1981.

Landsverk, T., and Nordstoga, K. Intestinal adenomatosis in pigs. A patho-morphological investigation. *Nord Vet Med* **33**: 77–80, 1981.

Lawson, G. H. K. *et al.* Proliferative haemorrhagic enteropathy. *Res Vet Sci* **27**: 46–51, 1979.

Lawson, G. H. K. *et al.* Some features of *Campylobacter sputorum* subsp. *mucosalis* subsp. nov., nom. rev. and their taxonomic significance. *Int J Syst Bacteriol* **31**: 385–391, 1981.

Lomax, L. G. Porcine proliferative enteritis: experimentally induced disease in Caesarean-derived colostrum-deprived pigs. *Am J Vet Res* **43**: 1622–1630, 1982.

Lomax, L. G., and Glock, R. D. Naturally occurring porcine proliferative enteritis: pathologic and bacteriologic findings. *Am J Vet Res* **43**: 1608–1614, 1982.

Love, D. N., and Love, R. J. Pathology of proliferative haemorrhagic enteropathy in pigs. *Vet Pathol* **16**: 41–48, 1979.

Manninen, K. I., Prescott, J. F., and Dohoo, I. R. Pathogenicity of *Campylobacter jejuni* isolates from animals and humans. *Infect Immun* **38**: 46–52, 1982.

Moon, H. W. *et al.* Intraepithelial *Vibrio* associated with acute typhlitis of young rabbits. *Vet Pathol* **11**: 313–326, 1974.

Olubunmi, P. A., and Taylor, D. J. Production of enteritis in pigs by the oral inoculation of pure cultures of *Campylobacter coli*. *Vet Rec* **111**: 197–202, 1982.

Prescott, J. F. *et al. Campylobacter jejuni* colitis in gnotobiotic dogs. *Can J Comp Med* **45**: 377–383, 1981.

Prescott, J. F., and Munroe, D. L. *Campylobacter jejuni* enteritis in man and domestic animals. *J Am Vet Med Assoc* **181**: 1524–1530, 1982.

Rahko, T., and Saloniemi, H. On the pathology of regional ileitis in the pig. *Nord Vet Med* **24**: 132–138, 1972.

Roberts, L. Natural infection of the oral cavity of young piglets with *Campylobacter sputorum* ssp *mucosalis*. *Vet Rec* **109**: 17, 1981.

Roberts, L. *et al.* Porcine intestinal adenomatosis and its detection in a closed pig herd. *Vet Rec* **104**: 366–368, 1979.

Rowland, A. C., and Rowntree, P. G. M. A haemorrhagic bowel syndrome associated with intestinal adenomatosis in the pig. *Vet Rec* **91**: 235–241, 1972.

Skirrow, M. B. *Campylobacter* enteritis in dogs and cats: a 'new' zoonosis. *Vet Res Commun* **5**: 13–19, 1981.

Skirrow, M. B. *Campylobacter* enteritis—the first five years. *J Hyg (Lond)* **89**: 175–184, 1982.

Smibert, R. M. The genus *Campylobacter*. *Annu Rev Microbiol* **32**: 673–709, 1978.

Taylor, D. J. *Campylobacter jejuni* infections in calves. *Vet Annu* **23**: 61–64, 1983.

Vandenberghe, J. *et al. Campylobacter jejuni* related with diarrhoea in dogs. *Br Vet J* **138**: 356–361, 1982.

Vandenberghe, J., and Hoorens, J. *Campylobacter* species and regional enteritis in lambs. *Res Vet Sci* **29**: 390–391, 1980.

Yates, W. D. G. *et al.* Proliferative hemorrhagic enteropathy in swine: an outbreak and review of the literature. *Can Vet J* **20**: 261–268, 1979.

Swine Dysentery

Andress, C. E., Barnum, D. A., and Thomson, R. G. Pathogenicity of *Vibrio coli* for swine. I. Experimental infection of gnotobiotic pigs with *Vibrio coli*. *Can J Comp Med* **32**: 522–528, 1968.

Argenzio, R. A., Whipp, S. C., and Glock, R. D. Pathophysiology of swine dysentery: colonic transport and permeability studies. *J Infect Dis* **142**: 676–684, 1980.

Beer, R. J. *et al.* Spirochaetal invasion of the colonic mucosa in a syndrome resembling swine dysentery following experimental *Trichuris suis* infections in weaned pigs. *Res Vet Sci* **13**: 593–595, 1972.

Burrows, M. R., and Lemcke, R. M. Identification of *Treponema hyodysenteriae* by a rapid slide agglutination test. *Vet Rec* **108**: 187–189, 1981.

Ferguson, H. W., Neill, S. D., and Pearson, G. R. Dysentery in pigs associated with cystic enlargement of submucosal glands in the large intestine. *Can J Comp Med* **44**: 109–114, 1980.

Glock, R. D., Harris, D. L., and Kluge, J. P. Localization of spirochetes with the structural characteristics of *Treponema hyodysenteriae* in the lesions of swine dysentery. *Infect Immun* **9**: 167–178, 1974.

Hamdy, A. H., and Glenn, M. W. Transmission of swine dysentery with *Treponema hyodysenteriae* and *Vibrio coli*. *Am J Vet Res* **35**: 791–797, 1974.

Harris, D. L. *et al.* Swine dysentery—I. Inoculation of pigs with *Treponema hyodysenteriae* (new species) and reproduction of the disease. *VM SAC* **67**: 61–64, 1972.

Harris, D. L. *et al.* Swine dysentery: studies of gnotobiotic pigs inoculated with *Treponema hyodysenteriae, Bacteroides vulgatus,* and *Fusobacterium necrophorum*. *J Am Vet Med Assoc* **172**: 468–471, 1978.

Harris, D. L., and Glock, R. D. Swine dysentery. *J Am Vet Med Assoc* **160**: 561–565, 1972.

Harris, D. L., and Kinyon, J. M. Significance of anaerobic spirochetes in the intestines of animals. *Am J Clin Nutr* **27**: 1297–1304, 1974.

Hughes, R. *et al.* Swine dysentery. Induction and characterization in isolated colonic loops. *Vet Pathol* **9**: 22–37, 1972.

Hughes, R., Olander, H. J., and Williams, C. B. Swine dysentery: pathogenicity of *Treponema hyodysenteriae*. *Am J Vet Res* **36**: 971–977, 1975.

Joens, L. A. *et al.* Location of *Treponema hyodysenteriae* and synergistic anaerobic bacteria in colonic lesions of gnotobiotic pigs. *Vet Microbiol* **6**: 69–77, 1981.

Kennedy, G. A., Strafuss, A. C., and Schoneweis, D. A. Scanning electron microscopic observations on swine dysentery. *J Am Vet Med Assoc* **163**: 53–55, 1973.

Kinyon, J. M., Harris, D. L., and Glock, R. D. Enteropathogenicity of various isolates of *Treponema hyodysenteriae*. *Infect Immun* **15**: 638–646, 1977.

Meyer, R. C. Swine dysentery: a perspective. *Adv Vet Sci Comp Med* **22**: 133–158, 1978.

Olson, L. D. Staining of histologic sections of colon with Victoria blue 4-R as an aid in the diagnosis of swine dysentery. *Am J Vet Res* **34**: 853–854, 1973.

Olson, L. D. Induction of swine dysentery in swine by the intravenous injection of filtered *Treponema hyodysenteriae*. *Can J Comp Med* **45**: 371–376, 1981.

Ritchie, A. E., and Brown, L. N. An agent possibly associated with swine dysentery. *Vet Rec* **89**: 608–609, 1971.

Songer, J. G. *et al.* Isolation of *Treponema hyodysenteriae* from sources other than swine. *J Am Vet Med Assoc* **172**: 464–466, 1978.

Taylor, D. J., and Alexander, T. J. L. The production of dysentery in swine by feeding cultures containing a spirochaete. *Br Vet J* **127**: lviii–lxi, 1971.

Taylor, D. J., and Blakemore, W. F. Spirochaetal invasion of the colonic epithelium in swine dysentery. *Res Vet Sci* **12**: 177–179, 1971.

Taylor, D. J., Simmons, J. R., and Laird, H. M. Production of diarrhoea and dysentery in pigs by feeding pure cultures of a spirochaete differing from *Treponema hyodysenteriae*. *Vet Rec* **106**: 326–332, 1980.

Teige, J., Jr. *et al.* Swine dysentery: a scanning electron microscopic investigation. *Acta Vet Scand* **22**: 218–225, 1981.

Teige, J., Jr. *et al.* Swine dysentery: the influence of dietary vitamin E and selenium on the clinical and pathological effects of *Treponema hyodysenteriae* infection in pigs. *Res Vet Sci* **32**: 95–100, 1982.

Turek, J. J., and Meyer, R. C. Studies on a canine intestinal spirochaete. *Can J Comp Med* **41**: 332–337, 1977.

Van Ulsen, F. W., and Lambers, G. M. Doyles dysentery in dogs. *Tijdschr Diergeneeskd* **98**: 577–579, 1973.

Wilcock, B. P., and Olander, H. J. Studies on the pathogenesis of swine dysentery. I. Characterization of the lesions in colons and colonic segments inoculated with pure cultures or colonic content containing *Treponema hyodysenteriae*. *Vet Pathol* **16**: 450–465, 1979.

Windsor, R. S. Swine dysentery. *Vet Annu* **19**: 89–96, 1979.

Diseases Associated with Enteric Clostridial Infections

Al-Mashat, R. R., and Taylor, D. J. Production of diarrhoea and enteric lesions in calves by the oral inoculation of pure cultures of *Clostridium sordellii*. *Vet Rec* **112**: 141–146, 1983.

Arbuckle, J. B. R. The attachment of *Clostridium welchii (Cl. perfringens)* type C to intestinal villi of pigs. *J Pathol* **106**: 65–72, 1972.

Breukink, H. J. *et al.* Voedselvergiftiging bij runderen veroorzaakt door het eten van bierbostel besmet met *Clostridium botulinum* type B. *Tijdschr Diergeneeskd* **103**: 303–311, 1978.

Bullen, J. J., and Batty, I. Experimental enterotoxaemia of sheep: the effect on the permeability of the intestine and the stimulation of antitoxin production in immune animals. *J Pathol Bacteriol* **73**: 511–518, 1957.

Burrows, C. F. Canine hemorrhagic gastroenteritis. *J Am Anim Hosp Assoc* **13**: 451–458, 1977.

Buxton, D., Linklater, K. A., and Dyson, D. A. Pulpy kidney disease and its diagnosis by histological examination. *Vet Rec* **102**: 241, 1978.

Buxton, D., and Morgan, K. T. Studies of lesions produced in the brains of colostrum deprived lambs by *Clostridium welchii (Cl. perfringens)* Type D toxin. *J Comp Pathol* **86**: 435–447, 1976.

Carman, R. J., and Lewis, J. C. M. Recurrent diarrhoea in a dog associated with *Clostridium perfringens* type A. *Vet Rec* **112**: 342–343, 1983.

Dalling, T. Lamb dysentery. *J Comp Pathol* **39**: 148–163, 1926.

Gardner, D. E. Pathology of *Clostridium welchii* type D enterotoxaemia. II. Structural and ultrastructural alterations in the tissues of lambs and mice. *J Comp Pathol* **83**: 509–524, 1973.

Gardner, D. E. Pathology of *Clostridium welchii* type D enterotoxaemia. III. Basis of the hyperglycaemic response. *J Comp Pathol* **83**: 525–529, 1973.

Greig, A. An outbreak of *C. welchii* type C enterotoxaemia in young lambs in south west Scotland. *Vet Rec* **96**: 179, 1975.

Hart, B., and Hooper, P. T. Enterotoxaemia of calves due to *Clostridium welchii* type E. *Aust Vet J* **43**: 360–363, 1967.

Hartley, W. J. A focal encephalomalacia of lambs. *NZ Vet J* **4**: 129–135, 1956.

Lauerman, L. H., Jensen, R., and Pierson, R. E. *Clostridium perfringens* type C enterotoxemia in feetlot cattle and sheep. *Proc Annu Meet Am Assoc Vet Lab Diagn* **20**: 363–364, 1977.

McEwen, A. D., and Roberts, R. S. Struck: enteritis and peritonitis of sheep caused by a bacterial toxin derived from the alimentary canal. *J Comp Pathol* **44**: 26–49, 1931.

McDonel, J. L. *Clostridium perfringens* toxins (type A, B, C, D, E). *Pharmacol Ther* **10**: 617–655, 1980.

McGowan, B., Moulton, J. E., and Rood, S. E. Lamb losses associated with *Clostridium perfringens* type A. *J Am Vet Med Assoc* **133**: 219–221, 1958.

Mason, J. H., and Robinson, E. M. The isolation of *Cl. welchii*, type B, from foals affected with dysentery. *Onderstepoort J Vet Sci* **11**: 333–337, 1938.

Moon, H. W., and Dillman, R. C. Comments on clostridia and enteric disease in swine. *J Am Vet Med Assoc* **160**: 572–573, 1972.

Niilo, L. *Clostridium perfringens* in animal disease: a review of current knowledge. *Can Vet J* **21**: 141–148, 1980.

Niilo, L., and Chalmers, G. A. Hemorrhagic enterotoxemia caused by *Clostridium perfringens* type C in a foal. *Can Vet J* **23**: 299–301, 1982.

Niilo, L., Harries, W. N., and Jones, G. A. *Clostridium perfringens* type C in hemorrhagic enterotoxemia of neonatal calves in Alberta. *Can Vet J* **15**: 224–226, 1974.

Oxer, D. T. Enterotoxaemia in goats. *Aust Vet J* **32**: 62–66, 1956.

Prescott, J. R. *et al.* Haemorrhagic gastroenteritis in the dog associated with *Clostridium welchii*. *Vet Rec* **103**: 116–117, 1978.

Rose, A. L., and Edgar, G. Enterotoxaemic jaundice of cattle and sheep. A preliminary report on the aetiology of the disease. *Aust Vet J* **12**: 212–220, 1936.

Corynebacterium equi

Barton, M. D., and Hughes, K. L. *Corynebacterium equi:* a review. *Vet Bull* **50**: 65–80, 1980.

Cimprich, R. E., and Rooney, J. R. *Corynebacterium equi* enteritis in foals. *Vet Pathol* **14**: 95–102, 1977.

Johnson, J. A., Prescott, J. F., and Markham, R. J. F. The pathology of experimental *Corynebacterium equi* infection in foals following intragastric challenge. *Vet Pathol* **20**: 450–459, 1983.

Woolcock, J. B., Mutimer, M. D., and Farmer, A.-M. T. Epidemiology of *Corynebacterium equi* in horses. *Res Vet Sci* **28**: 87–90, 1980.

Mycobacterial Enteritis

Allen, W. M., Berrett, S., and Patterson, D. S. P. A biochemical study of experimental Johne's disease. I. Plasma protein leakage into the intestine of sheep. *J Comp Pathol* **84**: 381–384, 1974.

Baker, J. R. A case of generalised avian tuberculosis in a horse. *Vet Rec* **93**: 105–106, 1973.

Bendixen, P. H. Immunological reactions caused by infection with *Mycobacterium paratuberculosis*. *Nord Vet Med* **30**: 163–168, 1978.

Buergelt, C. D. *et al.* Pathological evaluation of paratuberculosis in naturally infected cattle. *Vet Pathol* **15**: 196–207, 1978.

Cimprich, R. E. Equine granulomatous enteritis. *Vet Pathol* **11**: 535–547, 1974.

Doyle, T. M. Isolation of Johne's bacilli from the udder of clinically affected cows. *Br Vet J* **110**: 215–218, 1954.

Fodstad, F. H., and Gunnarsson, E. Post-mortem examination in the diagnosis of Johne's disease in goats. *Acta Vet Scand* **20**: 157–167, 1979.

Gilmour, N. J. L. The pathogenesis, diagnosis and control of Johne's disease. *Vet Rec* **99**: 433–434, 1976.

Goudswaard, J. *et al.* Diagnosis of Johne's disease in cattle: a comparison of five serological tests under field conditions. *Vet Rec* **98**: 461–462, 1976.

Gunnarsson, E., and Fodstad, F. H. Cultural and biochemical characteristics of *Mycobacterium paratuberculosis* isolated from goats in Norway. *Acta Vet Scand* **20**: 122–134, 1979.

Julian, R. J. A short review and some observations on Johne's disease with recommendations for control. *Can Vet J* **16**: 33–43, 1975.

Larsen, A. B., Moon, H. W., and Merkal, R. J. Susceptibility of swine to *Mycobacterium paratuberculosis*. *Am J Vet Res* **32**: 589–595, 1971.

Larsen, A. B., Moon, H. W., and Merkal, R. S. Susceptibility of horses to *Mycobacterium paratuberculosis*. *Am J Vet Res* **33**: 2185–2189, 1972.

McQueen, D. S., Russell, E. G. Culture of *Mycobacterium paratuberculosis* from bovine foetuses. *Aust Vet J* **55**: 203–204, 1979.

Morin, M. Johne's disease (paratuberculosis) in goats: a report of eight cases in Quebec. *Can Vet J* **23**: 55–58, 1982.

Patterson, D. S. P., and Barrett, S. Malabsorption in Johne's disease in cattle: an *in vitro* study of L-histidine uptake by isolated intestinal tissue preparations. *J Med Microbiol* **2**: 327–334, 1969.

Payne, J. M., and Rankin, J. D. A comparison of the pathogenesis of experimental Johne's disease in calves and cows. *Res Vet Sci* **2**: 175–179, 1961.

Pemberton, D. H. Diagnosis of Johne's disease in cattle using mesenteric lymph node biopsy: accuracy in clinical suspects. *Aust Vet J* **55**: 217–219, 1979.

Riemann, H. *et al.* Paratuberculosis in cattle and free-living exotic deer. *J Am Vet Med Assoc* **174**: 841–843, 1979.

Saitanu, K., and Holmgaard, P. An Epizootic of *Mycobacterium intracellulare*, serotype 8 infection in swine. *Nord Vet Med* **29**: 221–226, 1977.

Thoen, C. O., and Muscoplat, C. C. Recent developments in diagnosis of paratuberculosis (Johne's disease). *J Am Vet Med Assoc* **174**: 838–840, 1979.

Enteritis Due to Chlamydia psittaci

Dourhri, A. M. *et al.* Electron microscopic tracing of pathogenetic events in intestinal chlamydial infections of newborn calves. *Exp Mol Pathol* **18**: 10–17, 1973.

Doughri, A. M. *et al.* Ultrastructural changes in the *Chlamydia*-infected ileal mucosa of newborn calves. *Vet Pathol* **10**: 114–123, 1973.

Doughri, A. M., Young, S., and Storz, J. Pathologic changes in intestinal chlamydial infection of newborn calves. *Am J Vet Res* **35**: 939–944, 1974.

Ehret, W. J. *et al.* Chlamydiosis in a beef herd. *J S Afr Vet Assoc* **46**: 171–179, 1975.

Shewen, P. E. Chlamydial infection in animals: a review. *Can Vet J* **21**: 2–11, 1980.

Mycotic Diseases of the Gastrointestinal Tract

Angus, K. W., Gilmour, N. J. L., and Dawson, C. O. Alimentary mycotic lesions in cattle: a histological and cultural study. *J Med Microbiol* **6**: 207–213, 1973.

Cordes, D. O., Royal, W. A., and Shortridge, E. H. Systemic mycosis in neonatal calves. *NZ Vet J* **15**: 143–149, 1967.

Cordes, D. O., and Shortridge, E. H. Systemic phycomycosis and aspergillosis of cattle. *NZ Vet J* **16**: 65–80, 1968.

Miller, R. I., Qualls, C. W., Jr., and Turnwald, G. H. Gastrointestinal phycomycosis in a dog. *J Am Vet Med Assoc* **182**: 1245–1246, 1983.

Smith, J. M. B. Mycoses of the alimentary tract of animals. *NZ Vet J* **16**: 89–100, 1968.

Taylor, R. L., and Kintner, L. D. Phycomycosis of feedlot cattle. *J Am Vet Med Assoc* **174**: 371–372, 1979.

Candidiasis

Gilardi, G. L. Nutrition of systemic and subcutaneous pathogenic fungi. *Bacteriol Rev* **29**: 406–424, 1965.

Gross, T. L., and Mayhew, I. G. Gastroesophageal ulceration and candidiasis in foals. *J Am Vet Med Assoc* **182**: 1370–1373, 1983.

Mills, J. H. L., and Hirth, R. S. Systemic candidiasis in calves on prolonged antibiotic therapy. *J Am Vet Med Assoc* **150:** 862–870, 1967.

Osborne, A. D., McCrae, M. R., and Manners, M. J. Moniliasis in artificially reared pigs and its treatment with Nystatin. *Vet Rec* **72:** 237–241, 1960.

Smith, J. M. B. Candidiasis in animals in New Zealand. *Sabouraudia* **5:** 220–225, 1967.

Histoplasma capsulatum

Berry, C. L. The development of the granuloma of histoplasmosis. *J Pathol* **97:** 1–10, 1969.

Dade, A. W., Lickfeldt, W. E., and McAllister, H. A. Granulomatous colitis in a horse with histoplasmosis. *VM SAC* **68:** 279–281, 1973.

Mahaffey, E. *et al.* Disseminated histoplasmosis in three cats. *J Am Anim Hosp Assoc* **13:** 46–51, 1977.

Protothecal Enterocolitis

Chandler, F. W., Kaplan, W., and Callaway, C. S. Differentiation between *Prototheca* and morphologically similar green algae in tissue. *Arch Pathol Lab Med* **102:** 353–356, 1978.

Migaki, G. *et al.* Canine protothecosis: review of the literature and report of an additional case. *J Am Vet Med Assoc* **181:** 794–797, 1982.

Pore, R. S. *et al. Prototheca* ecology. *Mycopathologia* **81:** 49–62, 1983.

Sudman, M. S., and Kaplan, W. Antigenic relationships between *Chlorella* and *Prototheca* spp. *Sabouraudia* **12:** 364–370, 1974.

Gastrointestinal Helminthosis

General

Arundel, J. H. Parasitic diseases of the horse. "Veterinary Review," No. 18. University of Sydney Postgraduate Foundation in Veterinary Science, Sydney, N.S.W., 1978.

Arundel, J. H. Diseases caused by helminth parasites. *In* "Veterinary Medicine," D. C. Blood, O. M. Radostits, and J. A. Henderson (eds.), 6th ed., pp. 895–944. London, Baillière, 1983.

Bremner, K. C. The pathophysiology of parasitic gastroenteritis of cattle. *In* "Biology and Control of Endoparasites," L. E. A. Symons, A. D. Donald, and J. K. Dineen (eds.), pp. 277–289. Sydney, Academic Press, 1982.

Castro, G. A. Physiology of the gastrointestinal tract in the parasitized host. *In* "Physiology of the Gastrointestinal Tract," L. R. Johnson (ed.), pp. 1381–1406. New York, Raven Press, 1981.

Chitwood, M., and Lichtenfels, J. R. Identification of parasitic metazoa in tissue sections. *Exp Parasitol* **32:** 407–519, 1972.

Corwin, R. M., McDowell, A. E., and Talent, N. K. Internal parasites. *In* "Diseases of Swine," A. D. Leman *et al.* (eds.), 5th ed., pp. 560–578. Ames, Iowa State Univ. Press, 1981.

Dargie, J. D. The pathophysiological effects of gastrointestinal and liver parasites in sheep. *In* "Digestive Physiology and Metabolism in Ruminants," Y. Ruckebusch and P. Thivend (eds.), pp. 349–371. Lancaster, England, MTP Press, 1980.

Drudge, J. H., and Lyons, E. T. Pathology of infections with internal parasites in horses. *Blue Book* **27:** 267–275, 1977.

Dunn, A. M. "Veterinary Helminthology," 2nd ed. London, Heinemann, 1978.

Levine, N. D. "Nematode Parasites of Domestic Animals and of Man," 2nd ed. Minneapolis, Burgess, 1980.

Lichtenfels, J. R. Helminths of domestic equids. *Proc Helminthol Soc Wash* **42:** Spec Issue, 1–92, 1975.

Poynter, D. Some tissue reactions to the nematode parasites of animals. *Adv Parasitol* **4:** 321–383, 1966.

Soulsby, E. J. L. "Helminths, Arthropods and Protozoa of Domesticated Animals," 7th ed. London, Baillière, 1982.

Steel, J. W., and Symons, L. E. A. Nitrogen metabolism in nematodosis of sheep in relation to productivity. *In* "Biology and Control of Endoparasites," L. E. A. Symons, A. D. Donald, and J. K. Dineen (eds.), pp. 235–256. Sydney, Academic Press, 1982.

Sykes, A. R. Nutritional and physiological aspects of helminthiasis in sheep. *In* "Biology and Control of Endoparasites," L. E. A. Symons, A. D. Donald, and J. K. Dineen (eds.), pp. 217–234. Sydney, Academic Press, 1982.

Titchen, D. A. Hormonal and physiological changes in helminth infestations. *In* "Biology and Control of Endoparasites," L. E. A. Symons, A. D. Donald, and J. K. Dineen (eds.), pp. 257–275. Sydney, Academic Press, 1982.

Urquhart, G. M., and Armour, J. "Helminth Diseases of Cattle, Sheep and Horses in Europe." Glasgow, R. MacLehose, 1973.

Ostertagosis

Al Saqur, I. *et al.* Observations on the infectivity and pathogenicity of three isolates of *Ostertagia* spp *sensu lato* in calves. *Res Vet Sci* **32:** 106–112, 1982.

Anderson, N. *et al.* A field study of parasitic gastritis in cattle. *Vet Rec* **77:** 1196–1204, 1965.

Anderson, N. *et al.* Experimental *Ostertagia ostertagi* infections in calves: results of single infections with five graded dose levels of larvae. *Am J Vet Res* **27:** 1259–1265, 1966.

Anderson, N., Blake, R., and Titchen, D. A. Effects of a series of infections of *Ostertagia circumcincta* on gastric secretion of sheep. *Parasitology* **72:** 1–12, 1976.

Armour, J., Jarrett, W. F. H., and Jennings, F. W. Experimental *Ostertagia circumcincta* infections in sheep: development and pathogenesis of a single infection. *Am J Vet Res* **27:** 1267–1278, 1966.

Armour, J., and Ogbourne, C. P. Bovine ostertagiasis: a review and annotated bibliography. *Common Inst Parasitol Misc Publ* **7:** 1–93, 1982.

Coop, R. L., Sykes, A. R., and Angus, K. W. The effect of a daily intake of *Ostertagia circumcincta* larvae on body weight, food intake and concentration of serum constituents in sheep. *Res Vet Sci* **23:** 76–83, 1977.

Hilton, R. J., Barker, I. K., and Rickard, M. D. Distribution and pathogenicity during development of *Camelostrongylus mentulatus* in the abomasum of sheep. *Vet Parasitol* **4:** 231–242, 1978.

Holmes, P. H., and MacLean, J. M. The pathophysiology of ovine ostertagiasis: a study of the changes in plasma protein metabolism following single infections. *Res Vet Sci* **12:** 265–271, 1971.

Mcleay, L. M. *et al.* Effects on abomasal function of *Ostertagia circumcincta* infections in sheep. *Parasitology* **66:** 241–257, 1973.

Murray, M. Structural changes in bovine ostertagiasis associated with increased permeability of the bowel wall to macromolecules. *Gastroenterology* **56:** 763–772, 1969.

Murray, M., Jennings, F. W., and Armour, J. Bovine ostertagiasis. Structure function and mode of differentiation of the bovine gastric mucosa and kinetics of the worm loss. *Res Vet Sci* **11:** 417–427, 1970.

Parkins, J. J., Holmes, P. H., and Bremner, K. C. The pathophysiology of ovine ostertagiasis: some nitrogen balance and digestibility studies. *Res Vet Sci* **14:** 21–28, 1973.

Randall, R. W., and Gibbs, H. C. Effects of clinical and subclinical gastrointestinal helminthiasis on digestion and energy metabolism in calves. *Am J Vet Res* **42:** 1730–1734, 1981.

Ritchie, J. S. D. *et al.* Experimental *Ostertagia ostertagi* infections in calves: parasitology and pathogenesis of a single infection. *Am J Vet Res* **27**: 659–667, 1966.

Sommerville, R. I. The histology of the ovine abomasum, and the relation of the globule leukocyte to nematode infestations. *Aust Vet J* **32**: 237–240, 1956.

Sykes, A. R., Coop, R. L., and Angus, K. W. The influence of chronic *Ostertagia* infection on the skeleton of growing sheep. *J Comp Pathol* **87**: 521–529, 1977.

Haemonchosis

Allonby, E. W., and Urquhart, G. M. The epidemiology and pathogenic significance of haemonchosis in a Merino flock in East Africa. *Vet Parasitol* **1**: 129–143, 1975.

Andrews, J.S. Pathology from *Haemonchus contortus* in lambs. *J Agric Res* **65**: 1–18, 1942.

Bremner, K. C. The parasitic life cycle of *Haemonchus placei* (Place) Ransom (Nematoda: Trichostrongylidae). *Aust J Zool* **4**: 146–151, 1956.

Clark, C. H., Kiesel, G. K., and Goby, C. H. Measurements of blood loss caused by *Haemonchus contortus* infection in sheep. *Am J Vet Res* **23**: 977–980, 1962.

Coop, R. L. The effect of large doses of *Haemonchus contortus* on the level of plasma pepsinogen and the concentration of electrolytes in the abomasal fluid of sheep. *J Comp Pathol* **81**: 213–219, 1971.

Dargie, J. M., and Allonby, E. W. Pathophysiology of single and challenge infection of *Haemonchus contortus* in Merino sheep: studies on red cell kinetics and the 'self cure' phenomenon. *Int J Parasitol* **5**: 147–157, 1975.

Elek, P. *et al.* The reaction of calves to helminth infection under natural grazing conditions. II. Pathology of terminal disease. *Aust J Agric Res* **19**: 161–170, 1968.

Fernando, S. T. The life cycle of *Mecistocirrus digitatus,* a trichostrongylid parasite of ruminants. *J Parasitol* **51**: 156–163, 1965.

Jennings, F. W. The anaemias of parasitic infections. *In* "Pathophysiology of Parasitic Infections," E. J. L. Soulsby (ed.), pp. 41–67. New York, Academic Press, 1977.

Le Jambre, L. F. Hybridization studies of *Haemonchus contortus* (Rudolphi, 1893) and *H. placei* (Place, 1893) (Nematoda: Trichostrongylidae). *Int J Parasitol* **9**: 455–463, 1979.

Malczewski, A. Gastrointestinal helminths of ruminants in Poland. II. Pathogenesis and pathology in experimental *Haemonchus contortus* infection in lambs. *Acta Parasitol Pol* **18**: 399–415, 1971.

O'Sullivan, B. M., and Donald, A. Responses to infection with *Haemonchus contortus* and *Trichostrongylus colibriformis* in ewes of different reproductive status. *Int J Parasitol* **3**: 521–530, 1973.

Roberts, F. H. S. Reactions of calves to infestation with the stomach worm *Haemonchus placei* (Place, 1893) Ransom 1911. *Aust J Agric Res* **8**: 740–767, 1957.

Silverman, P. H., Mansfield, M. E., and Scott, H. L. *Haemonchus contortus* infection in sheep: effects of various levels of primary infections on nontreated lambs. *Am J Vet Res* **31**: 841–857, 1970.

Trichostrongylus axei

Leland, S. E. *et al.* Studies on *Trichostrongylus axei* (Cobbold, 1879). VII. Some quantitative and pathologic aspects of natural and experimental infections in the horse. *Am J Vet Res* **22**: 128–138, 1961.

Purcell, D. A., Ross, J. G., and Todd, J. R. The pathology of *Trichostrongylus axei* infection in calves and sheep. *In* "Pathology of Parasitic Diseases," S. M. Gaafar (ed.), pp. 295–302. Lafayette, Indiana, Purdue University, 1971.

Ross, J. G., Purcell, D. A., and Todd, J. R. Investigations of *Tri-*

chostrongylus axei infections in calves: observations using abomasal and intestinal cannulae. *Br Vet J* **125**: 149–158, 1970.

Gastric Parasitism in Horses

Drudge, J. H. *et al.* Occurrence of second and third instars of *Gasterophilus intestinalis* and *Gasterophilus nasalis* in stomachs of horses in Kentucky. *Am J Vet Res* **36**: 1585–1588, 1975.

Lyons, E. T. *et al.* Parasites in Kentucky thoroughbreds at necropsy: emphasis on stomach worms and tapeworms. *Am J Vet Res* **44**: 839–844, 1983.

Shefstad, D. K. Scanning electron microscopy of *Gasterophilus intestinalis* lesions of the equine stomach. *J Am Vet Med Assoc* **172**: 310–313, 1978.

Waddell, A. H. The pathogenicity of *Gasterophilus intestinalis* larvae in the stomach of the horse. *Aust Vet J* **48**: 332–335, 1972.

Gastric Parasites in Swine

Castelino, J. B., Herbert, I. V., and Lean, I. J. The live-weight gain of growing pigs experimentally infected with massive doses of *Hyostrongylus rubidus* (Nematoda) larvae. *Br Vet J* **126**: 579–582, 1970.

Connan, R. M. Observations on the epidemiology of parasitic gastroenteritis due to *Oesophagostomum* spp. and *Hyostrongylus rubidus* in the pig. *Vet Rec* **80**: 424–429, 1967.

Dey-Hazra, A. *et al.* Gastro-intestinal loss of plasma proteins in *Hyostrongylus* infected pigs. *Z Parasitenkd* **38**: 14–20, 1972.

Dodd, D. C. *Hyostrongylus* and gastric ulceration in the pig. *NZ Vet J* **8**: 100–103, 1960.

Kendall, S. B., and Small, A. J. *Hyostrongylus rubidus* in sows at pasture. *Vet Rec* **5**: 388–390, 1974.

Kendall, S. B., Thurley, D. C., and Peirce, M. A. The biology of *Hyostrongylus rubidus.* I. Primary infection in young pigs. *J Comp Pathol* **79**: 87–95, 1969.

Lean, I. S., Herbert, I. V., and Castelino, J. B. Studies on the pathogenesis of infection with *Hyostrongylus rubidus* (Nematoda). The effects of levels of infection of up to 150 000 infective stage larvae on the growing pig. I. Nutritional studies. *Br Vet J* **128**: 138–146, 1972.

Lean, I. S., Herbert, I. V., and Castelino, J. B. Studies on the pathogenesis of infection with *Hyostrongylus rubidus* (Nematoda). The effects of levels of infection of up to 150 000 infective stage larvae on the growing pig. II. Blood studies. *Br Vet J* **128**: 147–152, 1972.

Marti, O. G., Stewart, T. B., and Hale, D. M. Effect of diet, sex and *Hyostrongylus* on pigs. *J Anim Sci* **41**: 320, 1975.

Stockdale, P. H. G. Pathogenesis of *Hyostrongylus rubidus* in growing pigs. *Br Vet J* **130**: 366–373, 1974.

Stockdale, P. H. G. *et al.* Hyostrongylosis in Ontario. *Can Vet J* **14**: 265–268, 1973.

Titchener, R. N., Herbert, I. V., and Probert, A. J. Plasma protein loss in growing pigs during the prepatent and early patent periods of infection with high doses of *Hyostrongylus rubidus* larvae. *J Comp Pathol* **84**: 399–406, 1974.

Varma, S. *et al.* Pathology of *Ascarops strongylina, Physocephalus sexalatus* and *Simondsia paradoxa* the stomach worms of swine. *Arch Vet* **13**: 41–46, 1978.

Gastric Parasitism in Dogs and Cats

Beveridge, I., Presidente, P. J. A., and Arundel, J. H. *Gnathostoma spinigerum* infection in a feral cat from New South Wales. *Aust Vet J* **54**: 46, 1978.

Coman, B. J., Jones, E. H., and Driesen, M. A. Helminth parasites and arthropods of feral cats. *Aust Vet J* **57**: 324–327, 1981.

Greve, J. H., and Kung, F. Y. *Capillaria putorii* in domestic cats in Iowa. *J Am Vet Med Assoc* **182**: 511–513, 1983.

Hargis, A. M. *et al*. Chronic fibrosing gastritis associated with *Ollulanus tricuspis* in a cat. *Vet Pathol* **19:** 320–323, 1982.

Hargis, A. M., Haupt, K. H., and Blanchard, J. L. *Ollulanus tricuspis* found by fecal flotation in a cat with diarrhea. *J Am Vet Med Assoc* **182:** 1122–1123, 1983.

Hargis, A. M., Prieur, D. J., and Blanchard, J. L. Prevalence, lesions, and differential diagnosis of *Ollulanus tricuspis* infection in cats. *Vet Pathol* **20:** 71–79, 1983.

Nayak, B. C., and Rao, A. T. Pathology of gastric lesions in *Gnathostoma spinigerum* infection in a dog. *Indian Vet J* **49:** 750–753, 1972.

Strongyloides Infection

Dey-Hazra, A. *et al*. Protein synthesis changes in the liver of piglets infected with *Strongyloides ransomi*. *Vet Parasitol* **5:** 339–351, 1979.

Dey-Hazra, A., Enigk, K., and Kohn, H. P. Intestinal absorption of palmitate and 2-aminoisobutyric acid in piglets infected with *Strongyloides ransomi*. *Res Vet Sci* **22:** 353–356, 1977.

Enigk, K., and Dey-Hazra, A. Intestinal plasma and blood loss in piglets infected with *Strongyloides ransomi*. *Vet Parasitol* **1:** 69–75, 1975.

Enigk, K., Dey-Hazra, A., and Batke, J. Zur Klinischen Bedeutung und Behandlung des Galktogen erworbenen *Strongyloides*. Befalls der Fohlen. *Dtsch Tieraerztl Wochenschr* **81:** 605–607, 1974.

Etherington, W. G., and Prescott, J. F. *Corynebacterium equi* cellulitis associated with *Strongyloides* penetration in a foal. *J Am Vet Med Assoc* **177:** 1025–1027, 1980.

Garcia, F. T. *et al*. Intestinal function and morphology in strongyloidiasis. *Am J Trop Med Hyg* **26:** 859–865, 1977.

Giese, W., Dey-Hazra, A., and Enigk, K. Enteric loss of plasma proteins in *Strongyloides*-infection of pigs. *Int J Parasitol* **3:** 631–639, 1973.

Greer, G. J., Bello, T. R., and Amborski, G. F. Experimental infection of *Strongyloides westeri* in parasite-free ponies. *J Parasitol* **60:** 466–472, 1974.

Harmeyer, J. *et al*. Messung der intestinalen Resorptionsstorung durch *Strongyloides*-Befall bei Ferkeln. *Z Parasitenkd* **41:** 47–60, 1973.

Lyons, E. T., Drudge, J. H., and Tolliver, S. C. On the life cycle of *Strongyloides westeri* in the equine. *J Parasitol* **59:** 780–787, 1973.

Malone, J. B. *et al*. *Strongyloides tumefaciens* in cats. *J Am Vet Med Assoc* **171:** 278–280, 1977.

Malone, J. B. *et al*. *Strongyloides stercoralis*–like infection in a dog. *J Am Vet Med Assoc* **176:** 130–133, 1980.

Moncol, D. J. Supplement to the life history of *Strongyloides ransomi* Schwartz and Alicata, 1930 (Nematoda: Strongyloididae) of pigs. *Proc Helminthol Soc Wash* **42:** 86–92, 1975.

Nwaorgu, O. C., and Connan, R. M. The importance of arrested larvae in the maintenance of patent infections of *Strongyloides papillosus* in rabbits and sheep. *Vet Parasitol* **7:** 339–346, 1980.

Pande, B. P., and Rao, P. The nematode genus *Strongyloides* Grassi 1879 in Indian livestock. I. Observations on natural infections in the donkey (*Equus asinus*). *Br Vet J* **116:** 281–283, 1960.

Stewart, T. B., Stone, W. M., and Marti, O. G. *Strongyloides ransomi*: prenatal and transmammary infection of pigs of sequential litters from dams experimentally exposed as weanlings. *Am J Vet Res* **37:** 541–544, 1976.

Stone, W. M., and Simpson, C. F. Larval distribution and histopathology of experimental *Strongyloides ransomi* infection in young swine. *Can J Comp Med* **31:** 197–202, 1967.

Stone, W. M., and Smith, F. W. Infection of mammalian hosts by milkborne nematode larvae: a review. *Exp Parasitol* **34:** 306–312, 1973.

Turner, J. H. Experimental strongyloidiasis in sheep and goats. I. Single infections. *Am J Vet Res* **20:** 102–110, 1959.

Turner, J. H., and Shalkop, W. T. Larval migration and accompanying pathological changes in experimental ovine strongyloidiasis. *J Parasitol* **44:** 28–38, 1958.

Trichostrongylosis

Barger, I. A., Southcott, W. H., and Williams, V. J. Trichostrongylosis and wool growth. 2. The wool growth response of infected sheep to parenteral and duodenal cystine and cysteine supplementation. *Aust J Exp Agric Anim Husb* **13:** 351–359, 1973.

Barker, I. K. A study of the pathogenesis of *Trichostrongylus colubriformis* infection in lambs, with observations on the contribution of gastrointestinal plasma loss. *Int J Parasitol* **3:** 743–757, 1973.

Barker, I. K. Scanning electron microscopy of the duodenal mucosa of lambs infected with *Trichostrongylus colubriformis*. *Parasitology* **67:** 307–314, 1973.

Barker, I. K. Intestinal pathology associated with *Trichostrongylus colubriformis* infection in sheep: histology. *Parasitology* **70:** 165–171, 1975

Barker, I. K. Intestinal pathology associated with *Trichostrongylus colubriformis* infection in sheep: vascular permeability, and ultrastructure of the mucosa. *Parasitology* **70:** 173–180, 1975.

Barker, I. K., and Beveridge, I. Development of villus atrophy in the small intestine of sheep infected with *Trichostrongylus rugatus*. *Vet Parasitol* **13:** 67–75, 1983.

Barker, I. K., and Titchen, D. A. Gastric dysfunction in sheep infected with *Trichostrongylus colubriformis*, a nematode inhabiting the small intestine. *Int J Parasitol* **12:** 345–356, 1982.

Coop, R. L., and Angus, K. W. The effect of continuous doses of *Trichostrongylus colubriformis* larvae on serum electrolytes and intestinal enzyme activity in sheep. *Parasitology* **67:** v–vi, 1973.

Coop, R. L., and Angus, K. W. The effect of continuous doses of *Trichostrongylus colubriformis* larvae on the intestinal mucosa of sheep and liver Vitamin A concentration. *Parasitology* **70:** 1–9, 1975.

Coop, R. L., Angus, K. W., and Sykes, A. R. Chronic infection with *Trichostrongylus vitrinus* in sheep. Pathological changes in the small intestine. *Res Vet Sci* **26:** 363–371, 1979.

Coop, R. L., Sykes, A. R., and Angus, K. W. Subclinical trichostrongylosis in growing lambs produced by continuous larval dosing. The effect on performance and certain plasma constituents. *Res Vet Sci* **21:** 253–258, 1976.

Frandsen, J. C. Effects of concurrent subclinical infections by coccidia (*Eimeria christenseni*) and intestinal nematodes (*Trichostrongylus colubriformis*) on apparent nutrient digestibilities and balances, serum copper and zinc, and bone mineralization in the pigmy goat. *Am J Vet Res* **43:** 1951–1953, 1982.

Hennessey, D., and Pritchard, R. K. Functioning of the thyroid gland in sheep infected with *Trichostrongylus colubriformis*. *Res Vet Sci* **30:** 87–92, 1981.

Horak, I. G., Clark, R., and Gray, R. S. The pathological physiology of helminth infestations. III. *Trichostrongylus colubriformis*. *Onderstepoort J Vet Res* **35:** 195–224, 1968.

Jones, D. G. Intestinal enzyme activity in lambs chronically infected with *Trichostrongylus colubriformis*: effect of anthelmintic treatment. *Vet Parasitol* **12:** 79–89, 1983.

Prichard, R. K., Hennessey, D. R., and Griffiths, D. A. Endocrine responses of sheep to infection with *Trichostrongylus colubriformis*. *Res Vet Sci* **17:** 182–187, 1974.

Roseby, F. B. Effect of *Trichostrongylus colubriformis* (Nematoda) on the nutrition and metabolism of sheep. III. Digesta flow and fermentation. *Aust J Agric Res* **28:** 155–164, 1977.

Roseby, F. B., and Leng, R. A. Effects of *Trichostrongylus colubriformis* (Nematoda) on the nutrition and metabolism of sheep. II. Metabolism of urea. *Aust J Agric Res* **25:** 363–367, 1974.

Shayo, M. E., and Benz, G. W. Histopathologic and histochemic changes in the small intestine of calves infected with *Trichostrongylus colubriformis*. *Vet Parasitol* **5**: 353–364, 1979.

Steel, J. W., Symons, L. E. A., and Jones, W. O. Effects of level of larval intake on the productivity and physiological and metabolic responses of lambs infected with *Trichostrongylus colubriformis*. *Aust J Agric Res* **31**: 821–838, 1980.

Sykes, A. R., Coop, R. L., and Angus, K. W. Experimental production of osteoporosis in growing lambs by continuous dosing with *Trichostrongylus colubriformis* larvae. *J Comp Pathol* **85**: 549–559, 1975.

Sykes, A. R., Coop, R. L., and Angus, K. W. Chronic infection with *Trichostrongylus vitrinus* in sheep. Some effects on food utilisation, skeletal growth and certain serum constituents. *Res Vet Sci* **26**: 372–377, 1979.

Symons, L. E. A., and Hennessy, D. R. Cholecystokinin and anorexia in sheep infected by the intestinal nematode *Trichostrongylus colubriformis*. *Int J Parasitol* **11**: 55–58, 1981.

Symons, L. E. A., and Jones, W. O. *Nematospiroides dubius, Nippostrongylus brasiliensis,* and *Trichostrongylus colubriformis:* protein digestion in infected animals. *Exp Parasitol* **27**: 496–506, 1970.

Symons, L. E. A., and Jones, W. O. Skeletal muscle, liver and wool protein synthesis by sheep infected by the nematode *Trichostrongylus colubriformis*. *Aust J Agric Res* **26**: 1063–1072, 1975.

Taylor, S. M., and Pearson, G. R. *Trichostrongylus vitrinus* in sheep. II. The location of nematodes and associated pathological changes in the small intestine during clinical infection. *J Comp Pathol* **89**: 405–412, 1979.

Waller, P. J., Donald, A. D., and Dobson, R. J. Arrested development of intestinal *Trichostrongylus* spp in grazing sheep and seasonal changes in the relative abundance of *T. colubriformis* and *T. vitrinus*. *Res Vet Sci* **30**: 213–216, 1981.

Nematodirus and Cooperia Infection

Ahluwalia, J. S., and Charleston, W. A. G. Studies on the pathogenicity of *Cooperia curticei* for sheep. *NZ Vet J* **23**: 197–199, 1975.

Alicata, J. E., and Lynd, F. T. Growth rate and signs of infection in calves experimentally infected with *Cooperia punctata*. *Am J Vet Res* **22**: 704–707, 1961.

Benz, G. W., and Ernst, J. V. Alkaline phosphatase activities in intestinal mucosa from calves infected with *Cooperia punctata* and *Eimeria bovis*. *Am J Vet Res* **37**: 895–899, 1976.

Borgsteede, F. H. M., and Hendriks, J. Experimental infections with *Cooperia oncophora* (Railliet, 1918) in calves. Results of single infections with two graded dose levels of larvae. *Parasitology* **78**: 331–342, 1979.

Coop, R. L., Angus, K. W., and Mapes, C. J. The effect of large doses of *Nematodirus battus* on the histology and biochemistry of the small intestine of lambs. *Int J Parasitol* **3**: 349–361, 1973.

Coop, R. L., Mapes, C. J., and Angus, K. W. The effects of *Nematodirus battus* on the distribution of intestinal enzymes in lambs. *Res Vet Sci* **13**: 186–188, 1972.

Coop, R. L., Sykes, A. R., and Angus, K. W. The pathogenicity of daily intakes of *Cooperia oncophora* larvae in growing calves. *Vet Parasitol* **5**: 261–269, 1979.

Fabiyi, J. P., Oluyede, D. A., and Negedu, J. O. Late dry season outbreak of clinical haemonchosis and cooperiasis in cattle of northern Nigeria. *Vet Rec* **105**: 399–400, 1979.

Mapes, C. J., and Coop, R. L. The development of single infections of *Nematodirus battus* in lambs. *Parasitology* **64**: 197–216, 1972.

Mapes, C. J., Coop, R. L., and Angus, K. W. The fate of large infective doses of *Nematodirus battus* in young lambs. *Int J Parasitol* **3**: 339–347, 1973.

Martin, J., and Lee, D. L. *Nematodirus battus:* scanning electron micro-

scope studies of the duodenal mucosa of infected lambs. *Parasitology* **81**: 573–578, 1980.

Randall, R. W., and Gibbs, H. C. Effects of clinical and subclinical gastrointestinal helminthiasis on digestion and energy metabolism in calves. *Am J Vet Res* **42**: 1730–1734, 1981.

Rowlands, D.ap.T., and Probert, A. J. Some pathological changes in young lambs experimentally infected with *Nematodirus battus*. *Res Vet Sci* **13**: 323–329, 1972.

Samizadeh-Yazd, A., and Todd, A. C. Observations on the pathogenic effects of *Nematodirus helvetianus* in dairy calves. *Am J Vet Res* **40**: 48–51, 1979.

Seghetti, L., and Senger, C. M. Experimental infections in lambs with *Nematodirus spathiger*. *Am J Vet Res* **19**: 642–644, 1958.

Hookworm Infections

Ansari, Md.Z., Singh, Kr.S., and Iyer, P. K. R. A note on histological studies on the experimental infection of *Gaigeria pachyscelis* Railliet and Henry, 1910, in natural and laboratory animals. *Indian J Anim Sci* **49**: 491–493, 1979.

Areekul, S., Tipayamontri, U., and Ukoskit, K. Experimental infection of *Ancylostoma braziliense* in dogs and cats in Thailand. II. Blood loss. *Southeast Asian J Trop Med Public Health* **5**: 230–235, 1974.

Baker, K. P., and Grimes, T. D. Cutaneous lesions in dogs associated with hookworm infestation. *Vet Rec* **87**: 376–379, 1970.

Buelke, D. L. Hookworm dermatitis. *J Am Vet Med Assoc* **158**: 735–739, 1971.

Gibbs, H. C. On the gross and microscopic lesions produced by the adults and larvae of *Dochmoides stenocephala* (Railliet, 1884) in the dog. *Can J Comp Med* **22**: 382–385, 1958.

Hart, R. J., and Wagner, A. M. The pathological physiology of *Gaigeria pachyscelis* infection. *Onderstepoort J Vet Res* **38**: 111–116, 1971.

Jacobs, D. E. The epidemiology of hookworm infection of dogs in the UK. *Vet Annu* **18**: 220–224, 1978.

Kalkofen, U. P. Intestinal trauma resulting from feeding activities of *Ancylostoma caninum*. *Am J Trop Med Hyg* **23**: 1046–1053, 1974.

Lee, K. T., Little, M. D., and Beaver, P. C. Intracellular (muscle-fiber) habitat of *Ancylostoma caninum* in some mammalian hosts. *J Parasitol* **61**: 589–598, 1975.

McKenna, P. B., McPherson, W. B., and Falconer, G. J. Fatal ancylostomiasis in a dog. *NZ Vet J* **23**: 151–152, 1975.

Migasena, S., Gilles, H. M., and Maegraith, B. G. Studies in *Ancylostoma caninum* infection in dogs. I. Absorption from the small intestine of amino-acids, carbohydrates and fats. *Ann Trop Med Parasitol* **66**: 107–128, 1972.

Migasena, S., Gilles, H. M., and Maegraith, B. G. Studies in *Ancylostoma caninum* infection in dogs. II. Anatomical changes in the gastrointestinal tract. *Ann Trop Med Parasitol* **66**: 203–207, 1972.

Miller, T. A. Blood loss during hookworm infection, determined by erythrocyte labeling with radioactive ^{51}Chromium. I. Infection of dogs with normal and with X-irradiated *Ancylostoma caninum*. *J Parasitol* **52**: 844–855, 1966.

Miller, T. A. Blood loss during hookworm infection, determined by erythrocyte labeling with radioactive ^{51}Chromium. II. Pathogenesis of *Ancylostoma braziliense* infection in dogs and cats. *J Parasitol* **52**: 856–865, 1966.

Miller, T. A. Vaccination against the canine hookworm diseases. *Adv Parasitol* **9**: 153–183, 1971.

Onwuliri, C. O. E., Nwosu, A. B. C., and Anya, A. O. Experimental *Ancylostoma tubaeforme* infection of cats: changes in blood values and worm burden in relation to single infections of varying size. *Z Parasitenkd* **64**: 149–155, 1981.

Pacenovsky, J., and Brezanska, M. Penetration of *Bunostomum phle-*

botomum larvae into the body of cattle. *Vet Med (Praha)* **13:** 277–383, 1968.

Pearson, G. R. *et al.* Uncinariasis in kennelled foxfounds. *Vet Rec* **110:** 328–331, 1982.

Schad, G. A., and Page, M. R. *Ancylostoma caninum:* adult worm removal, corticosteroid treatment, and resumed development of arrested larvae in dogs. *Exp Parasitol* **54:** 303–309, 1982.

Smith, B. L., and Elliot, D. C. Canine pedal dermatitis due to percutaneous *Uncinaria stenocephala* infection. *NZ Vet J* **17:** 235–239, 1969.

Soulsby, E. J. L., Venn, J. A. J., and Green, K. N. Hookworm disease in British cattle. *Vet Rec* **67:** 1124–1125, 1955.

Spellman, G. G., Jr., and Nossel, H. L. Anticoagulant activity of dog hookworm. *Am J Physiol* **220:** 922–927, 1971.

Stoye, M. Üntersuchungen über die Moglichkeit pränataler und galaktogener Infektionen mit *Ancylostoma caninum* Ercolani 1859 (Ancylostomidae) beim Hund. *Zentralbl Veterinaermed [B]* **20:** 1–39, 1973.

Trichurosis

Batte, E. G. *et al.* Pathophysiology of swine trichuriasis. *Am J Vet Res* **38:** 1075–1079, 1977.

Batte, E. G., and Moncol, D. J. Whipworms and dysentery in feeder pigs. *J Am Vet Med Assoc* **161:** 1226–1228, 1972.

Beck, J. and Beverley-Burton, M. The pathology of *Trichuris, Capillaria* and *Trichinella* infections. *Helminthol Abstr* **37:** 1–26, 1968.

Beer, R. J. S. Studies on the biology of the life-cycle of *Trichuris suis* Schrank 1788. *Parasitology* **67:** 253–262, 1973.

Beer, R. J. S. The relationship between *Trichuris trichiura* (Linnaeus 1758) of man and *Trichuris suis* (Schrank 1788) of the pig. *Res Vet Sci* **20:** 47–54, 1976.

Beer, R. J. S., and Lean, I. J. Clinical trichuriasis produced experimentally in growing pigs. Part 1. Pathology of infection. *Vet Rec* **93:** 189–195, 1973.

Beer, R. J. S., Sansom, B. F., and Taylor, P. J. Erythrocyte losses from pigs with experimental *Trichuris suis* infections measured with a whole-body counter. *J Comp Pathol* **84:** 331–346, 1974.

Beveridge, I., and Green, P. E. Species of *Trichuris* in domestic ruminants in Australia. *Aust Vet J* **57:** 141–142, 1981.

Ewing, S. A., and Bull, R. W. Severe chronic canine diarrhea associated with *Balantidium–Trichuris* infection. *J Am Vet Med Assoc* **149:** 519–520, 1966.

Frechette, J. L. *et al.* Infection des jeunes bovins par *Trichuris discolor. Can Vet J* **14:** 243–246, 1973.

Georgi, J. R., Whitlock, R. H., and Flinton, J. H. Fatal *Trichuris discolor* infection in a Holstein–Friesian heifer. *Cornell Vet* **62:** 58–60, 1972.

Hall, G. A., Rutter, J. M., and Beer, R. J. S. A comparative study of the histopathology of the large intestine of conventionally reared, specific pathogen free and gnotobiotic pigs infected with *Trichuris suis. J Comp Pathol* **86:** 285–292, 1976.

Hass, D. K., and Meisels, L. S. *Trichuris campanula* infection in a domestic cat from Miami, Florida. *Am J Vet Res* **39:** 1553–1555, 1978.

Ruben, R. Studies on the common whipworm of the dog, *T. vulpis. Cornell Vet* **44:** 36–39, 1954.

Rutter, J. M., and Beer, R. J. S. Synergism between *Trichuris suis* and the microbial flora of the large intestine causing dysentery in pigs. *Infect Immun* **11:** 395–404, 1975.

Sansom, B. F., Beer, R. J. S., and Kitchenham, B. A. Changes in concentrations of serum urea nitrogen, albumin, globulin, sodium and inorganic phosphorus in weaner pigs infected with *Trichuris suis. J Comp Pathol* **84:** 409–415, 1974.

Smith, H. J., and Stevenson, R. G. A clinical outbreak of *Trichuris discolor* in stabled calves. *Can Vet J* **11:** 102–104, 1970.

Widmer, W. R., and Van Kruiningen, H. J. *Trichuris*-induced transmural ileocolitis in a dog—an entity mimicking regional enteritis. *J Am Anim Hosp Assoc* **10:** 581–585, 1974.

Oesophagostomum and Chabertia Infection

Bawden, R. J. Relationships between *Oesophagostomum columbianum* infection and the nutritional status of sheep. III. Serum and tissue protein changes. *Aust J Agric Res* **20:** 965–970, 1969.

Bremner, K. C. Pathogenetic factors in experimental bovine oesophagostomosis. IV. Exudative enteropathy as a cause of hypoproteinemia. *Exp Parasitol* **25:** 382–394, 1969.

Bremner, K. C. Pathogenetic factors in experimental bovine oesophagostomosis. V. Intestinal bleeding as cause of anemia. *Exp Parasitol* **27:** 236–245, 1970.

Bremner, K. C., and Fridemanis, R. *Oesophagostomum radiatum* in calves: intestinal hemorrhage associated with larval emergence. *Exp Parasitol* **36:** 424–429, 1974.

Bremner, K. C., and Fridemanis, R. A defibrination syndrome in calves caused by histotrophic larvae of *Oesophagostomum radiatum. J Comp Pathol* **85:** 383–390, 1975.

Bremner, K. C., and Keith, R. K. *Oesophagostomum radiatum:* adult nematodes and intestinal hemorrhage. *Exp Parasitol* **28:** 416–419, 1970.

Clark, R. G., Mason, P. C., and Fennessy, P. F. Nodular lesions in the absence of *Oesophagostomum columbianum. NZ Vet J* **26:** 33, 1978.

Dash, K. M. The life cycle of *Oesophagostomum columbianum* (Curtice, 1890) in sheep. *Int J Parasitol* **3:** 843–851, 1973.

Dobson, C. Changes in the protein content of the serum and intestinal mucus of sheep with reference to the histology of the gut and immunological response to *Oesophagostomum columbianum* infections. *Parasitology* **57:** 201–219, 1967.

Elek, P., and Durie, P. H. The histopathology of the reactions of calves to experimental infection with the nodular worm *Oesophagostomum columbianum* (Rudolphi, 1803). II. Reaction of the susceptible host to infection with a single dose of larvae. *Aust J Agric Res* **18:** 549–559, 1967.

Hale, O. M. *et al.* Influence of an experimental infection of nodular worms (*Oesophagostomum* spp.) on performance of pigs. *J Anim Sci* **52:** 316–322, 1981.

Herd, R. P. The pathogenic importance of *Chabertia ovina* (Fabricius, 1788) in experimentally infected sheep. *Int J Parasitol* **1:** 251–263, 1971.

McCracken, R. M., and Ross, J. G. The histopathology of *Oesophagostomum dentatum* infections in pigs. *J Comp Pathol* **80:** 619–623, 1970.

Pattison, H. D., Thomas, R. J., and Smith, W. C. The effect of subclinical nematode parasitism on digestion and performance in growing pigs. *Anim Prod* **30:** 285–294, 1980.

Poelvoorde, J., and Berghen, P. Experimental infection of pigs with *Oesophagostomum dentatum:* pathogenesis and parasitology of repeated mass infection. *Res Vet Sci* **31:** 10–13, 1981.

Shelton, G. C., and Griffiths, H. J. *Oesophagostomum columbianum:* experimental infections in lambs. Effects of different types of exposure on the intestinal lesions. *Pathol Vet* **4:** 413–434, 1967.

Stewart, M. *et al.* The energy and nitrogen metabolism and performance of pigs infected with *Oesophagostomum dentatum. Anim Prod* **36:** 137–142, 1983.

Stockdale, P. H. G. Necrotic enteritis of pigs caused by infection with *Oesophagostomum* spp. *Br Vet J* **126:** 526–530, 1970.

Equine Strongylosis

Duncan, J. L., and Dargie, J. D. The pathogenesis and control of strongyle infection in the horse. *J S Afr Vet Assoc* **46**: 81–85, 1975.

Duncan, J. L., and Pirie, H. M. The life cycle of *Strongylus vulgaris* in the horse. *Res Vet Sci* **13**: 374–379, 1972.

Duncan, J. L., and Pirie, H. M. The pathogenesis of single experimental infections with *Strongylus vulgaris* in foals. *Res Vet Sci* **18**: 82–93, 1975.

Enigk, K. On the development of *Strongylus vulgaris* (nematode) in the host animal. *Cornell Vet* **63**: 223–246, 1973.

Enigk, K. Further investigations on the biology of *Strongylus vulgaris* (Nematoda) in the host animal. *Cornell Vet* **63**: 247–263, 1973.

Georgi, J. R. The Kekuch-Enigk model of *Strongylus vulgaris* migrations in the horse. *Cornell Vet* **63**: 220–222, 1973.

Klei, T. R. *et al.* Morphologic and clinicopathologic changes following *Strongylus vulgaris* infections of immune and nonimmune ponies. *Am J Vet Res* **43**: 1300–1307, 1982.

McCraw, B. M., and Slocombe, J. O. D. *Strongylus vulgaris* in the horse: a review. *Can Vet J* **17**: 150–157, 1976.

McCraw, B. M., and Slocombe, J. O. D. *Strongylus edentatus:* development and lesions from ten weeks postinfection to patency. *Can J Comp Med* **42**: 340–356, 1978.

Ogbourne, C. P. Pathogenesis of cyathostome (*Trichonema*) infections of the horse. A review. *Commonw Inst Helminthol* **5**: 25, 1978.

Ogbourne, C. P., and Duncan, J. L. *Strongylus vulgaris* in the horse: its biology and veterinary importance. *Commonw Inst Helminthol* **4**: 1–40, 1977.

Patton, S., and Drudge, J. H. Clinical response of pony foals experimentally infected with *Strongylus vulgaris*. *Am J Vet Res* **38**: 2059–2066, 1977.

Smith, H. J. Experimental *Trichonema* infections in mature ponies. *Vet Parasitol* **4**: 265–273, 1978.

Ascarid Infection

Andersen, S. *et al.* Experimental *Ascaris suum* infection in piglets. *Acta Pathol Microbiol Scand* **81**: 650–656, 1973.

Barron, C. N., and Saunders, L. Z. Visceral larval migrans in the dog. *Pathol Vet* **3**: 315–330, 1966.

Bindseil, E. The tissue reaction to migrating larvae of *Ascaris suum*. *In* "Parasitic Zoonoses: Clinical and Experimental Studies," E. J. L. Soulsby (ed.), pp. 313–318. New York, Academic Press, 1974.

Clayton, H. M., and Duncan, J. L. The migration and development of *Parascaris equorum* in the horse. *Int J Parasitol* **9**: 285–292, 1979.

Clayton, H. M., and Duncan, J. L. The development of immunity to *Parascaris equorum* infection in the foal. *Res Vet Sci* **26**: 383–384, 1979.

Clayton, H. M., Duncan, J. L., and Dargie, J. D. Pathophysiological changes associated with *Parascaris equorum* infection in the foal. *Equine Vet J* **12**: 23–25, 1980.

Copeman, D. B. Immunopathological response of pigs in ascariasis. *In* "Pathology of Parasitic Diseases," S. M. Gaafar (ed.), pp. 135–145. Lafayette, Indiana, Purdue Univ. Stud., 1971.

DiPietro, J. A., Boero, M., and Ely, R. W. Abdominal abscess associated with *Parascaris equorum* infection in a foal. *J Am Vet Med Assoc* **182**: 991–992, 1983.

Enyenihi, U. K. Pathogenicity of *Neoascaris vitulorum* infection in calves. *Bull Epizoot Dis Afr* **17**: 171–178, 1969.

Fitzgerald, P. R., and Mansfield, M. E. Visceral larva migrans (*Toxocara canis*) in calves. *Am J Vet Res* **31**: 561–566, 1970.

Glickman, L. T., Schantz, P. M., and Cypess, R. H. Canine and human toxocariasis: review of transmission, pathogenesis, and clinical disease. *J Am Vet Med Assoc* **175**: 1265–1269, 1979.

Greve, J. H. Somatic migration of *Toxocara canis* in ascarid-naive dogs. *In* "Pathology of Parasitic Diseases," S. M. Gaafar (ed.), pp. 147–159. Lafayette, Indiana, Purdue Univ. Stud., 1971.

Hani, H., and Indermuhle, N. A. Esophagogastric ulcers in swine infected with *Ascaris suum*. *Vet Pathol* **16**: 617–618, 1979.

Hayden, D. W., and Van Kruiningen, H. J. Experimentally induced canine toxocariasis: laboratory examinations and pathologic changes, with emphasis on the gastrointestinal tract. *Am J Vet Res* **36**: 1605–1614, 1975.

Jones, K. Adult *Toxocara canis* in the pancreas and peritoneal cavity of a pup. *Aust Vet J* **57**: 349, 1981.

McCraw, B. M., and Greenway, J. A. *Ascaris suum* infection in calves. III. Pathology. *Can J Comp Med* **34**: 247–255, 1970.

McCraw, B. M., and Lautenslager, J. P. Pneumonia in calves associated with migrating *Ascaris suum* larvae. *Can Vet J* **12**: 87–90, 1971.

McLennan, M. W., Humphris, R. B., and Rao, R. *Ascaris suum* pneumonia in cattle. *Aust Vet J* **50**: 266–268, 1974.

Mia, S. *et al.* The route of infection of buffalo calves by *Toxocara* (*Neoascaris*) *vitulorum*. *Trop Anim Health Prod* **7**: 153–156, 1975.

Mitchell, G. B. B., and Linklater, K. A. Condemnation of sheep livers due to ascariasis. *Vet Rec* **107**: 70, 1980.

Nicholls, J. M. *et al.* A pathological study of the lungs of foals infected experimentally with *Parascaris equorum*. *J Comp Pathol* **88**: 261–274, 1978.

Smith, H. J. *Probstmayria vivipara* pinworms in ponies. *Can J Comp Med* **43**: 341–342, 1979.

Srihakim, S., and Swerczek, T. W. Pathologic changes and pathogenesis of *Parascaris equorum* infection in parasite-free pony foals. *Am J Vet Res* **39**: 1155–1160, 1978.

Stephenson, L. S. *et al. Ascaris suum:* nutrient absorption, growth, and intestinal pathology in young pigs experimentally infected with 15-day-old larvae. *Exp Parasitol* **49**: 15–25, 1980.

Taffs, L. F. Immunological studies on experimental infection of pigs with *Ascaris suum*, Goeze 1782. VI. The histopathology of liver and lung. *J Helminthol* **42**: 157–172, 1968.

Warren, E. G. Observations on the migration and development of *Toxocara vitulorum* in natural and experimental hosts. *Int J Parasitol* **1**: 85–99, 1971.

Cestode Infection

Allen, R. W. The biology of *Thysanosoma actinoides* (Cestoda: Anoplocephalidae) a parasite of domestic and wild ruminants. *Bull NM Agric Exp Stn* **69**: 69, 1973.

Amjadi, A. R. Studies on histopathology of *Stilesia globipunctata* infections in Iran. *Vet Rec* **88**: 486–488, 1971.

Arundel, J. H. A review of cysticercoses of sheep and cattle in Australia. *Aust Vet J* **48**: 140–155, 1972.

Bain, S. A., and Kelly, J. D. Prevalence and pathogenicity of *Anoplocephala perfoliata* in a horse population in South Auckland. *NZ Vet J* **25**: 27–28, 1977.

Barclay, W. P., Phillips, T. N., and Foerner, J. J. Intussusception associated with *Anoplocephala perfoliata* infection in five horses. *J Am Vet Med Assoc* **180**: 752–753, 1982.

Bearup, A. J. Life history of a spirometrid tapeworm, causing sparganosis in feral pigs. *Aust Vet J* **29**: 217–224, 1953.

Clegg, F. G., and Bayliss, J. B. Coenuriasis as a cause of hydrocephalus in the ox. *Vet Rec* **70**: 441–442, 1958.

Crellin, J. R., Marchiondo, A. A., and Anderson, F. L. Comparison of suitability of dogs and cats as hosts of *Echinococcus multilocularis*. *Am J Vet Res* **42**: 1980–1981, 1981.

Eckert, J., Muller, H., and Partridge, A. J. The domestic cat and dog as natural definitive hosts of *Echinococcus* (*Alveococcus*) multi-

locularis in southern Federal Republic of Germany. *Tropenmed Parasitol* **25**: 334–337, 1974.

Edwards, G. T. Small fertile hydatid cysts in British horses. *Vet Rec* **108**: 460–461, 1981.

Edwards, G. T., and Herbert, I. V. The course of *Taenia hydatigena* infections in growing pigs and lambs: clinical signs and postmortem examination. *Br Vet J* **136**: 256–264, 1980.

Fagbemi, B. O., and Dipeolu, O. O. *Moniezia* infection in the dwarf breeds of small ruminants in southern Nigeria. *Vet Q* **5**: 75–80, 1983.

Kates, K. C., and Goldberg, A. The pathogenicity of the common sheep tapeworm *Moniezia expansa*. *Proc Helminthol Soc Wash* **18**: 87–101, 1951.

Mueller, J. F. The biology of *Spirometra*. *J Parasitol* **60**: 3–14, 1974.

Oliver, D. F., Jenkins, C. T., and Walding, P. Duodenum rupture in a nine-month-old colt due to *Anoplocephala magna*. *Vet Rec* **101**: 80, 1977.

Poole, J. B., and Marcial-Rojas, R. A. Echinococcosis. *In* "Pathology of Protozoal and Helminthic Diseases," R. A. Marcial-Rojas (ed.), pp. 635–657. Baltimore, Williams & Wilkins, 1971.

Rausch, R. Studies on the helminth fauna of Alaska. 20. The histogenesis of the alveolar larvae of *Echinococcus* species. *J Infect Dis* **94**: 178–186, 1954.

Rees, G. Pathogenesis of adult cestodes. *Helminthol Abstr* **36**: 1–23, 1967.

Smyth, J. D. The biology of the hydatid organisms. *Adv Parasitol* **7**: 327–347, 1969.

Sweatman, G. K., and Henshall, T. C. The comparative biology and morphology of *Taenia ovis* and *Taenia krabbei*, with observations on the development of *T. ovis* in domestic sheep. *Can J Zool* **40**: 1287–1311, 1962.

Sweatman, G. K., and Plummer, P. J. G. The biology and pathology of the tapeworm *Taenia hydatigena* in domesic and wild hosts. *Can J Zool* **35**: 94–109, 1957.

Sweatman, G. K., Robinson, R. G., and Manktelow, B. W. Comparative observations on the scolex and germinal membrane of *Echinococcus granulosus* as a source of secondary hydatid cysts. *Am J Trop Med Hyg* **12**: 199–203, 1963.

Thompson, R. C. A. Hydatidosis in Great Britain. *Helminthol Abstr* [A] **46**: 837–861, 1977.

Thompson, R. C. A. Biology and speciation of *Echinococcus granulosus*. *Aust Vet J* **55**: 93–98, 1979.

Thompson, R. C. A., and Kumaratilake, L. M. Intraspecific variation in *Echinococcus granulosus:* the Australian situation and perspectives for the future. *Tran R Soc Trop Med Hyg* **76**: 13–16, 1982.

Verster, A. A taxonomic revision of the genus *Taenia* Linnaeus, 1758 *s. str. Onderstepoort J Vet Res* **37**: 3–58, 1969.

Wardle, R. A., McLeod, J. A., and Radinovsky, S. "Advances in the Zoology of Tapeworms, 1950–1970." Minneapolis, Univ. of Minnesota Press, 1974.

Williams, J. F., Westheimer, J., and Banman, W. R. *Mesocestoides* infection in the dog. *J Am Vet Med Assoc* **166**: 996–998, 1975.

Intestinal Fluke Infections and Salmon Poisoning Disease

Azzie, M. A. J. Pathological infection of thoroughbred horses with *Gastrodiscus aegyptiacus*. *J S Afr Vet Med Assoc* **46**: 77–78, 1975.

Boray, J. C. Studies on intestinal amphistomosis in cattle. *Aust Vet J* **35**: 282–287, 1959.

Boray, J. C. Studies on intestinal paramphistomosis in sheep due to *Paramphistomum ichikawai* Fukui, 1922. *Vet Med Rev* **4**: 290–308, 1969.

Boray, J. C. The pathogenesis of ovine intestinal paramphistomosis due to *Paramphistomum ichikawai*. *In* "Pathology of Parasitic Dis-

eases," S. M. Gaafer (ed.), pp. 209–216. Lafayette, Indiana, Purdue Univ. Stud., 1971.

Cordy, D. R., and Gorham, J. R. The pathology and etiology of salmon disease in the dog and fox. *Am J Pathol* **26**: 617–637, 1950.

Crusz, H. The nature, incidence and geographical distribution of amphistome infestations in meat cattle, buffaloes and goats in Ceylon. *Ceylon J Sci* [B] **25**: 59–73, 1952.

Dinnik, J. A., and Dinnik, N. N. The life cycle of *Paramphistomum microbothrium* Fischoeder, 1901 (Trematoda, Paramphistomidae). *Parasitology* **44**: 285–299, 1954.

Durie, P. H. The paramphistomes (Trematoda) of Australian ruminants. II. The life history of *Ceylonocotyl streptocoelium* (Fischoeder) Nasmark and of *Paramphistomum ichikawai* Fukui. *Aust J Zool* **1**: 193–222, 1953.

Durie, P. H. The paramphistomes (Trematoda) of Australian ruminants. 3. The life history of *Calicophoron calicophorum* (Fischoeder) Nasmark. *Aust J Zool* **4**: 152–157, 1956.

Edgar, G. Paramphistomiasis of young cattle. *Aust Vet J* **14**:27–31, 1938.

Farrell, R. K., Leader, R. W., and Johnston, S. D. Differentiation of salmon poisoning disease and Elokomin fluke fever: studies with the black bear (*Ursus americanus*). *Am J Vet Res* **34**: 919–922, 1973.

Fernandes, B. J. *et al.* Systemic infection with *Alaria americana* (Trematoda). *Can Med Assoc J* **115**: 1111–1114, 1976.

Frank, D. W. *et al.* Lymphoreticular lesions of canine neorickettsiosis. *J Infect Dis* **129**: 163–171, 1974.

Hadlow, W. J. Neuropathology of experimental salmon poisoning of dogs. *Am J Vet Res* **18**: 898–908, 1957.

Hayden, D. W. Alariasis in a dog. *J Am Vet Med Assoc* **155**: 889–891, 1969.

Herd, R. P., and Hull, B. L. *Paramphistomum microbothrioides* in American bison and domestic beef cattle. *J Am Vet Med Assoc* **179**: 1019–1020, 1981.

Horak, I. G. Host–parasite relationships of *Paramphistomum microbothrium* Fischoeder, 1901, in experimentally infected ruminants with particular reference to sheep. *Onderstepoort J Vet Res* **34**: 451–540, 1967.

Horak, I. G. Paramphistomiasis of domestic ruminants. *Adv Parasitol* **9**: 33–72, 1971.

Hussein, M. F., Taylor, M. G., and Dargie, J. D. Pathogenesis and immunology of ruminant schistomiasis in the Sudan. *Isot Radiat Parasitol 4 Proc Advis Group Meet 1979* pp. 75–82, 1981.

Knapp, S. E., and Milleman, R. E. Salmon poisoning disease. *In* "Infectious Diseases of Wild Mammals," J. W. Davis, L. H. Karstad, and D. O. Trainer (eds.), 2nd ed., pp. 476–387. Ames, Iowa State Univ. Press, 1981.

Lawrence, J. A. Bovine schistosomiasis in Southern Africa. *Helminthol Abstr* **47**: 261–270, 1978.

Millemann, R. E., and Knapp, S. E. Biology of *Nanophyetus salmincola* and 'Salmon poisoning' disease. *Adv Parasitol* **8**: 1–41, 1970.

Protozoal Enteritis

General and Other Protozoa

Anonymous. Battles against *Giardia* in gut mucosa. *Lancet* **2**: 527–528, 1982.

Arean, V. M., and Echevarria, R. Balantidiasis. *In* "Pathology of Protozoal and Helminthic Diseases," R. A. Marcial-Rojas (ed.), pp. 234–253. Baltimore, Williams & Wilkins, 1971.

Arundel, J. H. Diseases caused by protozoa. *In* "Veterinary Medicine," D. C. Blood, O. M. Radostits, and J. A. Henderson (eds.), 6th ed., pp. 867–893. London, Bailliére, 1983.

Barlough, J. E. Canine giardiasis: a review. *Small Anim Pract* **20**: 613–623, 1979.

Ewing, S. A., and Bull, R. W. Severe chronic canine diarrhea associated with *Balantidium–Trichuris* infection. *J Am Vet Med Assoc* **149:** 519–520, 1966.

Hartong, E. A., Gourley, W. K., and Arvanitakis, C. Giardiasis: clinical spectrum and functional–structural abnormalities of the small intestinal mucosa. *Gastroenterology* **77:** 61–69, 1979.

Jordan, H. E. Amebiasis (*Entamoeba histolytica*) in the dog. *VM SAC* **62:** 61–64, 1967.

Laufenstein-Duffy, H. Equine intestinal trichomoniasis. *J Am Vet Med Assoc* **155:** 1835–1840, 1969.

Levine, N. D. "Protozoan Parasites of Domestic Animals and of Man," 2nd ed. Minneapolis, Burgess, 1973.

Levine, N. D. *et al.* A newly revised classification of the Protozoa. *J Protozool* **27:** 37–58, 1980.

MacDonald, T. T., and Ferguson, A. Small intestinal epithelial cell kinetics and protozoal infection in mice. *Gastroenterology* **74:** 496–500, 1978.

Meyer, E. A., and Radulescu, S. Giardia and giardiasis. *Adv Parasitol* **17:** 1–47, 1979.

Nesvadba, J. *et al.* Giardiasis beim Rind. *Proc 12th World Congr Dis Cattle* pp. 237–241, 1982.

Perez-Tamayo, R., and Brandt, H. Amebiasis. *In* "Pathology of Protozoal and Helminthic Diseases," R. A. Marcial-Rojas (ed.), pp. 145–188. Baltimore, Williams & Wilkins, 1971.

Pittman, F. E., El-HasHimi, W. K., and Pittman, J. C. Studies of human amebiasis. II. Light and electron-microscopic observations of colonic mucosa and exudate in acute amebic colitis. *Gastroenterology* **65:** 588–603, 1973.

Pitts, R. P., Twedt, D. C., and Mallie, K. A. Comparison of duodenal aspiration with fecal flotation for diagnosis of giardiasis in dogs. *J Am Vet Med Assoc* **182:** 1210–1211, 1983.

Stevens, D. P. Giardiasis: host–pathogen biology. *Rev Infect Dis* **4:** 851–858, 1982.

Thorson, R. E., Seibold, H. R., and Bailey, W. S. Systemic amebiasis with distemper in a dog. *J Am Vet Med Assoc* **129:** 335–336, 1956.

Watson, A. D. J. Giardiosis and colitis in a dog. *Aust Vet J* **56:** 444–447, 1980.

Willson, P. J. Giardiasis in two calves. *Can Vet J* **23:** 83, 1982.

Coccidiosis

Barker, I. K., and Remmler, O. The endogenous development of *Eimeria leuckarti* in ponies. *J Parasitol* **58:** 112–122, 1972.

Catchpole, J., Norton, C. C., and Joyner, L. P. The occurrence of *Eimeria weybridgensis* and other species of coccidia in lambs in England and Wales. *Br Vet J* **131:** 392–401, 1975.

Chapman, H. D. The effects of natural and artificially acquired infections of coccidia in lambs. *Res Vet Sci* **16:** 1–6, 1974.

Chobotar, B., and Hammond, D. M. Development of gametocytes and second asexual generation stages of *Eimeria auburnensis* in calves. *J Parasitol* **55:** 1218–1228, 1969.

Chobotar, B., and Scholtyseck, E. Ultrastructure. *In* "The Biology of the Coccidia," P. L. Long (ed.), pp. 101–165. Baltimore, University Park Press, 1982.

Davis, L. R., and Bowman, G. W. Observations on the life cycle of *Eimeria bukidnonensis* Tubangui 1931, a coccidium of cattle. *J Protozool* **11:** Suppl, 17, 1964.

Davis, L. R., Bowman, G. W., and Boughton, D. C. The endogenous development of *Eimeria alabamensis* Christensen 1941, an intranuclear coccidium of cattle. *J Protozool* **4:** 219–225, 1957.

Desser, S. S. Extraintestinal development of eimeriid coccidia in pigs and chamois. *J Parasitol* **64:** 933–935, 1978.

Dubey, J. P. A review of *Sarcocystis* of domestic animals and of other coccidia of cats and dogs. *J Am Vet Med Assoc* **169:** 1061–1078, 1976.

Dubey, J. P. Taxonomy of *Sarcocystis* and other coccidia of cats and dogs. *J Am Vet Med Assoc* **170:** 778–782, 1977.

Dubey, J. P. Pathogenicity of *Isospora ohioensis* infection in dogs. *J Am Vet Med Assoc* **173:** 192–197, 1978.

Dubey, J. P., Weisbrode, S. E., and Rogers, W. A. Canine coccidiosis attributed to an *Isospora ohioensis*–like organism: a case report. *J Am Vet Med Assoc* **173:** 185–191, 1978.

Elibihari, S., and Hussein, M. F. *Eimeria kosti* sp. n., an abomasal coccidium from a cow. *Bull Anim Health Prod Afr* **22:** 105–107, 1974.

Eustis, S. L., and Nelson, D. T. Lesions associated with coccidiosis in nursing piglets. *Vet Pathol* **18:** 21–28, 1981.

Fernando, M. A. Pathology and Pathogenicity. *In* "The Biology of the Coccidia," P. L. Long (ed.), pp. 287–327. Baltimore, University Park Press, 1982.

Fitzgerald, P. R. The economic impact of coccidiosis in domestic animals. *Adv Vet Sci Comp Med* **24:** 121–143, 1980.

Fitzgerald, P. R., and Mansfield, M. E. Effects of bovine coccidiosis on certain blood components, feed consumption and body weight changes of calves. *Am J Vet Res* **33:** 1391–1397, 1972.

Foreyt, W. J., Gates, N. L., and Rich, J. E. Evaluation of lasalocid in salt against ovine coccidia. *Am J Vet Res* **42:** 54–60, 1981.

Friend, S. C. E., and Stockdale, P. H. G. Experimental *Eimeria bovis* infection in calves: a histopathological study. *Can J Comp Med* **44:** 129–140, 1980.

Gregory, M. W. *et al.* Ovine coccidiosis in England and Wales 1978–1979. *Vet Rec* **106:** 461–462, 1980.

Hammond, D. M., Sayin, F., and Miner, M. L. Über den Entwicklungszyklus und die Pathogenität von *Eimeria ellipsoidalis* Becker und Frye, 1929 in Kalbern. *Berl Muench Tieraerztl Wochenschr* **76:** 331–332, 1963.

Hani, H., and Pfister, K. Zur Kokzidiose des Schweines. *Schweiz Arch Tierheilkd* **121:** 421–424, 1979.

Hilali, M. Studies on globidial schizonts in the abomasum of Norwegian sheep. *Acta Vet Scand* **14:** 22–43, 1973.

Joyner, L. P. Coccidioisis in pigs. *Vet Annu* **22:** 140–144, 1982.

Joyner, L. P. Host and site specificity. *In* "The Biology of the Coccidia," P. L. Long (ed.), pp. 35–62. Baltimore, University Park Press, 1982.

Levine, N. D. Nomenclature of *Sarcocystis* in the ox and sheep and of fecal coccidia of the dog and cat. *J Parasitol* **63:** 36–51, 1977.

Levine, N. D., and Ivens, V. "The Coccidian Parasites (Protozoa, Sporozoa) of Ruminants," Ill. Biol. Monogr. No. 44. Urbana, Univ. of Illinois Press, 1970.

Levine, N. D., and Ivens, V. "The Coccidian Parasites (Protozoa, Apicomplexa) of Carnivores," Ill. Biol. Monogr. No. 51. Urbana, Univ. of Illinois Press, 1981.

Lima, J. D. Development of *Eimeria* species in mesenteric lymph nodes of goats. *J Parasitol* **65:** 976–978, 1979.

Lima, J. D. Prevalence of coccidia in domestic goats from Illinois, Indiana, Missouri and Wisconsin. *Int Goat Sheep Res* **1:** 234–241, 1980.

Lima, J. D. Life cycle of *Eimeria christenseni* Levine, Ivens & Fritz, 1962 from the domestic goat, *Capra hircus* L. *J Protozool* **28:** 59–64, 1981.

Lindsay, D. S. *et al.* Endogenous development of the swine coccidium, *Isospora suis* Biester 1934. *J Parasitol* **66:** 771–779, 1980.

Lindsay, D. S. *et al.* Diagnosis of neonatal porcine coccidiosis caused by *Isospora suis*. *VM SAC* **78:** 89–95, 1983.

McDougald, L. R. Attempted cross-transmission of coccidia between sheep and goats and description of *Eimeria ovinoidalis* sp. n. *J Protozool* **26:** 109–113, 1979.

McKenna, P. B., and Charleston, W. A. G. Coccidia (Protozoa: Sporozoasida) of cats and dogs. IV. Identity and prevalence in dogs. *NZ Vet J* **28:** 128–130, 1980.

McQuery, C. A., Worley, D. E., and Catlin, J. E. Observations on the life cycle and prevalence of *Eimeria leuckarti* in horses in Montana. *Am J Vet Res* **38**: 1673–1674, 1977.

Mason, P. Naturally acquired coccidia infection in lambs in Otago. *NZ Vet J* **25**: 30–33, 1977.

Matuschka, F.-R., and Heydorn, A. O. Die Entwicklung von *Isospora suis* Biester und Murray 1934 (Sporozoa: Coccidia: Eimeriidae) im Schwein. *Zool Beitr* **26**: 405–476, 1980.

Mesfin, G. M., and Bellamy, J. E. C. The thymic dependence of immunity to *Eimeria falciformis* var. *pragensis* in mice. *Infect Immun* **23**: 460–464, 1979.

Michael, E., and Probert, A. J. Histopathological observations on some coccidial lesions in natural infections of sheep. *Res Vet Sci* **11**: 441–446, 1970.

Norton, C. C., and Catchpole, J. The occurrence of *Eimeria marsica* in the domestic sheep in England and Wales. *Parasitology* **72**: 111–114, 1976.

Norton, C. C., Joyner, L. P., and Catchpole, J. *Eimeria weybridgensis* sp. nov. and *Eimeria ovina* from the domestic sheep. *Parasitology* **69**: 87–95, 1974.

Pellerdy, L. P. "Coccidia and Coccidiosis," 2nd rev. ed. Berlin, Parey, 1974.

Pout, D. D. Coccidiosis of sheep. *Vet Bull* **39**: 609–618, 1969.

Pout, D. D. Coccidiosis of lambs. III. The reaction of the small intestinal mucosa to experimental infections with *E. arloingi* "B" and *E. crandallis*. *Br Vet J* **130**: 45–53, 1974.

Prasad, R. S., Chabra, M. B., and Singh, R. P. Clinical coccidiosis in kids associated with *Eimeria christenseni*. *Indian Vet J* **58**: 330–332, 1981.

Radostits, O. M., and Stockdale, P. H. G. A brief review of bovine coccidiosis in western Canada. *Can Vet J* **21**: 227–230, 1980.

Robinson, Y., and Morin, M. Porcine neonatal coccidiosis in Quebec. *Can Vet J* **23**: 212–216, 1982.

Rose, M. E., and Hesketh, P. Coccidiosis: T-lymphocyte-dependent effects of infection with *Eimeria nieschulzi* in rats. *Vet Immunol Immunopathol* **3**: 499–508, 1982.

Ross, A. D., and Day, W. A. Intestinal polyps in a lamb. *NZ Vet J* **27**: 172–173, 1979.

Sanford, S. E., and Josephson, G. K. A. Porcine neonatal coccidiosis. *Can Vet J* **22**: 282–285, 1981.

Savin, F., Dincer, S., and Milli, U. The life cycle and pathogenicity of *Eimeria arloingi* (Marotel, 1905) Martin, 1909, in Angora kids and an attempt at its transmission to lambs. *Zentralbl Veterinaermed [B]* **27**: 382–397, 1980.

Shastri, U. V., and Krishnamurthi, R. A note on pathological lesions in clinical bubaline coccidiosis due to *Eimeria bareillyi*. *Indian J Anim Sci* **45**: 46–47, 1975.

Stockdale, P. H. G. Schizogony and gametogony of *Eimeria zuernii* (Rivolta, 1878) Martin, 1909. *Vet Parasitol* **1**: 367–376, 1976.

Stockdale, P. H. G. The pathogenesis of the lesions produced by *Eimeria zuernii* in calves. *Can J Comp Med* **41**: 338–344, 1977.

Stockdale, P. H. G. *et al.* Some pathophysiological changes associated with infection of *Eimeria zuernii* in calves. *Can J Comp Med* **45**: 34–37, 1981.

Stuart, B. P. *et al. Isospora suis* enteritis in piglets. *Vet Pathol* **17**: 84–93, 1980.

Stuart, B. P. *et al.* Coccidiosis in swine: dose and age response to *Isospora suis*. *Can J Comp Med* **46**: 317–320, 1982.

Sutoh, M. *et al. Eimeria leuckarti* infection in foals. *Natl Inst Anim Health Q* (Tokyo) **16**: 59–64, 1976.

Taylor, S. M. *et al.* Diarrhea in intensively-reared lambs. *Vet Rec* **93**: 461–464, 1973.

Vetterling, J. M. Coccidia (Protozoa: Eimeriidae) of swine. *J Parasitol* **51**: 897–912, 1965.

Wacha, R. S., Hammond, D. M., and Miner, M. L. The development of the endogenous stages of *Eimeria ninakohylakimovae* (Yakimoff and Rastegaieff, 1930) in domestic sheep. *Proc Helminthol Soc Wash* **38**: 167–180, 1971.

Wheeldon, E. B. *Globidium leuckarti* infection in a horse with diarrhoea. *Vet Rec* **100**: 102–104, 1977.

Yvore, P. *et al.* Experimental coccidiosis in the young goat: parasitic development and lesions. *Int Goat Sheep Res* **1**: 163–167, 1980.

Cryptosporidiosis

Anderson, B. C. Cryptosporidiosis in Idaho lambs: natural and experimental infections. *J Am Vet Med Assoc* **181**: 151–153, 1982.

Boch, V. J. *et al.* Kryptosporidien-Infektion bei Haustieren. *Berl Muench Tieraerztl* Wochenschr **95**: 361–367, 1982.

Moon, H. W. *et al.* Experimental fecal transmission of human cryptosporidia to pigs, and attempted treatment with an ornithine decarboxylase inhibitor. *Vet Pathol* **19**: 700–707, 1982.

Pearson, G. R. *et al.* Distribution of cryptosporidia within the gastrointestinal tract of young calves. *Res Vet Sci* **33**: 228–231, 1982.

Pohlenz, J. *et al.* Cryptosporidiosis as a probable factor in neonatal diarrhea of calves. *J Am Vet Med Assoc* **172**: 452–457, 1978.

Poonacha, K. B., and Pippin, C. Intestinal cryptosporidiosis in a cat. *Vet Pathol* **19**: 708–710, 1982.

Sanford, S. E., and Josephson, G. K. A. Bovine cryptosporidiosis: clinical and pathological findings in forty-two scouring neonatal calves. *Can Vet J* **23**: 343–347, 1982.

Tzipori, S. Cryptosporidiosis in animals and humans. *Microbiol Rev* **47**: 84–96, 1983.

Tzipori, S. *et al.* Cryptosporidiosis: evidence for a single-species genus. *Infect Immun* **30**: 884–886, 1980.

Tzipori, S. *et al.* Experimental infection of lambs with *Cryptosporidium* isolated from a human patient with diarrhoea. *Gut* **23**: 71–74, 1982.

Tzipori, S. *et al.* Experimental cryptosporidiosis in calves: clinical manifestations and pathological findings. *Vet Rec* **112**: 116–120, 1983.

Toxoplasma, Sarcocystis, and Related Protozoa

Averill, D. R., Jr., and De Lahunta, A. Toxoplasmosis of the canine nervous system: clinicopathologic findings in four cases. *J Am Vet Med Assoc* **159**: 1134–1141, 1971.

Beech, J., and Dodd, D. C. *Toxoplasma*-like encephalomyelitis in the horse. *Vet Pathol* **11**: 87–96, 1974.

Beverley, J. K. A., and Henry, L. Experimental toxoplasmosis in young piglets. *Res Vet Sci* **24**: 139–146, 1978.

Capen, C. C., and Cole, C. R. Pulmonary lesions in dogs with experimental and naturally occurring toxoplasmosis. *Pathol Vet* **3**: 40–63, 1966.

Dubey, J. P. Direct development of enteroepithelial stages of *Toxoplasma* in the intestines of cats fed cysts. *Am J Vet Res* **40**: 1634–1637, 1979.

Dubey, J. P. Clinical sarcocystosis in calves fed *Sarcocystis hirsuta* sporocysts from cats. *Vet Pathol* **20**: 90–98, 1983.

Dubey, J. P. *et al.* Equine encephalomyelitis due to a protozoan parasite resembling *Toxoplasma gondii*. *J Am Vet Med Assoc* **165**: 249–255, 1974.

Dubey, J. P. *et al.* Porcine toxoplasmosis in Indiana. *J Am Vet Med Assoc* **174**: 604–609, 1979.

Dubey, J. P. *et al.* Caprine toxoplasmosis: abortion, clinical signs, and distribution of *Toxoplasma* in tissues of goats fed *Toxoplasma gondii* oocysts. *Am J Vet Res* **41**: 1072–1076, 1980.

Dubey, J. P. *et al.* Sarcocystosis in goats: clinical signs and pathological and hematologic findings. *J Am Vet Med Assoc* **178**: 683–699, 1981.

Dubey, J. P. *et al.* Sarcocystosis in newborn calves fed *Sarcocystis cruzi* sporocysts from coyotes. *Am J Vet Res* **43**: 2147–2164, 1982.

Dubey, J. P., and Frenkel, J. K. Cyst-induced toxoplasmosis in cats. *J. Protozool* **19**: 155–177, 1972.

Dubey, J. P., and Frenkel, J. K. Immunity to feline toxoplasmosis: modification by administration of corticosteroids. *Vet Pathol* **11**: 350–379, 1974.

Dubey, J. P., and Hoover, E. A. Attempted transmission of *Toxoplasma gondii* infection from pregnant cats to their kittens. *J Am Vet Med Assoc* **170**: 538–540, 1977.

Dubey, J. P., and Johnstone, I. Fatal neonatal toxoplasmosis in cats. *J Am Anim Hosp Assoc* **18**: 461–467, 1982.

Dubey, J. P., and Williams, D. S. F. *Hammondia heydorni* infection in sheep, goats, moose, dogs and coyotes. *Parasitology* **81**: 123–127, 1980.

Frenkel, J. K. Toxoplasmosis: parasite life cycle, pathology, and immunology. *In* "The Coccidia. *Eimeria, Isospora, Toxoplasma,* and Related Genera," D. M. Hammond and P. L. Long (eds.), pp. 344–410. Baltimore, University Park Press, 1973.

Frenkel, J. K. *Besnoitia wallacei* of cats and rodents: with a reclassification of other cyst-forming isosporoid coccidia. *J Parasitol* **63**: 611–628, 1977.

Frenkel, J. K., and Dubey, J. P. *Hammondia hammondi:* a new coccidium of cats producing cysts in muscle of other mammals. *Science* **189**: 222–224, 1975.

Hansen, H. J. *et al.* On porcine toxoplasmosis in Sweden. *Nord Vet Med* **29**: 381–385, 1977.

Hartley, W. J. Sporozoa in animals. With particular reference to *Toxoplasma* and *Sarcocystis. NZ Vet J* **24**: 1–5, 1976.

Hartley, W. J., and Kater, J. C. Observations on diseases of the central nervous system of sheep in New Zealand. *NZ Vet J* **10**: 128–142, 1962.

Hirth, R. S., and Nielsen, S. W. Pathology of feline toxoplasmosis. *J Small Anim Pract* **10**: 213–221, 1969.

Hong, C. B. *et al.* Sarcocystosis in an aborted bovine fetus. *J Am Vet Med Assoc* **181**: 585–588, 1982.

Hutchinson, W. M. *et al.* The life cycle of the coccidian parasite, *Toxoplasma gondii,* in the domestic cat. *Trans R Soc Trop Med Hyg* **65**: 380–399, 1971.

Ito, S. *et al.* Pathogenicity for piglets of *Toxoplasma* oocysts originated from naturally infected cat. *Natl Inst Anim Health Q (Tokyo)* **14**: 182–187, 1974.

Ito, S. *et al.* Life cycle of the large type of *Isospora bigemina* of the cat. *Natl Inst Anim Health Q (Tokyo)* **18**: 69–82, 1978.

Jolly, R. D. Toxoplasmosis in piglets. *NZ Vet J* **17**: 87–89, 1969.

Levine, N. D., and Tadros, W. Named species and hosts of *Sarcocystis* (Protozoa: Apicomplexia: Sarcocystidae). *Syst Parasitol* **2**: 41–59, 1980.

McErlean, B. A. Ovine paralysis associated with spinal lesions of toxoplasmosis. *Vet Rec* **94**: 264–266, 1974.

Markus, M. B. *Sarcocystis* and sarcocystosis in domestic animals and man. *Adv Vet Sci Comp Med* **22**: 154–193, 1978.

Munday, B. L., and Mason, R. W. Toxoplasmosis as a cause of perinatal death in goats. *Aust Vet J* **55**: 485–487, 1979.

Parker, G. A. *et al.* Pathogenesis of acute toxoplasmosis in specific-pathogen-free cats. *Vet Pathol* **18**: 786–803, 1981.

Overdulve, J. P. Studies on the life cycle of *Toxoplasma gondii* in germfree, gnotobiotic and conventional cats. *Proc k Ned Akad Wet* [*C*] **81**: 19–59, 1978.

Quinn, P. J., and McCraw, B. M. Current status of *Toxoplasma* and toxoplasmosis: a review. *Can Vet J* **13**: 247–262, 1972.

Sasaki, Y. *et al.* Experimental *Toxoplasma* infection of pigs with oocysts of *Isospora bigemina* of feline origin. *Jpn J Vet Sci* **36**: 459–465, 1974.

Simpson, C. F., and Mayhew, I. G. Evidence for *Sarcocystis* as the etiologic agent of equine protozoal myeloencephalitis. *J Protozool* **27**: 288–292, 1980.

Smart, M. E. *et al.* Toxoplasmosis in a cat associated with cholangitis and progressive pancreatitis. *Can Vet J* **14**: 313–316, 1973.

Smith, D. D. The Sarcocystidae: *Sarcocystis, Frenkelia, Toxoplasma, Besnoitia, Hammondia,* and *Cystoisospora. J Protozool* **28**: 262–266, 267–270, 1981.

Smith, D. D., and Frenkel, J. K. *Besnoitia darlingi* (Protozoa: Toxoplasmatinae): cyclic transmission by cats. *J Parasitol* **63**: 1066–1071, 1977.

Stalheim, O. H. V. *et al.* Update on bovine toxoplasmosis and sarcocystosis, with emphasis on their role in bovine abortions. *J Am Vet Med Assoc* **176**: 299–302, 1980.

Teale, A. J. *et al.* Experimentally induced toxoplasmosis in young rams: the clinical syndrome and semen secretion of toxoplasma. *Vet Rec* **111**: 53–55, 1982.

Turner, G. V. S. Some aspects of the pathogenesis and comparative pathology of toxoplasmosis. *J S Afr Vet Assoc* **49**: 3–8, 1978.

CHAPTER 2

The Liver and Biliary System

W. ROGER KELLY
University of Queensland, Australia

General Considerations

The liver is central to the metabolic pathways and has a responsibility for the metabolic function and health of other organs and tissues. Disease of the liver may relate to local matters or to dysfunction and pathologic change in other tissues. In fact, the clinical manifestations of hepatic disease are usually remote from the liver itself, being expressed, in particular, in the brain, skin, peritoneal cavity, and alimentary canal. The pathogenesis of the remote changes is perhaps better understood than that of the hepatic disease. The anatomic connections of the liver, and certain structural and functional attributes, account for the frequency of lesions of the liver in diseases that are not primarily hepatic. Pathologic changes in the liver are much more common than the evidence of hepatic failure, but the lesions are important in terms of the assistance provided to the pathologist in the determination of the nature of many systemic diseases. They will be mentioned here, but the primary discussion will be directed at hepatic disease that can lead to hepatic failure with retention of ammonia, bile salts, and pigments, and failure of synthetic function.

Positioned as it is in the abdominal cavity, and connected to other viscera, the pathways of injury to the liver are variable. Transabdominal injury is common in traumatic incidents, and many parasites pass through it, including flukes, cysticerci, strongyles of horses, and kidney worms of pigs. The vena cava transmits backward the effects of increased central venous pressure. The lymphatics drain to the hilar lymph nodes as well as dorsally in the ligaments of the liver, to the cysterna chyli and the thoracic duct; these and the lymphatics in the capsule may be enormously increased but remain incompetent when lymph production is increased. At the hilus of the liver, the hepatic artery, portal vein, and bile duct come together, and within the liver, their radicles lie in a sheath of connective tissue in the portal triads. The integrity of the liver depends on the integrity of these conduits, and it is also via these that most noxious influences are conveyed; the analysis of pathologic changes in the liver requires a recognition of these facts.

The shape of the liver depends on blood flow and biliary arrangements. The ratio of blood flow to parenchymal mass is the same in all parts of the liver, and a similar relationship is deduced for biliary volume. If blood flow is impaired or biliary drainage impaired in part of the liver, the parenchyma of that part will atrophy; many alterations of gross form occur as responses to vascular or biliary disturbance. At the gross level there are also consistent differences in susceptibility between lobes, some of which are attributable to differences in blood supply, biliary architecture, and anatomic location.

Four consequences of the large size of the liver are sometimes overlooked. First, the mass of the organ, coupled with its relative fragility, has ballistic significance during episodes of abdominal violence (see Displacement and Rupture). Second, when there is widespread acute liver injury, a large mass of damaged tissue has immediate and intimate access to a large volume of blood. This has important effects on the homeostasis of the blood-clotting cycle, as well as releasing large amounts of the products of hepatocyte degeneration into the general circulation; this will be considered further under Hemorrhage and Liver Failure. Third, the large sinusoidal volume holds an important quantity of blood, and the liver can play an important part in modifying splanchnic blood flow in such states as hypovolemic shock and anaphylaxis. In severe congestive heart failure, the total body blood volume may increase by as much as 30%, and a large proportion of this increase is accommodated in the liver. Fourth, the mass of the liver represents an important reserve of readily metabolizable nutrients to tide the animal over episodes of malnourishment, so variations in liver size must be considered in the light of recent nutritional history.

The liver is probably unique in the extent to which its mass, when altered experimentally or in disease, can be returned to normal as a proportion of body mass. In this very general sense, the whole liver can be considered as the reactive unit even though in restoring the mass the gross configuration is greatly changed. Pathologic analysis, however, requires attention to units of smaller scale, such as intracellular organelles, cells, and cellular units or groupings, which would, if adequately repeated, constitute a liver. The traditional unit of liver structure is the hexagonal lobule, and it is still sometimes convenient to report pathologic changes in terms of the conventional lobule. However, descriptions in this chapter are based on the **acinus**. This unit stresses the dependence of the liver on its afferent blood vessels and efferent bile ducts. The acinus is oriented to these conduits, and consists in its smallest divisions, of acinar clumps of hepatic parenchyma served by terminal portal venules.

Selection of the acinus as the descriptive unit should not imply a rigidity in its structure, blood supply, biliary drainage, or lymphatic drainage. There is a vast potential for collateral circulation of blood, bile, and lymph through sinusoids, bile canaliculi and spaces of Disse, respectively, so that in disturbances of the steady state, adjacent acini may share the blood that flows through them and allow the passage of bile and lymph. If the steady state is permanently displaced, the parenchymal organization is rearranged, in particular, to new afferent vascular arrangements.

When the liver is viewed microscopically, each parenchymal cell in each cord appears to be exactly like its neighbors, and it is reasonable to consider each functioning as a miniature of the parenchymatous part of the liver, replicating the enormous complexity of the physiologic activities known for that tissue. There is a metabolic heterogeneity of cells, and there is a gradient of metabolic activities along the cord of cells from the portal vein to the hepatic venule. The gradient is probably dependent largely on the direction of blood flow and the oxygen tension in the plasma. Many hepatic diseases in animals are problems of acute metabolic assault, which injures cells selectively and in accordance with their position in the acinus. But it is possible to change the metabolic activities of hepatic cells and thereby to alter the sensitivity to injury of cells in different parts of an acinus. The metabolic differences between cells are quantitative rather than qualitative, and the differences are reflected in the different zonal patterns of acute injury.

There are, in addition to the accessory structures already mentioned (blood and lymph vessels, bile ducts), other differentiated tissues of the liver, including the cells that line the sinusoids. Best known of these are the Kupffer cells, representatives of the monocyte–macrophage system, which possess potent phagocytic functions. The adjacent parenchyma is not known to be specifically subservient to the Kupffer cells, but as a result of their natural activity, indirect injury to the parenchyma is common in patterns that are usually local but sometimes diffuse. The sinusoids are lined, incompletely, by specialized endothelial cells with special transport functions, subendothelial fat-storing cells, and occasional granulated cells in the space of Disse that presumably have some endocrine function. Most if not all of these cells are readily replaced after loss, which may occur during episodes of hepatocellular necrosis. The delicate lining of the sinusoids may be changed in chronic disease to acquire the characteristics of capillaries, possibly as part of developing fibrosis or as a result of acquired direct exposure to pulsatile arterial blood flow.

Emphasis in hepatic pathology must be placed on the parenchymal cells, which endow the organ with its specific functions. Being highly differentiated, they are also highly susceptible to injury. The degenerative changes consequent on injury include those reactions—hydropic degeneration, fatty change, and necrosis—that are well known from general pathology. Characteristic of the liver are the anatomic patterns of degeneration and their sequelae, and the physiologic disturbances resulting therefrom. These are discussed in more specific detail later, but certain general principles can be remarked on here.

General Reactions of the Liver to Injury

In spite of its high degree of differentiation, the liver retains to an almost embryonic degree the capacity to regenerate itself. A certain amount of **regeneration** to balance natural necrobiosis occurs continually, but the full regenerative capacity of the tissue is seen only after destruction of much of the parenchyma by noxious influences or its removal by surgery. As much as 70% of the liver can be removed surgically without particular upset, and in the course of a few weeks it is back to normal size; the regeneration may be even more rapid following a toxic injury that destroys that much parenchyma, because in this circumstance a framework remains on which regeneration can take place. Regeneration must be regarded as a natural response of the liver to injury, but there are certain limitations on the process: to be complete, the affected areas of tissue must be provided with an adequate supply of blood and free drainage of bile; to be architecturally normal, the regenerating columns of cells must have as guidelines the original fibrous and reticulin framework.

While regeneration is one characteristic reaction of the liver to injury, **fibrosis** is another, and it is the combination of these that is responsible for the coarse or fine nodularities of chronic acquired hepatic disease. Any hepatic insult severe enough to cause hepatocellular necrosis with subsequent regeneration will result in some local fibrogenesis. After recovery from mild insults, this immature collagen is removed by enzymatic degradation. The balance is tipped in favor of progressive fibrosis when the insult continues to act or when the initial damage is so severe that the scar that results is extensive enough to damage the parenchyma by progressive sclerosis. The fibrosis may develop in a number of ways. It is, as elsewhere, a response to inflammation of the connective tissues of the liver, which, for practical purposes, include only those of the portal triads; in the event of

inflammation in the portal triads, the fibrosis remains largely confined to these areas and is nominated as **biliary fibrosis** (Fig. 2.14A). Fibrosis is also a response to primary parenchymal injury, and its manner of development and degree, and therefore its pattern, depends on the pattern and duration of the antecedent injury. In massive necrosis (*massive* applies to events in individual units and not in the liver as a whole), all parenchymal cells of a number of adjacent acini are destroyed, and the reticulin network collapses and condenses with approximated surviving portal areas to produce broad, irregular bands of scar tissue. This form of fibrosis is called **postnecrotic scarring** and is due to condensation of preexisting stroma with some fibroplasia and scarification (Fig. 2.8). The third general type of fibrosis is known as **diffuse hepatic fibrosis**. This is the outcome of a chronic parenchymal process, such as prolonged infiltration, or of repeated parenchymal injury, such as many episodes of zonal necrosis. The fibrosis is generated slowly to link portal areas and central veins, intersecting the classical lobules to produce pseudolobulation.

Finally, fibrosis may develop around hepatic venules when the primary injury is in that region. The best examples are in prolonged congestive cardiac failure (Fig. 2.10A,B), but this is unusual in animals compared with extracardiac sources of increased venous pressure. Otherwise, **periacinar (cardiac) fibrosis** is a response to toxic injury; poisoning by pyrrolizidine alkaloids may cause it in ruminants, and extraordinary development of periacinar fibrosis may follow accidental exposure to nitrosamines in several species.

The third of the characteristic morphologic reactions in the injured liver is **hyperplasia** of **bile ducts**. Such involves the smaller interlobular bile ducts and the intralobular cholangioles. Much has still to be learned regarding the proliferative potentialities of these structures and the metabolic stimuli that provoke them. Bile duct proliferation often occurs quite independently of changes in the parenchyma. It can also be independent of other changes in the portal units (Fig. 2.25D), at least to the extent that there may be no more fibrosis than necessary to provide basement membranes for the new ducts. Such pure cholangiolar proliferation is the typical response to poisons, of which butter yellow is the classical example, and is observed after biliary obstruction before infection complicates the picture. When the insults are removed, the excess of bile ducts may disappear completely; how they do so is not known. Biliary hyperplasia also tends to accompany fibrosis in the liver, the new ducts following but lagging behind the increase of fibrous tissue. Whether biliary hyperplasia is ever a response simply to prolonged parenchymal injury is difficult to determine because it is difficult to dissociate the influence of the parenchymal injury from that of the fibrosis it tends to provoke. In some circumstances, such as in poisoning by the pyrrolizidine alkaloids or aflatoxin, biliary, or more specifically cholangiolar, hyperplasia may be an attempt to regenerate parenchyma when the parenchymal cells themselves have lost this capacity (Fig. 2.23C).

Chronic Liver Disease

Acute diseases of the liver and patterns of acute injury are reasonably understood or are becoming so. Single, acute injuries producing something less than massive necrosis can heal completely and without residue. Chronic liver disease remains very difficult to understand in terms of either cause or morphogenesis. In some chronic disease, the cause may be easily ascertainable or perhaps remain present, but it is more likely to have occurred long before the liver is examined. There are many, varied causes of hepatic injury. Their effects depend to a large extent on the relationship of dose to time, the degree of injury, and the persistence or repetitiveness with which they act. Chronic or repeated injury to the parenchyma produces eventually an organ distorted in shape and size, compounded of proliferated bile ducts, fibrosis, and nodular regenerative hyperplasia. The damage eventually becomes self-perpetuating.

Reference has been made to **bile duct proliferations**. Some of the ducts are composed of normal ductal epithelium, possess a lumen, and are often continuous with bile ducts. They probably are not continuous with liver-cell plates. In other patterns, the new ducts are more trabecular and without a lumen, and their lining cells resemble hepatocytes. These often have anatomic connection with hepatic laminae, but seldom with ducts of the portal triad. There are many patterns intermediate between these two. In any particular circumstance, it has not been determined whether these new ducts take origin from preexisting bile ducts, cholangioles (the intralobular canals of Hering), or hepatocytes. Generally, in the case of primary biliary disease, especially if obstructive, the new ducts form from preexisting interlobular ducts; in chronic hepatocellular disease they originate from preexisting intralobular cholangioles. They appear neither to have a useful purpose nor to contribute to the course of the disease. They must, however, be functionally abnormal and contribute to an altered local mesenchymal environment.

Fibrosis is usually part of the picture of chronic progressive hepatic disease. Chronic fatal liver disease with regenerative nodules does occur, in which the amount of fibrosis is insignificant. In these cases, any development of fibrosis is likely to follow, rather than precede, the development of regenerative nodules.

The patterns of fibrous tissue growth follow fairly well the patterns of parenchymal injury. Excepting obvious direct inflammation of mesenchymal tissue, as in chronic cholangitis, the progression of fibrosis to irreversibility must depend on interaction between fibrous tissue and parenchyma. Fibrosis from the portal areas removes the terminal plate of liver cells and progressively encroaches on the periportal parenchyma. Parenchymal degeneration in turn provokes more fibrosis. The liver cells may be further compromised by spreading changes in the sinusoid. Ordinarily this very delicate and widely fenestrated structure is loosely applied to the liver-cell cords and separated from them by the space of Disse, an arrangement that brings plasma into direct contact with the hepatic cells (Fig. 2.22A). As chronic fibrosis progresses, reticulin and then collagen is deposited in the space of Disse. Ultimately, the hepatic cells become isolated from sinusoidal blood by further fibrosis, and the sinusoid comes to resemble a capillary.

Regenerative liver in chronic disease is typically nodular. In chronic toxic or nutritional hepatic injury, a reduced life expectancy of hepatocytes and reduced ability to complete mitosis successfully may be part of an overall reduction of regenerative capacity. In some instances, such as biliary fibrosis, regenera-

tive capacity is probably not impaired and will continue as usual from the periportal zone. In diffuse toxic injury, the degree of regenerative nodularity is dose and time dependent. With high dosage and short time, regeneration is impaired, and the liver is decreased in size with distorted but otherwise preserved histoarchitecture. Later, regenerative nodularity develops (Figs. 2.1 and 2.27A). The nodular change is generalized in the organ but is not uniform. The nodules may be few and large or numerous and smaller, apparently as a matter of dose and time. The longer the course, the greater the opportunity for groups of liver cells to escape the toxic depression.

The origin of the regenerative nodules in chronic hepatic disease is not clear and may well be different for different injuries. Sometimes they may be derived from surviving hepatocytes around terminal portal venules, a site most favorably situated with respect to the original acinar distribution of blood supply. Alternatively, they may develop from whole acinar units that have escaped injury. Regenerative nodules for the most part appear to develop at random in the liver, the lobe, and the acinar conglomerate. They continue to grow and for a long time may not show the signs of degeneration that affected their fellows, even though the toxic agent is still present. This suggests that the regenerating cells may be different from normal hepatocytes in their metabolic activity.

The growing nodules compress and displace the original liver tissue, and the preexisting stroma is condensed to form capsules around the nodules and the irregular remnants between them. The vascular and biliary connections between the nodules and preexisting portal structures are of uncertain nature, but the main conduits of the portal tracts appear to bypass the nodules. The regenerative nodules may eventually be subdivided by ingrowth of septa to form structures of nearly normal architecture. It is in this manner that regenerative liver after diffuse injury may take on the architectural features of postnecrotic scarring.

The ratio of arterial to portal blood flowing in the regenerative nodules may be altered in favor of the hepatic artery, with a reduction in the total volume of flow traversing the parenchyma. Venous bypasses develop within the fibrous septa or the displaced portal areas at the periphery of nodules. Biliary drainage from regenerative nodules appears usually to be adequate since bile retention and staining of nodules are uncommon. These disturbances, coupled with the possibility of deviant metabolic patterns in the regenerated cells, can account for the progression of chronic liver disease.

Cirrhosis may be defined as nodular regeneration of the liver combined with fibrosis. The term is often used to describe livers that are tough due to postnecrotic collapse rather than de novo collagen synthesis. Livers distorted by fibrosis rather than by true nodular regeneration are also said to be cirrhotic. The term cirrhosis, then, has a certain convenience of usage that is often offset by imprecise application, and we prefer to use the various designations of fibrosis, combined with the addition of nodular regeneration where appropriate.

It is convenient to describe here a liver disease of dogs that is characterized by obvious nodular regeneration combined with equally obvious atrophy and eventual liver failure. The cause is unknown, but it is tempting to ascribe it, at least in part, to repeated exposure to a hepatotoxin such as aflatoxin.

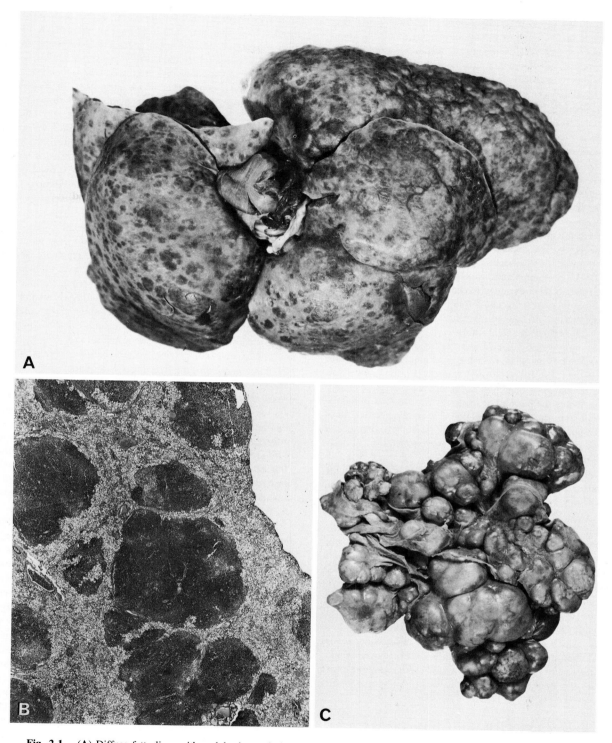

Fig. 2.1. (A) Diffuse fatty liver with nodular hyperplasia. Dog. (B) Section of (A), showing diffuse fatty change and large nonfatty nodules. (C) The end result of (A).

The gross impression of the liver is one of nodularity affecting most of the organ, most of the nodules being small but some measuring 2–3 cm. In extreme cases (Fig. 2.1C), some of the nodules are pedunculated and attached by stalks of capsular tissue, and they are easily dislodged. The capsule over the nodules is of ordinary thickness, but between them it appears thickened and opaque. The margins of the lobes, where these are not incorporated in a nodule, are thin and leaflike and quite tough; this is in consequence of atrophy and may result in complete dissociation of the lobes at the hilus, each lobe then appearing to hang on its own stalk of vessels. Neither through consistency, resistance to cutting, nor by gross inspection is there any suggestion of fibrosis. The nodules may be of normal color and of liver-like consistency, or they may be yellowish, greasy, and soft or even pultaceous. The whole may be bile stained.

The microscopic picture is dominated by nodular regenerative hyperplasia, which causes compression and atrophy of remnants of severely fatty hepatic parenchyma (Fig. 2.1B). The nodules may be microscopic in size and are then seen to be derived from portal units and of irregular distribution. They may be fatty from the outset or acquire fat later; compound nodules may be a mixture of units without fat and units moderately or severely fatty. There is a light fibrosis largely confined to portal areas. In the regenerative nodules, the fibrosis is irregular but has a tendency to originate from the axial parent portal unit and to link up the veins. In the residual, nonregenerative areas, there is a fine fibrosis, but its pattern is obscured by compression and atrophy. Where the margins of the lobes are atrophic so that the capsule condenses into a leaflet, there is collagenization. It is worth emphasizing that fibrosis is minimal in these organs and that they do not qualify for the designation cirrhosis, usually applied to them.

Livers of the type described are seen in animals dying after the age of at least 2 years, and because these are "end stage" livers, it is difficult to be sure of the stages of their development. Earlier stages of the disease may be discovered incidentally in animals that have shown no clinical sign of liver disease (Fig. 2.1A). In these cases the distribution of fatty change is very irregular, and the demarcation between original and regenerating parenchyma is quite difficult to discern; it may be more obvious on gross inspection than in sections.

Nodular hyperplasia of the liver, in which one or more nodules one to several centimeters in diameter project hemispherically from the surface, is common in old dogs. These nodules, which are always fatty, arise not in an organ that is otherwise normal, but in livers or portions of liver that are themselves the seat of fatty change and of mild chronic congestion of irregular distribution.

Liver Failure

It is appropriate to include here a consideration of the consequences of failure of liver functions. The discussion will be confined to those disturbances that lead to recognizable clinical syndromes. The physiologic functions of the liver can be broadly categorized into those concerned with the secretion of bile and the excretion of those few substances, such as phylloerythrin, that have a limited biliary circulation, metabolic functions of great diversity, and detoxifying functions that are also of much diversity. To understand the clinical manifestations of hepatic insufficiency, a number of features must be borne in mind. First, the liver is possessed of a very large reserve of function, which is potentially increased by the powers of regeneration. Signs of insufficiency do not develop until the reserve is exhausted, and by the time the lesions are far advanced and usually irreversible. Equivalent degrees of reserve for all functions should not be expected. Second, the liver is a composite organ, and lesions of its substance involve several tissues, each of which may contribute some component to the symptomatology. Third, the symptomatology of acute insufficiency differs from that of chronic insufficiency, although there is considerable overlapping. Fourth, the presenting signs may appear at first sight to be unrelated to hepatic disease and may be unaccompanied by other signs of hepatic failure.

CHOLESTASIS AND JAUNDICE.   Jaundice, or discoloration of tissues and body fluids by an excess of bile pigments, is traditionally regarded as having two basic causes: overproduction of bilirubin, as in hemolytic disease, or impaired excretion of the pigment. The latter, cholestasis, may be conveniently subdivided into failure of uptake or conjugation of unconjugated bilirubin, and inability to excrete conjugated bilirubin. It is usual for these causes of jaundice to be combined to varying degrees in any case of jaundice. In hemolytic disease, the large amount of bilirubin presented to the liver for excretion may overload both the hepatocellular bile uptake and bilirubin conjugation mechanisms, as well as the intracellular and canalicular transport process. In addition, the anemia usually associated with severe hemolytic disease will compromise hepatocellular function and further hamper bilirubin excretion. Hepatocellular accumulation of bile salts in obstructive jaundice interferes with bile conjugation and transport by the smooth endoplasmic reticulum. For these reasons, it is difficult to predict the ratio of conjugated to unconjugated bilirubin in hyperbilirubinemia in most cases of jaundice.

The hepatocellular injury that causes failure of bile salt excretion may be nonspecific, as in severe necrotizing hepatotoxicity, or conversely, the injury may inhibit this function alone, leaving the hepatocyte with most other functions intact. One of the best examples of the latter type of injury in domestic animals is that of *Lantana* poisoning. In humans, this type of cholestasis is most often associated with idiosyncratic reactions to a wide variety of drugs, but this cause is rarely implicated in animals.

The mechanism of the cholestasis in *Lantana* poisoning is discussed later, but the details of most of the cholestatic diseases of animals remain to be worked out. There are two components of the hepatocyte cytoplasm that are likely targets for specific cholestatic insults. One is the smooth endoplasmic reticulum, in which bile conjugation and intracellular bile salt transport takes place; attention will be drawn to the changes that occur in this organelle in a wide variety of toxicities. The other is the contractile filamentous apparatus in the pericanalicular cytoplasm, which seems to be involved in active propulsion of bile along the canaliculi. Cholestasis has been produced by administration of cytochalasin, a toxin capable of specifically disorganizing these filaments.

Rarely, jaundice may be due to congenital incompetence of

hepatocellular uptake or transport of bile salts. In mutant South-down sheep there is deficiency in the bile salt uptake mechanism, and these animals, while showing few liver lesions, eventually develop chronic renal disease, the reason for which is not clear. Unconjugated bilirubin levels in the plasma are consistently elevated, but sufficient bile salt excretion takes place to prevent them from becoming icteric. They become photosensitized, indicating that phylloerythrin excretion is less efficient than that of bilirubin.

A similar defect in mutant Corriedales is in conjugated bilirubin excretion. There is also elevation of plasma bilirubin (just over half of which is conjugated), but there is no obvious jaundice. Nevertheless, phylloerythrin excretion in these Corriedales is sufficiently impaired to produce photosensitization. There is impaired excretion of other conjugated metabolites, and there is pigmentation of the liver by polymerized residues of retained catecholamine metabolites. This pigment, resembling lipofuscin, accumulates in lysosomes in the pericanalicular cytoplasm.

The intensity of jaundice observed at autopsy is greatest in those diseases where more than one of the classical causes of cholestasis are operating, as in chronic copper poisoning. In this condition there is not only severe hemolysis but also widespread hepatocyte destruction, and some escape of bile into the sinusoids is likely as hepatocytes die and round up, thus rupturing the canaliculi.

Another factor influencing the intensity of jaundice is the duration of cholestasis. Maximum uptake of bile pigment by tissues takes a day or two, so cholestasis due to a single cause may be quite intense if the cause has been persistent.

PHOTOSENSITIZATION. Photosensitization is an almost invariable accompaniment of nonhemolytic cholestasis of more than a few days duration in herbivores that are kept in sunlight and that have been eating green feed. The term is applied to inflammation of skin (usually unpigmented) due to the action of ultraviolet light of wavelengths of 290 to 400 nm on fluorescent compounds that have become bound to dermal cells. These compounds may have been deposited unchanged in the skin after ingestion, the normal liver being incapable of excreting the native fluorescent compound. This is known as primary (type 1) photosensitivity and is seen, for example, after ingestion of hypericin in St. John's wort (*Hypericum perforatum*). Photodynamic agents may also be produced by aberrant endogenous metabolism (type 2 photosensitivity), the best example being congenital porphyria of cattle, which is due to accumulation of photodynamic porphyrins as a result of deficiency of uroporphyrinogen cosynthetase. The type of photosensitization we are concerned with here, and which is by far the most common, is hepatogeneous (type 3) photosensitization, in which the photodynamic agent, phylloerythrin, is derived from chlorophyll by microbial transformation in the gastrointestinal tract of herbivores. This conversion occurs in normal animals in which the phylloerythrin is excreted in the bile by the same mechanism as the bile pigments. Any instance of intrahepatic cholestasis or severe nonspecific hepatocellular injury in herbivores therefore is likely to result in photosensitivity if survival time is longer than a few days. It is possible, however, for mild

photosensitization to appear in the absence of gross or microscopic evidence of cholestasis. This occurs unpredictably in animals on such apparently wholesome pastures as alfalfa or *Paspalum*, or pangola and *Panicum* grasses. In some instances there is accumulation in bile ducts of a crystalloid lipophilic deposit similar to that seen in *Tribulus* poisoning (Fig. 2.24B). These deposits may be derived from the plant, or they may be complexes of cholesterol and phospholipid that have crystallized instead of forming normal micelles with bile salts. If no hepatic changes can be discerned in photosensitized animals, the possibility of primary photosensitization must be considered.

HEPATIC ENCEPHALOPATHY. The neurologic manifestations of hepatic failure are variable and nonspecific; they range from dullness, through complete unawareness and compulsive and aimless movement, to mania and generalized convulsions. These signs usually indicate imminent death, the exceptions being portosystemic shunting or deficiency of a urea-cycle enzyme. In these cases the less severe clinical syndrome of hepatic encephalopathy may occur intermittently for many months, and the clinical signs may disappear after appropriate dietary modification.

Ammonia retention is responsible for the major part of the clinical signs and the brain lesions (see diseases of the Nervous System, Volume 1). Ammonia accumulates in the general circulation and in the cerebrospinal fluid in both shunting and general liver failure, and the brain changes typical of hepatic encephalopathy have been reproduced by ammonia infusion. Nevertheless, the central nervous system derangement in liver failure is the result of a considerably more complex biochemical disorder than simple ammonia retention. A range of variably toxic amines, which are normally removed from the portal blood in one passage through the liver after production in the large bowel, may reach the brain, where possibly they act as false neurotransmitters. In cases of complete liver failure, hypoglycemic convulsions may result from failure of glucose synthesis.

HEMORRHAGE AND LIVER FAILURE. Spontaneous hemorrhage is not often part of the syndrome of slowly developing liver failure; the implication is that in chronic liver disease, loss of the ability to synthesize clotting factors does not have the significance of the other consequences of liver failure. In acute necrotizing liver damamge, however, a severe drain on soluble clotting factors is present as the result of rapid consumption because of sinusoidal intravascular coagulation. This is initiated by the huge area of damaged endothelial tissue presented to the blood in these livers. Consumption coagulopathies are discussed with the Cardiovascular System (Volume 3), and hemorrhage in liver disease with the Hematopoietic System (Volume 3).

Postmortem Changes in the Liver

The liver, rich in nutrient for bacteria and freely exposed to agonal invaders from the intestine, undergoes postmortem decomposition very rapidly. Gas bubbles form in the blood vessels. The vessels and adjacent parenchyma are stained by hemoglobin. The substance of the organ becomes soft and claylike, and the formation of putrefactive gases may make it foamy. On the capsular surface, irregular, pale foci are visible; they resemble infarcts or fatty areas but can be observed to increase in size and, microscopically, are without cellular reaction. Bacilli are present in large numbers in such foci. Greenish black pigmentation of the capsule and superficial parenchyma occur where the liver is in contact with gut. The lobes surrounding the gallbladder are stained brownish with bile.

There is much microscopic structural change in the liver approaching and immediately following death. In general, the confusing autolytic changes affect mainly the regions around the radicles of the hepatic veins. Indeed, cytologic criteria of necrosis in periacinar necrosis are more reliably found in animals that have been allowed to die or that are killed in extremis. Shrinkage of liver cells and disappearance of many with widening of periacinar sinusoids is seen after death with hepatic congestion. Dissociation of liver cells may be complete, with every cell in every cord separated and free from adjacent cells so architectural patterns are lost. The least expression of this change affects periacinar cells first, and they become detached, rounded in contour, condensed, and hyperchromatic. The dissociation is seen particularly in feline panleukopenia and leptospirosis. It is related somewhat to postmortem change.

Developmental Anomalies

Developmental anomalies occur, but most are not important. A variety of defects may accompany generalized malformations. As isolated defects, there may be absence or hypoplasia of one or more lobes, with corresponding hypertrophy of the others. Abnormal furrowing may produce additional lobes, and incisures of abnormal depth may isolate lobes. Accessory buttons of parenchyma may occur in the ligaments and in the thorax; these are frequently fibrotic and gray.

Congenital cysts of the liver occur in all species. Their origins are probably diverse. **Intrahepatic congenital cysts** are probably derived from embryonic bile ducts. The embryogenesis of the bile ducts has not been clearly determined. The short intralobular portions of the ducts, the cholangioles, may have a common origin with the hepatic parenchyma from the distal portion of the hepatic anlage. The main bile ducts and the interlobular branches in the portal triad are probably derived from the proximal portion of the hepatic anlage. It also seems that many more embryonic cholangioles are formed than are actually necessary. Accordingly, cystic bile ducts may rise by (1) failure of fusion of inter- and intralobular portions, (2) failure of superfluous cholangioles to involute, or (3) establishment of the duct system with subsequent development of localized zones of atresia. The number, size, and degree of loculation of the cysts are quite variable. The walls are of connective tissue and are lined by a flattened or cuboidal epithelium. The content is clear and serous.

Serous cysts are occasionally found attached to the capsule on the diaphragmatic surface in calves, lambs, and foals. The cysts are usually small and multiple, but some are isolated and very large (Fig. 2.4D). Their origin is not known, but it is variously postulated that they are serosal inclusion cysts, part of congenital polycystic (biliary) liver, or implanted cysts of enteric origin. They do not contain bile. The incidence of these anomalies related to age suggests that a large proportion of them

involutes with aging. To be distinguished are acquired cysts, parasitic cysts and biliary cystadenomas. Anomalies of the extrahepatic biliary system include absence of gallbladder, partial or complete duplication of the gallbladder, and absence and atresia of one or more ducts.

Another form of congenital hepatic cystic anomaly occurs in piglets and dogs, in which **multiple cysts** derived from **bile ducts** are found throughout the liver. The common bile duct is patent, communicates with the duodenum, yet is itself dilated. There are also polycystic renal anomalies in these animals, which may die of renal insufficiency; jaundice is not usually seen. The livers are often enlarged enough to cause abdominal distension and are riddled with large, softly fluctuant, irregular cysts that intercommunicate and whose content appears to be normal bile. An inherited basis for the disease has been proposed but not proven for dogs, and there is even less evidence for it in pigs, although the anomaly may appear in littermates.

In carnivores, bile duct atresia may lead to jaundice as well as vitamin D–deficiency rickets, due to inability to absorb fat-soluble vitamins.

Displacement and Rupture

The lie of the liver should be observed as soon as the abdomen is opened. Most displacements are caudal, so that the margins of the liver come to be much behind the costal arch. Caudal displacements are the result of enlargement of the organ or displacement of the diaphragm, the latter due to pleural effusion or other space-occupying lesion in the thorax. Congenital or acquired displacements in ventral and diaphragmatic hernias are common. Usually only one lobe goes into the thorax with other viscera; its blood supply may not be embarrassed, but usually it is severely congested and, in time, indurated. It may rupture. Torsion of individual lobes, usually the left lateral, occurs in swine and dogs, and the resultant infarction causes death due to shock or hemorrhage. If the lobe becomes infected by anaerobic bacteria and undergoes putrefaction, it is dry and crepitant.

Rupture of the liver occurs commonly as the result of trauma. It is quite common for fatal liver rupture to be produced by the sudden accelerations and pressures of road accidents, without significant evidence of trauma to other parts of the body; this testifies to the relative fragility of the organ, which, although protected to some degree by its location, nevertheless offers little resistance to blunt trauma, particularly in the neonate. Large tears may develop in the liver capsule and hepatic parenchyma after trauma. In some cases of hepatic rupture, anastomosing linear patterns of fine, capsular fissures form that are usually quite shallow, but from which severe hemorrhage may issue until clotting seals them shortly before death, obscuring their significance. Survival for a day or two may allow necrotic liver in the immediate vicinity of the rupture to take on a pallid, opaque appearance.

Diffuse hepatic disease with enlargement, in which the substance is friable and the capsule taut, provides a predisposition to rupture, which may occur spontaneously. Predisposing lesions include acute hepatitis, amyloidosis, severe congestion, fatty degeneration, and secondary neoplasms. Usually there is very little hemorrhage from spontaneous ruptures, which suggests that they occur in the terminal stages of the illness. Parasites that penetrate the capsule cause numerous small ruptures but seldom lead to significant hemorrhage.

Cytopathology of the Liver

Cells with a very specialized range of metabolic function, such as muscle fibers or osteoblasts, as a rule have only a limited repertoire of reaction to injury. It is not surprising, therefore, that hepatocytes, with their diverse metabolic capacity, should exhibit a rather wider range of changes in response to various insults. It is not easy to establish with the light microscope whether or not these changes are reversible, as much depends on the nature of the insult and the relative speed of onset of its effects on the cell.

The term **megalocytosis** was used first in the description of the changes of liver-cell cytoplasm and nucleus that occur in pyrrolizidine alkaloid poisoning (Fig. 2.25D). This form of meglocytosis has some rather specific features and is described under Pyrrolizidine Alkaloids. Very similar hepatocyte enlargement can be produced by other alkylating agents. Hepatocellular mitosis is preceded by enlargement of the cells, and some degree of nuclear enlargement will be seen in any process that induces hyperplasia in the liver. Increased amounts of nucleochromatin are present in prophase nuclei, which must be distinguished from those of megalocytosis. Mitoses may be rare even when expected, as in rapid regeneration following zonal necrosis, but may be frequent in other conditions, such as copper poisoning and lupinosis. Nuclei are normally diploid and uniform, but they may become tetraploid or even octoploid in cells that have large nuclei but that are otherwise normal.

Cytosegresome formations (Councilman bodies, acidophilic bodies) are spherical, refractile, eosinophilic structures seen in liver cells that have been sublethally injured by a variety of insults, ranging from hypoxia, through a variety of intoxications, to malnutrition, specific deficiencies, and some viral infections. They may be formed when masses of cytoplasmic organelles are gathered and condensed, and are sequestered from remaining cytoplasm by membranes that fuse with lysosomes (autolysosomes). They may also be derived from other hepatocytes that have undergone the form of shrinkage necrosis known as apoptosis and whose condensed fragments are taken up by remaining hepatocytes. These bodies can either be digested by lysosomal hydrolases (sometimes incompletely, to leave dense residual bodies) or extruded from the cytoplasm (exocytosis), to be taken up by Kupffer cells. Undigested remnants of these bodies may be observed at the light microscopic level as lipofuscin granules.

The volume of hepatocyte cytoplasm occupied by **smooth endoplasmic reticulum** varies with the location of the cell within the acinus; periacinar hepatocytes usually have the largest amount. Hypertrophy of smooth endoplasmic reticulum is readily induced over a few days by exposure to a wide spectrum of compounds that are, before excretion, degraded in the liver by mixed-function oxidases; phenobarbitone is perhaps the best known of these inducing agents. The phenomenon of microsomal enzyme induction has considerable significance in the reaction of the liver to many hepatotoxins and will be dealt with further under Toxic Liver Disease.

In some intoxications the smooth endoplasmic reticulum forms granular aggregates in the cytoplasm within a few hours of exposure to the toxin. Although the bulk of the organelle seems to have increased, this reaction probably represents clumping of the normally dispersed reticulum, the functions of which are more likely to be depressed than enhanced in these circumstances.

The aggregated smooth endoplasmic reticulum forms a large, semidiscrete, eosinophilic mass, which displaces the nucleus and other organelles to the periphery (Fig. 2.2C). In cells that survive, the deranged smooth endoplasmic reticulum may eventually be sequestered as a cytosegresome.

Besides the various **nuclear inclusions** associated with some virus infections, there are three types of inclusions that may be found in hepatocyte nuclei. The most common of these is the spherical, apparently hollow globule within the body of the nucleus (Fig. 2.23C); these are membrane bound, the result of cytoplasmic invagination, and have been shown to contain glycogen. These inclusions are seen infrequently in otherwise normal livers but are prone to occur in the same sort of circumstances as the cytoplasmic acidophilic bodies. Another sort of intranuclear inclusion is the eosinophilic blocklike structure in which a regular crystal lattice can be seen with the electron microscope, and which are also present in nuclei of renal proximal tubular epithelium, probably with greater frequency. Their precise structure and significance is obscure; there is no heavy-metal component, as was once suspected. These inclusions are sometimes large enough to distort the nucleus. They are more likely to be found in old animals, particularly dogs, and should be distinguished from the acid-fast, noncrystalline intranuclear inclusions of lead poisoning. Lead inclusions are again more frequently seen in the renal tubular epithelium; they consist of lead–protein complex and have a characteristic furry appearance in electron micrographs and are very electron dense.

Hepatocellular fusion is a rare phenomenon that may be found unexpectedly in cats; it has been produced in this species by experimental dioxin poisoning. The hepatocytes have a peculiar syncytial appearance due to fusion, then disappearance of adjacent cell membranes.

Pigmentations

Congenital melanosis occurs in calves and occasionally in lambs and swine. The deposits may be numerous and vary in size from flecks to irregular, bluish black areas 2.0 cm or more in diameter. The melanin is confined to the capsule and the stroma. These deposits are sharply defined at birth but become more diffuse and fade with age.

The most striking example of **acquired melanosis** is the massive accumulation of melanin in hepatocytes of mature sheep and, less frequently, cattle after prolonged grazing on extensive unimproved pastures in inland eastern Australia and the Falkland Islands. The color of the affected livers ranges from a dull gray to uniform jet black, and there is usually a prominent acinar pattern. In severe cases there is also dusky pigmentation of the hepatic lymph nodes, lungs and, renal cortex. Histologically, the pigment is present as granules in lysosomes in hepatocytes and macrophages of the liver, the proximal tubular

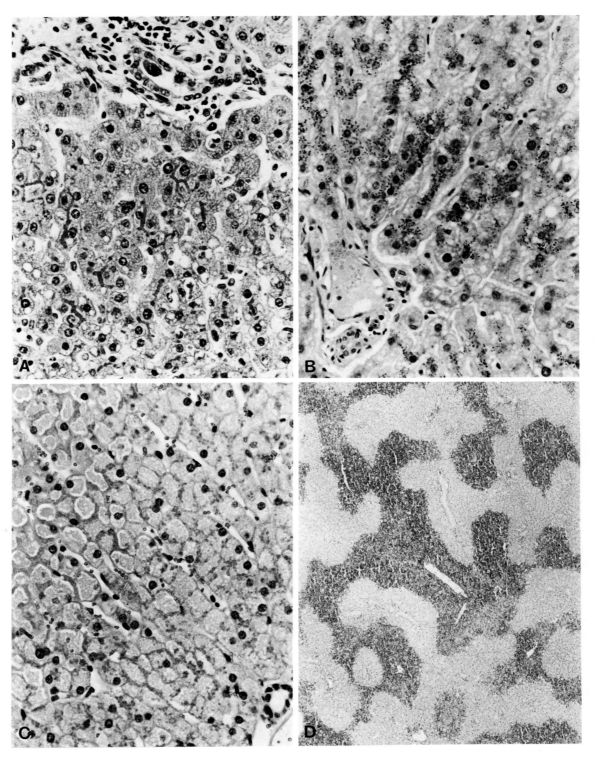

Fig. 2.2. (A) Bile lakes in canaliculi and bile duct. Hemolytic disease (babesiosis). Ox. (B) Lysosomal pigment in periportal hepatocytes. Environmental melanosis. Sheep. (C) Aggregation of smooth endoplasmic reticulum in hepatocyte cytoplasm in sublethal *Cestrum parqui* poisoning. Sheep. The reaction is most severe in the periacinar zone. (D) Acini outlined by periacinar hemorrhagic necrosis. *Cestrum* poisoning. Sheep.

epithelium of the kidneys, and in alveolar and interstitial macrophages in the lung. There is no evidence of liver dysfunction, even in the blackest livers. The source of this pigment is not known, but the epidemiologic features of its occurrence indicate that it is derived from a component of the diet that after biotransformation, polymerization, and condensation, leaves an insoluble residue. This residue is sequestered within lysosomes without interfering further with hepatocellular function. Another possibility is that some dietary component is capable of inhibiting the catabolic sequence normally responsible for complete degradation of melanin precursors. The pigment first appears in periportal and midzonal hepatocytes (Fig. 2.2B), which are probably the only cells to produce it. Release of pigment to other tissues may be through exocytosis or after normal necrobiosis. This environmental melanosis was originally characterized as a lipofuscin.

Lipofuscin-type pigment also accumulates in hepatocellular lysosomes of animals with deficiencies of enzymes involved with bile salt conjugation and transport, such as mutant Corriedale sheep, in which the liver becomes quite black.

The chemical relationship between some melanins, lipofuscin, and ceroid can be difficult to determine, and the latter two pigments tend to be distinguished more by their origins and associations than their structure. Ceroid is associated with peroxidation of fat deposits, and lipofuscin is the term given to small, golden, granular deposits derived from the lipid component of membranous organelles. Lipofuscin accumulates in hepatocellular lysosomes and indicates senility or some other cause of reduced membrane repair; the phenomenon is more obvious in cells near the periphery of the acinus and in atrophied cells.

Hemosiderin deposits are seldom sufficient to give gross discoloration, but if so, the color is dark brown. The pigment is detected microscopically as yellowish or brown crystals chiefly in the Kupffer cells, although small amounts may be found in hepatic cells. The nature of the pigment as iron containing can be demonstrated by staining with Prussian blue.

Diffuse hemosiderosis occurs quite commonly in all species, and its presence is suggestive of excess hemolytic activity relative to the rate of reutilization of iron. Thus it is seen in the hemolytic anemias, the anemia of copper deficiency, and in cachexia. It may be seen in the periacinar zones in severe chronic passive congestion of the liver. The pigment is normally present in the early neonatal period, when fetal hemoglobin is being replaced by mature hemoglobin. Hemosiderosis should be distinguished from hematin, which is produced by the action of formic acid on hemoglobin. Hematin is crystalline but darker brown than hemosiderin and occurs in irregular clumps, mainly within the blood vessels. Hematin may, however, be found in Kupffer cells and macrophages in small amounts. Localized hemosiderosis occurs in areas of hemorrhage. As well as being present in Kupffer cells, the pigment may be encrusted on the connective tissues.

Bile pigmentation may impart on olive green color to the liver in obstructive biliary disease. Lesser amounts may accumulate in diffuse hepatic disease as yellowish pigments, which should be differentiated from ceroid and hemosiderin. Conjugated bile pigments may distend bile canaliculi, which then stand out microscopically as greenish yellow stellate lakes between the hepatocytes (Fig. 2.2A). In this case, the identity of the pigment is obvious, but when it is present in granular form in hepatocyte or Kupffer-cell cytoplasm, it may be confused with hemosiderin and hematin.

The term feathery degeneration is applied to a type of hydropic change that occurs in hepatocytes in which there has been prolonged cholestasis. The cells are swollen and vacuolated and crisscrossed by a fine protoplasmic network that is brown with bile pigments (Fig. 2.23D).

Heavy deposits of black **iron–porphyrin** compound are formed about the cysts and migratory pathways of *Fascioloides magna*. Lesser amounts of similar pigment are deposited about bile ducts infested by *Fasciola hepatica*. The presence of this pigment in the hilar nodes should suggest otherwise inapparent infestations by flukes. In schistosomiasis, the liver may be grayish in color owing to the accumulation of black pigment in Kupffer cells.

Degenerations

Hydropic degeneration and **cloudy swelling** are terms that have been used for many years to describe cytoplasmic changes in cells prepared by conventional histologic techniques. It now seems agreed that cloudy swelling describes mitochondrial changes that are nonspecific for types of injury or disease, being reflections of ischemic or toxic injury. These changes are also present in the early stages of autolysis. The mitochondrial changes include swelling, coagulation, and calcification. Hydropic degeneration is a common change in hepatocytes in a number of diseases, ranging from mild intoxication to hypoxia, and is even seen in well-nourished animals that have recently fasted; in these it probably represents fluid in the cytosol left after glycogen has been metabolized either pre- or postmortem. Insults such as hypoxia, damage by a wide range of toxins, and overload by bile pigment can all produce hydropic degeneration, so there is little specificity to the change. Any of the membranous compartments of the cytoplasm can be involved; thus hypoxia may produce lysosomal and mitochondrial vacuolation, while toxins that bind to endoplasmic reticulum may cause that organelle to take up large volumes of water. Probably the most severe example of hepatocellular hydropic change is seen in dogs with hyperadrenocorticoidism due either to functional adrenal cortical or pituitary tumors, or to treatment with glucocorticoids (Fig. 2.3A). The cytoplasm of the cells contains spaces with poorly demarcated edges; the cells are swollen, and the nucleus, although normal in appearance, is often displaced from its central position. Careful examination usually serves to distinguish the cytoplasmic spaces from those seen in fat infiltration, which should be spherical and have sharp borders. It is sometimes impossible to distinguish hydropic from fatty change in routine sections, and special stains must be used; both changes may be present in the same cell. The severe hydropic change of hyperadrenocorticoidism seems to be completely reversible, and hydropic change due to other causes is usually regarded as such, but the change may progress to necrosis if the damage is severe enough.

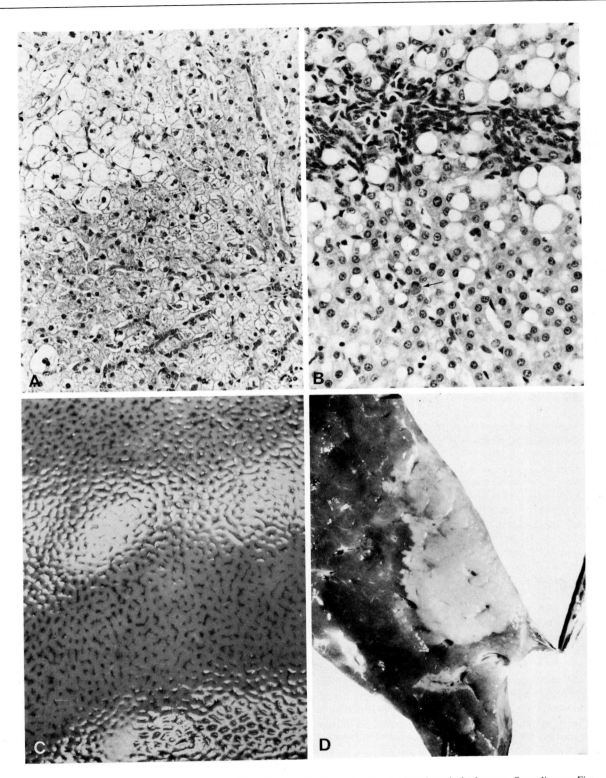

Fig. 2.3. (**A**) Severe hydropic degeneration. Dog. Hypercorticoidism, functional adrenal cortical adenoma. Same liver as Fig. 2.11B. (**B**) Fatty change and cholangiolar proliferation. Ovine white-liver disease. Ceroid in sinusoidal macrophage (arrow). (Courtesy of S. McOrist.) (**C**) Severe fatty liver with periacinar necrosis. Acute anemia in a fat goat. (**D**) Subcapsular focal fatty change associated with capsular adhesion. Ox.

Fatty Liver

Fatty liver is the term used to describe livers that contain more visible lipid, usually in hepatocytes, than one expects to see in that organ. This definition can include those examples of hepatocellular lipid accumulation that are more or less "physiologic," such as seen in late pregnancy or heavy lactation in ruminants. In these animals, nutritional stress may lead to clinical ketosis, but clinically normal animals may have very fatty livers, and there is little diagnostic significance in mild degrees of fatty change.

The liver plays a vital role in the lipid economy of the body. Tissues such as skeletal muscle can directly utilize fatty acids that have been mobilized from the fat depots, but a far greater proportion of fatty acids from this source are taken up by the liver and transformed into triglyceride or are used directly by the liver, which derives most of its energy from the oxidation of fatty acids. The bulk of hepatocellular triglyceride is destined for the synthesis of low-density lipoproteins, which are secreted into the plasma and are more readily utilized by most tissues than the fatty acids. Practically all the lipid absorbed from the gut is presented to the liver as chylomicrons, whose triglyceride has to be hydrolyzed (in part by the sinusoidal lining cells), absorbed by the hepatocytes, and resynthesized as low-density lipoproteins. The synthesis and transport of lipoprotein within the hepatocyte are processes requiring a small but indispensible energy input, thus any disturbance of protein and phospholipid synthesis or ATP synthesis has the potential to inhibit lipoprotein synthesis or secretion. Triglyceride synthesis from incoming fatty acid (from chylomicrons or fat depots), perhaps being independent of ATP synthesis, may continue; the result is the accumulation of excess triglyceride in the hepatocyte cytoplasm.

The assembly of lipoprotein takes place in the cisternae of the granular endoplasmic reticulum, and any damage to the membranes of this structure or the Golgi is likely to inhibit the rate of lipoprotein synthesis. This sort of disturbance seems to be the basis of the fatty liver of intoxication. Excessive intake or mobilization of triglyceride may cause fatty acids to be presented to the liver in excess of its capacity to utilize them; nevertheless, they will usually be taken up and stored as triglyceride.

Small droplets of fat, usually in a periportal and juxtasinusoidal position, can normally be found in the liver. In lipidosis, the amount is increased, most of the increment occurring in the more peripheral portion of the circulatory fields. The amount of fat present in the earlier stages of degeneration is usually much more than can be appreciated microscopically. The fat accumulates in small globules in the cytoplasm, and these show little tendency to fuse. The nucleus is not displaced but may be distorted. Fatty change that is the result of acute cell injury, such as may be produced by toxins and acute anoxia, may not develop past the stage of forming small globules, its course being either to restitution or to death of the cell. Such livers may be of normal or reduced size but are not enlarged. They are yellowish, especially at the periphery of circulatory fields, but the color may not be readily evident, except in those areas ischemic from pressure of an adjacent viscus. The consistency is softer than normal. On the cut surface, the architectural markings are obscure, although if there is some necrosis, the hepatic venules may be prominent and surrounded by a yellow halo.

In the more severe degrees of hepatic lipidosis, most of the parenchymal cells are involved. Probably as a result of fusion of globules, each cell usually contains one large globule, which alters the contour of the cell and displaces the nucleus (Fig. 2.3B). The sinusoids are compressed and appear anemic, and the tissue at low magnification resembles adipose tissue. Fat is also present in the epithelium of the bile ducts. Fatty change of this degree requires some time to develop and, therefore, implies a relatively mild cellular injury such as might result from nutritional and metabolic imbalances rather than from toxic or anoxic insult. With these severe degrees of degeneration, the liver is moderately or greatly enlarged, of a uniform light yellow color, and doughy. The edges are rounded, and the surface is smooth. The cut surface is uniform, greasy, and without acinar pattern unless there is also some congestion or zonal necrosis, in which event the cut surface is finely mottled red and yellow (Fig. 2.3C). The least equivocal evidence of severe fatty change is the ability of the liver to float in water or fixative.

Severe fatty liver may not necessarily produce severe hepatic dysfunction, and the liver can return to normal structure and function once the metabolic defect has been corrected, especially if the duration of the lipid accumulation has not been long. There is, however, a range of chronic hepatic changes often seen in livers that have presumably been fatty for a long time. The assumption is usually made that these changes, which include fibrosis, pigment accumulation, and nodular hyperplasia, are directly related to the long-term presence of excess lipid in the hepatocytes or sinusoidal fat-storage cells. Fatty livers are very vulnerable to a wide range of toxic and nutritional insults, and the necrogenic effects of these are likely to be more potent initiators of fibrosis and remodeling than the long-term presence of the fat per se. Nevertheless, some chronic changes can be ascribed to long-term presence of lipid. These are most commonly seen in the livers of old dogs and include fatty cysts, ceroid accumulation, and rarely, calcifying focal fibrous reactions to accumulations of cholesterol.

When lipid accumulates rapidly and in large amounts, there is a tendency for groups of the fat-laden cells to rupture or fuse and eventually form a multinucleate rim about a foamy mass of lipid. This epithelial structure is known as a fatty cyst as is the next stage, which occurs when released lipid is picked up by macrophages, which form foamy aggregations in sinusoids, the stroma of portal triads, and hepatic venules (Fig. 2.4A). These mesenchymal cells have only limited capacity for complete lysosomal digestion of neutral triglyceride; the result is progressive lipoperoxidation and disintegration of the less saturated fatty acids, followed by polymerization of the reactive residues. These form complex and variable compounds, known collectively as ceroid, which are only slightly soluble in lipid solvents and are periodic acid–Schiff (PAS) positive, acid fast, and autofluorescent. In histologic sections this pigment appears as colorless or yellow irregular fragments associated with the lipid globules in macrophages and, to a lesser extent, hepatocytes. Considerable amounts of lipid and ceroid may find their way into the lymphatics in the hepatic stroma and into the portal lymph nodes, which become slightly enlarged, yellow-green, and

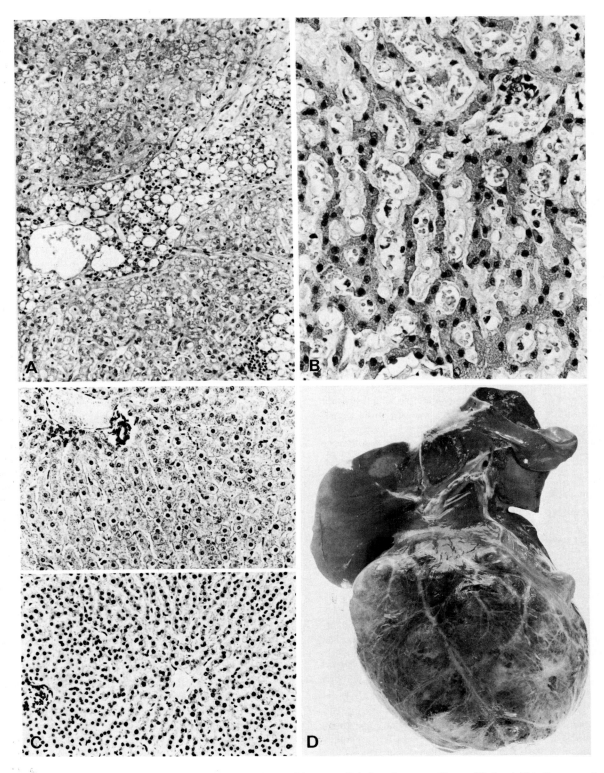

Fig. 2.4. (A) Accumulations of lipid-filled macrophages (''fatty cysts'') in hepatic stroma. Dog.   (B) Amyloid in the space of Disse compressing the hepatocellular plates. Cat.   (C) Normal (top) and atrophic (bottom) liver at same magnification. Starvation. Sheep.   (D) Hepatic cyst. Sheep.

rather oily on section. Most of the hepatocellular lipid may disappear from these livers, leaving the fatty cysts, and the result is a liver of relatively normal color, perhaps with a slightly nodular surface, with the stroma outlined by a delicate tracery of yellow ceroid deposit. It is difficult to distinguish between these livers and those developing more pronounced remodeling, nodular regeneration, and regional atrophy, which were described with nodular regeneration under Chronic Liver Disease.

Occasionally in the liver of old dogs there can be found sharply defined, fibrous, stony, hard masses, usually close to the surface, sometimes as much as 3 to 4 cm in diameter. These masses are usually sufficiently mineralized to show up distinctly on clinical radiographs. The mineral appears to be deposited on a matrix of degenerate collagen, laid down about perivascular foci of foamy macrophages and accumulations of cholesterol. The fibrous tissue may be laid down in response to the continued presence of fat, ceroid, or cholesterol, but no reason is apparent for the strictly localized distribution of the reaction. There are no recognizable hepatocytes in these lesions.

Physiologic fatty liver occurs in late pregnancy and heavy lactation, particularly in ruminants. Obvious fat infiltration is also seen in neonates, especially in those species whose milk is relatively rich in fat. These livers are fatty enough to be pale to the naked eye.

Fasting an animal with reasonable fat reserves rapidly depletes hepatocellular stores of glycogen and *de novo* lipogenesis ceases. There follows a heavy demand on adipose tissue fat stores, since the liver, dependent primarily on fatty acid oxidation for its own considerable energy needs must also provide a large amount of lipoprotein for export to other tissues. Under these circumsantces, it appears that the synthesis and transport of low-density lipoprotein acts as a bottleneck in the movement of lipid through the hepatocyte. Triglyceride accumulates in the cytoplasm, particularly if starvation reduces the availability of protein and cofactors such as choline, which are essential to the synthetic process.

Ketosis of **ruminants** typically is associated with fatty liver. It is rather unrealistic to try to separate discussion of starvation from that of ruminant ketosis, especially from the morphologic point of view, as the differences are really quantitative. In biochemical terms, the difference seems to be related to the added stimulus for fatty acid oxidation, which is occasioned by the added drain of heavy pregnancy or lactation and the enormous potential for ketogenesis. In ewes freshly dead of pregnancy toxemia, one may see indistinct patches of white discoloration of abdominal fat, which may reflect accelerated lipolysis. These patches tend to be obscured by postmortem solidification of the fat. The fatty infiltration of hepatocytes in these animals is often most severe in the periportal zone, whereas the distribution of lipid in ketosis of cattle is predominantly periacinar.

Fatty liver of **diabetes** occurs when insulin is deficient or inactive due to lack of functioning receptors. There is greatly accelerated lipolysis from adipose tissue. The liver is thus presented with a large load of fatty acid, the mitochondrial oxidation of which is hindered by the shortage of ATP occasioned by reduced glucose availability. Lipoprotein synthesis is also reduced, in part, because of the ATP limitation and, in part, as a result of reduced uptake by the liver of branched-chain amino

acids. Insulin deficiency alone will produce fatty liver, but most cases in carnivores are associated with exocrine pancreatic insufficiency as well, which further reduces the availability of amino acids as a result of protein malabsorption. All these factors may combine to produce very fatty livers in chronic uncontrolled diabetes mellitus. The periacinar hepatocytes usually show the greatest degree of fatty infiltration.

Lipoprotein synthesis and transport are dependent on oxidative metabolism, and **hypoxia** of **hepatocytes** leads to triglyceride accumulation. The two most common causes of hepatocellular hypoxia are anemia and reduced sinusoidal perfusion in passive venous congestion. The hepatocytes most severely affected are those in the periacinar zone.

Small, sharply demarcated patches of intense fatty infiltration are often seen in bovine livers at or adjacent to sites of **capsular fibrous adhesion** (Fig. 2.3D). These patches are neither swollen nor shrunken, extend usually less than a centimeter into the parenchyma, and are of the same consistency as normal liver. The acinar structure of these lesions is undisturbed, but the hepatocytes therein show pronounced lipidosis, presumably related to interference with local perfusion.

Fatty liver due to **intoxication** is common. There are several stages of the cycle of hepatic lipid metabolism that can be affected selectively by various toxins to produce fatty liver. For example, it is possible experimentally to cause triglyceride accumulation by interfering with mitochondrial fatty acid oxidation with sublethal doses of cyanide, or by inhibiting apolipoprotein synthesis by administration of orotic acid. Most toxins that cause fatty liver in naturally occurring situations, however, also produce a greater or lesser degree of hepatocellular necrosis. Fatty liver occurring as a manifestation of toxic liver disease will be further discussed in that section, but the generalization may be made here that most important veterinary hepatic intoxications cause widespread membrane damage and/or disturbance of protein synthesis. These cause lipid accumulation in the hepatocyte by interfering with lipoprotein synthesis and transport as well as with fatty acid oxidation.

While fatty liver is more frequently associated with shortage of metabolizable energy in domestic animals, there are some more specific **deficiencies** that will produce fatty liver; usually, they have been defined under experimental conditions and have no valid naturally occurring equivalent. Choline deficiency, for example, in the absence of other suitable methyl donors, soon produces fatty liver as a result of reduced synthesis of lecithin and consequent impairment of triglyceride binding and transport. It is unlikely, however, that choline deficiency uncomplicated by other forms of malnutrition would occur in domestic animals; the same may be said of essential fatty acid deficiency, which also produces fatty liver in experimental animals.

One naturally occurring example of fatty liver that appears to be at least partly due to a specific deficiency is **ovine white-liver disease**, first described in lambs in New Zealand and now known to occur in southern Australia and Europe. This is a syndrome of ill thrift, anorexia, mild normocytic, normochromic anemia with, occasionally, photosensitization and icterus. The condition is associated with low liver cobalt levels and low plasma concentrations of vitamin B_{12}. Lambs up to ~1 year of age are more commonly affected than ewes, and pastures are likely to be adequate at the times of peak incidence (late spring and early summer); these epidemiologic features clearly indicate a different pathogenesis from pregnancy toxemia. The disease has been shown to be cobalt and vitamin B_{12} responsive, and there is clearly a degree of overlap between this condition and the more conventional forms of cobalt deficiency; nevertheless, the liver pathology is sufficiently distinctive to allow classification as a separate entity.

In the early stages, the liver changes consist of vacuolar triglyceride accumulations in hepatocytes, usually most severe in the periacinar zones. In addition, ceroid pigment is present in all cases, early in hepatocytes and later also in sinusoidal cells and stromal macrophages. The fatty change may be very severe in the early stage, the liver being grossly swollen. A moderate degree of bile ductular proliferation is also a consistent feature (Fig. 2.3B). The explosive nature of some outbreaks suggests that a pasture toxin acts in concert with the deficiency of vitamin B_{12} to produce this disease. Whatever the factors in its initiation, the metabolic disturbances of starvation are invoked by the severe inappetance, and these will no doubt confuse attempts to define the condition biochemically.

Equine hyperlipemia is almost exclusively a disease of ponies, and among these the Shetland breed predominates. The pathogenesis is not known. The disease is usually fatal. Pregnant or lactating mares are most likely to develop the disease, particularly if they are excessively fat and have recently suffered reduced feed intake due to conditions such as laminitis or parasitism or other form of stress. The clinical course is marked by somnolence, complete anorexia, and colic, progressing to mania in some cases. Some ponies develop ventral subcutaneous edema, and most develop moderate diarrhea. All show marked increase in plasma triglyceride concentration, the lipid being predominantly very low density lipoprotein, but all other lipid fractions are elevated, and the concentration is sufficient to impart a striking milkiness to the serum and blood. Metabolic acidosis is a consistent feature in animals that die, and they also develop signs of disseminated intravascular coagulation. At autopsy, there is severe fatty liver, which may have ruptured; the lipidosis also extends to heart and skeletal muscle, kidney, and adrenal cortex. The hepatic lipidosis is remarkable only by its severity; there is little hepatocellular necrosis, although there is consistent prolongation of sulfobromophthalein retention time and elevation of serum alkaline phosphatase levels. Evidence of disseminated intravascular coagulation is seen as serosal hemorrhages and microscopic thrombi in various organs, and even gross infarction of myocardium and kidney.

Fatty liver syndrome in **cats** has some features in common with hyperlipemia of pones in that both occur in overfat, nutritionally stressed animals; there is hypertriglyceridemia, and the mortality rate is high. In the feline condition, however, there is no sex predilection, jaundice is frequently observed, and there may be severe periacinar hepatocellular necrosis, at least in the later stages. The liver has severe fatty accumulation in all hepatocytes; bile pigment accumulation, when seen, is mostly present in Kupffer cells and can be confused with polymerized lipid residues.

As with horses, the pathogenesis of this disease is obscure.

Since the excess lipid in liver and blood is in the form of triglyceride, the implication is that the liver is capable of esterifying fatty acid mobilized from depot fat. The triglyceride thus formed is presumably then exported to the plasma as low-density lipoprotein until the plasma transport mechanisms are saturated, at which stage fatty buildup in the hepatocyte begins. Another possibility is that there is an inability on the part of all tissues to utilize fatty acids or low-density lipoproteins at the normal rate, while triglyceride synthesis from fatty acids continues.

Amyloidosis

Amyloid infiltration of the liver occurs in cattle, horses, dogs, and cats. In the latter two species, the amyloidosis is primary, or at least not obviously secondary; in cattle it is secondary to some chronic tissue-destructive process; and in horses it occurs chiefly in those used for the production of hyperimmune serum. In each species, it is part of generalized amyloidosis. The amyloid is deposited between the sinusoidal reticulum and the hepatic cords (Fig. 2.4B) and is sometimes found in the walls of the afferent vessels. The surrounded hepatic cords atrophy. Affected livers are enlarged, with rounded edges, pale, and soft in horses, firm in cattle. The amyloid is deposited first in the parenchyma about the portal tracts and appears grayish and waxy. The liver is predisposed to rupture. Horses may develop icterus and other signs of hepatic failure, but cattle die first of the primary disease or from the uremia resulting from concurrent renal amyloidosis.

Hepatic Atrophy

The large mass of the liver allows a considerable reserve to be available for catabolism in starvation. This appears to be the basis of atrophy in severe malnutrition of slow onset and long duration, as seen, for example, in old grazing herbivores with poor teeth. In such cases the liver is dark and small, and the capsule may appear too large for the organ, showing fine wrinkles on handling. These livers may even appear to be firmer than normal, due to condensation of normal stroma. Sections give an impression of greatly increased numbers of hepatocytes; these are small, with scanty cytoplasm (Fig. 2.4C). Portal triads and hepatic venules are closer together than normal due to the small size of the acini.

Atrophy of part of the liver may be a response to pressure or impairment of blood or bile flow. Local pressure atrophy occurs adjacent to space-occupying lesions in the liver or as a result of chronic pressures from neighboring organs, such as distended rumen or colon. Chronic diffuse diseases of the biliary tract, such as sporidesmin poisoning and fascioliasis, are likely to cause atrophy of the left lobe in ruminants, probably as a result of the greater difficulty in maintaining adequate biliary drainage from this dependent lobe. The atrophy of biliary obstruction is complicated by some degree of inflammation and fibrosis superimposed on it.

Hepatotrophic factors are components of the portal blood. They are essential for the maintenance of normal hepatic mass, and atrophy of part or all of the liver occurs when portal blood is diverted or obstructed. The histologic features of this atrophy are similar to those of starvation atrophy.

Patterns of Hepatic Necrosis

The later stages of hepatocellular degeneration, which eventually produce the irreversible state of necrosis, are similar to those producing necrosis in other tissue, and reference to reviews of the subject in general pathology texts should be made for details of the ionic fluxes, disruption of cell and organelle membranes, and interference with energy metabolism that occur in the dying cell. Here, the various morphologic patterns of hepatic necrosis are described.

Single-Cell Necrosis

Necrobiosis is the term applied to the death of single effete cells in any tissue; it occurs more frequently in the liver than in many other organs, but the process is never obvious. The manner in which the cell disappears may not always be the same, but usually it is in the form of shrinkage necrosis known as apoptosis.

Apoptosis, shrinkage, and coagulative necrosis may be applied to different stages of the same process, which begins with sudden condensation of the cytoplasm and nucleus of a cell that is alive and still metabolically active; the process of apoptosis may in its earlier stages be energy dependent. Within a short interval, the cytoplasm is shredded away in membrane-bound fragments containing normal organelles (including fragments of nucleus) embedded in an electron-dense matrix. These fragments are rapidly engulfed by neighboring hepatocytes and by Kupffer cells and, if they contain no nuclear chromatin, may be recognized as the acidophilic bodies described earlier. Larger fragments containing nuclear remnants show nuclear pyknosis. If this pattern of necrosis involves many adjacent cells simultaneously, their removal may be delayed. The term **coagulative necrosis** may be applied to foci of intact shrunken hepatocytes.

In some circumstances, destruction of hepatocytes involves rapid swelling and disintegration of the cells, usually in groups. This pattern of **lytic necrosis** may be seen in some intoxications, such as beryllium toxicosis, but is usually associated with foci of inflammation (Figs. 2.5B and 2.19D). The lysis may result from the activity of neutrophil leukocytes and macrophages.

Models of immune-mediated hepatocyte necrosis have emerged from studies of human viral hepatitis and some forms of drug-induced chronic hepatitis. The mechanisms may involve either direct damage to hepatocytes by the uptake of antigen–antibody complexes, or cooperation between macrophages and T lymphocytes. These may cause cell-mediated destruction of hepatocytes that have taken up these complexes or, perhaps, native antigen or virus. Whether these models are valid for any spontaneous liver disease in domestic animals remains to be proven.

Focal Necrosis

Focal necrosis is very common in autopsy material. The lesions are microscopic or barely visible to the naked eye and are usually numerous. Their designation as focal depends on their size and on a random distribution in the acini. There is sometimes apparent a tendency for focal necroses to occur nearer to the axial portal vessels than the periphery of the circulatory fields and to be concentrated in some acinar agglomerates rather than others. Focal necrosis occurs in many infections, parasitic migrations, and instances of biliary obstruction. The infectious causes may be viral, such as equine herpesvirus-1 in the fetus, or bacterial. Many bacterial infections that are septicemic produce focal hepatic lesions consistently; examples are salmonellosis, tularemia, pseudotuberculosis, listeriosis in the fetus and newborn, and *Pasteurella haemolytica* septicemia in lambs. The focal necrosis may be the outcome of a Kupffer-cell reaction, as in salmonellosis, or of bacterial embolism, as in pasteurellosis. Usually, the approximate cause can be determined by histologic examination. This type of focal necrosis is usually attended by some degree of focal inflammation.

In cattle, especially, focal necrosis in few or many visible foci is common at postmortem and common enough to be important at slaughter; it is responsible for the descriptive appellation ''sawdust.'' The pathogenesis is not known and probably varies, but it may be caused by organisms from the gut that reach the liver in the portal blood. The lesion is not specific and consists of focal parenchymal necrosis with disruption of reticulin fibers and an infiltration of neutrophils and lymphocytes (Fig. 2.13B); suppuration does not occur.

Focal necrosis in biliary obstruction follows rupture of distended canaliculi and the formation of small bile lakes. The yellow pigment is readily visible microscopically and provokes small granulomas with giant cells.

Focal necroses are of very little significance for the liver and even when numerous produce no dysfunction. When they heal, there is some scarring, but this too probably disappears in time. They are of diagnostic importance in some diseases, such as salmonellosis, and of economic importance to the meat industry.

Periacinar Necrosis

The hepatocytes in the periacinar zone are particularly vulnerable to two types of necrotizing insult. They are furthest from the source of incoming portal and arterial blood and are therefore last in line for oxygen and essential nutrients. Also, they contain the greatest concentration of mixed-function oxidases, which are capable of transforming certain exogenous compounds into reactive metabolites, and these are sufficiently toxic to kill the cells that produce them.

Several viral infections, such as canine infectious hepatitis and Rift Valley fever can produce periacinar necrosis (centrilobular necrosis), and the reasons for the increased susceptibility of the hepatocytes in this zone in these diseases are not obvious. It is possible that hepatocellular swelling and sinusoidal damage reduce effective perfusion of the periacinar hepatocytes, but it is also possible that these cells have greater intrinsic susceptibility to the viruses.

Periacinar degeneration and necrosis are seen commonly in animals that have died rather slowly. It is assumed that in the agonal period the hepatocytes in this zone are disproportionately disadvantaged as a result of the failing circulation and that the damage is due to tissue hypoxia. This necrosis is more extensive if the animal is anemic. Periacinar necrosis is also seen in passive venous congestion of the liver and is described under Obstruction of the Efferent Hepatic Vessels.

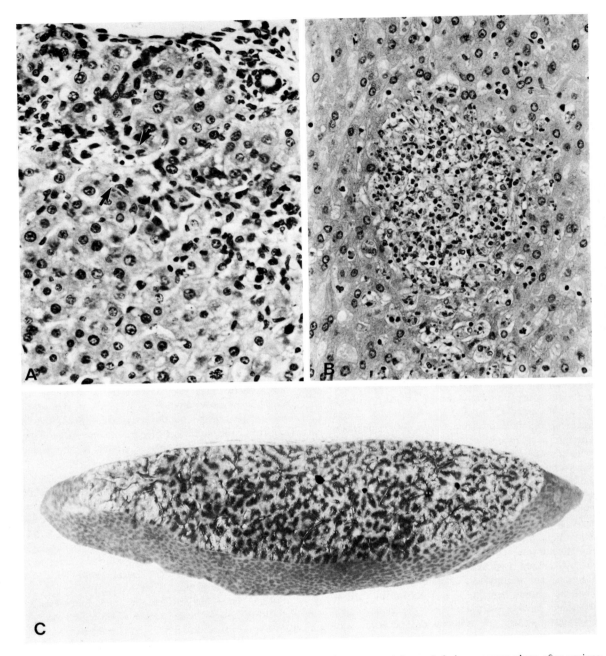

Fig. 2.5. (A) Midzonal necrosis. The necrotic hepatocytes have been removed (arrows) during recovery phase after ngaione poisoning. Sheep. (Courtesy of A. A. Seawright.)   (B) Focal inflammation and lytic necrosis in salmonellosis.   (C) Slice of liver from equine serum hepatitis. The reticular pattern suggests zonal necrosis.

The necrotic cells are usually replaced by stagnant blood, at least in the acute phase; therefore, in the liver with periacinar necrosis, there is usually a prominent acinar pattern, which takes the form of a fine, regular, pallid network of surviving, often fatty, hepatocytes in the periportal zone, which stands up above the red, collapsed areas adjacent to the hepatic venules (Fig. 2.9A,B). But fatty change in the liver may also have a zonal distribution, and such livers may show a marked acinar pattern without having significant necrosis.

The zones of necrosis are usually coagulative in nature and may be restricted to the hepatocytes immediately surrounding the hepatic venules; this pattern gave rise to the time-honored designation centrilobular necrosis. Frequently, however, the areas of necrosis are joined to one another, thus cutting the conventional lobules into segments, and at the same time outlining the periphery of the circulatory fields of the hepatic acini (Fig. 2.2D). Some of these areas of necrosis extend up to larger portal triads, because the periphery of acini may lie against the larger portal tracts. Often, the hepatocytes between the necrotic and more normal zones show hydropic degeneration or fatty change (Fig. 2.6A).

Quite extensive periacinar necrosis may be followed by repair (Fig. 2.22D) and complete restoration of normal structure and function within a few days if the necrotizing insult is of short duration. Severe periacinar necrosis may be followed shortly by cholangiolar-cell proliferation and bile duct proliferation; this reaction seems to be related to the stimulus for hepatocellular proliferation, to which the cells of the finest branches of the bile ducts also seem susceptible. With restitution of the normal complement of hepatocytes, the proliferative response in the biliary tract subsides unless the original insult is continuous or repeated.

Midzonal Necrosis

The rarity of midzonal necrosis has in the past led to the proposition that it was either an artifact or a stage on the way to periacinar necrosis. It is now established that some intoxications can produce midzonal necrosis that progresses no further, and the lesion has been reliably produced in experimental animals.

Acute midzonal necrosis may involve only a narrow, sharply defined band of hepatocytes or may be more diffuse within the acinus, so that periportal or periacinar degeneration may be superimposed on the more severe midzonal lesion. The acute phase of coagulative necrosis is followed by intense macrophage activity, which rapidly removes the dead cells and allows complete regeneration of normal structure.

Periportal Necrosis

The remarks just made about midzonal necrosis apply to coagulative periportal necrosis (Fig. 2.6C,D). It is a rare lesion, perhaps more often seen than midzonal necrosis, and is caused by the same sort of complex interaction between specific types of hepatotoxins and the hepatic microsomal apparatus. It is common to find in the same liver areas that show one or both of the patterns of zonal necrosis.

A different type of periportal necrosis may occur when inflammatory processes extend beyond the portal triad and involve the adjacent hepatocytes.

The various forms of zonal necrosis cannot reliably be distinguished grossly, but one may expect to see in periportal necrosis a reversal of the pattern seen in periacinar necrosis; that is, in periportal necrosis the surviving pale hepatocytes about the hepatic venules may appear as pale, raised islands in the meshes of a regular network of red, collapsed periportal tissue. Careful scrutiny may reveal the smallest hepatic venules at the center of the pale islands.

Paracentral Necrosis

Paracentral necrosis, a variant of coagulative necrosis, occurs when an isolated complete hepatic acinus dies and is viewed in transverse section. It is possibly an ischemic lesion or infarct produced by an occlusion of a terminal portal venule, such as may occur in disseminated intravascular coagulation.

Its appearance in certain of the acute hepatotoxicities (Fig. 2.6B) probably represents the death of a single complete acinus, as a result of local high microsomal enzyme activity, or of local deficiency of hepatocellular protective factors. Occlusion and

rupture of a bile ductule or cholangiole is another potential cause of paracentral necrosis.

Massive Necrosis

Massive necrosis refers to events in individual acini, not to events in the liver as a whole. By accepted definition, every cell in the affected acinus is dead, including the hepatocytes of the limiting plate (Fig. 2.7C). The definition is of some importance because the sequelae of this pattern of necrosis are quite distinct. There being no surviving parenchyma in the acinus, there is no source of cells for regeneration, and none to hold open the reticulin network of the acinus. The sequel to massive necrosis is collapse of the reticulin and fibrous framework so that portal areas and the hepatic venule are approximated, and the connective tissues are condensed and scarify. The definition is too restrictive, because about the periphery of such areas, it is possible to find acini showing necrosis of zonal distribution both paracentral and periacinar. The distribution of massive hepatic necrosis of dietary origin in experimental animals, and occasionally spontaneously in others, clearly relates the lesion to vascular distributions in the organ, and the microscopic finding of zonal patterns of necrosis in many acini, not entirely destroyed, relates the necrosis to smaller units in the vascular fields. Massive hepatic necrosis can thus be defined as a process that destroys acinar agglomerates, usually very many contiguous ones, and produces lesser zonal injury to the periphery of surrounding acini. Collapse, condensation, and heavy scarring are characteristic (Fig. 2.8), the end result being known as postnecrotic scarring. The liver is not uniformly involved. Large areas of parenchyma remain intact, and adjacent to the necrotic areas, isolated acini and acinar agglomerates survive. From these, regeneration takes place concentrically to form giant hypertrophic nodules on axial portal vessels. Successive bouts of massive necrosis may occur, each with collapse and scarring as an inevitable sequel.

Massive hepatic necrosis may develop in three ways. It may in some parts of the organ represent the extreme degree of a zonal (periacinar) necrosis that in the remainder of the liver remains uniformly zonal. Acute vascular accidents may produce massive necrosis in which not only the parenchyma, but the supporting tissue as well, dies. Or it may be of dietetic origin.

A liver that is the seat of massive necrosis is of about normal size or small. Fine red threads of fibrin may be present on the surface, especially in the grooves between the lobes. The organ presents a mosaic appearance of red, gray, or yellow areas intermingled with areas of dark redness. The mosaic pattern is occasionally broad, the intermingled colorful areas being some centimeters across, or the red hemorrhagic areas may be few and scattered. Usually, however, the mosaic pattern is finer (Fig. 2.7B), the yellow areas of parenchyma forming irregular, coalescing patches that may not be more than 1.0 cm in diameter. The gray or yellow areas represent surviving tissue; the intermingled red areas represent areas of necrosis, hemorrhage, and collapse, and these are depressed a few millimeters below the surface. The mosaic pattern is present also on the cut surface and is especially striking in pigs, in which the lobules in necrotic areas appear as partially emptied blood cysts. In the healing stage, the depressed areas of hemorrhage and necrosis are con-

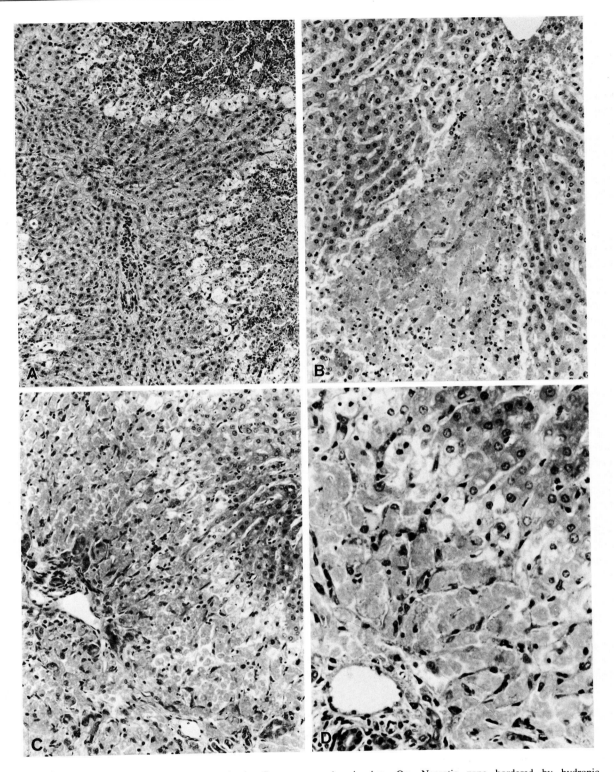

Fig. 2.6. (**A**) Acute periacinar necrosis in *Cestrum parqui* poisoning. Ox. Necrotic zone bordered by hydropic hepatocytes. (**B**) Paracentral necrosis in ngaione poisoning. Sheep. (**C** and **D**) Periportal necrosis in ngaione poisoning. Sheep. (Courtesy of A. A. Seawright.)

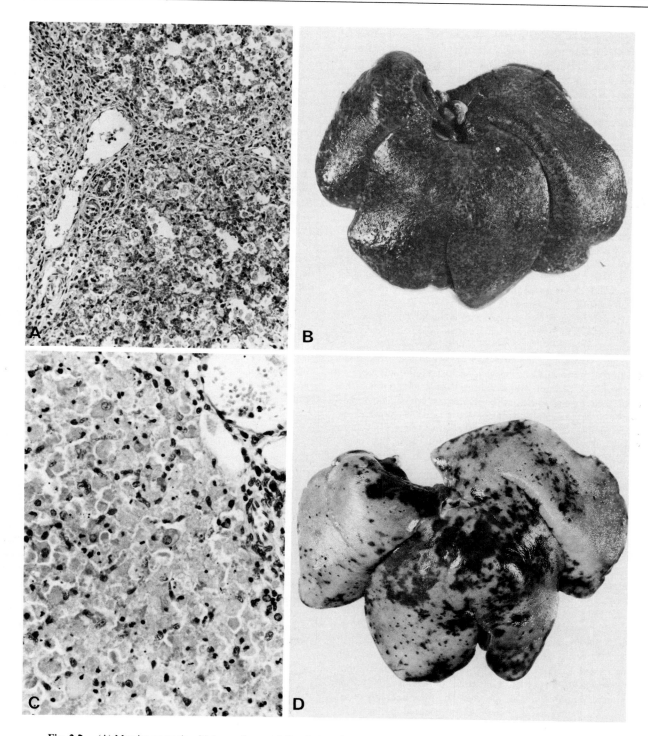

Fig. 2.7. (A) Massive necrosis with hemorrhage and dissolution of parenchyma. Hepatosis dietetica. Pig. (B) Massive necrosis with darkening and early postnecrotic collapse. Hepatosis dietetica. Pig. (Courtesy of C. A. Grant.) (C) Massive necrosis with destruction of the periportal limiting plate. Algal poisoning. Sheep. (Courtesy of A. R. B. Jackson.) (D) Early massive necrosis with random hemorrhage and pallor. Iron–dextran poisoning. Pig.

densed, shrunken, and scarified so that the surface of the liver is traversed by fine or heavy scars, which separate large nodules of regenerative hyperplasia. Further acute episodes may be superimposed so that the presented lesion may be a mixture of acute massive necrosis and postnecrotic scarring. Continuing acute necrosis in areas of scarring is also commonly present, either because of continuance of the initial insult or as a consequence of the scarring itself.

When cells die of massive hepatic necrosis, the death is sudden and complete, and there is no evidence that they have passed through an initial stage of vacuolar degeneration. Examination of the lesion in the early stage reveals hemorrhage and pooling of blood close about the axial portal vessels, a picture superficially resembling periportal necrosis. Later, there is hemorrhage to replace all the dead parenchyma (Fig. 2.7A), but the early lesion, with its sudden necrosis and damming back of blood in the portal vessels, is consistent with the idea that massive necrosis develops as a sudden swelling of all the cells in acinar agglomerates, with complete cessation of intrasinusoidal blood flow in the affected areas.

Massive necrosis may appear with apparent randomness in the organ, but there is a tendency for it, especially when not extensive, to involve the left lobe(s) of the liver; when the lesion is severe, portions of all lobes are involved. The relative restriction of some cases of massive necrosis to the left lobes is explained on the basis of streamlined portal flow. In rats, the usual experimental animal for producing dietary hepatic necrosis, the left lobes receive blood from the spleen and colon and are expected to be deficient in nutriment relative to the right lobe, which receives its blood from the small intestine. The occurrence of streamlining in domestic animals other than the dog is not established, but massive necrosis, or the scarring that results from it, is occasionally observed in sheep, cattle, and swine and is limited to, or most severe in, the left lobes.

HEPATOSIS DIETETICA. Hepatosis dietetica of swine is a polymorphous syndrome compounded of massive hepatic necrosis with its immediate or late effects, "yellow-fat disease," degeneration of skeletal and cardiac muscle, serous effusions, ulceration of the squamous mucosa of the stomach, and fibrinoid necrosis of arterioles. All these lesions seldom occur in one animal; in practice, they occur alone or in any combination. They are known to be of nutritional origin, and the fact that the various lesions can occur separately indicates the complexity of the pathogenesis, which is discussed with diseases of muscle (in Muscles and Tendons, Volume 1). Experimental observations have revealed the need for concurrent deficiencies of sulfur-containing amino acids, tocopherols, and trace amounts of selenium if hepatic necrosis is to develop. Selenium protects efficiently against the hepatic necrosis and massive effusions, and tocopherols are probably protective against all lesions of the syndrome.

Hepatosis dietetica occurs in rapidly growing pigs fed diets largely of grain and containing protein supplements lacking either in quality or quantity. There is some evidence that in pigs that are nutritionally predisposed, a cold, damp environment may precipitate the disease. Death usually occurs without signs of illness or after a short period of dullness. Melena, dyspnea,

weakness, and trembling may be observed in some cases. Jaundice is indicative of a relapsing course.

Affected pigs are usually in good condition. The carcass is anemic if ulceration of the gastric mucosa has occurred, and in these cases, free and digested blood may be found in the stomach and intestine. Jaundice is not common, but yellow staining of adipose tissues (yellow-fat disease) is. In relapsing cases, hemorrhagic diathesis may occur, manifested mainly by hemorrhage into and about joints. Fluid containing much protein collects in the serous cavities in small volume. Fine strands of fibrin are present in the peritoneum. Pulmonary edema accompanies myocardial lesions that consist of intramural and subendocardial hemorrhages with focal areas of hyaline degeneration. The changes in the liver dominate the autopsy findings. The massive hepatic necrosis is of the typical appearance described earlier (Fig. 2.7B), and in a number of cases, both acute and chronic lesions are found. The sites of severest injury are the dorsal parts on the diaphragmatic surface. The right lobe may escape and later undergo marked hypertrophy. The gallbladder is often edematous.

The histologic changes that occur in this syndrome are described elsewhere with the particular organs involved. Additionally, a fibrinoid degeneration of small arteries occurs in some cases. The arterial degeneration may occur in any organ or in most organs but is relatively common only in the small vessels of the mesentery, gut, and heart (see mulberry-heart disease, in Cardiovascular System, Volume 3).

Necrosis of Sinusoidal Lining Cells

When hepatocytes are being destroyed by the elaboration of toxic molecules within their cytoplasm, it is to be expected that the sinusoidal lining cells may also suffer should the products of these biotransformations spill into the spaces of Disse. Lytic necrosis of these cells is in fact seen very early in the course of hepatotoxicities such as acute algal and ngaione poisoning, but the pathogenesis proposed above remains unproven. The sinusoidal phagocytes are sometimes vulnerable by virtue of their role in clearing the portal blood of particulate or colloidal material; should these particles be toxic or infectious, Kupffer-cell necrosis may occur alone, but more usually there is damage to surrounding hepatocytes as well.

It is unusual for the bile duct epithelium to be singled out by specific necrogenic insults; usually there is accompanying portal inflammation.

Vascular Factors in Liver Injury

The dynamics of the liver-cell population in health and disease are interwoven with the dynamics of its blood supply. Hepatic parenchyma manifests the usual degenerative changes of hydropic change, fatty degeneration, and necrosis. But very characteristic of the liver is the extraordinary rapidity with which necrosis develops in response to a wide variety of insults. Part of the explanation lies in the action of the liver in accumulating toxic compounds or degrading them into even more toxic fragments. The frequency with which necrosis develops suggests that there is often, or even inevitably, some additional influence that may transform a mild primary injury to, in cellular terms, a

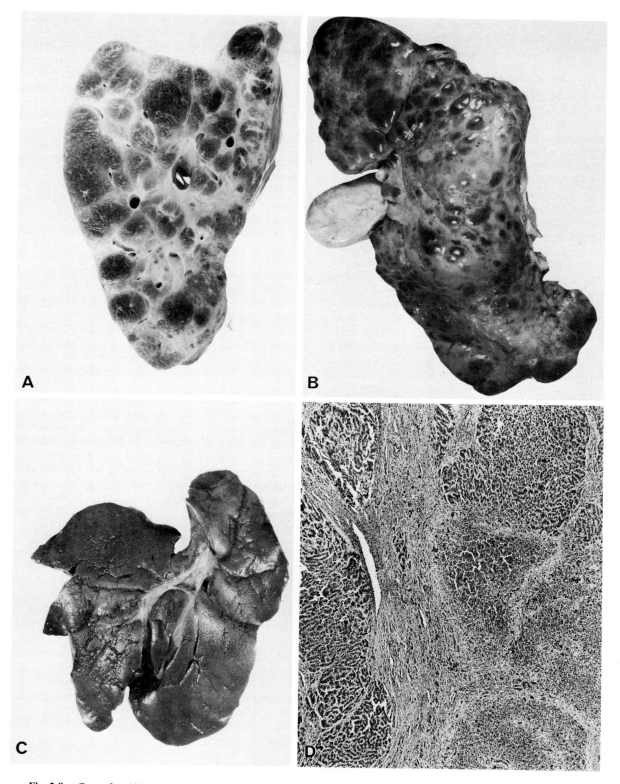

Fig. 2.8. Cut surface (**A**) and capsular surface (**B**), showing postnecrotic scarring. Ox. (**C**) Postnecrotic collapse of liver tissue in hepatosis dietetica. Pig. (**D**) Postnecrotic scarring and nodular regeneration. Ox.

fatal or necrotizing injury. If there is such a complicating influence, it is likely to reside in deranged circulation in the sinusoids.

Obstruction of the Hepatic Artery

The mammalian liver has a double blood supply, of which the hepatic artery is an important part. It distributes largely to the peribiliary capillary circulation of the portal triads, via which it also anastomoses with the portal vein. Its distribution of blood to the sinusoids is through these other vessels rather than directly. It is difficult to ascribe a function to the hepatic artery in terms of parenchymal function, and its role may be no more than that of providing a reserve supply of oxygen. It is doubtful that any mammalian liver can survive complete interruption of its arterial supply, a feat difficult to achieve because of the abundance of potential collaterals. Obstruction developing rapidly enough to prevent other collaterals from developing leads to parenchymal necrosis in dogs, cats, and horses and probably ruminants as well. The extent of necrosis depends on how completely the obstruction excludes collateral circulation and also on the oxygen tension of the portal blood. Oxygen tension varies between and within species and depends on the state of the general circulation, varying directly with blood pressure. In ischemic areas, bile flow ceases immediately, and a pattern of ischemic necrosis occurs that involves acinar agglomerates. The fate of animals with arterial occlusion and parenchymal ischemia is determined largely by bacteriologic factors; anaerobes, especially clostridia, proliferate rapidly, and intoxication can cause death.

Hepatic arterial occlusions occur rather commonly in animals but usually, as in parasitic infestations, involve small intrahepatic branches and are of little consequence. Large segments may be necrotic in cats as a result of thrombosis of the aorta and hepatic artery. Verminous arteritis may occlude the hepatic artery in horses.

Obstruction of the Portal Vein

The portal vein, draining the splanchnic viscera, contributes most of the large volume of blood perfusing the liver. Available estimates indicate that normally, approximately two-thirds of hepatic blood flow is portal in origin. An odd feature of the portal flow is that in some animals, including the dog, it is streamlined, blood from the stomach and duodenum passing preferentially to the left lobe and that from the jejunum and ileum passing to the right lobe. In the dog, under stable conditions, this streamlining is consistent. Frequent shifts in streamlining occur with altered disposition of viscera so that only slight differences are expected in the perfusates in right and left lobes of the liver. These differences may, however, be critical in some types of liver injury, as has been suggested for the patterns of dietary hepatic necrosis. Streamlining may account for the different regional distributions sometimes observed with metastatic tumors and infections (Figs. 2.13A and 2.18D). In the same sense, the umbilical vein usually delivers to the left lobe in preference to the right, and metastatic umbilical infections may be strictly localized to one lobe or the other.

The volume of portal blood flow is determined largely by events in the splanchnic circulation. From the hilus on, the portal vein demonstrates an extraordinarily high degree of branching, which tends to ensure an even distribution of portal blood flow while providing for a wide variety of flow patterns. The size of the liver or any segment of it is dependent on the volume of blood perfusing it, and the average blood flow per unit weight of tissue tends to be uniform. This emphasizes the correlation between portal flow and the shape and size of the liver or its lobes, but also that, ordinarily, hilar areas of the liver are no better perfused than the marginal areas. If the volume of hepatic blood is increased to a portion of the liver, that portion will hypertrophy. Reduction in the volume of hepatic flow leads to atrophy of deprived segments of liver.

Obstruction of the portal vein, if sudden and complete, produces a condition akin to strangulation of the gut, and death occurs quickly without significant hepatic change. Obstruction of a large branch of the portal vein leads in cattle, sheep, and cats to acute ischemia of a wedge of tissue in which necrosis may be zonal or massive. Obstruction to many small portal radicles is common, with necrosis of many acini. It is evident that if a collateral supply develops and oxygenation remains adequate, obstruction of portal radicles will have no immediate effect on the hepatic parenchyma, save perhaps to make it more sensitive to toxic injury. There is, however, a long-term effect, probably nutritional. The parenchyma in the affected lobe, deprived of hepatotrophic factors, loses much of its regenerative power and atrophies fairly rapidly, allowing condensation and scarification of the stromal tissues.

Acute increase in pressure in the portal vein may occur in any severe episode of widespread acute hepatic necrosis; the cause appears to be simple obstruction of the sinusoidal flow by thrombosis and actual sinusoidal disruption. In such animals there is severe acute congestion of the liver, slight ascites, free fibrin accumulations in the abdomen (not the firm capsular adhesions seen in passive congestion), and distended portal lymphatics. Chronic portal hypertension and ascites are discussed with the peritoneum.

Obstruction of the Efferent Hepatic Vessels

In essence, the sinusoidal bed of the liver is a vast, continuous meshwork of interconnected blood spaces in which, potentially, blood can move in any direction, at least within a lobe. Probably, with normal activity, the path of the red cell through the liver is devious and variable and responsive to the many factors influencing intrahepatic pressure. This should not obscure the fact, however, that there is a basic pattern of flow, fairly direct between portal areas and central vein and associated with a basic pattern of pressure gradients and streamlines. It is the basic pattern of flow that determines metabolic gradients within acini and that, in association with metabolic differences, influences the zonal susceptibility of the liver to injury. The immediate importance of sinusoidal flow rates and directions is probably determined largely by oxygen tension.

Severe respiratory hypoxemia can produce pathologic changes in the liver. Acute anemia may also do so, with periacinar necrosis as the result. Low levels of oxygen saturation, as in chronic passive congestion, are also responsible for periacinar lesions, although necrosis in this condition is not blatant. More debated is the contribution of reduced sinusoidal flow and oxygen saturation on the zonal distribution of many toxigenic liver lesions, especially those producing the common periacinar necrosis. It is self-evident that any reduced blood perfusion would further place at a disadvantage any parenchymal cells already injured by direct toxic action. Reduced sinusoidal flow some hours after carbon tetrachloride injury has been demonstrated. Whether this is due to swelling of injured parenchymal cells is not clear; other mechanisms, including altered properties of sinusoidal endothelium, have not been assessed.

The hepatic venules anastomose to form the hepatic veins and the efferent circulation. The structure of these vessels varies between species, but these are matters largely unexamined. Spiral sphincters of the hepatic vein are well developed in dogs, and sphincter spasm is invoked to explain the intense engorgement of the liver with certain anesthetics and in anaphylaxis in this species. It is likely that the rate and pattern of development of fibrosis in some types of liver injury are determined to some extent by the amount of stroma normally present in these vessels.

The principal problem of the efferent circulation is chronic obstruction of its outflow. Obstruction is seldom noted at the level of the hepatic veins, although this effect, due to suppurative phlebitis, is occasionally seen in cows, and space-occupying lesions in critical positions occur in all species. Caudal caval compression or thrombosis contributes some cases, but most cases by far are due to passive congestion as a result of cardiac failure or constrictive pericarditis, accompanied by ascites.

Passive venous congestion denotes an elevation of pressure in the hepatic veins and venules relative to the pressure in the portal venules. This may be due to congestive heart failure, or much less frequently, to partial obstruction of the larger hepatic veins or posterior vena cava by abscess or neoplasm. It is also seen when part of the liver is incarcerated as a result of diaphragmatic hernia, or when a lobe is subjected to chronic partial torsion. When the liver is simply engorged with blood as a result of anaphylaxis, shock, or other acute insult, it is simply said to be congested.

In the early stages, the liver is swollen, dark, and bloody on section, and there is little accentuation of the acinar pattern. There is usually excessive blood-tinged abdominal fluid, because the congested liver elaborates lymph at a vastly increased rate; this may be seen exuding from the capsule and distending hilar and gallbladder lymphatics in fresh carcasses. Because this lymph is rich in most clotting factors, it tends to clot on the liver capsule, and the lobes may be stuck together by wads of fibrin, which are often blood tinged (Fig. 2.9A).

In passive congestion of longer duration, the capsular surface takes on a finely nodular texture and becomes thick and gray, and the fibrin deposits may become organized into flat, tough, capsular plaques (Fig. 2.9C). In dogs and cats, the edges of the central lobes become rounded, while the margins of lateral and caudate lobes are sharpened by peripheral atrophy and fibrosis (Fig. 2.10A). If the cause of the congestion is still present, there is usually copious ascites at this stage. Slicing a chronically congested liver reveals a reticulated acinar pattern, which is often more obvious beneath the capsule than in deeper parenchyma. This pattern is known as ''nutmeg liver'' and is due to

the contrast of the red color of periacinar necrosis and blood replacement with the pallid, slightly raised periportal tissue consisting of surviving but fatty hepatocytes (Fig. 2.9B). This pattern may be mimicked by some forms of toxic periacinar necrosis or fatty change but should always be distinguishable from them by the presence of capsular fibrin or fibrous plaques in the passively congested liver.

The microscopic picture in acute passive congestion is one of fairly uniform sinusoidal engorgement, with accompanying distension of lymphatics in the stroma of hepatic veins, portal triads, and capsule. There follows rapidly fatty change, atrophy, and necrosis of periacinar hepatocytes; these cells are not replaced while poor sinusoidal circulation persists. The reticulum framework in the periacinar zone, however, remains, and erythrocytes tend to percolate into the spaces left by the hepatocytes and may be trapped there when blood drains from sinusoids and veins in freshly fixed sections (Fig. 2.9D). The intrahepatic network of lymphatics at this stage becomes very distended and may form extensive cavernous channels about hepatic veins and venules, in portal triads, and just beneath the capsule. Distension of the space of Disse may be seen, but rarely if ever in tissue well fixed soon after death, and is best regarded as a postmortem artifact. The parenchyma that lies against the larger portal areas is periportal in a geographic sense only, and not in a functional or circulatory sense. In fact, much of it is relatively peripheral in a circulatory sense, so there should be no surprise in finding that in a suitable plane of section, the zones of hemorrhage and necrosis cut back to involve the parenchyma against the larger portal tracts, thereby isolating small, viable clumps of tissue about the terminal portal venules.

Over longer periods, the stagnant blood and remnants of stroma in the periacinar zones are gradually replaced by fibrous tissue, which links hepatic venules with one another and with the larger portal triads; in other words, simple and compound acini are outlined by periacinar fibrosis. This pattern of hepatic fibrosis is known as cardiac fibrosis (Fig. 2.10B).

Portocaval Shunts

Portocaval shunts may be either congenital or acquired. Congenital shunts may be extra- or intrahepatic anomalous channels. They are usually large and single, and the extrahepatic shunts may occur between the portal vein and the abdominal posterior vena cava, or the portal vein may bypass the liver via a connection with the azygous vein.

The **intrahepatic congenital shunts** usually involve anomalous persistence of the fetal ductus venosus, which instead of closing at birth, forms a dilated, thin-walled, and somewhat sigmoid channel that directly connects the portal vein with the hepatic veins.

Congenital portosystemic shunts are seen in cats but are more frequent in dogs, which are mostly presented as adolescents with failure to thrive or with the nervous signs of hepatic encephalopathy (see Liver Failure).

The liver that has been bypassed by a congenital shunt is very small (Fig. 2.11A) because it has been deprived of primary perfusion by portal hepatotrophic factors such as insulin, glucagon, and amino acids. These livers may be smooth surfaced and normal in color and texture, but histologically, the

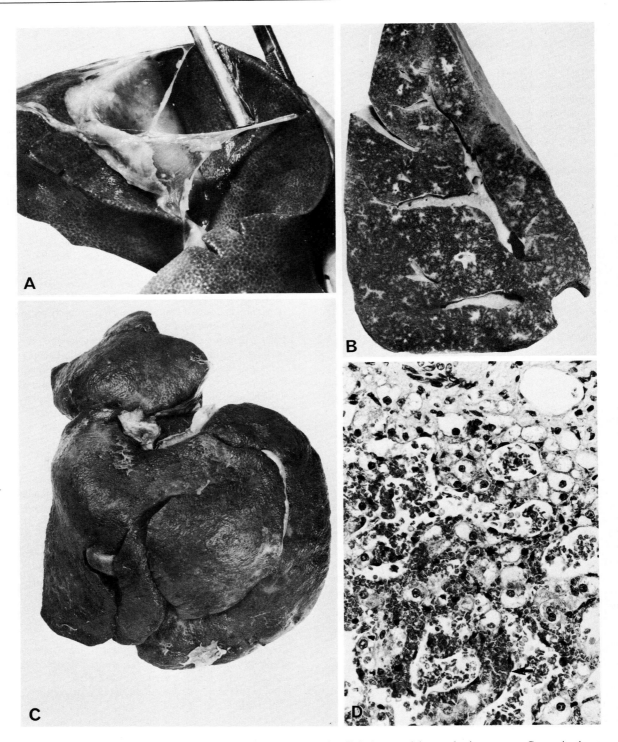

Fig. 2.9. (A) Severe subacute passive congestion of liver, showing fibrin between lobes, and acinar pattern. Congestive heart failure. Dog.   (B) Chronic passive congestion (''nutmeg liver''). Ox.   (C) Capsular irregularity and patchy fibrosis in chronic passive congestion. Dog.   (D) Atrophy and loss of periacinar hepatocytes (arrow) and replacement of them by erythrocytes within the remaining reticulin framework. Passive congestion. Dog.

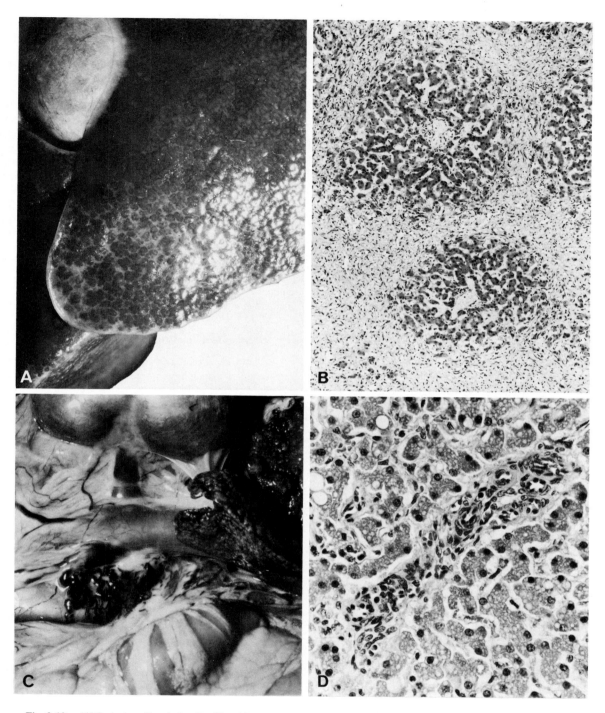

Fig. 2.10. (**A**) Periacinar fibrosis (cardiac fibrosis), most severe at the periphery of the lobe in chronic passive congestion. Chronic heartworm disease. Dog. (**B**) Section of (**A**). (**C**) Acquired portosystemic shunts (from mesentery to right renal vein) in chronic liver disease. The shunts are thin walled and plexiform. Dog. (**D**) Portal triad. Pup with congenital portocaval shunt (see Fig. 2.11A). The portal venule is indiscernible, there are several hepatic arterioles, and hepatocytes are atrophic.

hepatocytes are very small. Portal veins in the smaller triads are small or absent, and the hepatic arterioles are often prominent and multiple (Fig. 2.10D).

Acquired shunts may be difficult to identify postmortem, and they are likely to be overshadowed by rather more dramatic liver changes than is the case with congenital shunts. To be classified as *acquired,* the shunts should be associated with evidence of portal hypertension, such as distension of the portal veins and ascites. The shunts tend to develop between cranial mesenteric veins and the posterior vena cava, right renal vein, or gonadal veins and are multiple, taking the form of a plexus of tortuous, thin-walled vessels (Fig. 2.10C). Portosystemic diversion may take place via the veins of the caudal esophagus or hemorrhoidal veins, as in humans, but these shunts are even more difficult to demonstrate than the portocaval ones.

Livers associated with secondary shunting are also small but show variable nodularity and increase in proportion of fibrous tissue. The cause of the degeneration is rarely apparent; there may be chronic, diffuse, progressive inflammation, or simply nodular regeneration among bands of condensed stroma.

A distinctive form of congenital liver disease has been described in young dogs that develop extrahepatic shunts early in life as a result of portal fibrosis and deficiency of smaller radicles of the portal veins. These animals are presented with hepatic encephalopathy and ascites, and the shunts are multiple and resemble those seen in acquired liver disease. This condition has been designated as **hepatoportal fibrosis**. The only clear distinction from acquired hepatic disease is the pattern of portal fibrosis, the absence of small portal venules, distension of the larger intrahepatic branches of the portal vein, and the immaturity of the animals. Grossly, the livers are small, show irregular capsular depressions, or are finely nodular throughout. A few cases of congenital **portosystemic shunting** have been described in dogs with arteriovenous fistulas involving the hepatic artery and the portal vein. Retrograde flow of portal blood, portal hypertension, and portocaval shunts develop in these animals.

Telangiectasis

Telangiectasis is a cavernous ectasia of groups of sinusoids that occurs in all species but is particularly common in cattle. The lesion is not functionally significant.

Telangiectases occur throughout the liver as dark red areas, irregular in shape but well circumscribed, and ranging from pinpoints to many centimeters in size. Sectioned or capsular surfaces are depressed after death, and on cutting they appear as cavities from which the blood drains to reveal a delicate network of residual stroma and strands of atrophic hepatocytes.

Telangiectasis in feline liver is quite common in older animals. As with the bovine lesion, there is no evidence clinically of related liver dysfunction. In cats, the cavities are rather more frequent in the subcapsular zone (Fig. 2.11C) and rarely exceed 2–3 mm in size. There are often other senile changes in these livers, such as chronic fatty change, nodular hyperplasia, and chronic cholangiohepatitis, but there is no evidence that these changes have any causal relationship to the telangiectasis. In livers that bear early telangiectases, there are usually small foci of mononuclear cells that are intimately associated with a few

degenerate hepatocytes in the center of the cluster. The reaction is reminiscent of cell-mediated immune reactions and suggests the possible pathogenetic mode.

The term **peliosis hepatis** has been used for a long time to designate focal, blood-filled spaces in the liver in humans; these lesions are of unknown cause and were originally described in tuberculous patients and, more recently, in association with therapy by various steroids. There is a similarity between the changes of telangiectasis and peliosis, but to consider them identical is probably an error. One form of sinusoidal dilatation in cattle is named peliosis, specifically to differentiate it from bovine telangiectasis. This form, unlike telangiectasis, begins as a diffuse periportal sinusoidal dilatation (Fig. 2.11D) and develops in cattle poisoned by *Pimelea* spp. (members of the Thymelaeaceae). These changes appear to be adaptive to progressive and dramatic increases in total blood volume, which may actually double. In the late stages of the intoxication, the liver may resemble a huge, blood-filled sponge; other organs with sinusoidal circulation are affected to a lesser degree. The animals eventually die of a combination of hemodilutional anemia and circulatory failure.

Inflammation of the Liver and Biliary Tract

The term hepatitis is reserved for hepatic lesions, focal or diffuse, that are known or reasonably assumed to be caused by infectious agents, including parasites, or are lesions that reveal the full inflammatory response, irrespective of the cause. This definition allows us to include viral infections that are hepatotropic even though the lesions are necrotizing and not easily distinguishable, except by the presence of inclusion bodies, from toxic necrosis.

There are, in inflammations of the liver, some reactions that are specifically hepatic but not specifically inflammatory. Edema of the liver occurs in diffuse hepatitis or diffuse cholangitis, but also in severe toxic injury and passive congestion, and is directly related to hyperemia. Grossly, edema is not evident unless it involves the gallbladder, as it often does, or the large extrahepatic bile ducts. Microscopically, edema is evident in the portal triads and sometimes in the adjacent parenchyma as a clear separation of the sinusoidal lining cells from the hepatic cords by fluid that is often rich in protein.

Mobilization of the Kupffer cells and their related histiocytes in the portal units is a response to inflammation of the liver. This also occurs in many diseases of which hepatitis is not a part, the Kupffer cells merely participating in the monocyte–macrophage activity of engulfing circulating matter such as bacteria in subacute bacteremia, erythrocytes in the hemolytic anemias, or even breakdown products of hepatic cells in hepatic injuries of many causes. Active Kupffer cells increase in number and size, the nuclei become large and vesicular, and the cytoplasm is basophilic and may contain vacuoles or ingested particulate matter. In overwhelming infections, many of the Kupffer cells are dead, and only naked yeastlike nuclei may be present.

A diffuse sequestration of leukocytes (Fig. 2.19C) in the sinusoids (hepatic leukocytosis) occurs in many acute or subacute bacteremias just as they become sequestered in the pulmonary vessels to produce one anatomic form of interstitial pneu-

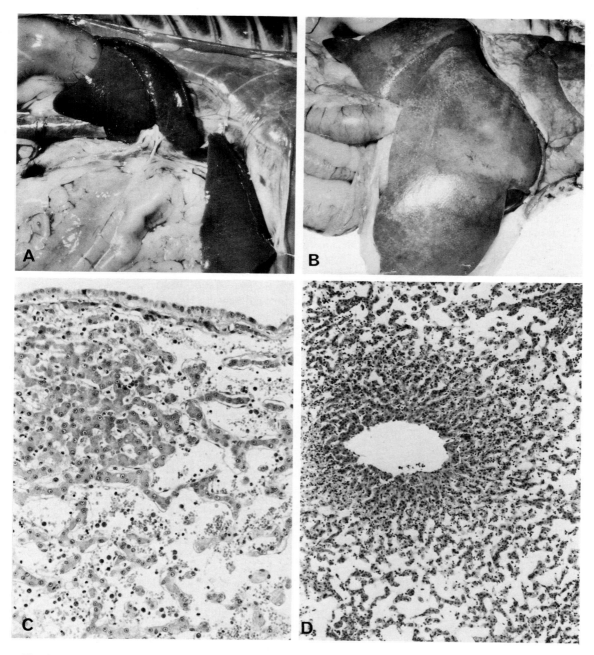

Fig. 2.11. (**A**) Small liver in a pup with congenital portocaval shunt (persistent sinus venosus). For histology, see Fig. 2.10D. (**B**) Extreme hepatomegaly due to steroid hepatopathy (functional adrenocortical adenoma). Dog. For histology, see Fig. 2.3A. (**C**) Subcapsular telangiectasis. Cat. (**D**) Periportal sinusoidal dilatation. Chronic *Pimelea* poisoning. Ox.

monia. While they are certainly of functional significance in the lung when numerous, they are probably not so in the liver. Hepatic leukocytosis may be very difficult to distinguish from myeloid metaplasia, which develops when the liver attempts to assume the functions of an incompetent bone marrow.

Agents capable of causing hepatitis include viruses, bacteria, spirochetes, fungi, and helminths. They will be discussed in this order, excepting the fungi and spirochetes. The systemic my-

coses frequently involve the liver, but these diseases have been discussed with other organs or systems. The spirochetal disease, leptospirosis, is discussed with the Hematopoietic System (Volume 3). Hepatitis is a particularly common lesion in autopsy material, and in the livers of almost all adult animals there are traces of inflammation, usually insignificant in degree and obscure in pathogenesis.

The conventional signs of acute inflammation are those that

occur in vascular connective tissue, which in the liver is restricted to portal triads and the surrounds of the bile duct. Inflammatory phenomena in these tissues are easily overlooked, but they are nonetheless important in hepatitis, which may be associated with subtle primary lesions in the parenchyma. This is often the case with viral infections. The capsule of the liver is well supplied with lymphatics, and exudation from these may be indicative of diffuse hepatic inflammation; the exudates are removed by normal visceral movements, and the residues on the surfaces of the liver must be looked for carefully. Within the parenchyma, the indicators of inflammation consist of aggregations of inflammatory cells in the sinusoids, lymphatic distension and edema in the portal triads, and the presence in the triads of a few leukocytes.

Acute diffuse hepatitis is a common pathologic change in animals. Its epidemiologic characteristics are those of the infecting agent, which is usually viral, and it is, grossly, difficult to recognize in the absence of visible necrosis. In the dog, acute diffuse hepatitis is best exemplified in infectious canine hepatitis and toxoplasmosis. The herpesvirus infections of neonatal calves and foals produce an acute hepatitis, as does Rift Valley fever in lambs.

The causes of focal hepatitis include those of focal necrosis, as discussed earlier. The foci may be few or numerous and may be acute or chronic in their characteristics, or granulomatous, and reaction may be sufficient to cause swelling of the organ. Foci of hepatitis that lack specificity are common incidental findings microscopically. They are assumed to reflect Kupffer-cell activity against enteric bacteria, but focal leukocyte reactions to cell death also occur in accelerated single-cell necrosis.

Cholangiohepatitis

Inflammation of the gallbladder is cholecystitis. Inflammation of the bile ducts is cholangitis. Inflammation of the smallest bile ducts, the intrahepatic cholangioles, almost never occurs in animals, but when it does, it can be labeled cholangiolitis. The divisions are largely artificial. Cholecystitis may occur alone if the neck of the bladder is obstructed. Cholangiolitis may occur alone, and in humans is thought to be associated with altered permeability of the cholangioles for bile. It is more usual for inflammation in the biliary system in animals to involve all of it. Involvement of the periportal hepatic parenchyma by extension of inflammation from the ducts is almost inevitable, and the lesions can quite accurately be regarded as cholangiohepatitis.

Cholangiohepatitis in animals is usually attributable to parasites, their effects aggravated by bacteria. It is also the specific lesion produced by the fungal toxin sporidesmin. Bacterial cholangiohepatitis is relatively uncommon.

The pathogenesis of bacterial cholangiohepatitis is similar to the pathogenesis of pyelonephritis, the main questions concerning whether the bacteria arrive hematogenously and descend in the ducts to produce inflammation or ascend the ducts from the intestine, and whether in either event there is some predisposition. If bacterial cholangiohepatitis is to develop, as opposed to the mere presence of organisms in bile, then stasis in the biliary system is required. It is sometimes possible to demonstrate a mechanical obstruction to the flow of bile. This may be a tumor of the pancreas, or scar tissue derived from an inflammatory process in an adjacent viscus, such as granulomatous or suppurative gastritis, suppurative lymphadenitis of the hilar nodes, or a primary hepatic abscess situated at the hilus. There may be no obvious mechanical obstruction save that produced by the cholangitis itself.

Several bacterial species that produce bacteremic disease are eliminated in the bile, the Salmonelleae being the best known example, and it may be assumed from this that there is a continuous normal portal–biliary circulation of enteric microorganisms. Bacterial cholangiohepatitis is usually caused by nonspecific organisms, such as coliforms and streptococci, which are probably of enteric origin. Descending infections of hematogenous origin are at least feasible, if there is relative stasis in the extrahepatic ducts.

What are clearly descending inflammations are occasionally observed in cattle. They take their origin in traumatic suppurative hepatitis and may extend directly from the suppurative focus or arise as "seedings" from inflamed intrahepatic lymphatics. Cholangiohepatitis of this origin may be restricted in its distribution to biliary fields, but it does in some cases become quite diffuse in the biliary system.

The course and pathologic changes in cholangiohepatitis vary greatly, from a fulminating suppurative infection to a persistent but mild inflammation that over a period of months or years leads to hepatic fibrosis of biliary distribution. Severe suppurative cholangiohepatitis may follow a short course to death, the effects being those of the infection itself, which may become septicemic, rather than of hepatic injury. At autopsy, the liver is swollen, soft, and pale, and its architecture is blurred. Few or many suppurative foci may be visible beneath the capsule and on the cut surface (Fig. 2.12A). They are small, sometimes miliary in distribution, and not encapsulated. Lesions in other organs may be those of septicemia and jaundice. Microscopically, the larger ducts contain purulent exudate, and the smaller ones are disintegrated. Dense masses of neutrophils, liquefied or not, are present in the portal triads and infiltrate the degenerate parenchyma.

In subacute and chronic cholangiohepatitis, the inflammation is more proliferative than exudative. The liver is enlarged and may be of normal shape, or distorted owing to irregular areas of atrophy and regenerative hyperplasia. Its surface may be smooth or finely granular; the capsule is thickened and may bear fibrous villi or be adherent to adjacent viscera. Eventually, jaundice develops, and the organ is pigmented with bile. On the cut surface, the enlarged portal tracts are easily visible and accentuate the architecture of the organ. Eventually, the new fibrous tissue replaces the parenchyma, and in chronic diffuse cases in which the original infection persists, continuous fibroplasia may produce hepatic enlargement, the organ becoming huge, gray, and gristly. Alternatively, the chronic fibrosis may occur in wedge-shaped areas oriented to a small bile duct. The enlarged interlobular ducts may be readily visible and frequently contain plugs of inspissated secretion and debris.

Microscopically, the reaction remains centered on portal tracts (Fig. 2.12D). These are expanded in subacute cases by infiltration of leukocytes and histiocytes and the proliferation of small ducts (Fig. 2.12C), and in chronic cases, chiefly by organizing fibrous tissue and proliferating bile ducts. Encroachment

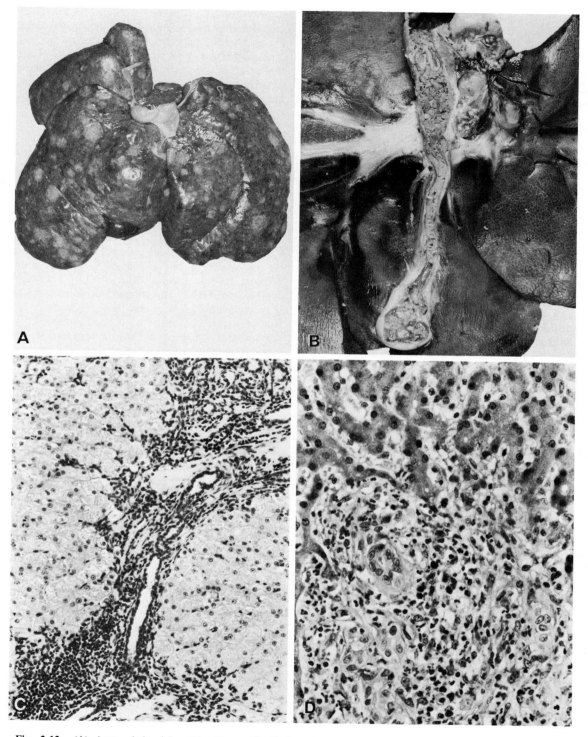

Fig. 2.12. (**A**) Acute cholangiohepatitis. Dog. (**B**) Cholangitis and cholecystitis secondary to *Ascaris suum* invasion. Pig. (**C**) Lymphocytic cholangiohepatitis. Cat. (**D**) Cholangiohepatitis. Dog. Destruction of limiting plate.

on the parenchyma is minimal but inevitable (Fig. 2.12D). Continued degeneration of the periportal parenchyma probably is an additional stimulus to local fibroplasia, which as well as thickening the smallest portal triads, extends along their length and links up with neighboring triads, thus subdividing the acini into segments. The hepatic venules and sublobular veins are involved. Regenerative nodules are not a prominent feature of cholangiohepatitis unless large areas of parenchyma have been destroyed, in which case the least damaged lobes are expanded by coarse nodules.

Chronic cholangitis and cholangiohepatitis of ill-defined cause occur in mature cats, often in conjunction with a low-grade interstitial pancreatitis. The inflammatory portal infiltrate is dominated by lymphocytes (Fig. 2.12C), but there is also scant participation by granulocytes, including eosinophils. These animals develop some portal fibrosis, bile ductular proliferation, and eventually, a degree of hepatic remodeling due to fibrosis. The condition has been observed to regress after prednisolone therapy and has been compared to primary biliary cirrhosis. In the cat and horse, however, the biliary and pancreatic ducts have a common entry to the duodenum, and simultaneous infectious inflammation of these systems is common.

Chronic active hepatitis is used to designate a pattern of chronic, progressive inflammation of the liver in humans, many cases of which follow hepatitis B virus infection. Identical liver changes, however, may occur in immune-mediated diseases, such as systemic lupus erythematosus, and in some idiosyncratic drug reactions. There is chronic inflammation of the portal tracts, extending into the periportal parenchyma, obliterating first the limiting plate and then more distant hepatocytes. In this process, known as piecemeal necrosis, individual and small groups of hepatocytes are isolated by fine, fibrous septa and small groups of inflammatory cells of various types. Piecemeal necrosis may eventually account for enough of the parenchyma to cause liver failure; nevertheless, nodular regeneration is not a regular feature, even of chronic cases.

There is considerable overlap between the morphologic features of chronic active hepatitis as described in humans and of chronic cholangiohepatitis. There is increasing interest in hepatic disease in dogs with features resembling the human disease (Fig. 2.13C), but stringent clinical, immunologic and pathologic criteria will need to be applied before chronic active hepatitis can be established as a separate entity in animals.

Cholelithiasis, Obstruction, and Rupture of the Biliary Tract

Cholelithiasis (gallstones) is seldom observed in animals. The stones usually form in the gallbladder and are composed of a mixture of cholesterols, bile pigments, salts of bile acids, calcium salts, and a proteinaceous matrix. Such stones of mixed composition are yellowish black or greenish black and are friable. There may be hundreds of small ones or a few large ones (Fig. 2.14B). The large stones are usually faceted. The origin of these mixed gallstones is uncertain, but their development is probably secondary to chronic mild cholecystitis and related to disturbances of the resorptive activities of the gallbladder, whereby the bile salts are removed faster than the stone-forming compounds. Calculi seldom form in the ducts, although cal-

careous stones may do so in distomiasis of cattle. Gallstones are usually asymptomatic. Occasionally, they lodge in and obstruct bile ducts to cause jaundice. The larger stones may cause pressure necrosis and ulceration of the mucosa, local dilatations of the bile ducts, and saccular diverticula of the gallbladder.

Occasionally, particles of solid ingesta may find their way into the gallbladder; sand has been seen in sheep, and seeds in pigs.

Biliary **obstruction** in animals is rarely due to impacted gallstones. Usually it is due to cholangitis, the obstruction being produced by masses of detritus and biliary constituents, parasites, or cicatricial stenosis of the ducts. Adult ascarids may cause mechanical obstruction (Fig. 2.12B). Tumors of the pancreas and duodenum, and tumors and abscesses of the hilus of the liver and portal nodes, may cause compression stenosis of the ducts.

Edematous swelling of the papilla in enteritis may also be of significance. The consequences of biliary obstruction depend on the site and duration of the obstruction. When the main duct is involved, there is jaundice. When one of the hepatic ducts is involved, there is no jaundice, and depending on the efficiency of biliary collaterals, there may be no pigmentation of the obstructed segments of liver. The ducts undergo progressive cylindric dilatation, which may be extreme. The smallest interlobular ducts and the cholangioles proliferate. There is inflammation in the walls of the ducts and the portal triads, and this is probably due in part to chemical irritation by bile acids but is due largely to secondary bacterial infections. These infections may be acute and purulent, or low grade; in these cases, bacteria may not be easily cultured. The cholangiohepatitis that almost inevitably follows has been described earlier.

Inflammatory stenoses of larger ducts may recanalize via mucosal glands, which can proliferate and link up to form a tortuous detour around the obstruction.

Rupture of the biliary tract or the gallbladder causes steady leakage of bile into the peritoneal cavity, the omentum being unable to seal even small defects. The bile salts are very irritating and may cause acute chemical peritonitis. The peritoneal effusion that follows may remain sterile; more often it is infected by enteric bacteria, and severe diffuse peritonitis ensues. This may be rapidly fatal, particularly if clostridia are involved. Most perforations of the biliary tract are traumatic in origin.

Virus Diseases of the Liver

Herpesvirus infections (Fig. 2.16C) are discussed with diseases of the fetus and newborn in the Female Genital System (Volume 3), feline infectious peritonitis is discussed with the Peritoneum, Retroperitoneum, and Mesentery (this volume) and the parvoviruses (Fig. 2.17A) of dogs and cats, with the Alimentary System (this volume).

INFECTIOUS CANINE HEPATITIS.   This virus can cause severe disease in dogs and other canids and is ubiquitous, being excreted in the urine for long periods by infected animals. Vaccination has greatly reduced the frequency with which the disease occurs, and it is now rare in many countries in which it was endemic. In areas where the disease is not controlled by vaccina-

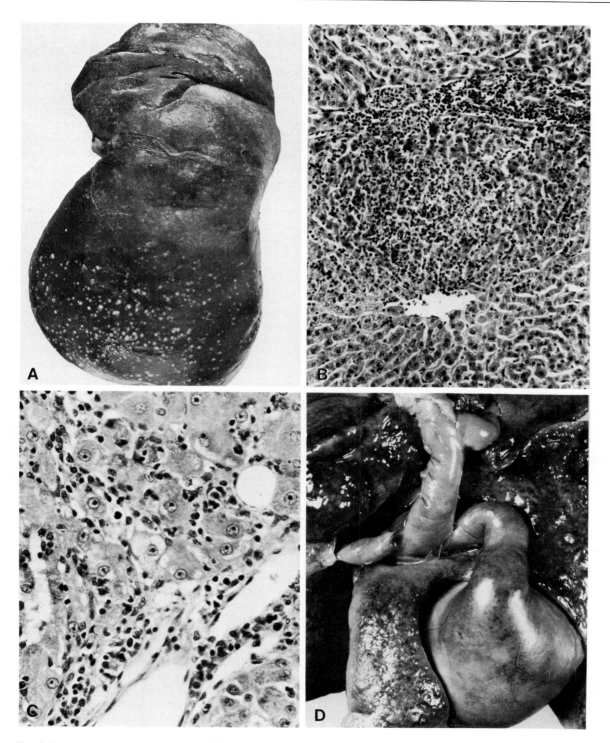

Fig. 2.13.   (**A**) Miliary abscesses in left lobe of liver. Neonatal listeriosis. Lamb.   (**B**) Focal hepatitis, the so-called sawdust of cattle.   (**C**) Periportal piecemeal necrosis and inflammation. So-called chronic active hepatitis. Dog.   (**D**) Common bile duct obstruction and ascending cholangiohepatitis. Dog.

tion, it is probable that most dogs in the general population contact the virus in the first 2 years of life and suffer either an inapparent infection or a mild febrile illness with pharyngitis and tonsillitis. In more severe cases there is vomiting, melena, high fever, and abdominal pain. There may be petechiae on the gums; the mucous membranes are blanched and only occasionally are they slightly jaundiced. Nervous signs of nonspecific character occur in a few cases. There is also a peracute form of the disease in which the animal is found dead without signs of illness, or after an illness of a few hours only. In convalescence, there may be a unilateral or bilateral opacity of the cornea caused by edema, which disappears spontaneously (Fig. 2.14C).

Deaths from infectious canine hepatitis are usually sporadic, although small outbreaks occur among young dogs in kennels. Fatalities seldom occur among dogs more than 2 years of age.

The virus of infectious canine hepatitis has special tropism for endothelium, mesothelium, and hepatic parenchyma, and it is injury to these that is responsible for the pathologic features, hemorrhages, and hepatic necrosis. The histologic specificity of the lesions depends on the demonstration of large, solid intranuclear inclusion bodies in endothelium or hepatic parenchyma (Fig. 2.14D). Inclusions are occasionally observed in other differentiated cells but always have the same morphologic and tinctorial features, being deeply acidophilic with a bluish tint.

The morbid picture of spontaneously fatal cases is usually distinct enough to allow a diagnosis to be made at gross postmortem. The superficial lymph nodes are edematous, slightly congested, and often hemorrhagic. Blotchy hemorrhages may be present on the serous membranes (Fig. 2.15D), and there is usually a small quantity of fluid, clear or blood-stained, in the abdomen. Hemorrhages on the serosa of the anterior surface of the stomach are usually linear, the so-called paintbrush type. Jaundice, if present, is slight. The mesenteries are slightly moist, and the serosa of the small intestine has a ground-glass appearance. The liver is slightly enlarged, with sharp edges, and is turgid and friable, sometimes congested, with a fine, uniform, yellowish mottling. Red strands of fibrin can be found on its capsule, especially between the lobes. In the majority of cases the wall of the gallbladder is edematous (Fig. 2.15C); when the edema is mild it may be detected only in the attachments of the gallbladder. In some cases in which the gallbladder is edematous, it may also be darkened by intramural hemorrhages.

Gross lesions in other organs are inconstant. Small hemorrhagic infarcts may be found in the renal cortices of young puppies. Hemorrhages may occur in the lungs, and occasionally there are irregular areas of hemorrhagic consolidation in the diaphragmatic lobe. Hemorrhages in the brain occur in a small percentage of cases. These are capillary and venular hemorrhages best appreciated when darkened by formalin, and then, depending on their concentration, the affected portions of brain appear grayish or dark brown. Microscopic hemorrhages occur in any part of the brain, but when numerous enough to be grossly visible, they are oddly confined to the midbrain and brain stem, avoiding the cerebral cortex and cerebellum (Fig. 2.15A). Hemorrhagic necrosis of medullary and endosteal elements occurs in the metaphyses of long bones in young dogs, and the hemor-

rhages are readily visible through the thin cortex of the distal ends of the ribs.

At low magnification, the histologic changes in the liver are quite reminiscent of the zonal necrosis of acute hepatotoxicities. There is an as yet unexplained susceptibility of the periacinar parenchyma to necrosis in this disease (Fig. 2.15B). Close to the portal triads, the hepatocytes may be near normal in appearance, except for loss of basophilia and the presence of a scattering of inclusion bodies. In spontaneously fatal cases, most of the parenchyma of the peripheral and central portions of the acini is dead, the hepatocytes having undergone granular acidophilic coagulation necrosis, and in some of these, ghosts of inclusion bodies may be detectable. The margin between necrotic parenchyma and viable tissue is usually quite sharp, although in the viable tissue there are many individual hepatocytes undergoing apoptosis, most of them without inclusion bodies. Fatty changes are common but not constant. The dead cells do not remain long, so the sinusoids become dilated and filled with blood. The reticulin framework remains intact, an observation in keeping with the fact that in recovered cases restitution of the liver is complete. Massive necrosis with collapse does not occur. As is typical of severe periacinar necrosis, the necrotic zones, initially eccentric areas about hepatic venules, extend and link up to isolate portal units. Intranuclear inclusions can be found in Kupffer cells in variable numbers. Many of the Kupffer cells are dead, others are proliferating, and others are actively phagocytic in the removal of debris. Leukocytic reactions in the liver are mild and are directed against the necrotic tissue; mononuclear cells are present, but neutrophils, many degenerating, predominate. There is some collection of bile pigment, but it is moderate, in keeping with the short course of the disease.

Microscopic lesions in other organs are due largely to injury to endothelium. Inclusion bodies in endothelial cells can be difficult to find and are looked for with most profit in renal glomeruli, where endothelium is concentrated. Occasionally, they are found in the epithelium of collecting tubules. When areas of hemorrhagic consolidation of the lungs are present, there is hemorrhage, edema, and fibrin formation in the alveoli, and in these consolidated areas, inclusions are often common in alveolar capillaries and even in dying cells of the bronchial epithelium. Changes in the brain are essentially secondary to vascular injury and may be absent. Hemorrhages, if present, are from capillaries and small venules, and inclusions in endothelial nuclei can usually be found in vessels that have bled. Other endothelial and adventitial cells are hyperplastic and mixed with a few lymphocytes. Small foci of softening or demyelination may be present in relation to the hemorrhages.

The lymphoreticular tissues are congested, and inclusions may be found in the primitive reticulum cells of follicles, in the red pulp of the spleen, and in histiocytes anywhere.

The detailed pathogenesis of infectious canine hepatitis has to be worked out. Many infections appear to be clinically silent, and other dogs recover after mild febrile disease with tonsillitis. The fulminating pattern of clinical disease and the possibility of convalescent phenomena need further examination. Some sudden deaths in this disease are associated with midbrain hemorrhage, and others occur with, at most, slight structural evidence

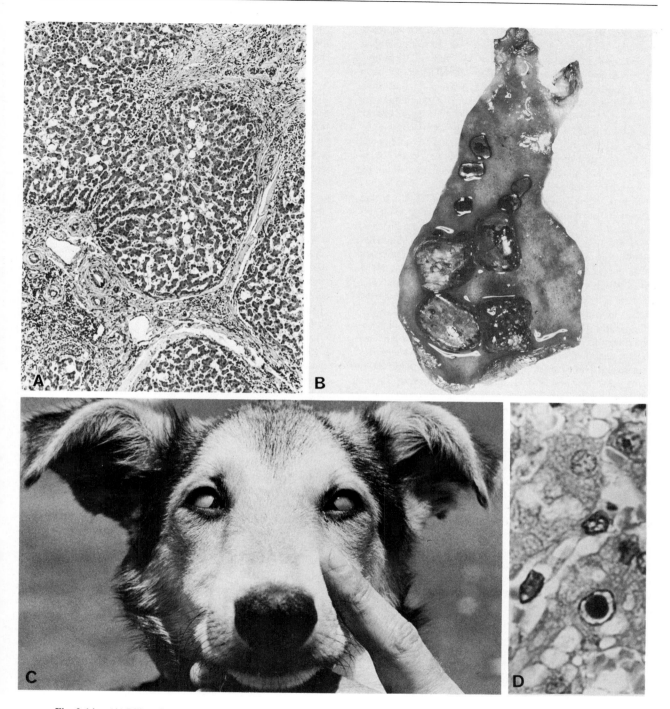

Fig. 2.14. (**A**) Biliary fibrosis secondary to chronic cholangitis. Dog. (**B**) Gallstones. Dog. (**C**) Corneal edema in convalescent stage of infectious canine hepatitis. (**D**) Infectious canine hepatitis. Intranuclear inclusion body in hepatocyte.

of liver injury. Following oral exposure, which is probably the natural route of infection, virus multiplication occurs in the tonsils and leads to tonsillitis. The tonsillitis is sometimes quite severe, with extensive clear edema of the throat and larynx. Fever accompanies the tonsillitis and apparently precedes the viremic phase, which is of short duration and accompanied by a severe leukopenia. Hepatic necrosis develops at about the seventh day of experimental infection. The sequence of developments in the liver is not clear, but it is possible that virus proliferation occurs first in Kupffer cells. In surviving animals, hepatic regeneration occurs rapidly, and there do not appear to be any significant residual lesions. Small foci of hepatocellular necrosis involving one to several liver cells may still be present at 2 weeks, and foci of proliferated Kupffer cells may be detectable for another week or two, but progressive hepatic injury does not occur in the natural disease. This is consistent with failure to demonstrate virus in the liver after about the tenth day of experimental infection. Focal interstitial nephritis occurs commonly, and the cellular infiltrates are persistent but not functionally significant. They consist of interstitial lymphocytic accumulations, especially about the corticomedullary junction and in the loose stroma of the pelvis.

Corneal edema is a late development (Fig. 2.14C). It may occur by the seventh day of infection but is usually delayed to between 14 and 21 days. Viral antigen can be detected in these eyes by fluorescent techniques, but not in the corneal structures. Inflammatory edema is present in iris, ciliary apparatus, and corneal propria, and inflammatory cells are abundant in the filtration angle and iris. The infiltrates are principally plasma cells, and there is evidence that the ocular lesion is a hypersensitivity reaction to viral antigen.

Originally it was assumed that the widespread tendency to hemorrhage in this disease was due to leakage from damaged vascular endothelium, coupled with an inability on the part of the damaged liver to replace clotting factors. While these effects play a role, it is now known that the exhaustion of clotting factors is in large part due to their accelerated consumption, as the widespread endothelial damage is a potent initiator of the clotting cascade.

WESSELSBRON DISEASE.   Wesselsbron disease is caused by an arthropod-borne virus that according to serological surveys is widespread in Africa in various species of animals and birds. Humans are also susceptible to clinical and inapparent infection. Rarely, the virus may produce outbreaks of abortion and perinatal death in sheep; susceptible adults rarely show clinical signs but may have a biphasic febrile response to infection.

The lesions in lambs dying within 12 hr of birth consist mainly of widespread petechiae and gastrointestinal hemorrhage; longer survival allows jaundice to develop, and the liver becomes orange-yellow, enlarged, friable, and patchily congested. The bile in the gallbladder becomes thick and dark in some cases, but this may be due more to hemorrhage into the gallbladder than to hemolysis. Lymph nodes are rather constantly enlarged, congested, and edematous.

The most characteristic histologic changes are seen in the liver. There is no zonal pattern of hepatocellular damage as in infectious canine hepatitis; rather, there are randomly scattered foci of necrosis, with apoptosis and proliferation of sinusoidal lining cells. Mononuclear cells and pigment-filled macrophages accumulate in the portal stroma as well as in the sinusoids. In a variable proportion of cases, hepatocyte nuclei may contain eosinophilic, irregular inclusions. These are not accompanied by as much margination of nuclear chromatin as that associated with conventional viral inclusions, and their significance at this stage is obscure. In jaundiced animals there may be considerable canalicular cholestasis; whether or not this is the result of hemolysis does not appear to have been determined. Hepatocellular

proliferation is apparent in the less acute cases. Lymphoid follicles in lymph nodes and spleen show pronounced lymphocyte necrosis and stimulation of lymphoblasts.

RIFT VALLEY FEVER.   Rift Valley fever is an arthropod-borne virus infection of ruminants in Africa and is in many respects similar to Wesselsbron disease. Rift Valley fever is, however, responsible for greater losses than the former infection. Morbidity and mortality may occur in adult sheep; death sometimes occur in adult cattle, but it is chiefly a disease of the young, causing heavy mortality among lambs and calves and abortion in ewes and cows.

As in Wesselsbron disease, the gross postmortem picture is dominated by widespread hemorrhage, ranging from serosal petechiae to severe gastrointestinal bleeding. The liver in the acute cases in neonatal lambs is similar to that in cases of Wesselsbron disease, being yellow, swollen, soft, and patchily congested or hemorrhagic. In older animals and in less acute cases, however, the liver tends to be darker and show scattered pale foci of necrosis 1–2 mm in diameter (Fig. 2.16A). There may be fibrinous perihepatitis, edema of the gallbladder wall, and a moderate, blood-tinged ascites.

Within 12 hr of experimental infection of lambs, there are randomly distributed foci of hepatocellular necrosis in the liver. These foci include knots of inflammatory cells and prominent apoptotic bodies and initially involve about half a dozen hepatocytes (Fig. 2.16B). Within a few hours, however, these primary foci enlarge and may become almost confluent. In the meantime, the remaining parenchyma may rapidly undergo necrosis that spares only a small rim of periportal hepatocytes. In naturally infected calves, the primary foci of necrosis undergo lysis more rapidly than the surrounding parenchyma; these foci thus have a striking "washed out" appearance. Where the expanding foci of necrosis include portal triads, there may follow fibrinous vasculitis and thrombosis. Fibrin deposition in sinusoids is common, and so is mineralization of necrotic hepatocytes. Cholestasis is apparent in sections but is not a prominent feature.

Eosinophilic intranuclear inclusion bodies, often elongated, are sometimes seen in degenerate hepatocytes; there is associated nuclear vesiculation and chromatin margination. There is necrosis in germinal centers of lymphoid follicles in lymph nodes and spleen similar to that seen in Wesselsbron disease. Renal glomerular hypercellularity and necrosis have been described in the experimental disease.

Ultrastructural studies have shown condensation of degenerate hepatocytes, abundant apoptosis, and the presence of mummified, membrane-bound fragments of hepatocellular cytoplasm, but sinusoidal lining cells are not notably damaged; the Kupffer cells instead participate in the uptake of the dying hepatocytes. There is abundant fibrin in sinusoids in the vicinity of the primary foci of necrosis and also within hepatocytes and macrophages. The intranuclear inclusions are not composed of recognizable virus particles but of filaments. Virus is discernible occasionally in the cytoplasm, associated with tubular membranes.

It seems that the primary infection of the liver produces the primary necrotic foci, from which more virus spreads to damage

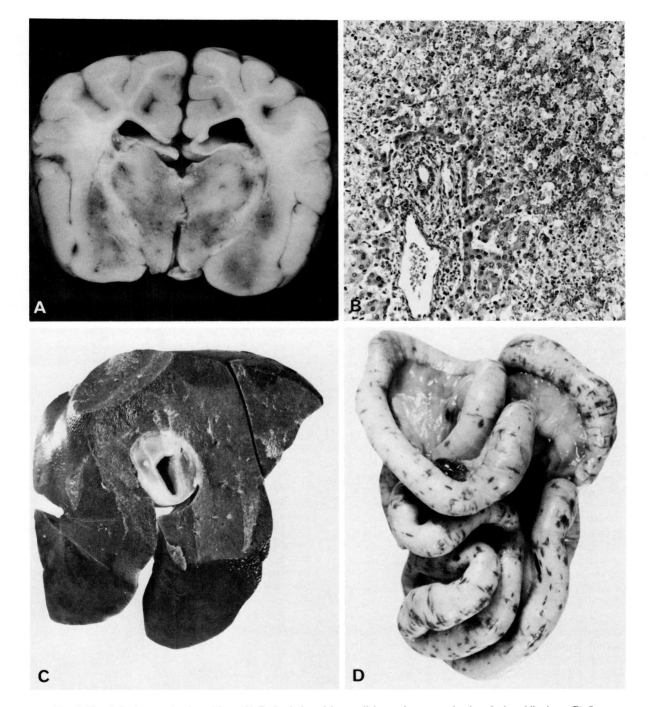

Fig. 2.15. Infectious canine hepatitis. **(A)** Brain darkened by small hemorrhages, predominantly in midbrain. **(B)** Severe periacinar necrosis with periportal survival. **(C)** Severe edema of gallbladder wall. **(D)** Serosal hemorrhages over intestine.

neighboring parenchyma; the virus clearly has a marked preference for hepatocytes over other tissues. The hemorrhagic component of the syndrome is probably related to consumption of clotting factors; there is no direct evidence for the endothelial damage seen in infectious canine hepatitis.

It is now evident that there has been some confusion in early reports from Africa of liver diseases of ruminants. Some cases of phyto- and mycotoxicosis and of chronic copper poisoning have probably been ascribed to virus infection, and vice versa. It is also understandable that Rift Valley fever and Wesselsbron disease may have been mistaken for one another, but it is now held that these two diseases may be distinguished by careful pathologic examination as well as by isolation of the viruses. In summary, Rift Valley fever is characterized by obvious focal hepatic necrosis, on which is superimposed an almost massive periacinar and midzonal necrosis; cholestasis is not as prominent as it is in Wesselsbron disease. The liver lesions in the latter disease consist of smaller, randomly distributed foci of hepatocellular necrosis, more active reaction by the sinusoidal lining cells, and more obvious cholestasis.

EQUINE SERUM HEPATITIS.   We are taking some liberty in including equine serum hepatitis under viral hepatitis, but we are impressed by its epidemiologic and pathologic similarities to so-called homologous serum jaundice, type B viral hepatitis of humans. The disease usually, but not invariably, occurs in horses that have been injected with equine serum or tissue emulsions and has a rather constant incubation period of 42 to 60 days, although this may be a few days shorter or up to a month longer. The disease was originally observed in horses passively immunized against African horse sickness and later in horses passively immunized against anthrax, tetanus, and equine encephalomyelitis. A high incidence has been observed in horses passively immunized against *Clostridium perfringens* toxins in an attempt to protect against grass sickness. Vaccines against equine viral rhinopneumonitis prepared from equine fetal tissue have produced the disease, and finally, the disease continues to be a problem where pregnant mare serum is routinely injected into mares at the time of breeding. In each of the above situations, the inoculated serum or tissue is of equine origin, and while such an association holds for the great majority of cases, there are many, but usually sporadic, cases that have certainly not been inoculated with anything. The origin of the infection, if it is such, in these latter cases is not known. The incidence of equine serum hepatitis among inoculated animals is very variable. Attempts to reproduce the disease by experimental transmission have rarely been successful. The disease is seldom diagnosed in the absence of acute neurologic disturbances, and at this stage is fatal. There are observations, however, that indicate that recovery after transient illness with jaundice is common, and that recovery is in some instances incomplete, such horses remaining stupid and intractable.

The onset of the clinical syndrome is usually sudden and the course short, death occurring in 6 to 24 hr or so. There is jaundice and neurologic disturbance, hyperexcitability, often with mania, continuous walking and pushing, apparent blindness, and ataxia. Death then occurs suddenly without a period of prostration.

At autopsy, icterus is present, there is moderate ascites, the spleen is normal or congested, and there may be petechial hemorrhages on serous membranes and renal cortices, and some congestion of the intestine with hemorrhage into its lumen. The characteristic lesions are hepatic. The liver usually is of normal size but may be slightly enlarged or shrunken, friable, and stained by bile pigments; its surface is mottled and may bear a few strands of fresh fibrin. The mottling is more evident on the cut surface, which appears as if severely congested and fatty (Fig. 2.5C).

The hepatic lesion is considerably older than the clinical course would suggest (Fig. 2.17B). There are a few swollen and fatty hepatocytes against the portal units, or there may be no normal parenchymal cells. Severe fatty changes, usually as single, very large globules, affect most of the cells of the acini. Acute necrosis is not in evidence, but in the periphery of the acini, severely fatty cells undergo dissolution to leave scattered fatty cysts, but most of them disappear to leave either sinusoids that are dilated and stuffed with blood or a condensed and distorted reticulin framework. There is no significant hemorrhage. Extensive deposits of bile pigments are present in Kupffer cells and hepatocytes. Leukocytes infiltrate diffusely but not in large numbers, lymphocytes, plasma cells, and histiocytes being present with a few neutrophils, many of which undergo necrobiotic changes. There is a diffuse but very slight fibroplasia, especially in the portal units. In some cases, there is attempted regeneration, small irregular columns of regenerating cells being present in the portal areas, apparently derived from cholangioles. Healed lesions have not been reported.

Bacterial Diseases of the Liver

Bacterial hepatitis is especially common, but except in some specific diseases or syndromes, it is not in itself often of much significance. Bacteria may gain entrance to the liver by direct implantation, as by foreign body penetrating from the reticulum; by invasion of the capsule from an adjacent focus of suppurative peritonitis; hematogenously via the hepatic artery, portal veins, and umbilical veins; or via the bile ducts.

Excepting peracute septicemias, there are few specific bacterial infections that have a sustained or repeated bacteremic phase without producing hepatic lesions, and there are, in addition, many cases of nonspecific bacteremia, especially portal in origin, in which focal hepatitis occurs. Because their differential diagnosis is of some importance, it is probably useful here to list those specific bacterial diseases in which focal hepatitis is expected or characteristic (but not constant). The specific infections may occur in the fetus, and it will be noted that many of these examples are fetal or perinatal infections. The list includes *Listeria monocytogenes* in fetal and neonatal lambs, calves, and piglets, *Campylobacter fetus* in fetal and neonatal lambs, *Actinobacillus equuli* in foals, *Yersinia pseudotuberculosis* in lambs and occasionally in dogs and cats, *Y. tularensis* in lambs, *Pasteurella haemolytica* and *Haemophilus agni* in lambs, *Salmonella* spp. in all hosts (Fig. 2.5B), *Nocardia asteroides* in dogs, and *Mycobacterium tuberculosis* in all hosts.

Hepatic Abscess

Hepatic abscesses, quite apart from the lesions of the specific infections just given, are common, especially in cattle. They may arise by direct implantation with a foreign body from the reticulum or by direct invasion of the capsule from a suppurative lesion of traumatic reticulitis and may be single or multiple, but in either case they are largely restricted to the extremity of the left lobe. They may be hematogenous from portal emboli or by direct extension of an omphalophlebitis (Fig. 2.18D). Arteriogenic abscesses via the hepatic artery may occur in pyemias but are quite uncommon.

Omphalogenic abscesses are more common in calves than in other species but occur in all. The bacterial flora is frequently

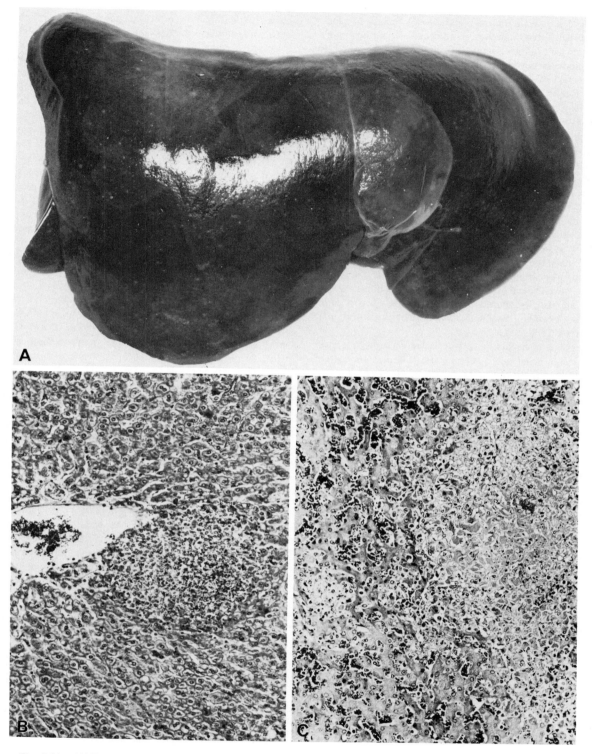

Fig. 2.16. (**A**) Experimental Rift Valley fever. Lamb. (Courtesy of B. C. Easterday.) (**B**) Random focal necrosis in early Rift Valley fever. Lamb. (**C**) Focal coagulative necrosis in equine herpesvirus type 1 infection. Foal.

mixed, but *Corynebacterium pyogenes,* streptococci, and staphylococci usually predominate or may be pure. Hepatic abscesses are not an inevitable sequel to omphalitis or even to omphalophlebitis, but they do not develop from navel infections in the absence of omphalophlebitis. There being no flow of blood in these vessels, involvement of the liver is by direct growth along the physiologic thrombus. Omphalophlebitis can be quite severe without extension to the liver. Hepatic abscesses of omphalogenic origin are often restricted to the left lobe (Figs. 2.13A and 2.18D), but they may be restricted to the right or be diffuse in their distribution.

Hepatic abscesses are also common and of much economic importance in cattle that have been fattened for slaughter. They are usually found at slaughter (Fig. 2.18C), but when numerous, may be fatal after a few days of vague digestive illness. Their pathogenesis and character are discussed with rumenitis (in the Alimentary System, this volume), to which they are a sequel.

Hepatic abscesses of biliary origin occur in all animals. They are perhaps most frequent in pigs in which ascarids have migrated into the bile ducts. Cholangitic abscesses in horses, dogs, and cats are usually caused by enterobacteria as part of a fulminating ascending cholangiohepatitis that is fatal after a short course (Fig. 2.12A).

The sequelae of hepatic abscessation are variable. Usually, they are insignificant and asymptomatic. Sterilization of the focus with either resorption and complete healing or encapsulation is common. Those near the surface of the liver regularly produce fibrinous and then fibrous inflammation of the capsule (Fig. 2.18C) and adhesion to adjacent viscera. They seldom perforate the capsule but do commonly break into hepatic veins to produce any one or combination of thrombophlebitis of the vena cava, endocarditis, or pulmonary abscesses or embolism. Generalization is common, especially from omphalogenic abscesses of young animals. In adults, death may occur if the abscesses are multiple and fresh, and especially if they are necrobacillary in origin; death is probably the result of toxemia.

Occasionally, *Fusobacterium necrophorum* infection of the liver is observed following omphalophlebitis in lambs and calves, or as a complication of rumenitis in adult cattle. The hepatic lesions are multiple and typical of necrobacillary infection, being slightly elevated, rounded, dry areas of coagulation necrosis, sometimes a few centimeters in diameter (Fig. 2.18B) and surrounded by a zone of intense hyperemia. Affected neonates seldom live long enough for the necrotic foci to liquefy and assume the appearance of ordinary abscesses, but this may be seen in adult cattle. The histologic appearance of the foci in the stage of coagulative necrosis is quite characteristic. The necrotic amorphous central area is bordered by a zone of wholesale destruction of leukocytes, whose nuclear chromatin is dissipated in a finely divided form, and among which the filamentous fusobacteria are mostly concentrated. Outside this zone there is severe hyperemia and hemorrhage, and thrombosis of local vessels is common. The lesion in neonatal lambs is to be distinguished from that caused by *Campylobacter fetus.*

BLACK DISEASE.   Organisms of the genus *Clostridium* are notably circuitous in their means of producing disease. This is true of *C. novyi,* the type B strains of which are the cause of black disease (infectious necrotic hepatitis). This particular type of *C. novyi* produces three potent exotoxins, namely, alpha (α), the classical lethal toxin of the species; beta (β), which is a necrotizing and hemolytic lecithinase; and zeta (ζ), which is hemolytic. Black disease is essentially an intoxication produced by these exotoxins, and its development requires a combination of circumstances, namely, a host that is not immune, a latent spore infection of tissue, (usually the liver), and some agency to injure the liver sufficiently to produce an anaerobic environment in which the spores can germinate and vegetate. This combination of circumstances takes place most commonly in sheep, in which an environment suitable for germination of the organism is produced by immature wandering *Fasciola hepatica.*

Clostridium novyi is widely distributed in soil. Its distribution is possibly related to the movements of animals and is, as judged by the distribution of black disease, increasing. The spores are continually being ingested by grazing animals in areas where black disease occurs, and some of them cross the mucous membranes, probably in phagocytes, and remain as latent infections in histiocytic cells, mainly in the liver, spleen, and bone marrow. The duration of latency in tissue is not known, but it can be many months, apparently. Many healthy sheep, cattle, and dogs harbor latent infections in their livers, the incidence of latent infections being much higher in animals that come from areas in which the disease is endemic than in animals from areas in which black disease does not occur endemically.

Black disease is principally a disease of sheep. It occurs in cattle, perhaps with a higher incidence than is generally appreciated. It is occasionally seen in horses. The distribution of black disease as an enzootic malady parallels the distribution of the common fluke *Fasciola hepatica,* which is in turn determined by the distribution of the snails that act as intermediate hosts for the flukes. In Bessarabia and France, it is endemically related to the distribution of *Dicrocoelium dendriticum,* the lancet liver fluke. Cases of sporadic distribution may be related to *Cysticercus tenuicollis,* or a provoking agency may not be detectable.

Deaths in sheep from black disease occur rapidly and usually without warning signs. Illness, if observed, is brief and characterized by reluctance to move, drowsiness, rapid respiration, and quiet subsidence. Affected animals are usually in good nutritional condition. Postmortem decomposition occurs rapidly.

The name of the disease is derived from the appearance of flayed skins, the dark coloration being caused by an unusual degree of subcutaneous venous congestion. Frequently, there is edema of the sternal subcutis. The serous cavities contain an abundance of fluid, which clots on exposure to air. The fluid is usually straw colored, but that in the abdomen may be tinged with blood. The volume of fluid in the abdomen and thorax may vary from about 50 ml to 1.5 liters. The pericardial sac is distended with similar fluid in amounts up to ~300 ml. Subendocardial hemorrhages in the left ventricle are almost constant. Patchy areas of congestion and hemorrhage may be present in the pyloric part of the abomasum and in the small intestine.

The typical and diagnostic lesions occur in the liver and are always present. They are usually clearly evident on the capsular surface, the diaphragmatic surface especially, but the organ may have to be sliced carefully to find them. The liver will be the seat of the acute traumatic hemorrhagic lesions of acute fascioliasis,

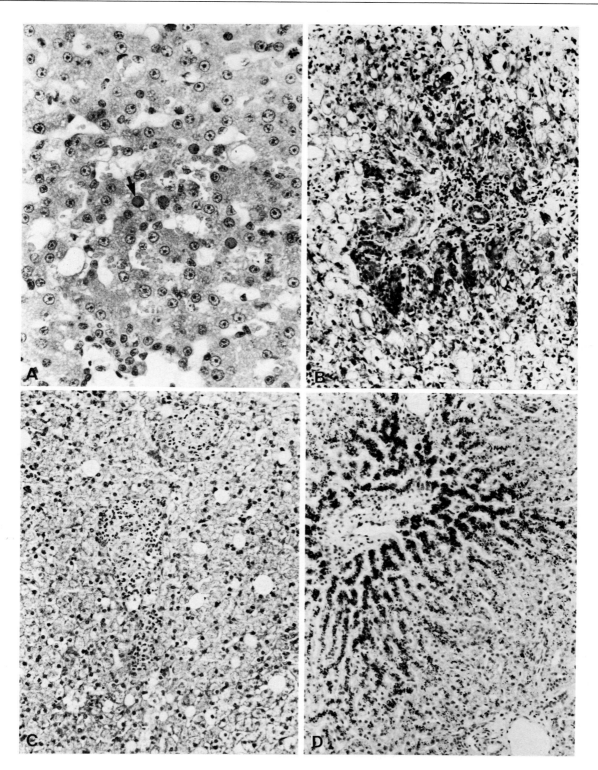

Fig. 2.17. (A) Parvovirus intranuclear inclusions (arrow) in feline panleukopenia. An uncommon finding in this disease. Kitten. (B) Equine serum hepatitis. Section of the liver in Fig. 2.5C, showing extensive periacinar degenerative changes, cellular infiltration, and periportal survival zone. (C) Liver of Bedlington terrier. Infiltrate of inflammatory cells and granular macrophages in portal stroma and random fatty change. (D) Section of the liver in (C), stained with rhodanine for copper. Predominantly periacinar distribution of lysosomal copper.

or the cholangiohepatitis of the chronic disease, or a mixture of both. It is also, in consequence of hydropericardium, congested. The lesion of black disease, and occasionally there are several, is a yellowish white area of necrosis 2–3 cm in diameter, surrounded by a broad zone of intense hyperemia, roughly circular in outline, and extending hemispherically into the substance of the organ (Fig. 2.19A). There may be a coagulum of fibrin on the capsular surface overlying the necrotic area. Occasionally, the essential lesions are rectilinear in shape or very irregular. The lesions appear homogeneous on the cut surface, but some contain poorly defined centers of soft or cheesy material.

The histologic evolution of the hepatic lesions begins with the necrotic and hemorrhagic tracts caused by wandering immature flukes. These are sinuous tunnels ~0.5 cm in diameter that contain blood, necrotic hepatic cells, and the leukocytes, chiefly eosinophils, attracted by the flukes. About the tunnels is a narrow zone of coagulative necrosis, also produced by the flukes. As usual, the necrotic tissue is demarcated by a thin zone of scavenger cells, chiefly neutrophils. If latent spores are present in the necrotic areas, they quickly vegetate and are visible in sections as large, Gram-positive bacilli. The vegetative organisms by means of their exotoxins cause necrosis of the surrounding tissue (Fig. 2.19B), including the eosinophils of the fluke tunnel. As the area of necrosis expands, the bacterial proliferation keeps pace so that bacilli can be found in all parts of the necrotic focus but not in the surrounding viable tissue. Usually they are concentrated at the advancing margin of the lesion, just inside a zone of infiltrated neutrophils. At about the time of death and immediately afterward, the bacilli scatter in the liver and to other organs.

BACILLARY HEMOGLOBINURIA. Bacillary hemoglobinuria is a counterpart of black disease. The cause is *Clostridium haemolyticum*, which may quite properly be regarded as a toxigenic type of *C. novyi*, both species producing the β toxin, which is a necrotizing and hemolytic lecithinase. The pathogenesis of the two diseases is comparable, both of them depending on a focus of hepatic injury within which latent spores can germinate. Bacillary hemoglobinuria as an endemic malady exists only in areas where *Fasciola hepatica* abounds, and it is probable that flukes are the main cause of the initiatory lesion. The disease does occur sporadically where there are no flukes and may be prompted by other parasites or other diverse focal lesions, which are smudged out in the expanding areas of necrosis. There is scant information on the ecology of the organism. Spores may persist in the bones of cadavers for 2 years. Spores of this and other sporulating anaerobes can frequently be demonstrated in the liver, where they are probably retained in Kupffer cells.

Bacillary hemoglobinuria occurs in cattle and rarely in other species. It is characterized clinically by intravascular hemolysis with anemia and hemoglobinuria, but, perhaps reflecting variety in exotoxins between strains of the organism, hemolysis may not be a feature. The essential lesion is hepatic and similar to that of black disease but is much larger and usually single. It has been described as an infarct secondary to portal thrombosis, and although this may occur in isolated cases, it is scarcely a creditable pathogenesis for a disease of endemic occurrence. Thrombosis

does occur in the affected areas but can be a result rather than a cause of the initial lesion and is found more frequently in the hepatic venules than in branches of the portal vein. There is severe anemia, the kidneys are speckled reddish or brown by hemoglobin, and the urine is of port wine color. The peritoneal vessels are injected, and in some cases there is severe, dry, fibrinohemorrhagic peritonitis.

BACILLUS PILIFORMIS INFECTION. *Bacillus piliformis* infection has been known for a long time as a cause of severe losses in laboratory rodents; however, it has also been reported in foals, dogs, and cats. Although the disease is probably initiated by an intestinal infection, lesions in the gut are less specific and constant than those in the liver, which consist of focal hepatitis and necrosis.

Affected foals usually die between the ages of 1 to 4 weeks; often they are found dead after a short illness. The liver shows pale foci up to a few millimeters across; these are represented microscopically by randomly distributed foci of coagulative necrosis with moderate polymorphonuclear inflammatory infiltrate. This lesion in itself is not diagnostic; its specificity depends on the presence of the causal organism in hepatocytes in the periphery of the necrotic zones. *Bacillus piliformis* can at present only be isolated with difficulty on artificial media, so diagnosis is usually based on the demonstration of the large, long bacilli in the cytoplasm of degenerate and also otherwise apparently normal hepatocytes at the periphery of the necrotic zones. The organisms are Gram-negative and are best delineated with silver-impregnation techniques such as that of Warthin–Starry, but they may be seen with routine stains, particularly when the material is fresh. The bacilli tend to lie in sheaves or bundles (Fig. 2.18A). There may also be colitis sufficiently severe to cause diarrhea, but not as severe as that seen in rabbits with this disease.

Only a few cases of Tyzzer's disease have been reported in dogs and cats, and it seems likely that some form of immunologic inadequacy is necessary to allow infection in these species. The liver lesions are essentially the same as those in foals and rodents, and there is also enteritis involving the small intestine.

Helminthic Inflammations of the Liver and Bile Ducts

A variety of helminths, cestodes, nematodes, trematodes, and even the degenerate arachnid *Linguatula serrata* produce inflammation of liver and bile ducts, and indeed, they are as a group the most common cause of hepatic inflammation. Some of these parasites have the biliary system as their final habitat, and these are the ones to be discussed in detail here. The others produce hepatic lesions in the course of their natural or accidental migrations, and the lesions are discussed with the parasites under the organ, for most of them the gut, that is their final habitat. It is useful to describe here the lesions produced by larvae in transit.

The initial lesion produced by wandering larvae is traumatic. Sinuous tunnels permeate the parenchyma and often breach the capsule. In the tunnel, there are hemorrhage, degenerating

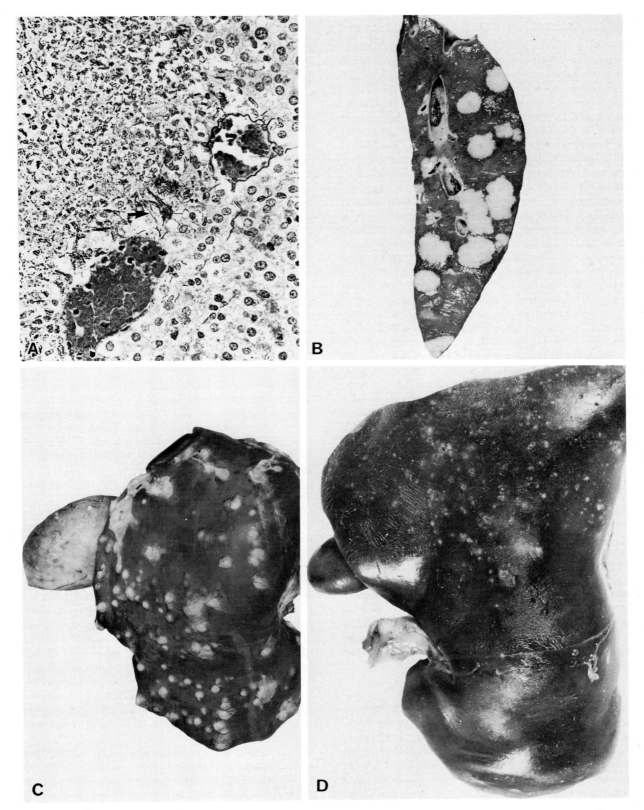

Fig. 2.18. (A) *Bacillus piliformis* infection (Tyzzer's disease). Foal. Focal hepatitis: organisms in bundles in hepatocytes at margin of lesion (arrow). Warthin–Starry stain. (B) Early hepatic necrobacillosis. *Fusobacterium necrophorum* infection. Ox. The pale areas of coagulative necrosis are bordered by acute inflammation. (C) Necrobacillosis of liver secondary to rumenitis. Ox. (D) Omphalophlebitis with miliary metastatic abscesses in right lobe. Calf.

hepatocytes, and leukocytes, chiefly eosinophils, which react to the parasites. Bordering the tunnel is a narrow zone of coagulation necrosis of parenchyma with infiltrated neutrophils at its margin. Eosinophils also infiltrate the portal triads. The necrotic parasitic tracts heal by scarification, and the fibroblastic tissue, infiltrated with eosinophils, is eventually incorporated into the portal units (interstitial hepatitis) (Fig. 2.20D). Most larvae escape from the liver but some eventually become encapsulated in the liver in abscesses containing numerous eosinophils. The abscesses may caseate and come to resemble tubercles, and eventually many are heavily mineralized to form permanent pearly nodules. In sheep, the most common cause of this type of hepatitis (aside from liver fluke) is *Cysticercus tenuicollis* in its wandering phase. Lambs may die of severe hemorrhagic hepatitis caused by very heavy infections of this parasite, and in pigs, an aberrant host, *C. tenuicollis* can produce a very intense inflammatory reaction.

In pigs, larvae of *Ascaris suum* and *Stephanurus dentatus* produce similar but distinct patterns of focal interstitial hepatitis. The ascarids produce their distinctive accentuation of the stroma (''milk spots'') when quite small larvae are immobilized by the host's inflammatory reaction; thus the foci are relatively small. The fibrotic lesion produced by *S. dentatus* larvae, on the other hand, is less focal and more in the nature of a track, and there are usually small, inflamed, capsular craters, where the larvae have emerged from the liver to migrate to their preferred perirenal site. There will be obvious portal phlebitis at the hepatic hilus when infection by *S. dentatus* has been by the oral route (Fig. 2.20C), and in these livers the parenchymal lesion is more severe in this vicinity.

Migration tracks left by larval strongyles are common under the liver capsule in young horses and are probably related to the dense, discrete fibrous tags that are an almost universal finding on the diaphragmatic surface of the liver of mature horses. The range of strongyle species capable of causing these lesions has not been defined. There are other and more devious means by which parasites produce hepatic lesions: the hydatid intermediate stages of *Echinococcus* encyst in the liver and may destroy much of it (Fig. 2.25A,B); the larvae of *Ascaris suum* in cattle add to the usual insult by causing portal phlebitis and small areas of infarction; the adults of *Ascaris* in all species, but especially in pigs, may migrate into the bile ducts (Fig. 2.12B); and the eggs of schistosomes float up in the portal blood to lodge in the liver and provoke granulomatous inflammation.

Cestodes

Stilesia hepatica and *Thysanosoma actinioides,* the ''fringed tapeworm,'' are the only cestodes that belong in the bile ducts. They are parasites of ruminants, *Stilesia* occurring in Africa, *Thysanosoma* in North America. The life cycles of the parasites are not completely known but probably involve oribatid mites as intermediate hosts. *Thysanosoma actinioides* may also be found in the pancreatic ducts and small intestine. Usually, the infestations are light but, even when heavy, are not of much significance. Very heavy infestations by *S. hepatica* occur without signs of illness, though the bile ducts may be nearly occluded, slightly thickened, and dilated. Saccular dilations of the ducts may occur and be filled with worms. The fringed tapeworm is

perhaps more pathogenic, and unthriftiness may accompany heavy infestations.

Nematodes

Capillaria hepatica (*Hepaticola hepatica*) is the one nematode that in the adult phase inhabits the liver. It is a slender worm, morphologically resembling the whipworms, and it lives in the parenchyma rather than in the bile ducts. The usual hosts of the adult stage are rodents, but sporadic infestations are observed in dogs. These worms are not highly pathogenic. The adults provoke some traumatic hepatitis, and the eggs, which are deposited in clusters, provoke the development of localized granulomas. The eggs are readily recognized by their ovoid shape and polar caps. The granulomas can be seen through the capsule or in the substance of the liver as yellowish streaks or patches. The eggs cannot escape from the liver unless they are eaten by a predator. Predators, however, act only as transport hosts, and the ingested eggs are passed in the feces. Larvae develop in the eggs only in the external environment, and the cycle is completed when the mature larvae in the eggs are eaten by a suitable host.

Trematodes

A variety of trematodes (flukes) are parasitic in the livers of animals. They belong to the families Fasciolidae (*Fasciola hepatica, F. gigantica, Fascioloides magna*), Dicrocoeliidae (*Dicrocoelium dendriticum, D. hospes, Platynosomum concinnum*), and Opisthorchiidae (*Opisthorchis tenuicollis, O. sinensis, Pseudamphistomum truncatum*). The diseases produced are known collectively as distomiasis.

Fasciola hepatica, the common liver fluke of sheep and cattle, is the most widespread and important of the group. Patent infestations can develop in other wild and domestic animals and in humans. These flukes are leaf-shaped and ~2.5 cm long in sheep and slightly larger in cattle. They are found in the bile ducts. Being hermaphroditic, only one fluke is necessary to establish a patent infestation, and each adult may produce 20,000 eggs per day. The longevity of the adult flukes is amazing and is potentially as great or greater than that of the host; they have been known to survive for 11 years, and it seems that they can produce eggs for all of this period. The eggs are eliminated in bile, and on pasture, in conditions of suitable warmth and moistness, hatch a larva (miracidium) in ~9 days. If the environmental temperature is low, the incubation period may be delayed for some months. The miracidium can survive only in moisture. It is actively motile and penetrates the tissues of the intermediate host, which is an aquatic snail. Different snails serve this purpose in different countries, but all of them belong to the genus *Lymnaea.*

Each miracidium, on penetrating a snail, develops into a mother sporocyst that reproduces, probably parthenogenetically, giving rise to a small number of the second generation, the redia. Each redia gives birth to either redia or cercaria, or to the two successively. Cercaria, the larval stage of the third (sexual) generation, first appear 1–2 months after the miracidium penetrates. Cercariae continue to escape daily for the life of the snail, but even so, total cercarial production is only 500–1000. They actively escape from the snail and are attracted to green

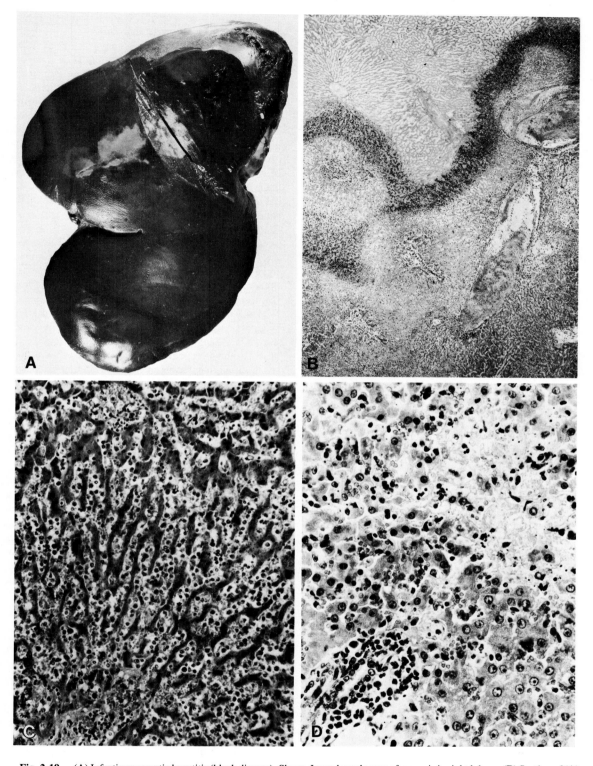

Fig. 2.19. (A) Infectious necrotic hepatitis (black disease). Sheep. Irregular pale area of necrosis in right lobe. (B) Section of (A). Vascular thrombosis, and area of coagulative necrosis, isolated by a zone of acute inflammatory infiltrate. (C) Sinusoidal leukocytosis in pyometra. Bitch. (D) Lytic necrosis. Toxoplasmosis. Kitten.

plants, where they encyst and become infective metacercariae in 1 day. These can remain infective for 1 month in summer and up to 3 months in winter. The developmental events from egg to this stage take 1–2 months under favorable conditions.

Infestation occurs by ingestion. Excystment occurs in the duodenum. The young flukes penetrate the intestinal wall and cross the peritoneal cavity, attaching here and there to suck blood and penetrate the liver through its capsule; a few no doubt pass in the portal vessels or migrate up the bile duct. They wander in the liver for a month or more before settling down in the bile ducts to mature, which they do in 2 to 3 months. Some may, by accident, enter the hepatic veins and systemic circulation to lodge in unusual sites; intrauterine infestations are on record. Lesions caused by aberrant flukes are quite common in bovine lung. They consist of resilient nodules just under the pleura of the peripheral parts of the lung. They range in diameter from about one to many centimeters and consist of thinly encapsulated abscesses situated at the ends of bronchi (Fig. 2.20A). The content is slightly mucoid, unevenly coagulated brown fluid; in some lesions the reaction is predominantly caseous. A careful search is sometimes necessary to find the fluke in this debris; it is usually quite small. The location of the lesion suggests that it begins as a peripheral bronchiectasis, which later becomes sealed off.

The essential lesions produced by *Fasciola hepatica* occur in the liver and may be described separately, as those produced by the migratory larvae, and those produced by the mature flukes in the bile ducts; the two often intermingle. There is the further incidence of peritonitis, which is produced by the young flukes on their way to the liver and, perhaps also, by some that break out through the capsule.

Usually there is no obvious reaction to the passage of young flukes through the intestinal wall and across the peritoneal cavity, except for small hemorrhagic foci on the peritoneum, where the flukes have been temporarily attached. Few or many parasites may be found in any ascitic fluid and attached to the peritoneum of the diaphragm and the mesenteries. When the infestations are heavy and repeated, such as may be observed in sheep, cattle, and swine, peritonitis occurs. The young flukes at this stage are less than 1.0 mm long. The peritonitis may be acute and exudative or chronic and proliferative. It is usually concentrated on the hepatic capsule (Fig. 2.21A), especially its visceral surface, but may be restricted to the parietal peritoneum or to the visceral peritoneum, including the mesenteries of the gut. In acute cases there are fibrinohemorrhagic deposits on the serous surfaces, and in chronic cases there may be fibrous tags, with adhesions or a more or less diffuse thickening by connective tissue. Many young flukes can be found microscopically in the fibrinous deposits, and in the diffuse peritoneal thickenings there are tortuous migration tunnels containing blood, debris, and the young parasites (Fig. 2.21B). In cases with involvement of the visceral peritoneum, young flukes can be found in enlarged mesenteric lymph nodes.

The acute lesions in the liver caused by the wandering flukes are basically traumatic, but there is an element of coagulation necrosis, which is possibly related to toxic excretions of the flukes. The migratory pathways are tortuous tunnels that appear on cross section as hemorrhagic foci 2–3 mm in diameter. If the tunnels are followed, a young fluke less than 1.0 mm long can be found at the ends. When the infestation is heavy, the liver may appear to be permeated by dark hemorrhagic streaks and foci. Older tunnels from which the debris has been cleared may appear as light yellow streaks due to infiltration of eosinophils (Fig. 2.21A). Microscopically, fresh tunnels are filled with blood and degenerate hepatocytes and are soon infiltrated by eosinophils. Later, histiocytes and giant cells arrange themselves about the debris and remove it, and healing occurs by granulation tissue, which is rich in lymphocytes and eosinophils. In light infestations the scars may disappear, but in heavy infestations they may fuse with each other and with portal areas to produce a moderate irregular fibrosis. There may, as yet, be no change in the bile ducts. Probably, most of the young flukes reach the bile ducts, but some do not, and they become encysted in the parenchyma. One or more flukes may be present in each cyst, which consists of a connective-tissue capsule and a dirty brown content of blood, detritus, and excrement from flukes. The cysts ultimately caseate and may mineralize or be obliterated by fibrous tissue. These cysts are most frequent on the visceral surface, where they cause bulging of the capsule.

Heavy infestations by immature flukes may cause death in the stage of acute hepatitis. Such an outcome is not common, but occurs in sheep. It is estimated that 10,000 metacercariae ingested over a short period are necessary to produce acute death in sheep. Death may occur suddenly or after a few days of fever, lassitude, inappetance, and abdominal tenderness. This is also the stage of the parasitism in which black disease occurs (see above).

The mature flukes are present in the larger bile ducts and cause cholangiohepatitis. The relative importance of different factors in their pathogenicity is not known, but they cause mechanical irritation by the action of their suckers and scales, cause obstruction of the ducts with some degree of biliary retention, predispose to bacterial infections, possibly suck blood, and probably produce toxic and irritative metabolic excretions.

The biliary changes occur in all lobes but are usually most severe in the left (Fig. 2.21C), and the right may be moderately hypertrophied. From the hilus, the bile ducts on the visceral surface stand out as whitish, firm, branching cords that in extreme instances may be an inch in diameter and allow detectable fluctuation over extended segments or in localized areas of ectasia (Fig. 2.21D). This dilatation of the ducts in sheep, swine, and horses is largely mechanical and is due to distension by masses of flukes and bile. It is permitted by the relative paucity of new connective-tissue formation in the walls of the ducts in these species; this in turn is probably related to the rather mild catarrhal type of inflammation in the lumina of the ducts. In cattle, desquamative and ulcerative lesions in the large bile ducts are more severe than in other species, and there is a correspondingly greater proliferation of granulation tissue in and about the walls of the ducts. The walls of the ducts in cattle are, in consequence, much thickened, and the lumen is irregularly stenotic and dilated and lined largely by granulation tissue. This contributes the typical "pipe stem" appearance to the ducts in cattle; the connective tissue may be, in addition, mineralized, sometimes so heavily that it cannot be cut with a knife. When the bile ducts are opened, their contents may pour out. They consist of

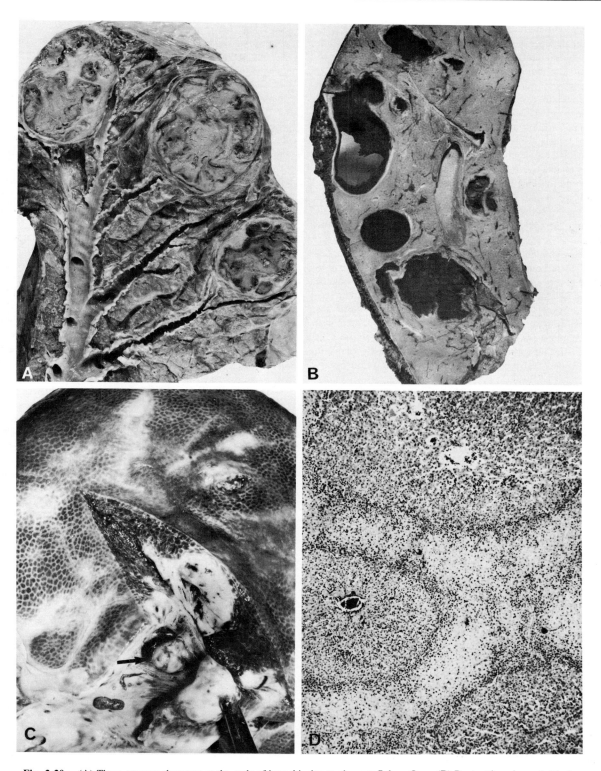

Fig. 2.20. (A) Three caseous abscesses at the ends of bronchi, due to aberrant flukes. Ox.   (B) Destructive pigmented lesions produced by *Fascioloides magna*. Ox.   (C) Portal phlebitis and interstitial hepatitis produced by *Stephanurus dentatus* larvae after oral infection. Fresh and organizing thrombi in portal vein (arrow). Pig.   (D) Subacute interstitial hepatitis. *Stephanurus dentatus* infection. Pig.

dirty dark brown fluid of a mucinous or tough consistency, containing degenerate bile, some of it in floccules, pus, desquamated cells and detritus, clumps of flukes, and small masses of eggs in dark brown granular agglomerates.

Although the lesions are most obvious in ducts large enough to contain the flukes, there is, with time and severe or repeated infestations, progressive inflammation in the smaller portal units due to direct irritation by the flukes, superimposed infections, and biliary stasis. The course of events is as described earlier for subacute and chronic cholangiohepatitis (Fig. 2.21C). The proliferating connective tissue and bile ductules in individual portal areas extend to join each other and the scars left over from the migratory phase, so that inflammatory fibrosis may obliterate parenchyma in many foci. In such livers, the left lobe, which is the one most severely affected, may be atrophied, indurated, and irregular.

The development of a cholangiohepatitis of the degree described depends on long-standing or heavy infestations. Lesions of lesser severity, or those less fully developed, are associated with light infestations of short duration. They may then be recognized only by local dilatations of the ducts, or even these may not be readily apparent. In such mild infestations, the fact of past or present parasitism may be suggested only by the detection of characteristic black iron–porphyrin pigments, grossly visible in the hilar nodes. It also contributes to the character of the biliary contents.

Chronic debility with vague digestive disturbances is common in chronic fascioliasis and, among sheep, deaths are common. Clinically and at postmortem there are, in addition to the essential lesions, more or less severe anemia, moderate anasarca, and cachexia. Jaundice is seldom seen.

Fasciola gigantica displaces *F. hepatic* as the common liver fluke in many parts of Africa and in nearby countries, the Far East, and the Hawaiian Islands. It is two or three times as large as *F. hepatica*, but its life cycle and pathogenicity are comparable.

Fascioloides magna is the large liver fluke of North America. It is a parasite of ruminants and lives in the hepatic parenchyma, not in the bile ducts, although in tolerant hosts, Cervidae, the cysts in which it localizes communicate with the bile ducts to provide an exit for ova and excrement. The life cycle of this parasite generally parallels that of *Fasciola hepatica*. The young flukes are very destructive as they wander in the liver. In cattle, they wander briefly, producing large necrotic tunnels before becoming encysted. The cysts, enclosed by connective tissue, do not communicate with bile ducts but form permanent enclosures for the flukes, their excreta, and ova. The cysts, which may be an inch or two in diameter, are remarkable for the large deposits of jet black, sooty iron–porphyrin pigment they contain (Fig. 2.20B), and except for the flukes and soft contents, they superficially resemble heavily pigmented melanotic tumors. Commonly, these flukes pass from the liver to the lungs of cattle, to produce lesions of similar character. In sheep, this parasite wanders continuously in the liver, producing black, tortuous tracts, which may be 2 cm in diameter, and extensive parenchymal destruction. Even a few flukes may kill sheep.

The dicrocoelid flukes inhabit both biliary and pancreatic ducts. *Eurytrema pancreaticum* prefers the pancreas (and is described with that organ, this volume) but in heavy infestations can be found in the bile ducts. *Dicrocoelium* and *Platynosomum*

prefer the bile ducts. These are small, narrow flukes 0.5–1.0 cm long and may easily be mistaken for small masses of inspissated bile pigment. They are not highly pathogenic, and even in heavy infestations there may be no signs of the toxemia observed in infestations by *Fasciola hepatica*. These flukes may occur as mixed infestations.

Platynosomum fastosum is a parasite of cats in North America and the Amazonian regions of South America. The life cycle involves snails and lizards and presumably an arthropod. The infested livers are enlarged, friable, and may be bile stained. There is catarrhal inflammation of biliary passages, but it is not severe, and the walls may not be much thickened. The ducts are dilated and easily visible. There are vague digestive disturbances, and heavy infestations may cause complete anorexia and death.

Dicrocoelium hospes is found in cattle in countries south of the Sahara. Little is known of it, but it is presumed to be comparable in all respects to the well-known *D. dendriticum*. *Dicrocoelium dendriticum* (the lancet fluke) is common in Europe and Asia, and sparsely distributed in the Americas and North Africa. This fluke is no more fastidious in its choice of final hosts than many other species of flukes, and depending on opportunity, it can infest all domestic species, with the possible exception of cats. It is, however, of most importance as a parasite of sheep and cattle, in which it inhabits the bile ducts. Other domestic species and rodents are important as reservoirs.

The life cycle of *Dicrocoelium dendriticum* differs in some details from that of *Fasciola hepatica*. The eggs are embryonated when laid and do not hatch until swallowed by one of the many genera of land snails that are the first intermediate hosts. In the snails, the mother sporocyst produces a second generation of daughter sporocysts, which in turn produce cercariae. The cercariae leave the snail in damp weather and are expelled from the snail's lung, clumped together in slime balls. The slime balls are not infective until the cercariae are swallowed by, and encyst in, the ant *Formica fusca*; other ants may be involved in different countries. The cycle is completed when the definitive hosts swallow the ants. The route of migration of the larvae from the gut to the liver is probably via the bile ducts from the duodenum.

The pathologic changes in the liver produced by *Dicrocoelium dendriticum* are those of a cholangiohepatitis that is less severe than that produced by *Fasciola hepatica*. The severity and diffuseness of the hepatic lesion is determined by the number of lancet flukes present, and they may be in the thousands. The dilated ducts are darkened by the flukes and their eggs. Even in early infestations, there may be some scarring of the organ at its periphery. In heavy infestations of long standing, there is extensive biliary fibrosis, producing an organ that is indurated, scarred, and lumpy and that at the margins may bear areas that are shrunken and completely sclerotic. The histologic changes are the same as those in fascioliasis, with perhaps a more remarkable hyperplasia of the mucous glands of the large ducts.

The opisthorchid flukes are parasites in the bile ducts of carnivores. They may also occur in swine and humans, and one species, *Opisthorchis sinensis* (≡ *Clonorchis sinensis*), is an important human parasite. There is some uncertainty regarding the proper classification of these flukes, and some of those given

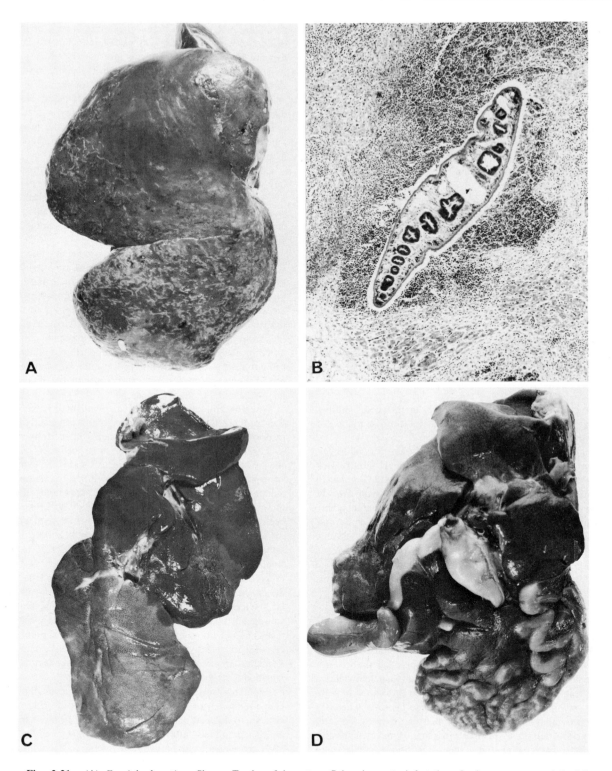

Fig. 2.21. (**A**) *Fasciola hepatica*. Sheep. Tracks of immature flukes in acute infestation. Lesions concentrated in left lobe. (**B**) Immature fluke, accompanied by acute inflammation. Sheep. (**C**) Subacute *Fasciola* infestation. Sheep. Early cholangiohepatitis and cholestasis in left lobe. (**D**) Chronic fascioliasis. Sheep. Bile duct ectasia, atrophy of left lobe, and hypertrophy of right lobe.

below may not be valid species. The life cycles, where known, include molluscs as the first intermediate hosts and freshwater fish as the second.

Metorchis conjunctus is the common liver fluke of cats and dogs in North America and is important as a parasite of sled dogs in the Canadian Northwest Territories. The first intermediate host is the snail *Amnicola limosa porosa,* and the second is the common sucker *Catostomus commersonii.* The cercariae actively burrow into the musculature of the fish to encyst and become infective. The immature flukes crawl into the bile ducts from the duodenum and mature in ~28 days. Infestations may persist for more than 5 years. *Metorchis albidis* has been described in a dog from Alaska, *Parametorchis complexus* in cats in the United States, and *Amphimerus pseudofelineus* in cats and coyotes in the United States and Panama; the life cycles are not known but are presumed to include fish.

Opisthorchis felineus is the lanceolate fluke of the bile ducts of cats, dogs, and foxes in Europe and Russia. It is particularly common in East Europe and Siberia and is more sparse in other areas. *Opisthorchis sinensis* is well documented as the Oriental or Chinese liver fluke; it is endemic in Japan, Korea, southern China, and Southeast Asia. There are additional species of *Opisthorchis* in humans and animals, but they are less well known than the species cited. The first intermediate hosts for the miracidia of *O. tenuicollis* and *O. sinensis* are snails of the genus *Bithynia,* and several genera of cyprinid fishes can act as second intermediate hosts.

Pseudamphistomum truncatum occurs in carnivores and humans sporadically in Europe and Asia. Its life cycle is as for *Opisthorchis.*

The opisthorchid flukes, so far as known, resemble *Dicrocoelium* in migrating up the bile ducts to their habitat. This may be the reason that they are more numerous in the left than in the right lobes of the liver. They can probably live in the liver for as long as the host lives. The pathologic effects are comparable to those of *D. dendriticum.* Light infestations may be asymptomatic, and heavy infestations may cause jaundice, chronic cholangiohepatitis, and severe biliary fibrosis. Both in humans and animals, adenomatous and carcinomatous changes of the biliary glands have occurred in association with these parasites; the association is probably more than coincidental.

Toxic Liver Disease

Here we are concerned primarily with those intoxications to which the liver seems more susceptible than other tissues. Immediately there arises a paradox: the liver has an acknowledged central role in detoxification and excretion of xenobiotic substances yet may undergo almost complete necrosis when exposed to compounds that leave the rest of the body virtually untouched. Attempts to resolve this paradox have, naturally, assumed an association between this susceptibility and the more unique aspects of liver function. The biotransformation of xenobiotics is itself a well-developed (although not unique) function of hepatocytes, and it is now known that a large class of toxins are hepatotoxic because, in its attempts to transform these substances into excretable metabolites, the liver converts them to intermediate reactive radicals that are much more toxic than

the parent molecules. If the original compound is of relatively low toxicity, as is the case with carbon tetrachloride, it follows that the liver will suffer much more damage than any other tissue, for the toxic metabolite, which is usually unstable and short-lived, tends only to damage the cytoplasm of the cell in which it is produced. The observation has been made earlier that the usual periacinar location of such liver injury is related to the relatively high concentration in this zone of the microsomal mixed-function oxidases responsible for this sort of biotransformation.

Compounds that are hepatotoxic after metabolism tend to be fat soluble rather than water soluble, as the latter are more readily excreted by the kidney. Many of the biotransformations effected by the microsomal enzymes are in fact directed to the task of rendering lipophilic substances more water soluble so as to increase their renal clearance rate.

When death follows severe acute toxic hepatic necrosis, severe acute pulmonary congestion and edema are often observed as well. A possible reason for this phenomenon is that sufficient toxic intermediate metabolites and fibrin degradation products are swept from the liver to damage the lung. Apart from the probable occurrence of "spillover" of toxic pyrrolic metabolites from the liver after large doses of pyrrolizidine alkaloids, however, there is little experimental support for this suggestion. Lung tissue has been shown to possess its own complement of mixed-function oxidases and is therefore capable of performing its own suicidal biotransformations.

When the role of intermediary metabolism in hepatotoxicity was recognized, it soon became apparent that the activity of the responsible enzymes could be increased (induced) by exposure to a range of nontoxic xenobiotics or to intrinsic compounds such as steroid hormones. This increase should lead to increased susceptibility to certain hepatotoxins. Some toxins have been demonstrated to depress these enzymes, thus conferring some protection against the acute hepatotoxicity of other toxins. It has been shown, for example, that a small dose of carbon tetrachloride will prevent death in rats given a normally lethal dose of the same toxin shortly afterward, carbon tetrachloride in this instance having the opposite of a cumulative effect. This protection is due to the small prior dose's binding with and inactivating the enzymes of the mixed-function oxidase system, in particular, the terminal heme cytochrome *P*-450. This inactivation and subsequent protection may explain the apparently anomalous results of some dosage trials, in which a larger amount of toxic material given in divided doses may cause less liver damage than a smaller amount given as a single dose. Other factors such as nutritional status may be involved. Prolonged starvation, for example, may result in the catabolism of microsomal protein and hence reduction of enzyme activity, thus conferring some resistance to this sort of hepatotoxicity. On the other hand, well-nourished animals, after a short fast sufficient only to deplete glycogen stores, may be very susceptible to hepatotoxicity. It has been suggested that glycogen in the cytoplasm may exert a protective effect against toxic reactive radicals by trapping them before they damage the more vital membranous components of the cell.

The importance of reduced glutathione and the selenium–vitamin E status of the liver cell in dietary hepatic necrosis is related to the ability of the membranes of the cell to cope with toxic endogenous free radicals. It is therefore reasonable to expect that livers deficient in these factors will be more susceptible to hepatotoxins.

With so many variables involved, it is not surprising that the outcome of naturally occurring exposure to this class of hepatotoxins is most unpredictable. The severity and pattern of the liver lesions depend on the sum of the variables and on the tempo of metabolic reactions triggered by the episodes of intoxication. The complexity of these interactions is exemplified by experimental manipuation of the pattern of necrosis produced by ngaione, a furanosesquiterpene component of essential oils from species of Myoporaceae. Administration of this toxin to normal animals at certain dose rates produces, in a high proportion of cases, a distinctive pattern of midzonal necrosis (Fig. 2.5A), a lesion described above. If prior to intoxication the animals have had their microsomal mixed-function oxidases induced by administration of barbiturate or DDT, the predominant distribution of necrosis produced by ngaione is periportal (Fig. 2.6C,D). On the other hand, if the activity of the enzymes has been chemically suppressed, the ngaione-induced lesion is predominantly periacinar. The explanation of this phenomenon rests on the fact that the activity of the microsomal enzymes is always greater in the periacinar zone, even after induction or suppression, and assumes that ngaione and related compounds are degraded by microsomes by rate-limited processes whose efficiency is proportional to the concentration of the mixed-function oxidases present in the cell. Accordingly, if the concentration of enzyme is high (as in the periacinar hepatocytes in the normal animal), the parent compound is completely degraded to nontoxic metabolites so rapidly that there will be accumulation of toxic intermediates sufficient to damage the cell. In the normal animal, then, necrosis will only occur in those midzonal hepatocytes that have enzyme sufficient to produce toxic intermediates, but insufficient to completely degrade these to safe levels. The periportal hepatocytes will not be damaged because they have not enough enzyme to produce sufficient toxic intermediates from the parent compound. In the induced animal, enough enzyme is present in periacinar and midzonal cells for complete detoxification, so the necrosis is periportal. In the enzyme-suppressed liver, only the periacinar hepatocytes retain enzyme activity sufficient to produce lethal concentrations of the toxic intermediate; the necrosis in this case is therefore periacinar. This explanation may explain those naturally occurring instances of periportal and midzonal toxic hepatic necrosis that appear from time to time.

Rarely, biotransforming enzymes may be more concentrated in the periportal than in the other zones, leading consistently to periportal necrosis on exposure to compounds that are degraded by them to toxic intermediates. The classic example of this is the effect of allyl formate or allyl alcohol on rat liver. Both these substances are metabolized to acrolein by alcohol dehydrogenase, a microsomal enzyme that is more concentrated in the periportal hepatocytes. Acrolein is an alkylating aldehyde capable of producing lethal membrane damage. The necrosis can be prevented by pretreatment with pyrazole, which inhibits alcohol dehydrogenase.

There are other reasons for the peculiar vulnerability of the liver to some toxins; these depend on the capacity of the organ to selectively concentrate certain intrinsic compounds and xenobiotics. There are transport systems that greatly facilitate the entry of bile acids into the hepatocytes, and it follows that if these mechanisms promote the uptake of toxins, then the liver will be preferentially damaged by such agents. This mechanism has been established as part of the basis of the hepatotoxicity of phalloidin, the toxic polypeptide from *Amanita*, but there is some evidence that the hepatotoxicity of blue-green algae may depend on similar mechanisms. The hepatotoxic component of chronic copper poisoning of ruminants is certainly the result of the peculiar avidity of the liver for this element, particularly in sheep. The underlying mechanism of the hepatic uptake in this case remains to be clarified.

The morphologic changes in acute toxic hepatic injury are rather stereotyped. They range from single-cell necrosis, through confluent coagulative and shrinkage zonal necrosis, to massive hemorrhagic destruction that includes sinusoidal lining cells. The characteristics of these injuries were described under Patterns of Hepatic Necrosis. Depending on the metabolic status of the animal, there may be variably severe fatty or hydropic change in hepatocytes adjacent to the necrotic zones (Figs. 2.6A and 2.22C), and the necrotic cells may accumulate calcium, but these variations on the general theme have little diagnostic specificity. In sublethally injured cells there may be spectacular clumping of smooth endoplasmic reticulum (Fig. 2.2C), particularly in the periacinar zones. This change is not specific.

The clinical and gross characteristics of fatal acute intoxications are rather consistent, regardless of the origin of the toxin. The animal dies after a brief period of dullness, anorexia, colic, and a variety of neurologic disturbances, including convulsions. Postmortem examination reveals petechial and ecchymotic hemorrhages under the serosa of abdomen and thorax. There is usually a slight excess of clear, yellow abdominal fluid, which contains sufficient fibrinogen to form a loose, nonadherent clot. The liver may be deep reddish purple and obviously swollen in very heavily intoxicated cases, with prominent edema of the gallbladder wall and its attachments, and there is distension of lymphatics of the serosa of the gallbladder and of the porta hepatis. In fatal cases where the toxic dose more nearly approaches the LD_{50}, there is less severe hemorrhage, and the liver is paler and shows more obvious acinar pattern.

The histology of these acute intoxications is usually characterized by severe periacinar necrosis (Fig. 2.6A). Rarely, the pattern of necrosis may be periportal (Fig. 2.6C) or midzonal (Fig. 2.5A); this is sometimes seen in algal poisoning and in intoxication by *Myoporum* spp. Reasons for this have been discussed above.

In acute fatal hepatotoxicities there is almost always widespread hemorrhage terminally; petechiae and ecchymoses are seen most consistently on serous membranes, especially on the epi- and endocardium. Diffuse hemorrhage into the gut, particularly the duodenum in ruminants, is also common, as are hemorrhages into the wall of the gallbladder. The hemorrhage in these organs is probably related to damage done by toxic metabolites excreted in the bile. Hemorrhages elsewhere have in the past often been taken as evidence of primary vascular damage by the toxin, but most of the bleeding is due to excessive consumption

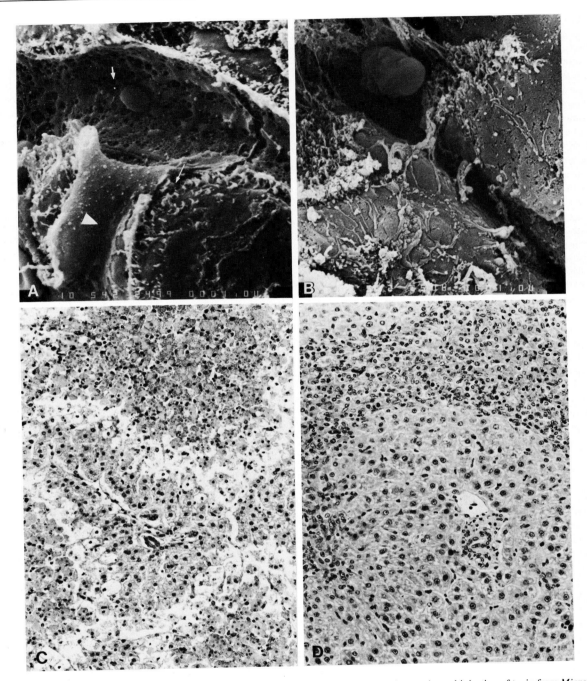

Fig. 2.22. (A) Scanning electron micrograph of mouse liver, perfused 15 min after intraperitoneal injection of toxin from *Microcystis aeruginosa*. Essentially normal structure of fenestrated endothelium (short arrow), sinusoidal lining cell (arrowhead), and space of Disse (long arrow). (B) As for (A), 30 min after injection. The endothelium has largely disintegrated; the underlying hepatocytes are still intact. (A and B courtesy of I. R. Falconer and the *Australian Journal of Biological Sciences*.) (C) Acute coagulative and hemorrhagic periacinar necrosis in *Cestrum parqui* poisoning. Ox. The periportal and the necrotic zones are separated by a margin zone of hydropic hepatocytes. (D) *Cestrum* poisoning. Ox. Repair of the periacinar injury 4 days after sublethal intoxication.

of clotting factors by the disrupted sinusoids on the one hand, and on the other, to failure of the damaged liver to replace those factors.

Photosensitization is not a feature of the acutely fatal hepatotoxicities, unless it occurs in the recovery phase in sublethally intoxicated animals; in these it is likely to be relatively mild and transient.

It is emphasized that the outcome of acute exposure to hepatotoxins is often an unpredictable product of many factors. The same factors operate in chronic hepatotoxicity but are compounded by variations in rates of exposure and by adaptive responses of the liver. Continuous exposure to a toxin may maintain detoxification mechanisms at such a pitch as to enable the liver to handle concentrations of toxin that would cause severe damage if administered intermittently.

In contrast to the acute intoxications, lesions with a fair degree of specificity are produced by many of the more chronic hepatotoxicities. In addition to the individually specific features, the chronic intoxications produce a range of changes common to them. These include accelerated necrobiosis, fibrosis of various patterns, bile duct hyperplasia, nodular regeneration, and some degree of cholestasis. Some of these hepatotoxins are potent carcinogens, but this is not an important consequence in domestic animals. Clinical signs of hepatic failure may include photosensitization, nervous dysfunction, and jaundice.

Most of the toxins responsible for chronic hepatotoxicity may produce acute nonspecific zonal or massive necrosis if exposure is at dose rates higher than those ordinarily acquired.

The causes of acute hepatotoxicity include administered drugs, but phytotoxins may produce spectacular losses in free-ranging herbivores; usually the victims are ruminants that are either under some nutritional stress or that have been introduced suddenly to new grazing; herds and flocks of traveling stock are particularly prone to this sort of accident. Other factors involving the plant, such as stage of growth, are of paramount importance in determining toxicity. An extreme example of this is poisoning by *Xanthium pungens* (Noogoorah burr), in which the toxin is greatly concentrated in the cotyledons. Since the seeds are never eaten, even by cattle, field intoxications only occur when this plant is eaten shortly after germination.

The botanical range of plants capable of producing acute hepatotoxicity is extremely broad, toxic genera being found in families as diverse as the relatively primitive Cycadaceae and blue-green algae, through the Compositae and Solanaceae. The toxic compounds are probably also as diverse, but in many cases these remain to be identified. An exhaustive review of the toxicity of these plants would be repetitive; instead, some of the better known and more representative examples are discussed, with comments on special features where appropriate.

Blue-green Algae

Blue-green algae growing as a waterbloom on lakes and ponds may be highly toxic. Outbreaks of poisoning are not common, but they occur in many countries and may be responsible for heavy mortality among animals or birds that take the algae when drinking. Most well-documented cases have involved *Microcystis aeruginosa*, a bloom that may poison stock after the algae have been piled by wind against the shores of expanses of

water that have accumulated phosphates and nitrates as runoff from fertilized soils (Fig. 2.22A,B). It is not known to what extent natural poisoning is caused by the algae themselves in their various stages of growth and decay, or to what extent it may be caused by saprophytic bacteria.

Some deaths are too sudden to be due to liver damage and are probably the result of the "fast-death factor" that has been found in some blooms. The syndrome is one of collapse and prostration, with hyperesthesia that may be manifested as convulsions; there are no specific lesions.

Most work has been done on the hepatotoxin, which is a polypeptide whose amino acid content seems to be variable. Mention has been made of the possibility that this toxin uses bile acid transport mechanisms to enter the hepatocyte, and that it may not need microsomal metabolism to exert its effect. Poisonings that are not very acute may be characterized by photosensitization and icterus. The distribution of the necrosis is usually periacinar to massive (Fig. 2.7C) but is occasionally periportal or, even more rarely, midzonal. The pattern may vary within the one liver.

Cycadales

Members of the order Cycadales have been responsible for chronic hepatotoxicity and neurotoxicity, but acute hepatotoxicity has been reported in sheep that have eaten the seeds or young leaves of species of Zamiaceae. The toxin responsible is methylazoxymethanol, which is the aglycone of various nontoxic glycosides in these plants. The toxin is split from the glycoside in the gut, and its hepatotoxicity is the result of further metabolism in hepatic microsomes; the pattern of necrosis is thus periacinar. The metabolites of the aglycone are apparently potent alkylating agents, and the chronic liver lesions reflect this. There is megalocytosis (which is not as persistent as that of pyrrolizidine alkaloid poisoning), nuclear hyperchromasia, cholestasis, fatty change, and varying degrees of diffuse fibrosis. Cytoplasmic invaginations into nuclei, and cytosegresome formation, are apparently not a prominent feature. There is fairly consistent tubular nephrosis.

Chronic cycad poisoning of cattle causes a chronic nervous disorder characterized by a progressive proprioceptive deficit. This is due to axonopathy in upper spinocerebellar and lower corticospinal tracts. The axonopathy, morphologically subtle at first, may progress eventually to frank Wallerian degeneration. Two neurotoxic agents have been isolated from cycads; neither is methylazoxymethanol.

Solanaceae

Cestrum parqui causes acute hepatotoxicity under field conditions in South America and Australia. Cattle are more frequently poisoned than other species, but sheep are susceptible, and fowl may be if they eat the fruit. There are no records of chronic liver disease caused by this plant, and photosensitization is rarely seen. The toxin is as yet unidentified. The pattern of necrosis is consistently periacinar (Figs. 2.6A and 2.22C).

Compositae

The toxin of *Xanthium pungens* is concentrated in the cotyledons. Pigs and cattle are the subject of most intoxications, usually after rain has allowed germination following a period of feed scarcity. The clinical signs and lesions are not specific, being those described for acute hepatotoxins in general. The toxin carboxyatractyloside is present in the achenes and cotyledons and appears to be responsible for the field intoxications.

Helichrysum blandowskianum is hepatotoxic to cattle and has caused sudden deaths with periacinar necrosis in the field in southern Australia. The toxin has not been identified.

Three species of Compositae in South Africa, *Asaemia axillaris*, *Athanasia trifurcata*, and *Lasiosperum bipinnatum*, have been associated with field outbreaks of acute hepatotoxicity, but it seems that they are more often responsible for more chronic disease with photosensitivity. Experimental intoxications by all three of these species have in some animals produced midzonal as well as periacinar necrosis.

Myoporaceae

The variation in pattern of zonal necrosis (Figs. 2.5A and 2.6B–D) seen in intoxication by Myoporaceae has been discussed under Toxic Liver Disease. Species so far incriminated are *Myoporum deserti*, *M. acuminatum*, *M. insulare*, and *M. tetrandum* of Australia, and *M. laetum* of New Zealand. The toxic oils are contained in the leaves and branchlets, but within the species there is variation in the chemical characters and toxicity of the oils; not all strains of toxic species are toxic. There is some delay between ingestion and absorption of the furanosesquiterpenoid oils, the best known of which is ngaione, which are responsible for intoxication, so 24–48 hr may elapse before signs of toxicity appear. Some animals live long enough to become photosensitized; others may die much more rapidly, with pulmonary edema. The edema appears to be a direct effect of the toxin after metabolism by alveolar lining cells.

Livers from intoxicated sheep may show a striking, broad pattern of variable congestion and even infarction, which is superimposed on the more regular acinar pattern of zonal necrosis. Sections of these livers reveal acute fibrinoid necrosis of portal vessels, which suggests that the coarser lesions may have a vascular basis.

Ulmaceae

Trema aspera has caused severe losses in cattle in Australia. The syndrome is acute, there is no photosensitization, and mildly intoxicated animals may recover completely. The toxic principle is a glycoside, designated trematoxin. The pattern of necrosis is consistently periacinar.

The gross and microscopic pathology of experimental poisoning by *Trema*, *Xanthium pungens*, and *Cestrum parqui* has been shown to be identical in all observable respects in the same group of sheep.

Carbon Tetrachloride

The toxin carbon tetrachloride has been mentioned already as the archetype of toxic metabolism, in which necrogenic membranous lipoperoxidation follows the evolution of a highly reactive radical from the parent molecule after microsomal transformation. Carbon tetrachloride has been intensively studied in the development of laboratory animal models of hepatic necrosis,

fatty liver and hepatic fibrosis, and remodeling, but it was also been used for many years as a fasciolicide. Under certain conditions there have been severe losses, usually sheep, following administration of recommended anthelmintic doses. Part of the early loss after drenching is due to respiratory dysfunction when the chemical is delivered into the pharynx or trachea. Much effort has been exerted to define the factors leading to increased susceptibility to delayed mortality from hepatic disease. Hepatic factors such as induced microsomal metabolism and impaired antioxidant capacity may be important in the toxicity in sheep under field conditions. Additional nutritional factors, however, may be involved; for example, high intake of protein after dosage may produce a concentration of ammonia in the portal blood that is too high for the damaged liver to detoxify, resulting in death from ammonia intoxication.

Very severe acute carbon tetrachloride poisoning produces severe periacinar to massive liver necrosis. In less severe intoxications there may be more obvious fatty change in hepatocytes surrounding the necrotic zones than that seen in other acute hepatotoxicities, so that, grossly, the liver may be very pale and swollen. In these animals there are degenerative changes in renal tubular epithelium. Photosensitization after intoxication is slight or does not occur, and survival beyond a few days should allow complete restoration of normal hepatic histology. Hexachlorethane, tetrachlorethylene, and chloroform are other chlorinated hydrocarbons with apparently similar hepatotoxic properties, but these agents are little used now as medicinal agents.

Phosphorus

White phosphorus is still used for vermin control. It is mixed with fat in order to promote absorption, and much of the dose is transported to the liver shortly after ingestion. A small amount may be lost by vomition, for elemental phosphorus is directly irritant to the gastrointestinal tract. The mechanism of phosphorus hepatotoxicity is uncertain; it is apparent that metabolism to a toxic intermediate is not necessary, but there is some dispute on the involvement of lipoperoxidation in the hepatocellular injury. There is evidence that protein synthesis is impaired early and that this is responsible for the lipid accumulation that is so prominent a feature.

A few hours after ingestion of phosphorus there is severe colic and vomition, due to the irritant nature of the element. If the animal survives this acute phase there may be apparent recovery for a few days, followed by jaundice and other signs of liver failure, and death by about the fifth day. At autopsy there is severe icterus and fatty liver, the latter sometimes being predominantly periportal in distribution. Hepatocellular necrosis is not often a prominent feature histologically, notwithstanding the evidence of liver failure. Fatty change is also seen in the myocardium and distal nephrons.

Cresols

The tarred walls and floors of piggeries and the "clay pigeons" used as targets by gun clubs are occasionally responsible, by virtue of contained cresols, for poisoning of pigs. The poisoning may be acute, with severe periacinar necrosis the only significant lesion; or it may be chronic, with jaundice, ascites, and severe anemia added to the pathologic picture.

Saccharated Iron

Iron–dextran complexes have been widely used in the treatment and prevention of anemia in suckling swine. Very occasionally, severe losses may occur in animals with marginal vitamin E–selenium deficiency; in these cases there is, apparently, iron-catalyzed lipoperoxidation in hepatocytes and muscle. The result of this, as far as the liver is concerned, is sudden massive necrosis similar in many respects to that of hepatosis dietetica. This releases large amounts of potassium into the circulation, and sudden death may result from the cardiotoxicity of this ion. At autopsy, there is staining of the subcutaneous tissues and lymph nodes near the site of injection, and there are lesions in the liver or skeletal muscles (see below). The liver is of normal size and of normal color or pale, depending on whether or not the animal is anemic. The presence of an underlying necrosis may be indicated only by the numerous small or large hemorrhages present on the capsular and cut surface (Fig. 2.7D). Insoluble iron compounds with the staining reactions of hemosiderin are found in mesenchymal cells in many tissues, the largest amounts being in macrophages of the local lymph nodes and in the Kupffer cells.

Saccharated iron may, in the same circumstances as above, produce acute widespread muscle necrosis rather than hepatic necrosis. The myocardium is not affected (see diseases of muscle, in Muscles and Tendons, Volume 1).

Sawfly Larvae

This acute hepatotoxicity of cattle and, to a lesser extent, sheep, is of particular interest in that the toxin is present in an insect, the larva of the sawfly *Lophyrotoma interruptus*. This larva is parasitic on the leaves of the tree *Eucalyptus melanophloia,* and heavy infestations may occur in parts of northeastern Australia. On completion of feeding, masses of larvae sometimes accumulate at the base of the tree, where they may die and decompose. Cattle in particular find these masses attractive, perhaps as a result of nutritional stress. The hepatotoxin is an octapeptide, which produces acute periacinar necrosis with no specific features. Whether or not the larvae synthesize the toxin, or concentrate it from the tree, has not been determined.

Idiosyncratic Drug-Induced Hepatotoxicity

Idiosyncratic drug-induced hepatotoxicity has not been reported in animals as frequently as it has in humans, in which the unexpected and atypical response to a drug is reputed to be the most common cause of massive hepatic necrosis. Severe periacinar hepatic necrosis has been associated with use of the anthelmintic mebendazole in dogs; signs of hepatic failure appear at any time up to 2 weeks after exposure. Drug-induced hepatotoxicity may be mediated by allergic phenomena, which are characterized by granulomatous infiltrates containing eosinophils; this does not seem to be the case with mebendazole. It is likely that susceptibility to this type of intoxication is related to production of atypical drug metabolites, but if this is the case, the delayed onset of some cases is not explained.

Aflatoxin

The association between illness and death in animals and the ingestion of moldy feed has been known by veterinary diagnosticians for a long time. Developments in commerce, science, and technology since the 1950s have enormously expanded the potential scale of mycotoxic disease and have provided the techniques necessary for identification and assay of toxic metabolites. The target organs for the action of mycotoxins vary with the toxic metabolite, and there are species differences in susceptibility. Some of the syndromes of intoxication are sufficiently distinctive in clinical signs and pathologic changes to allow firm diagnosis, but others are not, and the subclinical effects are not well defined for any of them. Reference to defined mycotoxicoses is made in relation to target organs in several other chapters in these volumes.

The aflatoxins are a group of bisfuranocoumarin compounds produced as metabolites mainly by *Aspergillus flavus, A. parasiticus,* and *Penicillium puberulum.* The metabolites are designated by spectral qualities, and the major ones are B_1, B_2, G_1, and G_2. Many others may be produced in minor amounts in fungal colonies or as metabolic products of the major toxins in animals. The most significant and best studied of the aflatoxins is B_1 because of its relative abundance and its potency as a hepatotoxin. Strains of *Aspergillus* differ in the varieties and amounts of individual toxins produced, indicating that the biosynthesis of the toxins is genetically determined. The production of toxins also varies under different conditions of fungal growth, being influenced by the quality of the substrate, temperature, relative humidity and moisture content of the substrate, and microbial competition. Thus the toxicity of moldy feedstuffs is impossible to assess without measurement of toxin production. Aflatoxins can be produced on growing crops in the field, but much greater significance attaches to fungal activity in stored grain commodities or on mature unharvested grains.

Aflatoxins are metabolized by the hepatic mixed-function oxidase system to a variety of toxic and nontoxic metabolites, the proportions of which vary with the species and age of animal involved. There is very much species variation in susceptibility to the toxin, and as much or more variation with age. The LD_{50} of aflatoxin B_1, in 2-day-old ducklings, for example, is reported to be double that for 1-day-old birds, and the same sort of variation seems to hold for mammals. This age susceptibility has important implications in suckling animals, for toxic metabolites of aflatoxins may be excreted in the milk. Sheep and adult cattle are quite resistant to the toxin, whereas dogs, pigs, and calves are sensitive and may be fatally intoxicated by a dose rate of less than 1.0 mg per kilogram body weight.

The toxic effects of aflatoxin B_1 are related principally to the binding of its toxic metabolites to macromolecules, in particular, to nucleic acids and nucleoproteins. It is not surprising, therefore, that the toxic effects include carcinogenesis, teratogenesis, mitotic inhibition, and immunosuppression. Less is known of the pathogenesis of the hepatocellular necrosis caused by high dose rates of aflatoxin.

Prolonged exposure to low concentrations of the toxin may merely produce reduced growth rates and moderate enlargement of the liver without any significant hepatic signs. The enlargement may be partly due to hypertrophy of hepatocellular smooth endoplasmic reticulum and some degree of fatty change. As the level of aflatoxin in the ration increases (in young pigs, e.g., to 1.0 mg per kilogram ration), the liver may show all or none of the following changes: pallor, enlargement, bile staining, increased firmness due to *de novo* fibrogenesis, and fine nodular regenerative hyperplasia. There may also be edema of the gall-bladder and bile-tinged ascites in more severe cases. Even under experimental conditions, some individuals may show minimal liver lesions, while their fellows, under the same levels of exposure, die of liver failure. Histologically, affected livers show obvious increase in size of some hepatocytes and their nuclei (megalocytosis), focal necrosis, and cytosegresome formation. Bile ductules proliferate early (Fig. 2.23C), and reticulin and collagen deposition occurs throughout the acinus according to no distinct pattern. Fatty change in affected livers is variable in extent and occurrence, and bile pigments accumulate in canaliculi and hepatocytes in more severely affected livers. Minor degrees of megalocytosis may be seen in proximal tubular epithelium in the kidney. The changes produced resemble those of pyrrolizidine alkaloid toxicosis.

At higher dose rates of aflatoxin, most periacinar hepatocytes disappear and are replaced by an ill-assorted mixture of inflammatory cells, fibroblasts, and primitive vascular channels (Fig. 2.23C). The liver may be much smaller than normal, particularly in young animals, due presumably to mitotic inhibition, and focal hepatocellular necrosis is more obvious or may be supplanted by zonal (periacinar) necrosis. Fatty change in these livers may be severe and uniformly distributed.

The pathology of acute, fulminating liver necrosis is described under Patterns of Hepatic Necrosis. It is sometimes seen in dogs that eat moldy bread, dog food, or garbage, which may contain very high concentrations of the toxin. Younger animals are much more susceptible and may die within a few hours, the postmortem picture dominated by widespread hemorrhage and massive hepatic necrosis.

Phomopsin

There are two distinct manifestations of toxicity associated with *Lupinus* spp.; discussed here is the condition formerly known as "lupinosis," which is a true mycotoxic liver disease. The teratogenic and neurotoxic effects of some of the isoquinoline alkaloids from the plants themselves are discussed with Bones and Joints and the Nervous System (Volume 1).

The fungus *Phomopsis leptostromiformis* is parasitic on green *Lupinus* plants, but it becomes saprophytic after the host dies. Phomopsins (A or B) are produced if the lupin stubble is moistened, and such stubbles may remain toxic for months. Severe acute liver damage has been described in sheep on very toxic stubbles in western Australia, but in many of these cases it has been difficult to separate the toxicity of the lupins from that of copper, which in this area is often concentrated in ovine livers (see Copper, below).

The usual syndrome of phomopsin poisoning is subacute to chronic. Inappetance occurs soon after experimental administration of the toxin is begun; liver damage is clinically inapparent for several days, although there is early hydropic change and accelerated necrobiosis among hepatocytes. An increase in mitotic activity is soon apparent, although the liver has by this time become smaller. The mitotic activity is in fact largely ineffectual, as close examination reveals that many mitotic figures are abnormal (Fig. 2.23B). There is either clumping or dispersal

of chromatin, and there appears to be mitotic arrest at late metaphase. Remaining hepatocytes swell, their cytoplasm becomes granular, and their nuclei vesicular. With progression, hepatic fibrosis occurs, predominantly diffuse in distribution, and by this stage there is usually clinical icterus and anorexia. There will be variably severe fatty change, dependent to a large degree on the fat reserves of the animal (Fig. 2.23A). There is also accumulation of complex pigment in macrophages in portal stroma and about hepatic venules; this granular material contains lipofuscin, ferric iron, and copper at least. Bile duct proliferation is also a prominent feature of the chronic disease.

The liver continues to shrink, presumably as a result of continued mitotic inhibition and progressive fibrosis. The organ is small, tough, and has a finely granular surface and texture. It is pale grayish orange but usually retains its shape. In naturally occurring cases, however, discontinuous intake of the toxin may produce a liver grossly distorted by asymmetric nodular regeneration and fibrosis. The atrophic changes are most severe in the left lobe.

Photosensitization occurs in phomopsin-poisoned sheep; it may be severe if the animals have access to green feed while under the influence of the toxin.

Phomopsin poisoning in cattle causes most losses when the animals are lactating or heavily pregnant; in these animals the syndrome is essentially one of ketosis, to which such cows would be predisposed by the anorexia that is an obvious clinical feature of this intoxication. Pregnant sheep are less likely to have access to toxic lupin roughage during late gestation, otherwise ketosis triggered by phomopsin would be expected just as often as in cattle.

Chronic hepatic fibrosis with fine, nodular regeneration may occur infrequently in cattle due to chronic phomopsin poisoning. Similar liver changes may also be seen in horses, in which there may also be hemolytic anemia of unknown pathogenesis.

Sporidesmin

The mycotoxin sporidesmin is produced by the fungus *Pithomyces chartarum;* the most important substrate is dead ryegrass (*Lolium perenne*) that has been moistened in warm weather. Intoxication causes chronic liver damage and severe hepatogenous photosensitivity ("facial eczema") and is a serious cause of loss of sheep and, to a lesser extent, cattle on the North Island of New Zealand. Sporadic and subclinical intoxication occurs irregularly on the South Island and in southern Australia and South Africa. Sporidesmin intake in conjunction with ingestion of *Tribulus terrestris* causes another hepatogenous photosensitivity (*geeldikkop*); this is similar to but distinct from facial eczema, and is described below.

Sporidesmin is concentrated in the fungal spores, and the toxigenicity of pasture is related to the density of the spores in it. Sporidesmin is not specifically hepatotoxic. Administration of the toxin does produce rapid disorganization of hepatic-cell organelles and triglyceride accumulation, but these are mild and nonspecific changes. If administered in suitable dosage, the toxin causes permeability alterations in many tissues and will, for example, produce corneal edema on local application. The hepatobiliary lesions are due to the excretion of unconjugated sporidesmin in bile and its concentration there. Sporidesmin is

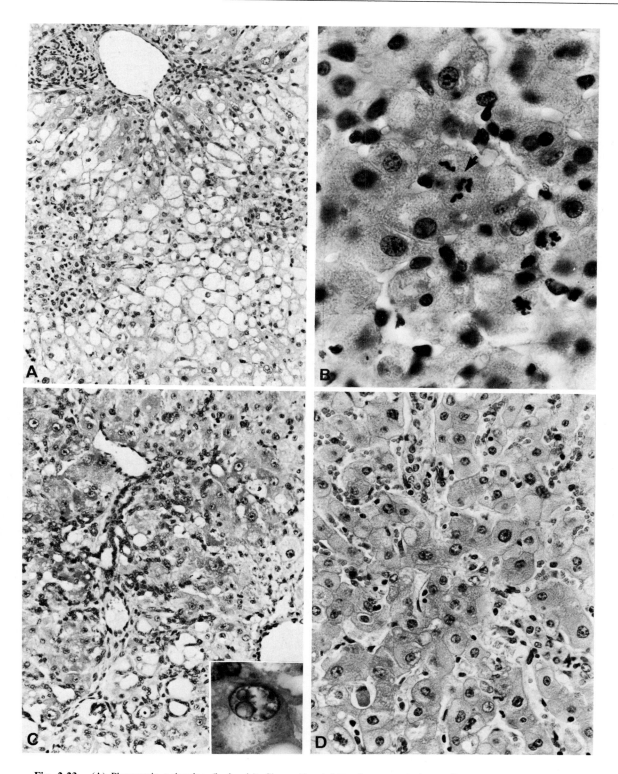

Fig. 2.23. (A) Phomopsin poisoning (lupinosis). Sheep. Zonal fatty change, periacinar collapse, and periportal megalocytosis. (B) Subacute phomopsin poisoning. Sheep. Numerous and abnormal mitotic figures (arrow). (A and B courtesy of J. G. Allen.) (C) Subacute aflatoxin poisoning. Calf. Bile ductule proliferation, megalocytosis, and nuclear vesiculation. (Inset) Intranuclear inclusions formed by invagination of cytoplasm into nucleus; seen in many subacute and chronic intoxications. (Courtesy of R. A. MacKenzie.) (D) *Lantana* poisoning. Ox. Hepatocellular swelling, hydropic (feathery) degeneration, and apoptosis.

also excreted in urine, and if the dose is high enough, edema and mucosal hemorrhage occur in the bladder. The hepatic lesion is due to irritation of mesenchymal tissues in the portal triads and surrounding the bile ducts. If the concentration of sporidesmin is high enough, the biliary epithelium undergoes necrosis, and diffusion of toxin produces irritative lesions in the adjacent blood vessels.

The liver in acute forms of the disease is enlarged, with rounded edges, and is finely mottled and discolored yellowish green by retained bile pigments, although the discoloration may be blotchy. There is mild edema and congestion of the wall of the gallbladder, and it may be distended with bile of normal quality or with mucin (white bile). The extrahepatic ducts are thickened and prominent, and there is edema of the adventitia. The ductal changes may extend to the papilla of Vater and can be traced by the naked eye deeply into the parenchyma. In more chronic cases, alterations of size and pigmentation of the liver are variable. Pale areas of capsular thickening, which may be elevated or depressed, are visible. On cut surface they extend deeply as wedge-shaped areas in which biliary fibrosis has produced an exaggerated lobular pattern, and the parenchyma is pale and atrophic; these areas are related to occluded bile ducts.

The liver is firm and cuts with increased resistance. The intrahepatic ducts are conspicuous. There is irregular stenosis of their lumens, some are occluded by cellular debris and inspissated bile or mucin, and in some, cicatrization of the new fibrous tissue causes complete atresia. Occlusion of the ducts causes the parenchyma served by them to undergo atrophy, necrosis, and fibrosis. The livers of animals that have survived an attack of cholangiohepatitis of this genesis are distorted in shape and size by large nodules of regeneration and persistent areas of atrophy and fibrosis. The atrophy and fibrosis may affect either lobe, but usually the left most severely (Fig. 2.24A).

Histologically, the changes are those of an acute cholangitis or cholangiohepatitis to which there is a minimum of leukocytic reaction. There is extensive necrosis of the lining of the larger intrahepatic ducts and the extrahepatic ducts, the epithelium being cast off as debris mixed with a few leukocytes. There is edema of the adventitia of the ducts, with active fibroplasia and scarring. Inflammatory cells are present, but not in large numbers, and they are chiefly lymphocytes and histiocytes. Injury to the smaller radicles of the bile ducts is less severe, but fibrosis and collagenization are active. The portal tracts are enlarged by fibrous tissue and by the active generation of new bile ducts that follows.

In more severe intoxications there may be coagulative necrosis of blood vessel walls in the portal triads; when this is incomplete, the most damaged segment of the vessel tends to be that adjacent to the nearest injured bile duct. Both arteries and veins may be affected, and it is possible that the so-called bile infarcts are related to vascular insufficiency as well as to impaired bile drainage.

Changes in the hepatic parenchyma are minimal and secondary to those in the portal triads. In acute cases, there may be extensive pigmentation of hepatocytes and Kupffer cells by bile pigments, but this is irregular in distribution in the liver. Inspissated bile can be found in the bile ducts and as plugs in the canaliculi. There is some necrosis of hepatocytes adjacent to inflamed portal areas, and other areas of necrosis, focal in type and distribution and probably the result of biliary obstruction, may be numerous. Other morbid alterations include great enlargement of the adrenals, produced by cortical hypertrophy, sclerotic intimal plaques in the arteries, veins, and lymphatics in the hilus of the liver, and a tendency for the newly formed bile ductules to recanalize occluded ducts.

Pyrrolizidine Alkaloids

The pyrrolizidine alkaloids have been found in plants belonging to various unrelated botanical families, principally the Compositae, Leguminosae, Boraginaceae, and particularly in the genera *Senecio, Crotalaria, Heliotropium, Cynoglossum, Amsinckia, Echium,* and *Trichodesma.* There are, widely distributed in the world, many hundreds of species within these genera. Contained in these species is a huge range of pyrrolizidine alkaloids; more than 100 have been chemically defined, and ~30 of these have been shown to be toxic. Most of the toxic plant species contain more than one of the alkaloids, the toxic varieties of which are all esters of one of three amino alcohol bases. These toxins all must be metabolized to highly reactive pyrroles before they can express their full effects, to which the nuclei of the target cell seems most susceptible.

The toxicity of an alkaloid for a given organ depends on three factors: the rate at which the parent alkaloid is converted to the pyrrolic derivative, the proportion of the alkaloid so converted, and the reactivity or binding capacity of the pyrrole. The rate, extent, and qualitative nature of these conversions vary with the species, age, and sex of the animal intoxicated as well as with the metabolic and mitotic status of its target cells; these variables in some measure explain the difficulty in predicting the outcome of pyrrolizidine alkaloid poisoning in an individual. In ruminants, an additional complicating factor may be the degree to which the toxins are degraded in the rumen before they have had a chance to be absorbed. Nevertheless, there are some consistent differences in species susceptibility to these toxins; pigs, for example, may be as much as 200 times more susceptible than sheep or goats, with cattle and horses being only ~15 times more resistant than pigs. These differences account for the fact that sheep can be used to graze out stands of *Senecio* that would be lethal to cattle.

The most characteristic effect of these toxins on the liver is the induction of nuclear and cytoplasmic gigantism ("megalocytosis") (Fig. 2.25D); this is related to an antimitotic effect, the mechanism of which is not yet known. It is not due to inhibition of DNA synthesis; indeed, continued nucleoprotein synthesis, combined with mitotic inhibition, accounts for the great increase in size of the nucleus and, probably, the basophilia of the cytoplasm that develops. Megalocytosis is not a change specific for pyrrolizidine alkaloidosis; it is seen in intoxication by other alkylating agents such as nitrosamines and aflatoxins. Nevertheless, the most florid examples of this change are produced by the pyrrolizidine alkaloids. The onset of megalocytosis is delayed by an interval determined by the mitotic activity of the organ. Thus experimentally, animals that have had hepatocytes removed by hepatectomy or by acute hepatotoxic insults will develop megalocytosis more rapidly and to a more severe degree than controls.

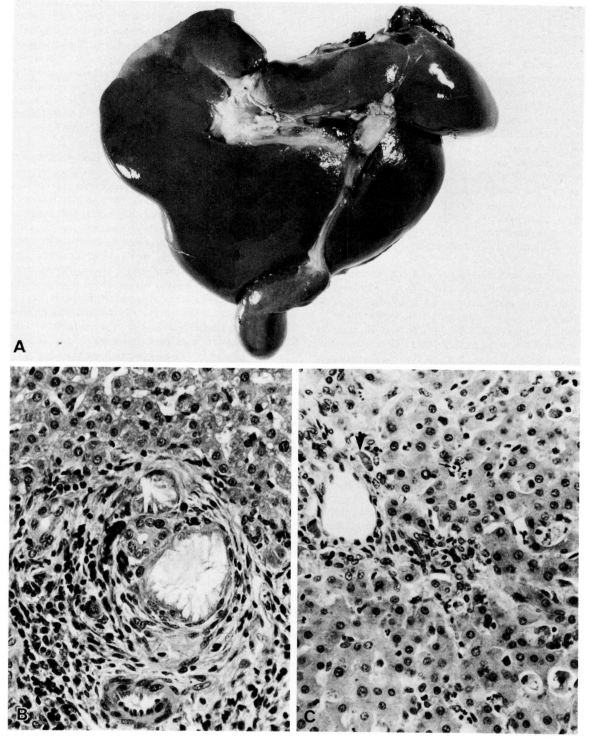

Fig. 2.24. (**A**) Chronic sporidesmin poisoning (''facial eczema''). Atrophy of left lobe, with hypertrophy of right and caudate lobes. Sheep. (Courtesy of W. J. Hartley.) (**B**) Chronic cholangitis and plugging of bile duct by lipophilic crystalloid material. Photosensitivity disease of sheep on pangola grass. Similar reaction to that seen in *geeldikkop*. (**C**) Liver in prehemolytic phase of chronic copper poisoning. Apoptosis (small arrow), focal leukocyte aggregation, and pigmented macrophages in sinusoids and stroma (large arrow). Sheep.

The volume of affected cells may be increased as much as 20 times (Fig. 2.25D). Their nuclei are enlarged and single, the nuclear membrane stains strongly with basic dyes and is sharp, the chromatin is scanty and fragmented, the nucleolus is enlarged, and frequently, there are globular cytoplasmic invaginations within the nuclei. The cytoplasmic volume is increased, the margins are condensed and sharp, the peripheral part of the cytoplasm is usually pale, and a diffuse central zone is rich in the basophilic granules of nucleic acids. Acidophilic spherical cytosegresomes are also a common but less specific finding. The enlarged cells are closely apposed, so sinusoids may not be evident. Small extravasations of bile may be present between them. Many of these megalocytes are in different stages of dying, but they die slowly, individually, and not as a tissue. These changes affect all the cells of the acinus, but in the early stages, periportal hepatocytes may be relatively spared. Occasionally, a whole acinus may escape, so a paracentral cluster of cells of normal size may be found adjacent to some hepatic venules.

In severe pyrrolizidine alkaloid poisoning, the liver becomes smaller while its hepatocytes get larger; cells must obviously be lost to balance this equation. They are not replaced, owing to the mitotic inhibition, and the remaining megalocytes suffer reduced function. The evidence that megalocytes are not very good hepatocytes lies in the fact that liver failure occurs long before the liver mass falls below the 30% theoretically necessary to sustain life.

The sequential hepatic changes in domestic species receiving small or intermittent doses of alkaloids have not been studied, but intermittent doses are probably responsible for the many livers in which nodular regenerative hyperplasia occurs. The nodules are diffusely but not uniformly distributed in the liver and consist of cells that are morphologically normal or that are small and contain fatty vacuoles. The origin of these cells and their relation to preexisting architecture are not clear. They may also fall victim to later alkaloid intoxication.

Concurrent with the development of megalocytosis, there is some fibroplasia and proliferation of bile ducts in the portal triads. The fibroplasia is minimal in sheep, moderate in horses, and may be marked in cattle (Fig. 2.26). As a rule, it is only in cattle that the fibrous tissue infiltrates along the sinusoids to dissect lobules, separate individual cells, and link up with the walls of efferent veins; the fibrosis can be regarded, as usual, as a response to chronic parenchymal degeneration. The amount of bile duct proliferation may be much greater than that of fibrosis. Its stimulus is not known, but it may be an abortive attempt at regeneration and it may in the terminal stages account for almost half the weight of the liver. In fatal cases in cattle, the primary hepatocyte injury is abetted by the vascular complications of chronic hepatic fibrosis and remodeling. The livers are very tough and nodular (Fig. 2.26B), and the nodules have variably efficient biliary drainage, so there may be a very striking color pattern, ranging from fatty yellow through green and brown. Ascites is present due to portal hypertension, which may also produce severe mesenteric edema and diarrhea; rectal prolapse may accompany the latter. Moderate jaundice and photosensitization are usual.

The disease in sheep is always protracted as a consequence of the relative resistance of this species; indeed, clinical signs may not be seen until after a second season's exposure. The shape of these failed livers is normal, but they are small, grayish yellow, fairly smooth, and toughened by condensation of normal stroma rather than by fibroplasia. If the liver copper content was high before intoxication, there will in the terminal stages of the disease probably be enough copper released to trigger an episode of intravascular hemolysis. In this case the carcass will be intensely jaundiced, and the urinary tract stained with hemoglobin. Chronic copper poisoning and its relationship to pyrrolizidine alkaloid poisoning are discussed below.

Liver failure produced in horses by these alkaloids is characterized pathologically by much the same sort of picture as that seen in cattle; clinically there is usually severe nervous disorder, such as head pressing and compulsive walking. In the past this gave rise to the colloquial names "walkabout" and "walking" disease. This is regarded as hepatic encephalopathy, rather than evidence of any specific neurotoxic property of the alkaloids.

Acute poisoning by the pyrrolizidine alkaloids is unusual; because of the unpalatability of the plants, the amount of toxin naturally ingested is usually too small to produce acute effects. It produces a periacinar necrosis with hemorrhage and laking of blood in the affected zones and endothelial damage to the hepatic venules and smaller hepatic veins. The morphology of the acute lesion is not clearly different from that produced by a variety of other hepatotoxins and is associated with biochemical disturbances similar to those produced by carbon tetrachloride. Small zones of necrosis and hemorrhage may occur in natural poisonings in horses especially, and less commonly in cattle, but necrosis of tissue can be entirely absent in these species, as it usually is in sheep, and it does not contribute to the natural evolution of the typical lesions. The injury to efferent veins may be of some significance in cattle, in which extensive fibrosis sometimes develops around smaller hepatic veins. Such perivenous fibrosis is spotty in distribution in horses and absent in sheep; its development in cattle is quantitatively related to fibrosis in portal areas, and although it may be in part due to the initial injury to the veins, it is largely a natural development of the extensive fibrosis that sometimes occurs in cattle. This perivenous fibrosis has been dignified with the name of a disease, "veno-occlusive disease of the liver," but this cannot be justified; the venous lesion is neither constant, characteristic, nor contributory to the course of the lesions in the liver as a whole.

The metabolites of pyrrolizidine alkaloids affect tissues other than the liver; death in some instances may be due to renal damage and in others to pulmonary vascular and interstitial lesions. Variation in the source of the toxin and in the species of target animal accounts for the differences in susceptibility of the different tissues, but as a generalization it may be stated that the alkaloids from *Crotalaria* affect the widest range of tissues in most animals.

The pulmonary toxicity of pyrrolizidine alkaloids in rats is well recognized, and lung lesions occur that are characterized by severe vascular engorgement and edema. It should not be assumed that all hepatotoxic pyrrolizidine alkaloids produce lung lesions or that all animal species are equally susceptible to this type of lung injury. *Jaagsiekte* has been described in horses eating *Crotalaria dura*, and *C. crispata* produces similar le-

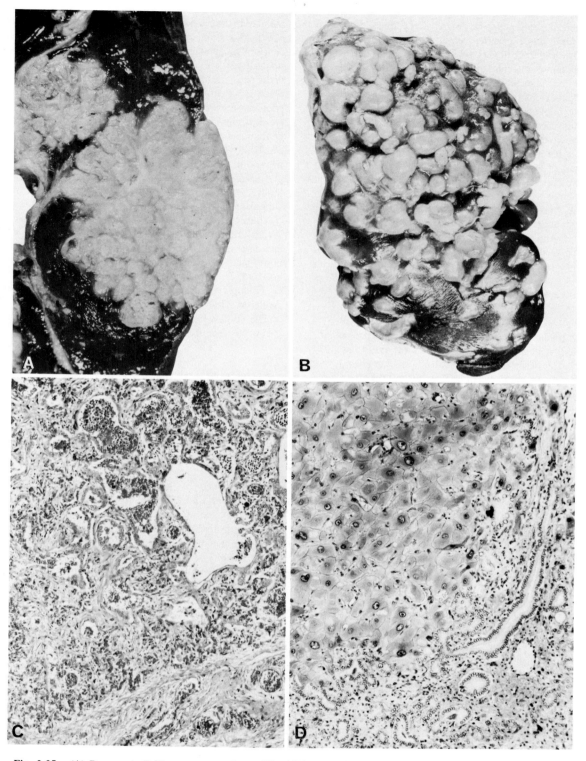

Fig. 2.25. (A) Degenerate *Echinococcus granulosus*. Mineralizing membranous debris and fibrosis. Ox. (B) *Echinococcus granulosus*. Severe hydatid liver disease. Sheep. (C) Pulmonary congestion and hemorrhage, septal fibrosis, and epithelial metaplasia. *Senecio* poisoning. Pig. (D) Megalocytosis and bile duct proliferation in *Crotalaria* poisoning. Horse.

sions. Sheep develop pulmonary signs after eating *C. globifera* and *C. dura,* and pigs after eating *Senecio jacobaea* (Fig. 2.25C). The reference to *jaagsiekte* implies a morphologic similarity to pulmonary adenomatosis of sheep that is not warranted. The experimental feeding of *C. spectabilis* to rats or the injection of the alkaloid monocrotaline, extracted from the plant, produces progressive pulmonary disease and cor pulmonale, with necrotizing vasculitis of the pulmonary arterioles. These lesions in the rat, which are of hypertensive nature, are secondary to changes in the alveolar septa, and this is probably the site of initial injury in domestic species. Monocrotaline produces septal edema and degeneration of all cells and the elastic tissue of rat alveolar septa.

There is considerable hyperemia, hemorrhage, and alveolar edema with migration of septal cells. There is progressive deposition of reticulin and collagen in the alveolar septa. Emphysema occurs in pigs and is an outstanding feature of the *jaagsiekte* of horses. The essential reactive lesion is diffuse fibrosis of alveolar and interlobular septa, with patchy epithelialization occurring more slowly (Fig. 2.25C).

Lantana

Lantana camara contains at least two cholestatic poisons, the triterpenes lantadene A and B, of which A is the more toxic. Like the other toxins described here, lantadene A will produce severe acute zonal necrosis of the liver if given in artificially large doses. The naturally occurring disease, however, is a subacute or chronic one characterized by anorexia, severe icterus, constipation, polyuria, dehydration, and photosensitization; this intoxication is most commonly seen in cattle, and rarely in sheep and goats. The latter species are quite susceptible to the toxin but are less likely to eat the plant.

Heavily intoxicated cattle can die within 2 days, but most fatal cases run a course of ~2 weeks. Ruminal statis and anorexia appear early, along with polyuria due to nephrosis. Photosensitization is usually severe after 2 days, and the animals become severely dehydrated as a result of the renal lesion and disinclination to drink. The static rumen is a reservoir of toxin, and should rumen activity recommence, more toxin is released to the lower alimentary tract, where it is absorbed and perpetuates the intoxication.

Bile retention is present in poisoned animals, the jaundice being more severe in chronic cases, which have had more time for bile pigments to bind to tissues. The liver is enlarged, pale, and stained yellow, orange, or greenish gray by bile pigment. The gallbladder is enlarged, often spectacularly so, and is filled with pale, sometimes slightly mucoid bile. The gallbladder distension is partly explained by specific paralysis of this organ by lantadene A. The large bowel contains dark, dry feces, and the kidneys are slightly enlarged and wet on section, and especially in the more chronic cases, the cortex is pale and the medulla hyperemic.

The most consistent histologic finding in the liver is hepatocellular enlargement and fine cytoplasmic vacuolation (Fig. 2.23D), together with some degree of bile accumulation in canaliculi, hepatocyte cytoplasm, and Kupffer cells. The canalicular cholestasis is usually more severe in the periacinar zones, while the cytoplasmic vacuolation is often more pro-

nounced in the periportal hepatocytes. There is usually some bile duct proliferation, and in some cases there will be a high incidence of focal coagulative necrosis or hepatocellular dissociation. There is also much apoptosis and cytosegresome formation in the periportal zone. The severity of the liver changes may be much less than expected from the intensity of the icterus and photosensitization; in these cases electron microscopy will show an apparent increase in volume of smooth endoplasmic reticulum and a quite characteristic form of collapse of many bile canaliculi. Other canaliculi are distended and have damaged microvilli. Since much of the bilirubin that accumulates in the plasma of such animals is conjugated, it seems that the cholestasis is due in large measure to direct interference with canalicular transport of bile.

The renal lesion is a nonspecific tubular nephrosis, ranging in severity from mild vacuolar change to patchy tubular necrosis and extensive tubular cast formation. The role of the hyperbilirubinemia in the production of the renal damage has not been assessed. Severe myocardial necrosis can be produced in sheep by *Lantana* poisoning and may be responsible for the early deaths in cattle.

The cholestatic agent in *Lippia rehmanni,* icterogenin, is chemically identical to lantadene A.

Tribulus terrestris

Photosensitizing liver diseases have caused enormous loss of sheep in South Africa, and it is now apparent that the most important of these, *geeldikkop,* is due to the interaction between sporidesmin and a component of *Tribulus terrestris.* The sporidesmin may be produced on a variety of substrates (including *Tribulus*); facial eczema, the disease it produces in the absence of *Tribulus,* has been described above. It seems that *Tribulus* by itself rarely if ever produces changes in the liver, but an unidentified component of the plant, together with the mycotoxin, produces liver lesions that are histologically distinct from those produced by sporidesmin alone.

The gross lesions of *geeldikkop* are similar to those of facial eczema in that there is generalized icterus, and the liver is discolored by bile pigment and either slightly swollen or distorted, according to the duration of the disease. In poisoning by sporidesmin alone, however, there is more obvious edema and fibrosis of bile ducts, and bile infarcts in the parenchyma are more common. In *geeldikkop,* the most characteristic gross finding is the presence of a white, semifluid accumulation of fine, crystalline material that can be expressed from the cystic duct and larger intrahepatic ducts. The gallbladder mucosa is also partly covered with a fine, crystalline deposit.

The most consistent histologic abnormality in *geeldikkop* is the presence in bile ducts of varying amounts of crystalline material, or rather, the demonstration of acicular clefts left after the cholesterol-like crystals have been dissolved during paraffin processing (Fig. 2.24B). The density of these accumulations varies but is often clearly sufficient to block the bile ducts, which may be distended and surrounded by a modest, low-grade inflammatory infiltrate. The severity of peribiliary fibrosis is more variable and probably depends on the relative contribution of sporidesmin to the intoxication. There is some hepatocellular degeneration, including cytosegresome formation and apop-

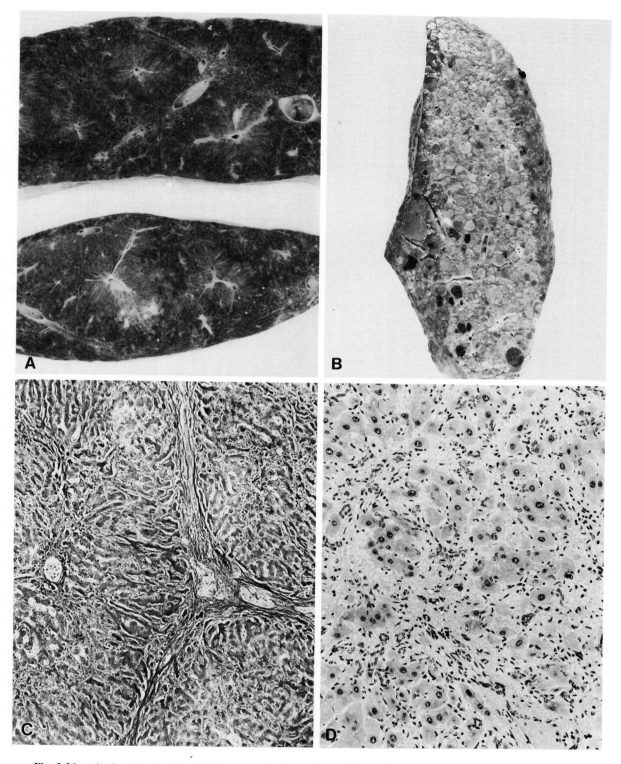

Fig. 2.26. (A) *Senecio* poisoning. Calf. Diffuse fibrosis, mimicking "nutmeg" liver of chronic congestion. (B) Liver. *Heliotropium* poisoning. Cow. Fibrosis and nodular regeneration. Some nodules stained by bile. (C) Diffuse fibrosis of liver in chronic *Senecio* poisoning. Ox. (D) Megalocytosis and diffuse fibrosis in *Crotalaria* poisoning. Ox. Fibrous septa have subdivided the acini.

tosis, and there is fairly uniform swelling of cytoplasm. Bile pigment accumulates in Kupffer cells and hepatocyte cytoplasm, but not to any marked extent in canaliculi. Focal necrosis of the gallbladder mucosa is often present.

The identity of the biliary crystals is not known; limited studies have shown that they are not cholesterol, cholic acid, glycocholate, or taurocholate. They are not likely to be specific for *Tribulus* intoxication, because very similar crystals are also seen in bile ducts of sheep intoxicated by *Agave* and *Nolina,* and in photosensitization seen sporadically in sheep grazing *Panicum* and other grass genera (Fig. 2.24B). The crystals are never seen in poisoning by sporidesmin alone, thus in *geeldikkop* they are clearly associated with *Tribulus* ingestion.

Nitrosamine

Epizootics of poisoning by dimethylnitrosamine occurred in Norwegian cattle, sheep, and fur-bearing animals, from 1957 to 1962. The toxin was present in herring meal and was thought to be a reaction product of trimethylamine and other lower amines with sodium nitrite, added as a preservative, the reacting amines being products of decomposition. Animals consumed several pounds of the toxic meal each day before becoming ill.

At autopsy, there was moderate anasarca and signs of hemorrhagic diathesis. Livers affected acutely were enlarged and firm, with mottled discoloration and sometimes a nutmeg appearance. In chronic intoxication, the liver was small, granular, and very firm. A number of cases recovered after a prolonged convalescence, and in these there was atrophy and fibrosis of the left and caudate lobes, and the right lobe was hyperplastic and hemispheric. Histologically, in acute cases, there was widespread hemorrhagic necrosis of periacinar distribution and an unusual degree of intimal and subendothelial reaction in sublobular and hepatic veins. The chronic lesion was dominated by extensive fibrosis of periacinar distribution, with obliterative changes in many central and sublobular veins.

The hepatocellular changes in chronic nitrosamine poisoning are not specific; they are essentially those described with the other alkylating agents. There is megalocytosis, nuclear vesiculation and nucleolar prominence, cytoplasmic intranuclear inclusions, and variable fatty change and cytoplasmic bile accumulation.

This intoxication has little veterinary importance now that it is easily prevented; most interest in these compounds is based on their use as research tools in molecular pathology. They have great carcinogenic potential, but this was not evident to any significant extent in the accidental poisonings.

Copper

Copper alone of the heavy metals seems to have a selectively toxic effect on the liver, and there is significant variation in species susceptibility. Sheep as a species are most prone to copper poisoning, with some breeds being more susceptible than others. Bedlington terriers are also unusually susceptible. In these dogs and sheep, toxic amounts of copper can accumulate in the liver while dietary copper levels are not excessive by standards for other species. Copper poisoning does occur in cattle and pigs, but in these species it is due to abnormally high intake of the element.

Chronic copper poisoning of sheep occurs as a result of the presence of three environmental factors acting alone or in concert. First, excessive copper intake may occur as a result of contamination of pasture or prepared feed; the latter is difficult to avoid when feed mills are preparing rations for different species and is probably partly responsible for the observation that housed sheep are more prone to copper poisoning than animals at pasture. Second, increased copper accumulation occurs as a result of increased availability of dietary copper; this happens when dietary levels of molybdenum are unusually low. Molybdenum, in the presence of sufficient sulfate, forms insoluble complexes with copper in the gut and liver, making the copper biologically inert. Subterranean clover growing on calcareous soils in southern Australia may be relatively deficient in molybdenum, and in these areas British breeds of sheep are known to be more susceptible than Merinos to chronic copper poisoning. A breed of sheep from the Hebridean island of North Ronaldsay has apparently adapted to a seaweed diet low in both copper and molybdenum but rich in zinc. Zinc is also capable of interfering with copper uptake, and these sheep, while avoiding copper deficiency, are exquisitely susceptible to chronic copper poisoning when transferred to normal pasture. Other hepatotoxins constitute the third environmental factor that predisposes sheep to outbreaks of chronic copper poisoning. The most important of these are pyrrolizidine alkaloids (from *Heliotropium* or *Echium*) in eastern Australia, and phomopsin from lupins in western Australia and, possibly, South Africa.

The basis for chronic copper poisoning in sheep is the peculiar avidity of the liver for copper, coupled with the very limited rate at which this species can excrete the element in the bile. After intraportal injection of a copper isotope, practically all the radioactivity is removed during the first passage through the liver. Most of the copper is sequestered in hepatocellular lysosomes, where it does little damage at concentrations of up to 200 to 300 ppm dry weight. As the concentration rises, there is presumably more interaction between other cell components and the copper. There is some evidence that lysosomal membranes lose integrity and allow copper and lysosomal hydrolases to damage the rest of the cytoplasm. By the time the liver copper concentration has reached ~300 ppm or more, there is a histologically apparent increase in hepatocellular turnover, with single hepatocytes undergoing apoptosis within a dense knot of neutrophils. At still higher copper levels, the apoptotic rate increases, while all cells become swollen and their nuclei vesicular. The mitotic rate increases, presumably to keep pace with the accelerated loss of hepatocytes, and large macrophages appear in the sinusoids and stromal spaces about the vessels (Fig. 2.24C). These cells contain eosinophilic, granular debris, which consists of copper-containing lipofuscins.

Sheep with liver copper concentrations in excess of 1000 ppm may be clinically and hematologically normal, so long as the increasing mitotic rate produces enough new hepatocytes to take up the copper released by dying cells. At this stage, however, there will be elevated levels of liver-specific enzymes in the plasma. As soon as the rate of hepatocellular loss exceeds the replacement rate, the plasma copper levels begin to rise. Eventually, the blood copper concentration is high enough to damage circulating erythrocytes, and intravascular hemolysis ensues. The effect of the hemolysis on the liver is to accelerate the rate of hepatocellular necrosis, thus copper enters the circulation at an increasing rate. The clinical syndrome then is one of paroxysmal intravascular hemolysis and liver failure, in which a sheep may pass from apparent good health to death within ~6 hr.

The association of chronic copper poisoning with phomopsin and pyrrolizidine alkaloid poisoning has already been noted. The relationship is understandable in the light of the critical role hepatocellular mitosis plays in sheep in delaying the onset of the hemolytic crisis. It is to be expected that any agent that interferes with the mitotic process will provoke the crisis at an earlier stage of copper accumulation. There is good field evidence that less specific stresses, such as brief starvation, may also precipitate the crisis in susceptible sheep.

The carcass is discolored by deep jaundice, superimposed on which is the reddish color imparted by free hemoglobin. Often there is a brownish hue as well, because a proportion of the hemoglobin is oxidized to methemoglobin. The kidneys are deep reddish brown and the urine deep red, as a result of hemoglobinuria. The liver is slightly soft and swollen, and deep orange. The bile is dark and granular, and the spleen is engorged, dark and soft. The histologic changes of the preclinical stages are present in the liver and are somewhat obscured by the periacinar necrosis of hypoxemia and the bile accumulations of hemolytic disease. The histology may be further confused by the presence of changes induced by other toxins, should these have been involved.

During the hemolytic crisis, some of the copper is lost from the disintegrating liver; some passes into the urine, and kidney copper concentration rises to 1000 ppm or more. Kidney copper levels therefore give a truer indication of a prior hemolytic crisis due to chronic copper poisoning than does elevation of liver copper alone.

The events described in sheep also occur in chronic copper poisoning in pigs and cattle, and acute intravascular hemolysis may be seen, especially in calves. Usually, however, there is less of the acute terminal chain reaction in these species, and there is more evidence of chronic liver damage with diffuse fibrosis.

Acute copper poisoning is most often seen in ruminants after accidental administration of single large doses of copper, by either the oral or parenteral routes. The liver lesion is a nonspecific acute periacinar necrosis, and intravascular hemolysis may occur if plasma copper levels are sufficiently elevated. Acute gastroenteritis will be produced by oral dosage and may also be seen after sufficiently large parenteral doses of copper.

Chronic copper toxicosis in **Bedlington terriers** differs from the disease in sheep in that the susceptibility to it is inherited within the breed as an autosomal recessive character. The canine disease is not characterized by a hemolytic finale, as in sheep; hemolysis, if it occurs, is never a prominent part of the disease.

Affected dogs are usually presented with signs of progressive liver failure; ill thrift, wasting, ascites, nervous signs, and less consistently, jaundice. Grossly, the livers are fibrotic and pale, and in later stages, finely nodular. The most characteristic feature of the histology is the presence of numerous golden brown,

refractile granules in most hepatocytes, and darker pigment in Kupffer cells. These granules are autophagolysosomes that contain ferric iron and copper (Fig. 2.17D), but their ultrastructure and other histochemical reactions suggest that they consist mostly of lipofuscin. The hepatic lesion has been described as chronic active hepatitis, because scanty periportal infiltrates of inflammatory cells (Fig. 2.17C) and prominent piecemeal necrosis are present. It seems likely that the inflammatory infiltrates are a reaction to accelerated hepatocyte turnover. The pattern of fibrosis is complex; it seems to be a mixture of portal and diffuse types. Most hepatocytes are swollen, and many contain fat.

Hepatic copper concentrations in these animals may be very high; as much as 12,000 ppm by dry weight has been recorded, and levels higher than 5000 ppm are not uncommon. Thus it would seem that these dogs have much more effective copper-binding mechanisms in their hepatocellular lysosomes than sheep. This disease has been proposed as a model of hepatolenticular degeneration (Wilson's disease) of humans, but there are differences between the two copper-storage diseases. In the human condition, there are lowered levels of plasma ceruloplasmin; this is not seen in Bedlingtons, nor are the fairly specific brain lesions of Wilson's disease.

Neoplastic and Like Lesions of the Liver and Bile Ducts

Hepatobiliary tumors are quite common in animals and are probably, excepting lymphomas, the most common of visceral tumors in cats, cattle, sheep, and dogs. It also seems, again excepting lymphomas, that primary tumors are more common than secondary tumors perhaps due to the infrequency of gastrointestinal neoplasms and to interruption of the life of animals before primary tumors elsewhere have disseminated as fully as they might.

The classification of tumors of the liver and bile ducts presents some difficulty in terms of deciding whether a tumor is benign or malignant, or of hepatocellular or cholangiocellular origin. With respect to the first difficulty, tumors of orderly and benign appearance may metastasize. The second difficulty is perhaps artificial, and a histogenetic classification requires a clearer statement than can presently be made on the embryogenic relationships of the hepatocytes, intralobular cholangioles, and interlobular bile ducts. There is no record of tumor of the extrahepatic bile ducts in animals, but it is possible that some carcinomas thought to arise from the pancreatic ducts may actually arise from the distal portions of the bile duct.

Hyperplastic nodules are common in old dogs in whose livers there are signs of prolonged but mild fatty changes and congestion (Fig. 2.27A). Hepatocellular carcinomas are occasionally observed in such livers; their relation to the hyperplasia is probably not fortuitous. Hyperplastic nodules also occur in fibrotic livers. The smaller ones do not always contain biliary radicles or hepatic venules, and these may be quite difficult to distinguish histologically from adenomas. The conservative diagnosis is justified because hepatocellular carcinomas seldom, if ever, are observed to arise in fibrotic livers in animals.

Cystic hyperplasia of the mucus-producing glands in the

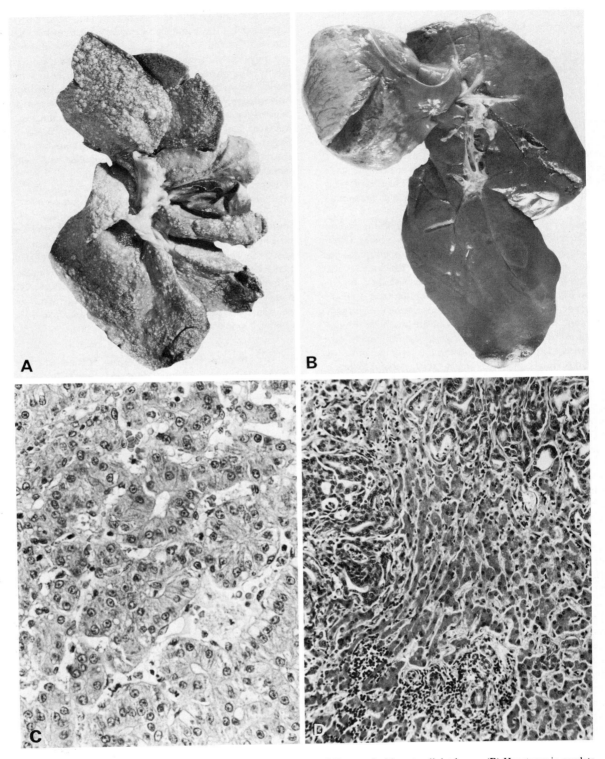

Fig. 2.27. (**A**) Early nodular regeneration. Dog. This lesion may follow gradual hepatocellular loss.   (**B**) Hepatoma in caudate lobe. Sheep.   (**C**) Hepatoma of glandular acinar form. Dog.   (**D**) Infiltrative biliary carcinoma compressing hepatocellular plates. Dog.

walls of the gallbladder and larger bile duct is occasionally observed in dogs. The hyperplastic nodules are sessile or polypoid, and the cysts contain mucin. Some of these may be the result of chronic inflammation. Mucosal hyperplasia in the large bile ducts is observed frequently in the long-standing mild cholangiohepatitis of fluke infestation. The hyperplasia is of microscopic dimensions, but in some instances it appears histologically to be atypical. Localized, polypoid foci of cystic hyperplasia are specific changes in cattle poisoned by highly chlorinated naphthalene.

True neoplasms of the liver and bile ducts are best designated as either hepatocellular or cholangiocellular. Hepatocellular tumors predominate in cattle and sheep, and cholangiocellular tumors predominate in dogs and cats. Other species rarely have primary hepatic tumors.

Hepatocellular Tumors

Hepatocellular adenomas (hepatomas) are usually single and they may be 15 cm or more in diameter. The smaller ones project as smooth nodes, but some of the larger specimens are lobate, and some pedunculated (Fig. 2.27B). They are soft and light brown or yellowish; some are pigmented by bile, the remainder of the liver not being pigmented. Demarcation is fairly sharp and sometimes provided by a connective-tissue capsule. Histologically, the cells do not differ clearly from normal hepatocytes, are arranged in cords or tubules (which may be irregular) (Fig. 2.27C), and often contain small amounts of fat. There are no portal tracts, bile ducts or cholangioles, or hepatic venules, and no suggestion of acini. Bile pigments may be present. In sheep and cattle, hematopoietic foci may be found in the adenomas.

Hepatocellular carcinomas are uncommon. As a general rule, hepatocellular tumors in dogs and cats are more likely to be malignant than benign; in the ox and sheep the opposite applies. The primary tumor is usually single. Small intrahepatic metastases may surround the primary, having developed in the portal lymph nodes. Malignant tumors cannot be clearly distinguished from adenomas. Several features suggest malignancy, including the absence of pedunculation or clear demarcation and the presence of a varied coloration of the cut surface produced by hemorrhage, necrosis, fatty change, and bile pigmentation. Invasion of portal vessels, sometimes clearly evident grossly, is decisive. Some of these tumors in cattle are scirrhous, hard, and white. Carcinomas occasionally penetrate the capsule to implant on the peritoneum. Hematogenous metastases occur first in the lungs, and some appear to arrive in masses to impact in relatively large vessels.

Hepatocellular carcinomas may be clearly composed of hepatocytes that have granular acidophilic cytoplasm, a large nucleus with a distinct membrane, and acidophilic nucleoli. Some tumors are composed of cells in which the cytoplasmic volume is small and its quality hard to determine, and these tumors are difficult to distinguish from those of cholangiocellular origin. Free venous invasion is typical of the hepatocellular tumors. These also tend to grow in diffuse sheets or as trabeculae, cords, or alveolar masses, a few to many cells thick. In some trabecular areas, canaliculi or acini are formed,

and these spaces may contain bile. A feature of some hepatocellular tumors is the presence of giant cells, quite conspicuous by virtue of a large nucleus, multilobed nuclei, or multiple nuclei.

Cholangiocellular Tumors

Cholangiocellular adenomas are seen mainly in old dogs and cats. The smaller specimens may be solid on the cut surface and white, but the large specimens, and many of the small ones, are cystic, forming small or large blisters that contain a clear watery fluid. Their volume may be greater than that of the lobe they occupy. Whether these are truly neoplasms or represent acquired or congenital cystic lesions can be argued with little confidence. If any bile is present in the fluid, the tumors should probably be regarded as cysts; if the content is clearly mucinous, the cysts are probably neoplastic.

The solid specimens are composed of a large number of tubules lined by a single layer of respectable biliary epithelium. The stroma varies in amount. There is no sign of active invasion of the parenchyma. The cystadenomas are multilocular and lined by a mucosa resembling that of the bile ducts; it may, however, be flattened by pressure, or it may in some areas be papillary. The septal stroma is collagenous. Adenomas of the gallbladder are seldom observed, and then chiefly in cattle.

Cholangiocellular carcinomas are a curious group because in dogs and cats, the species usually affected, the tumors are almost always multiple or diffuse, suggesting that whatever incites them acts diffusely (Fig. 2.28A). Solitary ones do occur. There is no suggestion as to their cause, and the livers so affected are usually otherwise normal. The multiple nodules of tumor must to some extent represent intrahepatic lymphogenous metastases. Hematogenous metastases are distinctly unusual, but deposits in the regional nodes are common. In cats especially, there is a tendency to invade Glisson's capsule and implant on the peritoneum.

Cholangiocellular tumors can usually be distinguished from the hepatocellular variety by their multiplicity, firmness, whitish color produced by more or less abundant stroma, and the typical umbilication of those that involve the capsule. Even multiple nodules may not cause much enlargement of the liver, but the diffuse variety may cause great enlargement, although with retention of shape, and severe bile pigmentation.

Microscopically, cholangiocellular carcinoma is usually distinctly adenocarcinomatous, producing ductules and acini, and sometimes papillary formations. The cells are cuboidal or columnar, with a small amount of clear or slightly granular cytoplasm. The nuclei are small and fairly uniform, and the nucleoli are not prominent. The tubules do not contain bile but in well-differentiated specimens may contain mucin.

Primary mesodermal tumors of the liver are quite uncommon. Benign tumors of smooth muscle are occasionally observed in the gallbladder of dogs and oxen. Malignant mesenchymal tumors of hemangiosarcomatous type, and possibly derived from Kupffer cells, are observed rarely in dogs and cattle. Some of these tumors are solitary, large, and grayish white, with scattered hemorrhagic areas, and others are ill defined and cavernous. The latter may rupture into the peritoneal

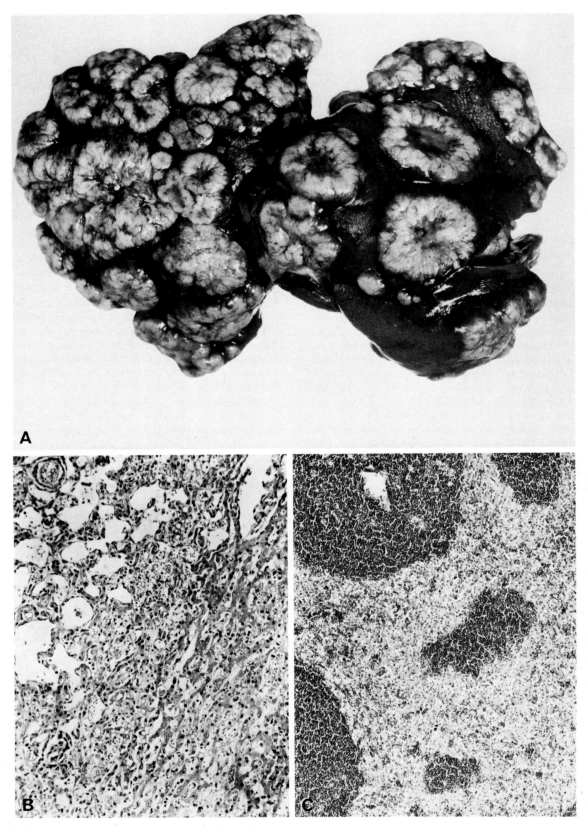

Fig. 2.28. (A) Multiple umbilicated foci of bile duct carcinoma. Cat. (B) Hemangiosarcoma. Dog. Attentuation and isolation of hepatocytes by invading cells. (C) Lymphoma. Dog. The malignant infiltrate is heaviest in the stroma of triads and hepatic venules.

cavity to produce severe hemorrhage. Microscopically, it may be impossible to find malignant cells in or lining cavernous areas. At the margins of the tumor, there is a distinctive pattern of growth in which small, solid nodules of malignant cells may be found, or these cells can be found forming capillary structures or invading along preexisting sinusoids. The latter phenomenon is particularly characteristic. As the cells invade along the sinusoids, perhaps in single file, they initially produce little distortion of the hepatic cords. Behind them the sinusoids are spread widely apart, and individual hepatocytes or portions of cords are isolated and appear to be floating freely, surrounded by a thin layer of connective tissue and neoplastic cells. Some of the malignant cells manifest phagocytic properties, and in some there is a suggestion of reproduction by amitosis.

Secondary neoplasms of the liver are of wide variety. Most of the carcinomas and sarcomas come via the lungs and hepatic artery so that although the metastases may be multiple, they are seldom numerous; some thyroid and mammary carcinomas are exceptions. Except for the pigment of melanomas and the blood of hemangiosarcomas, the type of metastatic tumor cannot be distinguished by its gross appearance. Sarcomas do tend to form a few large, smooth-surfaced nodules, and carcinomas do tend to form more nodules and to be umbilicate when in contact with Glisson's capsule. Hemangiosarcomas (Fig. 2.28B) come from the spleen, usually, and may virtually replace the liver with small, blood-filled caverns. Lymphomatosis is common (Fig. 2.28C), especially when the spleen is involved. The hepatic infiltration may be in discrete nodules 2 cm or more in size, but it is usually diffuse (see the Hematopoietic System, Volume 3). Diffuse infiltration of the liver in myeloproliferative disorders may cause extreme enlargement of the organ.

ACKNOWLEDGMENTS

Thanks are due to Dr. A. A. Seawright for reviewing part of this chapter, to Ms. R. Murray for typing, and to Mr. P. Fabbri for photography.

BIBLIOGRAPHY

General

Adler, M., Chung, K. W., and Schaffner, F. Pericanalicular hepatocytic and bile ductular microfilaments in cholestasis in man. *Am J Pathol* **98**: 603–616, 1980.

Arias, I. M. *et al.* "The Liver. Biology and Pathobiology." New York, Raven Press, 1982.

Badylak, S. F., and Van Vleet, J. F. Alterations of prothrombin time and activated partial thromboplastin time in dogs with hepatic disease. *Am J Vet Res* **42**: 2053–2056, 1981.

Badylak, S. F., and Van Vleet, J. F. Tissue γ-glutamyl transpeptidase activity and hepatic ultrastructural alterations in dogs with experimentally induced glucocorticoid hepatopathy. *Am J Vet Res* **43**: 649–655, 1982.

Bhathal, P. S., and Christie, G. S. A fluorescence microscopic study of bile duct proliferation induced in guinea pigs by 7-naphthyl isothiocyanate. *Lab Invest* **20**: 480–487, 1969.

Cameron, R., Murray, R. K., and Farber, E. Some patterns of response of liver to environmental agents. *Ann NY Acad Sci* **329**: 39–47, 1979.

De Saram, W., Gallagher, C. H., and Goodrich, B. S. Melanosis of sheep liver. I. Chemistry of the pigment. *Aust Vet J* **45**: 105–108, 1969.

Finckh, E. S., and Simpson, G. E. C. Changes in the pattern of cirrhosis after repeated partial hepatectomies in a rat. *J Pathol Bacteriol* **86**: 371–375, 1963.

Franken, P. *et al.* Biliary atresia in a Texelaar lamb. A case report. *Zentralbl Veterinaermed [A]* **28A**: 276–281, 1981.

Gemmell, R. T., and Heath, T. Fine structure of sinusoids and portal capillaries in the liver of the adult sheep and the newborn lamb. *Anat Rec* **172**: 57–69, 1972.

Hooper, P. T. Spongy degeneration in the central nervous system of domestic animals. III. Occurrence and pathogenesis—hepatocerebral disease caused by hyperammonemia. *Acta Neuropathol (Berl)* **31**: 343–351, 1975.

Jewell, S. A. *et al.* Bleb formation in hepatocytes during drug metabolism is caused by disturbances in thiol and calcium ion homeostasis. *Science* **217**: 1257–1258, 1982.

Kerr, J. F. R. A histochemical study of hypertrophy and ischaemic injury of rat liver with special reference to changes in lysosomes. *J Pathol Bacteriol* **90**: 419–435, 1965.

Kerr, J. F. R. Liver cell defaecation: an electron microscope study of the discharge of lysosomal residual bodies into the intercellular space. *J Pathol* **100**: 99–103, 1970.

Kerr, J. F. R. Shrinkage necrosis: a distinct mode of cellular death. *J Pathol* **105**: 13–20, 1971.

Kerr, J. F. R., Wyllie, A. H., and Currie, P. R. Apoptosis: a basic biological phenomenon with wide-ranging implications in tissue kinetics. *Br J Cancer* **26**: 239–257, 1972.

Klion, F. M., and Schaffner, F. The ultrastructure of acidophilic "Councilman-like" bodies in the liver. *Am J Pathol* **48**: 755–767, 1966.

McKenna, S. C., and Carpenter, J. L. Polycystic disease of the kidney and liver in the Cairn terrier. *Vet Pathol* **17**: 436–442, 1980.

Popper, H. Pathologic aspects of cirrhosis. A review. *Am J Pathol* **87**: 228–264, 1977.

Reid, I. M. Hepatic nuclear glycogenesis in the cow: a light- and electron-microscopic study. *J Pathol* **110**: 267–270, 1973.

Richards, R. B. *et al.* Bovine generalized glycogenesis. *Neuropathol Appl Neurobiol* **3**: 45–56, 1977.

Rogers, W. A., and Ruebner, B. H. Retrospective study of probable glucocorticoid-induced hepatopathy in dogs. *J Am Vet Med Assoc* **170**: 603–606, 1977.

Rogoff, T. M., and Lipsky, P. E. Role of the Kupffer cells in local and systemic immune responses. *Gastroenterology* **80**: 854–860, 1981.

Rudolph, R., McClure, W. J., and Woodward, M. Contractile fibroblasts in chronic alcoholic cirrhosis. *Gastroenterology* **76**: 704–709, 1979.

Russo, M. A., Kane, A. B., and Farber, J. L. Ultrastructural pathology of phalloidin-intoxicated hepatocytes in the presence and absence of extracellular calcium. *Am J Pathol* **109**: 133–144, 1982.

Scheuer, P. J., and Maggi, G. Hepatic fibrosis and collapse: histological distinction by orcein staining. *Histopathology* **4**: 487–490, 1980.

Schleger, A. V. Histopathology of melanotic sheep liver. I. Histology and non-enzymic histochemistry. *Aust Vet J* **46**: 48–54, 1970.

Schleger, A. V. Histopathology of melanotic sheep liver. II. Enzymic histochemistry. *Aust Vet J* **46**: 55–61, 1970.

Short, J. *et al.* Induction of deoxyribonucleic acid synthesis in the liver of the intact animal. *J Biol Chem* **247**: 1757–1766, 1972.

Simpson, G. E. C., and Finckh, E. S. The pattern of regeneration of rat liver after repeated partial hepatectomies. *J Pathol Bacteriol* **86**: 361–370, 1963.

Stein, R. J., Richter, W. R., and Brynjolfsson, G. Ultrastructural phar-
macopathology 1. Comparative morphology of the livers of the normal street dog and pure bred beagle (intranuclear crystalline inclusions). *Exp Mol Pathol* **5:** 195–224, 1966.

Strombeck, D. R. "Small Animal Gastroenterology," pp. 332–513.
Davis, California, Stonegate Publishing, 1979.

Strombeck, D. R., Meyer, D. J., and Freedland, R. A. Hyperammonemia due to a urea cycle enzyme deficiency in two dogs. *J Am
Vet Med Assoc* **166:** 1109–1111, 1975.

Strombeck, D. R., Weiser, M. G., and Kaneko, J. J. Hyperammonemia
and hepatic encephalopathy in the dog. *J Am Vet Med Assoc* **166:**
1105–1108, 1975.

Thompson, S. W., Sparano, B. M., and Diener, R. M. Vacuoles in the
hepatocytes of cortisone-treated dogs. *Am J Pathol* **63:** 135–148,
1971.

Thornburg, L. P. Diseases of the liver in the dog and cat. *Compend
Contin Edu Prac Vet* **4:** 538–546, 1982.

Thornburg, L. P., and Moody, G. M. Hepatic amyloidosis in a dog. *J
Am Anim Hosp Assoc* **17:** 721–723, 1981.

Webster, W. R., and Summers, P. M. Congenital polycystic kidney and
liver syndrome in piglets. *Aust Vet J* **54:** 451, 1978.

Wisse, E., and Knook, D. L. (eds.) "Kupffer Cells and Other Liver
Sinusoidal Cells." Amsterdam, Elsevier/North Holland Biomedical
Press, 1977.

Ying, T. S., Sarma, D. S. R., and Farber, E. The sequential analysis of
liver cell necrosis. *Am J Pathol* **99:** 159–174, 1980.

Fatty Liver

Barsanti, J. A. *et al.* Prolonged anorexia associated with hepatic
lipidosis in three cats. *Feline Pract* **7:** 52–57, 1977.

Caple, I. W. *et al.* Starvation ketosis in pregnant beef cows. *Aust Vet J*
53: 289–291, 1977.

Christoffersen, P. *et al.* Lipogranulomas in human liver biopsies with
fatty change. *Acta Pathol Microbiol Scand [A]* **79:** 150–158, 1971.

Collins, R. A., and Reid, I. M. A correlated biochemical and ster-
eological study of periparturient fatty liver in the dairy cow. *Res Vet
Sci* **28:** 373–376, 1980.

Gay, C. C. *et al.* Hyperlipemia in ponies. *Aust Vet J* **54:** 459–462, 1978.

Hartroft, W. S, Diagnostic significance of fatty cysts in cirrhosis. *Arch
Pathol* **55:** 63–69, 1953.

Henderson, G. D., Read, L. C., and Snoswell, A. M. Studies of liver
lipids in normal, alloxan–diabetic and pregnancy–toxemic sheep.
Biochim Biophys Acta **710:** 236–241, 1982.

McGarry, J. D., and Foster, D. W. Regulation of hepatic fatty acid
oxidation and ketone body production. *Annu Rev Biochem* **49:** 395–
420, 1980.

Morris, M. D., Zilversmit, D. B., and Hintz, H. F. Hyperlipoproteinemia in fasting ponies. *J Lipid Res* **13:** 383–389, 1972.

Lombardi, C. Considerations of the pathogenesis of fatty liver. *Lab
Invest* **15:** 1–20, 1966.

Pritchard, D. H. *et al.* Ceroid–lipidosis: an acquired storage-type disease of liver and hepatic lymph node. *Vet Pathol* **20:** 242–244, 1983.

Reid, I. M. *et al.* The pathology of post-parturient fatty liver in high-
yielding dairy cows. *Invest Cell Pathol* **3:** 237–249, 1980.

Richards, R. B., and Harrison, M. R. White liver disease in lambs. *Aust
Vet J* **57:** 565–568, 1981.

Schotman, A. J. H., and Wagenaar, G. Hyperlipemia in ponies.
Zentralbl Veterinaermed [A] **16A:** 1–7, 1969.

Sutherland, R. J., Cordes, D. O., and Carthew, G. C. Ovine white liver
disease—an hepatic dysfunction associated with vitamin B$_{12}$ deficiency. *NZ Vet J* **27:** 227–232, 1979.

Thornburg, L. P., Simpson, S., and Digilio, K. Fatty liver syndrome in
cats. *J Am Anim Hosp Assoc* **18:** 397–400, 1982.

Zaki, G. F. Fatty cirrhosis in the rat. XII. The cirrhotic nodules. *Arch
Pathol* **81:** 536–543, 1966.

Dietary Necrosis

Arpi, T., and Tollerz, G. Iron poisoning in piglets, autopsy findings in
experimental and spontaneous cases. *Acta Vet Scand* **6:** 360–373,
1965.

Cordy, D. R., and McGowan, B. The pathology of massive liver necrosis in sheep. *Cornell Vet* **46:** 422–438, 1956.

Grant, C. A., and Thafvelin, B. Selon och hepatosis diaetetica hos svin.
(Selenium und hepatosis diaetetica beim Schwein.) *Nord Vet Med*
10: 657–663, 1958.

Moir, D. C., and Masters, H. G. Hepatosis dietetica, nutritional myopathy, mulberry heart disease and associated hepatic selenium levels in
pigs. *Aust Vet J* **55:** 360–364, 1979.

Nafstad, I., and Tollersrud, S. The vitamin E deficiency syndrome in
pigs. I. Pathological changes. *Acta Vet Scand* **11:** 452–480, 1970.

Obel, A.-L. Studies on the morphology and aetiology of so-called toxic
liver dystrophy in swine. *Acta Pathol Microbiol Scand [Suppl]* **94:** 1–
118, 1953.

Piper, R. C. *et al.* Selenium–vitamin E deficiency in swine fed peas
(*Pisum sativum*). *Am J Vet Res* **36:** 273–281, 1975.

Schwarz, K., Porter, L. A., and Fredga, S. Some regularities in the
structure–function relationships of organoselenium compounds effective against dietary liver necrosis. *Ann NY Acad Sci* **192:** 200–
214, 1972.

Simesen, M. G., and Petersen, K. B. Selenium determinations in
Danish swine affected with hepatosis dietetica. *Acta Vet Scand* **16:**
137–139, 1975.

Van Vleet, J. F., Carlton, W., and Olander, H. J. Hepatosis dietetica
and mulberry heart disease associated with selenium deficiency in
Indiana swine. *J Am Vet Med Assoc* **157:** 1208–1219, 1970.

Obstruction and Inflammation
of Biliary Apparatus

Brown, J. M. M. The chemical pathology of ovine icteric states. Mechanical obstruction of the common bile duct. *J S Afr Vet Med Assoc*
38: 311–323, 1968.

Dickson, J., Nottle, M. C., and White, J. B. Sand impaction of the bile
ducts of a sheep. *Aust Vet J* **60:** 64, 1982.

Kelly, D. F., Baggott, D. G., and Gaskell, C. J. Jaundice in the cat
associated with inflammation of the biliary tract and pancreas. *J.
Small Anim Pract* **16:** 163–172, 1975.

Long, R. D. Rupture of the common bile duct in the dog: a case report.
Vet Rec **92:** 370, 1973.

Mullowney, P. C., and Tennant, B. C. Choledocholithiasis in the dog: a
review of a case with rupture of the common bile duct. *J Small Anim
Pract* **23:** 631–638, 1982.

Prasse, K. W. *et al.* Chronic lymphocytic cholangitis in three cats. *Vet
Pathol* **19:** 99–108, 1982.

Timbs, D. V., Durham, P. K., and Barnsley, D. G. C. Chronic cholecystitis in a dog infected with *Salmonella typhimurium*. *NZ Vet J*
22: 100–102, 1974.

Van Der Luer, R. J. T., and Kroneman, J. Three cases of cholelithiasis
and biliary fibrosis in the horse. *Equine Vet J* **14:** 251–253, 1982.

Chronic Hepatitis

Bennett, A. M. *et al.* Lobular dissecting hepatitis in the dog. *Vet Pathol*
20: 179–188, 1983.

Bishop, L. *et al.* Chronic active hepatitis associated with leptospires. *Am
J Vet Res* **40:** 839–844, 1979.

Doige, C. E., and Lester, S. Chronic active hepatitis in dogs—a review of fourteen cases. *J Am Anim Hosp Assoc* **17:** 725–730, 1981.

Johnson, G. F. *et al.* Chronic active hepatitis in Doberman pinschers. *J Am Vet Med Assoc* **180:** 1438–1442, 1982.

Meyer, D. J., Iverson, W. O., and Terrell, T. Obstructive jaundice associated with chronic active hepatitis in a dog. *J Am Vet Med Assoc* **176:** 41–44, 1980.

Scheuer, P. J. Chronic hepatitis: a problem for the pathologist. *Histopathology* **1:** 5–19, 1977.

Strombeck, D. R., and Gribble, D. Chronic active hepatitis in the dog. *J Am Vet Med Assoc* **173:** 380–386, 1978.

Thornburg, L. P. Chronic active hepatitis: What is it and does it occur in dogs? *J Am Anim Hosp Assoc* **18:** 21–22, 1982.

Circulatory Factors

Anderson, A. C. The pathogenesis of telangiectasis in the bovine liver. 2. Histopathological and microbiological studies. *Am J Vet Res* **16:** 217–236, 1955.

Branam, J. E. Suspected methionine toxicosis associated with a portocaval shunt in a dog. *J Am Vet Med Assoc* **181:** 929–931, 1982.

Ewing, G. O., Suter, P. E., and Bailey, C. S. Hepatic insufficiency associated with congenital anomalies of the portal vein in dogs. *J. Am Anim Hosp Assoc* **10:** 463–476, 1974.

Greenway, C. V., and Oshiro, G. Intrahepatic distribution of portal and hepatic arterial blood flow in anaesthetized cats and dogs and the effect of portal occlusion, raised venous pressure and histamine. *J Physiol (Lond)* **227:** 473–485, 1972.

Hamir, A. N. Torsion of the liver in a sow. *Vet Rec* **106:** 362–363, 1980.

Jensen, R. *et al.* Ischemia—a cause of hepatic telangiectasis in cattle. *Am J Vet Res* **43:** 1436–1439, 1982.

Johnson, E. R. An unusual cause of death in a sow (liver torsion). *Aust Vet J* **38:** 434–435, 1962.

Kaman, J. Morphology of functional relations between the arteria hepatica and the vena portae. *Zentralbl Veterinaermed [A]* **16A:** 323–329, 1968.

Kanel, G. C. *et al.* A distinctive perivenular hepatic lesion associated with heart failure. *Am J Clin Pathol* **73:** 235–239, 1980.

Kardon, R. H., and Kessel, R. G. Three-dimensional organization of the hepatic microcirculation in the rodent as observed in scanning electron micrographs of corrosion casts. *Gastroenterology* **79:** 72–81, 1980.

Kelly, W. R., and Seawright, A. A. *Pimelea* poisoning of cattle. *In* "Effects of Poisonous Plants on Livestock," R. F. Keeler, K. R. Van Kampen, and L. F. James (eds.), pp. 293–300. New York, Academic Press, 1978.

Lautt, W. W., and Greenway, C. V. Hepatic venous compliance and the role of liver as a blood reservoir. *Am J Physiol* **231:** 292–295, 1976.

Maddison, J. E. Porto-systemic encephalopathy in two young dogs—some additional diagnostic and therapeutic considerations. *J Small Anim Pract* **22:** 731–739, 1981.

Porter, R., and Whelan, J. (eds.) "Hepatotrophic Factors." Ciba Found. Symp. No. 55. Amsterdam, Elsevier, 1978.

Rappaport, A. M. Hepatic blood flow: morphologic aspects and physiologic regulation. *Int Rev Physiol* **21:** 1–63, 1980.

Rappaport, A. M., and Hiraki, G. Y. Histopathologic changes in the structural and functional unit of the human liver. *Acta Anat* **32:** 240–255, 1958.

Rogers, W. A. *et al.* Intrahepatic arteriovenous fistulae in a dog resulting in portal hypertension, portocaval shunts and reversal of portal blood flow. *J Am Anim Hosp Assoc* **13:** 470–475, 1977.

Rothuizen, J., and Van den Ingh, T. S. G. A. M. Arterial and venous ammonia concentrations in diagnosis of canine hepato-encephalopathy. *Res Vet Sci* **33:** 17–21, 1982.

Selman, I. E. *et al.* A respiratory syndrome in cattle resulting from thrombosis of the posterior vena cava. *Vet Rec* **94:** 459–466, 1974.

Starzl, T. E. *et al.* The effects of diabetes mellitus on portal blood hepatotrophic factors in dogs. *Surg Gynecol Obstet* **140:** 549–562, 1975.

Starzl, T. E. *et al.* Portal hepatotrophic factors, diabetes mellitus and acute liver atrophy, hypertrophy and regeneration. *Surg Gynecol Obstet* **141:** 843–858, 1975.

Van den Ingh, T. S. G. A. M., and Rothuizen, J. Hepatoportal fibrosis in three young dogs. *Vet Rec* **110:** 575–577, 1982.

Ware, A. J. The liver when the heart fails. *Gastroenterology* **74:** 627–628, 1978.

Cholestasis

Cornelius, C. E., Arias, I., and Osburn, B. I. Hepatic pigmentation with photophotosensitivity: a syndrome in Corriedale sheep resembling Dubin–Johnson syndrome in man. *J Am Vet Med Assoc* **146:** 709–713, 1965.

Cornelius, C. E., and Gronwall, R. R. Congenital photosensitivity and hyperbilirubinaemia in Southdown sheep in the United States. *Am J Vet Res* **29:** 291–295, 1968.

Clarke, N. T. Photosensitization in diseases of domestic animals. *Commonw Bur Anim Health Rev Ser* **3,** 1952.

Galitzen, S. J., and Oehme, F. W. Photosensitization: a literature review. *Vet Sci Commun* **2:** 217–230, 1978,

Gopinath, G., and Ford, E. J. H. Location of liver injury and extent of bilirubinemia in experimental liver lesions. *Vet Pathol* **9:** 99–108, 1972.

McGavin, M. D., Cornelius, C. E., and Gronwall, R. R. Lesions in Southdown sheep with hereditary hyperbilirubinemia. *Vet Pathol* **9:** 142–151, 1972.

Phillips, M. J. *et al.* Intrahepatic cholestasis as a canalicular motility disorder: evidence using cytochalasin. *Lab Invest* **48:** 205–211, 1983.

Popper, H., and Schaffner, F. Pathophysiology of cholestasis. *Hum Pathol* **1:** 1–24, 1970.

Tanikawa, J. Pathobiology of jaundice and cholestasis at the ultrastructural level. *In* "Pathobiology of Cell Membranes," B. F. Trump and A. V. Arstila (eds.), Vol. 2. New York, Academic Press, 1980.

Viral Diseases

Carmichael, L. E. The pathogenesis of ocular lesions of infectious canine hepatitis. I. Pathology and virological observations. *Pathol Vet* **1:** 73–95, 1964.

Carmichael, L. E. The pathogenesis of ocular lesions of infectious canine hepatitis. II. Experimental ocular hypersensitivity produced by the virus. *Pathol Vet* **2:** 344–359, 1965.

Coetzer, J. A. W. The pathology of Rift Valley fever. I. Lesions occurring in natural cases in new-born lambs. *Onderstepoort J Vet Res* **44:** 205–212, 1977.

Coetzer, J. A. W. The pathology of Rift Valley fever. II. Lesions occurring in field cases in adult cattle, calves and aborted foetuses. *Onderstepoort J Vet Res* **49:** 11–17, 1982.

Coetzer, J. A. W., and Ishak, K. G. Sequential development of the liver lesions in new-born lambs infected with Rift Valley fever virus. I. Macroscopic and microscopic pathology. *Onderstepoort J Vet Res* **49:** 103–108, 1982.

Coetzer, J. A. W., Ishak, K. G., and Calvert, R. C. Sequential development of the liver lesions in new-born lambs infected with Rift Valley fever virus. II. Ultrastructural findings. *Onderstepoort J Vet Res* **49:** 109–122, 1982.

Coetzer, J. A. W., Theodoridis, A., and Van Heerden, A. Wesselsbron disease: pathological, haematological and clinical studies in natural cases and experimentally infected new-born lambs. *Onderstepoort J Vet Res* **45**: 93–106, 1978.

Curtis, R., and Barnett, K. C. The "blue eye" phenomenon. *Vet Rec* **112**: 347–353, 1983.

Givan, K. F., and Jezequel, A.-M. Infectious canine hepatitis: a virologic and ultrastructural study. *Lab Invest* **20**: 36–45, 1969.

Gocke, D. J. *et al.* Experimental viral hepatitis in the dog: production of persistent disease in partially immune animals. *J Clin Invest* **46**: 1506–1517, 1967.

Gocke, D. J., Morris, T. Q., and Bradley, S. E. Chronic hepatitis in the dog: the role of immune factors. *J Am Vet Med Assoc* **156**: 1700–1705, 1970.

Hamilton, J. M. *et al.* Studies on the pathogenesis of canine virus hepatitis. *Br Vet J* **122**: 225–238, 1966.

Morris, T. Q., and Gocke, D. J. Modified acute canine viral hepatitis—a model for physiologic study. *Proc Soc Exp Biol Med* **139**: 32–36, 1972.

Robinson, M., Gopinath, C., and Hughes, D. L. Histopathology of acute hepatitis in the horse. *J Comp Pathol* **85**: 111–118, 1975.

Shahan, M. S. *et al.* Secondary disease occurring subsequent to infectious equine encephalomyelitis. *Vet Med* **34**: 354–358, 1939.

Wright, N. G. The relationship between the virus of infectious canine hepatitis and interstitial nephritis. *J Small Anim Pract* **8**: 67–70, 1967.

Wright, N. G. Experimental infectious canine hepatitis. IV. Histological and immunofluorescence studies of the kidney. *J Comp Pathol* **77**: 153–158, 1967.

Wright, N. G. Experimental infectious canine hepatitis. V. The effect of reticulo-endothelial blockade. *J Comp Pathol* **77**: 331–337, 1967.

Bacterial Diseases

Bagadi, H. O., and Sewell, M. M. H. Experimental studies on infectious necrotic hepatitis (black disease) of sheep. *Res Vet Sci* **15**: 53–61, 1973.

Dodd, S. The aetiology of black disease. *J Comp Pathol* **34**: 1–26, 1921.

Gay, C. C. *et al.* Infectious necrotic hepatitis (black disease) in a horse. *Equine Vet J* **12**: 26–27, 1980.

Getty, R. The histopathology of a focal hepatitis and of its termination ("sawdust" and "telang" liver) in cattle. *Am J Vet Res* **7**: 437–449, 1946.

Jamieson, S. The identification of *Clostridium oedematiens* and an experimental investigation of its role in the pathogenesis of infectious necrotic hepatitis ("black disease") of sheep. *J Pathol Bacteriol* **61**: 389–402, 1949.

Janzen, E. D., Orr, J. P., and Osborne, A. D. Bacilliary haemoglobinuria associated with necrobacillosis in a yearling feedlot heifer. *Can Vet J* **22**: 393–394, 1981.

Jensen, R. *et al.* The rumenitis–liver abscess complex in beef cattle. *Am J Vet Res* **15**: 202–216, 1954.

Jensen, R., Flint, J. C., and Griner, L. A. Experimental hepatic necrobacillosis in beef cattle. *Am J Vet Res* **15**: 5–14, 1954.

Olander, H. J., Hughes, J. P., and Biberstein, E. L. Bacillary hemoglobinuria: induction by liver biopsy in naturally and experimentally infected animals. *Pathol Vet* **3**: 421–450, 1966.

Qureshi, S. R., Carlton, W. W., and Olander, H. J. Tyzzer's disease in a dog. *J Am Vet Med Assoc* **168**: 602–604, 1976.

Thomson, G. W. *et al.* Tyzzer's disease in the foal: case reports and a review. *Can Vet J* **18**: 41–43, 1977.

Turk, M. A. M., Gallina, A. M., and Perryman, L. E. *Bacillus piliformis* infection (Tyzzer's disease) in foals in the northwestern United States: a retrospective study of 21 cases. *J Am Vet Med Assoc* **178**: 279–281, 1981.

Parasitic Diseases

Allen, R. W., and Kyles, P. M. The pathologic changes associated with *Thysanosoma actinioides*. *J Parasitol* **36**: 45, 1950.

Anderson, P. J., Berrett, S., and Patterson, D. S. P. Resistance to *Fasciola hepatica* in cattle. II. Biochemical and morphological observations. *J Comp Pathol* **88**: 245–251, 1978.

Arundel, J. H., and Hamir, A. N. *Fascioloides magna* in cattle. *Aust Vet J* **58**: 35–36, 1982.

Brown, P. J., and Clayton, H. M. Hepatic pathology of experimental *Parascaris equorum* infection in worm-free foals. *J Comp Pathol* **89**: 115–123, 1979.

Dawes, B. Hyperplasia of the bile duct in fascioliasis and its relation to the problem of nutrition in the liver-fluke, *Fasciola hepatica* L. *Parasitology* **53**: 123–133, 1963.

Fairley, N. H., and Wright-Smith, R. J. Hydatid infestation (*Echinococcus granulosus*) in sheep, oxen and pigs, with special reference to daughter cyst formation. *J Comp Pathol* **32**: 309–335, 1929.

Grice, H. C., Hutchinson, J. A., and Say, R. R. Obstructive jaundice ascribed to *Metorchis conjunctus* in a cat with a bifid gallbladder. *J Am Vet Med Assoc* **130**: 130–132, 1957.

Krull, W. H. The migratory route of the metacercaria of *Dicrocoelium dendriticum* (Rudolphi, 1819) Looss, 1899 in the definitive host: Dicrocoeliidae. *Cornell Vet* **48**: 17–24, 1958.

Mapes, C. R., and Krull, W. H. Studies on the biology of *Dicrocoelium dendriticum* (Rudolphi, 1819) Looss, 1899 (Trematoda: Dicrocoeliidae), including its relation to the intermediate host, *Cionella lubrica* (Müller). *Cornell Vet* **41**: 382–444, 1951. (Includes pathologic description.)

Ross, J. G., Todd, J. R., and Dow, C. Single experimental infections of calves with the liver fluke, *Fasciola hepatica* (Linnaeus 1758). *J Comp Pathol* **76**: 67–81, 1966.

Rushton, B., and Murray, M. Hepatic pathology of a primary experimental infection of *Fasciola hepatica* in sheep. *J Comp Pathol* **87**: 459–470, 1977.

Taylor, D., and Perri, S. F. Experimental infection of cats with the liver fluke *Platynosomum concinnum*. *Am J Vet Res* **38**: 51–54, 1977.

Watson, T. G., and Croll, N. A. Clinical changes caused by liver fluke *Metorchis conjunctus* in cats. *Vet Pathol* **18**: 778–785, 1981.

Weinbren, B. M., and Coyle, T. J. Uganda Zebu cattle naturally infected with *Fasciola gigantica* with special reference to changes in serum proteins. *J Comp Pathol* **70**: 176–181, 1960.

Wensvoort, P., and Over, H. J. Cellular proliferations of bile ductules and gamma-glutamyl transpeptidase in livers and sera of young cattle following a single infection with *Fasciola hepatica*. *Vet Q* **4**: 161–172, 1982.

Toxic Liver Disease

Miscellaneous

Allen, J. G., and Seawright, A. A. The effect of prior treatment with phenobarbitone, dicophane (DDT) and β-diethylaminoethyl phenylpropyl acetate (SKF 525A) on experimental intoxication of sheep with the plant *Myoporum deserti* Cunn. *Res Vet Sci* **15**: 167–179, 1973.

Bath, G. F. Enzootic icterus—a form of chronic copper poisoning. *J S Afr Vet Assoc* **50**: 3–14, 1979.

Bull, L. B. The histological evidence of liver damage from pyrrolizidine alkaloids. *Aust Vet J* **31**: 33–40, 1955.

Bull, L. B., Culvenor, C. C. J., and Dick, A. T. "The Pyrrolizidine Alkaloids." Amsterdam, North-Holland Publ. Co., 1968.

Bunch, S. E. *et al.* Hepatic cirrhosis associated with long-term anticonvulsant drug therapy in dogs. *J Am Vet Med Assoc* **181**: 357–362, 1982.

Elleman, T. C. *et al.* Isolation, characterization and pathology of the toxin from a *Microcystis aeruginosa* (= *Anacystis cyanea*) bloom. *Aust J Biol Sci* **31:** 209–218, 1978.

Falconer, I. R. *et al.* Liver pathology in mice in poisoning by the blue-green alga *Microcystis aeruginosa*. *Aust J Biol Sci* **34:** 179–187, 1981.

Freeman, B. A., and Crapo, J. D. Biology of disease: free radicals and tissue injury. *Lab Invest* **47:** 412–426, 1982.

Gooneratne, S. R., Howell, J. McC., and Cook, R. D. An ultrastructural and morphometric study of normal and copper-poisoned sheep. *Am J Pathol* **99:** 429–450, 1980.

Gorham, P. R. Toxic waterblooms of blue-green algae. *Can Vet J* **1:** 235–246, 1960.

Harding, J. D. J. *et al.* Experimental poisoning by *Senecio jacobaea* in pigs. *Pathol Vet* **1:** 204–220, 1964.

Hooper, P. T. Pyrrolizidine alkaloid poisoning—pathology with particular reference to differences in animal and plant species. *In* "Effects of Poisonous Plants on Livestock," R. F. Keeler, K. R. Van Kampen, and L. F. James (eds.), pp. 161–176. New York, Academic Press, 1978.

Hooper, P. T. Cycad poisoning in Australia—etiology and pathology *In* "Effects of Poisonous Plants on Livestock," R. F. Keeler, K. R. Van Kampen, and L. F. James (eds.), pp. 337–347. New York, Academic Press, 1978.

Hooper, P. T., and Scanlan, W. A. *Crotalaria retusa* poisoning of pigs and poultry. *Aust Vet J* **53:** 109–114, 1977.

Hunt, E. R. Hepatotoxicity of carbon tetrachloride in sheep. I. The influence of diet. *Aust Vet J* **47:** 272–274, 1971.

Ishmael, J., Gopinath, C., and Howell, J. McC. Experimental chronic copper toxicity in sheep. Histological and histochemical changes during the development of the lesions in the liver. *Res Vet Sci* **12:** 358–366, 1971.

Ishmael, J., Gopinath, C., and Howell, J. McC. Experimental chronic copper toxicity in sheep. Biochemical and haematological studies during the development of lesions in the liver. *Res Vet Sci* **13:** 22–29, 1972.

Jackson, A. R. B. *et al.* Clinical and pathological changes in sheep experimentally poisoned by the blue-green alga *Microcystis aeruginosa*. *Vet Pathol* **21:** 102–113, 1984.

Jerrett, I. V., and Chinnock, R. J. Outbreaks of photosensitization and deaths in cattle due to *Myoporum* aff. *insulare* R. Br. toxicity. *Aust Vet J* **60:** 183–186, 1983.

Kellerman, T. S. *et al.* Photosensitivity in South Africa. I. A comparative study of *Asaemia axillaris* (Thunb.) Harv. ex Jackson and *Lasiopermum bipinnatum* (Thunb.) Druce poisoning in sheep. *Onderstepoort J Vet Res* **40:** 115–126, 1973.

King, T. P., and Bremner, I. Autophagy and apoptosis in liver during the prehemolytic phase of chronic copper poisoning in sheep. *J Comp Pathol* **89:** 515–530, 1979.

Koppang, N. An outbreak of toxic liver injury in ruminants. Case reports, pathological–anatomical investigations and feeding experiments. (Dimethylnitrosamine.) *Nord Vet Med* **16:** 305–322, 1964.

Koppang, N. A severe progressive liver disease in fur animals. I. Symptoms and organ changes. (Dimethylnitrosamine.) *Nord Vet Med* **18:** 205–209, 1966.

Koppang, N. The toxic effects of dimethylnitrosamine in sheep. *Acta Vet Scand* **15:** 533–543, 1974.

Koppang, N., and Helgebostad, A. Toxic hepatosis in fur animals. II. The etiology elucidated by feeding experiments. III. Conditions affecting the formation of the toxic factor in herring meal. *Nord Vet Med* **18:** 210–215 and 216–225, 1966.

Lannek, N., Lindberg, P., and Tollery, G. Lowered resistance to iron in vitamin E–deficient piglets and mice. *Nature* **195:** 1006–1007, 1962.

Ludwig, J. *et al.* The liver in the inherited copper disease of Bedlington terriers. *Lab Invest* **43:** 82–87, 1980.

MacLachlan, G. K., and Johnston, W. S. Copper poisoning in sheep from North Ronaldsay maintained on a diet of terrestrial herbage. *Vet Rec* **111:** 299–301, 1982.

McLean, E. K. The toxic actions of pyrrolizidine (*Senecio*) alkaloids. *Pharmacol Rev* **22:** 429–483, 1970.

Nash, A. S., Thompson, H., and Bogan, J. A. Phenytoin toxicity: a fatal case in a dog with hepatitis and jaundice. *Vet Rec* **100:** 280–281, 1977.

Oelrichs, P. B. *et al.* Lophyrotomin, a new toxic octapeptide from the larvae of a sawfly, *Lophyrotoma interrupta*. *Lloydia* **40:** 209–214, 1977.

Pass, M. A. The relationship of drug metabolism to hepatotoxicity with some examples in sheep. *Vet Annu* **22:** 129–134, 1982.

Pass, M. A. *et al.* Lantadene A toxicity in sheep. A model for cholestasis. *Pathology* **11:** 89–94, 1979.

Pass, M. A., Gemmel, R. T., and Heath, T. J. Effect of *Lantana* on the ultrastructure of the liver of sheep. *Toxicol Appl Pharmacol* **43:** 589–596, 1978.

Patterson, D. S. P. *et al.* The toxicity of iron–dextran in piglets. *Vet Rec* **80:** 333–334, 1967.

Polzin, D. J. *et al.* Acute hepatic necrosis associated with the administration of mebendazole to dogs. *J Am Vet Med Assoc* **179:** 1013–1016, 1981.

Recknagel, R. O. Carbon tetrachloride hepatotoxicity. *Pharmacol Rev* **19:** 145–208, 1967.

Rees, K. R., and Tarlow, M. J. The hepatotoxic action of allyl formate. *Biochem J* **104:** 757–761, 1967.

Reid, W. D. Mechanism of allyl alcohol–induced hepatic necrosis. *Experientia* **28:** 1058–1061, 1972.

Russo, M. A., Kane, A. B., and Farber, J. L. Ultrastructural pathology of phalloidin-intoxicated hepatocytes in the presence and absence of extracellular calcium. *Am J Pathol* **109:** 137–144, 1982.

Seawright, A. A. Studies on the pathology of experimental lantana (*Lantana camara* L.) poisoning of sheep. *Pathol Vet* **1:** 504–529, 1964.

Seawright, A. A. *et al.* Toxicity of *Myoporum* spp. and their furanosesquiterpenoid essential oils. *In* "Effects of Poisonous Plants on Livestock," R. F. Keeler, K. R. Van Kampen, and L. F. James (eds.), pp. 241–250. New York, Academic Press, 1978.

Seawright, A. A., and Allen, J. G. Pathology of the liver and kidney in *Lantana* poisoning of cattle. *Aust Vet J* **48:** 323–331, 1972.

Seawright, A. A., Filippich, L. J., and Steele, D. P. The effect of carbon disulphide used in combination with carbon tetrachloride on the toxicity of the latter drug for sheep. *Res Vet Sci* **15:** 158–166, 1973.

Seawright, A. A., and Hrdlicka, J. The effect of prior dosing with phenobarbitone and β-idethylaminoethyl diphenylpropyl acetate (SKF 525A) on the toxicity and liver lesion caused by ngaione in the mouse. *Br J Exp Pathol* **53:** 242–252, 1972.

Seawright, A. A., and McLean, A. E. M. Induced susceptibility of sheep to carbon tetrachloride intoxication. *Aust Vet J* **43:** 354–358, 1967.

Sissons, C. H., Watkinson, J. H., and Byford, M. J. Selenium deficiency, the drug metabolizing enzymes and mycotoxicoses in sheep. *NZ Vet J* **30:** 9–12, 1982.

Slater, T. F. (ed.) "Biochemical Mechanisms of Liver Injury." New York, Academic Press, 1978.

Su, L.-C. *et al.* A defect of biliary excretion of copper in copper laden Bedlington terriers. *Am J Physiol* **243:** G231–G236, 1982.

Thorpe, E., and Ford, E. J. Development of hepatic lesions in calves fed with ragwort (*Senecio jacobea*) [*sic*]. *J Comp Pathol* **78:** 195–205, 1968.

Twedt, D. C., Sternlieb, I., and Gilbertson, S. R. Clinical, morphological and chemical studies on copper toxicosis of Bedlington terriers. *J Am Vet Med Assoc* **175:** 269–275, 1979.

Valdivia, E. *et al.* Alterations in pulmonary alveoli after a single injection of monocrotaline. *Arch Pathol* **84**: 64–76, 1967.

Zimmerman, H. J. "Hepatotoxicity: The Adverse Effects of Drugs and Other Chemicals on The Liver." New York, Appleton, 1978.

Mycotoxins

Allen, J. G. An evaluation of lupinosis in cattle in Western Australia. *Aust Vet J* **57**: 212–215, 1981.

Done, J., Mortimer, P. H., and Taylor, A. Some observations on field cases of facial eczema: liver pathology and determinations of serum bilirubin, cholesterol, transaminase and alkaline phosphatase. *Res Vet Sci* **1**: 76–83, 1960.

Gagne, W. E., Dungworth, D. L., and Moulton, J. E. Pathologic effects of aflatoxin in pigs. *Pathol Vet* **5**: 370–384, 1968.

Gardiner, M. R. Cattle lupinosis. A clinical and pathological study. *J Comp Pathol* **77**: 63–69, 1967.

Gardiner, M. R., and Parr, W. H. Pathogenesis of acute lupinosis of sheep. *J Comp Pathol* **77**: 51–62, 1967.

Jago, M. V. *et al.* Lupinosis: response of sheep to different doses of phomopsin. *Aust J Exp Biol Med Sci* **60**: 239–251, 1982.

Kellerman, T. S. *et al.* Photosensitivity in South Africa. II. The experimental production of the ovine hepatogenous photosensitivity disease *geeldikkop* (tribulosis ovis) by the simultaneous ingestion of *Tribulus terrestris* plants and cultures of *Pithomyces chartarum* containing the mycotoxin sporidesmin. *Onderstepoort J Vet Res* **47**: 231–261, 1980.

Ketterer, P. J. *et al.* Field cases of aflatoxicosis in pigs. *Aust Vet J* **59**: 113–117, 1982.

McFarlane, D., Evans, J. V., and Reid, C. S. W. Photosensitivity diseases in New Zealand. 14. The pathogenesis of facial eczema. *NZ J Agric Res* **2**: 194–200, 1959.

McGavin, M. D., and Knake, R. Hepatic midzonal necrosis in a pig fed aflatoxin and a horse fed moldy hay. *Vet Pathol* **14**: 182–187, 1977.

Miller, D. M., Crowell, W. A., and Stuart, B. P. Acute aflatoxicosis in swine: clinical pathology, histopathology and electron microscopy. *Am J Vet Res* **43**: 273–277, 1982.

Mortimer, P. H. The experimental intoxication of sheep with sporidesmin, a metabolic product of *Pithomyces chartarum*. III. Some changes in cellular components and coagulation properties of the blood, in serum and in liver function. *Res Vet Sci* **3**: 269–286, 1962.

Mortimer, P. H. The experimental intoxication of sheep with sporidesmin, a metabolic product of *Pithomyces chartarum*. IV. Histological and histochemical examinations of orally-dosed sheep. *Res Vet Sci* **4**: 166–185, 1963.

Mortimer, P. H., and Taylor, A. The experimental intoxication of sheep with sporidesmin, a metabolic product of *Pithomyces chartarum*. I. Clinical observations·and findings at postmortem examination. *Res Vet Sci* **3**: 147–160, 1962.

Mortimer, P. H., Taylor, A., and Shorland, F. B. Early hepatic dysfunction preceding biliary obstruction in sheep intoxicated with sporidesmin. *Nature* **194**: 550–551, 1962.

Newberne, P. M. Chronic aflatoxicosis. *J Am Vet Med Assoc* **163**: 1262–1267, 1973.

Newberne, P. M., and Butler, W. H. Acute and chronic effects of aflatoxin on the liver of domestic and laboratory animals: a review. *Cancer Res* **29**: 236–250, 1969.

Newberne, P. M., Carlton, W. W., and Wogan, G. N. Hepatomas in rats and hepatorenal injury in ducklings fed peanut meal or *Aspergillus flavus* extract. *Pathol Vet* **1**: 105–132, 1964.

Newberne, P. M., Russo, R., and Wogan, G. N. Acute toxicity of aflatoxin B_1 in the dog. *Pathol Vet* **3**: 331–340, 1966.

Peterson, J. E. *Phomopsis leptostromiformis* toxicity (lupinosis) in nursling rats. *J Comp Pathol* **88**: 191–203, 1978.

Shank, R. C. (ed.) "Mycotoxins and *N*-Nitroso Compounds: Environmental Risks," Vols. I and II. Boca Raton, Florida, CRC Press, 1981.

Thompson, K. G., Lake, D. E. and Cordes, D. O. Hepatic encephalopathy associated with chronic facial eczema. *NZ Vet J* **27**: 221–223, 1979.

Wieland, T. Poisonous principles of mushrooms of the genus *Amanita*. *Science* **159**: 946–952, 1968.

Neoplastic and Like Lesions

Anderson, W. A., Monlux, A. W., and Davis, C. L. Epithelial tumors of the bovine gall bladder. A report of eighteen cases. *Am J Vet Res* **19**: 58–65, 1958.

Becker, F. F. Hepatoma—nature's model tumor. A review. *Am J Pathol* **74**: 179–210, 1974.

Fabry, A., Benjamin, S. A., and Angleton, G. M. Nodular hyperplasia of the liver in the beagle dog. *Vet Pathol* **19**: 109–119, 1982.

Feldman, W. H. Primary carcinoma of the liver: two cases in cattle. *Am J Pathol* **4**: 593–600, 1928.

Mulligan, R. M. Primary liver-cell carcinoma (hepatoma) in the dog. *Cancer Res* **9**: 76–81, 1949.

Patnaik, A. K. *et al.* Canine hepatocellular carcinoma. *Vet Pathol* **18**: 427–438, 1981.

Patnaik, A. K. *et al.* Canine bile duct carcinoma. *Vet Pathol* **18**: 439–444, 1981.

Patnaik, A. K. *et al.* Canine hepatic carcinoids. *Vet Pathol* **18**: 445–453, 1981.

Patnaik, A. K., Hurvitz, A. I., and Lieberman, P. H. Canine hepatic neoplasms: a clinicopathologic study. *Vet Pathol* **17**: 553–564, 1980.

Trigo, F. J. *et al.* The pathology of liver tumors in the dog. *J Comp Pathol* **92**: 21–39, 1982.

Trotter, A. M. Primary adenocarcinoma of the liver. *J. Comp Pathol* **17**: 129–139, 1904. [Ox]

CHAPTER 3

The Pancreas

General Considerations

The pancreas is tucked away with the duodenum in the upper abdomen, where it is relatively well protected against trauma and where it is not readily accessible to the clinician. For these reasons, destructive processes of the pancreas, with the exception of acute pancreatic necrosis, which can be shockingly painful, are revealed as metabolic disturbances, digestive abnormalities, or biliary retention. There are large reserves of endocrine and exocrine function in the pancreas, and metabolic disturbances do not become manifest until a large proportion of the organ or of the islets of Langerhans is lost. Pancreatic disease not associated with pain can therefore remain clinically silent for long periods.

The exocrine pancreas is formed from two anlagen that develop from the foregut on opposite sides of the duodenum. Eventually they fuse to form the mature organ; there may be some fusion of ducts, but separate openings into the duodenum are retained. The dual primordia suggest that there may be functional differences between the two parts of the pancreas, and there are, in some species, regional differences in the number and cellular content of islets, the density being greater in the dorsal than in the ventral derivatives.

The embryologic derivation of acinar cells from ductal anlagen is accepted. Only a limited amount of regeneration, of either ducts or acini, occurs as a result of injury or resection. The pancreas contains cells of intermediate type, which are similar to cholangiolar lining cells of the liver and which have a capacity to differentiate as ductular cells or acinar cells, according to local circumstances. The limitations identified for regeneration of liver, and in particular the requirements for retention of a stromal arrangement to guide regeneration, retention of an adequate blood supply, and retention of efficient drainage probably apply equally to regeneration of the pancreas. Impaired exocrine drainage of the pancreas, following experimental ligation or obstruction of the ducts, leads to exocrine atrophy, with retention of endocrine structures, but the studies so far have not adequately considered the frustrated regenerative attempts or the dynamic processes of regeneration and atrophy that follow duct obstruction. Obstruction of the pancreatic duct leads to progressive atrophy of acinar tissue, with slight fibrosis but without evidence of inflammatory change; the islets remain intact. Incomplete or intermittent obstruction may be accompanied by active interstitial inflammation and fibrosis if infection is superimposed, but in the absence of inflammatory damage, acinar and ductular regeneration may follow relief of obstruction.

Protein synthetic activity in the pancreas is of a high order, directed to the production of large volumes of exocrine secretion, and the size and histologic appearance of the pancreas reflect changes in function. Hypertrophy may occur on diets high in protein and energy, and atrophy if the diet is deficient or unbalanced. The acinar capillary circulation is a portal circulation derived from the large-caliber capillaries of the islets. This arrangement indicates that islet hormones have trophic and functional influences on the acinar tissues, and such influences have been demonstrated; they have not been incorporated into schemes for pathologic evaluation of the pancreas.

The islets of Langerhans constitute a dispersed endocrine organ within the pancreas. They are thought to be derived in common with acinar cells from the ductules of the pancreatic anlagen. They are, however, to a large extent independent of the exocrine gland; they do not regenerate when the acinar pancreas does, they do not atrophy when the exocrine tissue does following duct obstruction, and they can continue to perform some at least of their physiologic functions after separation from the pancreas.

The great complexity of endocrine control systems involving polypeptide hormones and their diffuse regulatory responsibilities bear on understanding of dysfunction of the islets. The present concepts would see the peptide hormones as belonging to a neuroendocrine system and as being produced by cells of wide distribution although of common origin from cells genetically programmed in ectoblast. The gastroenteropancreatic cells, which produce peptide hormones, are responsible for coordinating the physiologic processes of digestion and carbohydrate metabolism; some of these peptide-producing cells remain in the gut epithelium and some have, in evolution, come to form aggregates as the islets of Langerhans. Islets vary in their distribution in different parts of the pancreas, and in the cells that constitute them, although cellular composition has not been fully surveyed in animals. The peptide hormones, which are native to the islets, are glucagon from α cells, insulin from β cells, somatostatin from δ cells, and "pancreatic polypeptide" from F cells; enterochromaffin cells produce the amine serotonin. Diseases of the islets in domestic animals are most common in dogs and manifest either as a deficiency or excess of insulin effect. Dysfunction arising from dysplasia of islet cells, other than β cells, is likely to very subtle, with the exception of the rare gastrin-producing islet tumors.

Anomalies of the Pancreas

A variety of anomalies occur in the pancreas, but with the exception of hypoplasia and congential aplasia of islets of Langerhans, they are of no significance. Variations of the disposition of the ducts are common in dogs. Accessory or ectopic portions of pancreas have been observed in dogs. These are probably produced by dislocation of portions of the duodenal buds and are found as small nodules in the submucosa or muscularis of the stomach, intestine, and gallbladder and in the mesentery. The ectopic tissue is of normal integrity and presumably functional, though the entry of ducts into an adjacent viscus cannot always be demonstrated. Islet-cell tissue may or may not be present. In cats, pancreatic bladders that resemble gallbladders and that are formed by dilation of a duct have been recorded. More severe malformations of the pancreas occur as part of generalized malformations incompatible with life. Cystic pancreatic ducts may occur with polycystic kidneys and cystic bile ducts in various species. Animals affected die in uremia.

Hypoplasia of the pancreas occurs in dogs and calves. The defect is of the acinar tissue; the islet-cell tissue may be quantitatively and qualitatively normal, although in some canine cases that are not diabetic, islets may be difficult to demonstrate, even with special stains. The hypoplastic pancreas in the **calf** is small, pale, loosely textured, and has indefinite margins. Microscopically, the islets are normal, but the acinar tissue is present as small, separated groups of cells in glandular arrangement. Some of these cell groups are well differentiated with zymogen granules and no acinar lumen, but in most of them the cells are small, dark, and of indifferent type, arranged as glands with a patent lumen. The ducts are normal. Clinically, steatorrhea and diarrhea are observed.

In **dogs**, hypoplasia of the pancreas usually is not revealed until the affected animals are ~1 year of age. These animals then develop steatorrhea and quickly become emaciated in spite of a voracious appetite. The late onset of signs of pancreatic insufficiency is probably to be attributed to decompensation, and it is perhaps noteworthy in this respect that the onset of steatorrhea is often preceded by an intercurrent illness. At postmortem, these dogs are potbellied because the intestines are greatly dilated. Of those that are allowed to die, many have intestinal accidents. The intestinal veins are congested, and the intestinal lumen contains bulky, fatty stool. The abdomen is devoid of fat, and the clearness of the mesenteries allows the flimsy tissue of the hypoplastic pancreas to be recognized (Fig. 3.1A). The main ducts and their larger tributaries can be seen and recognized by the naked eye. Many of the smaller ducts are recognizable grossly with the aid of transillumination. The ducts are of normal size, length, and configuration. Surrounding the axial ducts is a narrow thin veil or sheet of pink acinar tissue. In a small proportion of dogs the pancreas may appear normal, but microscopically it contains nodules of acinar tissue in a gland with abundant fat. The relationship of this lesion to the more common type is unclear. Usually the acinar tissue is seen to form small fasciculi, each of which would probably correspond to a lobule in a normoplastic gland (Fig. 3.1B,C). The cells are small, of an indifferent nature, stain darkly, and do not assume a glandular interstitial tissue. Cases of hypoplasia of the pancreas in dogs tend to be anatomically of comparable degree, but histologically there is evidence of continuing regression of ducts and acini. Others have interpreted this condition as pancreatic atrophy because of the degeneration present in acinar cells. However, it is not clear whether this degeneration develops in a normal pancreas or represents secondary change in an hypoplastic gland.

Pancreatic hypoplasia has been observed in several breeds of dogs. It is most frequent in the German shepherd, in which there is good evidence for a genetic basis, but the causes and pathogenesis may not be the same in all cases.

Aplasia of **islet tissue**, causing diabetes mellitus, has been reported in dogs aged 2–3 months. The distribution of islets in the normal pancreas is irregular, and it is necessary to examine tissue from many parts of the organ in order to establish the diagnosis.

Regressive Changes in the Pancreas

The exocrine pancreas is a labile organ, which shares with the other parenchymatous tissues a susceptibility to many adverse influences. The classical morphologic types of cellular degeneration occur in many febrile, toxic, and cachectic illnesses; these appear to be of little clinical importance, but the point is not clear because the pancreas is seldom examined systematically at autopsy. Degenerative changes should not be confused with postmortem autolysis. Autolysis occurs rapidly after death. Advanced autolysis with a patchy distribution is rather common in histologic material and is produced by rough handling of the organ at postmortem, with rupture of cells and liberation of enzymes. The autolyzed tissue stains a slate gray color with hematoxylin, resists eosin, and has a washed-out appearance.

A **lipofuscin pigment** is responsible for khaki color sometimes observed in the canine pancreas. It has been produced by prolonged tocopherol deficiency. The intestinal musculature is similarly pigmented. The pigment, in the form of small brown granules, is present in the basal portions of the cytoplasm and the acinar cells, in the myocytes of the intestine, and in a number of other locations, such as the pigment epithelium of the retina, where it is distinguishable from pigments normally present.

Lipomatosis of the pancreas is occasionally observed in cats and swine. It is usually part of a general adiposity but may be restricted to the pancreas. The adipose tissue accumulates in the interstitium and disperses the parenchyma, creating a false impression, microscopically, of a severe reduction in glandular tissue. There may be some pressure atrophy, but lipomatosis is without clinical significance for the pancreas.

Atrophy of the pancreas occurs commonly but is seldom appraised. It may be a primary cellular atrophy or it may be secondary to other pancreatic lesions. Cellular atrophy is a diffuse change that does not produce any alteration of the gross form of the organ. The acinar cells progressively lose their zymogen granules, and there is, at the same time, a progressive shrinkage of the cytoplasm and dissociation of cells to produce, finally, a microscopic picture in which there is no acinar or glandular arrangement, but instead, a diffuse sheet of small, dark-staining cells that lack polarity (Fig. 3.2A,B). This form of pancreatic atrophy, the full sequential history of which is not known, is a product of malnutrition, especially protein depletion, and as such is seen in cases of starvation, chronic gastroenteritis, and cachexia of a variety of causes.

Secondary pancreatic atrophy is lobular, or multilobular, in distribution, a complication of pancreatic fibrosis or obstruction of the ducts. Ligation of the ducts was the method used to obtain complete exocrine atrophy, to permit insulin to be extracted from the remnants; the islets are completely spared when the duct is ligated, but the exocrine tissues undergo atrophy. Spontaneous obstruction of the ducts, with the exception of the developmental stenosis that is occasionally seen in cats, is in animals usually accompanied by some degree of inflammation and interstitial fibrosis so that the diffuse atrophy of duct obstruction usually has added to it the atrophy of pressure and ischemia induced by interstitial scar tissue. For this reason, the islet tissue is involved as well as the zymogenic tissue. Cicatricial change in the interstitium unaccompanied by obstruction of ducts is a healing change in relapsing pancreatic necrosis and leads to atrophy of pressure and ischemia.

Secondary atrophy may involve either a portion of the pancreas or the whole organ, although not uniformly. The affected parts of the organ are reduced in size, misshapen, coarsely nodular, and tough. On section, the affected portions consist largely of fibrofatty tissue in which accessory structures, such as nerves, vessels, ducts, and islets of Langerhans, are condensed. The islets, except for being concentrated in smaller areas, may appear normal.

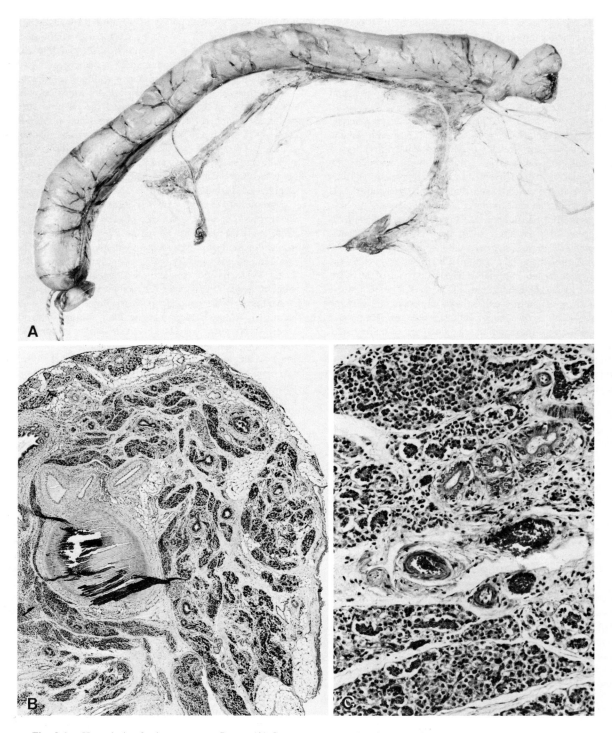

Fig. 3.1.   Hypoplasia of acinar pancreas. Dog.   (A) Gross appearance, showing normal duct system with condensed endocrine tissue.   (B and C) Microscopic appearance of pancreatic hypoplasia. Islet tissue, and intercalated and interlobular ducts are condensed (C).

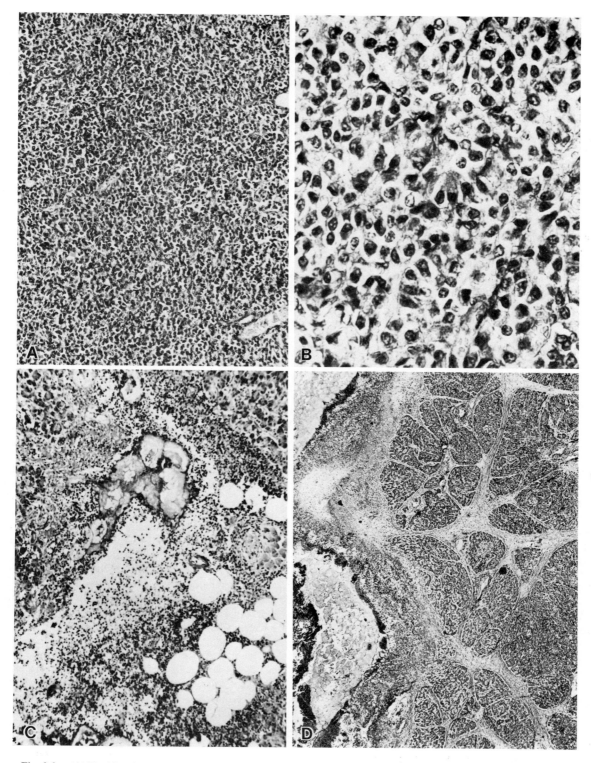

Fig. 3.2.   (**A**) Nutritional atrophy of pancreas. Pig.   (**B**) Detail of (**A**), showing absence of cytoplasmic granularity with vacuolation.   (**C**) Acute pancreatic necrosis. Dog. The severe inflammatory reaction is centered on pancreatic fat, with relative sparing of acinar tissue (upper right).   (**D**) Acute necrosis in pancreas which also shows postnecrotic scarring. Dog.

Acute Pancreatic Necrosis

Acute pancreatic necrosis (acute hemorrhagic pancreatitis, necrotizing pancreatitis, acute hemorrhagic necrosis) is an important disease of dogs and also occurs rarely in horses and swine. It is unknown in other domestic species but is an important disease in humans. For reasons that are quite obscure, the potent arsenal of pancreatic enzymes is turned on its parent tissue and progressively destroys it. The designation of pancreatic necrosis is preferred to one of pancreatitis, to indicate more precisely the basic necrotizing character of the lesion. Even this designation is not wholly satisfactory because the major morphologic changes are not in the parenchyma of the organ, but rather in the interstitial and peripancreatic adipose tissue.

It is doubtful whether recovery from acute pancreatic necrosis ever occurs. The term chronic relapsing pancreatitis is sometimes applied by the pathologist to the prolonged disease, but there is doubt as to whether this is really a relapsing disease. Rather, it appears that if the animal survives the initial acute episode, as it usually does, the necrotizing process smolders continuously and often asymptomatically, until there is almost no pancreas left. There is seldom any difficulty in finding microscopic areas of acute necrosis in these chronically affected organs, even in the terminal stage when the dog dies or is destroyed because it has diabetes mellitus, or steatorrhea and cachexia. Whether the apparently relentless course of the affection is due to persistence of the primary pathogenetic mechanism or to a self-perpetuating property of the lesion is not known. In favor of the former possibility are the facts that the initial lesion is often localized to one portion of the gland and that the smoldering foci are often multiple, of random distribution, affect the periphery of the remnants, and tend to avoid the parenchyma, which survives in the original focus and undergoes fibrous enclosure and atrophy.

The initial acute episode of pancreatic necrosis may or may not be clinically apparent. It occurs mainly in obese females and is characterized by signs of severe abdominal pain and cardiovascular collapse in shock. Death usually follows in 2 or 3 days. Of diagnostic significance is the small volume of turbid fluid with droplets of fat, which can be aspirated from the abdomen. The onset of the disease often passes unnoticed or unremembered, so that progressive pancreatic necrosis may be detected incidentally in dogs that have died from some other cause, or it may not be revealed until the terminal stages, when there are signs of both endocrine and exocrine insufficiency. Pancreatic necrosis is a common cause of diabetes mellitus in dogs since the acute reactions destroy islets as well as acinar tissue.

The pathogenesis of acute pancreatic necrosis in dogs is obscure, excepting perhaps those cases following surgical manipulation of the pancreas and those, usually with basic neurologic disease, given steroid therapy over a long period. Pancreatic necrosis can be produced by a wide variety of experimental manipulations in dogs as well as in other species. It is not always clear that the results, although described as acute pancreatic necrosis or one of its synonyms, are comparable, one with the other or with the natural disease in dogs. There is even more uncertainty about whether any of the experimental procedures has a natural counterpart; an exception is provided by the observations that dogs fed diets high in fat and low in protein will develop acute pancreatic necrosis that is, histogenetically, comparable to the natural disease. For the reasons given, there is little dividend in reviewing once more the experimental production of pancreatic necrosis in dogs or the theories concerning the disease in humans. Of the models available for producing this type of pancreatic injury, those involving dietary manipulations may be the most rewarding.

Irrespective of the primary mechanism of pancreatic necrosis, there is general agreement on the plausible suggestion that the visible lesions are produced by the proteolytic enzymes of the organ. In what manner remains hypothetical. The enzymes may become activated while within the acini, or there may be rupture of canaliculi or acini, with release of enzymes into the stroma. The latter is the likely possibility because in some cases the earliest lesions are edema and necrosis of the pancreatic adipose tissue. Once the process is initiated, the recruitment of other enzymes, including the activation of trypsinogen and chymotrypsinogen by inflammatory products, is probable.

In fatal cases of acute pancreatic necrosis, there is, at postmortem, a small quantity of fluid in the abdominal cavity. The fluid contains droplets of fat and is often bloodstained. Hemorrhages may be present in the omentum, but extensive hemorrhage is not a feature of the lesion. Numerous chalky areas of fat necrosis surrounded by a halo of reddening are present adjacent to the pancreas and in the mesentery. At a greater distance from the pancreas, areas of fat necrosis may be found as far away as the ventral mediastinum, to which, presumably, the enzymes are conveyed in lymphatics. The whole of the pancreas may be edematous, swollen, and soft, or the edematous swelling may be confined to the areas of more severe change. The necrotizing process may occur in the midportion of the gland opposite the ducts, or in one of the branches. Yellowish or hemorrhagic fibrinous adhesions pass from the affected surface of the pancreas to the omentum and visceral surface of the liver. The cut surface presents a variegated appearance due to merging of whitish areas of fat necrosis and grayish yellow areas of parenchymal necrosis and hemorrhage; one or the other appearance may predominate. The texture is unusually greasy. The areas of parenchymal necrosis are softened and may be liquefied to appear as pus, and in cases of some days duration, secondary infection with enteric organisms may, in fact, produce abscesses.

The microscopic picture is compounded of necrosis of adipose tissue, necrosis of parenchymal tissue, edematous separation of stroma, necrosis and thrombosis of blood vessels of all divisions, and reactionary inflammatory infiltrate (Fig. 3.2C,D). The infiltrating leukocytes form a border zone at the boundary of necrotic and viable tissue. The necrotic fat has the usual histologic characters. Necrosis of the pancreatic parenchyma begins from within the lobules, but near the periphery. Small foci of acinar tissue, separate from the stroma, become shrunken and acidophilic and undergo coagulative necrosis. The collagenous stroma resists digestion for some time. With the onset of parenchymal necrosis, the septal tissues are further distended with fluid in which much fibrin may be precipitated. Occlusion of capillaries by fibrin thrombi occurs at the margin of the necrotic areas. Venous thrombosis, sometimes with inflammation or necrosis of the wall of the vessel, occurs adjacent to, and distant from, the lesion; similar changes may occur in the small arteries, but these, as a rule, are less susceptible to injury. Widespread venous and arterial thrombosis is observed as a terminal development in many organs (see disseminated intravascular coagulation, in the Cardiovascular System, Volume 3).

The end result of the necrotizing process, provided that the acute episodes are not fatal, is almost complete destruction of the organ (Fig. 3.3A). Depending on the stage at which the pancreas is observed, it may be irregular in conformation and knobby, or reduced to a few distorted lobules adjacent to where the ducts enter the duodenum. In some cases, the remnants of the organ are too small to be visible, but they may still be palpable in areas indicated by a slight puckering of the mesentery. In spite of the severity of the active process, scar tissue is insignificant in amount, and adhesions are absent or minor. When the remnants are examined microscopically, a few small, rounded lobules remain that are compressed and atrophic. The interstitial tissue is increased, but this is probably due as much to condensation of stroma as to fibroplasia. The vessels and nerves are also condensed into the small area of the pancreatic remnant. Islets of Langerhans often cannot be identified.

In the terminal stages, other changes may be present at autopsy, their nature depending on whether the animal has steatorrhea or diabetes mellitus.

Inflammation of the Pancreas

Pancreatitis is of much lesser importance than pancreatic necrosis in animals. **Acute pancreatitis**, in which there is suppuration or the formation of abscesses, is seldom seen, but it can arise by direct extension from a neighboring focus of infection, as it occasionally does from peritonitis and from perforated esophagogastric ulcers of swine. Suppurative lesions of lymphohematogenous origin are rare. Generalized granulomatous infections have a lesser tendency to avoid the pancreas, but the metastatic lesions are usually microscopic and minor. Acute interstitial pancreatitis is common in systemic toxoplasmosis in cats. Grossly, the organ is slightly swollen by diffuse interlobular edema.

Chronic interstitial pancreatitis is the form of inflammation usually seen in animals. It is seldom of clinical significance but is occasionally responsible for death. The lesion is not common but is most often seen in cats, is occasionally observed in horses, and is rarely observed in other species. It arises usually by spread to the interstitial tissue of an inflammatory process that begins in the ducts (Fig. 3.3C). When of this pathogenesis, the causes are, with the exception of some parasitic trematodes, nonspecific, the microbes present being normal inhabitants of the gut. As an alternative to ascending inflammation of the ducts, pancreatitis that begins in the interstitial tissue is common in horses but of no significance; these lesions are produced by the larvae of *Strongylus equinus,* which pass part of their developmental cycle in and about the pancreas. *Stephanurus dentatus* may encyst in the pancreas of pigs following its intrahepatic migration. The ab-

scess-like lesions produced apparently are of no significance. With the exception of parasitic infestations and the predispositions offered by metaplastic changes in the epithelium of the ducts in vitamin A deficiency (Fig. 3.3B), the primary causes of chronic interstitial pancreatitis are not known. In cats, in which the pancreatic and biliary ducts fuse before entering the duodenum, cholangitis frequently and perhaps always coexists with inflammation of the pancreatic ducts. The same combination is seen in horses, but with what consistency cannot be said.

In chronic interstitial pancreatitis, the organ may be reduced in size or enlarged. In horses, the tendency is for enlargement to occur and the organ to be replaced by a tough mass of scar tissue that merges with surrounding attachments. Flattened remnants of pancreatic tissue may be present near the surface of the mass. When incised, the tortuous and eccentrically dilated ducts are readily apparent. In some of them there is an inflammatory exudate or pus, and in others a large amount of slightly opaque mucus, which makes the cut surface slimy and difficult to handle.

In cats, the pancreas is usually reduced in size and is firm, gray, and irregular. Through the capsule, but particularly on the cut surface, clear retention cysts are often visible. Fibrosis may not be recognizable on gross inspection, but there are exceptional cases in which the whole organ is converted into a shrunken, distorted, fibrous remnant. Histologically, the ducts contain a catarrhal exudate and are surrounded by heavy fibrosis (Fig. 3.3D). Localized stenoses occur and, in other segments, microcysts. The epithelium of the ducts is hyperplastic or metaplastic and may be squamous. The fibrous tissue spreads from around the ducts to the interlobular stroma and subdivides many of the lobules (Fig. 3.4A). As a response to enveloping fibrosis, the acinar tissues atrophy. The islets of Langerhans are well preserved. The stromal tissues are permeated by leukocytes, chiefly mononuclear. The chronically inflamed ducts are a potential site for the development of pancreatic **calculi,** but these are rarely seen; they are, perhaps, more frequent in cattle than in other species. The calculi are small, seldom larger than 4 or 5 mm, white, hard, composed of carbonates and phosphates, and thousands may be present.

Parasitic Diseases of the Pancreas

Ascarids may invade the pancreatic ducts from the intestine in swine and dogs. A variety of trematodes, including *Dicrocoelium dendriticum, Opisthorchis felineus, O. (Clonorchis) sinensis,* and *Metorchis conjunctus,* occur in the pancreatic ducts. Their presence there in numbers large enough to provoke interstitial pancreatitis indicates an overflow from the biliary ducts, where they normally occur (see the Liver and Biliary System, this volume).

Flukes of the genus *Eurytrema* accept the pancreatic ducts as their primary habitat although they may simultaneously infest the biliary tract. A number of species have been named in the genus, but their distinction as species is uncertain. *Eurytrema pancreaticum* of ruminants is probably the most important species, as it is common in parts of Asia, Madagascar, and South America; *E. coelomaticum* is common in cattle in Brazil; *E. fastosum* infests carnivorous animals in the same geographic

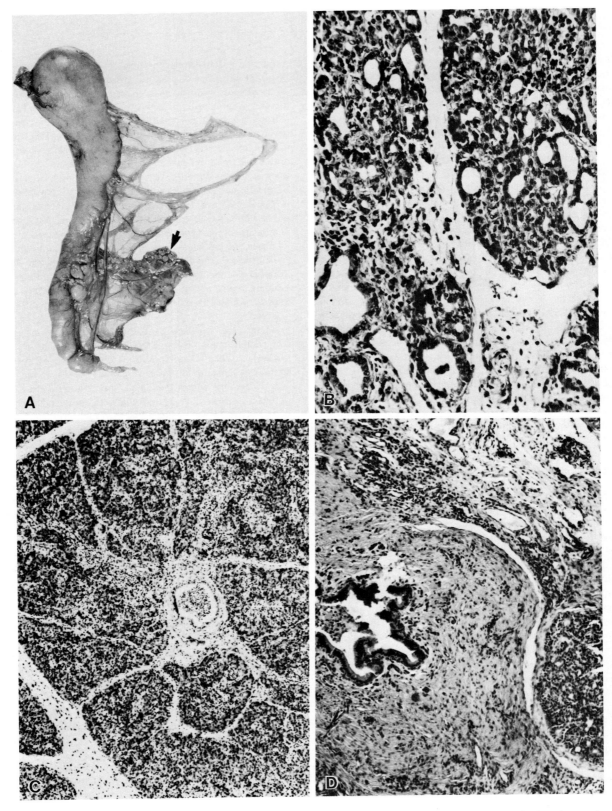

Fig. 3.3. (A) Postnecrotic scarring of pancreas. Dog. Only nodular remnants remain (arrow). (B) Atrophy of acinar tissue and dilatation of ducts in vitamin A deficiency. Calf. (C) Acute interstitial pancreatitis. Cat. Reaction is centered on duct. (D) Chronic interstitial pancreatitis. Cat. Note heavy fibrosis around duct.

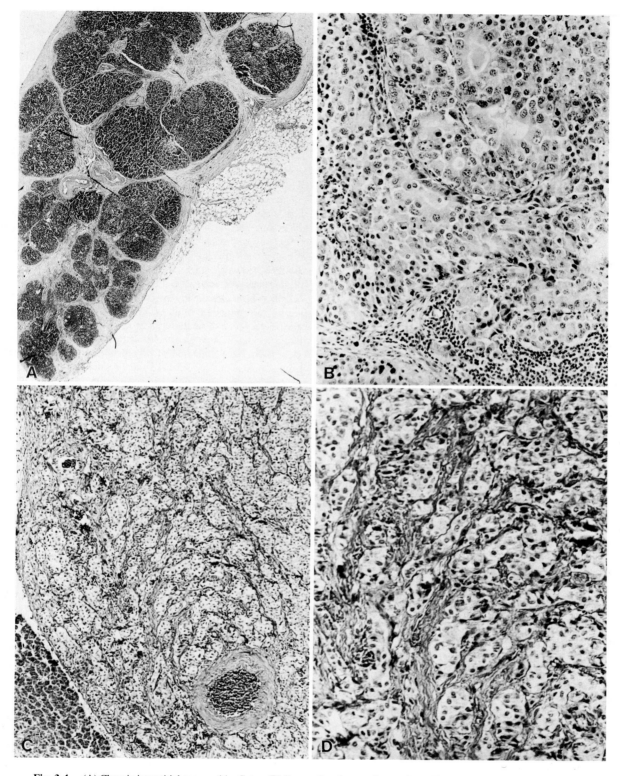

Fig. 3.4. (A) Chronic interstitial pancreatitis. Cat. (B) Pancreatic adenocarcinoma. Dog. There is necrosis of acinar tissue and a mononuclear-cell infiltration. Tumor is forming tubular structures. Karyomegaly and mitotic figures are present. (C) Islet-cell tumor compressing acinar pancreas. Dog. (D) Detail of (C).

areas as *E. pancreaticum*. Pigs can be infested with the species from either herbivores or carnivores.

Infestation of the pancreatic ducts by these trematodes leads to chronic interstitial pancreatitis. *Eurytrema pancreaticum* has some preference for the left lobe of the pancreas. The acinar tissue may be almost destroyed and replaced by fibrofatty tissue; the islets survive much better. *Eurytrema* (*Concinnum*) *procyonis* is found in the main pancreatic duct of small carnivores and is usually associated with some periductal fibrosis but with minimal changes in the parenchyma of the gland. In areas in which the fluke occurs, up to 10% of cats may be infested, and with heavy infestations the main duct may be greatly dilated and much of the gland shrunken, pale, and fibrotic.

Neoplastic and Like Lesions of the Exocrine Pancreas

Nodular hyperplasia of the pancreas is a common finding in old dogs, cats, and cattle, sometimes as a compensatory or regenerative hyperplasia. following pancreatic injury, but in most instances there is no sign of an antecedent injury. The hyperplasia involves the exocrine tissue only, occurs in many foci, and may involve whole lobules or only portions of them. Grossly, the hyperplastic lobules project as flat elevations from the contour of the organ, are whiter than the surrounding tissue, and are palpably hard. The histologic picture provides a mosaic and should be interpreted cautiously because the hyperplastic nodules cannot always be readily distinguished from adenomas. The hyperplasia seldom involves a whole lobule uniformly; instead, there are one or more nodules in the lobules. The hyperplastic nodules are not encapsulated and do not compress the surrounding parenchyma. The morphology of the cells in each nodule is rather uniform, and there is always some resemblance to acinar structure. The cells may appear as enlarged counterparts of normal exocrine cells with a bulky, brightly acidophilic cytoplasm; they may be of indifferent character, producing a low cuboidal lining for glandular spaces; or they may form small, indifferent clusters without a lumen. The mosaic appearance is due to the irregular admixture of nodules of diverse architecture.

Neoplasms of the pancreatic connective tissues are quite rare; **carcinoma** of the pancreas is somewhat less rare, the designation of carcinoma always implying an origin from the exocrine tissues or excretory ducts. Carcinomas are observed in cats, and more frequently in dogs. It is expected that some of those seen in cats may have arisen from the distal end of the bile duct. Benign epithelial tumors are seldom diagnosed, and they appear to be truly rare when allowance is made for the hyperplastic nodules that are occasionally accepted to be adenomas.

There is, perhaps, a greater tendency for pancreatic carcinomas in dogs and cats to arise in the central portion of the gland or in the duodenal wing. Those of central location may soon draw attention to themselves by obstructing the bile duct and causing jaundice. The neoplasms may be more or less spherical and circumscribed, or they may have some resemblance to masses of scar tissue. On cross section, the yellow, lobulated structure of normal glands is replaced by grayish scirrhous tissue in which there may be some areas of necrosis and hemorrhage. Some of these tumors may contain cysts with a mucinous content

and, histologically, localized ductular arrangements that may be well differentiated and difficult to distinguish from the duct response to incomplete obstruction.

Pancreatic carcinomas have a tendency to invade the wall of the duodenum and metastasize to the liver, either as many small nodules or a few larger ones. The local lymph nodes contain deposits of the tumor, and it is sometimes implanted as many nodules on the peritoneum.

Histologically, the tumors are adenocarcinomas that have a tendency to provoke much scirrhous stroma. It is not possible to correlate closely the histologic structure with behavior. Some well-differentiated specimens may metastasize widely. The whole spectrum of adenocarcinomatous structure, from diffuse groups of anaplastic cells to well-differentiated structures that mimic normal acini or ducts, can be found (Fig. 3.4B). An attempt is usually made to distinguish tumors of acinar origin from those arising from ducts. The distinction is rather arbitrary because the degree and direction of dedifferentiation are unpredictable. However, there are some tumors in which the neoplastic glandular structures are lined by cuboidal or columnar cells that have clear cytoplasm and secrete mucus and that resemble the epithelium of ducts. Tumors of probable acinar origin are composed of small hyperchromatic cells that tend to form distorted glandular arrangements. Clearly of acinar origin are those tumors that cannot be quickly distinguished histologically from normal acinar tissue; these may produce areas of fat necrosis both within, and adjacent to, the primary tumor and the metastases.

Islets of Langerhans

Reference was made earlier in this chapter to certain properties of the islets of interest to the pathologist. However, it is the β cells and their responsibilities in carbohydrate metabolism that are the matters of prime concern. Tumors of islet-cell type, which produce excessive gastrin effects, are rare in domestic animals. The β cells appear to be uniformly distributed in the islets, at variance with the distribution of other cell types.

The cells of pancreatic islets normally release amines and polypeptides that serve to regulate intermediary metabolism either in the conventional hormonal mode or as local trophic or paracrine influences. The syndromes that may result from dysplastic islet cells reflect either quantitative changes in the secretion of individual polypeptides, the aberrant secretion of more than one peptide, or the secretion of peptides of abnormal functional characteristics.

Degenerative Lesions of the Islets of Langerhans

Necrosis of the islets occurs in acute pancreatic necrosis. Their progressive destruction, along with the acinar tissue, is a common cause of diabetes mellitus in dogs. Atrophy of the islets occurs as a result of fibrosis in chronic interstitial pancreatitis, but because the islet tissue is more resistant to atrophy of this cause than the acinar tissue, diabetes mellitus is seldom a complication of pancreatitis. Insular insufficiency is possible from extensive neoplastic destruction of the pancreas. Amyloidosis of the islets, causing remarkable enlargement of them, is occasionally observed in cats (Fig. 3.5A). The amyloid is restricted to the islets and may not be found in other tissues. Amyloidosis of the islets is regularly associated with diabetes in cats, but whether the amyloid deposits cause or result from the diabetic state is not known. In dogs with diabetes mellitus that is not the result of pancreatic necrosis, varying degrees of sclerosis of the islets can sometimes be readily seen. Sclerosis is, however, occasionally observed in minor degrees in old nondiabetic dogs, so its significance is difficult to assess. The sclerotic process in diabetic dogs may replace whole islands or parts of them and may be so condensed as to assume to some extent the appearance of hyaline. It may be said of sclerosis, as of amyloidosis, that whether cause or effect has not been determined.

A number of viruses are known to replicate in the pancreas but, with the exception of the diabetes mellitus, which may be seen in chronic foot and mouth disease of cattle, are not known to be significant in islet disease. The occasional observation of lymphocytes in relation to a few islets in animals with diabetes mellitus is probably not of specific significance. Congenital aplasia of islet tissue is referred to under Anomalies of the Pancreas.

Diabetes Mellitus

Diabetes mellitus is characterized by a persistent rise in the level of blood sugar, with glycosuria. The glycosuria causes osmotic diuresis, polyuria, dehydration, and thirst. Secondary derangements of the intermediary metabolism of fat and protein lead to wasting, ketosis, and coma. As currently conceived, the primary metabolic defect is due either to deficient secretion of insulin by the β cells (insulin-dependent diabetes) or to a diminished effectiveness of secreted insulin (insulin-independent diabetes). In the latter type, which accounts for 80% of human diabetes, insulin receptors are often decreased. It is not clear whether this is a primary genetic defect or a secondary effect of the metabolic derangement. These are, at best, very broad concepts, which admit that diabetes mellitus is a syndrome that can result from diverse causes.

Deficient secretion of insulin may result from spontaneous destructive diseases of the pancreas. The pathogenesis of diabetes mellitus in these cases is clear. Fairly selective destruction of the β cells and diabetes can be produced experimentally by alloxan, streptozotocin, and other drugs; whether any normal or endogenously altered metabolic by-products are toxic to β cells is not known.

Diminished production of insulin as a result of insular exhaustion can be provoked by methods that cause prolonged antagonism to the efficient utilization of the secreted hormone. In some cases of diabetes, the islets are microscopically normal, and the granulation of β cells is not appreciably less than in a range of nondiabetic animals; this implies that insulin is synthesized by the β cells but for some reason not released, the implication based on the reasonable correlation between the granulation of β cells and the amount of extractable insulin; the granules are presumed to represent insulin in precursor or storage form.

There are several factors that are potentially diabetogenic by antagonizing the peripheral action of circulating insulin; as mentioned above, prolonged antagonism may result in exhaustion of

the supply of insulin. It is advisable to discuss briefly the function and fate of insulin before discussing the antagonists. The secretion of insulin may be constant in the "resting state," but increased secretion is a response to hyperglycemia, an adaptive mechanism for maintaining blood sugar within the normal range. Of lesser importance is the nervous control of secretion; insulin may be released under conditions of severe stress, but its effect is then overshadowed by the hyperglycemic activity of the epinephrine simultaneously released. Insulin is rapidly removed from the blood, partially by entry into cells and partially by the action of the proteolytic enzyme "insulinase."

There is experimental support for more than one mode of action or locus of activity for insulin. The hormone facilitates the transport of glucose and other hexoses across cell membranes and into cells, especially muscle cells and adipose tissue. The entry of glucose into a cell is not quite equivalent to its entry into the metabolic activities. Glucose, to enter the metabolic pool, must first be phosphorylated to glucose 6-phosphate, a process catalyzed by glucokinase and stimulated by insulin. These two functions of insulin are thus directed to propelling glucose into the cell and into the intracellular metabolic pool; keeping it there is the third probable function of the hormone, and this depends on the inhibition, by insulin, of the activity of hepatic glucose-6-phosphatase, which otherwise causes the overproduction of glucose.

Among the antagonists of insulin, "insulinase" has already been mentioned. Glucagon and epinephrine are glycogenolytic and hyperglycemogenic by virtue of their stimulating action on hepatic phosphorylase. Growth hormone of the anterior hypophysis is diabetogenic. It directly antagonizes the influence of insulin on hexokinase, and on permeability of cell membranes to glucose, and may stimulate the activity of "insulinase." The administration of growth hormone to normal dogs will cause hyperglycemia and hyperplasia of the islets, to be followed in many cases by atrophy. If diabetes occurs, it is qualified as metahypophyseal; it is more readily produced if a portion of the pancreas is removed surgically before growth hormone is administered. Metahypophyseal diabetes occurs naturally in humans, in association with active hyperplasia or tumor of the acidophil cells of the pituitary gland; diabetes of this pathogenesis has been seen in dogs, cats, and horses. A condition characterized by slight to severe hyperglycemia and glucose intolerance (hyperinsulinemia) and elevated levels of growth hormone is seen in female dogs shortly after estrus or during treatment with progestagens. It is apparently due to insulin resistance induced by the elevated levels of growth hormone. The syndrome may be reversed by the early removal of the sources of progestagens, or it may become permanent, with absence of peripheral insulin, if the islets are functionally exhausted. The adrenal glucocorticoids are diabetogenic, and hyperglycemia and reduced glucose tolerance may be found in 50% or more of spontaneous cases of adrenal hyperfunction.

The clinical diagnosis of diabetes mellitus depends on the demonstration of the end products of the metabolic disturbance, namely, persistent hyperglycemia and glycosuria with fluctuating or intermittent ketonemia and ketonuria. The principal clinical signs of the disease in dogs, the species most frequently affected, include polyuria, polydipsia, emaciation, and in

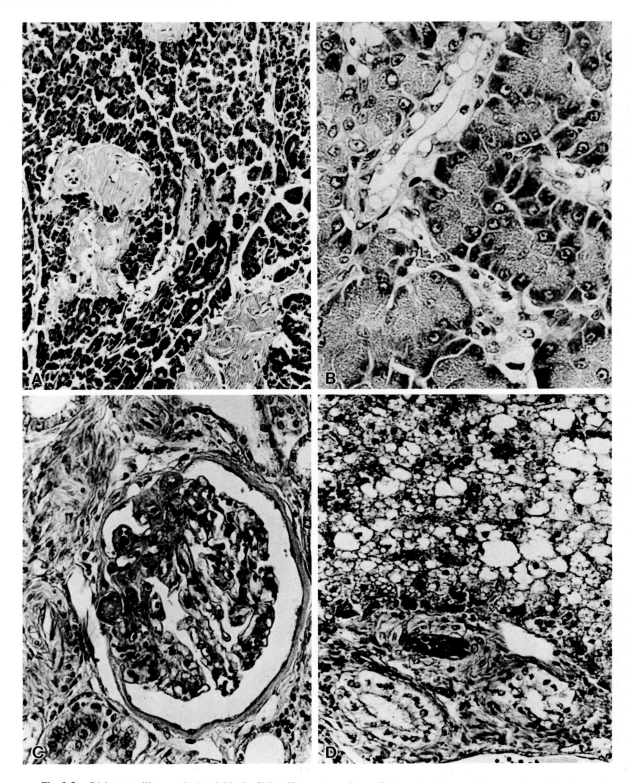

Fig. 3.5. Diabetes mellitus. **(A)** Amyloidosis of islet of Langerhans. Cat. **(B)** Vacuolar (glycogen) degeneration of islet (arrows) and ductal epithelium. Dog. **(C)** Diffuse and nodular hyalinization of glomerulus. Dog. Basement membranes are thickened, and there is a capsular adhesion. **(D)** Severe hepatic lipidosis with vacuolation of bile duct epithelium. Dog.

~70% of cases, rapidly developing lenticular opacities (see the Eye and Ear, Volume 1). Dogs are rather resistant to ketosis and diabetic coma, but when it develops, death follows in a few hours without response to treatment.

Diabetes mellitus in dogs usually affects females. It is a disease of the older age groups, the peak incidence being in animals about 8–9 years of age. A short familial history of the disease is sometimes obtained. The incidence in cats is much lower than in dogs, and castrated males appear to be affected more frequently than sexually entire males or females. There are rare reports of diabetes mellitus in herbivores, fewer in horses than in cattle, and some cases in cattle are reported to be a sequel to foot and mouth disease. Hyperglycemia and glycosuria occur in clostridial enterotoxemia of sheep and in some cases of acute cerebral injury. There is occasionally observed in cows a hyperglycosuria of remarkable degree, the basis of which has not been determined; such cases are fatal in a few days.

The lesions of diabetes mellitus in cats and dogs are comparable. Apart from emaciation, and possibly dehydration, the principal lesion at autopsy is a remarkably yellow, fatty liver. The pancreas may appear normal or reveal the lesions of postnecrotic scarring or pancreatitis. Lipemia may be evident as a milkiness of the serum.

Microscopic lesions can usually, but not always, be found in the pancreas. In addition to the insular changes described earlier, there may be vacuolation of the islet cells and, with it, vacuolation of the epithelium of the smaller ducts (Fig. 3.5B). The vacuolation in routine sections is due to the accumulation of glycogen and is a specific lesion for diabetes mellitus but is thought to be present only in acutely developing severe cases. Glycogen nephrosis, which is present as a vacuolar change in the renal epithelium, is also highly specific for diabetes. The glycogen is deposited chiefly in Henle's loop and the distal convoluted tubule, and mainly in the nephrons of the inner cortex. There is fatty degeneration of the epithelium of the proximal convoluted tubules. Fat emboli are occasionally present in the glomerular capillaries. In long-standing diabetes, diffuse or nodular (Kimmelstiel–Wilson nodules) glomerulosclerosis may develop. Periodic acid–Schiff (PAS) -positive basement membrane material accumulates, causing hyaline thickening of the capillary basement membranes and sclerosis of lobules in the glomerular tufts. Diffuse thickening of the mesangium develops and may lead to glomerular obliteration (Fig. 3.5C). The increased accumulation of basement membrane, at least in insulin-dependent diabetics, may be related to an inherent defect in somatic cells that leads to an increased rate of cell turnover with duplication of basement membranes. The lesion that is most obvious in glomerular capillaries also involves capillaries in other tissues and other basement membranes of Bowman's capsule and convoluted tubules. There is severe but nonspecific periacinar fatty degeneration of the liver (Fig. 3.5D), and vacuolation of bile duct epithelium may be prominent.

The complicating vascular lesions and infections so important in humans are very rare in animals, although emphysematous cystitis develops occasionally (see the Urinary System, this volume). This lack of complications is probably related to the severity and duration of the disease. The course of the disease in dogs is ordinarily fairly short, but the exceptional natural case and some experimental ones may survive for 2 years of more, and show, in addition to diffuse glomerulosclerosis, retinal capillary aneurysms. The latter are suitably demonstrated only in retinal spreads.

Neoplasms of the Islet Cells

Tumors of the pancreatic islets are observed mainly in dogs, and although few have been reported, they should not be regarded as extremely rare. They occur in older dogs. Islet-cell tumors may be adenomas or carcinomas as based on the usual criteria. There is the usual difficulty in differentiating hyperplastic from adenomatous islets. Size can be a criterion, but in the early stages, encapsulation and compression of surrounding tissue are more valuable in making the distinction. The distinction may be purely artificial because diffuse hyperplasia of the islets is quite rare, and when it is detected there is good reason for looking once more for a nodule of tumor. This statement is prompted by the observation that tumors of the islets, although usually reported as solitary, may be multiple, and that in some cases many, and perhaps most, of the islets are hyperplastic or enlarged when viewed microscopically. This should not be surprising because the islet tissue is endocrine tissue and although widely dispersed it is still, functionally, one organ.

Tumors of the islets are usually discrete nodules readily distinguished from the glandular pancreas by their firm to hard consistency, homogeneous cut surface, and their distinct grayish purple color. They tend to be encapsulated and easily "shelled out," but neither feature is a reliable distinction between benign and malignant characters. Even though the primary tumor is small and apparently encapsulated, it may have progeny in the pancreatic lymph nodes and liver.

Microscopically, these tumors, whether apparently benign or obviously malignant, are well differentiated, and the cells may not differ significantly, except in chromatic intensity, from those of normal islets. The cells are regular in form and tend to form branching cords supported by a moderate fibrous stroma, but they may produce a pseudoacinar or glandular arrangement (Fig. 3.4C,D). Most of the tumors are composed of β cells, or contain a proportion of β cells, distinguishable by their special granules.

The cellular composition of islet-cell tumors as well as their functional state will determine the nature of the clinical signs. The best known syndrome is that associated with hyperinsulinism and hypoglycemia. The hypoglycemia is of fluctuating severity, the troughs appearing in relation to fasting or exercise. The signs of hypoglycemia are neurologic and consist of confusion, stupor, loss of consciousness, and convulsions, and they should respond rapidly to the injection of glucose. Even small tumors can be responsible for profound neurologic disturbances, a fact indicating that care should be taken in searching for the tumor. Surgical removal of the tumor effects a remission of signs, but operation is attended by threat of acute pancreatic necrosis, and a return to hyperinsulinism, if the tumor has metastasized or is multiple.

Islet-cell tumors are, rarely, responsible for the production of excessive gastrin in dogs. Gastrin-producing cells are normally present in the gastroduodenal mucosa, but not in the normal adult islets. Tumors may arise in the gastroduodenal mucosa or in the islets, and the production of gastrin by the islet tumors may be a functional aberration. The clinical syndrome is associated with vomiting, diarrhea, anorexia, and weight loss, and with hyperplasia of the antral mucosa and gastroduodenal ulceration (see peptic ulcer in dogs, in the Alimentary System, this volume).

BIBLIOGRAPHY

Exocrine Pancreas

Baggenstoss, A. H. Dilatation of the acini of the pancreas: incidence in various pathological states. *Arch Pathol* **45:** 463–473, 1948.

Barron, C. N. Ectopic pancreas in the dog. A report of three cases *Acta Anat (Basel)* **36:** 344–352, 1959.

Bolydreff, E. B. Report of an accessory pancreas on the ileum of a dog. *Anat Rec* **43:** 47–51, 1929.

Burggraaf, H. Pancreas-distomatose. (Fascioliasis of the pancreas.) *Tijdschr Diergeneeskd* **62:** 399–407 and 469–481, 1935. [*Eurytrema*]

Christenson, N. O., and Schambye, P. Om diabetes mellitus hos kvaeg. *Nord Vet Med* **2:** 863–900, 1950. [Refers to all the previously recorded cases of diabetes mellitus in herbivores]

Coffin, D. L., and Thordal-Christensen, A. The clinical and some pathological aspects of pancreatic disease in dogs. *Vet Med (Kansas City, Mo)* **48:** 193–198, 1953.

Dalgaard, J. B. Pancreolithiasis in cattle. *Skand Vet Tidskr* **35:** 362–364, 1945.

Doeglas, A., and Teunissen, G. H. B. Pancreas-deficientie (atrophie) bij de hond. [Pancreatic deficiency (atrophy) in the dog.] *Tijdschr Diergeneeskd* **81:** 233–241, 1956.

Fitzgerald, P. J. The problem of the precursor cell of regenerating pancreatic acinar epithelium. *Lab Invest* **9:** 67–85, 1960.

Florence, R. Existence chez les bovins de Madagascar de l'*Eurytrema pancreaticum*. *Bull Soc Pathol Exot Filiales* **32:** 446–447, 1939.

Fox, J. J. *et al.* Pancreatic function in domestic cats with pancreatic fluke infection. *J Am Vet Med Assoc* **178:** 58–60, 1981.

Hashimoto, A. *et al.* Juvenile acinar atrophy of the pancreas of a dog. *Vet Pathol* **16:** 74–80, 1979.

Holzworth, J.: and Coffin, D. L. Pancreatic insufficiency and diabetes mellitus in a cat. *Cornell Vet* **43:** 502–512, 1953.

Joubert, L. *et al.* Pancréatite aigue necrosante stéatorrhéique d'allure enzootique, chez le porc d'engrais. *Rev Med Vet* **115:** 453–490, 1964.

Lindsay, S., Entenman, C., and Chaikoff, I. L. Pancreatitis accompanying hepatic disease in dogs fed a high fat, low protein diet. *Arch Pathol* **45:** 635–638, 1948.

Lombardi, B., Estes, L. W., and Longnecker, D. S. Acute hemorrhagic pancreatitis (massive necrosis) with fat necrosis induced in mice by DL-ethionine fed with a choline-deficient diet. *Am J Pathol* **79:** 465–478, 1975.

Mann, F. C. Accessory pancreas in the dog. *Anat Rec* **19:** 263–268, 1920.

Mann, F. C. An accessory pancreas in the wall of the gallbladder of a dog. *Anat Rec* **23:** 351–353, 1922.

Nielsen, S. W., and Bishop, E. J. The duct system of the canine pancreas. *Am J Vet Res* **15:** 266–271, 1954.

Panabokke, R. G. An experimental study of fat necrosis. *J Pathol Bacteriol* **75:** 319–331, 1958.

Perry, T. T. Role of lymphatic vessels in the transmission of lipase in disseminated fat necrosis. *Arch Pathol* **43:** 456–465, 1947.

Pinto, C. Variacoes morfologicas observadas no ''*Eurystrema fastosum*'' (Kossack, 1910). *Campo, Rio de J* **6:** 50–52, 1935. [Morphological types of *E. fastosum* (cats)]

Pound, A. W., and Walker, N. I. Involution of the pancreas after ligation of the pancreatic ducts. I. Histological changes. *Br J Exp Pathol* **62:** 547–558, 1981.

Prentice, D. E., James, R. W., and Wadsworth, P. F. Pancreatic atrophy in young beagle dogs. *Vet Pathol* **17:** 575–580, 1980.

Purves, G. B. The species of *Eurytrema* in domestic ruminants. *Vet Rec* **11:** 583–584, 1931.

Purves, G. B. Further parasites of domestic animals in Malaya. *Vet Rec* **11:** 761, 1931. [Includes *Eurytrema rebelle* from cat]

Rimaila-Parnanen, E., and Westermarck, E. Pancreatic degenerative atrophy and chronic pancreatitis in dogs. *Acta Vet Scand* **23:** 400–406, 1982.

Ruddick, H. B., and Willis, R. A. Malignant tumors in dogs. *Am J Cancer* **33:** 205–217, 1938.

Scott, E., and Moore, R. A. A case of pancreatic carcinoma in a cat. *J Cancer Res* **11:** 152–157, 1927.

Tang, C. C. Studies on the life history of *Eurytrema pancreaticum*, Janson, 1889. *J. Parasitol* **36:** 559–573, 1950.

Thordal-Christensen, A., and Coffin, D. L. Pancreatic diseases in the dog. *Nord Vet Med* **8:** 89–114, 1956.

Westermarck, E. The hereditary nature of canine pancreatic degenerative atrophy in the German shepherd dog. *Acta Vet Scand* **21:** 389–394, 1980.

Endocrine Pancreas

Bencosme, S. A., and Leipa, E. Regional differences of the pancreatic islet. *Endocrinology* **57:** 588–593, 1955.

Bencosme, S. A., Mariz, S., and Frei, J. Studies on the function of the alpha cell of the pancreas. Dogs with a low beta/alpha cell ratio. *Lab Invest* **7:** 139–144, 1958.

Bloodworth, J. M. B. Experimental diabetic glomerulosclerosis. II. The dog. *Arch Pathol* **79:** 115–125, 1965.

Bloom, F. Diabetes mellitus in cat. *N Engl J Med* **217:** 395–398, 1937.

Cello, R. M., and Kennedy, P. C. Hyperinsulinism in dogs due to pancreatic islet cell carcinoma. *Cornell Vet* **47:** 538–557, 1957.

Dohan, F. C., and Lukens, F. D. W. Lesions of the pancreatic islets produced in cats by administration of glucose. *Science* **105:** 183, 1947.

Ehrlich, J. C. Amyloidosis of the islets of Langerhans. *Am J Pathol* **38:** 49–59, 1961.

Eigenmann, J. E. Diabetes mellitus in elderly female dogs: recent findings on pathogenesis and clinical implications. *J Am Anim Hosp Assoc* **17:** 805–812, 1981.

Field, J. B. On the nature of the metabolic defect(s) in diabetes. *Am J Med* **26:** 662–673, 1959.

Fitzgerald, P. J., Carol, B. M., and Rosenstock, L. Pancreatic acinar cell regeneration. *Nature* **212:** 594–596, 1966.

Friesen, S. R. Tumors of the endocrine pancreas. *N Engl J Med* **306:** 580–589, 1982.

Gomori, G. Pathology of the pancreatic islets. *Arch Pathol* **36:** 217–232, 1943.

Groen, J. J., Frenkel, H. S., and Offerhaus, L. Observations on a case of spontaneous diabetes mellitus in a dog. *Diabetes* **13:** 492–499, 1964.

Hansen, H.-J. Insulom hos hund. *Nord Vet Med* **1:** 363–376, 1949.

Happe, R. P. *et al.* Zollinger–Ellison syndrome in three dogs. *Vet Pathol* **17:** 177–186, 1980.

Hausler, H. R., Sibay, T. M., and Campbell, J. Retinopathy in a dog following diabetes induced by growth hormone. *Diabetes* **13:** 122–126, 1964.

Huxtable, C. R., and Farrow, B. R. H. Functional neoplasms of the canine pancreatic-islet B-cells: a clinicopathological study of three cases. *J Small Anim Pract* **20:** 737–748, 1979.

Jarrett, I. G. Alloxan diabetes in sheep. *Aust J Exp Biol Med Sci* **24:** 95–102, 1946.

Lazarus, S. S., and Volk, B. W. Glycogen infiltration (''hydropic degeneration'') in the pancreas. A review. *Arch Pathol* **66:** 59–71, 1958.

McGrath, J. T. Convulsions in dogs with some clinico-pathologic observations. *Proc 89th Annu Meet Vet Med Assoc* pp. 220–223, 1952.

Marmor, M. *et al.* Epizootiologic patterns of diabetes mellitus in dogs. *Am J Vet Res* **43:** 465–470, 1982.

Patz, A., and Maumenee, A. E. Studies on diabetic retinopathy. I. Retinopathy in a dog with spontaneous diabetes mellitus. *Am J Ophthalmol* **54:** 532–541, 1962.

Rubarth, S. The degeneration of amyloid in the Langerhans' cell islands as the cause of diabetes mellitus in the cat. *Skand Vet Tidskr* **25:** 750–761, 1935.

Slye, M., and Wells, H. G. Tumors of islet tissue with hyperinsulinism in a dog. *Arch Pathol* **19:** 537–542, 1935.

Tasker, J. B., Whiteman, C. E., and Martin, B. R. Diabetes mellitus in the horse. *J Am Vet Med Assoc* **149:** 393–399, 1966.

Toreson, W. E. Glycogen infiltration (so-called hydropic degeneration) in the pancreas in human and experimental diabetes mellitus. *Am J Pathol* **27:** 327–348, 1951.

Vracko, R., and Benditt, E. P. Manifestations of diabetes mellitus—their possible relationships to an underlying cell defect. *Am J Pathol* **75:** 204–222, 1974.

Wachstein, M., and Meisel, E. Relation of dietary protein levels to pancreatic damage in the rat. *Proc Soc Exp Biol Med* **85:** 314–317, 1954.

Walker, D. Diabetes mellitus following steroid therapy in a dog. *Vet Rec* **74:** 1543–1545, 1962.

Wilkinson, J. S. Spontaneous diabetes in domestic animals. *Vet Rev Annot* **3:** 69–96, 1957; **4:** 93–117, 1958.

Wilkinson, J. S. Spontaneous diabetes mellitus. *Vet Rec* **72:** 548–555, 1960.

CHAPTER 4

The Peritoneum, Retroperitoneum, and Mesentery

RICHARD J. JULIAN
Ontario Veterinary College, Canada

General Considerations

The peritoneal cavity is a single unit incompletely divided into compartments by the mesentery, omentum, and ligaments of double peritoneal membrane. This, with the assistance of fibrin in inflammatory reactions, can result in localization of lesions within the abdomen, although peritonitis can also be more or less generalized. Omental bursitis is an example of peritonitis localized within a compartment, and the peritonitis of traumatic reticulitis is frequently localized by fibrin and adhesions. Blood or fluid in the abdomen can occasionally be localized within a cystic structure but is usually generalized. The peritoneal membrane forms "ligaments" between organs surrounded by it, and in some cases these ligaments are involved in bowel entrapments, particularly the nephrosplenic ligament in the horse. Normal holes, such as the epiploic foramen, and congenital or acquired defects in the double layer of peritoneum making up the mesentery can also be involved in entrapments.

The retroperitoneum is the areolar and adipose tissue immediately outside the peritoneal lining of the abdominal cavity. Its volume is small except when adipose tissue accumulates, as it normally does in the dorsal retroperitoneum, pelvic cavity, and mesenteries.

The normal peritoneum is a smooth, shiny membrane with just enough fluid present to keep it moist. It becomes dry in animals that die of, or with, severe dehydration and is then clammy, sticky, and slightly opaque. It seems that a horse's peritoneum dries out shortly after death because if examination is postponed for a few hours, apposed serous surfaces stick to each other so that when separated the serosa is drawn into tags; this is especially evident on the diaphragm and viscera touching it. These changes should not be taken as residue of peritoneal inflammation or confused with the fibrous tags of scar tissue that occur on the diaphragmatic surface of livers that have been traversed by many larval nematodes. Distinction should also be made between antemortem and postmortem effusions and discolorations. Some lymph accumulates in the peritoneal cavity after death, and this becomes stained with hemoglobin as soon as erythrocytes in the serosal vessels begin to undergo lysis. Such fluid does not clot and is also present in other serous cavities. Its nature is usually evident because gaseous changes of putrefaction accompany the lysis of erythrocytes. Diffusion of bile pigments through the wall of the gallbladder, the biliary ducts, or the duodenum will stain adjacent viscera. Where hydrogen sulfide from the intestine meets hemoglobin from lysed erythrocytes, greenish black sulfmethemoglobin is produced to discolor the tissues.

Congenital Anomalies

Congenital anomalies of the peritoneal membranes are rare and when present are most frequently associated with embryonic remnants of vitelline structures. A **persistent vitelline duct** may form a fibrous ligament between the intestine and the umbilicus, or a Meckel's diverticulum and the umbilicus. The remnant may be partial, not reaching the umbilicus, and attached to the mesentery or a loop of intestine to form a band that could act as an internal hernial ring. Either form of band may become involved in strangulation of the intestine.

A **persistent vitelline artery** results in an anomaly, classified as a mesodiverticular band. This is a fold of mesentery, occasionally carrying a patent vitelline artery in its free edge, that extends from the cranial mesenteric artery to the antimesenteric side of the intestine (to the site of Meckel's diverticulum). The pocket formed between this fold and the normal mesentery may entrap intestine, or defects may develop in it that allow passage of intestinal loops and strangulation. Occasionally, double (both left and right) mesodiverticular bands are present. Occasionally, fibrous cords of mesenteric tissue may be found that do not appear to be part of embryonic remnants of vitelline structures.

Abnormal Contents of the Peritoneal Cavity

Foreign bodies occur commonly in the peritoneal cavity, and obviously, there is potentially a wide variety in both objects and circumstances. Foreign materials of endogenous origin are important because their presence requires an abnormality of another organ.

Ingesta is frequently found in the peritoneal cavity of horses, cattle, and swine, seldom in sheep and goats, and rarely in dogs and cats. The origin of the ingesta is the stomach or intestine, and the site of leakage is usually easy to find, especially when the animal dies before there is time for peritonitis to develop; such is the case, for instance, in gastric rupture in the horse. Once peritonitis has developed and matted the intestines and mesenteries, the site of perforation may be very difficult to find, especially as severe peritonitis devitalizes segments of the intestinal wall and, occasionally, causes perforation of the bowel from the serosal surface.

Digestion of the abomasal wall postmortem will release gastric contents in calves and lambs fed on milk-replacement diets, especially if the amounts ingested are excessive. The margins of the abomasal defect and the peritoneum do not show evidence of reactionary changes. In horses, cecal rupture following impaction usually occurs on the medial side of the dorsal cecum following ischemic pressure necrosis. Perforation of the colon or rectum following impaction probably has a similar pathogenesis. Rectal perforation may be secondary to accidental injury, or occasionally in foals, to focal ischemic necrosis from adherent meconium.

Hemoperitoneum is the presence of blood in the peritoneal cavity. The amount present at death is not an indication of the volume of bleeding during life because the blood is removed quite rapidly by diaphragmatic lymphatics. The blood in the cavity may be fluid or partially clotted. Animals occasionally die from bleeding into the peritoneal cavity, but the outcome will depend on the rate and volume of bleeding, the site of hemorrhage, the cause, and the initial health of the animal.

Hemoperitoneum is seen most commonly in the dog and cat as a result of traumatic injury to the liver, spleen, and kidney. Rupture of the liver and hemorrhage occur in infectious canine hepatitis. Manual efforts at artificial resuscitation, especially if vigorous, will rupture the liver, particularly in anesthetized dogs, if the anesthetic is one causing hepatic congestion and turgidity. Repeated splenic ruptures at the site of hemangiomas are well known in dogs past middle age. Spleen and liver enlarged and tensed by infiltrating leukemic cells, fat, or amyloid are predisposed to rupture; the volume of hemorrhage in these cases may be very small.

Warfarin poisoning in several species may result in nonclotting blood in the abdomen. Manual squashing of a corpus luteum is a source of hemorrhage in cattle. In cattle and horses, laceration of the uterus or rupture of a uterine artery can result in a sometimes fatal hemorrhage. Calves born of cows fed moldy sweet-clover hay bleed from the umbilical vessels into the peritoneal cavity (as well as elsewhere).

Hemorrhage on or beneath the peritoneum without free blood in the cavity is commonly observed in many acute infectious toxemias and noninfectious conditions that interfere with vascular integrity or the hemostatic mechanisms. Peritoneal hemorrhage must be differentiated from hemorrhagic peritonitis, which is an important lesion in many diseases. Hemorrhage into an omental or mesenteric cyst can cause sudden abdominal enlargement without free blood in the abdomen.

Hydroperitoneum

Hydroperitoneum (ascites), is the accumulation of noninflammatory transudate in the peritoneal cavity. It is arguable that the term ascites should be reserved for peritoneal lymphedema of hepatic origin, whether the issue is primarily hepatic, as in hepatic fibrosis, or secondary to a sustained increase in central venous pressure with chronic hepatic congestion. The fluid of ascites is watery, clear, or straw colored and will contain few leukocytes but large numbers of desquamated mesothelial cells. The serosal lining is normal unless fluid has been present for some weeks, when the serosa acquires a flat, whitish semiopacity.

The principles governing the transfer of fluid (lymph) between blood vessels and lymphatics across the peritoneal membrane are, so far as known, basically the same as those governing fluid exchange in tissues, and there is normally a very rapid turnover of peritoneal fluid. In tissues generally, there is a small excess of filtration at the arteriolar end of the capillary bed over absorption at the venous end of the capillary bed; the excess of fluid is drained from the tissue spaces by lymphatics. These mechanisms are operative in abdominal viscera, but it is to be noted that free fluid in the peritoneal cavity drains through the ventral diaphragm and the sternal lymphatics. The accumulation of excess peritoneal fluid can be viewed most simply as the result of diminished removal or overproduction of fluid.

The relative importance of the various pathways for the **removal** of **fluid** from the peritoneal cavity has not been studied in detail for the various species, but the following schema is generally applicable. In spite of the large area of peritoneum, fluid absorption from the cavity is virtually limited to those diaphragmatic lymphatics that form an abundantly anastomotic plexus in the muscular portion of the right side of the diaphragm. Vessels penetrate the diaphragm to form a corresponding pleural plexus from which the lymph is conveyed in the sternal ducts to the anterior sternal node, and then via the right lymphatic duct to the vena cava. There are subsidiary pathways that will deliver some peritoneal lymph to the cisterna chyli or thoracic duct, but 80% or more of peritoneal lymph will follow sternal lymphatics. The smallness of the area of lymphatic absorption provides an explanation for the ease and rapidity with which peritoneal drainage can be obstructed.

Obstruction to **diaphragmatic lymphatics** leading to ascites is best exemplified in peritoneal carcinomatosis. Implantation metastasis of carcinomas usually and perhaps always, if given time, implant most extensively on the diaphragm in the region of the lymphatic exits, and there, permeation of the lymphatic vessels is easily demonstrated microscopically. It is probable that the neoplastic cells are carried to the anterior abdomen by the same forces that propel the lymph in that direction, namely, normal intestinal movements and normal respiratory excursions. The restriction of the area through which lymphatic absorption can take place is compensated by the high efficiency of the mechanism, a level of efficiency not satisfactorily explained.

Carcinomatous implants on the peritoneum, in addition to obstructing diaphragmatic lymphatics, may provoke fluid production. This has been argued for papillary adenocarcinoma of the ovary, which in the bitch provides the best example of implantation and ascites. It will be apparent that ascites may develop if there is obstruction to sternal pathways anterior to the diaphragm, and this condition seems often to be provided in lymphomatosis of adult cattle when there is massive neoplastic involvement of the anterior mediastinal lymph nodes.

The **overproduction** of **peritoneal lymph** is related to the mesenteric circulation and the hepatic circulation. This excludes the rare chylous ascites, which results when the cisterna chyli is ruptured, the chylous origin of the fluid indicated by the high content of chylomicron fat and the milkiness of the fluid.

The filtration pressures in mesenteries and omentum appear to differ quantitatively from those in other tissues, with the effective filtration occurring along the entire capillary bed. That all of the filtered fluid must return to the circulation via the lymphatics attests to the capacity for lymphatic drainage. Increased venous pressure in the portal venous system is not in itself expected to lead to ascites. Acute portal vein obstruction leads rapidly to death. Chronic obstruction to prehepatic portal flow leads quickly to the development of collateral venous circulation, with connections to the abdominal vena cava. The interstitial tissues of the mesentery and omentum are, as are interstitial tissues generally, rather noncompliant, and small increases in interstitial fluid volume produce marked increases of tissue hydrostatic pressure, which limit transudation.

The balance of oncotic and hydraulic pressure that regulates fluid exchange between blood vessels and interstitial tissue depends on the integrity of vascular structures and on the maintenance of their permeability characteristics. Vascular injury that allows increased permeability to plasma protein substantially alters the balance of forces and favors transudation. Small amounts of ascitic fluid may be generated under these circumstances in a variety of systemic illnesses, such as the clostridial intoxications, acute uremic syndromes in ruminants and pigs, and exudative diathesis of pigs deficient in vitamin E.

Ascites resulting from overproduction of fluid is usually an expression of hepatic lymphedema. It appears that the *sine qua non* of hepatic ascites is that there should be obstruction to the intrahepatic veins or the suprahepatic veins with congestion and edema of the liver; obstruction to the portal veins with increased portal venous pressure will not do, except perhaps if there is concurrently a critical degree of hypoproteinemia. The usual conditions providing obstruction to the efferent hepatic vessels are fibrosis of the liver and congestive heart failure. There is, of course, a variety of additional causes, including primary neoplasms of the liver, principally those of cholangiocellular type, which tend to be diffuse; secondary tumors, especially those of lymphocytic type; extensive infestation with hydatid cysts; chronic fascioliasis; and so on.

When the liver is congested, there is, as in any acutely congested tissue, an increased turnover of protein and fluid and an increased flow of hepatic lymph with a high concentration of protein. The bulk of hepatic lymph comes from the space of Disse, which is separated from the capillary lumen by a fenestrated endothelium that is freely permeable to plasma constituents, including protein of high molecular weight. Oncotic pressures, normally dependent on proteins of low molecular weight, are not as important in the liver as they are elsewhere in the regulation of fluid exchange. Instead, the formation of hepatic lymph is sensitive to small changes in hydraulic pressure in the sinusoids, which accounts for the frequency with which ascites is associated with those diseases leading to increased central and hepatic venous pressure.

If the ordinary capacity of the hepatic lymphatics is not equal to the challenge provided in hepatic venous stasis, then lymph high in protein oozes from the hepatic capsule, presumably from the rich lymphatic plexus there, and spills from the efferent lymphatics that pass from the porta hepatis to the cisterna chyli; in hepatic ascites, these efferent lymphatics become very large, numerous, and thick walled, and presumably, the same changes take place in all efferent hepatic lymphatics, some of which follow different routes, for example, through the suspensory ligaments.

The fluid that accumulates in the peritoneal cavity is not static but dynamic, continually produced and removed. The efficiency of normal removal has already been indicated, and it will be evident therefrom that it is only in instances of severe increased pressure in the hepatic vessels that gross ascites will develop. In all considerations of hepatic ascites, the thoracic duct, which is the main channel for removal of hepatic lymph, is assumed to be completely permissive. The conducting capacity of the duct is, however, probably quite limited, even though the duct is quite distensible. Concurrent increase of venous pressure at the thoracic inlet may impair lymph drainage; of greater importance may be altered configuration, when the duct is distended, of the opening between duct and vein.

In experimental ascites, the flow of lymph in the hepatic lymphatics can be increased in rate to five or more times the normal, and since only a part of this flow oozes into the peritoneal cavity, some additional factors would seem to be necessary before the drainage capacity is overwhelmed, if indeed it is overwhelmed, an event that seems unlikely in view of calculations purporting to show a complete turnover of the albumin in the ascitic fluid in ~2 days and a turnover of ~80% of the volume of ascitic fluid each hour. Thus it seems clear that although severe obstruction to the intrahepatic circulation is necessary to initiate hepatic ascites, the gross and persistent accumulation of fluid depends on additional factors. Chief among these is the retention, by diminished urinary excretion, of salt and therefore also of water.

There is much evidence connecting the retention of sodium and water, and the resultant expansion of plasma volume, with the development of edema and ascites in congestive heart failure and hepatic venous obstruction. The mechanisms remain obscure but may involve receptor sites for sensing volume–pressure changes in the systemic circulation. The effector mechanisms are renal and probably regulated by a variety of neural and humoral pathways that influence renal hemodynamics, the composition of tubular fluid, and ionic gradients.

The principal diseases of animals in which ascites occurs have been indicated in the foregoing discussion, but there are some others that ought to be mentioned. The ascites of congestive heart failure is presumably of the same pathogenesis as in humans, whatever that might be, and as indicated above, it may be related in part to the hepatic congestion that is part of the syndrome of cardiac failure. There is the additional possibility of retarded lymphatic flow, and although there appear to be no measurements of this, the tortuous dilatation of lymphatics in some cases of congestive heart failure are quite suggestive. Ascites occurs in congestive heart failure without edematous transudations elsewhere, especially in dogs and cats, but it should be pointed out that only a minority of cases of congestive failure in dogs and cats is associated with ascites. Excess peritoneal fluid is also part of a generalized dropsical condition in cachectic diseases, anemia, and starvation. Although the mechanisms have not been intensively studied, hypoproteinemia has been given consideration as one of the principal factors. Very probably it is also in those diseases that are known, or presumed, to result in chronic protein leakage and loss, such as gastrointestinal trichostrongylosis and Johne's disease. Hypoproteinemia appears not, however, to be of initiating significance in the edema and ascites of chronic starvation without other accompanying disease; it is suggested in such cases that the fluid-retention serves largely to replace wasted tissues, especially adipose tissue.

Effusion of fluid, sometimes massive, occurs in the peritoneal cavity, thorax, and ventral body wall in some instances of uremia in sheep and cattle. It is part of the postmortem picture in sheep and cattle dying of urethral obstruction by calculus, and the fluid may have a distinct uriniferous odor. The pathogenesis of this fluid accumulation has not been examined, and although in a few cases there is a rupture of the lower urinary tract (which might provide the fluid by leakage), in many cases a rupture cannot be demonstrated. Renal uremia also is associated with similar fluid accumulations in cattle; this is evident in some dying with renal amyloidosis, and the contributing factor here is probably hypoproteinemia consequent on prolonged massive proteinuria. Acute toxic nephrosis, of which certain plant poisonings and mycotoxicoses provide the best examples in ruminants and pigs, may also be accompanied by massive effusions, and as is usually the case with ascites of urinary tract disease, the mesenteries and retroperitoneum are also saturated.

Degenerative Conditions of the Peritoneum, Retroperitoneum, and Mesentery

Abdominal Fat Necrosis

Necrosis of the omental or other abdominal or retroperitoneal fat is a frequent finding at autopsy. The pathogenesis is poorly understood, but there appear to be a number of causes. In pancreatic necrosis, **enzymatic necrosis** of **fat** occurs constantly, and indeed, peripancreatic necrosis of fat may be the initial morphologic change. Enzymatic necrosis of fat may extend throughout the abdomen. The acute lesions are discrete foci or confluent masses of yellow, necrotic adipose tissue surrounded by a zone of intense hyperemia with fibrin deposited on the surface. Free droplets of fat can be found in the peritoneal fluid.

The lesion has been attributed to lipolytic enzymes from the acinar pancreas, but there is no agreement on which enzymes initiate the reaction. Pancreatic amylase, elastase, lipase, trypsin, and phospholipase A are examples of enzymes that may be involved, but some of these would have to overcome local enzyme inhibitors before becoming activated. Kinins, Hageman factor, and complement have been suggested as possible causes of fat necrosis once the process has been initiated. Neutrophils respond in large numbers, and their degeneration may aid the ongoing process. Lipase released from degenerating fat cells also contributes to fat necrosis.

Microscopically, the acute lesion is made up of necrotic fat cells containing acidophilic, opaque, amorphous or lacy substance or basophilic fibrillar or granular mineralized material. Masses of degenerating neutrophils and necrotic debris are present. Fibroplasia and vacuolated macrophages are features of the chronic lesion, along with necrotic fat and, occasionally, dystrophic mineralization.

Widespread or isolated **focal necrosis** of abdominal and retroperitoneal fat is frequently found in sheep and sometimes in horses, pigs, and other animals. This necrotic fat is usually seen only at the chronic stage in the form of small, dry, firm or gritty plaques. A flat white color gives the plaques clear distinction from surrounding normal fat. There is no grossly apparent inflammatory reaction, and histologically the lesions resemble the chronic lesion described above, with occasional large lipid vacuoles containing necrotic debris encapsulated by connective tissue. The pathogenesis of this form of fat necrosis has not been explained. The focal lesion may be due to avascular necrosis of fat from pressure ischemia, perhaps due to differences in the texture or composition of the fat, or some other circulatory deficit in the small capillaries that nourish the large masses of fat, since the lesion does appear more frequently in excessively fat animals. It is also possible that the lesions are initiated by intracellular lipolytic disturbances in circumstances in which there is accelerated mobilization of fat to meet acute metabolic demands.

The third form, not uncommon and perhaps the most curious, is **massive fat necrosis** in **cattle**. Although this condition has been reported to occur more frequently in Channel Island breeds, there is more evidence for herd than breed predisposition. It does appear to be associated with excessively fat and fattening cattle. Both sexes are affected, but probably not clinically before the second year of life. The disease has two significant features. First, although it is seen more often in the slaughterhouse than in the postmortem room, it is frequently fatal, perhaps always progressive and potentially fatal, and second, the hard masses of necrotic fat have been, and will be, mistaken for fetal prominences in the diagnosis of pregnancy by perrectal palpation. The fatal outcome in this disease is usually by intestinal obstruction, the intestine compressed by the expanding lumps of necrotic fat (Fig. 4.1B), but other complications also occur, such as compression and stenosis of the ureters. Affected animals may exhibit a variety of clinical signs such as anorexia, diarrhea, constipation, colic, or bloat. They may become emaciated prior to death.

The pathologic process occurs in any portion or all of the omental, mesenteric, and retroperitoneal fat. In the early stage of development there is evidence of acute inflammation, and the hard necrotic masses are surrounded by a zone of hyperemia, the overlying peritoneum may be necrotic, and the necrotic margins umbilicate. The masses may vary from small nodules to large solid masses encapsulated by fibrous tissue and that on cut section are firm, dry and caseous, or moist, and deep yellow. The inner surfaces of such masses are firmly molded to the contours of enclosed organs. Because of the unusual bulk of the necrotic tissue, and because fat is sometimes found in unusual locations, such as under the serosa of the intestine, the condition has been called lipomatosis, but there is no indication that the lesions are neoplastic.

On microscopic examination the tissue resembles a mixture of acute and chronic enzymatic fat necrosis with fewer neutrophils, some lymphocytes, plasma cells, and eosinophils, and more macrophages and giant cells. Crystal-shaped clefts are present in fat cells and in macrophages and giant cells.

The pathogenisis of this diffuse lipogranulomatosis in cattle is not clear, but there is accumulating evidence of a dietary cause somewhat similar to that of steatitis as it occurs in horses, pigs, and other species. The different lesions in cattle may be due to the different chemical composition of fat or to a different host response to material recognized as ''foreign'' (which might also allow for breed predisposition, as might breed differences in texture and amount of abdominal fat). The lesion is possibly related to ingestion, or production in the rumen, of high levels of saturated fatty acids, which form long-chain compounds that are solid at normal body temperature. Chemical change or avascular necrosis may initiate a reaction that results in the formation of insoluble salts, cholesterol, or other material recognized by the body as foreign. This material provokes the inflammatory response, with fibrosis, collagen formation, and the accumulation of materials in fat cells, giant cells, and macrophages.

Steatitis (yellow-fat disease) occurs in many species of animals except ruminants, affecting the abdominal and retroperitoneal fat along with other body fat. The condition is described (as panniculitis) with the Skin and Appendages (Volume 1) and is caused by a diet high in polyunsaturated fat and low in tocopherols, allowing oxidation of body fatty acids. Peroxidation creates free radicals, which damage tissue and provoke the characteristic inflammatory response in the adipose tissue. Several types of steatitis, all vitamin E responsive, occur in newborn or young, as well as in mature animals. Lipofuscin, which is not present in all forms of steatitis, is responsible for the yellow color and often fills the macrophages, which are a feature of this form of steatitis.

Inflammation of the Peritoneum: Peritonitis

Peritonitis is very common in the large domestic animals but uncommon in dogs and cats. It may be serofibrinous, fibrinopurulent, purulent, or hemorrhagic, and whatever the type, it may be localized or more or less generalized. Differences in type and distribution can be more or less anticipated from the origin and the causes; the latter are numerous and

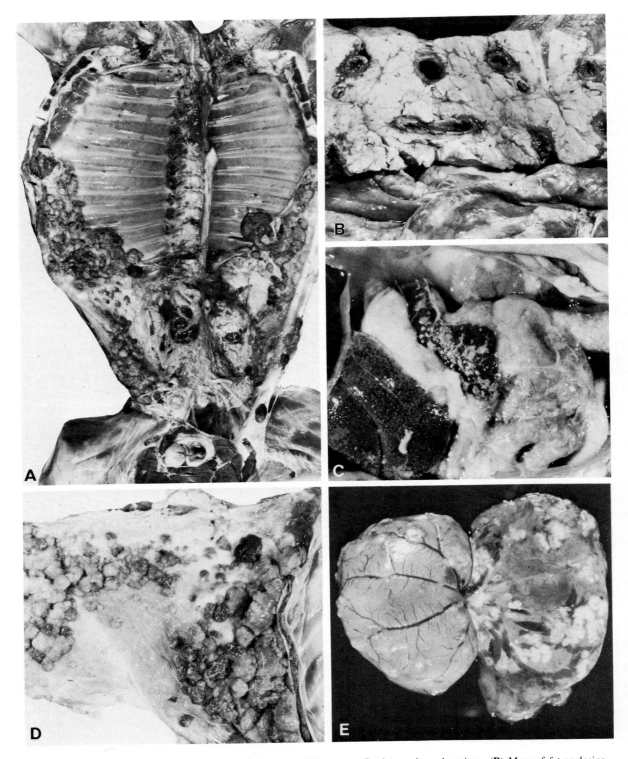

Fig. 4.1. (A) Congenital mesothelioma. Calf. Tumor nodules are confined to peritoneal cavity. (B) Mass of fat enclosing intestinal loops in abdominal fat necrosis. Ox. (C) Feline infectious peritonitis. Exudative lesion with fibrin on mesentery and viscera, and granulomas in liver, spleen, kidney, and wall of large and small intestine. (D) Close-up of (A), showing nodules of mesothelioma on peritoneum. (E) Feline infectious peritonitis. Focal pyogranulomatous lesions involving renal cortex and reflected capsule.

varied, so only some of the more common and important of them will be considered.

Most cases of peritonitis are caused by bacteria and their toxins, some by helminth infestations, a few are viral, and a few chemical. The intraperitoneal injection of a number of therapeutic agents causes a mild, and usually inconsequential, peritonitis. The most devastating forms of chemical peritonitis are endogenous and are caused by bile and pancreatic enzymes. The peritonitis caused by bile is intense, shock inducing, and may be rapidly fatal. There is very little exudate unless the leakage is minor and infected, and then it may become purulent. Biliary peritonitis is readily recognized by the typical staining. The peritonitis of pancreatic necrosis is also acute and is rather common in dogs, rare in horses, and virtually never occurs in other species. The reaction about the pancreas, particularly its head, is liquefactive and purulent, and the exudate mats the lesser omentum to the pancreas and the adjacent liver and other organs. This local peritoneal reaction resolves completely if the animal survives, and only very minor adhesions or slight puckering of the mesentery persist. The peritoneal exudate is usually scant but is distinctive because, as well as pus, it contains white droplets of fats and soaps released from the surrounding adipose tissues by the pancreatic enzymes.

Bacterial peritonitis may be regarded as primary in the sense that the bacteria are implanted directly on the peritoneum by perforating lesions from a contaminated surface, either a hollow viscus or the skin. It is secondary when it reaches the peritoneum from an adjacent focus by direct extension, or when the organisms are carried there in the blood or lymph streams.

Primary peritonitis need not be discussed further; it is most commonly associated with the lesions described above as being the source of peritoneal contamination by ingesta but may also rise from parasites penetrating the intestinal wall in some species. In females, the abdominal cavity is open to the exterior through the reproductive tract, and infection may enter the abdomen through the oviduct as well as by rupture of the uterus or laceration of the vagina.

Secondary bacterial peritonitis is also common either as an extension from localized inflammation in an abdominal viscus or as a typical part of the morbid picture in a number of specific diseases. Acute serofibrinous peritonitis occurs by extension through the wall of a gangrenous intestine or uterus prior to rupture, or death from toxemia may intervene before rupture occurs. Secondary peritonitis occasionally results by extension from retroperitoneal infection or, in ruminants, from omental bursitis. In those cases in which the peritonitis develops by direct extension, there is little difficulty in ascertaining its origin, even when the process becomes diffuse. The sources of secondary peritonitis are so varied that detailed consideration cannot be given to them here. Instead, some of the features of peritonitis in the different species are given with an indication of the specific diseases in which peritonitis is a feature, although not necessarily a consistent one. The incidence and nature of peritonitis in specific infections are discussed more fully with the specific diseases.

Horses

Diffuse peritonitis is usually fatal in horses, chronic diffuse peritonitis virtually never occurring. In almost all cases it is caused by rupture or perforation of the stomach or intestine. Acute or chronic local peritonitis does occur occasionally from castration wounds or other penetration from the skin, or streptococcal abscess in the mesentery. It may be due to local verminous lesions, suppurative gastritis in habronemiasis, or from perforating *Gasterophilus*. Abscesses or ulcerations attributable to *Strongylus* are more common in the colon than elsewhere. Migrating *S. equinus* or *S. edentatus* larvae cause retroperitoneal lesions in the flank, perirenal fat, and diaphragm, perihepatitis with fibrin tags on the liver capsule, and a chronic diffuse thickening and inflammation in the mesentery, omentum, and hepatorenal ligament, with occasional caseous nodules. Copious purulent peritonitis is often seen in infections of foals by *Corynebacterium equi*. Intestinal infection of foals by *Actinobacillus equuli* causes fibrinous mesenteric lymphadenitis and peritonitis.

Cattle

Acute diffuse purulent peritonitis in cattle is common and usually the result of perforation of a viscus, especially the reticulum or uterus. Both may also result in local acute, and then chronic, peritonitis. Perforation of the abomasum or intestine is more likely to give fibrinohemorrhagic peritonitis. A serofibrinous peritonitis, sometimes with very copious exudate (and with similar lesions on other serous membranes), is typical of sporadic bovine encephalomyelitis. A diffuse fibrinohemorrhagic peritonitis occurs in most cases of clostridial hemoglobinuria and in some cases of blackleg and septicemic pasteurellosis; a more localized peritonitis of this type occurs in some cases of clostridial enterotoxemia caused by *Clostridium perfringens* types B and C. Tuberculosis causes white, nodular granulomas (pearls), and actinobacillosis, although rather rare, produces the usual heavily scarified granulomas, especially about the peritoneum of the forestomachs. Extension of infection from the umbilicus of the newborn produces a fibrinopurulent peritonitis not localized but most severe along the ventral abdominal wall, or up the urachus to the bladder.

Sheep

Peritonitis of specific cause is uncommon in sheep except for the very local variety that accompanies penetration of the intestine by the larvae of *Oesophagostomum columbianum*. The uterus is probably the usual site in adults from which local spread occurs to the peritoneum, the antecedent lesion in most cases either a postpartum septic metritis or so-called blackleg of the fetus; in either event the peritonitis is fibrinosuppurative and hemorrhagic. A serofibrinous peritonitis is a feature of contagious agalactia, or any variant of it, caused by *Mycoplasma*.

Goats

Mycoplasma mycoides may cause an acute fibrinous peritonitis in goats, although acute death from septicemia or joint and mammary gland disease is more common. Paratuberculosis (Johne's disease) frequently produces a nodular granulomatous lymphangitis in the mesentery, and sometimes caseous or calcified lymphadenitis.

Swine

A few filmy strands of fibrin frequently overlie the intestine and the borders of the mesentery in many acute infectious diseases of swine, and in conditions that result in vascular damage such as edema disease and vitamin E/selenium-responsive conditions; this does not qualify as peritonitis. A diffuse suppurative and adhesive peritonitis is common in pigs; in these cases the intestines are so matted that they cannot be dissected. *Corynebacterium pyogenes, Escherichia coli,* or a miscellany of organisms are frequently present in these, and in some the extension of the inflammatory process can be traced up the inguinal canals from castration wounds; in other cases of similar type, the peritonitis is localized to the inguinal and pelvic regions, is adhesive, and causes death from intestinal obstruction. Occasionally, *C. pyogenes* produces discrete encapsulated abscesses as profuse implants on both visceral and parietal peritoneum. A serofibrinous peritonitis, more fibrinous than serous, and with similar lesions on other serous membranes, is almost pathognomonic for Glasser's disease caused by *Haemophilus suis. Mycoplasma hyorhinis* and possibly other mycoplasmas may produce a serofibrinous peritonitis that becomes fibrous, with adhesions to a thickened serous membrane; this disease is to be distinguished from Glasser's disease. Small, firm, lemon yellow nodules and flattened disks of inspissated fibrin often are found free in the peritoneal cavity in chronic *Mycoplasma* infections. Rectal strictures in swine cause a very dilated colon and cecum full of ingesta. The serosa is frequently thickened, white, and covered with fibrin tags, resembling infectious serositis. The thickening is probably caused by subserosal edema and fibrosis but may be due to passage of bacteria or by-products through the intestinal wall. *Stephanurus dentatus* larvae cause subserosal focal hepatitis and a mild reaction with edema in the perirenal fat and retroperitoneal tissue, and sometimes in the mesentery and local lymph nodes as they move to the kidney. In intestinal anthrax in swine there is an acute gelatinous hemorrhagic peritonitis very typically localized to the mesentery between the intestine and the mesenteric node. The distribution of the lesion is due to the lymphatic spread of the infection from the intestine. Tuberculous peritonitis in swine is localized and characterized by adhesions to the spleen.

Dogs

A fibrinohemorrhagic peritonitis, slight in degree and easily overlooked, is common in infectious canine hepatitis. The peritoneum, especially that covering the intestine, is gray and granular like ground glass, and there are a few reddish strands of fibrin, most of them about the liver. There is edema of the intestinal subserosa and, frequently, petechiae or larger hemorrhages. In parvovirus infection, similar lesions may be present on the serosa of the affected portion of intestine. Putrid peritonitis occurs when the uterus ruptures either as a result of pyometra or septic metritis with fetal putrefaction. Nocardiosis, which may be infection by bacteria of the genera *Nocardia* or *Actinomyces,* produces very characteristic lesions on the peritoneum (Fig. 4.2B). It is, however, more common on the pleura. Sometimes there are purulent granulomas, but most frequently there is a profuse, pink mush. The color is from admixture of copiously exuded cells and blood; the blood is derived from a tremendous proliferation of thin-walled capillaries from serous surfaces. Purulent peritonitis in the dog is rare; it has been observed as an extension from umbilical and hepatic abscesses in puppies and is caused by *Streptococcus canis.*

Cats

Putrid peritonitis occurs when the uterus ruptures in consequence of pyometra or fetal putrefaction. Peritonitis also occurs from penetrating wounds or by extension from retroperitoneal tissues. Nocardiosis similar in appearance to the disease in dogs frequently complicates myelodysplastic disease in cats.

FELINE INFECTIOUS PERITONITIS. Feline infectious peritonitis is a relatively recently recognized coronavirus infection of Felidae, particularly domestic cats. It has a worldwide distribution, but the incidence of disease is low and sporadic even in the countries where it is most common. The disease is in part immune mediated, and the lesions are for the most part the result of deposition of immune complexes leading to Arthus-type reactions. The naturally occurring disease tends to be chronic and results in death after one to several months, although there may be nonclinical carriers. Most cases have a relatively easily recognized clinical course with typical gross and histologic findings. Close contact appears to be necessary for the spread of the disease and is likely to occur by way of ingestion or inhalation of infective material from body secretions and excretions. Cats in catteries, pet shops, and households with multiple cats are at greatest risk. Cats of all ages can be affected, but there may be a higher incidence in two groups; young, entire adults and aged cats.

Feline infectious peritonitis has an insidious onset, and since cats have a propensity to mask serious illness, the disease may be well advanced before clinical signs are recognized. The early signs are nonspecific, consisting of decreased activity, depression, anorexia, or diarrhea. The increasing abdominal distension present in the effusive form of the disease may hide the progressive weight loss. A variety of mild to severe neurologic signs develop in up to 30% of affected cats, and it is these signs, and panophthalmitis (which is also relatively common), that are likely to attract attention. Affected cats are usually pyrexic and often hypergammaglobulinemic, with total serum protein increased and the albumin/globulin ratio lowered. Feline infectious peritonitis is unresponsive to antibiotics but may show a temporary response to corticosteroids. Occasionally, respiratory signs with cough or dyspnea are present, and in atypical or noneffusive forms, neurologic or ophthalmic signs may be the first noted. A variety of serologic tests are available to detect feline infectious peritonitis antibody. Antibody levels are usually high (titer > 1:400) in cats with clinical infectious peritonitis, but interpretation is complicated because current tests do not distinguish between antibodies formed in response to the virus and those stimulated by the feline enteric coronavirus.

For descriptive purposes, the disease has been divided into effusive "wet" and noneffusive "dry" forms, but since the only distinction between these forms is the extent of fibrinous peritonitis and exudate, the division serves little useful purpose. All serous surfaces throughout the body may be involved in the inflammatory response, and pleurisy with pleural effusion is

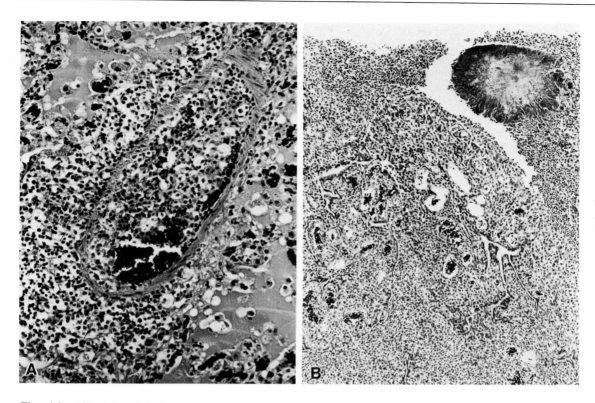

Fig. 4.2. (A) Feline infectious peritonitis. Vasculitis and perivasculitis in the lung. There is severe pulmonary edema. (B) Proliferative peritonitis in nocardial infection. Dog. Bacterial colony (top right) is attracting a stream of leukocytes.

present in ~40% of cases. Peritonitis is present in most natural cases, although this may be obvious grossly in only 60 to 70%. The tunica vaginalis is affected, resulting in periorchitis in entire males. Up to 1 liter of abdominal exudate may be present.

The fluid is usually clear and pale to deep yellow, although it may be flocculent and contain strands of fibrin. The serosal surfaces may be covered with fibrin exudate, giving them a granular appearance. Fibrin is frequently prominent over the visceral peritoneum (Fig. 4.1C), and fragile adhesions may be present. There are white foci of necrosis or raised granulomatous cellular infiltrations on the serosa and extending into the organs or wall of the intestine from the serosa. These vary in size from a few millimeters to a centimeter in diameter. The kidneys may be enlarged and nodular with single or multiple, small to large, white, granulomatous nodules protruding from the cortex (Fig. 4.1E). Severe or mild granulomatous hepatitis and pancreatitis may also be present. Small white foci of inflammation may be found in the organs. Fibrin is usually less prominent in the thorax, but white foci may be visible under the pleura, and the lungs may be dark, firm, and rubbery. Hydropericardium and fibrinous epicarditis occur less frequently but are similar in type to other serosal reactions. Abdominal and thoracic lymph nodes are enlarged and have a lobulated pattern. In the effusive form of the disease, visceral lesions are sometimes minimal, and in the noneffusive form, peritonitis may be mild or not obvious on gross examination, and in these cats the lesions can be in the abdominal or thoracic organs, as described above, or in the eyes or nervous system. The lesions in the eyes begin as a diffuse

uveitis progressing to a panophthalmitis, with fibrin usually seen in the anterior chamber. Lesions in the central nervous system can involve the leptomeninges, spinal cord, or brain but usually are visible grossly only on the leptomeninges as thickenings or white streaks.

A subacute form of feline infectious peritonitis with a shorter clinical course is seen occasionally, primarily in weaned kittens. It occurs as a generalized systemic infection, and the lesions are more fibrinonecrotic than granulomatous. An acute hepatic form of the disease resembling suckling mouse hepatitis (coronavirus infection of mice) has been described in experimentally infected kittens.

The basic histopathological lesion of the disease is a generalized vasculitis and perivasculitis (Fig. 4.2A) and focal pyogranulomatous reaction that occurs in the serous membranes, the meninges, and in the connective tissue of the parenchymatous organs. This results in the serofibrinous and cellular exudate on the visceral and parietal serosal surfaces of the body cavities, and the fibrinonecrotic and pyogranulomatous reaction around affected vessels. The small, random, necrotic foci in organ parenchyma may be part of the same process and due to thrombophlebitis, or they may develop as a result of a separate mechanism, such as disseminated intravascular coagulation, or as the direct effect of the virus.

The vascular lesion begins as a proliferation and desquamation of vessel endothelium followed by medial necrosis, narrowed vascular lumina, and thrombophlebitis. There are accumulations of neutrophils, lymphocytes, plasma cells, and macrophages in and around the affected vessels. Occasionally, adventitial fibrosis occurs with little cellular infiltrate. The changes in the omentum, mesentery, and serosal tissues may be mild or severe. The mild changes are proliferation of mesothelial cells, slight fibrin exudate with fibroblast proliferation, and scattered neutrophils and mononuclear cells. The severe changes result in a thick layer of fibrin adherent to the serosa, with necrosis and cuboidal metaplasia with syncytial cell formation of the serosa. Large numbers of neutrophils and mononuclear cells and necrotic debris are embedded in the fibrin. The focal necrosis and pyogranulomatous reaction may be present in the parenchyma of the organs and extend into the intestine, affecting the muscularis, peripheral nerve ganglia, submucosa, and mucosa.

Lesions in the various organs are caused by the vascular damage that occurs in the capsule and connective-tissue stroma. They may be found throughout the body. Subcapsular infiltrations occur particularly in the liver, lung, and pancreas, and the pyogranulomatous reaction can develop deep in the parenchyma, particularly of the kidney. In the spleen and lymph nodes there are histiocytic and fibroblastic proliferation and either depletion or hyperplasia of lymphoid follicles. In addition to focal lung lesions, there may be a diffuse interstitial pneumonia, sometimes most severe close to the visceral pleura. Similarly, a severe focal or generalized lymphocytic and plasmacytic interstitial nephritis may develop. Cellular infiltrations in the spinal or cerebral meninges and perivascular spaces tend to be more mononuclear and diffuse, with only occasional focal pyogranulomatous lesions. Degenerative and necrotic lesions in the parenchyma of the central nervous system appear to be related to the prominent vasculitis.

Experimental studies have clarified the pathogenesis of the disease and the role that the immunopathologic mechanisms play in the production of the lesion. The sequence of events proposed is as follows. The virus is phagocytized after introduction and transported to the regional node, where the primary viral replication takes place, with the generation of a primary viremia. This results in generalized infection of the monocyte–macrophage system and a secondary cell-associated viremia. The development of nonneutralizing antibody results in deposition of antigen–antibody complexes that fix complement and trigger the vascular and pyogranulomatous changes.

Complications of Peritonitis

Acute generalized peritonitis is a catastrophic development in many local diseases of the abdominal cavity, but it may be an inconsequential feature of the generalized infections because, obviously, peritonitis does not significantly affect the outcome of a strangulated loop of intestine or clostridial infections such as blackleg, hemoglobinuria, or braxy. Toxins from peritonitis may be absorbed directly through the peritoneum into retroperitoneal venules and lymphatics or may be carried from the peritoneal cavity via the diaphragmatic lymphatics. Death from toxemia may result before obvious peritonitis develops. The peculiarly efficient diaphragmatic lymphatics remove not only fluid but also particulate matter, including bacteria, and in this way the inflammation may spread via the lymphatics to the

pleura and the mediastinal nodes. Of all the abdominal viscera, the intestine is most affected by inflammation of its serosa.

The typical clinical syndrome includes, within the first few hours of generalized peritonitis, intestinal hypermotility with diarrhea. By 24 hr there is absence of bowel movement and, on auscultation, complete abdominal silence; by this time the serosal irritation has caused reflex paralysis of the gut, so-called ileus. The development of ileus has the advantage that exudates are no longer distributed by intestinal movements, but there is also the disadvantage that fibrinous adhesions develop between loops of intestine, and if the animal recovers, they scarify and produce fibrous adhesions that may cause intestinal stenosis. Assessing the age of peritonitis may have significance, such as in iatrogenic rectal perforation, and requires careful gross and microscopic examination of the serosal surface and the adherent fibrin. The proliferation and age of fibroblastic components in the fibrin, on the serosa, and in the edge of the wound will give some indication of the age of the lesion.

Not all cases of generalized peritonitis are immediately fatal; depending on the nature of the exudate, the lesions may resolve completely, be converted to diffuse adhesions, or persist in some localized areas as active or adhesive peritonitis. It is remarkable how adhesions may become attentuated and even removed under the stress of continual tension.

The main defenses in the usual sorts of peritonitis are cellular, and this seems to be equally true whether or not the animal has an acquired immunity to the bacteria present. The removal and destruction of any particulate matter, including bacteria, from the abdominal cavity is one function of the lowly omentum; it is so generously endowed with phagocytes that their clusters are often visible to the naked eye as small milky spots. These fixed histiocytes are very efficient at ingesting bacteria and, if exposed to opsonins, of destroying them. In the case of Johne's disease, the organisms may be ingested by the macrophages but protected from destruction. When the bacteria are sufficiently virulent, they may proliferate in and destroy the phagocytes. This, no doubt, is why in many instances of acute peritonitis the omentum is first and most severely involved in the inflammatory reaction. It is also a "purpose" of the omentum to seal off foci of inflammation, and this it does with exceptional efficiency. The omentum is continually moved about the abdominal cavity by bodily and intestinal movements, and it sticks to areas of inflamed peritoneum. Such local omental adhesions may persist indefinitely.

Parasitic Diseases of the Peritoneum

Most of the parasites found in the peritoneal cavity have their final habitat elsewhere, and entry on to the peritoneum occurs in the normal course of migrations or as an accident. Thus various cysticerci may be found on the peritoneum during their normal development, *Dioctophyma renale*, the young *Fasciola hepatica*, and a variety of nematode larvae pass this way, and an example of accidental entry is that of *Ascaris equorum* through an intestinal perforation. Their significance and the lesions they produce are described in other chapters in these volumes with the parasite in question, and for the most part they are readily recognized at autopsy. Filariae, which are occasionally found as young or adult worms in the abdomen of dogs, may be assumed to be *Dirofilaria immitis.*

Two parasites are unusual and deserve special attention. Young liver flukes, **Fasciola hepatica,** can cause acute and chronic peritonitis in cattle and sheep, and the inflammation involves the parietal peritoneum and sometimes the visceral peritoneum, especially that of liver, spleen, and omentum. The changes may consist of many tags of fibrin or a more diffuse, crusty thickening, and the young flukes may be found in the inflammatory lesions both on and beneath the peritoneum. *Stephanurus dentatus* larvae may produce severe peritonitis in the course of their migration across the peritoneal cavity of swine (see the Urinary System, this volume).

Plerocercoids, larval forms of *Mesocestoides* (dithyridium–tetrathyridium) or *Spirometra* (sparganum), occur as bladder worms or solid, straplike bodies in the peritoneal cavity of some carnivores, rodents, and reptiles in some countries. A local reaction may occur around these intermediate forms in tissues and in the peritoneal cavity, and ascites may be present. Some of these larvae can multiply by transverse division or budding, so very large numbers may be present.

Some parasites use the peritoneal cavity as their final habitat. Parasites of the subfamily Setariinae, family Onchocercidae, superfamily Filarioidea inhabit the peritoneal cavity of many domestic and wild ungulates, such as horses, cattle, buffalo, camels, sheep, goats, swine, deer, and antelope. They are commonly found at autopsy, particularly in cattle. There are only two genera, *Papillosetaria*, a monotypic genus found in *Thagulas,* which will not be referred to again, and *Setaria* (= *Hyraconema* = *Artionema*), in which there are many species.

Some species of *Setaria* have a cosmopolitan distribution and may be found in several species of wild and domestic ungulates within the same family (*S. equina* in Equidae, and *S. labiatopapillosa* in cattle, buffalo, and perhaps deer and antelope), while others are restricted geographically (*S. digitata,* Asia) perhaps by the distribution of intermediate hosts. All members of the genus live as well-adjusted symbionts as adults in their normal host and do not cause peritoneal lesions. The larval form of *S. digitata* can produce a mild fibrous peritonitis and granulomas in the retroperitoneum and bladder of cattle, and the larvae of *S. equina* and perhaps others that may normally spend part of their time in the central nervous system may occasionally penetrate the parenchyma and cause lesions.

Adults in the peritoneal cavity are oviparous, and the microfilariae can be found in the blood. The intermediate host may be one of a variety of genera of mosquitoes, or for some *Setaria* species, biting flies (*Hemotobia* spp.). The microfilariae develop into infective larvae in 2 to 3 weeks, depending on ambient temperatures, and may survive another 3 to 6 weeks in the intermediate host. They are released from the mosquito and penetrate the final host.

Setaria digitata is normally found as an adult in the peritoneal cavity of cattle and buffalo in Asia. The migration of immature forms in aberrant hosts, such as horses, camels, sheep, and goats, is an important cause of neurologic disease called **kumri** in Asia. The migratory pattern of the larvae is not known, but sensitive organs receive little or no damage in the natural host. In some aberrant hosts, however, infective larvae may invade the brain and spinal cord, usually about 2–6 weeks after infection. The sites of penetration and subsequent cerebral migrations are variable, as are the clinical signs produced. Characteristically, neurologic signs are of ataxia, weakness, or paralysis. The severity of the clinical signs varies from slight weakness to quadriplegia, depending on the number and location of the wandering parasites; however, affected animals may remain bright and alert. The lesions produced are fundamentally traumatic; the inflammatory component is less conspicuous. A careful gross examination of brain and spinal cord may show the areas of damage as brown foci or streaks. These are more prominent as black spots in formalin-fixed tissue. The lesions are apt to be confined to relatively small foci, so it is important that the examination be made carefully and the material for microscopic examination taken from suspicious areas. The clinical signs may suggest which parts of the brain and cord should receive the most attention. Apart from the foci of malacia, the remainder of the nervous system may be normal.

At low power, the most obvious feature of the lesions is the microcavitation that is caused mechanically by the migration of the larvae; hemorrhage is variable. Surrounding the areas of cavitation, there is loss of myelin, *Gitter*-cell formation, and fragmentation and beading of axons. In cross section this beading may appear as swollen basophilic masses, or alternatively as loss of axis cylinders. Gemastocytic astrocytes are present in older lesions. Occasionally the parasites can be found in section and made available for proper identification, but the cerebral lesions produced by aberrant parasitic migration, irrespective of the parasite, are distinctive and suggest the diagnosis. They differ from more conventional lesions in that all neural structures (myelin, axis cylinders, nerve cells, and glia) are involved, the patterns of damage are completely random, and frequently, eosinophils are the most common inflammatory cell. Neutrophils and macrophages are also frequently present, along with a mild meningitis and vascular cuffing.

The term **cerebrospinal nematodiasis** has been applied to the group of nervous diseases resulting from aberrant larval migrations (see the Nervous System, Volume 1); many parasites such as *Strongylus vulgaris* may be occasional culprits, but only *Setaria digitata* and a few other nematodes, such as *Pneumostrongylus tenuis* in moose, *Elaphostrongylus cervi* in deer, and *Baylissascaris procyonis* in rodents, have tropism for the nervous system and produce the syndrome in epizootic proportions. *Setaria cervi,* which may occur normally in deer and a variety of other cloven-hoofed animals, has been reported as causing cerebrospinal nematodiasis in deer, although *Elaphostrongylus* larvae produce similar signs and lesions, and differentiation may be difficult.

Setaria digitata larvae frequently invade the eyes of horses, as do the microfilariae of *S. equina.*

Neoplastic Disease of the Peritoneum

Primary tumors of the peritoneum may arise from the serosa itself, from the subserous connective tissues, and from the various differentiated special tissues, such as nerve sheaths. Tumors arising from the serosa are called **mesotheliomas**, sometimes qualified as malignant. The qualification is unnecessary as virtually all are malignant, although the malignant capability is nearly always exhibited as implantation rather than metastasis.

Mesotheliomas are not common. They occur with greatest frequency in cattle and dogs but occasionally in other species. Interest in mesotheliomas has increased since the association between asbestos fiber and mesothelioma was discovered in humans. This association has not been made in animals, in which the tumor has the distinction of occurring most frequently as a congenital neoplasm in fetal or young cattle (Fig. 4.1A,D).

Mesotheliomas arise from the cells of the serous linings of pericardial, pleural, and peritoneal cavities, frequently involving all three locations. They appear as multiple small firm nodules or villous projections on a thickened mesentery or serosal surface, although fibrous or sclerosing forms have occasionally been reported. The tumor frequently is associated with a milky effusion, and in sclerosing tumors in which adhesions occasionally occur, the lesion might resemble chronic granulomatous peritonitis. Ascites as the result of effusion and blocked lymphatics is nearly always present with peritoneal tumors.

Mesotheliomas of the pleura, pericardium, or peritoneum may assume a variety of histologic patterns. This is not surprising given the diverse potentialities of the tissue that lines the embryonic celomic cavity. The tumors usually take either of two histologic forms, the one predominantly fibrous and resembling fibrosarcoma, and the other papillary and resembling adenocarcinoma. The most common tumor is a solid mass made up of single layers of dark, plump, cuboidal or columnar, neoplastic mesothelial cells with a distinct border and abundant pink cytoplasm, over a proliferating fibrocellular stroma. The mesothelial cells form loops and festoons in a papillary pattern, or line cystic spaces and tubular structures. There may be a mucinous matrix in this acinar pattern. Such malignant mesotheliomas, that is, those resembling adenocarcinoma, can mimic implantation of a true carcinoma so completely that an adequate differentiation may rest on very careful examination and exclusion of some primary focus of carcinoma. Special stains or electron microscopic examination may be required to identify the cell type.

In mesotheliomas that are predominantly fibrous, the cells may be spindle-shaped and resemble a fibrosarcoma. In the sclerosing forms there may be a thick, fibrous serosa with adhesions, and large anaplastic cuboidal cells may be found in clusters or lining cystic spaces within the fibrous tissue.

Of the retroperitoneal tumors, the **lipoma** is most frequent. These benign tumors are well known in horses, in which they originate usually in the mesenteries. They may reach enormous size, but their special significance is that they tend to become pedunculated and occasionally cause acute intestinal obstruction when the pedicle winds about a loop of intestine. In the dog, these tumors arise in the omentum rather than the mesenteries and settle on the abdominal floor. They may attain a very large size but tend not to be pedunculated. They do not, therefore, cause acute distress, and although they may be histologically malignant, metastases are unusual. They develop a pseudocapsule and central areas of necrosis. Tumors of the subserosal connective tissues, myxomas, fibromas, and their malignant counterparts, are rare, although fibrosarcomas are observed in

dogs. Tumors of differentiated retroperitoneal tissues are also uncommon. Involvement of the abdominal nerves and plexuses occurs in **neurofibromatosis** of cattle, and ganglioneuromas have also been observed in this species. Extramedullary pheochromocytomas have been observed in cattle and dogs, and nonchromaffin paragangliomas occur in dogs, the latter usually in association with similar tumors elsewhere. Occasional adenocarcinomas of high malignancy, but of obscure histogenesis and origin, have been discovered in the dorsal retroperitoneum in dogs.

Secondary tumors of the peritoneum are not common but are to be expected in any abdominal neoplasia. These arise as direct implantations or as lymphogenous or hematogenous metastases. They are more usually carcinomas than sarcomas. Secondary carcinomas may be very scirrhous and, when accompanied by ascites, may closely resemble chronic peritonitis, although a relative or complete absence of adhesions is often a helpful distinguishing feature at autopsy. There are obviously many possibilities for the origin of secondary tumors; several common types are listed below. The cholangiocellular and ovarian carcinomas have already been mentioned. Those of bile duct tend to be scirrhous, as do intestinal adenocarcinomas in cattle and sheep. Squamous-cell carcinomas of the equine stomach form rather discrete implants, which may be partially caseated, but they are likely to be differentiated enough to be recognizably keratinized on gross inspection. Implants of ovarian carcinoma tend to be papillary. Vesical tumors developing in cattle in enzootic hematuria implant locally on pelvic epithelium, and rectal adenocarcinoma in dogs tends to confine its implants to the pelvic peritoneum. Malignant melanomas of perineal origin in horses produce flattish, black smudges on the peritoneum.

Miscellaneous Lesions

Cysts of the peritoneum are rather common but insignificant. Those associated with genital adnexa are described with those systems, and those associated with intermediate-stage tapeworms have been mentioned, except for *Echinococcus*, which, following the rupture of a mature hydatid into the abdomen, may develop cysts on the peritoneum. Small cysts, sometimes multiple, which are observed in the omentum, may be either inclusion cysts or local lymphatic ectasias. They are inert.

The normal flat, pavement-type cells of the serosa may undergo **metaplasia** to a cuboidal or columnar type resembling epithelium. Such metaplasia is probably the mildest response of the peritoneum to irritation but may also be a response to estrogen. Inflammatory metaplasia leading to ossification can occur in peritoneal scars, especially in swine, but may also be found in the mesenteries and the dorsal retroperitoneum without obvious antecedent change, although ossification may occur following fat necrosis as well. The newly formed bones are flat and of variable size and shape and are usually found in adipose tissue.

ACKNOWLEDGMENTS

The assistance of Jean Middlemiss, Sandra Brown, and E. W. Eaton in the preparation of the manuscript and illustrations is gratefully acknowledged. We thank Dr. Louise Laliberte for information obtained from her M.Sc. thesis "Epidemiological Study of Coronavirus Infection in Cats with Special Reference to Feline Infectious Peritonitis" and her supervisor, Dr. R. C. Povey, for advice on the section on that topic.

BIBLIOGRAPHY

General

Brownlow, M. A., Hutchins, D. R., and Johnston, K. G. Reference values for equine peritoneal fluid. *Equine Vet J* **13**: 127–130, 1981.

Chaimovitz, C., Alon, U., and Better, O. S. Pathogenesis of salt retention in dogs with chronic bile-duct ligation. *Clin Sci* **62**: 65–70, 1982.

Crowe, D. T., Jr., and Crane, S. W. Diagnostic abdominal paracentesis and lavage in the evaluation of abdominal injuries in dogs and cats: clinical and experimental investigations. *J Am Vet Med Assoc* **168**: 700–705, 1976.

Epstein, M. Renal sodium handling in cirrhosis: a reappraisal. *Nephron* **23**: 211–217, 1979.

Freeman, D. E., Kock, D. B., and Boles, C. L. Mesodiverticular bands as a cause of small intestinal strangulation and volvulus in the horse. *J Am Vet Med Assoc* **175**: 1089–1094, 1979.

Levy, M., and Wexler, J. J. Renal sodium retention and ascites formation in dogs with experimental cirrhosis but without portal hypertension or increased splanchnic vascular capacity. *J Lab Clin Med* **93**: 520–536, 1978.

Raftery, A. T. Mesothelial cells in peritoneal fluid. *J Anat* **115**: 237–253, 1973.

Schaffner, T. *et al.* Macrophage functions in antimicrobial defense. *Klin Wochenschr* **60**: 720–726, 1982.

Whitaker, D., Papadimitriou, J. M., and Walters, M. N.-I. The mesothelium: its fibrinolytic properties. *J Pathol* **136**: 291–299, 1982.

Abdominal Fat Necrosis: Steatitis

Danse, L. H. J. C., and Steenbergen-Botterweg, W. A. Enzyme histochemical studies of adipose tissue in porcine yellow fat disease. *Vet Pathol* **11**: 465–476, 1974.

Danse, L. H. J. C., and Verschuren, P. M. Fish oil induced yellow fat disease in rats. 1. Histologic changes. *Vet Pathol* **15**: 114–124, 1978.

Freeman, B. A., and Crapo, J. D. Biology of disease. Free radicals and tissue injury. *Lab Invest* **47**: 412–426, 1982.

Ito, T. A pathological study on fat necrosis in swine. *Jpn J Vet Sci* **35**: 299–310, 1973.

Ito, T. *et al.* Pathological studies on fat necrosis (lipomatosis) in cattle. *Jpn J Vet Res* **30**: 141, 1968.

Kirby, P. S. Steatitis in fattening pigs. *Vet Rec* **109**: 385, 1981.

Kroneman, J., and Wensvoort, P. Muscular dystrophy and yellow fat disease in Shetland pony foals. *Neth J Vet Sci* **1**: 42, 1968.

Maeda, T. Studies on fat necrosis of beef cattle in Japan. I. Occurring aspects. II. An area study of the outbreak of fat necrosis. *Bull Fac Agric Tottori Univ* **30**: 205–210 and 211–217, 1978.

Moreau, P. M. *et al.* Disseminated necrotizing panniculitis and pancreatic nodular hyperplasia in a dog. *J Am Vet Med Assoc* **180**: 422–425, 1982.

Platt, H., and Whitwell, K. E. Clinical and pathological observations on generalized steatitis in foals. *J Comp Pathol* **81**: 499–506, 1971.

Rumsey, T. S. *et al.* Chemical composition of necrotic fat lesions in beef cows grazing fertilized 'Kentucky-31' tall fescue. *J Anim Sci* **48**: 673–682, 1979.

Shimada, Y., and Morinaga, H. Studies on bovine fat necrosis. I. Epidemiological observations. *J Jpn Vet Med Assoc* **30**: 584–588, 1977.

Vanselow, B. A., and McCausland, I. P. Steatitis in two donkey foals. *Aust Vet J* **57**: 304–305, 1981.

Vitovec, J., Proks, C., and Valvoda, V. Lipomatosis (fat necrosis) in cattle and pigs. *J Comp Pathol* **85**: 53, 1975.

Wensvoort, P., and Steenbergen-Botterweg, W. A. Non-extractable lipids in the adipose tissue of horses and ponies affected with generalized steatitis. *Tijdschr Diergeneeskd* **100**: 106–112, 1975.

Feline Infectious Peritonitis

Evermann, J. F. *et al.* Characterization of a feline infectious peritonitis virus isolate. *Vet Pathol* **18**: 256–265, 1981.

Gouffaux, M. *et al.* Feline infectious peritonitis—proteins of plasma and ascitic fluid. *Vet Pathol* **12**: 335–348, 1975.

Hayashi, T. *et al.* Systemic vascular lesions in feline infectious peritonitis. *Jpn J Vet Sci* **39**: 365–377, 1977.

Hayashi, T. *et al.* Enteritis due to feline infectious peritonitis virus. *Jpn J Vet Sci* **44**: 97–106, 1982.

Horzinek, M. C., and Osterhaus, A. D. M. E. The virology and pathogenesis of feline infectious peritonitis: brief review. *Arch Virol* **59**: 1–15, 1979.

Jacobse-Geels, H. E. L., Daha, M. R., and Horzinek, M. C. Antibody, immune complexes and complement activity fluctuations in kittens with experimentally induced feline infectious peritonitis. *Am J Vet Res* **43**: 666–670, 1982.

Pedersen, N. C. *et al.* An enteric coronavirus infection of cats and its relationship to feline infectious peritonitis. *Am J Vet Res* **42**: 368–377, 1981.

Ward, J. M., Gribble, D. H., and Dungworth, D. L. Feline infectious peritonitis: experimental evidence for its multiphasic nature. *Am J Vet Res* **35**: 1271–1275, 1974.

Weiss, R. C., and Scott, F. W. Pathogenesis of feline infectious peritonitis: nature and development of viremia. *Am J Vet Res* **42**: 382–390, 1981.

Weiss, R. C., and Scott, F. W. Pathogenesis of feline infectious peritonitis: pathologic changes and immunofluorescence. *Am J Vet Res* **42**: 2036–2048, 1981.

Wolfe, L. C., and Griesemer, R. A. Feline infectious peritonitis. *Vet Pathol* **3**: 255–270, 1966.

Wolfe, L. G., and Griesemer, R. A. Feline infectious peritonitis: review of gross and histopathologic lesions. *J Am Vet Med Assoc* **158**: 987–993, 1971.

Parasitic Diseases

Anderson, R. C. The pathogenesis and transmission of neurotropic and accidental nematode parasites of the central nervous system of mammals and birds. Review article. *Helminthol Abstr* **37**(pt 3): 191–210, 1968.

Anderson, R. C., and Bain, O. "Keys to Genera of the Order Spirurida," No. 3. Part 3. Filarioidea, Aproctoidea and Diplotriaenoidea. CIH Keys to the Nematode Parasites of Vertebrates. Commonwealth Agricultural Bureaux, Farnham Royal, Bucks, England, 1976.

Baharsefat, M. *et al.* The first report of lumbar paralysis in sheep due to nematode larvae infestation in Iran. *Cornell Vet* **63**: 81–86, 1973.

Frauenfelder, H. C., Kazacos, K. R., and Lichtenfels, J. R. Cerebrospinal nematodiasis causes by a filariid in a horse. *J Am Vet Med Assoc* **177**: 359–362, 1980.

Innes, J. R. M., and Pillai, C. P. *Kumri*—so-called lumbar paralysis—of horses in Ceylon (India and Burma), and its identification with cerebrospinal nematodiasis. *Br Vet J* **111**: 223–235, 1955.

McCraw, B. M., and Slocombe, J. O. D. *Strongylus edentatus:* development and lesions from ten weeks postinfection to patency. *Can J Comp Med* **42:** 340–356, 1978.

Wardle, R. A., and McLeod, J. A. "The Zoology of Tapeworms." Minneapolis, Univ. of Minnesota Press, 1952.

Neoplastic Diseases

Dubielzig, R. R. Sclerosing mesothelioma in five dogs. *J Am Anim Hosp Assoc* **15:** 745–748, 1979.

Grant, C. A. Congenital tumors of calves (mesothelioma). *Zentralbl Veterinaermed* **5:** 231–244, 1958.

Scully, R. E. Smooth muscle differentiation in genital tract disorders. Editorial. *Arch Pathol Lab Med* **105:** 505–507, 1981.

Thrall, D. E., and Goldschmidt, M. H. Mesothelioma in the dog: six case reports. *J Am Vet Radiol Soc* **19:** 107–115, 1978.

Trigo, F. J., Morrison, W. B., and Breeze, R. G. An ultrastructural study of canine mesothelioma. *J Comp Pathol* **91:** 531–539, 1981.

CHAPTER 5

The Urinary System

M. G. MAXIE
Ontario Ministry of Agriculture and Food, Canada

THE KIDNEY

General Considerations

The kidney is an elaborate filtration–resorption device, intricate in its structural and functional details but relatively simple in its mode of operation. This simplicity allows the substitution of mechanical dialysis units to perform the most essential renal functions during renal failure. The primary responsibilities of the kidney are the maintenance of a constant quality and quantity of plasma and tissue fluids, and the excretion of waste products. It is also involved in the production of the hormones erythropoietin, renin, prostaglandin, and 1,25-dihydroxycholecalciferol, the latter the principal active form of vitamin D.

Water and salt are quantitatively and in an evolutionary sense the most important constituents of body fluids. The assumption during evolution of a terrestrial existence and homeothermy by mammals imposed a need to conserve water and simultaneously excrete large quantities of metabolites. Homeothermy, with sustained high body temperatures, imposed a sustained high metabolic rate, a need for control of the peripheral circulation, and structural modifications to the integument. Carbon dioxide is very soluble in water and highly diffusible, and responsibility for its excretion has been transferred from the integument of aquatic and amphibian ancestors to the respiratory system of mammals; as the end product of fat and carbohydrate metabolism, carbon dioxide presents no problem of elimination to the renal excretory mechanism. Nitrogenous wastes, and a multitude of other organic compounds and inorganic substances, impose a substantial load on the renal mechanism. Insoluble uric acid, necessary in oviparous species, spared birds and reptiles from using water in excreting nitrogenous end products. Mammals, however, have persisted in excreting urea, which is highly soluble, diffusible, and osmotically active; excretion of wastes and conservation of water in mammals require concentrating mechanisms capable of raising the osmotic pressure of urine above that of blood.

The extracellular fluid and plasma of the body are dialyzed through the kidney many times in a day, producing copious amounts of primary urine, of which almost all is reabsorbed. A unique feature of renal blood flow is that it varies little over a wide range of arterial pressures, thus ensuring stable glomerular filtration rates. The kidneys possess intrinsic mechanisms by which they vary their vascular resistance in order to maintain constant glomerular filtration.

Renal blood flow is normally high, up to 25% of the cardiac output. The kidneys are not given to reactive hyperemia, although blood flow may be increased by the action of pyrogens in febrile states. Pathologists are concerned particularly with the causes and consequences of reduced perfusion. Related to this concern is the fact that renal oxygen consumption, relatively small in relation to renal blood flow, is high relative to that of the other tissues and is equal to ~10% of whole body consumption. Most of the oxygen consumed by the kidney is expended in the interests of resorption of essential solutes, a predominantly cortical function, and the consequences of reduced perfusion are largely borne by the cortex.

The kidneys may be regarded as having two circulations, one cortical and one medullary, which in adversity may function independently of each other, or at least become unbalanced. The vascular volume of the medulla per unit of weight is about the same as for the cortex, but medullary blood flow is much slower. In the long capillary vasa recta, short-circuits are available that may be used, depending on the tonicity of distal urine and the medullary interstitium. If cortical vascular resistance is increased, blood may be shunted through the juxtamedullary glomeruli to the medulla. The converse may also hold. It appears that medullary blood flow is maintained more effectively than cortical flow and that under conditions of reduced renal blood flow, blood may be directed from the cortex to the medulla. Rather than distinguish between cortical and medullary flow in gross terms, it may be more appropriate to consider shunting as between two groups of nephrons: those almost wholly cortical, with short loops of Henle; and those juxtamedullary, with long loops of Henle.

Reduction in perfusion is a common occurrence in the kidney; it mainly affects the cortex and it may be due to cardiac abnormality with inadequate output, to reduced vascular volume and systemic pressure, or to physical obstruction to intrarenal blood flow. Reduced perfusion may lead to atrophy of tubular epithelium and tubular dilation, to necrosis of tubular epithelium, or to more or less extensive necrosis of the renal cortex.

The primitive kidney possessed a dual vascular arrangement, somewhat comparable to that of the mammalian liver, and it is retained in reptiles and birds; the glomeruli are perfused with arterial blood, and the tubules are supplied with venous blood in the renal portal system derived from the venous systems in the caudal part of the body. Mammals have discarded the portal system, and the tubules are supplied with blood that has first passed through their respective glomeruli. This is essential for the harmony existing between the glomerulus and its tubule.

The glomerulus is considered to be a filtration bed, but this is not strictly correct. Filtration is important, but so is diffusion. Complete dependence on filtration would require vascular pressures that would be impossibly high to overcome the osmotic pressures of plasma. The membrane is semipermeable, and dissolved substances and particles in suspension move across the glomerular capillaries at rates determined by size, shape, and electrical charge, and their presence in the glomerular spaces encourages transfer of water. Malfunction of the glomerulus may be due to inadequate glomerular blood flow and/or structural alterations that decrease or increase its permeability. For glomerular injury to occur, injurious substances must localize in the glomeruli. The outcome is influenced by the limited capacity in the glomerulus for enzymatic disposal of deposits, the capillary obstruction resulting from swelling of endothelial and mesangial cells, and the production of basement membrane–like material by injured mesangial cells and permeability changes in basement membranes.

The principal function of the kidney is the regulation of salt and water balance; this requires a system of monitors and feedbacks in order to achieve fine regulation. In particular, the renin–angiotensin system regulates sodium balance, and the hypothalamus and antidiuretic hormone controls osmotic and volume regulation. The structural basis of the renin–angiotensin system is provided by the juxtaglomerular apparatus: to maintain glomerulotubular balance, the glomerular filtration rate is adjusted locally and continually to changes in the chloride concentration of tubular fluid; generally, and over longer terms, the renin–angiotensin system stimulates the adrenal glands to produce aldosterone to assist in the retention of sodium and therefore, water. Primary pathologic changes have not been described in the juxtaglomerular apparatus, but all or portions of it are altered in conditions of glomerular injury or sustained hypertension. Sustained loss of the capacity for fine regulation of glomerular blood flow leads to functional imbalance between the glomerulus and its tubule, and to degeneration of the nephron.

The formation of primary urine requires that substances from plasma must pass freely across the glomerular membrane and into the tubules. Once within the tubules, the substances are, in a strict sense, outside the body. Many of the filtered substances are retrieved by a system of selective reabsorption that requires special machinery and energy. The function may be defective, allowing essential substances to be wasted in the urine. This occurs when enzymes are genetically deficient, the cortical epithelial cells are injured, or because plasma levels of filterable substances are unusually high or the glomerulus is unusually permeable, the quantity of the material to be reabsorbed exceeds the transport capacity of the epithelial cells.

Virtually all that is filtered is reabsorbed, and this in general is the function of the cortex. In addition to straightforward retrieval, the kidney must, with the guidance of aldosterone and antidiuretic hormone, precisely handle the balance of salt and water within its limits to dilute or concentrate. The distal tubules add precision with regard to salt and water and contribute to acid–base balance. The myriad functions are carried out sequentially, and the arrangement and structure of the tubule vary along its length, corresponding to the function to be performed. There are seven zones or segments to the mammalian tubule, and the patterns and zonation are basically the same in all species, with some important differences in the loops of Henle.

Terrestial mammals have a need to conserve water while eliminating high loads of waste, and a need therefore to concentrate urine above the tonicity of plasma. This function is provided by the loop of Henle: the wall of the loop is thin, to allow rapid diffusion of urea and water; the loop is elongated always in the same direction, toward the pelvis; and the limbs of the loop lie parallel and adjacent to each other and the long capillary vasa recta. This arrangement is suitable for the countercurrent multiplier system of concentration. The extent of elongation of the loop is variable. Juxtamedullary nephrons have long loops, and other cortical nephrons short loops, and some species have predominantly long loops, and some predominantly short loops. Those animals with a preponderance of long loops have greater concentrating ability. The volume of the medulla is determined largely by the number of long loops, and a simple index of concentrating ability is the ratio of cortical volume to medullary volume. When the ratio is wide, as in the pig, where it approximates 7:1 (in neonates), and part of the medulla is destroyed in disease, there is a high level of susceptibility to serious imbalances of fluid and electrolytes.

Harmony in urinary function depends on the correlated sequences of perfusion, filtration, resorption, secretion, and discharge. Failure of the urinary mechanism occurs if there is inadequate perfusion (prerenal failure), inadequate processing (renal failure), or inadequate discharge (postrenal failure). The outcome so far as the composition of body fluids is concerned is always approximately the same: there is imbalance of salt and water and of acids and bases, and there is retention of wastes. The most useful single index of failure is the amount of urea retained. Urea itself is rather harmless, but if other urinary functions are sufficiently disturbed, a fairly consistent set of clinical signs emerges and the syndrome is called uremia.

Reduced renal perfusion is quite common and is based on a contraction of circulating blood volume or diminished cardiac output. Although the kidney is to a large degree independent of variations in systemic blood pressure, there is a point at which it yields to the more vital priorities of brain and heart. Postrenal disturbances are also common and are based on obstruction or rupture of the lower urinary tract. Renal failure may be due to a temporary overload, especially of nitrogenous wastes, or it may be due to diffuse renal disease. Uremia occurs when the functional reserve of the kidney is destroyed. In acute disease, this is at the point where only ~30% of the nephrons remain; in chronic failure, which allows time for compensatory changes to occur, it is at the point where ~30% of potential function remains.

According to the ''intact nephron'' or ''adaptive nephron'' hypothesis, nephron function is an all-or-none phenomenon. In progressive renal disease, the remaining nephrons respond by hypertrophy, since new nephrons cannot be formed following renal maturation. Glomerular filtration and tubular function then increase concomitantly, and glomerulotubular balance and homeostasis are maintained. All of the renal components are interdependent, and if one component is irreversibly damaged, function of the other components is impaired. Glomerular disease can cause decreased peritubular perfusion and tubular atrophy; tubulointerstitial disease can cause glomerular obsolescence. There is a tendency for all forms of chronic renal disease to destroy all four components of the kidney, resulting in chronic renal failure and shrunken, scarred end-stage kidneys; differentiation of the initiating cause may be impossible.

Anatomy

The renal collecting system is derived from the ureteral bud (metanephric duct), a diverticulum of the mesonephric (Wolffian) duct, and consists of the ureter, pelvis, calyces, and collecting ducts. Nephrons develop from the metanephric blastema and attach to the growing ends (ampullae) of the collecting system. The uriniferous tubule consists of the nephron and the collecting tubule. The renal calyces are the cup-shaped recesses of the pelvis that enclose conical masses of medulla, the pyramids. The apex of a pyramid is referred to as a papilla, and its tip is fenestrated by collecting ducts (area cribrosa). The fornix is the uppermost blind end of a calyx or pelvis.

The kidneys of domestic animals can be classified as unipyramidal (unilobar) or multipyramidal (multilobar). Cats, dogs, small ruminants, and horses have unipyramidal kidneys. In cats, one lobe is present, and papillary ducts open into a calyx on a single renal papilla. In dogs, small ruminants, and horses, there is complete or partial fusion of several lobes and a single crestlike papilla (renal crest).

Pigs have multipyramidal kidneys in which there are several distinct renal lobes, each with a pyramid and its respective papilla. Extensions of renal cortex between the pyramids are known as the renal columns of Bertin. Simple papillae occur in central pyramids, and compound papillae in pyramids at the renal poles; this is of pathogenetic significance because compound papillae are more susceptible to ascending infection.

The kidneys of cattle are also multipyramidal, but have distinct external lobation, each lobe with one pyramid. The renal calyces of cattle join directly to form the ureter without forming a pelvis.

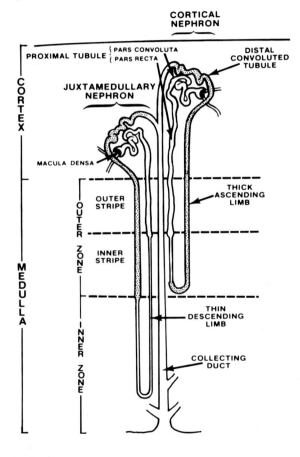

On sagittal section of a kidney, subdivisions of cortex and medulla may be distinguished, particularly in dogs and sheep; the arrangements are illustrated schematically in the accompanying diagram. The subdivisions correspond to segments of tubules and may be particularly evident in acute renal disease. The cortex has a darker outer zone and a paler inner zone, which in mature dogs often has prominent pale streaks due to the presence of fat in collecting ducts. Outer and inner zones may be seen in the medulla of canine kidneys, and the outer zone may be further subdivided into outer and inner bands (stripes), due to the presence of the thick segments of the descending and ascending limbs of the loop of Henle, respectively. The inner zone of the

medulla (papilla) contains the thin segments of the loop of Henle. Mucous glands are large and prominent in the pelvis of equine kidneys, and mucus and crystals are normally present in the equine renal pelvis.

The functional unit of the kidney is the nephron, which consists of the renal corpuscle, proximal tubule, loop of Henle, and distal tubule. The glomerulus and Bowman's capsule comprise the renal corpuscle. The following approximate numbers of nephrons are present in each kidney: human, 1,000,000; dog, 400,000; cat, 200,000. The number of nephrons is fixed at birth in most mammals, although nephrogenesis may continue for several weeks after birth in animals, such as dogs, cats, and pigs, that have a short gestation period.

In multilobed kidneys, the renal artery divides in the pelvic region to form interlobar arteries that run in the renal columns between lobes up to the corticomedullary junction, where they branch to form arcuate arteries. These arteries run along the corticomedullary junction parallel to the capsule and terminate as radiating interlobular arteries in the cortex. Glomerular afferent arterioles are given off by the interlobular arteries and give rise to several lobules of capillary loops within the glomerulus. The capillaries later rejoin to form the glomerular efferent arteriole, and then divide again to form a peritubular capillary plexus. The efferent arterioles of the juxtamedullary nephrons branch to form descending vasa recta (straight vessels), which enter the medulla. The ascending vasa recta reform from the medullary capillary plexus and form a countercurrent exchange system with their closely associated descending vasa recta.

Because the renal artery and its branches are end arteries, occlusion of any branch leads to infarction. Interference with glomerular capillary flow markedly alters peritubular blood flow, especially in the medulla. The medulla is particularly sensitive to ischemia because of its relative avascularity and the low hematocrit in medullary capillaries.

The renal venous system begins with formation of venules from the peritubular vasa recta and then closely parallels the arterial system. Veins in the outer cortex drain into stellate veins, which in cats are present on the capsular surface and prominent, and thence into interlobular veins. Veins within the kidney have very thin walls and are susceptible to compression.

Lymphatics occur in the renal cortex but not in the medulla. One set of lymphatics drains the cortical interstitium and follows the pattern of the vascular system; another set of lymphatics drains the capsular area. Lymphatic flow increases after urinary obstruction and in interstitial disease.

The interstitium normally contains peritubular capillaries and a few fibroblasts, and cortical interstitial tissue is usually only obvious around interlobar, arcuate, and interlobular arteries. Expansion of the cortical interstitium is abnormal and may occur due to edema, cellular infiltration, or fibrosis. The mucopolysaccharide content of the medullary interstitium increases with age and ischemia. Specialized interstitial cells produce prostaglandins, particularly PGE_2 and $PGF_{2\alpha}$.

Examination of the Kidneys

The systematic gross examination of a kidney includes observation of its size, shape, color, and consistency. The kidneys are usually equal in size and about three vertebrae long. Renal enlargement may occur due to addition of blood, edema fluid, fat, or urine in the pelvis or tubules, or to swelling or hypertrophy of nephrons. Acute renal disease causes renal enlargement due to addition of fluid and cells, whereas chronic renal disease causes scarring and loss of substance. Focal lesions, such as those caused by infarction or pyelonephritis, may markedly distort the renal outlines, whereas more generalized diseases such as glomerulonephritis do not. The normal renal color is brown-red, except in mature cats, in which the cortices are yellow due to their high lipid content. The lipid content in cats is apparently hormonally determined; pregnant females and sexually inactive old males have the most fat, pseudopregnant females and castrated males have somewhat less, estrous females and sexually active males have moderate amounts, and anestrous females have little or no renal fat. Autolysis occurs rapidly.

Each kidney is cut in the sagittal plane for examination. The normal cortex:medulla ratio in this plane is about 1:2 or 1:3, although the cortex normally accounts for 80% of the renal mass, a fact better appreciated in a coronal section. Diffuse diseases of the kidney usually respect the integrity of the medulla. Pyelonephritis is peripelvic with involvement of the medulla. A pale cut surface suggests the deposition of fat or acute early nephrosis, whereas if the surface is pale and wet, there is edema and diffuse tubular dilatation. Focal glomerular lesions do not cause glomerular prominence, but diffuse lesions, such as amyloidosis or diffuse glomerulitis, very often do. The normal glomeruli of horses are visible with the naked eye. Removal of the renal capsule is essential for examination of the outer surface of the cortex. The capsule should strip easily and leave a smooth surface underneath. Tearing of the cortex may indicate fibrous adhesions or scarring, except in the horse, which normally has trabeculae attached to the capsule.

RENAL BIOPSY.   Percutaneous needle biopsy of kidneys is useful to evaluate renal disease in domestic animals and is of particular use in cases of acute glomerulonephritis, nephrotic syndrome, asymptomatic proteinuria, and acute renal failure. It is usually possible to obtain 10–20 glomeruli using a Franklin–Silverman biopsy needle in an adult dog; a minimum of ~5 glomeruli is thought necessary to characterize a glomerular lesion. The main hazard of the technique is arterial puncture and hemorrhage, which on rare occasions is fatal.

In addition to the usual hematoxylin and eosin staining of paraffin sections of kidney, several other techniques are useful:

1. The periodic acid–Schiff (PAS) stain, which stains glomerular and tubular basement membranes and mesangial matrix magenta; thin sections (3 μm) must be used; the PAS–methenamine–silver technique is an improvement of this stain
2. Silver impregnation of basement membranes and of leptospires
3. Immunofluorescence studies for localization of immunoglobulins, complement, fibrin-related compounds, and foreign antigens, especially in glomeruli
4. Electron microscopy, particularly for characterizing glomerular basement membrane deposits
5. Other special stains for fibrin, amyloid, and lipids

Microscopic resolution of glomerular lesions is markedly improved by the use of 1-μm-thick methacrylate-embedded sections.

Uremia

Uremia literally means urine in the blood. It is a clinical syndrome of renal failure, caused by biochemical disturbances, and is often accompanied by extrarenal lesions. Azotemia, which is sometimes used synonymously, is a biochemical abnormality characterized by elevation of blood urea and creatinine, but without obligatory clinical manifestations of renal disease.

The biochemical disturbances of uremia reflect changes in the normal renal functions directed to regulation of fluid volume, regulation of electrolyte and acid–base balance, excretion of waste products, and metabolism of hormones. The clinical signs may be related to the renal disease itself, as with pyuria or renal pain; to the effects of reduced renal function, as with metabolic acidosis or dehydration; or to the compensatory responses to renal dysfunction, as with hyperparathyroidism.

Interference with **fluid volume** regulation may result in either dehydration or anasarca. Dehydration due to reduced renal concentrating ability may be related to lesions of the renal medulla and juxtamedullary nephrons. Vomition, and sometimes diarrhea, often exacerbates the dehydration. Anasarca, caused by reduction in the volume of glomerular filtrate in diffuse renal disease or by activation of the renin–angiotensin system, occurs infrequently. A more common cause of edema is hypoproteinemia due to loss of protein through injured glomeruli.

Disturbances in **electrolyte balance** include excesses and deficits of plasma sodium, potassium, and calcium. The handling of these substances by the kidney is complex, even in health; in disease it is often paradoxical and involves disordered tubular function, compensatory mechanisms, and endocrine imbalances. Excesses of plasma sodium, potassium, and calcium contribute to anasarca, cardiotoxicity, and calcium nephropathy, respectively, while deficits may cause dehydration, muscular weakness, and tetany, or osteodystrophy.

Several aspects of the uremic syndrome contribute to **acid–base imbalance** and metabolic acidosis. Compensatory hyperventilation may occur. The main factors leading to acidosis in uremia are a reduced capacity of distal and collecting tubules to produce ammonia, increased retention of hydrogen ions, and increased utilization, with impaired reabsorption, of bicarbonate ions.

Failure to **excrete metabolic wastes**, such as urea and creatinine, is the basis for tests of renal function; elevated levels indicate reduced glomerular filtration.

Disturbances in **endocrine function** are important causes of signs and lesions in uremic animals. Retention of phosphate, due to reduced glomerular filtration, causes depression of ionized calcium and development of secondary hyperparathyroidism (see renal osteodystrophy, in Bones and Joints, Volume 1). Reduced renal catabolism of parathyroid hormone, and end-organ resistance to the hormone, may contribute to hyperparathyroidism. Most uremic animals have hyperphosphatemia, and normocalcemia or hypocalcemia. Sometimes hypercalcemia and hypophosphatemia occur in uremic dogs, possibly because of lack of feedback inhibition of parathyroid hormone release. Similar changes occur in some uremic horses and may be related to decreased renal excretion of calcium.

Nonregenerative anemia in uremic animals may result from a combination of factors, including decreased renal production of erythropoietin (see the Hematopoietic System, Volume 3). Coagulopathy associated with a defect in thrombocyte function may exacerbate the anemia. Renal metabolism of vitamin D is sometimes impaired in animals with diffuse renal disease and may add an element of osteomalacia to renal osteodystrophy as well as augmenting the hypocalcemia. Abnormal glucose metabolism occurs occasionally in uremic dogs and may be a result of peripheral resistance to insulin-mediated uptake of glucose, and to reduced breakdown of insulin by diseased kidneys.

As well as the metabolic disturbances attributable to particular biochemical derangements, there is in uremic animals a nonspecific effect of "uremic toxins." This is probably due to the combined action of toxic products of protein catabolism and the various chemical and endocrine imbalances described above. These toxins include phenols, indoles and guanidines, potassium, sulfate and phosphate ions, absorbed degradation products of intestinal bacteria, and parathyroid hormone. They are thought to be responsible for the profound malaise that characterizes the uremic syndrome.

The cause of death in uremia probably varies from case to case. Metabolic acidosis, hyperkalemia, or hypocalcemia may be severe enough to be fatal.

Gross lesions in uremia are divisible into those causing uremia and those resulting from it. The former are usually intrarenal, but may not be in prerenal and postrenal azotemia. Lesions that are the result of uremia are mainly, but not exclusively, extrarenal.

Most forms of prerenal azotemia have a common basis of reduced renal blood flow and glomerular filtration. This occurs in a variety of circumstances, including severe dehydration, massive hemorrhage (especially into the upper intestinal tract), congestive heart failure, and shock of any cause. Reduced renal flow in these conditions is part of an adaptational mechanism that diverts blood to vital organs such as brain and heart. When the diversion is severe or prolonged, intrarenal mechanisms that channel renal flow away from cortical nephrons to juxtamedullary nephrons may produce patchy or diffuse cortical ischemia and necrosis (see Renal Cortical Necrosis and Acute Tubular Necrosis). In such cases, if the animal survives, prerenal azotemia may be superseded by uremia of renal origin originating in cortical necrosis.

Postrenal azotemia is always due to obstruction to the outflow of urine and hence is oliguric or anuric. The causes are those that if intermittent or incomplete may lead to hydronephrosis, or if sudden and complete may lead to rupture or leakage of the lower urinary tract.

A form of extrarenal uremia, distinct from those mentioned, occurs in newborn animals, especially pigs, and is characterized by very high levels of blood urea. The kidneys of newborn pigs, dogs, and cats are "immature" and incapable of producing hypertonic urine. Normally this is of no consequence, because milk provides enough fluid to excrete, in hypotonic urine, the small amount of waste produced. When these newborn animals are anorectic, however, they lack both nutrients and fluid and begin to catabolize tissue proteins. Being unable to excrete the excess solute from protein breakdown, their blood urea reaches very high levels. Since anorexia is usually associated with fever, vomition, or diarrhea, fluid loss is very rapid. In pigs, the excess solute is deposited in the inner medulla as streaks of light yellow urate precipitates (Fig. 5.18A), which disappears during histologic processing. Pigs apparently are unique among mammals in that they do not reabsorb urates from glomerular filtrate; this accounts for their concentration in the medulla. It is not clear whether baby pigs also have an "immature" liver that fails to convert uric acid to allantoin.

The **nonrenal lesions** of uremia occur inconstantly and unpredictably, though they tend to be seen most often in dogs, especially those with chronic rather than acute renal failure. Many animals dying with uremia are cachectic. This is probably caused by the anorexia, vomition, and diarrhea, which often occur, necessitating body tissue catabolism to supply energy. Besides this general lack of condition, several distinctive lesions may develop in the gastrointestinal, cardiovascular, respiratory, and skeletal systems (see also the chapters on these systems).

Ulcerative necrotic stomatitis occurs in dogs and cats, and there is usually a foul-smelling brown film coating the tongue (Fig. 5.1D) and buccal mucosa. Like the gastrointestinal changes, oral lesions are more common in chronic than in acute uremia. The pathogenesis of the ulcers is not always clear, but some are associated with fibrinoid necrosis of arterioles, and some are related to bacterial production of ammonia from urea in the saliva. Large areas of the gastric mucosa are often swollen, suffused with red-black blood, and partly ulcerated. This lesion, often called gastritis, is initially noninflammatory, though opportunist bacteria may infect the ulcerated mucosa. Mucosal infarction secondary to arteriolar necrosis occurs. Mineralization of the middle and deep zones of the gastric mucosa is common, but its cause is not known. Necrosis and mineralization of the muscular coats are sometimes present. Intestinal lesions resemble those in the stomach, but they are less frequent, less severe, and without mineralization. Gastrointestinal lesions probably account for much of the vomition, diarrhea, and melena of uremic dogs. Intestinal intussusceptions sometimes develop in dogs with gastrointestinal lesions. Cats may have gastrointestinal lesions similar to dogs, but in uremic cattle, colitis is more common, and the stomach and proximal intestine are edematous. The liver shows inconstant degenerative changes, and there may be acinar dilatation of the pancreas, with inspissation of secretion. The hyperamylasemia that occurs in some uremic dogs is probably related to reduced renal clearance of the enzyme.

The "myoarteritis" that occurs quite often in the stomach and to a lesser extent in the gut in dogs is rare in other organs. A "mucoarteritis" occurs in the atria, however, especially the left, in the proximal aorta, and less often in the pulmonary trunk. There may be a light yellow, roughened plaque on the endocardium, and ulceration of the endocardium in these areas (Fig. 5.1A), which is due to fibrinoid degeneration of the subendocardial connective tissue. Sometimes arteriolar lesions in the myocardium cause ischemia and degeneration. Arterial degeneration is most frequent in acute uremia due to tubular necrosis. In

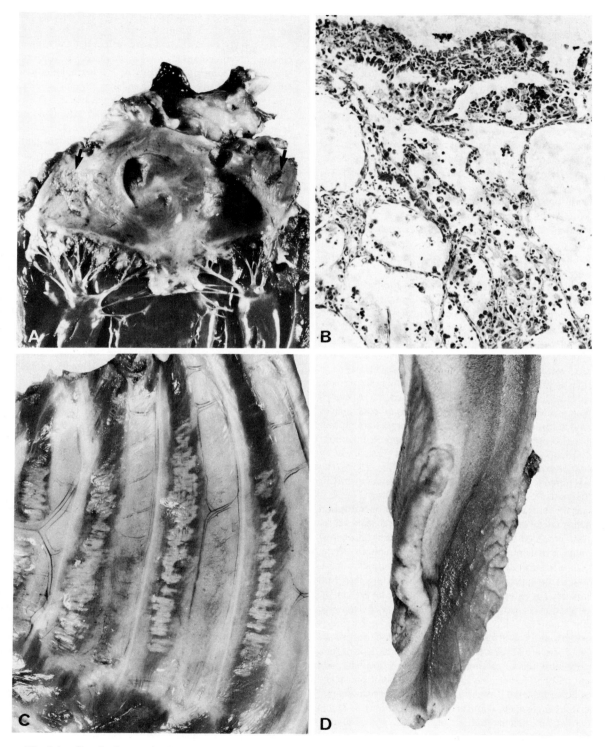

Fig. 5.1. Uremia. Dog.   (**A**) Ulceration and roughening (arrows) of endocardium of left atrium.   (**B**) Mineralization of alveolar and bronchiolar walls, mild edema, and intraalveolar cellular exudate.   (**C**) Necrosis and mineralization beneath intercostal pleura between cranial ribs.   (**D**) Ulceration of lateral margins and tip of tongue.

chronic uremia the left ventricle is often hypertrophied and di-lated. Hypertension is common in canine nephritis, and ven-tricular hypertrophy may be initiated or exaggerated by the hy-pertension. Lesions in the circulatory system are unusual, except in the dog, but myoarteritis may occur in intestinal vessels in cattle with acute nephrosis and contribute to the colonic lesions of acute uremic syndromes in this species. In cattle with urethral calculi, a pericardial effusion may be part of the anasarca. In dogs, hydropericardium with dull granulation of the pericardium may occur. Edematous distension of retroperitoneal tissue, ex-pressed particularly as perirenal edema, occurs in pigs and cat-tle. The underlying renal lesion is usually acute tubular necrosis caused by ochratoxin or *Amaranthus retroflexus* (Figs. 5.10D and 5.11) in pigs and cattle, and oak poisoning in cattle (see Nephrotoxic Acute Tubular Necrosis).

Most animals dying in uremia develop terminal pulmonary edema. The mechanism is obscure, and the edema is not always associated with significant pulmonary congestion. In a few ani-mals, acute pneumonia develops terminally. It may be associ-ated with aspiration of gastric content, and its fulminant nature possibly is related to the immunosuppression that develops in uremia. Pulmonary mineralization occurs in chronically uremic dogs. Mineral is deposited in the walls of the alveolar ducts and pulmonary arterioles. Dull granulations of the visceral pleura may be present over the cranial lobes. Occasionally in uremia, spectacular pulmonary lesions develop. They may be visible in radiographs as lines of increased density spreading out from the hilus, and these features are those of interstitial edema. At autop-sy the lung is edematous and resilient, and the alveolar spaces contain much fibrin in the edema fluid. Leukocytes are present but may be a response to accidental superimposed infection. Mineralization is extensive, with impregnation particularly on reticulin of alveolar walls, which are widened (Fig. 5.1B). The lesion is referred to as uremic lung or uremic pneumonopathy; it is not common, and when it occurs may be patchy.

Perhaps the most constant lesion in the dog is mineralization beneath the parietal pleura in the cranial intercostal spaces (Fig. 5.1C). It is preceded by necrosis of the subpleural connective tissue, with extension to intercostal muscle and overlying pleura. Once mineralization has occurred and the pleura is re-paired, the lesion appears as gray-yellow thickenings, horizon-tally wrinkled. The anterior intercostal spaces are involved first; when deposition is extensive, many more spaces may be affected.

The pathogenesis of diffuse tissue mineralization in uremia is not clear. There are at least two types of mineral deposit, and serum concentrations of calcium, magnesium, phosphate, and carbonate probably determine the type of calcium phosphate compound that is formed. When calcium is higher than magne-sium, apatites are formed, while the opposite relationship favors deposition of amorphous calcium phosphate. The regularity with which certain tissues and organs are mineralized is no doubt related to local characteristics such as tissue glycosaminogly-cans, local acidosis, and cellular factors.

The effects of chronic uremia on the skeleton are discussed with renal osteodystrophy (in Bones and Joints, Volume 1) and the parathyroid glands (in the Endocrine Glands, Volume 3).

Enlarged parathyroids are common in dogs with chronic renal failure; osseous lesions are less so.

The **renal lesions** of uremia are varied, but if the syndrome is chronic, certain common changes tend to occur. The end result is a fibrosed, mineralized kidney with sclerosed glomeruli, and sometimes areas of hyperplastic and hypertrophic tubules. Often this can only be diagnosed as end-stage kidney. Severe miner-alization occurs late in the course of renal failure and may dif-fusely involve glomerular and tubular basement membranes, or be deposited at the corticomedullary junction. In the latter case, temporary ischemia with reflow involving the straight part of the proximal tubule, which is at the periphery of the postglomerular circulation, may be responsible. Interstitial fibrosis and glomerulosclerosis are slowly progressive lesions that are com-mon in the end stages of many renal diseases. Hyperplasia and hypertrophy of tubules are inconstant changes that probably pre-cede the onset of renal failure. Azotemia develops when glomerular filtration is reduced to 60 to 70% of normal. Until that time, adaptive changes in intact nephrons maintain renal function at an adequate level as other nephrons are incapaci-tated. The glomerulus is probably the limiting factor in this compensatory mechanism, since it has a relatively limited abil-ity to increase its function. It seems unlikely that uremia pro-vides a suitable environment to permit or encourage compen-satory hyperplasia, and it is likely that enlargement of nephrons is an early response to a reduction in renal mass rather than an adaptation to uremia.

Anomalies of Development

The embryology of mammalian kidneys involves the sequen-tial development of three successive but overlapping structures, the pronephros, mesonephros, and metanephros. The first two become vestigial but act as inducers of the definitive kidney, the metanephros. Pronephric tubules, arising in the intermediate mesoderm of the cervical region, form the pronephric duct by fusion and extension of their caudal ends. This duct opens into the cloaca, and although the pronephric tubules are not func-tional in mammalian embryos, the utilization of their duct by the mesonephric tubules gives them potential significance in the genesis of renal anomalies. Mesonephric tubules develop from thoracic mesoderm caudal to the pronephros. The mesonephros is functional in mammalian embryos but degenerates before birth. In males, some of the caudal tubules persist as efferent ducts of the epididymis, and the duct itself is utilized as the vas deferens. In females, cystic remnants of mesonephric tubules in the mesovarium may form the epoophron and paroophoron, and remnants of the duct are known as Gartner's duct.

The formation of the metanephros, the definitive kidney, be-gins with the development of a ureteral bud from the meso-nephric duct immediately cranial to its junction with the cloaca. The bud, accompanied by vessels and nerves, grows into a mass of mesenchymal cells, the metanephric blastema, and it is on the interaction of these two structures that normal renal and ureteral development depend. As the bud grows into the blastema, it makes a specific number of successive, dichotomous divisions. The tubes formed by early divisions of the ureteral bud dilate and become the pelvis and calyces of the kidney. Tubes formed by later divisions develop into collecting ducts, and the last divisions give rise to collecting tubules. As the blind end of each collecting tubule, the ampulla, grows into the metanephric blastema, it induces compact masses of cells to form about it. These masses soon cavitate, become S-shaped, and unite with the side of the ampulla, which continues to advance and divide.

The cavitated cell masses develop into nephrons. Connection of the lumens of the nephron and the collecting tubule occurs very soon after the cell mass cavitates. Glomerular development involves the formation of a lateral invagination in the S-shaped mass by mesenchymal cells, which differentiate into endothelial and mesangial cells and become linked with the renal vasculature.

The complicated formation of the kidney provides for many patterns of malformation. The interaction of ureteral bud and metanephric blastema involves mutual inductions, and malformations of renal tissue often are accompanied by ureteral anomalies.

The incidence of urinary tract anomalies is not known for most species. Survey results from large numbers of lambs suggest that anomalies occur much more often than commonly believed.

Abnormalities in the Amount of Renal Tissue

Lack of renal tissue may be complete or partial and is called agenesis or hypoplasia, respectively.

Renal agenesis may be caused by developmental failure of the pronephros, mesonephros, or ureteral bud, by absence or complete unresponsiveness of the metanephric blastema, or by complete degeneration of the metanephric blastema. Partial degeneration, or partial responsiveness of the blastema to the inductive influences of the ureteral bud, probably produces renal dysplasia. The presence of even a fragment of recognizable metanephric tissue necessitates this diagnosis.

Agenesis may be unilateral or bilateral. As is the case with all renal anomalies, agenesis may be associated with other urogenital deformities. Unilateral renal agenesis is compatible with normal life if the other kidney is normal; however, contralateral dysplasia, or even hypoplasia, may be present, in which case renal failure ultimately develops. The ureter may be absent, or malformed with a blind end that terminates in connective tissue at the renal site. Bilateral agenesis is inconsistent with postnatal life. Renal agenesis occurs infrequently in all species, except when there is a familial incidence, as in some beagle and Doberman pinscher dogs. Bilateral agenesis may account for some stillbirths, but this can be assessed only by careful examination of fetuses.

Hypoplastic kidneys are small, but most abnormally small kidneys, even in young animals, are not hypoplastic. The limited size of hypoplastic kidneys is associated with a reduced number of histologically normal lobules and calyces. Renal hypoplasia is a quantitative defect caused by reduced mass of metanephric blastema or by incomplete induction of nephron formation by the ureteral bud. When the amount of blastema is normal, but there is malfunction of the ureteral bud, renal dysplasia

probably develops. Most of the small kidneys diagnosed as hypoplastic are probably dysplastic or scarred. The term "cortical hypoplasia" should be avoided since it is inconsistent with established concepts of renal embryology and anatomy. Renal hypoplasia is rare. It may be unilateral or bilateral. When unilateral, contralateral hypertrophy is expected.

Bilateral hypoplasia probably always leads to renal failure, and this often complicates or precludes the diagnosis because of the secondary changes that develop. Several forms of renal hypoplasia occur in humans, but because of the confusion of terminology, the variations and incidence of the condition in animals cannot be assessed. Kidneys suspected of being hypoplastic should be weighed along with their mate and examined for evidence of dysplasia and hypertrophy. In humans, in the absence of acquired disease, a decrease in size of one kidney by more than 50%, or reduction of total renal mass by more than one-third, is taken as evidence of hypoplasia.

Details regarding **excess renal tissue** are not well documented. Duplication of ureters and kidneys occurs in cattle, pigs, and dogs, but it is not clear whether total renal mass is increased.

Anomalies of Renal Position, Form, and Orientation

The kidneys develop in the pelvis and migrate to their sublumbar location, meanwhile rotating so that the ureter attains its normal orientation. During this movement, the blood supply shifts from the iliac arteries to the aorta. Various disruptions of this procedure may occur. Vitamin A deficiency in sows may cause anomalies such as those described below.

Malposition of the kidneys, observed more frequently in swine than in other species, is usually caudal, with the kidney in the pelvic or inguinal position. One or both kidneys may be misplaced. The kidneys are normal. The renal arteries arise close to the bifurcation of the aorta or from the iliacs. The ureter is short but may be kinked and thereby predispose to hydronephrosis and pyelonephritis.

Fetal lobulations, normal in embryos and cattle, may persist owing to failure of fusion of individual renal segments. They are not of pathologic significance.

Horseshoe kidney, seen in all species, results from a fusion of the anterior or posterior poles of the kidneys (Fig. 5.3A). The fusion may involve only a small portion of the capsule or parenchyma or be sufficient to produce a common pelvis. The ureters are not involved, and their disposition depends on whether the anterior or posterior poles are fused. Such kidneys function normally.

Renal Dysplasia

Renal dysplasia is disorganized development of renal parenchyma due to anomalous differentiation. Lesions may be gross or microscopic (Fig. 5.2A,C,D). Renal dysplasia is usually congenital, but in cats, dogs, and pigs, which have an active subcapsular nephrogenic zone at birth, dysplasias may be caused by disease in the early neonatal period until differentiation of the

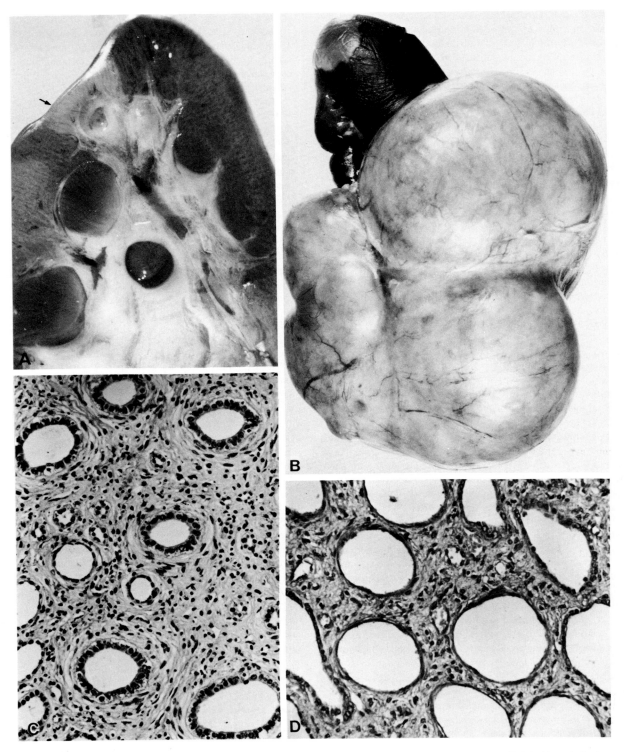

Fig. 5.2. (A) Focal renal dysplasia (arrow). Pig.   (B) Renal cysts involving each pole of the kidney. Pig.   (C) Primitive tubules in renal cortex. They are lined by cuboidal epithelium and surrounded by concentric layers of mesenchymal cells. Pig.   (D) Loose intertubular mesenchyme and dilated medullary tubules in renal dysplasia. Calf.

nephrogenic tissue is completed. The quantitative changes that continue until maturity are not susceptible to dysplastic influences.

The causes of renal dysplasia are ill defined, but there are indications that inheritance is not important if the familial renal diseases of dogs and the polycystic diseases are excluded. Most human cases are associated with intrauterine ureteral obstruction, and some cases in pigs and calves probably have the same cause. Renal dysplasia in kittens is caused by fetal infection with panleukopenia virus, in puppies by neonatal infection by canine herpesvirus, and in calves, associated with fetal infection by bovine virus diarrhea virus. Other teratogenic agents undoubtedly can produce renal dysplasia in these and other species.

There is considerable variation in the appearance of those dysplastic kidneys that are grossly abnormal. Most of them are small, which accounts for their frequent misdiagnosis as hypoplastic. They are usually misshapen and fibrosed, with thick-walled cysts and dilated tortuous ureters. One or both kidneys may be affected. If the lesion is unilateral, the ipsilateral ureter should be examined for anomalous valves or diverticuli. If both kidneys are involved, scrutiny of the bladder and lower urinary tract is indicated. Some dysplastic kidneys may be only slightly irregular in contour (Fig. 5.2A) or may appear normal, in which case microscopic examination is required for diagnosis. Dysplasias caused by teratogenic viruses usually are included in this group. Considerable emphasis has been placed on the size of renal arteries in dysplasias, but changes should be interpreted with caution since degenerative lesions in the renal parenchyma may be accompanied by vascular atrophy.

The microscopic criteria of renal dysplasia are the presence of structures inappropriate to the stage of development of the animal or the development of structures that are clearly anomalous. Among the former are areas of undifferentiated mesenchyme in cortex or medulla (Fig. 5.2C,D), and groups of immature glomeruli in the cortex of adolescent or adult animals. Anomalous structures include collecting tubules ending blindly in cortical connective tissue, or primitive ducts lined by cuboidal or columnar epithelium and surrounded by concentric layers of mesenchyme (Fig. 5.2C). Cartilage nodules, which are found in some dysplastic human kidneys, are rarely if ever present. This absence is probably a function of the stage of development at which metanephric injury occurs. Cartilage nodules imply injury to uncommitted mesenchyme, that is, to nephrogenic cord before its interaction with the ureteral bud. Other anomalous structures clearly are nephrogenic and represent improper interaction of ureteral bud and mesenchyme. There is some support for the opinion that only primitive ducts and cartilage nodules are prima facie evidence of dysplasia, on the grounds that all other lesions may be produced by acquired renal disease. Some of the more prominent gross lesions of dysplastic kidneys, such as fibrous cysts, dense medullary fibrosis, and fibrous wedges extending from pelvis to cortex, probably are regressive changes due to obstruction or infarction. Because ureteral anomalies are often concomitant, dysplastic kidneys are abnormally susceptible to pyelonephritis. Otherwise there is little or no evidence of infection in the renal parenchyma. The dark nuclei of improperly differentiated nephrogenic tissue should not be misinterpreted as lymphocytes.

Renal dysplasia with gross changes usually causes uremia. When lesions are bilateral, this is explicable in terms of reduced functional renal mass. With unilateral dysplasia, systemic hypertension induced by constriction of arteries in the affected kidney may be responsible.

Renal Cysts

Cystic diseases of the kidney include various conditions characterized by one or more grossly visible cystic cavities in the renal parenchyma. No satisfactory classification of renal cysts exists, but an acceptable compromise would be based on mode, or lack of inheritance, the presence of lesions in other organs, and the clinical course in affected animals.

Some prefatory remarks about renal cysts are in order. Cysts can arise during organogenesis and may be associated with histologic criteria of renal dysplasia. In humans, most dysplastic kidneys are cystic, and most cystic diseases of childhood are dysplasias. Cysts can arise in nephrons and collecting tubules after the end of nephrogenesis. Examples are provided by steroid-induced cysts in various species, and atypical cysts in patients undergoing long-term hemodialysis. Cysts can develop in any part of the nephron, including the glomerular space, or in the collecting system. In glomerulocystic disease, they develop only in Bowman's space, but this exclusivity is exceptional. There is no evidence that cysts are caused by failure of nephrons to unite with the collecting system. Analyses of their content indicate that they are part of functional nephrons and that their activity is consistent with their location in the nephron. Most renal cysts are not caused by obstructive lesions; exceptions are the acquired retention cysts of chronic renal disease, some dysplastic cysts, and possibly, those of glomerulocystic disease. The fundamental change that allows cyst development probably occurs in the tubular basement membrane and results in formation of saccular or fusiform dilatations of the tubules. Its nature is not known.

Renal cysts vary in size from the barely visible (Fig. 5.3C) to structures that exceed the size of the organ itself (Fig. 5.2B). Most lie within these limits, and although they are more numerous in the cortex than medulla, this may simply reflect the relative volumes of the two regions. The cyst wall is clear or opaque, depending on the amount of surrounding connective tissue. The content is watery. Cysts are lined by flattened or cuboidal epithelium, which grossly is smooth and shiny. A few cysts are more or less divided by thin trabeculae, but most are unilocular and roughly spherical, ovoid, or fusiform.

Renal cysts occur in all species but are most common in pigs and calves. There are different patterns of occurrence in pigs, but it is not clear whether patterns exist in other animals. The usual finding in pigs is one or a few unilocular cortical cysts, about 1–2 cm across, bulging from the renal surface or exposed when the kidney is sliced. They are usually bilateral, and are incidental findings in young pigs. Affected kidneys are discarded in abattoirs. Although usually regarded as sporadic occurrences, these lesions may be examples of a cystic renal disease inherited as an autosomal dominant trait. Polygenic inheritance may determine the number of cysts in animals with the dominant gene. In this condition few cysts are present at

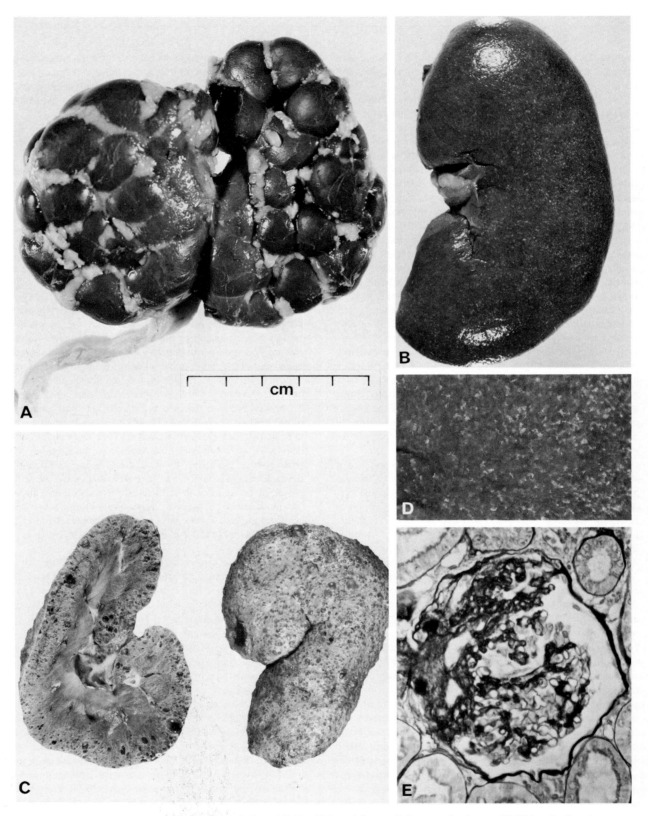

Fig. 5.3. (A) Horseshoe kidney. Calf. (B, D, and E) Familial renal disease. Doberman pinschers. (B) White stippling due to protein-filled tubules and lipid in tubular epithelium. (D) Close-up of cortical surface, showing details of lesion. (E) Membranoproliferative glomerulonephritis, with adhesions to Bowman's capsule. (C) Polycystic kidney. Horse 8 years old.

birth, but they gradually increase in number, and there may be 80–90 by 1 year of age. Cysts occur in different parts of the kidney and nephron. Signs of renal failure are not seen, but the condition has similarities to a human cystic disease in which renal failure develops in adults; a similar course in mature swine is not inconceivable.

Congenital forms of polycystic kidney disease associated with cystic bile ducts, bile duct proliferation, and sometimes, pancreatic cysts occur in pigs, lambs, calves, puppies, kittens, and foals. A genetic cause has been proposed in some species but rejected in others, and the role of inheritance is not established. A similar syndrome in humans is inherited, probably as an autosomal recessive trait.

In all species the disease is manifest by stillbirths or death in renal failure during the first few weeks of life. Grossly, the kidneys are large and pale and contain numerous 1- to 5-mm cysts that involve both cortex and medulla. Bile duct cysts range from barely visible up to 3 cm across, and the gallbladder and biliary system often are distended with bile, which discolors the liver.

Glomerulocystic disease is seen occasionally in stillborn foals and collie dogs. Cysts, barely visible, are present only in Bowman's spaces. Their significance in foals is not known. In dogs, uremia develops.

Occasionally, areas containing many small cysts occur in one lobe of a bovine kidney or one pole of an equine kidney. They are not significant clinically.

Many chemicals, such as long-acting corticosteroids, diphenylamine, 5,6,7,8,-tetrahydrocarbazole-3-acetic acid, alloxan, diphenylthiazole, and nordihydroguaiaretic acid, cause renal cysts in experimental animals. Corticosteroids induce hypokalemia, and cyst formation is prevented by injections of some potassium salts, but in general, the mechanisms of cyst development are not known. It seems possible that some of the therapeutic, prophylactic, and pollutant chemicals to which animals are exposed could be responsible for sporadic cases of renal cysts.

Acquired cysts of the kidney develop when tubules are obstructed by scar tissue. They are multiple and small, rarely exceeding 1.0 cm in diameter. Most are located in convoluted tubules and Bowman's spaces. Hyperplastic collecting tubules sometimes are grossly visible as elongated cysts in the medulla of dogs with renal failure. These acquired cysts are distinguishable from primary cysts in that they occur in kidneys with extensive scarring.

Familial Renal Disease

Familial renal diseases are documented or suspected in many dog breeds, and they are a major cause of renal failure in young animals. Familial diseases occur in the cocker spaniel, Norwegian elkhound, Samoyed, and Doberman pinscher breeds and probably exist in the Keeshond, Alaskan malamute, German shepherd, Lhasa Apso, Shih Tzu, miniature schnauzer, and beagle. Familial glomerulonephritis of Finnish Landrace sheep is discussed with other glomerulonephritides. Progressive renal fibrosis occurs in mutant Southdown sheep with hyper-

bilirubinemia. Specific tubular dysfunctions in dogs are discussed under Diseases of Tubules.

The canine familial renal diseases are characterized by renal failure, mostly in immature or young adult dogs, which is not associated with primary renal inflammation. For most breeds, only terminal clinical signs and end-stage lesions are described; inheritance, pathogenesis, and early morphologic changes have not been reported. The age of onset of renal failure varies from a few weeks to several years but in most cases is 4–18 months. This wide age range and the lack of morphologic specificity hinder the definition of these diseases since there is a danger that any noninflammatory renal lesion in a dog of an appropriate breed will be diagnosed as familial.

It is probable that some of the chronic interstitial nephritides formerly attributed to leptospirosis were familial renal diseases. The possibility that these diseases are examples of renal dysplasia seems unlikely since primitive ducts are not present. Glomeruli with the appearance of immaturity must be interpreted cautiously, particularly when they are found in areas of scarring.

Available evidence suggests that lesions primarily involve either glomeruli or interstitium around glomeruli. Interstitial lesions are fibrous and may be segmental or generalized. The fibrotic segments often contain apparently immature glomeruli, and this pattern is found frequently, but not exclusively, in Lhasa Apso and Shih Tzu dogs. Brief descriptions of some of the more clearly defined syndromes are given below.

SAMOYED DOGS. Familial renal disease occurs in both sexes but is much more common and severe, and has an earlier onset and more rapid course, in males than in females. In males, signs of renal failure with marked proteinuria begin at 4 to 13 months, and animals die in 3 to 6 weeks. In breeding trials, over half the males in affected litters have the disease. Females first show signs of renal disease in middle or old age, but these may be preceded by mild, persistent proteinuria lasting for several years. The disease appears to be transmitted by bitches to some of their sons regardless of the sire, but the mode of transmission is not known.

This disease is similar to Alport's syndrome in humans, which is inherited either as an autosomal dominant or as a sex-linked dominant trait. Glomerular lesions are prominent and consist of segmental proliferation and/or sclerosis of the tufts. Electron microscopic changes consisting of focal thickening, or attenuation with splitting, of the lamina densa of the glomerular basement membrane occur in many cases. The glomerular lesions are found in Samoyed dogs, but not the nerve deafness and ocular abnormalities that sometimes occur in the human syndrome.

DOBERMAN PINSCHERS. Doberman pinschers of both sexes are affected with familial glomerulonephritis, and signs, including polyuria, polydipsia, and weight loss, first develop at a few weeks to several years of age. Most animals are less than 1 year old. Prolonged survival is possible, dogs showing signs at a few months may live for many years.

Grossly, the kidneys are light brown, slightly small, and have diffuse, fine, subcapsular pits that appear as radial streaks on cut surface. There may be fine white stippling of the subcapsular surface due to the protein-filled tubules and lipid in epithelial cells in the subacute stage of the disease (Fig. 5.3B,D). A few bitches have concomitant agenesis of the right ureter and kidney, with or without contralateral compensatory hypertrophy. The association of renal agenesis is probably coincidental.

Microscopically, there is membranoproliferative glomerulonephritis, which begins as focal segmental mesangial thickening and accentuation of glomerular lobulation (Figs. 5.3E and 5.9B). These early lesions are sometimes present at birth, sometimes at several months. Glomerular changes progress to segmental or diffuse mesangial proliferation with increased mesangial matrix and glomerular adhesions and sclerosis. Sclerotic glomeruli appear as shrunken tufts at the vascular pole of cystic Bowman's spaces. The cysts may be visible grossly; they are associated with the progressive tubulointerstitial disease and are secondary to glomerular lesions. The interstitial lesions consist of fibrosis and monocyte infiltrations around diseased nephrons and in the medulla. In severely affected kidneys, compensatory hypertrophy and hyperplasia of tubules occur in adaptive nephrons.

This disease occurs in Doberman pinschers in North America. The variability in the rate of progression of the disease could indicate degrees of expressivity of the defect or reflect differences in exposure to exogenous or endogenous factors that injure the genetically predisposed kidney. Immune complexes have been identified in glomeruli of some dogs.

NORWEGIAN ELKHOUNDS. Familial renal disease occurs in both sexes of Norwegian elkhounds. Signs of renal failure begin as early as 3 months, but dogs with lesions may be clinically normal at 5 years of age. Animals showing early onset and rapid progression of renal failure may be dwarfed. There are no specific biochemical characteristics. Dwarfism in Norwegian elkhounds may be chondrodysplastic (see Bones and Joints, Volume 1).

Grossly, there are light gray streaks, and occasionally wedge-shaped lesions, in the cortex. As the disease progresses, the kidneys become contracted, pale, and tough from abundant cortical and medullary fibrosis.

Histologic changes begin as periglomerular fibrosis with hypertrophy and hyperplasia of parietal epithelium and progress to more or less diffuse fibrosis of cortex and medulla. The lesion is generalized, but not all glomeruli are necessarily involved. Wedge-shaped areas containing severe lesions are consistent with vascular injury, but there is no evidence of vascular abnormalities. As fibrosis progresses, constriction of normal nephrons occurs, and there is a progressive loss of glomeruli. In microdissected kidneys, small saccular dilatations are demonstrable in distal tubules and collecting ducts in the early phase of the disease. Late in the course, marked dilation and hyperplasia of collecting ducts occurs; this is a nonspecific lesion in chronic renal disease. There is no evidence of inflammation until renal disease is well established, at which time occasional, randomly distributed foci of mononuclear cells develop.

The disease is reproducible in breeding trials using dogs from appropriate strains, but the mode of transmission is not known.

Circulatory Disturbances and Diseases of the Blood Vessels

Renal Hyperemia

Active hyperemia is seen in acute nephritis, but especially in the acute septicemias and bacterial intoxications. The kidney is swollen and uniformly dark, although in some cases the hyperemia may be largely restricted to the medulla. Microscopically, all vessels, especially capillaries, are filled with blood. Very acute congestion with intertubular hemorrhages occurs in clostridial enterotoxemia of lambs and calves.

Passive hyperemia (congestion) follows the usual principles. Affected kidneys are enlarged and dark, and the capsular vessels are injected. On section, the corticomedullary junctional zone is dark and prominent, and there is engorgement of visible tributaries.

Renal Hemorrhages

Hemorrhages are especially common in the renal cortex in a variety of bacteremias and viremias, and sometimes in healthy slaughtered animals. Petechiae are very common in piglets dead of any cause (Fig. 5.4B). Many or few pinpoint hemorrhages occur beneath the capsule in hog cholera and porcine salmonellosis. In porcine erysipelas, the hemorrhages tend to be larger and more irregular in size and shape. Severe hemorrhage in the wall of the renal pelvis and the medulla sometimes occurs in hog cholera, in other acute infections of swine, and in the hemorrhagic diatheses; the hemorrhage occurs from the congested medullary vessels. Extensive subcapsular hemorrhage is not uncommon in clostridial enterotoxemia of calves; it produces a black cast molded to the shape of the cortex.

Renal Infarction

Infarcts of the kidney are common lesions of localized coagulation necrosis, produced by embolic or thrombotic occlusion of the renal artery or of one of its branches. The sequelae depend on whether the obstructing material is septic or bland and on the size and number of the vessels obstructed. Bland thrombi produce typical infarcts, and septic thrombi produce abscesses that may heal, sequestrate, or discharge into the pelvis. Thrombosis of a trunk of a renal artery will produce total or subtotal necrosis of the kidney, the extent of the latter depending on the presence and efficiency of parahilar and capsular collaterals. If an arcuate artery is obstructed, there is necrosis of a wedge of both cortex and medulla; if an interlobular vessel is involved, infarction is limited to the cortex. The ease and the frequency with which the kidneys are infarcted depend on their vascular architecture's being of the "end artery" type and on the large volume of blood that continually traverses them.

Soon after total obstruction of a vessel, the related wedge of tissue is swollen and intensely cyanotic, and it is congested by the blood that oozes into the vessels from collaterals. There is no sharp line between the infarcted zone and the adjacent normal tissue because in the narrow boundary zone there is an outer part in which blood continues to ooze slowly, and an inner part that is more or less well served by diffusion from the viable tissue. In

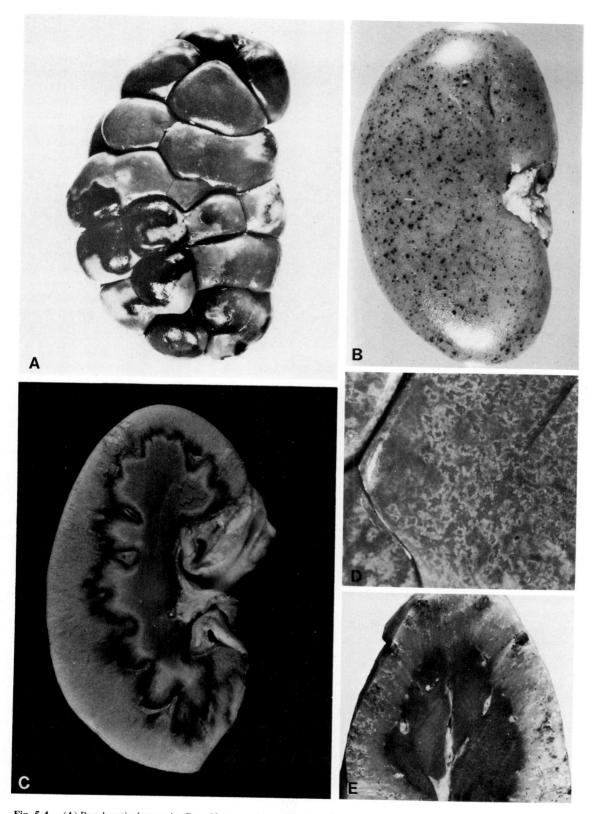

Fig. 5.4. **(A)** Renal cortical necrosis. Cow. Note recent hemorrhagic and older dehemoglobinized areas of infarction. **(B)** Renal cortical petechiae. Pig. Thrombocytopenic purpura. **(C)** Renal cortical necrosis. Pig. Pale cortex is delineated by hemorrhagic zone, which emphasizes the vascular supply. **(D and E)** Capsular and cut surfaces of kidney. Renal cortical necrosis associated with metritis and mastitis. Cow. Note predominance of lesions in outer cortex in **(E)**.

the outer part of the marginal zone, the red cells survive, and circulation may be reestablished, but this zone persists for the first 2 or 3 days; it is usually referred to, apparently erroneously, as the zone of reactive hyperemia. The limit of useful diffusion determines the actual limit of the infarct, and it is here that dehemoglobinization begins, neutrophils accumulate, and the area of total necrosis begins. The dehemoglobinization begins from the periphery at ~24 hr and may be complete in 2 or 3 days, the infarcted area then being white (Fig. 5.5A). Before decoloration begins, the area that will be affected is outlined by a thin but distinct white line of leukocytes.

The sequence of degenerative changes in the infarcted tissue reflects the specialization and sensitivity of the various structures. At the outer margins, only a few proximal tubules show epithelial necrosis. More centrally, every proximal tubule is dead, and inside the zone of diffusion everything is dead (Fig. 5.5B). In the peripheral dead zone there may in a week or so be some revascularization along preformed channels. The necrotic zone is progressively scarified, and healed infarcts persist as pale, gray-white scars, wedge-shaped and much depressed below the surface. The scars may be difficult or impossible to distinguish grossly from focal healed pyelonephritis.

Minute emboli lodging in the glomerular or intertubular capillaries may produce small infarcts not detectable macroscopically. Because of the small size of such infarcts, there may be adequate diffusion across the infarcted zone so that leukocytes do not accumulate, epithelial necrosis is minimal and soon repaired, and circulation is reestablished. Commonly, infarcts of varying age in a kidney indicate recurrent embolic episodes.

Renal Cortical Necrosis and Acute Tubular Necrosis

Acute tubular necrosis and renal cortical necrosis can be grouped together for purposes of discussion, although acute tubular necrosis is also discussed under Diseases of Tubules. These lesions occur infrequently in animals but may, if severe, cause acute renal failure and death. Outbreaks of renal cortical necrosis occur in kennels of dogs, but the causative circumstances have not been traced. Sporadic cases occur in cats, some of them due to thrombosis of the renal artery. Renal cortical necrosis and acute tubular necrosis occur in cattle in a variety of endotoxemic conditions, such as mastitis or metritis, and in gastrointestinal diseases, such as severe enteritis and grain overload. In horses, this often provides the fatal outcome to "azoturia." Bilateral cortical necrosis is a rare complication of esophagogastric ulceration in swine and apparently results from hemorrhagic shock.

In acute tubular necrosis, there is a patchy necrosis of segments of both proximal and distal tubules, with involvement also of the basement membranes. In renal cortical necrosis, the whole or part of both cortices is involved, and there is both tubular and glomerular destruction. It appears probable, from analogy with experimental results, that these lesions represent differences in degree and that they result from patchy or complete renal ischemia.

The mechanisms of renal ischemia are not completely understood. During hypotension, perfusion of outer cortical nephrons is reduced while perfusion of inner cortical nephrons is maintained, that is, intrarenal blood flow is redistributed toward the inner cortex and medulla. This reaction occurs because the vasoconstrictive effects of angiotensin II and adrenergic stimulation are unopposed in the outer cortex, while in the inner cortex, prostaglandins modulate vasoconstriction; PGE_2 is produced in the medulla in response to ischemia, travels in tubular fluid to the area of the juxtaglomerular apparatus, and has a local vasodilatory effect on efferent arterioles of juxtamedullary nephrons. The duration of ischemia is of obvious importance for the pathogenesis of necrosis. Complete ischemia of duration less than 2 hr can be expected to be followed by good reflow if cardiac output and blood pressure are restored to normal, whereas total ischemia of longer duration may be followed by patchy reflow or complete failure of reflow in the cortex, medulla, or both. Reflow is inhibited by ischemia-induced swelling of endothelial cells of glomeruli, vasa recta, and peritubular capillaries, by intravascular trapping of blood cells, and by swelling of parenchymal cells. This "no reflow" phenomenon may make an important contribution to renal ischemia and acute renal failure.

Another mechanism by which renal cortical necrosis occurs is via the generalized Shwartzman reaction, an example of disseminated intravascular coagulation, which is often due to Gram-negative endotoxemia. Endothelial injury in glomerular and peritubular capillaries leads to microthrombosis and hemorrhagic renal cortical necrosis. This severe degree of renal damage is usually rapidly fatal, but minimal lesions of this pathogenesis are common in a number of bacteremic diseases and visible as petechial or larger hemorrhages in the cortex.

The gross appearance of the kidneys other than those with hemorrhagic renal necrosis varies considerably from case to case; it is probably determined by the severity, distribution, and duration of the ischemia, and the quality of the reflow. In acute tubular necrosis, the cortices are finely mottled or flecked by small yellow foci of necrosis. In renal cortical necrosis, the cortices may be totally affected (Fig. 5.4C), or the injury may be patchy (Fig. 5.4A); pigs tend to develop a "turkey egg" pattern marked by hemorrhagic glomeruli but die before marked necrosis is evident, while cattle sometimes develop a distinctive patchy cortical necrosis (Fig. 5.4D,E). The reaction is the same as for infarction, given above. A narrow subcapsular rim of viable tissue may remain. The affected areas of cortex are pale, almost white, slightly swollen, and stop sharply at the corticomedullary junction. The irregular areas of cortical infarction may be outlined by hemorrhage. The medulla may be normal, but in some cases there is severe stasis and congestion at the corticomedullary junction or involving the whole of the medulla so that it is swollen and resembles a blood clot.

The histologic appearance of a kidney with acute tubular necrosis includes irregular necrosis of the proximal tubules, often with disruption of the tubular basement membranes. Hyaline and granular casts may be present, particularly in distal tubules and collecting ducts. There may be interstitial edema as a result of tubular leakage. If the animal survives the ischemic episode, evidence of regeneration may be seen in ~1 week, namely, tubules lined by flattened epithelial cells with hyperchromatic nuclei and occasional mitoses. In cases of severe

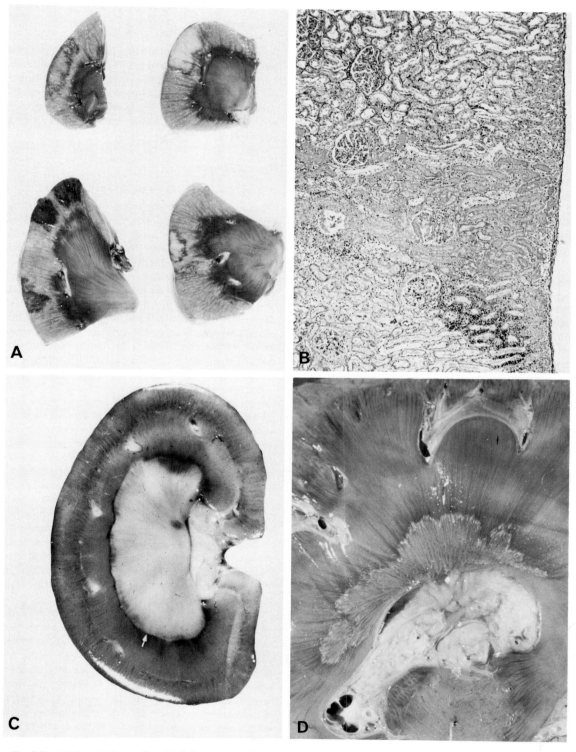

Fig. 5.5.   (A) Renal infarcts. Cow. Dark (hemorrhagic) infarcts are ∼1 day old. Those with dehemoglobinized centers are 2 or 3 days old.   (B) Renal infarct. Sheep.   (C) Renal medullary necrosis. Dog. Necrotic inner zone of medulla is outlined by a thin line of hemorrhage (arrow).   (D) Papillary necrosis. Horse. Lesion developed following intestinal resection and treatment with nonsteroidal antiinflammatory agents.

ischemia and renal cortical necrosis, various patterns of infarction may be seen, with glomeruli and vessels, as well as tubules, being necrotic. Microthrombi may be seen in capillaries, and hemorrhage may be present in glomeruli. The medulla is usually preserved.

Renal Medullary Necrosis

Under certain circumstances, medullary necrosis is the primary manifestation of renal injury. The conditions required to produce medullary necrosis are still being elucidated. As noted above, when renal hypotension occurs, cortical necrosis usually predominates due to redistribution of arterial flow to juxtamedullary nephrons. Medullary vessels are damaged by greater than 2 hr of ischemia, however, and there may hence be failure of both medullary and cortical reflow after temporary ischemia, both medullary and cortical necrosis resulting. In the case of venous occlusion, the elevated intrarenal blood pressure maintains the patency of lower-resistance cortical vessels but not of higher-resistance medullary vessels, and hence medullary infarction predominates. Prostaglandin synthetase, which occurs in the kidney primarily in the medulla, may be inhibited by nonsteroidal antiinflammatory agents, such as aspirin, phenacetin, and phenylbutazone, resulting in decreased production of PGE_2 and loss of its vasodilatory effect on arterioles of juxtamedullary nephrons. This pathogenetic sequence causes the papillary necrosis characteristic of "analgesic nephropathy" in humans, which also occurs in animals, especially if they are dehydrated when treated (Fig. 5.5D). Papillary necrosis occurs in lambs and calves that are dehydrated when treated with phenothiazine, and the necrosis is again apparently due to ischemia. Dehydration is also involved in the pathogenesis of papillary necrosis in racing greyhounds. Diabetes mellitus is not the important pathogenetic factor in animals that it appears to be in humans.

Papillary necrosis is a common consequence of urinary obstruction in animals. Pyelonephritis is also a common cause of papillary necrosis in animals, and fulminating pyelonephritic infections may produce necrosis of the papilla with scant inflammatory reaction in the early stages. The long, thin-walled vessels supplying the medulla are easily occluded by compression, and edema of the papillary interstitium alone could do this. Compression of vessels is probably the mechanism by which amyloidosis causes papillary necrosis in cats. Deposition of amyloid mainly in the renal medulla without, or with little concomitant glomerular deposition occurs often in cats and occasionally in cattle (see Amyloidosis).

The gross lesions of medullary necrosis vary greatly in their extent and stage of development (Fig. 5.5C,D). Acute papillary infarction may be an incidental finding in an animal dead of other causes, such as dehydration and electrolyte imbalances in neonatal diarrhea. Massive medullary infarction would no doubt be part of acute renal failue leading to death. In an animal surviving an episode of medullary necrosis, medullary scarring occurs, the papilla may slough, and secondary cortical scarring is seen. The sloughed papilla may remain in the pelvis and may become mineralized. Microscopic lesions cover the usual range of necrosis and scarring. Sequelae to medullary necrosis are based on the loss of the ability to concentrate urine and include chronic renal failure and uremia.

Primary vascular disease of the kidneys in animals is of little significance. Renal arteriosclerosis is not rare as an incidental finding in cattle, and arteritis is occasionally observed as "periarteritis nodosa" or in systemic disease such as malignant catarrhal fever. A variety of degenerative proliferative arterial changes occur in chronic diffuse inflammatory disease, but they are probably secondary, although exaggerated by the hypertension expected to develop.

Hydronephrosis

Hydronephrosis is dilation of the renal pelvis and calyces associated with progressive atrophy and cystic enlargement of the kidney. The cause is some form of urinary obstruction, existing at any level from the urethra to the renal pelvis, which may be complete or incomplete. The obstruction may be caused by anomalous development of the lower urinary passages, or it may be acquired. Acquired causes include urinary calculi in any location, prostatic enlargement in the dog, cystitis (especially if it is hemorrhagic), compression of the ureters by surrounding inflammatory or neoplastic tissue, displacement of the bladder in perineal hernias, and acquired urethral strictures. Depending on the site of obstruction, hydronephrosis may be unilateral or bilateral, and there may be some degree of hydroureter and dilation of the bladder.

The pathogenesis of hydronephrosis is based on the persistence of glomerular filtration in the presence of urinary obstruction, plus the development of ischemic lesions. Even with sudden complete obstruction, glomerular filtration continues since filtrate diffuses into the renal interstitium and perirenal spaces, where it is drained by lymphatics and veins. Continued filtration creates increased pressure throughout the nephrons, collecting ducts, and calyces and pelvis, and shearing forces develop between the compressible parenchyma and the resistant connective tissues of the trabeculae. Pressure atrophy of tubular epithelium occurs, hence tubular function and concentrating ability diminish. As well, blood vessels are compressed, particularly hilar veins and inner medullary vessels, leading to papillary ischemia and necrosis. Eventually, glomerular filtration decreases as nephrons atrophy and are replaced by scar tissue.

The degree of development of hydronephrosis depends on whether or not it is bilateral, the completeness of the obstruction, and on other complications of obstruction. The development of an extensive degree of hydronephrosis requires that it be unilateral. Bilateral obstruction, which includes obstruction localized to the bladder or urethra, results in early death from uremia. Unilateral obstruction will produce the greatest degree of hydronephrosis, especially if the obstruction is incomplete or intermittent, because glomerular filtration will be little suppressed, and such kidneys may be massively enlarged. If an obstruction is removed within ~1 week, renal function returns. After ~3 weeks of complete obstruction or several months of incomplete obstruction, irreversible renal damage occurs. If hydronephrosis is unilateral, the remaining kidney, if normal, compensates adequately. Urinary stasis predisposes to infection, hence pyelonephritis may be superimposed on hydronephrosis or vice versa.

Early gross changes consist of progressive dilation of the pelvis and calyces, with blunting of the apices of the pyramids (Fig. 5.6A,C). Eventually these may become excavated to form multilocular cysts communicating with the pelvis and separated by an intricate series of ridges, which represent original septa (Fig. 5.6B,D). In advanced cases, the kidney may be transformed into a thin-walled sac with only a thin shell of atrophic cortical parenchyma.

The microscopic changes begin with dilation of the proximal convoluted tubules, and shortly there is dilation also of the distal and straight segments. The latter persists, with atrophy of the epithelium, but the dilation of the proximal tubules subsides; these portions then atrophy, become separated, and are replaced by a light, diffuse cortical fibrosis. The glomeruli persist for a long time, flattened and spread apart. Various degrees of ischemia up to infarction may develop patchily in the cortex if the obstruction is sudden and complete; the infarcts are venous in origin. There is progressive destruction of the pyramids by liquefaction necrosis, which spares the pelvic epithelium and tissue in a narrow zone immediately beneath. The necrotic tissue, to which there is no reaction, is liquefied and removed, and the pyramids are gradually destroyed.

Glomerular Diseases

The specific glomerular diseases discussed below are glomerulonephritis, amyloidosis, and glomerular lipidosis. Glomerular disease is of importance because, first, interference with glomerular blood flow, as well as decreasing the formation of ultrafiltrate, impairs peritubular perfusion and hence may cause loss of the entire nephron, and second, glomerular permeability may be altered, leading particularly to proteinuria. The terms glomerulonephritis and glomerulonephropathy are used interchangeably and imply that secondary tubulointerstitial and vascular changes accompany the primary glomerular disease. The term glomerulitis is used when the inflammation is restricted to glomeruli, as may occur in acute septicemias. Glomerulonephritis, which is usually of immune origin, is a common form of renal disease in domestic animals and is a common antecedent of end-stage kidneys and renal failure, particularly in dogs and cats.

The clinical presentations of any renal disease are of limited variety, and clinicopathologic findings in animals with glomerular disease usually have no specificity. Thus hematuria, proteinuria, oliguria, hyposthenuria, and azotemia occur in glomerular and other renal diseases; only proteinuria, occurring in the absence of urinary tract inflammation, is particularly indicative of glomerular damage, namely, increased glomerular permeability. Marked proteinuria, as occurs in chronic glomerulonephritis and in amyloidosis, can lead to development of the nephrotic syndrome, which is a clinical syndrome characterized by hypoalbuminemia, generalized edema, and hypercholesterolemia. The edema is the result of decreased plasma colloid osmotic pressure, stimulation of the renin–angiotensin–aldosterone system, and release of antidiuretic hormone in response to hypovolemia. The hepatic response to hypopro-

teinemia is apparently a generalized increase in protein production, including lipoproteins, leading to hyperlipoproteinemia and hypercholesterolemia. Proteinuria due to glomerular disease may be highly selective or poorly selective, that is, albumin or albumin plus globulins respectively appear in the urine. In summary, glomerulonephritis can be expressed clinically as acute or chronic renal failure, or as the nephrotic syndome.

TERMINOLOGY. The following terms are generally accepted for the description of glomerular disease and are often appended to the histologic diagnosis:

Generalized: involves all glomeruli to some extent
Focal: involves only some glomeruli
Diffuse (global): involves the whole glomerulus
Segmental (local): involves only part of the glomerulus
Mesangial: affects primarily the mesangial area

Classification of glomerulonephritis in humans is relatively advanced and complex, based on extensive clinicopathologic correlations, clinical outcomes, and responses to therapy. The following simple classification system is currently in use for glomerulonephritis in domestic animals:

Membranous: basement membrane thickening predominates
Proliferative: cellular proliferation prodominates (Fig. 5.9B)
Membranoproliferative (mesangiocapillary): both changes are present (Figs. 5.7D and 5.8D)
Glomerulosclerosis: progressive hyalinization sometimes resulting in glomerular obsolescence, in which the glomerulus is a shrunken, eosinophilic, hypocellular mass (Fig. 5.8E)

Glomeruli at different stages of lesion development may occur in the same kidney, and the type of glomerular reaction may not be uniform among glomeruli.

Histologic Changes in Glomerulonephritis

Glomeruli commonly exhibit a spectrum of histologic changes. In view of the large renal reserve, it is important to correlate clinical and histologic findings in order to determine the clinical importance of glomerular changes. For example, in sheep and goats, glomerulonephritis is often generalized and well developed histologically but is usually of little functional significance. Conversely, histologic glomerular changes may be slight, but clinical disease may be marked, as occurs in minimal change disease, wherein a mild ultrastructural lesion is accompanied by marked proteinuria.

Glomeruli may be nonspecifically involved in renal reactions such as renal cortical necrosis, discussed above, and may be secondarily involved in tubulointerstitial diseases such as pyelonephritis. Septic emboli frequently lodge in the glomerular and peritubular capillary beds and cause focal glomerulitis and focal interstitial nephritis in diseases such as porcine erysipelas and in actinobacillosis of foals (Fig. 5.7A). Generalized glomerulitis, not necessarily associated with other renal change, is seen in acute septic disease and is characterized by increased glomerular cellularity involving either or both epithelial and endothelial cells. Inclusions are common in glomerular endothelium in infectious canine hepatitis (Fig. 5.7C).

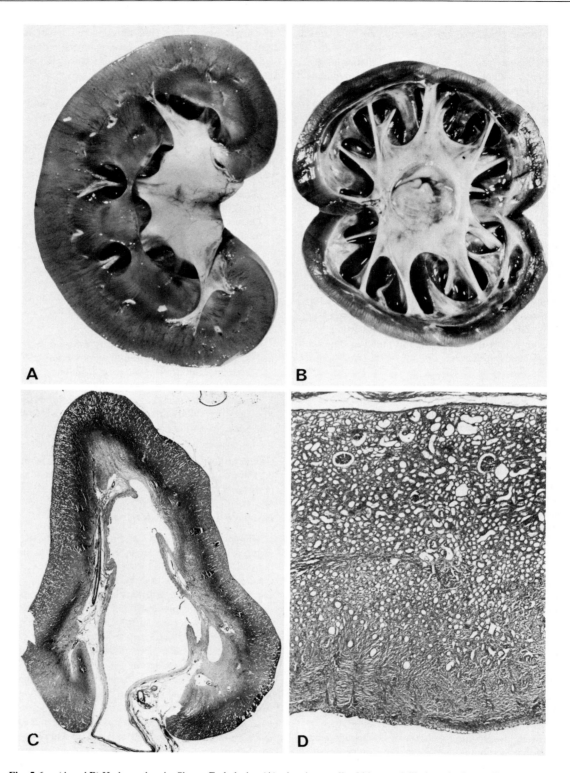

Fig. 5.6. (**A** and **B**) Hydronephrosis. Sheep. Early lesion (**A**), showing swollen kidney and dilation of calyces. Chronic lesion (**B**), showing loss of medulla, and cortical atrophy.   (**C**) Early hydronephrosis. Pig. Pelvis and cortical tubules are dilated. There is a discontinuous zone of congestion at corticomedullary junction.   (**D**) Section through cortex and medulla of kidney with chronic hydronephrosis. Note fibrosis of medulla (below) and dilation of tubules.

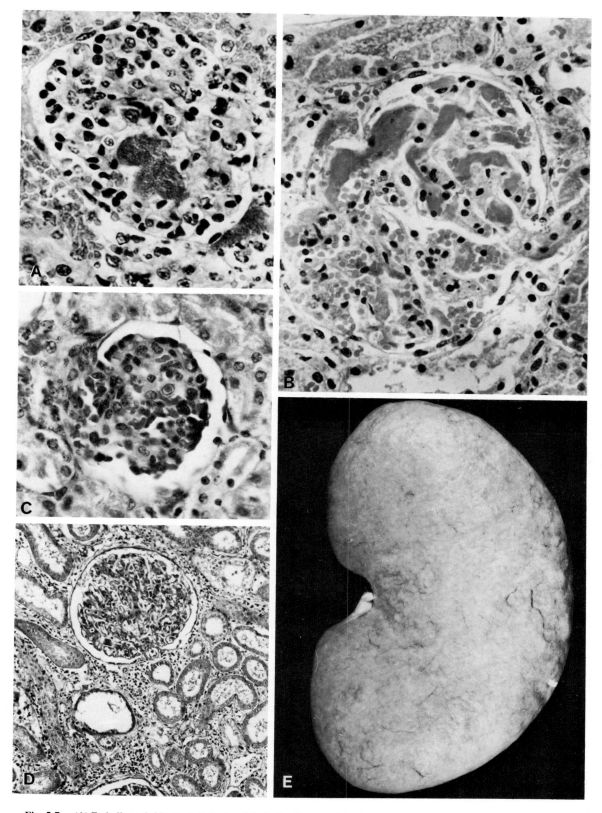

Fig. 5.7. (A) Embolic nephritis. Foal. Colonies of *Actinobacillus equuli* in glomerular and intertubular capillaries. (B) Fibrinoid thrombi in glomerular capillaries. Calf. Colibacillosis. (C) Glomerulus. Infectious canine hepatitis. Intranuclear inclusion body in endothelial cell. (D) Membranoproliferative glomerulonephritis and interstitial nephritis. Horse. Equine infectious anemia. (E) Pale, granular kidney of subacute–chronic glomerulonephritis. Dog.

Basic inflammatory reactions of exudation, necrosis, and thrombosis occur in glomeruli as elsewhere, but some changes are typically glomerular.

Cellularity of the glomerular tuft may be increased by proliferation of endothelial, epithelial, or mesangial cells. This assessment is usually subjective. Proliferation of endothelial versus mesangial cells may be difficult to distinguish, and the term endocapillary glomerulonephritis is then applied. Mesangial cells in glomeruli of dogs usually occur singly or in pairs, hence at least three mesangial cells must be in close proximity before the term mesangial hyperplasia is applied. In response to fibrin exudation into the urinary space in severe glomerular damage, monocytes invade, parietal epithelial cells proliferate, and epithelial crescents are formed. Some of the cells, possibly monocytes, undergo metaplasia to fibroblasts and produce collagen. In humans, crescents are most commonly seen in cases of rapidly progressive extracapillary glomerulonephritis, but they are only indicative of severe glomerular damage and not pathognomonic of one disease.

Intravascular accumulations of neutrophils and monocytes may accompany cellular proliferation in glomerulonephritis.

The swelling ("fusion") of foot processes and their subsequent retraction is a reversible reaction of the visceral epithelial cells, apparently occurring in response to basement membrane damage and protein leakage.

Glomerular capillary walls may be thickened in routine hematoxylin- and eosin-stained sections due to endothelial or epithelial swelling and/or thickening of the basement membrane. The basement membrane itself is not visible unless special stains, such as PAS or PAS–methenamine–silver, are employed on thin (1–3 μm) sections. Electron microscopy is required to characterize morphology of the thickening properly, which may be regular, as occurs in diabetic glomerulosclerosis, or irregular, as with deposition of electron-dense material in subendothelial, intramembranous, or subepithelial (epimembranous) locations. These electron-dense deposits are usually immune complexes. Thickened peripheral capillary walls are particularly prominent in cases of membranous glomerulonephritis and are referred to as "wire loops"; subepithelial immune complexes (humps) may become separated by projections (spikes) of basement membrane, and eventually are surrounded by and incorporated within the membrane. This marked thickening of the basement membrane is somewhat paradoxially associated with marked proteinuria, probably as a result of changes in the charge and pore size. In membranoproliferative glomerulonephritis, thickening of the membrane may be due to infiltration and splitting by mesangial processes and matrix and is seen with silver stains as a characteristic double-contoured glomerular basement membrane or "tram tracks," a change also termed "reduplication."

As seen by light microscopy, accumulations of homogeneous, eosinophilic, PAS-positive, basement membrane–like material are common in the mesangial areas in glomerulonephritis, especially in chronic cases. This mesangial sclerosis may be reversible but, if irreversible and progressive, may lead to obsolescence of the glomerulus. Hyaline material is commonly deposited in the mesangium in diabetes mellitus and amyloidosis; in diabetes mellitus, diffuse (Fig. 5.8B) or occa-

sionally nodular hyaline (Kimmelstiel–Wilson nodules) deposits may be seen in glomeruli.

Thickening of Bowman's capsule may occur due to various combinations of hyperplasia of parietal epithelial cells in crescents, thickening of the basement membrane, and periglomerular fibrosis. These changes may be particularly marked in glomerular ischemia due to vascular occlusion.

Glomerular tuft atrophy may occur subsequent to scarring, which causes tubular constriction, inhibits or stops tubular fluid flow, and causes dilation of Bowman's capsule and secondary atrophy of the glomerular tuft ("glomerulocystic" change).

Nonglomerular histologic changes in glomerulonephritis include tubular proteinuria, which is prominent in membranous glomerulonephritis but most marked in glomerular amyloidosis. Other histologic changes include those of ischemic origin due to decreased glomerular, hence efferent arteriolar and peritubular, blood flow, and acute and chronic interstitial inflammation. Hence, tubular atrophy, interstitial fibrosis, and scarring occur in advanced lesions, eventually producing the nonspecific histologic picture of end-stage kidney. Tubulointerstitial and glomerular damage may be coincident and due to the same mechanism rather than either one's being primary.

Pathogenesis of Generalized Glomerulonephritis

Glomerulonephritis may result from the deposition in glomeruli of immune complexes unrelated to glomerular components, from formation of antibodies against glomerular basement membrane (anti-GBM disease), or from activation of the alternate pathway of complement. Some types of glomerulonephritis are of unknown pathogenesis. By far the most commonly identified pathogenesis of glomerulonephritis in domestic animals is immune-complex deposition.

In immune-complex glomerulonephritis, nonglomerular antigen–antibody complexes localize in glomeruli and are visible by immunofluorescence or electron microscopy as granules within, or on either side of, the glomerular basement membrane. Causative antigens may be exogenous (e.g., serum sickness) or endogenous, (e.g., nucleic acid in systemic lupus erythematosus). Immune-complex deposition may cause acute or chronic, membranous or proliferative lesions. The classical example of immune complex glomerulonephritis is acute, or "single shot," serum sickness. When a large quantity of foreign protein is injected intravenously into an experimental animal, immune complexes occur in glomeruli in a characteristic "lumpy–bumpy" pattern as seen by immunofluorescence (Fig. 5.8C). By electron microscopy, the complexes are seen as irregular electron-dense deposits in a subendothelial or subepithelial location or within the mesangium. The immune complexes usually contain complement as well as antigen and antibody. In general, it has been believed that immune-complex deposition, hence glomerular damage, occurs during the period of equivalence of antigen and antibody concentrations or during slight antigen excess. However, an alternate view has received support; in this view, antigens capable of penetrating the basement membrane localize in a subepithelial position and then bind antibody of low avidity. This antigen localization may be charge dependent. As

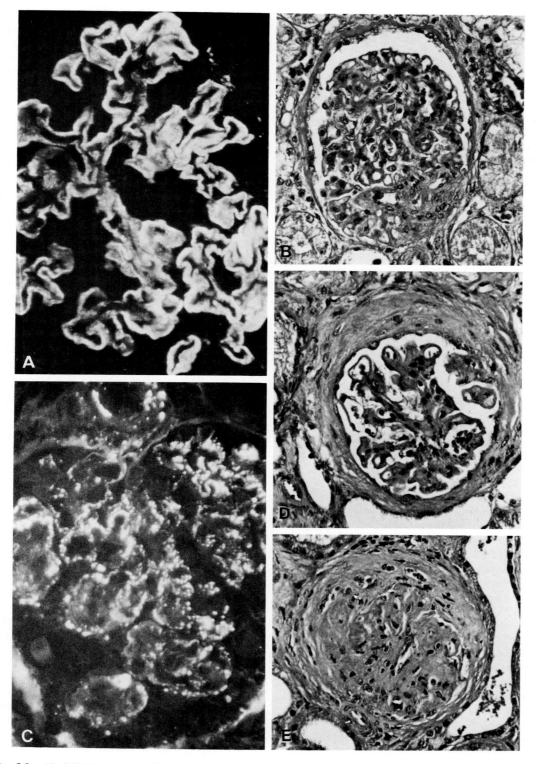

Fig. 5.8. (A) IgG linear immunofluorescence in membranous glomerulonephritis. (Courtesy of B. N. Wilkie.) (B) Glomerulosclerosis and glycogen nephrosis in diabetes mellitus. Dog. (C) C3 granular ("lumpy–bumpy") immunofluorescence. Postinfectious glomerulonephritis. (Courtesy of B. N. Wilkie.) (D) Membranoproliferative glomerulonephritis. Dog. Marked thickening of Bowman's capsule. (E) Obsolescent glomerulus in chronic glomerulonephritis. Dog.

well as taking part in the usual immune-complex glomerulone-phritis, dirofilarial antigens, for example, can apparently be deposited directly in basement membrane, inducing *in situ* formation of immune complexes and producing linear fluorescence, which is usually a characteristic of antiglomerular basement membrane disease (Fig. 5.8A). The relative importance of circulating soluble immune complexes versus *in situ* formation of complexes in causing immune complex glomerulonephritis is not resolved. Another modification of the classical soluble-immune-complex disease model is that insoluble or poorly soluble complexes play a major role in subendothelial and mesangial deposit diseases.

Chronic serum sickness occurs when repeated small doses of foreign protein are given to an animal, and circulating immune complexes are continually present. This condition of continued antigenemia occurs during various microbial and parasitic infections, such as feline leukemia virus infection and canine dirofilariasis, as well as during continued release of endogenous antigens, such as nucleoprotein in systemic lupus erythematosus or tumor-specific or tumor-associated antigens.

It is not completely straightforward to ascribe the cause of glomerulonephritis to immune complexes since the presence of immunoglobulins and complement in a lesion does not necessarily indicate that they are responsible for the lesion; certain components of complement (C3 and C1q) and immunoglobulin M (IgM) are sticky molecules that may adhere to previously injured tissue. As well, the significance of circulating soluble immune complexes is controversial, since they may be present in the absence of glomerulonephritis, and even if present, they may more be markers for the disease than actual causative agents, since glomerular damage may be caused by various combinations of insoluble, soluble, and *in situ*–formed immune complexes.

The reasons for localization of immune complexes in various glomerular sites, namely, subendothelial, intramembranous, subepithelial, or mesangial, are not clear. Localization may be affected by the size, shape, charge, and chemical composition of the complexes. Thus large complexes tend to localize in the mesangium and cause mesangiopathic glomerulonephritis, while small complexes (or antigens) penetrate the glomerular loop to produce the membranous or proliferative form. Antibody avidity may affect localization; complexes containing high-avidity antibody localize in the mesangium, while those with low-avidity antibody may localize subepithelially. Penetration of the basement membrane by complexes may be aided by products of inflammation, such as IgE-mediated release of histamine and serotonin from platelets and basophils, which is induced by antigen.

Modification of glomerular immune complexes occurs; they may be eliminated or may enlarge. Complexes may be eliminated by solubilization by excess antigen; phagocytosis by neutrophils, macrophages, or mesangial cells; passage through mesangial channels and egress at the vascular pole; excretion by mesangial cells through epithelial cells into the urinary space; degradation within the mesangial matrix; extracellular degradation by proteases; or solubilization by complement. Thus, for example, removal of the source of persistent antigenemia in pyometra of dogs by ovariohysterectomy results in resolution of

glomerulonephritis and cessation of proteinuria. Conversely, complexes may enlarge due to combination with various blood-borne reactants, such as small amounts of antigen, free antibody, immune complexes of the same or different specificity, complement components, or antibodies against immunoglobulins or complement components (immunoconglutinin or C3 nephritic factor).

In antiglomerular basement membrane glomerulonephritis, antibodies are formed against basement membrane antigens, resulting in a linear pattern of immunofluorescence reflecting the uniform distribution of immunoglobulins and complement along the basement membrane. There is a notable lack of dense or other deposits on electron microscopic examination. This lesion was the first recognized immune-mediated nephritis and was induced in rats by injection of anti-rat kidney antibodies obtained from rabbits or ducks immunized with rat kidney tissue; this experimental model is also referred to as Masugi or nephrotoxic nephritis. It occurs as a component of Goodpasture's syndrome in humans but occurs much less frequently than immune complex glomerulonephritis. In domestic animals, antiglomerular basement membrane disease is apparently rare, having been reported once in horses and suspected, but not proved, in several dogs.

While the above descriptions of immune complex glomerulonephritis and antiglomerular basement membrane disease are conceptually useful, the mechanisms operative in clinical cases are often less well defined and more complex. Thus, in the well-recognized acute poststreptococcal disease of humans, factors implicated in glomerular injury include immune-complex deposition, damage by antibodies that cross-react with streptococci and basement membrane, activation of the alternate complement pathway, and cell-mediated reactivity to altered glomerular basement membrane.

Mechanisms of Immunologic Glomerular Injury

Several mechanisms are effectors of glomerular injury once immune complexes are formed or deposited in glomeruli in either immune complex glomerulonephritis or in antiglomerular basement membrane disease. The best established mechanism is that of complement fixation with resultant chemotaxis of neutrophils. Complement components C3a, C5a, and C567 attract neutrophils that, in the process of ingesting complexes, release lysosomal enzymes and hence cause glomerular basement membrane damage. This is the complement/leukocyte-dependent mechanism. Complement fragments cause release of histamine from mast cells and hence caused increased capillary permeability, which may be important in allowing deposition of further immune complexes in the capillary wall. Since damage also occurs in the absence of complement or neutrophils, complement/neutrophil-independent mechanisms also exist but are less well understood.

It is paradoxical that while complement participates in glomerular injury, it also is capable of solubilizing immune complexes and accelerating their removal. Hence, hereditary hypocomplementemia, as occurs in Finnish Landrace lambs, may contribute to persistence of immune complexes and facilitate damage.

Interaction of complement fragments with platelets can initiate coagulation, thrombosis, and fibrinolysis; Hageman factor links the complement, coagulation, and kinin-forming systems. Fibrin and its degradation products are often present in glomeruli in glomerulonephritis, and fibrinogen that leaks into the urinary space is a stimulus to monocyte infiltration, proliferation of parietal epithelial cells, and crescent formation.

Monocytes are thought to play a role in glomerular damage also. Monocytes may be beneficial in removing immune complexes but may cause enzymatic damage, as do neutrophils. There is evidence that they transform to cells of fibroblastic type in glomerular crescents.

Cell-mediated hypersensitivity reactions occur in some people with progressive glomerulonephritis and may help cause glomerular damage.

Prevalence of Glomerulonephritis in Domestic Animals

The frequency of diagnosis of glomerulonephritis in domestic animals has increased dramatically since the early 1970s, mostly due to increased awareness and understanding of glomerulonephritis by clinicians and pathologists. There may also be a real increase in prevalence caused by poorly understood factors such as the increased use of modified live-virus vaccines, which may result in persistent antigenemia and predispose to immune-complex disease. Immune complexes commonly circulate throughout life, but few individuals develop significant lesions, so various factors such as genetic susceptibility or defective immune or other mechanisms may be operative in affected animals. Many associations of infectious and other diseases with glomerulonephritis have been identified (Table 5.1). In essence, any infec-

TABLE 5.1

Causes of Immune-Mediated Glomerulonephritis in Domestic Animals

Viral	Canine adenovirus-1 (infectious canine hepatitis)
	Feline leukemia virus
	Feline infectious peritonitis
	Equine infectious anemia
	Hog cholera
	African swine fever
	Bovine virus diarrhea
	Feline progressive polyarthritis
Bacterial	Canine pyometra
	Campylobacter fetus
	Subacute valvular endocarditis
Protozoal	African trypanosomiasis
Helminthic	Canine dirofilariasis
Neoplastic	Various
Autoimmune	Antiglomerular basement membrane disease
	Immune-mediated hemolytic anemia
	Systemic lupus erythematosus
	Polyarteritis
Hereditary	Hypocomplementemia in Finnish Landrace lambs
	Canine familial renal disease

tion of low pathogenicity that is able to produce persistent antigenemia has the potential to cause immune-complex disease. Most of the animal glomerulonephritides characterized to date are of immune-complex origin and of the membranoproliferative type. The morphology of the glomerular lesion is of little assistance in identifying its cause, however, since many agents cause the same type of lesion, and conversely, one agent can produce a spectrum of glomerular changes. Most cases in animals are idiopathic and hence may be referred to as primary; those occurring in association with other diseases or in which glomerular lesions contain known antigens are referred to as secondary.

Associations of particular types of glomerulonephritis with specific clinical presentations, clinical course, and outcome are rare in veterinary medicine but common in human medicine. An exception is membranous glomerulonephritis, which is often associated with the nephrotic syndrome. Most other forms of glomerulonephritis are associated with chronic renal failure.

The prevalence and importance of glomerulonephritis vary with species. In general, mild glomerular lesions (hypercellularity and occasional glomerular adhesions) are common, chronic lesions leading to renal failure are less common, and the acute disease is rare. Glomerulonephritis is a common finding in dogs and is a leading cause of renal failure; it is usually membranoproliferative. In cats, glomerulonephritis is also common but is predominantly membranous and a major cause of the nephrotic syndrome and/or renal failure. In ruminants, immunologic evidence of glomerulonephritis is common, but clinical disease is not. Glomeruli of sheep and goats are often hypercellular and have membranous changes, but the changes appear to have little clinical significance. An interesting exception is the membranoproliferative glomerulonephritis of Finnish Landrace sheep, discussed below. In horses, glomerulonephritis is fairly common, but renal failure is rare. Glomerulonephritis often occurs in horses with equine infectious anemia (Fig. 5.7D), and the renal lesions may be important. *Streptococcus equi* and herpesvirus infections have been suggested as causes of glomerulonephritis in horses. Acute fatal glomerulonephritis occurs sporadically in swine but is of little economic importance.

GLOMERULONEPHRITIS IN FINNISH LANDRACE SHEEP.   Glomerulonephritis, which is present at birth in Finnish Landrace sheep, is characterized by recessive inheritance of a deficiency of the complement component C3; in affected lambs, blood levels of C3 are ~5% of normal. This congenital deficiency contributes to the development of membranoproliferative (mesangiocapillary) glomerulonephritis, probably due to impaired complement-mediated solubilization of immune complexes in glomeruli. Affected lambs are clinically normal at birth but die between 1 and 3 months of age due to renal failure. At autopsy, the kidneys are enlarged, have pale cortices, and glomeruli grossly visible as red spots. The glomerular lesion is characterized by mesangial proliferation, capillary wall thickening, and, occasionally, formation of glomerular crescents. Subendothelial electron-dense deposits are present and consist of C3, smaller amounts of IgM and IgA, and with prolonged survival, progressively larger amounts of IgG. These changes begin *in utero* and develop progressively after birth. Choroid plexus lesions also occur due to immune-complex deposition and lead to encephalopathy.

Morphology and Chronology of Glomerulonephritis

Acute glomerulonephritis may not significantly alter the gross appearance of the kidney. The organ may be slightly or markedly enlarged, pale, soft, and edematous. The glomeruli may be visible as fine red dots. Petechial hemorrhages may be visible if bleeding has occurred from the inflamed glomeruli. In subacute glomerulonephritis, the kidney is enlarged, perhaps greatly, and pale with a smooth surface and nonadherent capsule (there may be numerous cortical petechiae, indicating recurrent acute episodes). The capsule is tense, and the cut surface bulges; the cortex is wide and yellow-gray, which demarcates it from a normal colored medulla. This subacute phase is anatomically and developmentally arbitrary and grades into the chronic phase, in which the kidney is shrunken and contracted with a generalized fine granularity of the capsular surface (Fig. 5.7E). The capsule may be adherent. On the cut surface the cortex is rather uniformly narrowed, and corticomedullary markings are obscured. Fine cysts may be present, developed from obstructed tubules. This stage, when contraction is severe, is grossly indistinguishable from chronic interstitial nephritis. It can usually be distinguished from the end result of pyelonephritis, which tends to produce more irregular contraction and scarring, often with intervening areas of normal parenchyma.

The histologic features of the acute phase are those of exudative inflammation. Initially hyperemic, the glomeruli soon become ischemic as a result of edematous thickening of the capillary walls and swelling of endothelial and epithelial cells. Neutrophils marginate in the capillaries and with the swollen and proliferated native cells of the glomerulus give a distinct impression of hypercellularity. The tuft swells and occupies most of the capsular space; any remaining space may contain migrated leukocytes, precipitated protein, or extravasated erythrocytes. Occasionally, fibrin thrombi form in the capillaries and cause focal necrosis and hemorrhage into the capsular space (Fig. 5.7B). This form of hemorrhagic glomerulonephritis with the formation of fibrin thrombi is the usual picture seen in swine with petechial hemorrhages as a gross manifestation. Concomitantly, interstitial edema develops. The tubular epithelium may contain hyaline droplets, and casts of protein, erythrocytes, and leukocytes form in the urine.

Although functional changes vary greatly, some can be anticipated. The swelling and resultant ischemia of the glomeruli reduce filtration, so there is oliguria. The concentrating capacity of the tubules is unimpaired, as yet, so the urine is of high specific gravity. It also contains protein, and hyaline, granular, and red-cell casts.

In the subacute phase, either mesangial hyperplasia or glomerular crescent formation may predominate. Fatty degeneration of the tubular epithelium may occur in this stage, as may hyaline-droplet formation or necrosis. Casts of protein, leukocytes, and necrotic epithelial cells are present in the tubules.

In the chronic phase, fibrous scarring of glomeruli occurs. There may be a reduction in the apparent number of glomeruli as

sclerotic glomeruli blend with surrounding scar tissue. If the original proliferative phase was mesangial, scarification may obliterate the tufts, transforming them to large or small masses of collagen and preserving the capsular space. If the proliferation was initially epithelial, fibrosis may completely obliterate the capsular space, but since the two forms usually coexist, obliteration of both glomerulus and capsule is usual. Although all glomeruli are usually involved, the degree varies somewhat so that many retain some function. The interstitial reaction initiated during the edematous exudative phase develops prominently with fibrosis and lymphocytic infiltration. Large numbers of tubules undergo disuse, ischemic, or pressure atrophy and are replaced by scar tissue, and the fibrosis becomes slowly self-perpetuating. Tubules that remain connected to functioning glomeruli may become dilated and develop epithelial hypertrophy and hyperplasia; these are in part responsible for the fine granularity of the surface and streakiness of the cut surface.

In chronic glomerulonephritis at the stage of decompensated renal failure, there is an increased volume of urine with a fixed, low specific gravity. Albuminuria may be only slight, and casts may be absent. Death occurs in uremia. Acute glomerulonephritis does not inevitably lead to fatal chronic glomerulonephritis. In fact, healed mild glomerular lesions with full renal function are much more common than debilitating or fatal chronic generalized glomerulonephritis. The only evidence of previous injury may be mild mesangial sclerosis and the presence of occasional small adhesions between peripheral capillary loops and the parietal epithelium.

Amyloidosis

Amyloidosis is a systemic disease in which amyloid, an eosinophilic, homogeneous, hyaline material, is deposited extracellularly in a variety of sites, particularly in renal glomeruli. Amyloidosis is currently classified as immunocytic (primary), in which case amyloid AL is produced from immunoglobulin light chains in plasma-cell dyscrasias, or reactive systemic (secondary), in which amyloid AA is derived from serum protein SAA, an immunoregulant product of hepatic and other cells that is produced in excess as a result of chronic antigenic stimulation. Most cases of amyloidosis in domestic animals are idiopathic but appear to be of the reactive systemic type. The deposits of amyloid may be found in many organs and may emphasize one or another of them, such as the liver or spleen, but the kidney is the organ most commonly involved in amyloidosis; localization of amyloid is usually glomerular, but medullary localization predominates often in cats and occasionally in cattle.

Amyloidosis is most common in dogs and is usually idiopathic, although some cases do occur in association with chronic suppurative and granulomatous lesions in other tissues; affected dogs develop progressive renal insufficiency and proteinuria, which may be sufficiently severe to cause the nephrotic syndrome. Amyloidosis is less common in cats than dogs, and marked proteinuria is a less prominent finding. In cattle, glomerular amyloidosis can cause severe proteinuria; medullary amyloidosis is reported as a common subclinical disease. A chronic suppurative or tissue-destructive process is occasionally demonstrable in affected cattle. Amyloidosis occurs in horses used for antiserum production; pigs rarely develop amyloidosis.

With small deposits of amyloid, the gross appearance of the kidney may be normal except for a slight increase in size and a peculiar translucence of the glomeruli. The characteristic renal change is one of paleness, enlargement, and increase in consistency. In cattle, the kidneys may be very large. The capsule strips smoothly to reveal a cortical surface with a finely stippled appearance due to numerous fine yellow spots, which are glomeruli, and gray points of translucence, which are dilated tubules. On cut surface, the cortex is widened and presents the same appearance as the capsular surface, rather like pumice stone. Affected glomeruli stain brown-red when exposed to an iodine solution; subsequent exposure to dilute sulfuric acid changes the color to purple.

Histologically, amyloid is first deposited in the mesangial area and in the subendothelium of glomerular capillaries. Nodules of amyloid gradually develop until the glomeruli, when uniformly involved, are enlarged and converted to homogeneous spheres with loss of endothelial and epithelial nuclei (Fig. 5.9C). Similarly, amyloid is deposited in tubular basement membranes, and eventually broad cuffs of amyloid appear around the tubules. The physical presence of amyloid causes ischemia and pressure atrophy of nephrons, and resultant scarring. The tubules contain a striking number of pink hyaline casts of protein and are dilated, sometimes to such an extent that normal renal structure is not recognized ("thyroidization"). Urinalysis reveals a high level of protein, and the loss of protein from this source may cause hypoproteinemic edema.

Thrombosis of the pulmonary arteries or renal veins is occasionally a prominent finding in dogs with the nephrotic syndrome due to amyloidosis; they are in a hypercoagulable state due to stimulation of production of acute-phase proteins, such as fibrinogen, and simultaneous loss of low molecular weight anticoagulants, such as antithrombin III, due to increased glomerular permeability.

The cat differs somewhat from other species in that amyloid is deposited mainly in the papilla and outer medulla, with relative sparing of the glomeruli. The kidneys are very firm, shrunken, and coarsely nodular. The papilla in cats dying in renal failure is necrotic, or excavated in some that survive. The nodularity is due to scarring extending from medulla to capsular surface. The capillary and tubular basement membranes in the medulla are thick and hyaline, and this is presumed to produce capillary occlusion with papillary necrosis on the one hand, and occlusion of collecting ducts with obstructive atrophy and fibrosis in the medullary rays on the other. The prevalence of amyloidosis in cats is much increased on diets providing excess vitamin A.

Amyloid is nonspecifically eosinophilic in routine sections and weakly birefringent in polarized light. The diagnosis is thus usually confirmed with special stains. Amyloid is stained a light orange-red with Congo red, and then exhibits green birefringence in polarized light. Amyloid exhibits a bright yellow fluorescence after staining with thioflavine-T, which may be required in cats due to poor staining of amyloid with Congo red in this species. These staining patterns of amyloid are due to its characteristic β-pleated pattern, which also confers on it resistance to proteolysis and its insolubility, hence its resistance to removal from tissues. The characteristic nonbranching fibrils of amyloid may be seen by electron microscopy. Because all amyloid fibrils have a β-pleated sheet structure, the term β-fibrilloses has been proposed as a more appropriate description of amyloid deposits and amyloidosis.

GLOMERULAR LIPIDOSIS. Large foam cells, which by appropriate techniques are seen to contain sudanophilic droplets, may be found in one or more lobules of glomerular tufts in many dogs (Fig. 5.9A). In paraffin preparations, the cells are closely packed and finely vacuolated, and the cell boundaries distinct. These large cells appear to arise from mesangial cells. This lesion is not associated with glomerulonephritis and has no functional significance.

Diseases of Tubules

Diseases of tubules are primarily reflected in morphologic changes in lining epithelial cells, although specific defects of function due to enzyme deletions may not have a morphologic representation. Degenerations are best regarded as homeostatic disturbances of intracellular functions that may become balanced at new levels or be sufficiently severe that the cell or part of it dies. As noted above, the tubules and interstitium are intimately associated, and damage to one affects the other, thus a number of disorders are termed tubulointerstitial diseases and are discussed later. Regeneration of tubular epithelium can occur (Fig. 5.11A,B), but postnatal development of new nephrons is limited to a short period of time, depending on species. The response of the kidney to destruction of tubules is limited to compensatory hypertrophy of remaining nephrons. Thus the tubules remaining in damaged kidneys are often large and dilated.

Degeneration and swelling of tubular cells cause the kidney to enlarge and bulge on cut surface. Hydropic degeneration occurs due to damage to mitochondrial membranes and formation of vacuoles and is potentially reversible. Necrotic tubular cells are eosinophilic, have pyknotic nuclei, and slough into the tubular lumen, where they are seen as cellular or coarsely granular casts (Figs. 5.10A,D and 5.11A). Tubules filled with proteinaceous fluid usually indicate increased glomerular permeability in that nephron; extreme proteinuria may indicate the presence of the nephrotic syndrome clinically. Tamm–Horsfall mucoprotein, which is produced in the ascending limb of the loop of Henle and the distal tubules, and/or autolytic tubular epithelial cytoplasm may appear as a granular pink substance in many cortical tubules, but this is not a lesion. Hyaline droplets, which are pink homogeneous globules of protein, appear in the cytoplasm of proximal tubular cells in nephrons with increased glomerular permeability. The hyaline droplets are lysosomes swollen with protein undergoing proteolysis and will be returned to the circulation as amino acids. Protein reabsorption by proximal tubules is a physiologic process; hyaline droplets indicate that this mechanism is saturated.

Fatty degeneration is difficult to evaluate in swine, dogs, and cats, which normally have considerable quantities of fat in the renal epithelium; infiltration fat accumulates in the loop of Henle in the outer medulla in starved animals. In fatty degeneration, the fat is usually found in the cells of the convoluted tubules.

Thickening of the basement membrane is seen in a variety of

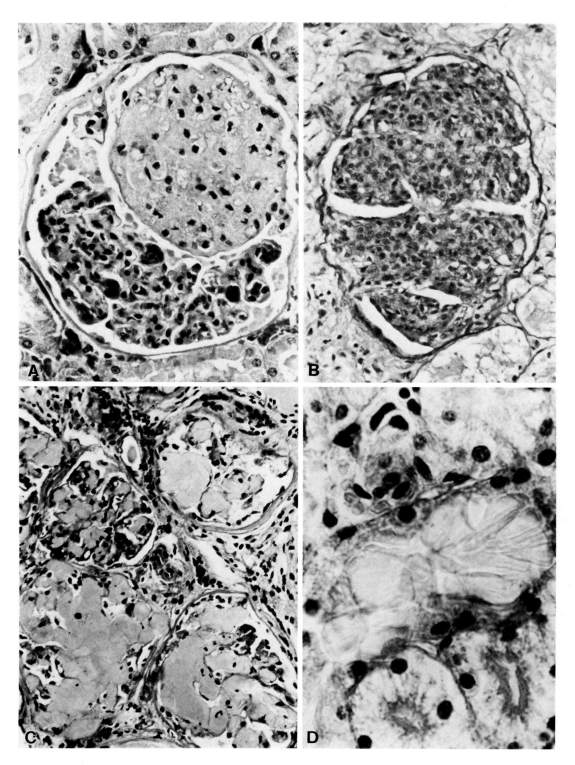

Fig. 5.9. (**A**) Glomerular lipidosis. Dog. (**B**) Proliferative glomerulonephritis. Doberman pinscher, 12 weeks old. (**C**) Amyloidosis. Dog. Severe lesions in glomeruli have caused atrophy of tubules and aggregation of tufts. (**D**) Oxalate crystals in proximal tubule. Dog.

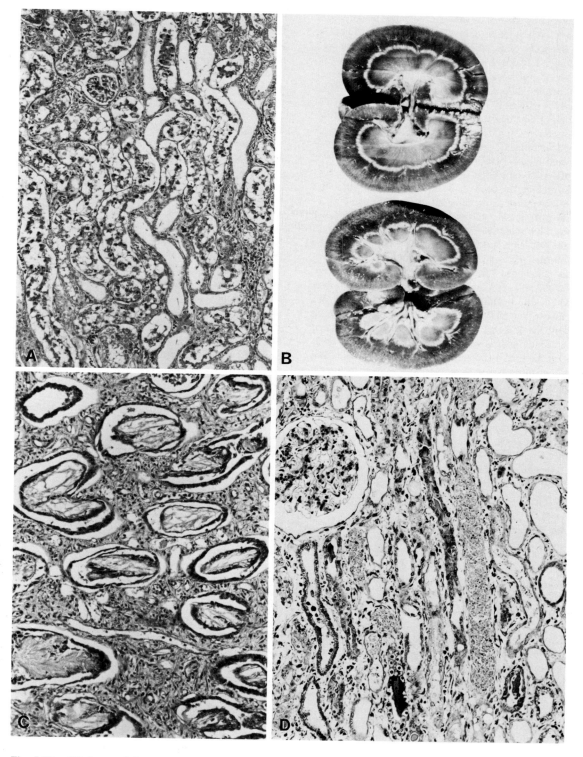

Fig. 5.10. (**A**) Acute tubular necrosis due to mercuric chloride poisoning. Necrosis, fragmentation, and shedding of tubular epithelium. Dog. (**B**) Hypercalcemic nephropathy. Dog. (**C**) Sulfonamide nephrosis. Calf. Sulfa crystals (removed in processing) have been covered by epithelium from collecting tubules. (**D**) Subacute nephrosis. Calf. *Amaranthus retroflexus*. Granular and hyaline casts, dilation of Bowman's spaces, interstitial edema, and tubules lined by flattened epithelium.

situations involving chronic tubule damage and is usually associated with atrophic tubular epithelium. In renal amyloidosis, amyloid is deposited on the tubular basement membrane as well as in glomeruli. Disruption of the tubular basement membrane occurs in ischemic necrosis and frequently in focal renal lesions and may allow herniation of tubular epithelial cells, with some of these cells persisting as interstitial foam cells.

In addition to the standard patterns of parenchymal cell degeneration, there are several miscellaneous histologic changes that may be found in renal epithelium. Some of the pyrrolizidine alkaloids cause megalocytosis in the proximal tubules. The lesion is similar in type to that in hepatocytes but is much less conspicuous and has not been observed to cause functional disturbance. Some pyrrolizidine alkaloid–containing plants, particularly *Crotalaria* spp., can produce significant glomerular megalocytosis and sclerosis in pigs that may lead to death from renal failure. Occasional nuclei in tubules of old dogs may be polyploid. In the proximal tubules, eosinophilic, crystalline, intranuclear inclusions (''brick inclusions'') are commonly encountered in old dogs. Similar inclusions occur in the liver, their source is unknown, and although they resemble the inclusions produced in experimental animals by heavy metals such as bismuth, they do not contain heavy metals. In cells in the same location, subacute lead poisoning produces amorphous, acid-fast inclusion material in nuclei, which are large, pale, and vesicular. Acute intravascular hemolysis results in the formation of hyaline droplets of hemoglobin in proximal tubular cells, and hemoglobin casts. Hemosiderin deposits are commonly found in animals and indicate previous intravascular hemolysis. Bile pigments may be present in hyperbilirubinemic animals. Renal pigmentation is considered in greater detail below. Glycogen is deposited in tubular cells in diabetes mellitus in dogs. As well as epithelial, granular, and hyaline casts, noted above, red-cell (hematuria) or white-cell (pyuria) casts may be recognized in sections.

Acute Tubular Necrosis

Acute tubular necrosis, or nephrosis, is a condition in which tubular degeneration is the primary process, and it is an important cause of acute renal failure. ''Nephrosis'' is an imprecise term applied to noninflammatory renal disease, particularly tubular degeneration; acute tubular necrosis is a more accurate descriptor of the changes to be discussed here. Affected animals are oliguric or anuric and die within a few days unless given appropriate therapy. The principal causes of acute tubular necrosis are ischemia and nephrotoxins. Another major cause of acute renal failure is postrenal, namely, complete urinary outflow obstruction. Severe acute glomerulonephritis can also cause acute renal failure but is uncommon in domestic animals. The renal tubules, particularly the proximal tubules, are metabolically very active and hence the renal components most susceptible to ischemia or nephrotoxins. ''Lower nephron nephrosis'' was a term applied in the past to acute tubular necrosis but is no longer used.

Ischemic or **tubulorrhectic acute tubular necrosis** follows a period of hypotension (shock) that causes marked renal isch-

emia. Prolonged renal ischemia causes renal cortical necrosis, that is, all cortical structures are affected. Massive hemolysis is a cause of acute tubular necrosis and produces an ischemic pattern known as hemoglobinuric nephrosis. Hemoglobin and myoglobin are not primary nephrotoxins, but they contribute to renal failure produced by other causes, such as hypotension. Ischemic tubular necrosis is characterized histologically by focal necrosis along nephrons, particularly the proximal tubules, and distal tubules to some extent, plus disruption of tubular basement membranes (tubulorrhexis) and occlusion of lumina by casts. Eosinophilic hyaline and granular casts occur commonly in the distal tubules and collecting ducts and consist of Tamm–Horsfall mucoproteins, degenerate epithelial cells, hemoglobin, myoglobin, and other plasma proteins. Interstitial edema may be present. Glomeruli are usually normal. After ~1 week, epithelial regeneration may be seen as tubules lined by flattened epithelium with hyperchromatic nuclei and mitoses (Fig. 5.11A,B). The renewed cells are smaller than normal initially and may appear close packed on the basement membrane. Their relationship with each other is also abnormal, and they tend frequently to pile up in small clusters, which eventually disappear. If the initial injury is mild and/or supportive therapy is adequate, recovery of architecture may be complete within about 2 to 3 weeks.

Nephrotoxic acute tubular necrosis, or exogenous toxic nephrosis, is contrasted here with ischemic necrosis, and specific examples are given below. Renal tubules, especially proximal tubules, are particularly susceptible to a wide variety of toxic agents as a consequence of their great metabolic activity and their exposure to agents in the large volume of ultrafiltrate they resorb in the process of urine formation. Their enzyme systems are thus exposed to, and inactivated by, agents such as heavy metals, which bind to sulfhydryl groups. Nephrotoxic acute tubular necrosis is usually characterized histologically by extensive necrosis of proximal tubules, but with preservation of tubular basement membranes (Fig. 5.10A). These two features distinguish toxic from ischemic nephrosis. Preservation of tubular basement membrane is necessary to provide the framework for epithelial regeneration, hence ischemic damage to tubules often has a worse prognosis for the kidney and the animal than toxic damage. Ischemia often complicates toxic nephrosis because the swelling of tubular epithelial cells caused by the toxin impairs intrarenal blood flow.

The pathogenesis of acute renal failure and oliguria in either ischemic or toxic necrosis remains controversial. Obstruction of tubular flow by cellular debris and casts appears to be an important factor (Fig. 5.10D). Other mechanisms proposed include preglomerular vasoconstriction, possibly due to activation of the renin–angiotensin system, leakage of tubular fluid into the interstitium, and decreased glomerular filtration, which occurs for unknown reasons. Oliguria is probably the result of various combinations of these factors. At the oliguric stage of acute renal failure, hyperkalemia is a life-threatening event. If the animal survives the oliguric phase, diuresis occurs, and electrolyte imbalances, such as hypokalemia, may contribute to death. As tubular regeneration proceeds, azotemia resolves and tubular function slowly returns.

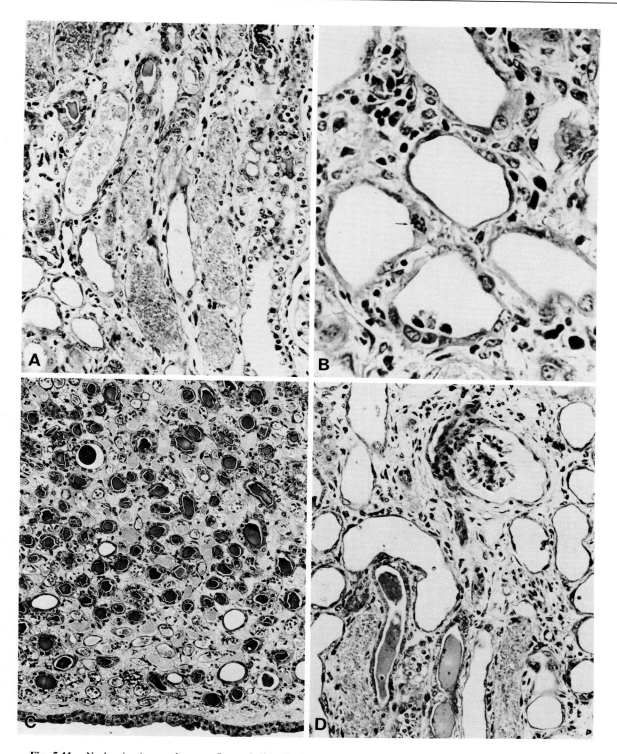

Fig. 5.11. Nephrosis. *Amaranthus retroflexus*. Calf. (A) Granular and hyaline casts. Tubules lined by flattened epithelium. Regenerating epithelial cells in tubules (arrows). (B) Mitotic figure in regenerating tubule (arrow). (C) Protein casts in medulla. (D) Fibrosis beginning around glomerulus and between tubules.

TABLE 5.2

Agents That Are Nephrotoxic in Domestic Animals

Exogenous	Antibiotics
	Aminoglycosides (neomycin, kanamycin, gentamicin, streptomycin, tobramycin)
	Tetracyclines
	Sulfonamides (sulfapyridine, sulfathiazole, sulfadiazine)
	Antifungals
	Amphotericin B
	Metals
	Arsenic
	Bismuth
	Cadmium
	Lead
	Mercury
	Thallium
	Paraquat
	Monensin
	Ethylene glycol
	Chlorinated hydrocarbons
	Methoxyflurane
	Oxalates (various plants)
	Mycotoxins (ochratoxin A, citrinin)
	Amaranthus retroflexus (pigweed)
	Tannins (*Quercus* spp., oaks)
	Lantana camara
	Isotropis
	Sodium fluoride (superphosphate fertilizer)
Endogenous	Bile
	Hemoglobin
	Myoglobin

Nephrotoxic Acute Tubular Necrosis

Numerous toxic substances may cause acute tubular necrosis in domestic animals (Table 5.2). Some are no longer important as nephrotoxins; for example, organomercurials were often used as fungicides on seed grains that were occasionally fed inadvertently to animals and humans with disastrous results. This use of mercury has been banned in many countries. Similarly, highly chlorinated naphthalenes, which cause hyperkeratosis and nephrosis in cattle, have been excluded from the farm environment. Sulfonamides were formerly important as nephrotoxins, but newer formulations are more soluble and less toxic. Some newly introduced agents have nephrotoxicity as a side effect (e.g., aminoglycosides). Numerous additional antibiotics that are toxic to humans (e.g., penicillin, semisynthetic penicillins, and polymixins) may also prove toxic to domestic animals. The toxicity of many of the exogenous agents is exacerbated by various systemic states, such as dehydration or shock, which concomitantly impair renal function in the affected animal. Discussion of specific examples of nephrotoxins follows.

Aminoglycosides

The group of aminoglycoside (aminocyclitol) drugs includes, in decreasing order of nephrotoxicity, neomycin, kanamycin, gentamicin, streptomycin, and tobramycin. Aminoglycosides are excreted primarily by glomerular filtration and selectively accumulate in, and cause damage to, proximal tubules; changes in tubular cells include formation of cytosegrosomes and myeloid bodies, and eventually necrosis. The pathogenesis of nephrotoxicity is not well established. Damage is dose related and enhanced by preexisting renal impairment. Toxicity is manifest clinically by inability to concentrate urine and by polyuria, proteinuria (due to degeneration and necrosis of proximal tubular cells), hematuria, cylindruria, and azotemia. Acute renal failure may result. Recovery from the nephrosis may occur even in the face of continued therapy, however, because the regenerating cells have increased resistance to aminoglycoside toxicity.

Tetracyclines

Tetracyclines cause several syndromes of renal disease in humans: progressive azotemia due to their antianabolic effect, a reversible Fanconi syndrome due to the use of outdated tetracycline-containing degradation products, and a reversible nephrogenic diabetes insipidus. An overdose of oxytetracycline may produce acute tubular necrosis and renal failure in dogs. Tetracycline administration has been reported to cause acute nephrosis and death in calves due to the presence of tetracycline degradation products. Use of tetracyclines is contraindicated in animals in renal failure.

Sulfonamides

Severe nephropathy may follow the ingestion of excessive doses of sulfonamides, especially if treated animals are dehydrated. Toxicity was much more common previously when only less soluble forms of the drug were available (e.g., sulfapyridine, sulfathiazole, and sulfadiazine). Crystalline nephropathy is now rare as the newer, shorter-acting sulfonamides have greater solubility. Affected kidneys are slightly enlarged and congested, and the sulfonamide crystals are grossly visible in the medulla, pelvis, and in some cases even in heavy deposits in the bladder. The deposits are yellow and form pale radial lines in the medulla. Crystals are not observed in section as they are dissolved during processing. The epithelium of the proximal convoluted tubules and of Bowman's capsule undergoes severe hydropic degeneration. There is little evidence of necrosis in the distal and convoluted tubules, but epithelial proliferation and swelling are prominent, and the tubules become densely populated with large, dark-staining cells. Some papillary formations into the lumen may even be present, and commonly in the collecting tubules there is more or less complete duplication of the epithelium, the inner epithelium enclosing a faintly basophilic hyaline precipitate (Fig. 5.10C). There is a diffuse but mild interstitial reaction about the corticomedullary junction. It appears that the renal lesions are due to both local toxic and mechanical effects and that hypersensitivity does not play a role in animals, as it apparently does in humans.

Amphotericin B

Amphotericin B is an antifungal agent, a polyene antibiotic, whose most important toxic effect is renal dysfunction. It causes decreased renal blood flow and glomerular filtration due to renal vasoconstriction. Necrosis of proximal and distal tubules occurs, and there is intratubular calcium deposition.

Ethylene Glycol

Dogs and cats are commonly poisoned by ingestion of ethylene glycol (antifreeze). The seasonal incidence of this poisoning coincides with the changing of engine antifreeze solutions in the spring and autumn. Cattle are also occasionally poisoned. Ethylene glycol, which is present in 95% concentration in antifreeze solutions, has a sweet taste and is usually voluntarily ingested, especially by young male dogs. Cats are more susceptible, but less commonly affected, than dogs; the minimum lethal dose is 1.5 ml/kg for cats and 6.6 ml/kg for dogs.

Ethylene glycol, which is itself nontoxic, is rapidly absorbed from the gastrointestinal tract, and most is excreted unchanged in the urine. A small percentage is oxidized by alcohol dehydrogenase in the liver to glycoaldehyde, which is in turn oxidized to glycolic acid, glyoxalate, and finally, oxalate. Glycolic acid (glycolate) is the primary toxic metabolite of ethylene glycol. Other end products of metabolism are lactic acid, hippuric acid, and carbon dioxide.

Central nervous system signs develop 30 min to 12 hr after ingestion of ethylene glycol. Although oxalate crystals are deposited around cerebral vessels and in perivascular spaces, nervous signs are due to the effect of aldehydes and possibly to the severe metabolic acidosis that develops as a result of accumulation of lactic acid, glycolate, and glyoxylate. Over the next 12 hr, pulmonary edema, tachypnea, and tachycardia occur. If the animal survives for 1 to 3 days after ingestion, acute renal failure develops, primarily due to renal tubular damage by glycoaldehyde, glycolic acid, glyoxylic acid, and oxalate. Severe renal edema impairs intrarenal blood flow and contributes to nephrosis and renal failure. Soluble calcium oxalates in the blood precipitate in the ultrafiltrate of the renal tubules as the pH of the fluid decreases. Calcium oxalate crystals may be found in tubular lumina (Fig. 5.9D), tubular cells, and the interstitium; they are light yellow, arranged in sheaves, rosettes, or prisms, and are birefringent in polarized light. Tubular lesions range from hydropic degeneration, to necrosis, to regeneration. In animals surviving the acute toxic insult, calcium oxalate crystals are thought to be of importance in causing renal failure. Large numbers of crystals in tubules are virtually pathognomonic of ethylene glycol poisoning; a few crystals may be seen with chronic tubular obstruction. Occasional calcium oxalate crystals are normally seen in urine sediment of dogs; large numbers of these crystals are highly suggestive of poisoning. Hypocalcemia due to the formation of crystals is usually mild in dogs. Animals that survive the acute exposure toxicity may have renal interstitial fibrosis. Few crystals may be left in the tubules; they tend to be removed in the weeks following their deposition. As well, hippuric acid crystals are found in the urine of dogs with ethylene glycol poisoning.

Oxalate

Plants are the usual source of oxalate poisoning in sheep and cattle. Plants that may contain toxic amounts of oxalate are *Halogeton glomeratus*, halogeton; *Sarcobatus vermiculatus*, greasewood; *Rheum rhaponticum*, the common garden rhubarb; *Oxalis cernua*, soursob; *Rumex* spp., sorrel, dock. Additional plants of lesser importance are *Portulacca oleracea*, *Trianthema portulacastrum*, and *Threlkeldia proceriflora* as well as some cultivated species such as mangel and sugar beet. Young plants may contain the equivalent of 7% or more of potassium oxalate; the amount decreases with maturity and drying of the plant. The above-listed plants are only eaten in unusual circumstances and not readily. Species of grasses in the genera *Cenchrus, Panicum,* and *Setaria,* which are widely cultivated in tropical and subtropical areas and which accumulate large amounts of oxalate, have been associated with renal oxalosis in cattle and skeletal disease in horses, the latter due to conditioned calcium deficiency.

Mortality rates of 10% may occur in sheep when, as frequently happens in some areas, these animals graze on almost pure stands of halogeton or soursob. It is more usual, however, for fatalities to be sporadic. Under natural conditions, sheep may ingest up to 75 g of oxalate a day, thus the ovine rumen must degrade the salt efficiently. Depending on the diet before exposure to oxalate-containing plants and, therefore, on the microbial composition of the rumen, some variation is to be expected in the ability of ruminal contents to degrade the salt. Cattle are less commonly affected under range conditions than sheep, but cattle and sheep are equally susceptible to experimental poisoning. Horses are resistant to oxalate-induced nephrosis and succumb to acute gastroenteritis only after receiving unnaturally large amounts of the chemical; they may develop osteodystrophia fibrosa with prolonged exposure (see Bones and Joints, Volume 1).

Chelation of calcium by unmetabolized oxalate in the ingesta contributes to hypocalcemia. Following absorption, oxalates combine with calcium to form insoluble calcium oxalate; hypocalcemic tetany may result. Calcium oxalate may crystallize in vessel lumens or walls, causing vascular necrosis and hemorrhage, or in renal tubules, causing tubular obstruction and acute renal failure. The nephrotoxicity of oxalates involves more than mechanical obstruction and may be due in part to intracellular chelation of calcium and magnesium and hence interference with oxidative phosphorylation. Clinically, weakness, prostration, and death may follow within 12 hr of ingestion of oxalate-containing plants.

Oxalates are produced endogenously in the degradation of glycine, an important constituent amino acid of collagen and elastin. A few crystals can frequently be found in fetal kidneys and in scarred tubules in any species; these oxalate crystals are without significance.

Mycotoxins

Aspergillus and *Penicillium* produce a number of nephrotoxic mycotoxins, namely, ochratoxins, citrinin, oxalate, and viridicatum toxin, which can contaminate feed grains. Ochratoxins have the general structure of β-phenylalanine linked to dehydroisocoumarin. Ochratoxin A is the only member of the group that is significant in disease. In pigs, ochratoxin A and citrinin produce tubular degeneration and atrophy, cortical interstitial fibrosis, and glomerular hyalinosis; the renal insufficiency produced is usually subclinical. Acute renal disease occurs very rarely and is manifested by severe perirenal edema resembling that produced by redroot pigweed (*Amaranthus retroflexus*, see below). Moldy feed also produces mycotoxic nephropathy in horses. Citrinin produces tubular degeneration in swine, horses, and sheep. Ochratoxins normally are degraded in the rumen, thus toxicity is unlikely to occur in ruminants.

Amaranthus retroflexus

Ingestion of redroot pigweed (*Amaranthus retroflexus*) causes perirenal edema and acute renal failure due to toxic nephrosis in swine and cattle, and uncommonly, in horses. The nephrotoxic principle of *A. retroflexus* has not yet been identified; the plants often contain high levels of nitrate and oxalate, but neither nitrate nor oxalate poisoning usually occur and do not produce perirenal edema. Lush growth of the plant occurs in early summer, and this plant often dominates the weed growth in disused lots and yards to which animals are moved when other pasture is depleted. Weakness, recumbency, and often death follow 5–10 days after grazing begins. Grossly, there is marked perirenal edema, which may be blood stained and accompanied by edema of mesenteries, bowel wall, and ventral abdominal wall, with moderate ascites and hydrothorax. The kidneys are pale but not usually enlarged. Histologically, there is degeneration and coagulation necrosis of proximal and distal tubules (Fig. 5.11), sometimes with mild glomerular epithelial injury and hypercellularity. Tubules contain granular casts. Animals that survive have cortical interstitial fibrosis and tubular dilation. The perirenal edema seen in acute cases is apparently due to tubular back-leak, with subsequent lymphatic drainage and leakage into perirenal connective tissue. The probable cause of death is heart failure due to hyperkalemia.

Oak

Poisoning of ruminants and occasionally of horses by acorns, leaves, and buds of oak shrubs and trees (*Quercus* spp.) occurs throughout the northern hemisphere, in some parts of which the acorns are accepted as a dietary staple in late autumn and early winter. There are many species and varieties of oaks, but not all are palatable. They are all potentially poisonous by virtue of the tannins they contain, but for the most part, they appear to be eaten with impunity. Simple indigestion occurs fairly frequently in cattle eating large amounts of the material, but gastroenteritis and acute tubular necrosis occur in a small number of animals only. The toxic substances are tannins; they are hydrolyzed to gallic acid and pyrogallol, which appear to be the active toxic metabolites and are capable of producing the same syndrome as tannic acid.

In acute oak poisoning, there is marked perirenal edema and hemorrhage, the kidneys are swollen and pale and, in cattle, are rather uniformly sprinkled with cortical hemorrhages 2–3 mm in diameter. The glomeruli are ischemic but otherwise normal, except for dilation of the urinary space after several days. There may be microscopic hematuria. Necrosis of the epithelium of the proximal tubules can be complete, to produce within the base-

ment membrane dense homogeneous casts. In less severe injury, adjacent groups of tubules may vary considerably in the extent of degeneration. Some animals may recover, and in others the renal lesion progresses with shrinkage and diffuse fibrosis and scattered collections of mononuclear cells. The completeness of the necrosis in groups of tubules with intratubular hemorrhage distinguishes the nephrosis of acute oak poisoning from that of other causes, although poisoning by the yellow-wood tree (*Terminalia oblongata*) in Australia, is reputed to produce similar lesions. The nonrenal lesions in cattle are those seen in acute renal uremia in this species, particularly the anasarca, severe perirenal edema, and hemorrhage ulcerative colitis.

Isotropis

Several species of the genus *Isotropis* are toxic to ruminants. In both cattle and sheep, reference is made to abomasitis and enteritis, petechial hemorrhages throughout the gastrointestinal tract, and accumulation of fluid in the body cavities and subcutis. The renal lesions are dominated by necrosis of proximal tubular epithelium. In many acute poisonings, there is abundant proteinaceous fluid in Bowman's space.

Specific Tubular Dysfunctions

Renal tubular dysfunction may occur secondary to other conditions; for example, glucosuria occurs when the tubular transport maximum for glucose is exceeded in diabetes mellitus and acute enterotoxemia, and heavy-metal toxicity causes glucosuria and aminoaciduria due to tubular degeneration. The primary tubular transport defects identified in domestic animals are hyperuricosuria in Dalmatian dogs, essential cystinuria, the syndrome of multiple resorptive defects in basenji dogs, and renal glucosuria. Hyperuricosuria and cystinuria are of importance because they predispose to urolithiasis, and are discussed in the section on that condition.

Basenjis and several other breeds of dogs may develop a proximal tubular disorder similar to the Fanconi syndrome in humans; the condition appears to be hereditary in basenjis. The syndrome in dogs is characterized by polyuria, polydipsia, hyposthenuria, glycosuria, normoglycemia, hyperphosphaturia, proteinuria, and aminoaciduria. The aminoaciduria may be generalized or limited to cystinuria. Affected dogs have impaired renal rubular reabsorption of glucose, phosphate, sodium, potassium, uric acid, and amino acids. Polyuria results from the glycosuria and natriuresis. The syndrome develops in adult dogs and is usually slowly progressive. Dehydration and acidosis result in renal papillary necrosis and death due to renal failure. Histologic renal changes are nonspecific and include interstitial fibrosis and tubular atrophy. Affected basenjis usually have karyomegaly in occasional tubular cells. Ultrastructural abnormalities have not been noted in tubular cells.

Renal glycosuria may occur as a singular transport abnormality without other defects. This defect is an inherited disorder in Norwegian elkhounds.

Hepatorenal Syndromes

The term hepatorenal syndrome is vague, and more specific diagnoses should be sought, but a number of more or less distinct associations of renal disease can occur in animals with hepatic disease. They may be the result of hypovolemia, failure of clearance of gastrointestinal bacteria and endotoxins from the portal blood with development of disseminated intravascular coagulation, or the result of various hepatic metabolites. Concentrations of bilirubin and bile acids may be greatly elevated in the blood, especially in obstructive jaundice, and the pigment accumulates in tubular epithelium, which is frequently swollen and hydropic ("cholemic nephrosis"). Some nephrotoxins are also (or mainly) hepatotoxic (e.g., carbon tetrachloride and *Lantana camara*).

Glycogen Nephrosis

In diabetes mellitus in dogs and cats, glycogen is deposited in the tubular epithelium (Fig. 5.8B), producing marked vacuolation of the epithelium in the outer medulla and innermost cortex. Glycogen can be readily demonstrated by appropriate techniques. The deposition occurs in the ascending limb, disappears following insulin administration, and has no effect on renal function. Often in diabetes mellitus of long duration there is hyaline thickening of the afferent arteriole, which may extend to the capillary basement membranes of the glomerulus.

Nephrogenic Diabetes Insipidus

This condition has been reported in several dogs with polyuria, polydipsia, and hyposthenuria. Affected dogs are unresponsive to water deprivation, exogenous administration of antidiuretic hormone, and infusion of hypertonic saline. The basis of the defect is a lack of responsiveness of the cells of the distal tubules and collecting ducts to the hormone. The defect may be congenital, or acquired as the result of tubulointerstitial diseases such as pyelonephritis or hypercalcemic nephropathy.

Hypokalemic Nephropathy (Vacuolar)

Chronic potassium depletion in humans, caused by diarrhea, adrenal overactivity, and some renal diseases, can result in impaired urine concentration and polyuria. Coarse vacuolation of the proximal convoluted tubules is due to reversible dilation of intercellular spaces. A vacuolar degeneration of proximal tubular cells has been reported in ewes deliberately given 11–17 times the recommended dose of thiabendazole. Many of the ewes developed hypokalemia, hypoproteinemia, and uremia before death; potassium loss was thought to occur through the kidneys. In a proposed case of hypokalemic nephropathy in a dog, chronic vomition due to a gastric foreign body was thought to be the cause of potassium depletion. Corticosteroids produce hypokalemia and reversible vacuolar degeneration of tubular cells. Hypokalemia may be related to the tubular dilation commonly seen in baby pigs with diarrhea and is related to experimental production of renal cysts.

Pigmentary Changes in the Kidney

Following acute hemolytic crises of any cause, the kidneys may by very dark, almost black, as a consequence of concentrated **hemoglobin**. Initially, the discoloration is uniform, but shortly thereafter most of the hemoglobin is dispersed, except from scattered clusters of nephrons in which it persists for many days to produce a diffuse brown speckling of the cortices. The color alone provides a good distinction between this pigmentary change and the red or blue speckling that occurs in acute hemorrhagic glomerulitis. It is particularly characteristic of the hemolytic crisis of chronic copper poisoning in sheep. Microscopically, the hemoglobin appears as fine red granules in the epithelial cells of the tubules and as red casts in the lower reaches of the nephron, especially Henle's loop and the collecting tubules. The same histologic picture occurs following incompatible blood transfusions and in paralytic myoglobinuria of horses, in which disease the pigment is **myoglobin**. Nutritional muscular degeneration of young animals does not produce this renal lesion because the myoglobin content of their muscle is very low. Hemoglobin and myoglobin pigmentation persist after the hemoglobin or myoglobin are no longer detectable grossly in urine samples.

Hemosiderosis occurs in the course of chronic hemolytic anemia and as residue from acute hemoglobinuric episodes. The pigment is found in epithelial cells of proximal tubules where it is produced by the degradation of resorbed hemoglobin, and it may be sufficient to produce a distinctive brown coloration of the cortex.

Lipofuscinosis of the kidneys of adult cattle, also referred to as hemochromatosis and xanthomatosis, consists of the deposition of brown iron-free pigments with staining characteristics of lipofuscin (Fig. 5.12A). The pigmentation also affects striated muscles, giving them too a dark-brown appearance. On the cut surface of the kidney, the pigmentation occurs in radial dark lines in the cortex but spares the medulla. Microscopically, it is present as fine, brown granules in the epithelial cells of the convoluted tubules. An environmental lipofuscinosis of the liver, kidney and other organs is discussed with the Liver and Biliary System (this volume).

Cloisonné kidney is a nonclinical pigmentary condition in goats. The renal cortices are uniformly brown or black, due to thickening and brown pigmentation of basement membranes restricted to the convoluted portions of the proximal tubules (Fig. 5.12B). The basement membrane thickening is due to the deposition of ferritin and hemosiderin, presumably the result of repeated episodes of intravascular hemolysis. A similar renal discoloration and basement membrane thickening has been reported in a horse, but was found to be due to lipofuscinosis.

In congenital **porphyria** of cattle, swine, and cats, brown pigmentation affects the cortex. Histologically, the pigment is present in the tubular epithelium and the interstitial tissue. The pigment is excreted in the urine, which, if allowed to stand in light, develops a port wine color due to photic activation of porphyrins. The urine and tissues fluoresce blue-green in ultraviolet light.

A green-yellow pigmentation of swollen kidneys is common in **icterus** of hepatic origin, and less notable in hemolytic icterus unless there is concomitant hepatic injury. It has been described under Hepatorenal Syndromes. Olive green coloration of the renal cortex is common in newborn lambs, calves, and foals. The pigment is bilirubin, and its presence is probably due to immaturity of hepatic conjugating mechanisms.

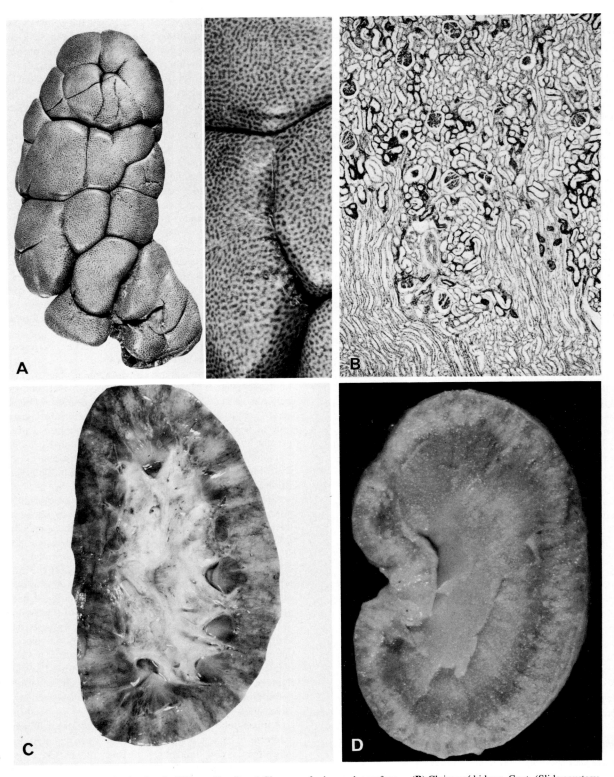

Fig. 5.12.   (**A**) Lipofuscinosis. Kidney. Ox. (Inset) Close-up of subcapsular surface.   (**B**) Cloisonné kidney. Goat. (Slide courtesy of A. Zubaidy.)   (**C**) Acute interstitial nephritis. Pig.   (**D**) Chronic renal fibrosis and mineralization (end-stage kidney) in Shih Tzu dog.

Tubulointerstitial Diseases

Tubulointerstitial diseases are those that involve primarily the interstitium and tubules. The term acknowledges that inflammatory and degenerative diseases of the interstitium almost always impair tubular function. Hence interstitial nephritis, which may be acute or chronic, focal or generalized, suppurative, or nonsuppurative, and pyelonephritis are classified as tubulointerstitial diseases. There is obvious overlap with the previous category of acute tubular necrosis, since animals that survive acute tubular necrosis often develop interstitial inflammation and fibrosis. Also included as tubulointerstitial disease may be nephropathy due to hypercalcemia, hypokalemia, analgesics, and oxalates as well as immunologically mediated tubulointerstitial disease.

Interstitial inflammation and fibrosis are the two predominant features of these diseases (Fig. 5.12C,D). Interstitial nephritis is usually hematogenous and part of systemic disease, while pyelonephritis is usually urogenous; both are usually due to infectious agents, although agents are often not identified, especially in chronic cases. Injury to glomeruli and vessels is usually secondary in tubulointerstitial disease, although they are eventually involved because of the interdependence of renal structures. The hallmark of glomerular disease is persistent proteinuria, while tubulointerstitial diseases are more likely to demonstrate defects of concentrating ability or specific tubular defects of resorption or secretion. However, the end point of both classes of renal disease, and the usual clinical presentation, is decompensated renal failure with isosthenuria and uremia.

Immunologically mediated tubulointerstitial disease has been identified in humans, and suspected, but not proved, in domestic animals. Hypersensitivity reactions occur to a variety of drugs (e.g., methicillin). Tubular immune-complex disease occurs in some patients with lupus nephritis and glomerulonephritis, indicating that autoantibodies may cross-react with glomerular and tubular basement membranes.

Nonsuppurative Interstitial Nephritis

Focal inflammation with slight scarring and some lymphoreticular cells is common in kidneys. The causes are seldom known and probably not specific; some lesions may be primarily inflammatory, and some may be foci of antigen persistence in scars of other origins.

This form of nephritis may be acute or chronic, and multifocal or generalized, probably depending on the intensity of the insult and the efficiency of the host's responses. Acute interstitial nephritis is characterized by acute clinical onset, and histologically by interstitial edema, leukocytic infiltration, and focal tubular necrosis. In chronic interstitial nephritis, there is mononuclear-cell infiltration, interstitial fibrosis, and generalized tubular atrophy. Many infectious agents are capable of causing nonsuppurative interstitial nephritis, and some are discussed here, but agents are often not identified in naturally occurring cases, especially in the chronic stages. Interstitial nephritis is common in dogs and cats, both as a primary disease and secondary to glomerular diseases. Acute generalized interstitial nephritis can be caused by *Leptospira canicola* infection in dogs. *Leptospira canicola* is commonly associated with in-

terstitial nephritis in the United Kingdom, although its importance is declining because of the efficacy of vaccination; *L. icterohemorrhagiae* and canine adenovirus-1 (infectious canine hepatitis) are also commonly involved.

According to serologic evidence, leptospirosis is common in domestic animals, and in severe cases, interstitial nephritis often occurs. The most severe infections are usually caused by *Leptospira pomona* in cattle and swine, and *L. canicola* and *L. icterohemorrhagiae* in dogs. When inflammation gradually subsides, marked interstitial fibrosis and loss of nephrons cause contracture of the kidney, and chronic interstitial nephritis results. Diffuse interstitial nephritis is less common in large domestic animals than in dogs; the usual end result of leptospirosis in cattle and swine is a focal interstitial nephritis. Leptospirosis is discussed with the Hematopoietic System (Volume 3).

Encephalitozoon cuniculi, an obligate intracellular protozoan parasite, causes diffuse nonsuppurative to granulomatous interstitial nephritis and granulomatous encephalitis in dogs. The renal lesion is characterized by heavy, almost pure interstitial infiltrates of plasma cells. The Gram-positive organisms occur in tubular epithelial cells, tubular lumina, and in vessel walls. The disease is discussed with the Nervous System (Volume 1).

The best known form of focal nonsuppurative interstitial nephritis is the "white-spotted kidney" of calves. This is common; it appears to be of little significance because it is largely an incidental finding in young calves and is probably obliterated with advancing age. The cause is usually undetermined but is most likely the result of bacteremia; *Escherichia coli* can occasionally be recovered from the lesions. *Salmonella* and *Brucella* are other suggested causes. Affected kidneys contain multiple small white nodules of up to 1 cm diameter throughout the cortex. The larger nodules may bulge from the capsular surface of the kidney and adhere to the capsule (Fig. 5.13A). Histologically, the initial lesion is a microabscess, which is usually replaced by many lymphocytes and occasional plasma cells and macrophages. Progressive fibrosis results in healing by scar tissue. The inflammation and scarring may cause tubular obstruction and/or atrophy (Fig. 5.13D).

Focal interstitial nephritis also occurs in cattle in the course of malignant catarrhal fever, theileriosis, and lumpy-skin disease; in sheep, in sheeppox; and in the horse, in equine infectious anemia. The renal lesions do not contribute significantly to the course of these diseases but are of some diagnostic importance; their gross and histologic features are given elsewhere. Focal pyogranulomatous lesions are a rather consistent finding in the kidneys of cats with feline infectious peritonitis. Canine herpesvirus produces a severe necrotizing nephritis as part of the systemic disease in puppies (see the Female Genital System, Volume 3).

Suppurative Interstitial Nephritis

Bacterial infection of the kidneys may be either hematogenous (Fig. 5.13B,C) and cause embolic suppurative nephritis, or urogenous and cause pyelonephritis. Pyelonephritis means inflammation of both the pelvis and renal parenchyma, and while pelvic inflammation may result from septic renal foci

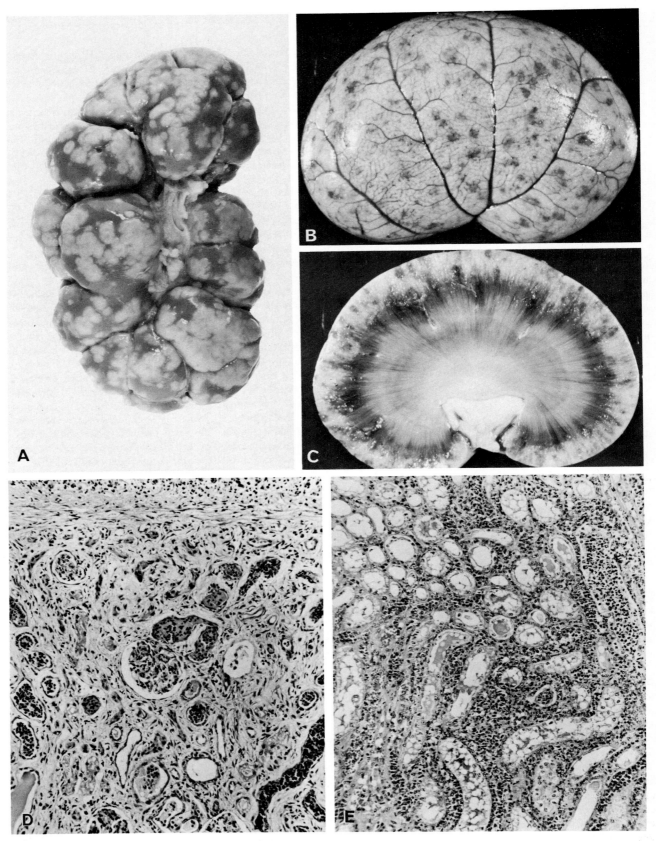

Fig. 5.13. (A) ''White-spotted kidney.'' Calf. (B and C) Multifocal embolic nephritis. Cat. *Pasteurella multocida*. (D) Section of cortex in (A), showing interstitial reaction. (E) Hematogenous interstitial nephritis. Dog. *Klebsiella pneumoniae*.

(Fig. 5.14A), most cases of pyelonephritis arise from ascending urinary infections.

Embolic Suppurative Nephritis

This is analogous to abscess formation in any organ and occurs when any of a wide variety of bacteria are seeded in the kidneys in the course of bacteremia or septic thromboembolism. Bacteria alone or in small clumps, and small septic emboli, lodge mainly in glomerular and peritubular capillaries (Figs. 5.7A and 5.13E) and may produce multiple small abscesses or fewer large ones. Larger emboli lodge in afferent vessels and produce septic infarcts, which may be unilateral. Many bacteria undoubtedly pass through the glomerular capillary walls into the tubules, where they are probably harmless unless there is stasis of urine. Developed abscesses are generally cortical rather than medullary, but in bacteremia caused by Gram-negative enterobacteria, microscopic suppurative foci may be scattered in the medulla. If healing of the suppurative lesions occurs, it is by scar formation. The healed lesions of isolated abscesses are occasionally seen, but extensive renal scarring as a sequel to multiple abscessation is rare as the animal is likely to die of the primary disease or from renal insufficiency early in the course of the disease.

In horses, the most common cause of embolic suppurative nephritis is *Actinobacillus equuli*, which is acquired *in utero*, during parturition, or shortly after birth; it is probably an umbilical infection. Death may occur due to fulminating septicemia. In foals that survive for several days, typical microabscessation is seen in the kidneys and other organs, and polyarthritis is present. The abscesses are usually green-yellow foci of up to 3 mm in diameter and contain a small droplet of pus. The most common cause of embolic nephritis in swine is probably *Erysipelothrix rhusiopathiae*. Embolic glomerulonephritis may be seen grossly as glomerular hemorrhages; microabscesses form in the interstitium. In adult cattle, most cases are caused by *Corynebacterium pyogenes* from valvular endocarditis, the septic emboli often producing large, randomly distributed abscesses and infarcts. In sheep and goats, renal abscessation caused by *C. pseudotuberculosis* is common.

Pyelonephritis

Pyelonephritis is inflammation of the pelvis and renal parenchyma, usually resulting from infection ascending from the lower urinary tract. It is characterized by inflammation, necrosis, and eventually, deformity of the calyces, in association with areas of tubulointerstitial inflammation and necrosis, and is hence distinguishable from other forms of nephritis. It is usually accompanied by ureteritis and cystitis. In acute pyelonephritis, cellular infiltration and necrosis predominate, with pelvic and medullary involvement more severe and advanced than involvement of the cortex. In chronic pyelonephritis, fibrosis replaces inflammation. In both cases, the disease process is asymmetric within the kidney, and chronic pyelonephritis may produce very irregular contracture of the kidneys with pelvic deformities. Pyonephrosis is the term applied to severe suppuration of the kidney in the presence of complete or nearly complete ureteral obstruction; the infected hydronephrotic kidney is converted to a sac of pus.

The pathogenesis of pyelonephritis begins with establishment of infection in the lower urinary tract, and this is dealt with below under Inflammation of the Lower Urinary Tract. Organisms involved in urinary tract infection are usually endogenous bacteria of the bowel and skin, such as *Escherichia coli*, staphylococci, streptococci, *Enterobacter, Proteus*, and *Pseudomonas*, and more specific urinary pathogens such as *Corynebacterium renale* in cattle, and *C. suis* in pigs. Infection is often mixed, and while *C. renale* may be present in bovine pyelonephritis and is an obligate parasite of urinary mucosae, various enteric pathogens may be of more pathogenetic importance. Virulence of bacteria in the urinary tract, as elsewhere, is enhanced by the presence of pili on their surface. Pili assist adhesion of *C. renale* to urinary epithelium; this process is pH dependent. One of the urinary tract defenses against bacterial infection and colonization is shedding of mature epithelial cells with attached bacteria. Normal voiding of urine, plus immune and other mechanisms, usually maintains sterility of the bladder, but once bacteria enter the bladder (e.g., via catheterization), they grow well in urine of low osmolality or alkaline pH. Stasis of urine is an important predisposing factor in the pathogenesis of cystitis and pyelonephritis. Urinary obstruction may be caused by ureteral anomalies in young animals, kinked ureters in pigs, pregnancy, urolithiasis, and prostatic hypertrophy. Females are predisposed to urinary tract infection because of their short urethras, urethral trauma, and possibly, hormonal effects. Clinically, infection is indicated by bloody or cloudy urine, with pyuria and bacteriuria. The presence of antibody-coated bacteria in urine, as detected by the fluorescent-antibody technique, indicates that the bacteria are of renal rather than bladder origin and is indicative of pyelonephritis.

Once infection is established in the bladder, probably the most significant mechanism in causing renal infection is **vesicoureteral reflux**. This retrograde flow of urine up the ureters may carry bacteria as far as the urinary space of glomeruli (intrarenal reflux). Reflux may occur during micturition, especially if there is urinary obstruction, or as a result of external compression of the bladder, as occurs during manual compression of the bladder in dogs and cats for collection of urine samples. Vesicoureteral reflux is very common in puppies and is a function of the short intravesical length of the ureters and hence an easily overcome vesicoureteral valve; reflux decreases with age and the development of greater intravesical length of the ureter and its more oblique entry through the bladder wall. Vesicoureteral reflux of sterile urine does little renal damage; the ureteral muscular layers may hypertrophy. Cystitis may alter normal ureteral peristalsis, perhaps causing reversed peristaltic waves. Hence persistent renal infection may result from vesicoureteral reflux, and possibly from reversed peristalsis, in animals with bladder infection and thus contribute to chronic active pyelonephritis. Progression of pyelonephritis probably depends on persistence of bacterial infection, or at least of bacterial antigens. Protoplasts (L forms) may be produced after antibacterial therapy and persist in the medulla; their significance is unknown.

For a number of reasons, the medulla is the part of the kidney most susceptible to infection. It is relatively hypoxic because of

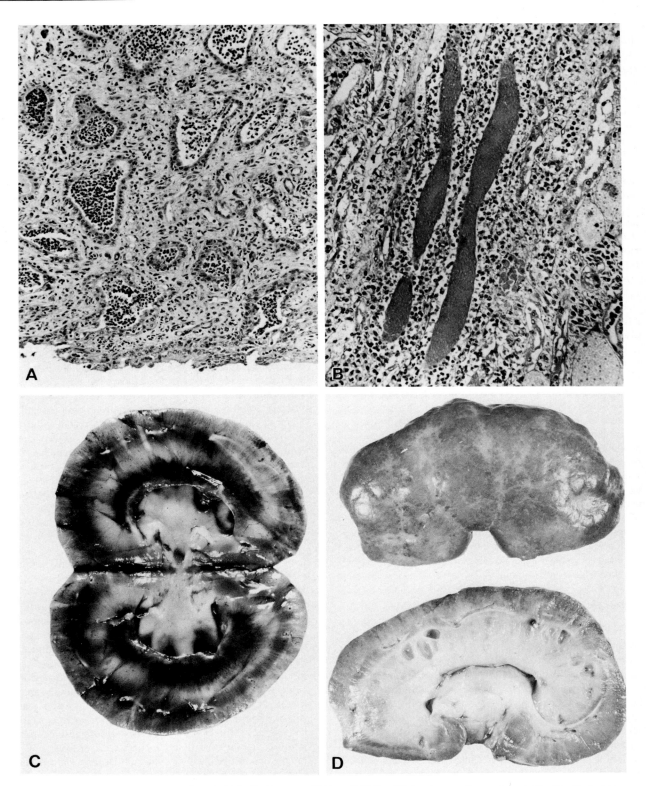

Fig. 5.14.   (**A**) Descending pyelonephritis in ''white-spotted kidney.'' Calf.   (**B**) Acute ascending pyelonephritis. Ox. Bacterial colonies in collecting tubules with suppuration.   (**C**) Acute pyelonephritis. Dog. There is ulceration of the renal crest and hemorrhage in medulla. Pale streaks extend to cortical surface.   (**D**) Chronic pyelonephritis. Dog. Ulceration of renal crest and deep, irregular scars, which are most prominent at the poles.

the low hematocrit in the vasa recta; hypertonicity depresses the phagocytic activity of leukocytes, and ammonia may interfere with activation of complement. In pigs, the renal poles are more susceptible to infection because the collecting ducts of their compound papillae do not collapse as readily as those of the simple papillae of the central lobes when exposed to the increased pelvic pressure of vesicoureteral reflux; hence intrarenal reflux is more common at the poles. Invasion of the kidney from the pelvis probably progresses by way of the collecting ducts, as suggested by the early development of lines of suppuration along the straight tubules and the presence of bacterial colonies in the tubules, and by direct invasion across the degenerate eroded pelvic epithelium.

Pyelonephritis is often bilateral but not necessarily symmetric. Acute disease is seen most commonly in sows, and chronic pyelonephritis in cows and dogs. A general description will be given of acute and chronic pyelonephritis before species differences are noted in more detail. Acute disease characteristically begins with necrosis and inflammation of papilla or renal crest ("necrotizing papillitis") in an irregular pattern (Fig. 5.14C). Bacteria may be abundant in the collecting tubules (Fig. 5.14B). Associated wedge-shaped areas of parenchyma are swollen, dark red and firm. Hyperemia subsides, and suppurative tubulointerstitial nephritis and tubular necrosis then predominate in these radially distributed wedges. Tubules are obliterated by the inflammation, tubular obstruction and dilation occur, and glomeruli, although initially resistant, may be obliterated. Leukocytic casts are present in tubules. As the process becomes chronic, mononuclear cells replace neutrophils, and fibrosis proceeds and eventually predominates. Contraction of the scars and loss of renal substance result in a wide variety of patterns of renal scarring, usually with deep cortical depressions. The scars in pyelonephritis extend from capsule to pelvis and are distinguished from those of other nephritides and infarcts by the associated fibrosis and deformities of the renal papilla and dilation of calyces and pelvis. The pelvis often contains exudate and debris. The papillary defects may be small and difficult to detect in mild cases. More or less total involvement of the kidney may produce a firm pale shrunken kidney with an irregular surface (Fig. 5.14D), which may be difficult to differentiate from other end-stage kidneys resulting from ischemic lesions.

In **dogs** and **cats**, acute pyelonephritis is not often detected, but scars attributed to chronic pyelonephritis are common. In dogs, accumulation of colloid-like material in tubules and glomerular capsules dilated due to scarring may produce a thyroid-like histologic appearance (Fig. 5.15C). Calculi may form in the pelvis on the nidi provided by cellular debris.

In **swine**, acute pyelonephritis is seen occasionally, but the chronic disease is rare. Acute pyelonephritis occurs in sows postpartum or 3 to 4 weeks postbreeding; young males are occasionally affected, and some of these have urinary tract anomalies. Bloodstained urine or discharge may be seen, but it is not unusual for prostration and death to occur in 12 hr or so. Severe cystitis and ureteritis are usually present with yellow-brown or bloody mucoid exudate. The renal poles are preferentially involved, and the infection may be fulminant and erupt through the renal capsule to produce retrorenal hemorrhage and inflammation. Less severe examples of tubulointerstitial nephritis also

occur and are seen as pale areas of cellular infiltration involving wedges or entire lobes.

In **cattle**, chronic pyelonephritis is a significant sporadic disease in cows, but acute pyelonephritis (Fig. 5.15A) is usually only an incidental finding. Tubulointerstitial nephritis in affected cows may be minimal, and a slowly progressive suppurative destructive papillitis may predominate. The medulla of each lobe is fairly uniformly destroyed. Eventually the cortex remains as a narrow capsule surrounding large amounts of pus in the calyces (Fig. 5.15B,D). Alternatively, and perhaps more commonly, the pattern of radially distributed tubulointerstitial nephritis develops as described above. Enlarged tan lobes are granular due to interstitial inflammation, and interstitial fibrosis may become extensive. Rupture of the kidney occurs in males with obstructive urolithiasis that develop fulminant pyelonephritis, but rupture is less common in cattle than in swine. Pyelonephritis is uncommon in sheep and horses.

Hypercalcemic Nephropathy and Renal Mineralization

Hypercalcemia occurs often in dogs and may be sufficiently severe to cause renal failure (hypercalcemic nephropathy). The leading cause is pseudohyperparathyroidism, a paraneoplastic syndrome, in which a nonendocrine tumor, usually a lymphoma, is a source of ectopic substances that stimulate bone resorption (see the Endocrine Glands and the Hematopoietic System, Volume 3). Other less common causes of hypercalcemia are primary hyperparathyroidism, hypervitaminosis D and like diseases, osteolytic neoplasms, acute or chronic renal failure, and hypoadrenocorticism. Hypercalcemia results in inactivation of adenyl cyclase, hence decreased cyclic adenosine monophosphate formation; sodium transport is impaired in the ascending limb of the loop of Henle, the distal tubule, and collecting ducts. Natriuresis results. As well, hypercalcemia interferes with antidiuretic-hormone receptors in the collecting ducts, resulting in renal diabetes insipidus. The resultant polyuria and compensatory polydipsia are reversible if the primary cause of the hypercalcemia is removed. If hypercalcemia persists, progressive renal mineralization occurs, beginning with tubular basement membranes and epithelium, particularly in the outer zone of the medulla (Fig. 5.10B), and eventually involving glomeruli. Tubular epithelial mineralization and cast formation causes tubular obstruction, and eventually loss of nephrons.

Other less significant examples of renal mineralization also occur. The deposition of calcium salts in the form of clumps of granules in the lumen and lining of collecting tubules and in the adjacent interstitium is rather common. They are associated with hypomagnesemia in some species; they are not significant.

Mineralization is very common in dogs, most unusual in other species, and occurs very quickly in casts, dead and degenerate epithelium, and injured basement membranes. In uremia, it may also involve the glomeruli and small blood vessels. Mineralization is a frequent result of secondary hyperparathyroidism induced by chronic renal insufficiency and coexists with similar deposits in the lungs, gastric mucosa, and other organs. Dogs fed a high-phosphorus diet similarly develop diffuse renal mineralization.

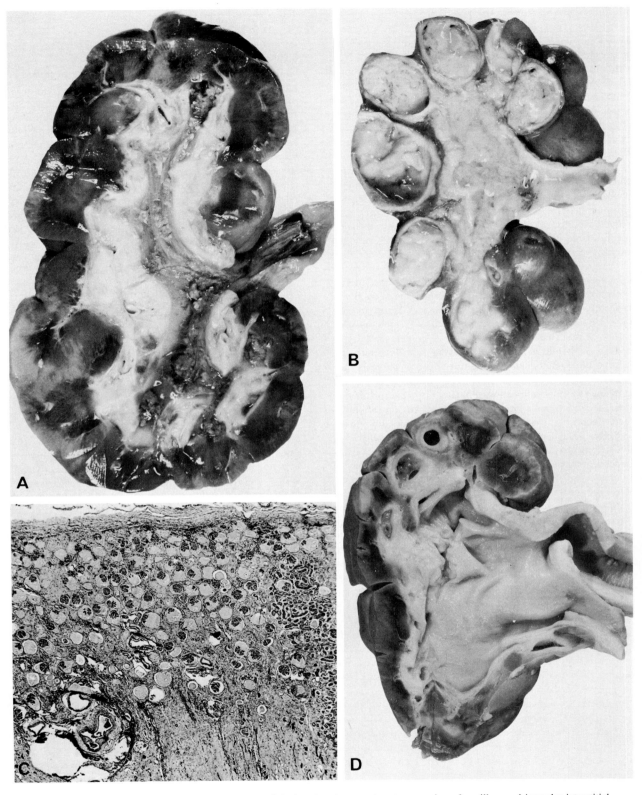

Fig. 5.15. (**A**) Acute pyelonephritis. Ox. Casts of detritus in calyces and ureters, erosion of papillae, and irregular interstitial inflammation of parenchyma. (**B**) Chronic pyelonephritis. Ox. Renal parenchyma is scarred and atrophic. Exudate fills the distended, thickened calyces. (**C**) Cortical and medullary scarring in pyelonephritis. Dog. Note inflammatory cells at corticomedullary junction and beneath capsule. (**D**) Chronic pyelonephritis. Ox. Renal parenchyma is scarred. Calyces and ureter are dilated and thickened.

Miscellaneous Renal Lesions

Extramedullary hematopoiesis occurs in the kidneys of dogs under a variety of circumstances, all of which probably have a common denominator of bone marrow depression or injury. When the kidneys are the site of hematopoiesis, it is usual that the liver, lymph nodes, spleen, adrenals, and lungs are also. The most pronounced hematopoiesis occurs in canine pyometra. **Bone** occasionally develops in association with urinary tract tissue, for example, following urinary tract surgery or in hydronephrotic kidneys. Transitional epithelium stimulates transformation of mesenchymal cells to osteoblasts.

Parasitic Lesions in the Kidney

Ascarid Granulomas

The most common parasitic lesion in the kidneys is the focal scar of reaction to the larvae of *Toxocara canis* in dog kidneys (Fig. 5.16A). These small granulomas, 2–3 mm in diameter, are found on the surface and cross section of the cortex. In the early stages of development, the lesions are gray-yellow and have soft centers; later they become firm and white, and the superficial ones cause dimpling of the cortex. These granulomas each surround an entrapped larva (Fig. 5.16B), which usually is hard to find in sections, and they are composed largely of epithelioid cells and lymphocytes, with an occasional eosinophil. Healing of the lesions occurs after the death and removal of the larvae; the residual scars are typical and consist of dense, concentrically arranged fibrous tissue. Similar lesions are produced in calves by the migratory larvae of *T. cati* and *T. canis,* acquired by fecal contamination of feed.

THE KIDNEY WORM OF SWINE.   *Stephanurus dentatus* is the kidney worm of swine. It is widely distributed in tropical and subtropical countries, and the incidence in grazing swine in such areas can be very high. The worms encyst in perirenal fat and adjacent tissues, the cysts communicating with the renal pelvis.

The life cycle of *Stephanurus dentatus* can be direct or, experimentally, involve earthworms as transport hosts. The latter mechanism has not been shown to occur naturally. Eggs are passed in the urine of the pig, sometimes in immense numbers, and the larvae hatch in 2 or 3 days. The infective stages are vulnerable to sunlight and drying. Infection may occur by penetration through the skin or by ingestion, and prenatal infections occur. Following oral infection, third-stage larvae migrate from the small and large intestine via the portal circulation and mesenteric lymphatics to the liver. A few migrate across the peritoneal cavity. After skin infection, most larvae migrate to the lungs and reach the intestines following tracheal migration. Deaths due to peritonitis and intestinal intussusception occur in some pigs 20 to 30 days after heavy infections and are associated with larval migration from the mesenteric nodes to the liver. The infective larvae migrate in the tissues of the pig, especially in the liver, where they may stay for several months. The hepatic migrations provoke considerable injury and a severe interstitial hepatitis, with lesions of the same character but much more severe than those produced by the larvae of *Ascaris suum. Stephanurus dentatus* also produces portal phlebitis with thrombosis, in some pigs (see the Liver and Biliary System, this volume). The liver is usually enlarged and may be very hard. It is pale, and the lobulation is remarkably emphasized by the perilobular fibrosis that develops. Many lobules are obliterated by contracting and proliferating scar tissue in the portal areas, and all lobules are more or less reduced in size in the diffuse hepatitis of heavy or prolonged larval infestation.

Many larvae are destroyed in the liver, being encapsulated in small abscesses that are eventually obliterated. From the liver, the larvae migrate across the peritoneal cavity to the perirenal region. Many become encysted in abscesses in adjacent tissue, especially the pancreas, and it is not unusual for some to invade the vertebral canal and cause posterior paralysis. The definitive site is the tissue around the renal pelvis and ureter, wherein the adults encyst (Fig. 5.16C). Occasionally, the cysts may be found in the kidney itself. The cysts communicate with the lumen of the ureter, allowing escape of eggs. Developmental stages in the definitive host take a long time, and patency may not be established for 9 months or more. Once patency is established, the mature females may lay eggs for 3 years or longer.

THE GIANT KIDNEY WORM.   *Dioctophyma renale* is the giant kidney worm, the largest of parasitic nematodes. The worm is red and cylindric, and in dogs the females measure 20–100 cm long and 4–12 mm in diameter. Males are 14–45 cm long and 4–6 mm in diameter. *Dioctophyma renale* is usually found in dogs, mink, cats, and other fish-eating mammals but is recorded in the pig, ox, and horse. It has a worldwide distribution, but its incidence is unknown.

The life cycle involves one intermediate and often one paratenic host. Eggs passed in the urine are very resistant to the external environment and may survive 2–5 years. Embryonation requires 1–7 months, depending on the climatic conditions. The embryonated eggs are ingested by the intermediate hosts, which are aquatic oligochetes ("mud worms"), *Lumbriculus variegatus,* and encyst in their body cavities. The paratenic hosts are fish and frogs, of which the northern black bullhead (*Ictalurus melas*) and the green frog (*Rana clamitans*) are known to serve in North America. Other fish and frogs may also act as paratenic hosts, but *L. variegatus* is the only known intermediate host. Following ingestion of infective larvae, they penetrate the gut wall and migrate across the peritoneal cavity to the kidney. The life cycle from egg to adult requires $3\frac{1}{2}$–6 months but may take 2 years.

The adult worms live in the renal pelvis but may encyst in a body cavity, the uterus, mammary gland, or bladder. The adults are very destructive, causing initially a hemorrhagic pyelitis that shortly becomes suppurative, and the parenchyma is progressively destroyed until only the tunic contains the worm and exudate.

Dogs, the domestic species usually affected by *Dioctophyma renale,* are regarded as abnormal hosts because usually only one or a very small number of worms is present, and worms of both sexes are found in only about one-third of infections. Intrarenal parasites in dogs are more common in the right kidney than the left, but in ~60% of infected dogs, parasites are in the peritoneal cavity only. Simultaneous renal and peritoneal infections occur in ~15% of dogs. Thus most canine infections are not patent.

In the peritoneal cavity, *Dioctophyma renale* often entwines a

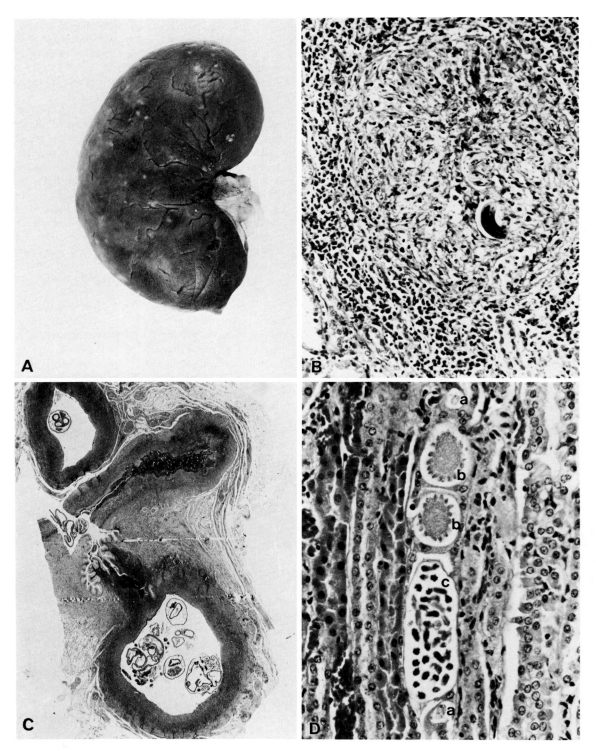

Fig. 5.16. (A) Cortical granulomas caused by *Toxocara canis*. Kidney. Dog. (B) Section from (A), showing larva in granuloma. (C) Encysted *Stephanurus dentatus* in hilus of kidney. Pig. (D) *Klossiella equi*. Horse. Within tubular epithelial cells are gamonts (a), sporonts (b), and sporocysts (c).

lobe of the liver and may cause erosion of the hepatic capsule and hemoperitoneum, or produce infarction and rupture. On occasion they rear up to startle surgeons engaged in exploratory laparotomy.

The definitive hosts are wild, fish-eating carnivores, mink in particular, in which the worms are smaller and usually located in the kidney.

Capillaria plica may be found in the lumen of the renal pelvis, ureter, or bladder of dogs, foxes, and smaller carnivores. Although widely distributed, it is not a common parasite. The life cycle is not clearly known but is probably indirect, earthworms being intermediate hosts. Ingestion of earthworms from infected premises causes patent infections in 61 to 68 days. Pathogenic effects usually are not attributed to *C. plica* infection, but hematuria and dysuria are produced occasionally.

Other species of *Capillaria* occur in the urinary bladder of other animals, such as *C. micronata* in mink and *C. feliscati* in the cat. The latter may be the same as *C. plica*. Light infestations are common but harmless, the anterior end of the worm embedded in the surface layer of epithelium, provoking at most a light cellular infiltration of the lamina propria.

KLOSSIELLOSIS OF EQUIDAE. *Klossiella equi* is a sporozoan parasite of the kidney of the horse and its relatives, including the zebra, donkey, and burro. It is apparently quite rare and harmless. The life cycle is not fully known. It is thought that following infection with sporocysts from the environment, sporozoites are released and enter the circulation. One schizont generation develops in the glomerular endothelium and another in proximal tubular epithelium. Sporogony occurs in the epithelium of the thick limb of Henle's loop, and sporocysts are probably passed in the urine (Fig. 5.16D).

Granulomas may be found in the renal pelvis in schistosomiasis of cattle and sheep (see the Cardiovascular System, Volume 3), and larvae of *Setaria digitata* may produce granulomas in the bladder of cattle in Asia (see the Peritoneum, Retroperitoneum, and Mesentery, this volume).

Micronema deletrix, a saprophagous nematode that may produce granulomatous masses in the nasal cavity of horses and occasionally is responsible for cerebral vasculitis and hemorrhagic necrosis, also localizes in the kidney. Renal infections are characterized by granulomatous inflammation with production of cream-colored masses that resemble neoplasms macroscopically.

Renal Neoplasia

Primary renal tumors are uncommon. One abattoir survey in the United Kingdom found 8.5, 0.9, and 4.3 cases per million animals in cattle, sheep, and pigs, respectively. Comparable figures are unavailable for horses. Primary renal tumors comprise ~1% of all canine neoplasms and probably ~0.5% of feline neoplasms.

Renal Adenoma

Renal adenomas are rare; they are said to occur more often in cattle and horses than in other species. In dogs they comprise ~15% of primary renal epithelial tumors. Renal adenomas, and

carcinomas also, arise from epithelium of the proximal convoluted tubules. Adenomas usually are incidental autopsy findings. Grossly, they tend to be solitary nodules less than 2 cm across but occasionally are huge. They grow expansively. Microscopically, the tumor cells usually are cuboidal, with moderate to abundant acidophilic cytoplasm. They form solid sheets, or papilliform or tubular structures, and stromal tissue is scant. Tumors with mixed architectural patterns occur. Histologic differentiation of adenoma and renal carcinoma sometimes is impossible; a few "adenomas" may be small, well-differentiated carcinomas.

Renal Carcinoma

Carcinomas are the most common primary renal tumors of dogs, cattle, and sheep. They occur in mature and old animals, thus their incidence is relatively low in some species. The average age of affected dogs is ~8 years. Males are affected about twice as often as bitches. Common presenting signs are hematuria, palpable abdominal mass, and weight loss. Polycythemia associated with erythropoietin production is very rarely seen. Grossly, renal carcinomas are spherical or ovoid masses, usually located in one pole of the kidney (Fig. 5.17A). Usually they are well demarcated from the remainder of the kidney, which is atrophic and compressed. Often the tumor is much larger than the original size of the host kidney but still has a discrete border. The tumor is usually gray or light yellow, often with darker areas of necrosis and hemorrhage. Invasion of the renal pelvis, ureter, renal vein, and hilar lymphatics may be visible (Fig. 5.17C).

Histologically, there are a variety of cell types and architectures, but if examined carefully, small or large areas composed of renal "clear cells" are often found. These cells have vacuolated cytoplasm, and only the basal nucleus and cytoplasmic outline are visible. The vacuoles contain fat. The presence of clear cells, even in metastases, should suggest renal carcinoma but is not pathognomonic—similar cells occur in certain endocrine tumors and other carcinomas. In other areas, the cells are cuboidal, with denser acidophilic or basophilic cytoplasm. They may be arranged in sheets or papillary or tubular structures, and occasionally they line small cystic spaces. All of these patterns may occur in a single tumor, and apparently there is no prognostic value associated with any pattern. The stroma of renal carcinomas is scant but highly vascularized, which predisposes to the extensive necrosis often seen grossly.

Renal carcinomas tend to grow expansively, but satellite nodules often develop from local permeation. Invasion of the renal vein is always likely but may not result in metastases. Peritoneal implantation sometimes occurs. Usually by the time a dog is presented for examination, widespread metastases are present, especially in lungs and liver, but also in brain, heart, and skin. Such behavior is not invariable, and in some cases unilateral nephrectomy is curative.

NEPHROBLASTOMA. Nephroblastoma (embryonal nephroma, Wilms' tumor) is the most common primary renal tumor of pigs and chickens. Abattoir surveys of pigs in the United Kingdom found 3.5 per million swine slaughtered, and in the United States, 43.5 per million, with an incidence of 197 cases per

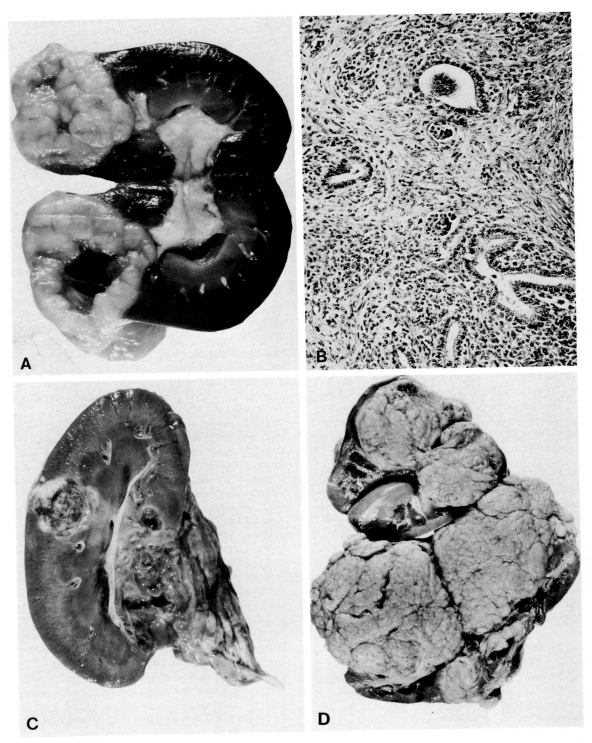

Fig. 5.17. (A) Renal carcinoma, showing cystic degeneration. Sheep. (B) Nephroblastoma. Pig. Note tubular and glomerular structures. (C) Renal carcinoma. Dog. There is extension to pelvis and pelvic structures. (D) Nephroblastomas. Pig. Lobulated tumors distort and replace renal parenchyma.

million in one area. Nephroblastomas occur far less often in calves and puppies and are very uncommon in other species. They are seen almost always in young animals and sometimes in fetuses, but also in mature sows.

Nephroblastomas are true embryonal tumors, which arise in primitive nephrogenic blastema and in foci of renal dysplasia. The presence in them of tissues such as cartilage and skeletal muscle, which normally are not associated with the kidney, indicates an origin in pluripotential mesenchyme before it becomes metanephrogenic. These tumors establish the important principle that all component tissues of the kidney arise from a common blastema.

Grossly, nephroblastomas may attain a huge size and cause abdominal enlargement. They are often multiple in the affected kidney, growing expansively and compressing the adjacent parencyma, and they are encapsulated. They are usually unilateral, but a few are bilateral (Fig. 5.17D), and these sometimes unite across the midline to form a single large mass. Widespread metastases to lung and liver occur in over half the canine cases but are rare in pigs and calves. The cut surface of nephroblastomas is variegated or lobulated, and the larger ones have extensive areas of hemorrhagic necrosis. The characteristic cut surface reveals a myxomatous, soft, gray-white or tan tissue that feels spongy. Histologically, the characteristic features are primitive glomeruli with primitive Bowman's spaces, abortive tubules, and a loose spindle-cell stroma (Fig. 5.17B), which may show some differentiation to a variety of mesenchymal tissues, including striated muscle, collagen, cartilage, bone, and adipose tissue. The mesenchymal components may predominate in certain tumors, especially in ruminants.

Transitional-cell papilloma and **carcinoma** of the renal pelvis are very rare tumors that occur in the dog, cow, pig, and horse. Squamous and glandular metaplasia develop in the carcinomas. Transitional-cell tumors are discussed under Urinary Bladder.

Primary mesenchymal tumors of the kidney occur but may be diagnosed only after very careful examination, to exclude a primary focus in some other tissue. Fibrous and vascular tumor are the most common types.

Metastatic tumors are common in the kidneys, and disseminated neoplasms of any type are likely to localize there, especially in the cortices, and be bilateral. Many such metastases are of microscopic size, and they are of hematogenous origin. Retrograde lymphatic invasion along the renal lymphatics may occur from carcinomas in adjacent organs.

Renal involvement in lymphoma is common in those species in which the neoplasm is common. The involvement may be diffuse or nodular. When the nodular lesions are grossly visible, they are numerous, poorly defined, fatty in appearance, and project hemispherically above the surface. The capsule is not adherent. When lymphomatous involvement is diffuse, the organ is enlarged and has a uniform white, fatty appearance. The differentiation of lymphomatous metastases from interstitial nephritis often requires microscopic examination, and indeed, metastases may sometimes be discovered, especially in cats, only by microscopic examination. Peripelvic and periureteral infiltrates that cause hydronephrosis are common in cattle.

In dogs, primary pulmonary adenocarcinoma with renal me-tastases may be difficult or impossible to distinguish from primary renal carcinoma with pulmonary metastases since their microscopic appearances are quite similar.

THE LOWER URINARY TRACT

General Considerations

The lower urinary tract consists of ureters, urinary bladder, and urethra. The ureters and bladder, and also the renal pelvis, are lined by transitional stratified epithelium—the urothelium. The ureters are of uniform diameter throughout and usually course directly to the bladder, although they may be tortuous and dilated distally in baby pigs. The ureters enter the bladder wall obliquely and are covered by a mucosal flap. Histologically, the ureteral mucosa is present in longitudinal folds, there are poorly defined internal and external longitudinal muscle layers and a prominent middle circular layer, and either adventitia or peritoneal serosa. Peritonitis may involve the ureters and interfere with their peristalsis. Ureters of horses have simple branched tubuloalveolar mucous glands in the propria–submucosa. The male urethra has a thin lining of transitional epithelium; the female's is similar but has stratified squamous epithelium at its termination. Histologically, the bladder is an expanded ureter. Lymphoid nodules are commonly found in the lamina propria of all domestic animals. The transitional epithelium varies from 3 to 14 cells thick, depending on species and degree of distension. Theliolymphocytes are common in ruminants. The urothelium of the renal pelvis, ureter, and perhaps the trigone of the bladder originates from mesoderm, whereas in the rest of the bladder it has an endodermal origin. This urothelium responds to chronic irritation from infections, calculi, excreted chemicals, etc. by proliferation and metaplasia, and metaplasia of squamous or mucous types often is superimposed on predominantly proliferative lesions. Both proliferative and metaplastic lesions of the urothelium are regarded as premalignant changes, thus papillary growths may give rise to transitional, squamous, or adenocarcinoma, and squamous or adenocarcinoma may develop in metaplastic lesions of the corresponding type. Downward proliferation of urothelium, a common reactive change, results in the formation of Brunn's nests when groups of proliferating cells are isolated in the submucosa. If the center of the nest undergoes liquefaction, cystitis cystica, ureteritis cystica, or pyelitis cystica results. Pyelitis, ureteritis, or cystitis glandularis develops if the epithelium lining the cyst undergoes mucous metaplasia. (Mucous glands are normal in the horse renal pelvis.) Most of the adenomas and adenocarcinomas of the lower urinary tract develop in these areas of mucous metaplasia. A few may arise in submucosal glands or mesonephric and urachal remnants. Urothelium not exposed to urine has a tendency to undergo metaplasia to an intestinal-type epithelium; such is the fate of some cystic urachal remnants, which normally are lined by transitional epithelium.

The function of the ureter is to propel urine from the kidney to the bladder by peristalsis; in this it is assisted by the renal pelvis. Ureteral peristalsis is controlled by one or more pacemakers, which are located in the recesses of the renal pelvis, and by the activity of the ureteropelvic junction, which determines whether a pacemaker stimulus initiates a peristaltic wave. At low urine production rates, peristalsis may occur with every fifth pacemaker stimulus, but during diuresis every stimulus initiates a peristaltic wave. The ureters pass obliquely through the muscular wall of the bladder at the ureterovesical junction. The segment of ureter in the bladder wall, the intravesical ureter, forms the basis of the **vesicoureteral valve**, which prevents reflux of urine from bladder to ureter. When the length of the intravesical ureter is short, as is often the case in puppies, reflux frequently occurs. Thus the competence of the valve is influenced by the angle of the ureteral entry and the thickness of the bladder wall. The urinary bladder stores urine and, in concert with the urethra, expels it. During continence, the bladder is relatively flaccid and the urethra acts as a valve. During micturition, the contracting bladder pumps urine through the relaxed urethra. The bladder also has a role, probably of minor significance in domestic animals, in conservation of water and salt.

Embryologically, the ureters are formed by buds from the mesonephric ducts, which develop cranial to their entrance into the cloaca. The cloaca is divided into a dorsal rectum and ventral urogenital sinus by the urorectal fold in such a way that the urogenital sinus is continuous with the allantois. (The allantois originates as an evagination of the hindgut.) At this stage of development the mesonephric duct and ureteral bud form a Y shape; one arm of the Y is the ureteral bud, and the other arm plus the stem of the Y are formed by the mesonephric duct. As the allantois and urogenital sinus develop, the stem of the Y is absorbed, and the mesonephric duct and ureteral bud enter the urogenital sinus independently. In females the entire urethra, plus the vaginal vestibule, is derived from the urogenital sinus, but in males only the prostatic urethra is so derived. The penile urethra forms by closure of a groove, the urethral groove, on the posterior face of the penis. The bladder, which is formed from the cranial part of the urogenital sinus and the caudal part of the allantoic diverticulum, communicates with the allantois via the urachus, which forms from the cranial part of the intraembryonic allantoic diverticulum. The communication is severed at birth, and the urachus closes but remains as the umbilical ligament of the bladder.

Most ailments of the lower urinary tract are associated with obstruction and infection, which often are concomitant. Unlike the gastrointestinal tract, which has a normal microbial flora through its length, only the most distal part of the male urethra, and the female vagina, normally host microorganisms. The operation of sphincter-like mechanisms in the urethra and vesicoureteral valves, and the intermittent pulsatile flow of urine from the kidneys and bladder, normally prevent the movement of organisms higher up the tract. The susceptibility of the urinary bladder of the female to severe infections is undoubtedly related to its short, distensible urethra and its proximity to the external environment and, especially, the rectal flora. On the other hand, the anatomy of the male urethras, with their flexures, ossa, and appendages, make them prone to obstruction, particularly by calculi. Specific factors concerned in the establishment and maintenance of infections in the urinary bladder and their spread to the kidney are discussed under Inflammation of the Lower Urinary Tract, and Pyelonephritis. The causes and effect of obstruction are considered under Urolithiasis and Hydronephrosis.

Urine may be obtained for urinalysis or culture by cystocentesis at autopsy. The bladder may be dilated in "downer" animals, even in states of dehydration, due either to the absence of the correct posture needed for urination or to decreased medullary tonicity due to hypoproteinemia (low urea production) that has led to polyuria. Dog bladders are often constricted at necropsy and hence have a thick wall. If the bladder can be dilated by pulling it between the fingers, the thickening is not pathologic. Horse urine normally contains mucus and crystals.

Anomalies of the Lower Urinary Tract

Ureters

Agenesis of the ureters is due to failure of the ureteral bud to form and may be unilateral or bilateral. It occurs in dogs accompanied by renal agenesis (see Anomalies of Development). Duplication of a ureter is caused by formation of two ureteral diverticula from the mesonephric duct. The posterior ureter drains the posterior part of the kidney, and the anterior one drains the anterior part. Usually the posterior ureter empties normally while the other is ectopic. Duplication is rare but occurs in dogs and pigs. Ureteral dysplasia occurs in association with renal dysplasia. Ureteral valves are seen occasionally in dogs.

Ectopic ureter is the most important ureteral anomaly. The affected ureter may empty into the vas deferens, vesicular gland, or urethra of the male, or the bladder neck, urethra, or vagina of the female. There are two possible causes: either the ureteral bud arises too far cranial to be incorporated into the urogenital sinus, or the differential growth of the sinus is abnormal and the ureter fails to migrate to its usual location. Ectopic ureters occasionally empty into the rectum because of anomalous cloacal division by the urorectal fold. Very rarely they empty into the cervix, uterus, or uterine tube, possibly as a result of aberrant origin from the paramesonephric (Müllerian) duct.

Ectopic ureter is most common in dogs and appears to affect females about nine times more often than males. This sex difference may be apparent or exaggerated, however, since affected females are usually incontinent, whereas affected males may not be. Ectopia can be unilateral or bilateral and is often associated with other urinary tract abnormalities, either congenital or acquired. Usually in bitches, the ureter terminates in the vagina or urethra. Certain dog breeds, especially the Siberian husky, have a high risk for the defect, but the West Highland white terrier, fox terrier, and miniature and toy poodle are also over represented. Ectopic ureter also occurs in white shorthorn bulls and tends to involve the region of the seminal vesicles.

Ureteral anomalies often predispose to pyelonephritis or urinary incontinence.

Urinary Bladder

Duplication of the urinary bladder occurs in dogs and causes dysuria, incontinence, and sometimes abdominal distension and cryptorchidism. The extra bladder originates dorsally between the urinary tract and uterus or rectum. Cystic remnants of the urorectal fold may be responsible for the defect.

Patent or **pervious urachus** is the most common malformation of the urinary bladder and is seen more often in foals than in other animals. Animals with this defect dribble urine from the umbilicus because the urachal lumen fails to close and remains as an open channel between the apex of the bladder and the umbilicus. Rupture of the urachus causes uroperitoneum. The condition must be differentiated from perinatal rupture of the bladder. Occasionally, urachal obliteration is partial, and rests of epithelium remain intact to develop into cysts at any point between the umbilicus and the bladder. These cysts may become quite large but usually are small, multiple, and are attached to the midline of the bladder. Occasionally they adhere to the intestinal serosa. The urachus is normally lined by transitional epithlium, but metaplasia is common in urachal cysts and sinuses, which are then lined by squamous or mucus-secreting columnar epithelium. Urachal remnants in the bladder wall may give origin to neoplasms.

Diverticula of the bladder may be acquired secondary to partial obstruction to the outflow of urine, or they may result at an abnormally weak area of the wall from the pressure of normal contractions. Diverticula are usually seen at the vertex, where they represent incomplete closure of the urachus, with an area of discontinuity in the muscle. Contraction of the bladder tends to distend the diverticulum, but rupture does not occur. Stasis of urine in the diverticulum eventually leads to persistent infection and inflammation. Calculi may form in the diverticulum.

Urethra

Urethral agenesis, duplicated urethra, ectopic urethra, and imperforate urethra occur rarely in dogs. Hypospadias is described with the Male Genital System (Volume 3). The most common urethral anomaly is **urethrorectal** or **rectovaginal fistula**, which is caused by incomplete division of the cloaca into rectum and urogenital sinus by the urorectal fold. In males, the communication involves the pelvic urethra, and affected dogs urinate from the rectum. In females, the opening is in the vagina and may be associated with imperforate anus. These defects occur in dogs, pigs and horses and usually predispose to urogenital tract infections but sometimes are incidental autopsy findings.

Acquired Anatomic Variations

Displacements of ureters and urethra are sometimes caused by local inflammatory and neoplastic swelling. Their main significance to the urinary system relates to obstruction of urine flow. Ureteral and urethral displacements may also occur with variations of position of the bladder. Torsion of the bladder is uncommon; it may be partial or complete about the long axis of the organ.

Dorsal retroflexion occurs in male dogs with tenesmus in response to prostatic enlargement or constipation. The normal position is assumed following emptying. A more serious type occurs in prolapse of the vagina in cows and sows, and occasionally in perineal hernia of dogs. In these cases, the bladder may be present in the hernial sac, and because of the retroflexion, there is obstructive kinking of the neck of the bladder and sometimes of the urethra and ureters. If the ureters are patent, the accumulation of urine in the bladder contributes to the size of the hernia. Hydronephrosis or rupture of the bladder may occur if the condition is not corrected.

Inversion of the bladder (invagination into and through the urethra) occurs in females and is permitted by the short, wide urethra in this sex. The bladder may arrive in the vagina. It can occur in any of the larger species and is perhaps most common in mares. Inversion is predisposed to by circumstances in which straining occurs, often after parturition.

Dilation of **ureters** may be due to obstruction by calculi, neoplasms, or inflammatory debris. Dilation without physical obstruction occurs in association with peritonitis and may be due to loss of muscle tone. Dilation of ureters is often present in neonatal pigs with enteric infections. Congenital hydroureter and hydronephrosis often occur in piglets in association with epitheliogenesis imperfecta.

Dilation of **bladder** may be of local obstructive or neuroparalytic origin. The wall is thin and almost transparent, and the distended organ may extent almost to the liver. Brief periods of distension may allow quick return of normal contractility, but severe or prolonged distension may result in loss of tone that is not restored before bacterial complications terminate the condition. The causes of obstruction include calculi, prostatic enlargement in dogs, accumulated inflammatory detritus or blood clots in the urethra, urethral strictures, and tumors of the neck of the bladder or urethra.

Neurogenic distension follows spinal injury with loss of tonic parasympathetic outflow from the sacral plexus. Spinal myelitis, as in canine distemper and rabies, may also cause paralysis of the bladder. Perhaps it most commonly follows herniation of intervertebral disks in the dog. Cystitis is the usual complication.

Distension of the bladder occurs in calves fed indigestible milk-replacer that starve to death. They are usually recumbent for several hours before death, but this is probably due to weakness rather than nervous disease. Renal concentrating ability is depressed by starvation because of lack of urea and a partial insensitivity to antidiuretic hormone and mineralocorticoids. Possibly the bladder distension is caused by overproduction of dilute urine.

Hypertrophy of the bladder is fairly common in dogs and less so in other species. It is a response to longstanding partial obstruction to the outflow of urine.

Rupture of **bladder** often occurs following urethral obstruction but rarely following pelvic trauma. The interval between obstruction and rupture depends somewhat on the competence of the vesicoureteral valve and whether hydronephrosis develops. Rupture of the bladder occurs in newborn foals, affecting either the dorsal or ventral aspect of the viscus. Males are most often affected. Some ruptures are congenital, but most are probably caused by birth trauma. Twists in the amniotic portion of the umbilical cord may compress the urachus, causing distension of both bladder and urachus and predisposing to rupture.

Circulatory Disturbances

Hemorrhages are the most important and common of circulatory disturbances. In the ureters and urethra they are associated with obstructive calculi, and ureteral hemorrhage is part of acute ascending infections. In the bladder they are located in the propria mucosa and may occur in any septicemia. Small hemorrhages with the shape of tiny hematomas are common and considered diagnostically significant in hog cholera, African swine fever, porcine salmonellosis, and equine purpura hemorrhagica. Larger hemorrhages are present in bracken fern poisoning of cattle. Hemorrhage occurs with acute cystitis and neoplastic diseases, and hemorrhage with hematoma formation is seen with rupture of the bladder.

Urolithiasis

Urolithiasis is the presence of calculi in the urinary passages. Calculi are grossly visible aggregations of precipitated urinary solutes, urinary proteins, and proteinaceous debris. Many have a laminated structure and are hard spheres or ovoids with a small amount of organic matrix impregnated with inorganic salts. Others are masses of sandy sludge with a much higher organic component, the form largely determined by the shape of the cavity they fill. Even densely mineralized calculi of the same type may have quite a different appearance, depending on whether they are located in renal pelvis or urinary bladder. Many calculi contain significant quantities of "contaminants," such as calcium oxalates in "silica" calculi; a few are relatively pure.

The diseases caused by uroliths are among the most important urinary tract problems of domesticated animals. Several factors are important in predisposing to calculus formation, and several are important in precipitating disease. These are not the same for all diseases. Obviously, calculogenic material must occur in urine in quantities sufficient to be precipitated. Sometimes this concentration is achieved because a substance is metabolized in an unusual way, as is uric acid in Dalmatian dogs; or it may be processed abnormally by the kidney, as is cystine in cystine stone-formers; or abnormally high levels of a substance in the diet, such as silicic acid in native pastures, may produce potentially dangerous urinary levels. Regardless of the type of calculus, certain factors are more or less important: urinary pH, in terms of its optimum for solute precipitation, and reduced water intake, in relation to the degree of urine concentration. Deficiency of vitamin A is frequently suggested as a predisposing factor, but the evidence is equivocal; it may contribute in exceptional circumstances by producing metaplastic changes in the urinary epithelium.

Urine is often supersaturated with respect to the components of stone-forming salts. Supersaturation may be in the unstable region where spontaneous precipitation occurs, or in the metastable range where precipitation occurs by epitaxy or heterogeneous nucleation. Although it was thought that urinary proteins (e.g., uromucoid), which make up 5–20% or more of most calculi, were preeminent initiators of crystal formation in the metastable range, it is now believed that in many cases either coprecipitation of proteins and minerals occurs or that proteins are absorbed onto formed crystals. It is possible that crystals of one salt, for which urine is supersaturated in the unstable range, cause epitactic induction of crystals of another salt, for which supersaturation is metastable.

Crystals are much more common than calculi in urine. The factors that promote crystal growth and crystal aggregation or, more importantly, prevent them in some animals are poorly understood. Experimentally, high levels of urinary inorganic pyrophosphate and magnesium are important inhibitors of calcium phosphate and calcium oxalate crystallization, and

TABLE 5.3

Composition and Importance of Calculi

Species	Common types	Uncommon types
Dog	Struvite Oxalate Urate Cystine	Xanthine Silica
Cat	Struvite	Urate Cystine
Ox	Silica Struvite Carbonate	Xanthine
Sheep	Silica Struvite Oxalate "Clover stones" Carbonate	Xanthine
Horse	—	Carbonate
Pig	—	Urate

pyrophosphate also inhibits aggregation of calcium phosphate crystals. Certain urinary macromolecules, probably glycosaminoglycans, are also strong inhibitors of crystal aggregation in experimental systems. Nothing of substance is known about why calculi stay in the renal pelvis and urinary bladder until they are large enough to cause disease.

The important and less important types of urinary calculi are given above according to species (Table 5.3). Brief discussions of some of these follow a discussion of their pathologic effects.

The division indicated in Table 5.3 is arbitrary. Obviously, silica calculi are not important where ruminants are not pastured, and clover stones are unimportant where subterranean clover does not grow. In general, calculi are important in cattle, sheep, dogs, and cats and unimportant in horses and pigs. In pigs, uroliths are found occasionally in the renal pelvis of old animals and, more often, in the pelvis of dehydrated sucklings (Fig. 5.18A) (see Uremia). In horses they occur sometimes as single or several, spherical or faceted carbonate stones in the bladder. Urethral obstructions are rare.

Calculi may form in any part of the urinary duct system, from the renal pelvis (Fig. 5.18B,C,E) to the urethra. Some uroliths clearly originate in the lower urinary tract, but the point for embryogenesis of most is not known. In experimental urolithiasis produced by oxalates or calcium phosphate in laboratory animals, the calculi, initially microscopic, form in the collecting tubules and encrust on the renal papilla. They may grow large enough to make voidance impossible. It is not known whether this is a general phenomenon. The tubular microlithiasis may simply represent crystallization in the highly concentrated urine of the medulla, or alternatively, it may indicate the production there of an abnormal or excessive matricial substance.

Small calculi may be voided in the urine, but impaction in the urethra is common in males. The common sites of urethral impaction are the ischial arch, the sigmoid flexure of ruminants, the vermiform appendage of rams (Fig. 5.18C), the proximal

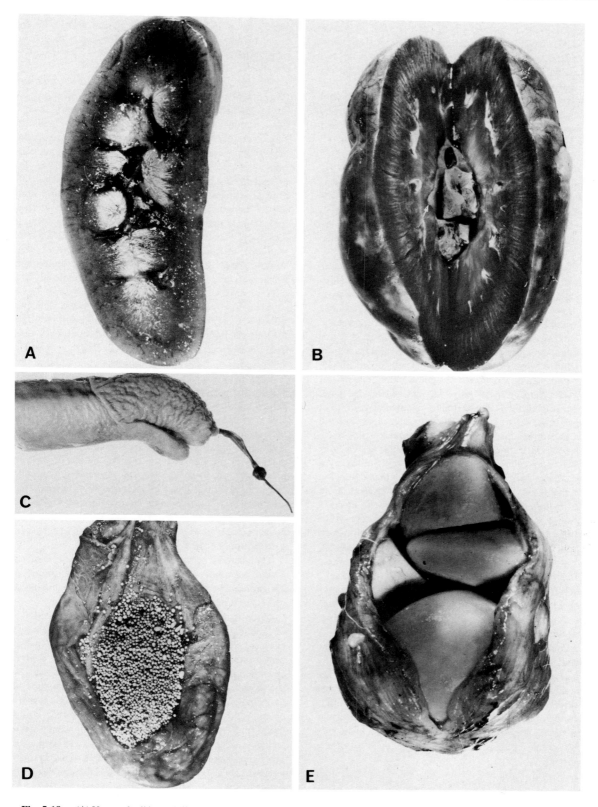

Fig. 5.18. **(A)** Urate calculi in medulla and pelvis of dehydrated piglet. Some calculi were transferred to the cortical surface when the kidney was sliced. **(B)** Calculus. Renal pelvis. Dog. Renal crest is ulcerated (arrow). Cortex is irregularly scarred. **(C)** Calculus impacted in vermiform appendage. Ram. **(D)** Struvite calculi in urinary bladder. Cow. **(E)** Faceted calculi filling bladder. Dog.

end of the os penis is dogs, and anywhere along the urethra of male cats. At the point of impaction, there is local pressure necrosis with ulceration of the mucosa, and because the urinary stasis favors bacterial growth, an acute hemorrhagic urethritis develops and often ascends to the bladder and even to the kidney. Hydronephrosis is not a prominent development with urethral calculi, and rupture of the urethra with leakage of urine into the surrounding tissues, often associated with infection and acute cellulitis, terminates the condition fairly quickly.

Silica Calculi

In ruminants, silica calculi are hard, white to dark brown, radio-opaque, often laminated, and up to 1 cm across. In the bladder of ruminants they are spherical, ovoid, or mulberry-shaped and have smooth surfaces, but in the kidney they are angular and irregular, having the shape of the minor calyces, where they are located almost exclusively.

"Pure" silica stones contain ~75% silica, as silica dioxide. Mixed calculi contain some calcium oxalate or carbonate. Silica calculi contain ~20% organic matter. Most have a friable core that is high in amorphous silica and low in organic matter. The core is surrounded by a layer of organic matter that separates it from the outer concentric laminations, which are high in silica.

Silica calculi are very common in pastured ruminants and are a major cause of urinary tract obstruction. They occur rarely in horses and dogs. Silica calculi are present in more than 50% of steers on native (unimproved) range in western Canada; fewer than 5% develop urethral obstruction. The singularity of adjacent laminae in the calculi is consistent with intermittent deposition as urine composition changes. Certain grasses contain 4–5% or more of silica; the level increases through the growing season. Most of it is relatively insoluble, but that in the cell sap is relatively soluble, unpolymerized silicic acid. Rumen fluid becomes saturated with respect to silicic acid. After absorption, some is returned to the gut in digestive secretions; less than 1% of dietary silica is excreted in urine, and up to 60% is resorbed from the filtrate. When urine production is very low, however, either because of the nature of the diet or because of high insensible fluid losses in hot climates, the concentration of silicic acid in urine may reach five times the saturation level. Even so, precipitation from solution requires other substances, probably proteins of renal or serum origin, in the urine. Calculus formation is reduced to subclinical levels by adding salt to the ration, thereby ensuring high water consumption.

Silica calculi have been reported in dogs in Kenya and the United States. In Kenya, they occur in both sexes and are mainly renal and asymptomatic. In the United States, male dogs are affected in most cases, and the stones, located in the bladder and urethra, often cause urinary obstruction. Unlike cystic silica calculi in ruminants, bladder stones in dogs have very irregular shapes. Dietary factors probably are involved in calculus formation in dogs, as they are in ruminants. Urine pH does not appear to be important.

Struvite Calculi

Struvite stones are white or gray, radio-opaque, chalky, usually smooth, and easily broken. They may be pure struvite but usually contain other compounds, such as calcium phosphate,

ammonium urate, oxalate, or carbonate. They may be single and large, or numerous and sandlike. Struvite is magnesium ammonium phosphate hexahydrate. Formerly it was called triple phosphate.

Struvite calculi are important in dogs, cats, and ruminants (Fig. 5.18D). In dogs they are the most common type; females are particularly susceptible, perhaps because they develop bladder infections more often than males. Struvite calculi are often single, rapidly forming masses that mold to the shape of the cavity they occupy. They are called infection calculi in recognition of their common association with infection. Bacterial ureases from staphylococci and *Proteus* induce supersaturation of urine with struvite by increasing urinary pH and ammonium ions. Alkaline urine decreases struvite solubility and increases ionization of trivalent phosphate, both of which favor calculus formation. Factors other than urease production that are associated with infection probably are important in the genesis of struvite stones. A high incidence of struvite calculi in miniature schnauzers may be related to a familial susceptibility to urinary tract infections.

In cats, struvite calculi often develop in the bladder of both sexes. The combination of inflammation and calculi produces the feline urologic syndrome, which is probably the most common urinary tract disease of cats. It is characterized by dysuria and hematuria, and by urethral obstruction in male cats.

Struvite crystalluria is seen often in cats with and without calculi; the reason for crystal aggregation is obscure. Unconfirmed reports suggest that virus infections may produce a suitable environment in the bladder. Other suggested predisposing factors, such as inhibition of urethral growth by early castration, and exclusive use of dry food, are also unconfirmed. Addition of magnesium and phosphate to the diet caused disease in some, presumably predisposed, cats, and conversely, reduction of dietary magnesium reduced the incidence. The apparent increased incidence during cold winter months may be due to decreased fluid consumption or increased intervals between urinations. None of these observations explains why struvite crystals aggregate to form calculi.

The obstructive material in male cats may be either struvite "sand" or rubber-like protein matrix, or a mixture of the two. The protein apparently is unique to feline calculi but has not been characterized.

In ruminants, struvite calculi usually occur in feedlot animals on high grain rations, and obstruction may develop in up to 10% of steers. As in cats, calculi usually form a gritty sludge with a high proportion of matrix. Inhibition of urethral growth by early castration predisposes to obstruction, and increased water consumption tends to prevent obstruction. Animals with crystalluria often have crystals adhering to preputial hairs. Diets high in phosphate can cause a very high incidence of calculi in sheep; a calcium:phosphorus ratio of 1:2 or wider appears to be the critical factor, but the form in which they are fed and the balance of other constituents such as sodium, potassium, and magnesium are probably also important. Additional potassium tends to promote phosphate urolithiasis. Magnesium deficiency leads to renal mineralization and tubular microlithiasis, at least in laboratory species, and both sodium and magnesium are competitive with calcium and increase the solubility of calcium salts in urine.

Oxalate Calculi

Oxalate calculi are hard, dense, white or yellow, and are typically covered with jagged spines, though some are smooth. They tend to be large and solitary in the bladder.

Oxalate calculi occur as the calcium oxalates whewellite and weddellite. Their development is not well understood, but obviously hypercalciuria and hyperoxaluria are involved. There are several causes of hypercalciuria (see Hypercalcemic Nephropathy and Renal Mineralization). Oxalic acid is synthesized from glyoxylic and ascorbic acid and may be ingested in certain foods; the relevance of these facts is obscure. Hyperuricosuria may be involved in oxalate precipitation, since sodium hydrogen urate may act as a heterogeneous nucleator.

Oxalate (and silica) calculi may be important in sheep grazing grain stubble, but the source of the oxalate is not known. Oxalate-containing plants apparently are not a source, since oxalate is metabolized in the rumen; nonetheless, occasional exceptions to this general rule do seem to occur. High magnesium intakes inhibit formation of oxalate calculi, while low levels induce formation in some species.

In dogs, oxalate calculi are of some importance, but little is known of their origins.

Uric Acid and Urate Calculi

Uric acid and urate calculi are usually multiple, hard, concentrically laminated, yellow to brown, and often radiolucent. In the bladder they are frequently spherical and less than 5 mm across. Most contain ammonium urate with some uric acid and phosphate; in others, sodium urate is the predominant salt.

Urate stones are most common in dogs, especially Dalmatians, but also occur in pigs (see Uremia) and rarely in cats. Dalmatians excrete high levels of uric acid in their urine. This is due to defective hepatocellular uptake of uric acid, which results in incomplete conversion of uric acid to more soluble allantoin; this defect is an inherited autosomal recessive trait. Hepatic uricase levels are normal. It is not clear whether the defective transport system also involves renal tubules and prevents reabsorption of uric acid from glomerular filtrate. Dogs with portosystemic shunts have ammonium biurate crystals in their urine and may have urate-containing calculi in kidneys and bladder.

Urates exist in supersaturated urine as lyophobic colloids that are flocculated by high levels of ammonium ion and, to a lesser extent, low pH. Urea-splitting organisms may be important in the development of urate calculi, since production of ammonium ion favors calculus formation. Also, although higher pH inhibits precipitation of uric acid, it favors precipitation of ammonium urate as well as phosphates, which are often found in urate calculi.

Cystine Calculi

Cystine calculi are small and irregular, soft and friable, waxy, and yellow, turning to green on exposure to daylight. They consist almost entirely of cystine; they may contain some calcium and then are slightly radio-opaque.

Cystine stones occur in dogs, especially dachshunds, and rarely in cats. They comprise ~10% of canine calculi, being second to phosphate calculi in incidence. Cystine calculi occur in males only, but cystinuria has been recorded in females.

Many dogs have high levels of urinary cystine because of defective tubular reabsorption from glomerular filtrate. Blood cystine levels are normal, demonstrating that this is a transport defect rather than an inborn error of metabolism. Many dogs with cystinuria also have high levels of other amino acids in their urine, but these are more soluble than cystine. Cystine precipitates in acid urine, but factors other than urinary pH probably are important in the genesis of cystine stones, since dogs with crystalluria do not always form them. The genetics of cystinuria is poorly understood; a familial tendency has been suggested in Irish terriers, and inheritance as an autosomal recessive trait with sex-modified expression has been postulated.

Clover Stones

Sheep grazing estrogenic pastures, particularly subterranean clover, or sheep injected or implanted with estrogens may have an incidence of fatal urinary obstruction as high as 10%. There are probably three separate developmental patterns, and in each, the obstructing material is soft or pulpy and scantily mineralized. Probably the most common pattern is urethral obstruction by desquamated cells and secretions of accessory glands originating in the pelvic urethra under the influence of estrogen. The second type, the so-called clover stone, is usually found in the renal pelvis as a yellow soft material, which leads eventually to fibrosis and shrinkage of the kidney. It affects both sexes equally. These calculi contain benzocoumarins, which may be metabolites of phytoestrogens. Third, sudden and serious mortalities may occur in male sheep grazing subterranean clover during its period of rapid maturation. The urethral process becomes impacted with a soft, white paste consisting mainly of calcium carbonate and an unidentified organic material probably related to isoflavones.

Xanthine Calculi

Xanthine stones are yellow to brown-red, often concentrically laminated, friable, and irregularly shaped. They are radiolucent. Xanthine is a metabolite of purines that seldom appears in urine because normally it is degraded by xanthine oxidase to uric acid.

Xanthine calculi occur occasionally in sheep and calves and have been reported in a dog. A high incidence in sheep was circumstantially related to deficiency of molybdenum in unimproved pasture; molybdenum is a component of xanthine oxidase. Several cases in calves in Japan were also associated with deficiency of xanthine oxidase. Xanthine precipitates in acid urine. Calculi usually form in the collecting ducts and calyces of the kidney and may cause hydronephrosis.

Other Types of Calculi

Several other types of calculi develop in animals; they may be important locally or simply be curiosities. Tetracycline and barium stones, iatrogenic and rare, fall into the latter category. Other chemical compounds are more common but often constitute a minor part of certain uroliths. Stones with a high carbonate content are associated with very alkaline urines and are seen in ruminants consuming high-oxalate plants or clover-dominated pastures. Calcium carbonate calculi are the most common type in horses but nevertheless are very rare.

Inflammation of the Lower Urinary Tract

Inflammation of the lower urinary tract revolves around inflammation of the bladder. Ureteritis is rare in the absence of cystitis, and clinical urethritis in animals usually is associated with obstruction by a calculus from the bladder. Under normal circumstances, the bladder is resistant to infection, and bacteria are quickly eliminated by the normal flow of normal urine. Predisposition to infection occurs when there is stagnation of urine due to obstruction, incomplete voiding at micturition, or urothelial trauma. Of itself, normal voiding is not sufficient to prevent and eliminate bladder infection. Defense mechanisms in the bladder and urethra that prevent bacterial adhesion to mucosal surfaces are essential if bacteria are to be removed by urine flow. Local production of IgA and surface mucins probably are important in preventing attachment of organisms to the normal urothelium, and IgG may have similar activity in specific infections.

Unlike human urine, which tends to be a good medium for bacterial growth, animal urines, especially those of dogs and cats, usually have antibacterial activity. This activity is related to urine pH and particularly to urine osmolality. In general, the further the pH from the optimum range 6–7, the less likely it is to support bacterial growth. The antibacterial effect of acid urines is related to their concentration of undissociated organic acids. High concentrations of urea and other solutes increase urine osmolality and contribute significantly to its bacteriostatic effect. Incomplete voiding at micturition may be a result of diverticula of the urinary bladder or vesicoureteral reflux. The presence of residual urine can maintain a bladder infection, allowing organisms to take advantage of any opportunity to invade the urothelium.

The usual causes of cystitis are bacteria from the urethra that are almost always from the rectal flora. When bacteria breach the surface defenses of the urothelium and attach to or penetrate the epithelial cells, the cells are desquamated and shed in the urine. When the urothelium is penetrated, neutrophils and macrophages in the submucosa respond in the usual way. Leukocytes in urines usually are not phagocytic. A variety of bacteria may be involved in bladder infections (see Pyelonephritis), and these include, in all hosts, *Escherichia coli, Proteus vulgaris,* streptococci, and staphylococci. *Corynebacterium renale* is important in cows (*C. suis* in sows), less so in other species, and is usually mixed with other organisms. In young animals with patent urachus, cystitis is common and the bacterial flora is mixed.

Cystitis does occur without obvious predispositions of the types described above. There is a higher incidence in females, which is probably associated with the short urethra. Pathologic urine may be a better medium for bacterial growth than normal urine, and although the glycosuria of diabetes mellitus promotes bacterial growth, the influence of other reducing substances and of even slight levels of proteinuria may be significant in the development of cystitis with this disease. Decreased leukocyte efficiency may also be involved. Emphysematous cystitis develops in some dogs and cats with diabetes mellitus and is thought to be caused by fermentation of sugar by glucose-fermenting bacteria. Emphysematous cystitis occurs less commonly in non-

diabetics (Fig. 5.20A). Hormone-induced changes, as in hyperestrogenism, may also affect the functional integrity of the urethral and vesicular epithelium, and the role of hormones in the production of glycosaminoglycans in the urogenital tract may also change the susceptibility to infection.

As well as the opportunistic bacterial infections that develop in all species, there are a few diseases of which inflammation of the lower urinary tract is often a part. Hemorrhagic cystitis sometimes occurs in malignant catarrhal fever in cattle and deer and occasionally is the dominant gross feature in the disease. Linear granulomas occur in the renal pelvis, ureter, and bladder of cattle with *Schistosoma mattheei* infections. Cystitis in horses and cattle grazing *Sorghum* is associated with ataxia caused by degenerative encephalomyelopathy; the bladder lesions are almost certainly neurogenic in origin. The cause of an epizootic cystitis of horses in Australia is not known.

Urogenital infections causing prostatitis, orchitis, nephritis, and cystitis may occur in canine blastomycosis.

Hemorrhagic cystitis may occur in dogs and cats treated for neoplastic or immunologic diseases with cyclophosphamide. Activated metabolites of the drug cause mucosal ulceration, hemorrhage, and edema. Signs of cystitis may follow an 8-week course of therapy. Concurrent treatment with other drugs, the degree of diuresis, and preexisting cystitis may influence the prevalence of cyclophosphamide-induced lesions. Transitional-cell carcinoma may develop in the bladder of dogs in association with prolonged cyclophosphamide therapy.

Cystitis is differentiated into acute and chronic forms, but there is considerable overlap in both the lesions and the causes. In simple acute catarrhal inflammation, there is moderate hyperemia and submucosal edema, and the surface is covered with a layer of tenacious catarrhal exudate. The urine is cloudy. Histologically, there is degeneration and desquamation of the epithelium and a prominent leukocytic infiltration. The submucosal vessels are dilated and cuffed by leukocytes. In somewhat more severe grades of inflammation, leukocytes may infiltrate all layers of the bladder wall, and hemorrhage from the dilated vessels may be severe enough to produce large clots in the bladder. These hemorrhagic complications are common in cystitis (Fig. 5.19A) following urethral obstruction, especially in cats and cattle. When the inflammatory process is severe, the cystitis may be of superficial fibrinous or deep diphtheritic type (Fig. 5.19C). In both, there is a thick, dirty yellow, friable encrustation that may peel with difficulty. A large portion of the mucosa may become necrotic, in addition to deep layers of the bladder wall. Ulcerations may penetrate the wall to the serosa or predispose to rupture.

Chronic cystitis may also take a number of anatomic forms. The simplest occurs in association with vesical calculi. The mucosa is irregularly reddened and usually thickened. There is some epithelial desquamation, and the submucosa is heavily infiltrated with inflammatory cells of mononuclear type. There are few neutrophils. In addition, there is often connective-tissue thickening of the submucosa and hypertrophy of the muscularis.

There are also some special anatomic forms of chronic cystitis. In follicular cystitis, which is common in dogs, the mucosa is studded with gray-white nodules ~1 mm across (Fig. 5.19D), which may be confluent or surrounded by a zone of

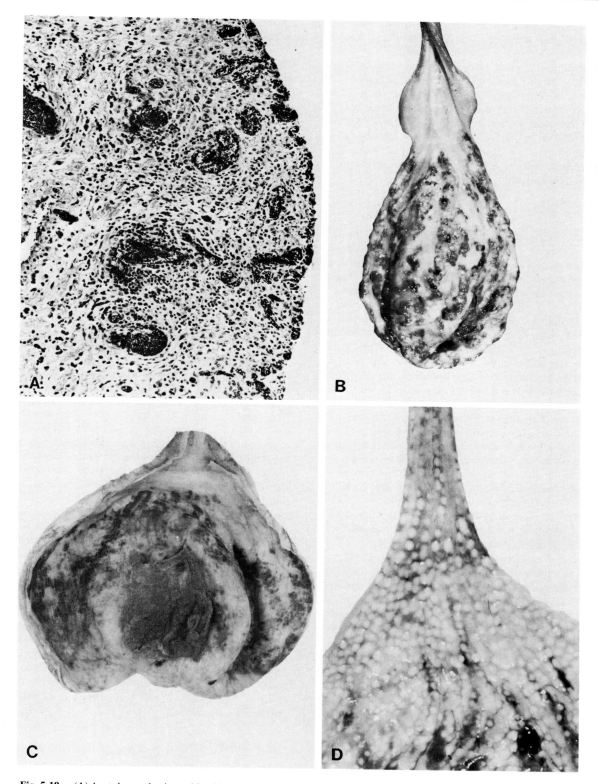

Fig. 5.19. (A) Acute hemorrhagic cystitis with complete loss of epithelium. Ox. (B) Polypoid cystitis. Dog. (C) Acute fibrinous cystitis. Dog. (D) Follicular cystitis. Dog.

hyperemia. Histologically, the nodules are proliferating aggregations of lymphocytic cells. These are immediately beneath the epithelium, which may be normal or ulcerated.

Chronic polypoid cystitis is common in any species (Figs. 5.19B and 5.20B). In this, the mucosa is thrown into many folds or villus-like sessile projections. The polyps are covered by epithelium over a core of proliferated connective tissue densely infiltrated with mononuclear leukocytes. The polyps often undergo mucoid degeneration in cattle or the epithelium may undergo metaplasia to a mucus-secreting, glandular type. Such polyps may break down and cause intermittent hematuria. Biopsy is required to differentiate them from neoplasms.

Enzootic Hematuria

Enzootic hematuria is a syndrome of mature cattle characterized by persistent hematuria and anemia, and associated with hemorrhages or neoplasms in the lower urinary tract. In more than 90% of cases, the hematuria originates from tumors of the urinary bladder. Outbreaks of the disease have been reported in sheep.

Enzootic hematuria occurs on all continents but is restricted to particular locations. In endemic areas, up to 90% of adult cattle may be affected. The syndrome is attributed to chronic ingestion of bracken fern and is reproducible experimentally; there are some apparent inconsistencies since enzootic hematuria occurs in areas devoid of bracken and does not occur in many areas where bracken is present. There are two subspecies of bracken fern, however, *Pteridium aquilinum* subsp. *aquilinum,* with eight varieties, and *P. aquilinum* subsp. *caudatum,* with four varieties, and it is not known whether all varieties are toxic. Also, the extent and persistence with which toxic ferns are grazed probably influence the incidence of bladder lesions. In areas where bracken does not grow, other plants, such as *Cheilanthes sieberi* (mulga or rock fern from Australia), appear capable of producing enzootic hematuria. In Kenya, a high incidence of bladder tumors in Zebu cattle is associated neither with ingestion of bracken nor with enzootic hematuria.

Bracken fern contains several toxic substances, including a thiaminase, a known carcinogen quercetin, and a "bleeding factor" of unknown structure; it also contains at least one other (unidentified) oncogen. The principle responsible for enzootic hematuria has not yet been identified, but it is not the thiaminase. The relationship of oncogenic viruses to bracken is discussed with the Alimentary System (this volume).

Cattle fed low levels of bracken fern develop microscopic, followed by macroscopic, hematuria. Microhematuria usually is associated with petechial, ecchymotic, or suffusive hemorrhages in the urothelium of the renal calyces, pelvis, ureter, and bladder. These lesions appear to be a manifestation of the hemorrhagic syndrome characteristic of acute bracken fern poisoning (see the Hematopoietic System, Volume 3). In some cases, microscopic hematuria occurs before gross lesions are visible. Diffuse or patchy areas of pink discoloration develop in the bladder mucosa and, microscopically, ectasia and engorgement of capillaries are present. These altered vessels are prone to hemorrhage into the bladder wall or lumen, and nodular hemangiomatous lesions develop in affected areas. In a few animals, macroscopic hematuria is associated solely with these nonneoplastic changes, but usually it is caused by development of tumors that ulcerate and bleed into the lumen (Fig. 5.20C). Occasionally, tumors also develop in the renal pelvis and ureter, and hepatic hemangiomas accompany bladder tumors in a few patients.

Several types of epithelial and mesenchymal neoplasms may develop, including transitional- and squamous-cell carcinoma, papilloma, adenoma, hemangioma, hemangiosarcoma, leiomyosarcoma, fibroma, and fibrosarcoma. Multiple tumors of more than one type may be present, and in more than 50% of affected cattle, mixed epithelial–mesenchymal neoplasms develop. Papillomas, fibromas, and hemangiomas with carcinomas are the most common types. Malignant types may invade locally, and ~10% of epithelial malignancies metastasize to iliac nodes or lungs. Chronic cystitis usually accompanies the neoplastic changes. The gross and microscopic appearance of the inflammatory and neoplastic lesions is conventional. Epithelial neoplasms appear to develop from the hyperplastic and metaplastic (squamous and mucous) changes in the urothelium, which often accompany the vascular lesions described above.

Neoplasms of the Lower Urinary Tract

Neoplasia of the lower urinary tract is most common in cattle (see Enzootic Hematuria) and dogs (Fig. 5.20B,C). There are few data for other animals, thus the following discussion concerns mainly these two species; almost all bovine tumors are from enzootic hematuria patients. Tumors of the **urinary bladder** account for less than 1% of all canine neoplasms. They occur somewhat more often in females than males, and the Scottish terrier, Shetland sheep dog, beagle, and collie seem to be at greater risk than other breeds. The greater susceptibility of females possibly is due to their decreased frequency of urination, which prolongs the exposure of the bladder mucosa to urinary oncogens. With the exception of rhabdomyosarcoma, neoplasia of the lower urinary tract usually occurs in old dogs.

Most, if not all, tumors of the **renal pelvis** and **urethra** are malignant, and except in cats are far less common than bladder tumors. This distribution in cats, admittedly based on limited data, seems to depend on the frequency of transitional-cell carcinomas in the renal pelvis and their infrequency in the urinary bladder in this species. The low incidence of bladder tumors in cats, compared to dogs, may be related to differences in their metabolism of tryptophan, which in dogs is a precursor of several aromatic amines with possible oncogenic activity. In dogs, tumors of the urethra are more common in females than males, and the beagle appears to be more prone than other breeds. They occur in old dogs, and about one-third of patients also have a tumor in the bladder.

Mesenchymal Tumors

Mesenchymal tumors comprise less than 20% of tumors of the lower urinary tract. Neoplasms causing enzootic hematuria in cattle are ~10% mesenchymal and ~55% mixed; most of the nonepithelial tumors in these mixtures are hemangiomas. A few vascular tumors also occur in the bladder and about the urethra of

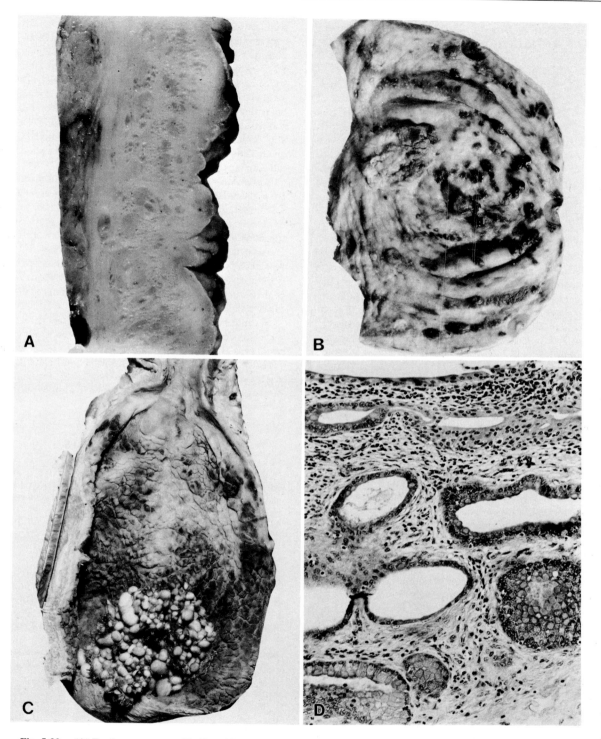

Fig. 5.20. (A) Emphysematous cystitis. Dog. Not associated with diabetes mellitus. (B) Chronic polypoid cystitis with multiple sessile and papillary areas of carcinoma. Cow. (C) Enzootic hematuria. Cow. Dark angiomatoid lesions and confluent nodular tumors involving most of the bladder mucosa. (D) Mucous adenocarcinoma of urinary bladder in enzootic hematuria. Cow. There is ulceration and inflammation of the bladder surface (above, right).

dogs, but most mesenchymal tumors in dogs are leiomyomas or fibromas. **Leiomyomas** originate in the muscular coats of the urinary bladder and form well-defined, projecting, spherical white nodules. The nodules may be multiple and seem to have a predilection for the neck of the bladder, where they may interfere with urinary outflow. Histologically, they are typical of smooth muscle tumors. **Leiomyosarcomas** are very rare and generally do not metastasize. **Fibromas** probably arise from subepithelial connective tissue, are usually solitary, and have a typical gross and microscopic appearance. **Fibrosarcomas** are rare; they are likely to metastasize, often widely. **Rhabdomyosarcoma** is a rare tumor in any location (see diseases of muscle, in Muscles and Tendons, Volume 1). Botryoid (shaped like a bunch of grapes) rhabdomyosarcoma occurs in the urinary bladder and occasionally in the urethra of young dogs; large breeds, particularly the St. Bernard, seem to be overrepresented. The youthfulness of the victims (younger than 18 months in most cases) raises the possibility that these tumors arise in rests of embryonic myoblasts. Grossly, the tumors usually project into the bladder near the neck as botryoid masses. They infiltrate the wall and may metastasize but usually draw attention to themselves before this occurs. Microscopically, there is usually a mixture of fusiform and pleomorphic cells, with some strap cells and multinuclear cells. Cytoplasmic cross-striations are sometimes present.

Epithelial Tumors

Epithelial tumors comprise ~80% of the lower urinary tract neoplasms. They occur as adenomas, papillomas, and carcinomas, and most of them develop in the bladder of old animals.

Adenomas are rare in all species; they originate from areas of mucous metaplasia of the urothelium and may be single or multiple with a papilliform or pedunculated appearance. Microscopically, they form glandular structures, some of which contain mucin. **Papillomas** constitute ~17% of primary tumors of the urinary bladder. They tend to be multiple and may be pedunculated or sessile, occasionally involving most of the mucosa. They are covered by well-differentiated transitional epithelium that is demarcated by basement membrane from a delicate supporting stroma. Squamous metaplasia of the epithelium may develop. Papillomas are susceptible to superficial necrosis, which results in hematuria. In dogs, some papillomas undergo malignant transformation to form transitional-cell or adenocarcinomas.

Carcinomas of the lower urinary tract are of four histologic types, namely, transitional-cell, squamous-cell, adeno-, and undifferentiated carcinoma. Together they make up ~60% of primary bladder tumors in dogs; approximately three-quarters of these are transitional-cell tumors. Carcinomas may be solitary or multiple and usually do not reach a large size before they cause hematuria or death from urinary complications.

Transitional-cell carcinomas may be papillary, polypoid, or sessile. Occasionally they are not visible on the vesical mucosa even though the bladder wall is infiltrated diffusely. Although there is some variation in structure, the papillary tumors, or parts of them, often are clearly transitional in type, whereas the non-

papillary tumors are usually more anaplastic and invasive. Both patterns, however, may be repeated in the metastases. A few transitional-cell carcinomas contain areas of squamous metaplasia. About 50% of transitional-cell carcinomas metastasize, sometimes in a rampant or unpredictable manner. The usual pattern is for late metastasis to regional lymph nodes and lungs, but peritoneal implantation or retrograde lymphatic spread to the soft tissue and bones of the hind limbs are common. Occasionally, solitary metastasis to bone occurs. Transitional-cell carcinoma sometimes develops in association with cyclophosphamide therapy in dogs.

Squamous-cell carcinomas and **adenocarcinomas** usually are nonpapillary infiltrative growths that grossly are nodular or sessile and often ulcerated. They develop in areas of squamous or mucous metaplasia. Histologically they are "pure," without transitional-cell areas (Fig. 5.20D). Squamous-cell carcinomas and adenocarcinomas occur in dogs and cattle, and also in cats. Apparently they are less likely to metastasize than transitional-cell tumors. **Undifferentiated carcinomas** are those very rare primary neoplasms that do not conform to one of the histologic types mentioned above.

Secondary tumors of the lower urinary tract are rare in animals but occasionally involve the bladder, comprising ~5% of neoplasms affecting the viscus. Most arrive by direct extension from the prostate (occasionally from rectum or uterus) or by implantation during peritoneal carcinomatosis. Hematogenous metastases are rare; localization of bovine lymphoma is the most common.

ACKNOWLEDGMENTS

We thank Jean Middlemiss and Sandra Brown for typing the manuscript, Jo Boyle and Pat Wallace for histologic sections, Dan Vautour for photography, and the pathologists of the Veterinary Laboratory Services and the Ontario Veterinary College for case material.

BIBLIOGRAPHY

General

Banks, W. J. Urinary system. *In* "Applied Veterinary Histology." Baltimore, Williams & Wilkins, 1981.

Barsanti, J. A., and Finco, D. R. Protein concentration in urine of normal dogs. *Am J Vet Res* **40:** 1583–1588, 1979.

Benitez, L., and Shaka, J. A. Cell proliferation in experimental hydronephrosis and compensatory renal hyperplasia. *Am J Pathol* **44:** 961–972, 1964.

Berliner, R. W. Mechanisms of urine concentration. *Kidney Int* **22:** 202–211, 1982.

Bernstein, L. M. "Renal Function and Renal Failure." Baltimore, Williams & Wilkins, 1965.

Bialestock, D. The extraglomerular arterial circulation of the renal tubules. *Anat Rec* **129:** 53–57, 1958.

Bradley, S. E., and Wheeler, H. O. On the diversities of structure, perfusion and function of the nephron population. *Am J Med* **24:** 692–708, 1958.

Brenner, B. M., Hostetter, T. H., and Humes, H. D. Molecular basis of proteinuria of glomerular origin. *N Engl J Med* **298:** 826–833, 1978.

Brown, E. M. Urinary system. *In* "Textbook of Veterinary Histology,"

H.-D. Dellman and E. M. Brown (eds.), 2nd ed. Philadelphia, Lea & Febiger, 1981.

Bulger, R. E., Cronin, R. E., and Dobyan, D. C. Survey of the morphology of the dog kidney. *Anat Rec* **194:** 41–66, 1979.

Burkholder, P. M. Functions and pathophysiology of the glomerular mesangium. *Lab Invest* **46:** 239–241, 1982.

Cheville, N. F. Kidney. *In* "Cell Pathology." Ames, Iowa State Univ. Press, 1976.

Chew, R. M. Water metabolism of desert-inhabiting vertebrates. *Biol Rev* **36:** 1–31, 1961.

Christensen, G. C. Circulation of blood through the canine kidney. *Am J Vet Res* **13:** 236–245, 1952.

Darmady, E. M., and MacIver, A. G. "Renal Pathology." London, Butterworth, 1980.

De Wardener, H. E., and Clarkson, E. M. The natriuretic hormone: recent developments. *Clin Sci Mol Med* **63:** 415–420, 1982.

Ericsson, J. L. E., Trump, B. F., and Weibel, J. Electron microscopic studies of the proximal tubule of the rat kidney, II. Cytosegresomes and cytosomes: their relationship to each other and to the lysosome concept. *Lab Invest* **14:** 1341–1365, 1965.

Eriksson, L. Renal corticopapillary concentration gradient in calves. *Acta Vet Scand* **13:** 197–205, 1972.

Francisco, L. L., Sawin, L. L., and DiBona, G. F. On the signal for activation of tubuloglomerular feedback. *J Lab Clin Med* **99:** 722–730, 1982.

Golden, A., and Maher, J. F. "The Kidney: Structure and Function in Disease," 2nd ed. Baltimore, Williams & Wilkins, 1977.

Goodwin, W. E., and Kaufman, J. J. Renal Lymphatics. 1. Review of some of the pertinent literature. *Urol Surv* **6:** 305–329, 1956.

Grauer, G. F., and Kunze, R. S. Potassium depletion nephropathy and renal medullary washout: a case report. *Calif Vet* **33:** 8–10, 1979.

Hay, D. A., and Evan, A. P. Maturation of the glomerular visceral epithelium and capillary endothelium in the puppy kidney. *Anat Rec* **193:** 1–22, 1979.

Heptinstall, R. H. "Pathology of the Kidney," 2nd ed., Vols. I and II. Boston, Little, Brown, 1974.

Hoffman, E. O., and Flores, T. R. High resolution light microscopy in renal pathology. *Am J Clin Pathol* **76:** 636–643, 1981.

Jamison, R. L., and Maffly, R. H. The urinary concentrating mechanism. *N Engl J Med* **295:** 1059–1067, 1976.

Jeraj, K., Osborne, C. A., and Stevens, J. B. Evaluation of renal biopsy in 197 dogs and cats. *J Am Vet Med Assoc* **181:** 367–369, 1982.

Kaufman, J. J., and Goodwin, W. E. Renal lymphatics. 3. Clinical implications and experiments of nature. *Ann Intern Med* **49:** 109–118, 1958.

Layton, J. M. The structure of the kidney from gross to the molecular. *J Urol* **90:** 502–515, 1963.

Leaf, A., and Cotran, R. "Renal Pathophysiology." London and New York, Oxford Univ. Press, 1976.

Levinsky, N. G. The renal kallikrein–kinin system. *Circ Res* **44:** 441–451, 1979.

Lobban, M. C. Some observations on the intracellular lipid in the kidney of the cat. *J Anat* **89:** 92–99, 1955.

Lucke, V. M. Renal disease in the domestic cat. *J Pathol Bacteriol* **95:** 67–91, 1968.

Maher, J. F. Pathophysiology of renal hemodynamics. *Nephron* **27:** 215–221, 1981.

Mayer, E., and Ottolenghi, L. A. Protrusion of tubular epithelium into the space of Bowman's capsule in dogs and cats. *Anat Rec* **99:** 477–510, 1947.

Oparil, S., and Haber, E. The renin–angiotensin system. *N Engl J Med* **291:** 389–401 and 446–457, 1974.

Osborne, C. A., Finco, D. R., and Low, D. G. Pathophysiology of renal disease, renal failure, and uremia. *In* "Textbook of Veterinary Inter-

nal Medicine," S. J. Ettinger (ed.), 2nd ed. Philadelphia, Saunders, 1983.

Peart, W. S. Renin 1978. *Johns Hopkins Med J* **143:** 193–206, 1978.

Potter, E. L. Development of the human glomerulus. *Arch Pathol* **80:** 241–255, 1965.

Robbins, S. L., and Cotran, R. S. The kidney. *In* "Pathologic Basis of Disease," 2nd ed. Philadelphia, Saunders, 1979.

Schmidt-Nielsen, B. Excretion in mammals: role of the renal pelvis in the modification of the urinary concentration and composition. *Fed Proc* **36:** 2493–2503, 1977.

Spangler, W. L. Pathophysiologic response of the juxtaglomerular apparatus to dietary sodium restriction in the dog. *Am J Vet Res* **40:** 809–819, 1979.

Walker, F. The origin, turnover, and removal of glomerular basement membrane. *J Pathol* **110:** 233–244, 1973.

Yadava, R. P., and Calhoun, M. L. Comparative histology of the kidney of domestic animals. *Am J Vet Res* **19:** 958–968, 1958.

Zins, G. R. Renal prostaglandins. *Am J Med* **58:** 14–24, 1975.

Zollinger, H. U., and Mihatsch, M. J. "Renal Pathology in Biopsy. Light, Electron, and Immunofluorescent Microscopy and Clinical Aspects." New York, Springer-Verlag, 1978.

Kidney

Uremia

Black, D. A. K. A perspective on uremic toxins. *Arch Intern Med* **126:** 906–909, 1970.

Brenner, B. M., Meyer, T. W., and Hostetter, T. H. Dietary protein intake and the progressive nature of kidney disease: the role of hemodynamically mediated glomerular injury in the pathogenesis of progressive glomerular sclerosis in aging, renal ablation, and intrinsic renal disease. *N Engl J Med* **307:** 652–659, 1982.

Bricker, N. S. On the pathogenesis of the uremic state. An exposition of the "trade-off hypothesis." *N Engl J Med* **286:** 1093–1099, 1972.

Cheville, N. F. Uremic gastropathy in the dog. *Vet Pathol* **16:** 292–309, 1979.

Comty, C. M., Cohen, S. L., and Shapiro, F. L. Pericarditis in chronic uremia and its sequels. *Ann Intern Med* **75:** 173–183, 1971.

Finco, D. R., and Rowland, G. N. Hypercalcemia secondary to chronic renal failure in the dog: a report of four cases. *J Am Vet Med Assoc* **173:** 990–994, 1978.

Gottschalk, C. W. Function of the chronically diseased kidney. The adaptive nephron. *Circ Res* **28** and **29:** Suppl II, 1–13, 1971.

LeGeros, R. Z., Contiguglia, S. R., and Alfrey, A. C. Pathological calcifications associated with uremia. Two types of calcium phosphate deposits. *Calcif Tissue Res* **13:** 173–185, 1973.

Massry, J. G., and Goldstein, D. A. Role of parathyroid hormone in uremic toxicity. *Kidney Int* **13:** Suppl 8, S39–S42, 1978.

Massry, S. G., and Ritz, E. The pathogenesis of secondary hyperparathyroidism of renal failure. Is there a controversy? *Arch Intern Med* **138:** 853–856, 1978.

Osborne, C. A., Finco, D. R., and Low, D. G. Pathophysiology of renal disease, renal failure, and uremia. *In* "Textbook of Veterinary Internal Medicine," S. J. Ettinger (ed.), 2nd ed. Philadelphia, Saunders, 1982.

Tennant, B., Bettleheim, P., and Kaneko, J. J. Paradoxic hypercalcemia and hypophosphatemia associated with chronic renal failure in horses. *J Am Vet Med Assoc* **180:** 630–634, 1982.

Renal Anomalies

Bernstein, J. The morphogenesis of renal parenchymal maldevelopment (renal dysplasia). *Pediatr Clin North Am* **18:** 395–407, 1971.

Bernstein, J. The classification of renal cysts. *Nephron* **11**: 91–100, 1973.

Burk, D., and Beaudoin, A. R. Arsenate-induced renal agenesis in rats. *Teratology* **16**: 247–259, 1977.

Cordes, D. O., and Dodd, D. C. Bilateral renal hypoplasia of the pig. *Pathol Vet* **2**: 37–48, 1965.

Crocker, J. F. S., Brown, D. M., and Vernier, R. L. Development defects of the kidney. A review of renal development and experimental studies of maldevelopment. *Pediatr Clin North Am* **18**: 355–376, 1971.

Dennis, S. M. Urogenital defects in sheep. *Vet Rec* **105**: 344–347, 1979.

Evan, A. P. *et al.* Evolution of the collecting tubular lesion in diphenylamine-induced renal disease. *Lab Invest* **38**: 244–252, 1978.

Jacobsson, L. *et al.* Fluid turnover in renal cysts. *Acta Med Scand* **202**: 327–329, 1977.

Johnson, C. A. Renal ectopia in a cat. A case report and literature review. *J Am Anim Hosp Assoc* **15**: 599–602, 1979.

Kilham, L., Margolis, G., and Colby, E. D. Congenital infections of cats and ferrets by feline panleukopenia virus manifested by cerebellar hypoplasia. *Lab Invest* **17**: 465–480, 1967.

Mack, C. O., and McGlothlin, J. H. Renal agenesis in the female cat. *Anat Rec* **105**: 445–450, 1949.

O'Handley, P., Carrig, C. B., and Walshaw, R. Renal and ureteral duplication in a dog. *J Am Vet Med Assoc* **174**: 484–487, 1979.

Palludan, B. The teratogenic effect of vitamin A deficiency in pigs. *Acta Vet Scand* **2**: 32–59, 1961.

Percy, D. H. *et al.* Lesions in puppies surviving infection with canine herpesvirus. *Vet Pathol* **8**: 37–53, 1971.

Pitts, W. R., and Muecke, E. C. Horseshoe kidneys: a 40-year experience. *J Urol* **113**: 743–746, 1975.

Risdon, R. A. Renal dysplasia. *J Clin Pathol* **24**: 57–71, 1971.

Robbins, G. R. Unilateral renal agenesis in the beagle. *Vet Rec* **77**: 1345–1347, 1965.

Story, H. E. A case of horseshoe kidney in the domestic cat. *Anat Rec* **86**: 307–319, 1943.

Webster, W. R., and Summers, P. M. Congenital polycystic kidney and liver syndrome in piglets. *Aust Vet J* **54**: 451, 1978.

Wells, G. A. H., Hebert, C. N., and Robins, B. C. Renal cysts in pigs: prevalence and pathology in slaughtered pigs from a single herd. *Vet Rec* **106**: 532–535, 1980.

Wijeratne, W. V. S., and Wells, G. A. H. Inherited renal cysts in pigs: results of breeding experiments. *Vet Rec* **107**: 484–488, 1980.

Wulfson, M. A. Pyelocaliceal diverticula. *J. Urol* **123**: 1–8, 1980.

Familial Renal Diseases

Bernard, M. A., and Valli, V. E. Familial renal disease in Samoyed dogs. *Can Vet J* **18**: 181–189, 1977.

Bloedow, A. G. Familial renal disease in Samoyed dogs. *Vet Rec* **108**: 167–168, 1981.

Chew, D. J. *et al.* Juvenile renal disease in Doberman pinscher dogs. *J Am Vet Med Assoc* **182**: 481–485, 1983.

Cuppage, F. E., Shimamura, T., and McGavin, M. D. Nephron obstruction in mutant Southdown sheep. *Vet Pathol* **16**: 483–485, 1979.

Finco, D. R. *et al.* Familial renal disease in Norwegian elkhound dogs: morphologic examinations. *Am J Vet Res* **38**: 941–947, 1977.

Hill, G. S., Jenis, E. H., and Goodloe, S. The nonspecificity of the ultrastructural alterations in hereditary nephritis. *Lab Invest* **31**: 516–532, 1974.

Lucke, V. M. *et al.* Chronic renal failure in young dogs—possible renal dysplasia. *J Small Anim Pract* **21**: 169–181, 1980.

McKenna, S. C., and Carpenter, J. L. Polycystic disease of the kidney and liver in the Cairn terrier. *Vet Pathol* **17**: 436–442, 1980.

O'Brien, T. D. *et al.* Clinicopathologic manifestations of progressive renal disease in Lhasa Apso and Shih Tzu dogs. *J Am Vet Med Assoc* **180**: 658–664, 1982.

O'Neill, W. M., Atkin, C. L., and Bloomer, H. A. Hereditary nephritis: a re-examination of its clinical and genetic features. *Ann Intern Med* **88**: 176–182, 1978.

Wilcock, B. P., and Patterson, J. M. Familial glomerulonephritis in Doberman pinscher dogs. *Can Vet J* **20**: 244–249, 1979.

Circulatory Disturbances

Alexander, N., Heptinstall, R. H., and Pickering, G. W. The effects of embolic obstruction of intrarenal arteries in the rabbit. *J Pathol Bacteriol* **81**: 225–237, 1961.

Baum, N. H., Moriel, E., and Carlton, C. E. Renal vein thrombosis. *J. Urol* **119**: 443–448, 1978.

Byrom, F. B., and Pratt, O. E. Oxytocin and renal cortical necrosis. *Lancet* **1**: 753–754, 1959.

Conger, J. D., and Schrier, R. W. Renal hemodynamics in acute renal failure. *Annu Rev Physiol* **42**: 603–614, 1980.

Davies, D. J. The patterns of renal infarction caused by different types of temporary ischaemia. *J Pathol* **102**: 151–162, 1970.

Diethelm, A. G., and Wilson, S. J. Obstruction to the renal microcirculation after temporary ischemia. *J Surg Res* **11**: 265–276, 1971.

Dunn, M. J., and Hood, V. L. Prostaglandins and the kidney. *Am J. Physiol* **233**: F169–F184, 1977.

Frega, N. S. *et al.* Ischemic renal injury. *Kidney Int* **10**: S17–S25, 1976.

Gavan, T. L., and Kaufman, N. Experimental renal infarction. 2. Histochemical, fatty, and morphologic changes. *Arch Pathol* **62**: 386–390, 1956.

Hall, G. A. Renal cortical necrosis in a cat. *Vet Pathol* **9**: 122–130, 1972.

Hani, H., and Indermuhle, N. A. Bilateral renal cortical necrosis associated with esophagogastric ulceration in pigs. *Vet Pathol* **17**: 234–237, 1980.

Johnston, W. H., and Latta, H. Glomerular mesangial and endothelial cell swelling following temporary renal ischemia and its role in the no-reflow phenomenon. *Am J Pathol* **89**: 153–166, 1977.

Kreisberg, J. I. *et al.* Effects of transient hypotension on the structure and function of rat kidney. *Virchows Arch [Cell Pathol]* **22**: 121–133, 1976.

Lauler, D. P., and Schreiner, G. E. Bilateral renal cortical necrosis. *Am J Med* **24**: 519–528, 1958.

Miyazaki, M., and McNay, J. Redistribution of renal cortical blood flow during ureteral occlusion and renal venous constriction. *Proc Soc Exp Biol Med* **138**: 454–461, 1971.

Montgomery, S. B. *et al.* The regulation of intrarenal blood flow in the dog during ischemia. *Circ Shock* **7**: 71–82, 1980.

Nordstoga, K. Spontaneous bilateral renal cortical necrosis in animals. *Pathol Vet* **4**: 233–244, 1967.

Nordstoga, K., and Fjolstad, M. The generalized Shwartzman reaction and *Haemophilus* infection in pigs. *Pathol Vet* **4**: 245–253, 1967.

Nordstoga, K., and Fjolstad, M. Necrotizing angiitis produced by the Shwartman mechanism. *Acta Pathol Microbiol Scand [A]* **81**: 775–783, 1973.

Plakke, R. K., and Pfeiffer, E. W. Blood vessels of the mammalian renal medulla. *Science* **146**: 1683–1685, 1964.

Raij, L., Keane, W. F., and Michael, A. F. Unilateral Shwartzman reaction: cortical necrosis in one kidney following *in vivo* perfusion with endotoxin. *Kidney Int* **12**: 91–95, 1977.

Rashid, H. A. *et al.* Renal cortical necrosis: a model for the study of juxtamedullary nephron physiology. *J Appl Physiol* **37:** 228–234, 1974.

Richman, A. V., Gerber, L. I., and Balis, J. U. Peritubular capillaries. A major target site of endotoxin-induced vascular injury in the primate kidney. *Lab Invest* **43:** 327–332, 1980.

Sevitt, S. Pathogenesis of traumatic uraemia. *Lancet* **2:** 135–140, 1959.

Sheehan, H. L., and Davis, J. C. Patchy permanent renal ischaemia. *J Pathol Bacteriol* **77:** 33–46, 1959.

Sheehan, H. L., and Davis, J. C. Renal ischaemia with failed reflow. *J Pathol Bacteriol* **78:** 105–120, 1959.

Sheehan, H. L., and Davis, J. C. Renal ischaemia with good reflow. *J Pathol Bacteriol* **78:** 351–377, 1959.

Sheehan, H. L., and Davis, J. C. Intermittent complete renal ischaemia. *J Pathol Bacteriol* **79:** 77–87, 1960.

Sheehan, H. L., and Davis, J. C. Minor renal lesions due to experimental ischaemia. *J Pathol Bacteriol* **80:** 259–270, 1960.

Skinner, D. G., and Hayes, M. A. Effect of staphylococcal toxin on renal function: irreversible shock. *Ann Surg* **162:** 161–180, 1965.

Stein, J. H. *et al.* Mechanism of the redistribution of renal cortical blood flow during hemorrhagic hypotension in the dog. *J Clin Invest* **52:** 39–47, 1973.

Steinmetz, P. R., and Kiley, J. E. Renal tubular necrosis following lesions of the brain. *Am J Med* **29:** 268–276, 1960.

Summers, W. K., and Jamison, R. L. The no reflow phenomenon in renal ischemia. *Lab Invest* **25:** 635–643, 1971.

Thal, A. Selective renal vasospasm and ischaemic renal necrosis produced experimentally with staphylococcal toxin. *Am J Pathol* **31:** 233–256, 1955.

Wardle, E. N. Endotoxinaemia and the pathogenesis of acute renal failure. *Q J Med* **44:** 389–398, 1975.

Wells, J. D., Margolin, E. G., and Gall, E. A. Renal cortical necrosis. *Am J Med* **29:** 257–267, 1960.

Papillary Necrosis

Burry, A. Pathology of analgesic nephropathy: Australian experience. *Kidney Int* **13:** 34–40, 1978.

Duggin, G. G. Mechanisms in the development of analgesic nephropathy. *Kidney Int* **18:** 553–561, 1980.

Eknoyan, G. *et al.* Renal papillary necrosis: an update. *Medicine (Baltimore)* **61:** 55–73, 1982.

Gunson, D. E. Renal papillary necrosis in horses. *J Am Vet Med Assoc* **182:** 263–266, 1983.

Lucke, V. M., and Hunt, A. C. Interstitial nephropathy and papillary necrosis in the domestic cat. *J Pathol Bacteriol* **89:** 723–728, 1965.

Salisbury, R. M. Mortality of lambs and cattle following the administration of phenothiazine. 1. Field cases. NZ Vet J **17:** 187–191, 1969.

Salisbury, R. M., McIntosh, I. G., and Staples, E. L. J. Mortality in lambs and cattle following the administration of phenothiazine. 2. Laboratory investigations. NZ Vet J **17:** 227–233, 1969.

Zenser, T. V. *et al.* Effect of aspirin on metabolism of acetaminophen and benzidine by renal inner medulla prostaglandin hydroperoxidase. *J Lab Clin Med* **101:** 58–65, 1983.

Hydronephrosis

Breitschwerdt, E. B. *et al.* Bilateral hydronephrosis and hydroureter in a dog associated with congenital urethral stricture. *J Am Anim Hosp Assoc* **18:** 799–803, 1982.

Dominguez, R., and Adams, R. B. Renal function during and after acute hydronephrosis in the dog. *Lab Invest* **7:** 292–327, 1958.

Greene, J. A., Thornhill, J. A., and Blevins, W. E. Hydronephrosis and hydroureter associated with a unilateral ectopic ureter in a spayed bitch. *J Am Anim Hosp Assoc* **14:** 708–713, 1978.

Hall, M. A., Osborne, C. A., and Stevens, J. B. Hydronephrosis with heteroplastic bone formation in a cat. *J Am Vet Med Assoc* **160:** 857–860, 1972.

Holmes, M. J., O'Morchoe, P. J., and O'Morchoe, C. C. C. The role of renal lymph in hydronephrosis. *Invest Urol* **15:** 215–219, 1977.

Nagle, R. B., and Bulger, R. E. Unilateral obstructive nephropathy in the rabbit. II. Late morphologic changes. *Lab Invest* **38:** 270–278, 1978.

Sheehan, H. L., and Davis, H. C. Experimental hydronephrosis. *Am Med Assoc Arch Pathol* **68:** 185–225, 1959.

Skye, D. V. Hydronephrosis secondary to focal papillary hyperplasia of the urinary bladder of cattle. *J Am Vet Med Assoc* **166:** 596–598, 1975.

Wilson, D. R. Pathophysiology of obstructive nephropathy. *Kidney Int* **18:** 281–292, 1980.

Yarger, W. E., Schocken, D. D., and Harris, R. H. Obstructive nephropathy in the rat. Possible roles for the renin–angiotensin system, prostaglandins, and thromboxanes in postobstructive renal function. *J Clin Invest* **65:** 400–412, 1980.

Glomerular Diseases

Abramowsky, C. R. *et al. Dirofilaria immitis*. 5. Immunopathology of filarial nephropathy in dogs. *Am J Pathol* **104:** 1–12, 1981.

Angus, K. W. *et al.* Mesangiocapillary glomerulonephritis in lambs: the ultrastructure and immunopathology of diffuse glomerulonephritis in newly born Finnish Landrace lambs. *J Pathol* **131:** 65–74, 1980.

Banks, K. L., and Henson, J. B. Immunologically mediated glomerulitis of horses. II. Antiglomerular basement membrane antibody and other mechanisms in spontaneous disease. *Lab Invest* **26:** 708–715, 1972.

Banks, K. L., Henson, J. B., and McGuire, T. C. Immunologically mediated glomerulitis of horses. I. Pathogenesis in persistent infection by equine infectious anemia virus. *Lab Invest* **26:** 701–707, 1972.

Biewenga, W. J., Gruys, E., and Hendriks, H. J. Urinary protein loss in the dog: nephrological study of 29 dogs without signs of renal disease. *Res Vet Sci* **33:** 366–374, 1982.

Cameron, J. S. Glomerulonephritis: current problems and understanding. *J Lab Clin Med* **99:** 755–787, 1982.

Casey, H. W., and Splitter, G. A. Membranous glomerulonephritis in dogs infected with *Dirofilaria immitis. Vet Pathol* **12:** 111–117, 1975.

Cohen, A. H. Morphology of renal tubular hyaline casts. *Lab Invest* **44:** 280–287, 1981.

Crowell, W. A., Duncan, J. R., and Finco, D. R. Canine glomeruli: light and electron microscopic change in biopsy, perfused, and *in situ* antolysed kidneys from normal dogs. *Am J Vet Res* **35:** 889–896, 1974.

Cutlip, R. C., McClurkin, A. W., and Coria, M. F. Lesions in clinically healthy cattle persistently infected with the virus of bovine viral diarrhea–glomerulonephritis and encephalitis. *Am J Vet Res* **41:** 1938–1941, 1980.

DiBartola, S. P. *et al.* Urinary protein excretion and immunopathologic findings in dogs with glomerular disease. *J Am Vet Med Assoc* **177:** 73–77, 1980.

Fillit, H. M., and Zabriskie, J. B. Cellular immunity in glomerulonephritis. *Am J Pathol* **109:** 227–243, 1982.

Gaffney, E. F. Prominent parietal epithelium: a common sign of renal glomerular injury. *Hum Pathol* **13:** 651–660, 1982.

Glick, A. D., Horn, R. G., and Holscher, M. Characterization of feline glomerulonephritis associated with viral-induced hematopoietic neoplasms. *Am J Pathol* **92:** 321–332, 1978.

Hamilton, J. M., Naylor, J., and Weatherley, A. Glomerular lesions associated with infestation with *Toxocara cati*. *Vet Rec* **111:** 583–584, 1982.

Hayashi, T., Ishida, T., and Fujiwara, K. Glomerulonephritis associated with feline infectious peritonitis. *Jpn J Vet Sci* **44:** 909–916, 1982.

Holdsworth, S. R., Neale, T. J., and Wilson, C. B. The participation of macrophages and monocytes in experimental immune complex glomerulonephritis. *Clin Immunol Immunopathol* **15:** 510–524, 1980.

Isaacs, K. L., and Miller, F. Role of antigen size and charge in immune complex glomerulonephritis. I. Active induction of disease with dextran and its derivatives. *Lab Invest* **47:** 198–205, 1982.

Kashgarian, M., Hayslett, J. P., and Spargo, B. H. Renal disease. *Am J Pathol* **89:** 187–272, 1977.

Kurtz, J. M. *et al.* Naturally occurring canine glomerulonephritis. *Am J Pathol* **67:** 471–482, 1972.

Lerner, R. A., and Dixon, F. J. Spontaneous glomerulonephritis in sheep. *Lab Invest* **15:** 1279–1289, 1966.

Lerner, R. A., Dixon, F. J., and Lee, S. Spontaneous glomerulonephritis in sheep. II. Studies on natural history, occurrence in other species, and pathogenesis. *Am J Pathol* **53:** 501–512, 1968.

Lewis, R. J. Canine glomerulonephritis: results from a microscopic evaluation of fifty cases. *Can Vet J* **17:** 171–176, 1976.

McCluskey, R. T. Modification of glomerular immune complex deposits. *Lab Invest* **48:** 241–244, 1983.

MacIver, A. G. Diagnosis and classification of primary glomerulonephritis: a review. *Diag Histopathol* **5:** 231–281, 1982.

Magil, A. B., and Wadsworth, L. D. Monocyte involvement in glomerular crescents. A histochemical and ultrastructural study. *Lab Invest* **47:** 160–166, 1982.

Morrison, W. I., Nash, A. S., and Wright, N. G. Glomerular deposition of immune complexes in dogs following natural infection with canine adenovirus. *Vet Rec* **96:** 522–524, 1975.

Morrison, W. I., and Wright, N. G. Immunopathological aspects of canine renal disease. *J Small Anim Pract* **17:** 139–148, 1976.

Mostofi, F. K., Antonovych, T. T., and Limas, E. Patterns of glomerular reaction to injury. *Hum Pathol* **2:** 233–252, 1971.

Müller-Peddinghaus, R., and Trautwein, G. Spontaneous glomerulonephritis in dogs. I. Classification and immunopathology. *Vet Pathol* **14:** 1–13, 1977.

Müller-Peddinghaus, R., and Trautwein, G. Spontaneous glomerulonephritis in dogs. II. Correlation of glomerulonephritis with age, chronic interstitial nephritis and extrarenal lesions. *Vet Pathol* **14:** 121–127, 1977.

Murray, M., and Wright, N. G. A morphologic study of canine glomerulonephritis. *Lab Invest* **30:** 213–221, 1974.

Osborne, C. A. *et al.* Natural remission of nephrotic syndrome in a dog with immune-complex glomerular disease. *J Am Vet Med Assoc* **168:** 129–137, 1976.

Osborne, C. A. *et al.* The glomerulus in health and disease: comparative review of domestic animals and man. *Adv Vet Sci Comp Med* **21:** 207–285, 1977.

Rouse, B. T., and Lewis, R. J. Canine glomerulonephritis: prevalence in dogs submitted at random for euthanasia. *Can J Comp Med* **39:** 365–370, 1975.

Simpson, C. F. *et al.* Glomerulosclerosis in canine heartworm infection. *Vet Pathol* **11:** 506–514, 1974.

Slauson, D. O., and Lewis, R. M. Comparative pathology of glomerulonephritis in animals. *Vet Pathol* **16:** 135–164, 1979.

Spencer, A. J., and Wright, N. G. Glomerular lesions in chronic interstitial nephritis in the dog: histological and ultrastructural features. *J Comp Pathol* **91:** 393–408, 1981.

Spencer, A. J., Wright, N. G., and MacMillan, I. Liquoid-induced renal lesions in the dog. *Vet Pathol* **18:** 92–109, 1981.

Stuart, B. P., Phemister, R. D., and Thomassen, R. W. Glomerular lesions associated with proteinuria in clinically healthy dogs. *Vet Pathol* **12:** 125–144, 1975.

Tornroth, T., and Skrifvars, B. The development and resolution of glomerular basement membrane changes associated with subepithelial immune deposits. *Am J Pathol* **79:** 219–236, 1975.

Wimberley, H. C., Antonovych, T. T., and Lewis, R. M. Focal glomerulosclerosis-like disease with nephrotic syndrome in a horse. *Vet Pathol* **18:** 692–694, 1981.

Wiseman, A., Spencer, A., and Petrie, L. The nephrotic syndrome in a heifer due to glomerulonephritis. *Res Vet Sci* **28:** 325–329, 1980.

Wright, N. G. *et al.* Chronic renal failure in dogs: a comparative clinical and morphological study of chronic glomerulonephritis and chronic interstitial nephritis. *Vet Rec* **98:** 288–293, 1976.

Wright, N. G. *et al.* Membranous nephropathy in the cat and dog. A renal biopsy and follow-up study of sixteen cases. *Lab Invest* **45:** 269–277, 1981.

Wright, N. G., Thompson, H., and Cornwell, H. J. C. Canine nephrotoxic glomerulonephritis. *Vet Pathol* **10:** 69–86, 1973.

Young, G. B. *et al.* Genetic aspects of mesangiocapillary glomerulonephritis in Finnish sheep. *Br Vet J* **137:** 368–373, 1981.

Amyloidosis

Chew, D. J. *et al.* Renal amyloidosis in related Abyssinian cats. *J Am Vet Med Assoc* **181:** 139–142, 1982.

Cohen, A. S. *et al.* Amyloid proteins, precursors, mediator, and enhancer. *Lab Invest* **48:** 1–4, 1983.

Crowell, W. A. *et al.* Generalized amyloidosis in a cat. *J Am Vet Med Assoc* **161:** 1127–1133, 1972.

DiBartola, S. P., and Meuten, D. J. Renal amyloidosis in two dogs presented for thromboembolic phenomena. *J Am Anim Hosp Assoc* **16:** 129–135, 1980.

Glenner, G. G. Amyloid deposits and amyloidosis. The β-filbrilloses. *N Engl J Med* **302:** 1283–1292 and 1333–1343, 1980.

Green, R. A., and Kabel, A. L. Hypercoagulable state in three dogs with nephrotic syndrome: role of acquired antithrombin III deficiency. *J Am Vet Med Assoc* **181:** 914–917, 1982.

Gruys, E. Amyloidosis in the bovine kidney. *Vet Sci Commun* **1:** 265–276, 1977.

Gruys, E., and Timmermans, H. J. F. Diagnosis of secondary amyloid in bovine renal amyloidosis. *Vet Sci Commun* **3:** 21–37, 1979.

Monaghan, M. Renal amyloidosis in slaughter cattle in Ireland. *Ir Vet J* **36:** 88–90, 1982.

Osborne, C. A. *et al.* Clinicopathologic progression of renal amyloidosis in a dog. *J Am Vet Med Assoc* **157:** 203–219, 1970.

Slauson, D. O., Gribble, D. H., and Russell, S. W. A clinicopathological study of renal amyloidosis in dogs. *J Comp Pathol* **80:** 335–343, 1970.

Glomerular Lipidosis

Fisher, E. R., and Fisher, B. Glomerular lipoidosis in the dog. *Am J Vet Res* **15:** 285–286, 1954.

Zayed, I. *et al.* A light and electron microscopical study of glomerular lipoidosis in beagle dogs. *J Comp Pathol* **86:** 509–517, 1976.

Diseases of Tubules

General

Baker, S. B. de C., and Davies, R. L. F. Experimental haemoglobinuric nephrosis. *J Pathol Bacteriol* **87:** 49–56, 1964.

Benson, J. A., and Williams, B. M. Acute renal failure in lambs. *Br Vet J* **130:** 475–481, 1974.

Bourdeau, J. E., and Carone, F. A. Protein handling by the renal tubule. *Nephron* **13:** 22–34, 1974.

Breitschwerdt, E. B., Verlander, J. W., and Hribernik, T. N. Nephrogenic diabetes insipidus in three dogs. *J Am Vet Med Assoc* **179:** 235–238, 1981.

Bryant, S. J. Hyaline droplet formation in the renal epithelium of patients with haemoglobinuria. *J Clin Pathol* **20:** 854–856, 1967.

Buck, W. B., Osweiler, G. D., and Van Gelder, G. A. *In* "Clinical and Diagnostic Veterinary Toxicology," G. A. Van Gelder (ed.), 2nd ed. Dubuque, Iowa, Kendall/Hunt Publ. Co., 1976.

Carroll, R., Kovacs, K., and Tapp, E. The pathogenesis of glycerol-induced renal tubular necrosis. *J Pathol Bacteriol* **89:** 573–580, 1965.

Clark, R. G., and Lewis, K. H. C. Deaths in sheep after overdosage with thiabendazole. *NZ Vet J* **25:** 187–190, 1977.

Davies, D. J., and Kennedy, A. The excretion of renal cells following necrosis of the proximal convoluted tubule. *Br J Exp Pathol* **48:** 45–50, 1967.

Diamond, J. R., and Yoburn, D. C. Nonoliguric acute renal failure. *Arch Intern Med* **142:** 1882–1884, 1982.

DiBartola, S. P. Acute renal failure: pathophysiology and management. *Compend Contin Educ* **2:** 952–958, 1980.

Divers, T. J. *et al.* Acute renal disorders in cattle: a retrospective study of 22 cases. *J Am Vet Med Assoc* **181:** 694–699, 1982.

Dobyan, D. C., Nagle, R. B., and Bulger, R. E. Acute tubular necrosis in the rat kidney following sustained hypotension. Physiologic and morphologic observations. *Lab Invest* **4:** 411–422, 1977.

Ericsson, J. L. E. Transport and digestion of hemoglobin in the proximal tubule. I. Light microscopy and cytochemistry of acid phosphatase. II. Electron microscopy. *Lab Invest* **14:** 1–15 and 16–39, 1965.

Fajers, C. M. Experimental studies in hemoglobinuric nephrosis. 3. The effect of acute hemolytic anemia (hemoglobinemia) combined with ten minutes' unilateral renal ischemia on the morphology and function of the rabbit's kidneys. *Acta Pathol Microbiol Scand* **46:** 177–196, 1959.

Faragalla, F. F. *et al.* Vitamin B$_6$ deficiency and oxalate nephrocalcinosis in the cat. *Am J Med* **27:** 72–80, 1959.

Finn, W. F. Nephron heterogeneity in polyuric acute renal failure. *J Lab Clin Med* **98:** 21–29, 1981.

Finn, W. F., Arendshorst, W. J., and Gottschalk, C. W. Pathogenesis of oliguria in acute renal failure. *Circ Res* **36:** 675–681, 1975.

Gardiner, M. R., and Royce, R. D. Poisoning of sheep and cattle in western Australia due to species of *Isotropis* (Papilionaceae). *Aust J Agric Res* **18:** 505–513, 1967.

Grauer, G. F., and Kunze, R. S. Potassium depletion nephropathy and renal medullary solute washout: a case report. *Calif Vet* **33:** 8–10, 1979.

Hook, J. B. (ed.) "Toxicology of the Kidney," Target Organ Toxicol. Ser. New York, Raven Press, 1981.

Levinsky, N. G. Pathophysiology of acute renal failure. *N Engl J Med* **296:** 1453–1458, 1977.

Lowe, M. B. Effects of nephrotoxins and ischaemia in experimental haemoglobinuria. *J Pathol Bacteriol* **92:** 319–323, 1966.

Mason, J., and Thiel, G. (eds.) Workshop on the role of renal medullary circulation in the pathogenesis of acute renal failure. *Nephron* **31:** 289–323, 1982.

Migone, L. (ed.) "Toxic Nephropathies," Contrib. Nephrol., Vol. 10. Basel, Karger, 1978.

Oliver, J., MacDowell, M., and Tracy, A. The pathogenesis of acute renal failure in association with traumatic and toxic injury. Renal ischemia, nephrotoxic damage and the ischemuric episode. *J Clin Invest* **30:** 1307–1440, 1951.

Osvaldo, L. *et al.* Reactions of kidney cells during autolysis. Light microscopic observations. *Lab Invest* **14:** 603–622, 1965.

Schneeberger, E. E., and Morrison, A. B. The nephropathy of experimental magnesium deficiency. *Lab Invest* **14:** 674–686, 1965.

Spangler, W. L., and Muggli, F. M. Seizure-induced rhabdomyolysis accompanied by acute renal failure in a dog. *J Am Vet Med Assoc* **172:** 1190–1194, 1978.

Sutton, R. H., and Atwell, R. B. Renal haemosiderosis in association with canine heartworm disease. *J Small Anim Pract* **23:** 773–777, 1982.

Thompson, S. W. *et al.* The protein nature of acidophilic crystalline intranuclear inclusions in the liver and kidney of dogs. *Am J Pathol* **35:** 1105–1115, 1959.

Wellington, J. *et al.* Myeloid bodies in drug-induced acute tubular necrosis. *J Pathol* **139:** 33–40, 1983.

Specific Tubular Dysfunctions

Bovee, K. C. *et al.* The Fanconi syndrome in basenji dogs: a new model for renal transport defects. *Science* **201:** 1129–1131, 1978.

Bovee, K. C. *et al.* Characterization of renal defects in dogs with a syndrome similar to the Fanconi syndrome in man. *J Am Vet Med Assoc* **174:** 1094–1099, 1979.

Easley, J. R., and Breitschwerdt, E. B. Glucosuria associated with renal tubular dysfunction in three basenji dogs. *J Am Vet Med Assoc* **168:** 938–943, 1976.

MacKenzie, C. P., and van den Broek, A. The Fanconi syndrome in a whippet. *J Small Anim Pract* **23:** 469–474, 1982.

Toxic Nephrosis

Ethylene Glycol and Oxalate

Anderson, W. A., and Huffman, W. *Halogeton* poisoning in a ewe. *J Am Vet Med Assoc* **130:** 330–331, 1957.

Beasley, V. R., and Buck, W. B. Acute ethylene glycol toxicosis: a review. *Vet Hum Toxicol* **22:** 255–263, 1980.

Crowell, W. A. *et al.* Ethylene glycol toxicosis in cattle. *Cornell Vet* **69:** 272–279, 1979.

Dickie, C. W. *et al.* Oxalate (*Rumex venosus*) poisoning in cattle. *J Am Vet Med Assoc* **173:** 73–74, 1978.

Dodson, M. E. Oxalate ingestion studies in the sheep. *Aust Vet J* **35:** 225–233, 1959.

Grauer, G. F., and Thrall, M. A. Ethylene glycol (antifreeze) poisoning in the dog and cat. *J Am Anim Hosp Assoc* **18:** 492–497, 1982.

Lincoln, S. D., and Black, B. *Halogeton* poisoning in range cattle. *J Am Vet Med Assoc* **176:** 717–718, 1980.

Mueller, D. H. Epidemiologic considerations of ethylene glycol intoxication in small animals. *Vet Hum Toxicol* **24:** 21–24, 1982.

Riley, J. H. *et al.* Urine and tissue oxalate and hippurate levels in ethylene glycol intoxication in the dog. *Vet Hum Toxicol* **24:** 331–334, 1982.

Stewart, J., and MacCallum, J. W. The anhydraemia of oxalate poisoning in horses. *Vet Rec* **56:** 77–78, 1944.

Van Kampen, K. R., and James, L. F. Acute halogeton poisoning of sheep: pathogenesis of lesions. *Am J Vet Res* **30:** 1779–1783, 1969.

Waltner-Toews, D., and Meadows, D. H. Urolithiasis in a herd of beef cattle associated with oxalate ingestion. *Can Vet J* **21:** 61–62, 1980.

Watts, P. S. Decomposition of oxalic acid *in vitro* by rumen contents. *Aust J Agric Res* **8:** 266–270, 1957.

Oaks and Acorns

Camp, B. J., Steel, E., and Dollahite, J. W. Certain biochemical changes in blood and livers of rabbits fed oak tannin. *Am J Vet Res* **28:** 290–292, 1967.

Dixon, P. M. *et al.* Acorn poisoning in cattle. *Vet Rec* **104:** 284–285, 1979.

Dollahite, J. W., Housholder, G. T., and Camp, B. J. Effect of calcium hydroxide on the toxicity of post oak (*Quercus stellata*) in calves. *J Am Vet Med Assoc* **148:** 908–912, 1966.

Dollahite, J. W., Pigeon, R. F., and Camp, B. J. The toxicity of gallic acid, pyrogallol, tannic acid and *Quercus havardi* in the rabbit. *Am J Vet Res* **23:** 1264–1266, 1962.

Fowler, M. E., and Richards, W. P. C. Acorn poisoning in a cow and sheep. *J Am Vet Med Assoc* **147:** 1215–1220, 1965.

Legg, L., Moule, G. R., and Chester, R. D. The toxicity of yellow-wood (*Terminalia oblongata*) to cattle. *Queensl J Agric Sci* **2:** 199–208, 1945.

Mullins, J. Acorn poisoning in sheep. *NZ Vet J* **3:** 159, 1955.

Pigeon, R. F., Camp, B. J., and Dollahite, J. W. Oral toxicity and polyhydroxyphenol moiety of tannin isolated from *Quercus havardi* (shin oak). Am J Vet Res **23:** 1268–1270, 1962.

Sandusky, G. E. *et al.* Oak poisoning of cattle in Ohio. *J Am Vet Med Assoc* **171:** 627–629, 1977.

Amaranthus retroflexus (Pigweed)

Buck, W. B. *et al.* Perirenal edema in swine: a disease caused by common weeds. (*Amaranthus*). *J Am Vet Med Assoc* **148:** 1525–1531, 1966.

Osweiler, G. D., Buck, W. B., and Bicknell, E. J. Production of perirenal edema in swine with *Amaranthus retroflexus*. *Am J Vet Res* **30:** 557–566, 1969.

Stuart, B. P., Nicholson, S. S., and Smith, J. B. Perirenal edema and toxic nephrosis in cattle, association with ingestion of pigweed. *J Am Vet Med Assoc* **167:** 949–950, 1975.

Metals

Angevine, J. M. *et al.* Renal tubular nuclear inclusions of lead poisoning, a clinical and experimental study. *Arch Pathol* **73:** 486–494, 1962.

Bank, N., Mutz, B. F., and Aynedjian, H. S. The role of "leakage" of tubular fluid in anuria due to mercury poisoning. *J Clin Invest* **46:** 695–704, 1967.

Beaver, D. L., and Burr, R. E. Electron microscopy of bismuth inclusions. *Am J Pathol* **42:** 609–617, 1963.

Cuppage, F. E., and Tate, A. Repair of the nephron following injury with mercuric chloride. *Am J Pathol* **51:** 405–429, 1967.

Davis, J. W. *et al.* Experimentally induced lead poisoning in goats: clinical observations and pathologic changes. *Cornell Vet* **66:** 489–496, 1976.

Fujimoto, Y. *et al.* Pathological studies on mercury poisoning in cattle. *Jpn J Vet Res* **4:** 17–32, 1956 [in English].

Gunson, D. E. *et al.* Environmental zinc and cadmium pollution associated with generalized osteochondrosis, osteoporosis, and nephrocalcinosis in horses. *J Am Vet Med Assoc* **180:** 295–299, 1982.

Harber, M. H., and Jennings, R. B. Renal response of the rat to mercury. *Arch Pathol* **79:** 218–222, 1965.

Kelly, D. F., Amand, W. B., and Fein, D. A. Acute nephrosis in a cat *J Am Vet Med Assoc* **159:** 413–416, 1971. [Bismuth]

Morgan, J. M., Hartley, M. W., and Miller, R. E. Nephropathy in chronic lead poisoning. *Arch Intern Med* **118:** 17–29, 1966.

Sun, C. N. *et al.* The renal tubule in experimental lead intoxication. *Arch Pathol* **82:** 156–163, 1966.

Antimicrobials

Appel, G. B., and Neu, H. C. The nephrotoxicity of antimicrobial agents. *N Engl J Med* **296:** 663–670, 722–728, and 784–787, 1977.

Crowell, W. A. *et al.* Neomycin toxicosis in calves. *Am J Vet Res* **42:** 29–34, 1981.

Dobyan, D. C., Cronin, R. E., and Bulger, R. E. Effect of potassium depletion on tubular morphology in gentamicin-induced acute renal failure in dogs. *Lab Invest* **47:** 586–594, 1982.

Elliott, W. C. *et al.* Gentamicin nephrotoxicity. II. Definition of conditions necessary to induce acquired insensitivity. *J Lab Clin Med* **100:** 513–525, 1982.

Gattone, V. H. *et al.* The morphology of the renal microvasculature in glycerol- and gentamicin-induced acute renal failure. *J Lab Clin Med* **101:** 183–195, 1983.

Houghton, D. C. *et al.* Gentamicin and tobramycin nephrotoxicity. A morphologic and functional comparison in the rat. *Am J Pathol* **93:** 137–152, 1978.

Pyle, R. L. Clinical pharmacology of amphotericin B. *J Am Vet Med Assoc* **179:** 83–84, 1981.

Riviere, J. E., and Coppoc, G. L. Dosage of antimicrobial drugs in patients with renal insufficiency. *J Am Vet Med Assoc* **178:** 70–72, 1981.

Riviere, J. E., Traver, D. S., and Coppoc, G. L. Gentamicin toxic nephropathy in horses with disseminated bacterial infection. *J Am Vet Med Assoc* **180:** 648–651, 1982.

Spangler, W. L. *et al.* Gentamicin nephrotoxicity in the dog: Sequential light and electron microscopy. *Vet Pathol* **17:** 206–217, 1980.

Stevenson, S. Oxytetracycline nephrotoxicosis in two dogs. *J Am Vet Med Assoc* **176:** 530–531, 1980.

Teuscher, E. *et al.* Une néphrose toxique chez des veaux traités par un médicament contenant des produits de dégradation des tétracyclines. *Can Vet J* **23:** 327–331, 1982.

Wedeen, R. P. *et al.* Transport of gentamicin in rat proximal tubule. *Lab Invest* **48:** 212–223, 1983.

Whelton, A., and Solez, K. Aminoglycoside nephrotoxicity—a tale of two transports. *J Lab Clin Med* **99:** 148–155, 1982.

Ziv, G. Clinical pharmacology of polymixins. *J Am Vet Med Assoc* **179:** 711–713, 1981.

Mycotoxins

Krogh, P. Mycotoxic nephropathy. *Adv Vet Sci Comp Med* **20:** 147–170, 1976.

Krogh, P. *et al.* Porcine nephropathy induced by long-term ingestion of ochratoxin A. *Vet Pathol* **16:** 466–475, 1979.

Thornton, R. H., Shirley, G., and Salisbury, R. M. A nephrotoxin from *Aspergillus fumigatus* and its possible relationship with New Zealand mucosal disease–like syndrome in cattle. *NZ J Agric Res* **11:** 1–14, 1968.

Interstitial Nephritis

Bloom, F. The histopathology of canine leptospirosis. *Cornell Vet* **31:** 266–288, 1941.

Burdin, M. L. Renal histopathology of leptospirosis caused by *Leptospira grippotyphosa* in farm animals in Kenya. *Res Vet Sci* **4:** 423–430, 1963.

Bush, B. M., and Evans, J. M. Infectious canine hepatitis and chronic renal failure. *Vet Rec* **90:** 33–34, 1972.

Cheville, N. F., Huhn, R., and Cutlip, R. C. Ultrastructure of renal lesions in pigs with acute leptospirosis caused by *Leptospira pomona*. *Vet Pathol* **17:** 338–351, 1980.

Cole, J. R. *et al.* Infections with *Encephalitozoon cuniculi* and *Leptospira interrogans,* serovars *grippotyphosa* and *ballum,* in a kennel of foxhounds. *J Am Vet Med Assoc* **180:** 435–437, 1982.

Hanson, L. E. Leptospirosis in domestic animals: the public health perspective. *J Am Vet Med Assoc* **181:** 1505–1509, 1982.

Hartley, W. J., and Done, J. T. Cytomegalic inclusion-body disease in sheep. A report of two cases. *J Comp Pathol* **73:** 84–87, 1963.

Krohn, K. *et al.* Immunologic observations in canine interstitial nephritis. *Am J Pathol* **65:** 157–172, 1971.

Krohn, K., and Sandholm, M. Myxovirus-like structures in the glomerular endothelial cell cytoplasm in canine nephritis. *Acta Pathol Microbiol Scand [A]* **83:** 355–359, 1975.

Lucke, V. M. Renal disease in the domestic cat. *J Pathol Bacteriol* **95:** 67–91, 1968.

McCluskey, R. T., and Klassen, J. Immunologically mediated glomerular, tubular and interstitial renal disease. *N Engl J Med* **288:** 564–570, 1973.

McIntyre, W. I. M., and Montgomery, G. L. Renal lesions in *Leptospira canicola* infection in dogs. *J Pathol Bacteriol* **44:** 145–160, 1952.

Monlux, A. W. The histopathology of nephritis in the dog. *Am J Vet Res* **14:** 425–447, 1953.

Monlux, A. W. *et al.* Leptospirosis in hogs. *North Am Vet* **33:** 467–469, 1952.

Morrison, W. I., and Wright, N. G. Canine leptospirosis: an immunopathologic study of interstitial nephritis due to *Leptospira canicola*. *J Pathol* **120:** 83–89, 1976.

Morrison, W. I., and Wright, N. G. Immunopathological aspects of canine renal disease. *J Small Anim Pract* **17:** 139–148, 1976.

Morrison, W. I., Wright, N. G., and Cornwell, H. J. C. An immunopathologic study of interstitial nephritis associated with experimental canine adenovirus infection. *J Pathol* **120:** 221–228, 1976.

Rudofsky, U. H., Dilwith, R. L., and Tung, K. S. K. Susceptibility differences of inbred mice to induction of autoimmune renal tubulointerstitial lesions. *Lab Invest* **43:** 463–470, 1980.

Shadduck, J. A., Bendele, R., and Robinson, G. T. Isolation of the causative organism of canine encephalitozoonosis. *Vet Pathol* **15:** 449–460, 1978.

Shirota, K., and Fujiwara, K. Nephropathy in dogs induced by treatment with antiserum against renal basement membrane. *Jpn J Vet Sci* **44:** 767–776, 1982.

Smith, T. Focal interstitial nephritis in the calf, following interference with the normal intake of colostrum. *J Exp Med* **41:** 413–426, 1925.

Taylor, P. L., Hanson, L. E., and Simon, J. Serologic, pathologic, and immunologic features of experimentally induced leptospiral nephritis in dogs. *Am J Vet Res* **31:** 1033–1049, 1970.

Timoney, J. F., Sheahan, B. J., and Timoney, P. J. *Leptospira* and infectious canine hepatitis (ICH) virus antibodies and nephritis in Dublin dogs. *Vet Rec* **94:** 316–319, 1974.

Wright, N. G. *et al.* Chronic renal failure in dogs: a comparative clinical and morphological study of chronic glomerulonephritis and chronic interstitial nephritis. *Vet Rec* **98:** 288–293, 1976.

Wright, N. G., Cornwell, H. J. C., and Thompson, H. Canine adenovirus nephritis. *J Small Anim Pract* **12:** 657–664, 1971.

Pyelonephritis

Andriole, V. T. Factors of obstruction and renal infection. *J Urol* **95:** 154–163, 1966.

Appleton, J. A., Munnell, J. F., and DeBuysscher, E. V. Scanning electron microscopy of experimentally induced pyelonephritis in the rat. *Am J Vet Res* **42:** 351–355, 1981.

Beeson, P. B. Factors in the pathogenesis of pyelonephritis. *Yale J Biol Med* **28:** 81–104, 1955.

Belman, A. B. The clinical significance of vesicoureteral reflux. *Pediatr Clin North Am* **23:** 707–720, 1976.

Biertuempfel, P. H., Ling, G. V., and Ling, G. A. Urinary tract infection resulting from catheterization in healthy adult dogs. *J Am Vet Med Assoc* **178:** 989–991, 1981.

Braude, A. I., Shapiro, A. P., and Siemienski, J. Hematogenous pyelonephritis in rats. 2. Production of chronic pyelonephritis by *Escherichia coli*. *Proc Soc Exp Biol Med* **91:** 18–24, 1956.

Brumfitt, W., and Heptinstall, R. H. Experimental pyelonephritis: the influence of temporary and permanent ureteric obstruction on the localisation of bacteria. *Br J Exp Pathol* **39:** 610–617, 1958.

Brumfitt, W., and Heptinstall, R. H. Experimental pyelonephritis: the relationship of bacterial virulence to the establishment of the renal lesion. *Br J Exp Pathol* **41:** 552–558, 1960.

Bush, B. M. A review of the aetiology and consequences of urinary tract infections in the dog. *Br Vet J* **132:** 632–641, 1976.

Christie, B. A. The occurrence of vesicoureteral reflux and pyelonephritis in apparently normal dogs. *Invest Urol* **10:** 359–366, 1973.

Christie, B. A. Vesicoureteral reflux in dogs. *J Am Vet Med Assoc* **162:** 772–776, 1973.

Cohen, M. S., Davis, C. P., and Warren, M. M. The response of the renal pelvis to infection. A scanning electron microscopic study. *Invest Urol* **16:** 360–364, 1979.

Cotran, R. S. *et al.* Retrograde *Proteus* pyelonephritis in rats. Bacteriologic, pathologic and fluorescent-antibody studies. *Am J Pathol* **43:** 1–31, 1963.

Crow, S. E., Lauerman, L. H., and Smith, K. W. Pyonephrosis associated with *Salmonella* infection in a dog. *J Am Vet Med Assoc* **169:** 1324–1326, 1976.

Ekman, H. *et al.* High diuresis, a factor in preventing vesicoureteral reflux. *J Urol* **95:** 511–515, 1966.

Feeney, D. A., Osborne, C. A., and Johnston, G. R. Vesicoureteral reflux induced by manual compression of the urinary bladder of dogs and cats. *J Am Vet Med Assoc* **182:** 795–797, 1983.

Guze, L. B., and Kalmanson, G. M. Persistence of bacteria in "protoplast" form after apparent cure of pyelonephritis in rats. *Science* **143:** 1340–1341, 1964.

Heptinstall, R. H. Experimental pyelonephritis: a comparison of bloodborne and ascending patterns of infection. *J Pathol Bacteriol* **89:** 71–80, 1965.

Hutch, J. A., Miller, E. R., and Hinman, F. Vesicoureteral reflux, role in pyelonephritis. *Am J Med* **34:** 338–349, 1963.

Jarvinen, A.-K. Urogenital tract infection in the bitch. *Vet Res Commun* **4:** 253–269, 1981.

Jurusik, R. J. *et al.* Experimental rat model for *Corynebacterium renale*-induced pyelonephritis. *Infect Immun* **18:** 828–832, 1977.

Kalmanson, G. M., Sommer, S. C., and Guze, L. B. Pyelonephritis. VII. Experimental ascending infection with progression of lesions in the absence of bacteria. *Arch Pathol* **80:** 509–516, 1965.

Kelly, D. F., Lucke, V. M., and McCullagh, K. G. Experimental pyelonephritis in the cat. 1. Gross and histological changes. *J Comp Pathol* **89:** 125–139, 1979.

Kelly, D. F., Lucke, V. M., and McCullagh, K. G. Experimental pyelonephritis in the cat. 2. Ultrastructural observations. *J. Comp Pathol* **89:** 563–579, 1979.

Kincaid-Smith, P., and Becker, G. Reflux nephropathy and chronic atrophic pyelonephritis: a review. *J Infect Dis* **138:** 774–780, 1978.

King, L. R., and Idriss, F. S. The effect of vesicoureteral reflux in renal function in dogs. *Invest Urol* **4:** 419–427, 1967.

Kivisto, A.-K., Vasenius, H., and Sandholm, M. Canine bacteruria. *J Small Anim Pract* **18:** 707–712, 1977.

Lovell, R. Bovine pyelonephritis. *Vet Rec* **63:** 645–646, 1951.

McCullagh, K. G. *et al.* Experimental pyelonephritis in the cat. 3. Collagen alterations in renal fibrosis. *J Comp Pathol* **93:** 9–25, 1983.

Morse, E. V. An ecological study of *Corynebacterium renale*. *Cornell Vet* **40:** 178–187, 1950.

Nicolet, J., and Fey, H. Antibody coated bacteria in urine sediment from cattle infected with *Corynebacterium renale*. *Vet Rec* **105:** 301–303, 1979.

Ransley, P. G., and Risdon, R. A. Renal papillae and intrarenal reflux in the pig. *Lancet* **2:** 1114, 1974.

Sato, H., Yanagawa, R., and Fukuyama, H. Adhesion of *Corynebacterium renale, Corynebacterium pilosum,* and *Corynebacterium cystitidis* to bovine urinary bladder epithelial cells of various ages and levels of differentiation. *Infect Immun* **36:** 1242–1245, 1982.

Shimono, E., and Yanagawa, E. Experimental model of *Corynebacterium renale* pyelonephritis produced in mice. *Infect Immun* **16:** 263–267, 1977.

Soltys, M. A., and Spratling, F. R. Infectious cystitis and pyelonephritis of pigs: a preliminary communication. *Vet Rec* **69:** 500–504, 1957.

Sommer, J. L., and Roberts, J. A. Ureteral reflux resulting from chronic urinary infection in dogs: long-term studies. *J Urol* **95:** 502–510, 1966.

Thomas, J. E. Urinary tract infection induced by intermittent urethral catheterization in dogs. *J Am Vet Med Assoc* **174:** 705–707, 1979.

Thorp, F. *et al.* The pathology of bovine pyelonephritis. *Am J Vet Res* **4:** 240–249, 1943.

Vivaldi, E. *et al.* Ascending infection as a mechanism in pathogenesis of experimental non-obstructive pyelonephritis. *Proc Soc Exp Biol Med* **102:** 242–244, 1959.

Yanagawa, R., and Honda, E. *Corynebacterium pilosum* and *Corynebacterium cystitidis*, two new species from cows. *Int J Syst Bacteriol* **28:** 209–216, 1978.

Renal Mineralization and Hypercalcemic Nephropathy

Carrillo, J. M., Burk, R. L., and Bode, C. Primary hyperparathyroidism in a dog. *J Am Vet Med Asoc* **174:** 67–71, 1979.

Drazner, F. H. Hypercalcemia in the dog and cat. *J Am Vet Med Assoc* **178:** 1252–1256, 1981.

Finco, D. R., and Rowland, G. N. Hypercalcemia secondary to chronic renal failure in the dog: a report of 4 cases. *J Am Vet Med Assoc* **173:** 990–994, 1978.

Ganote, C. *et al.* Acute calcium nephrotoxicity. An electron microscopical and semiquantitative light microscopical study. *Arch Pathol* **99:** 650–657, 1975.

Lucke, V. M., and Hunt, A. C. Renal calcification in the domestic cat. A morphological and X-ray diffraction study. *Pathol Vet* **4:** 120–136, 1967.

Meuten, D. J. *et al.* Hypercalcemia of malignancy. Hypercalcemia associated with an adenocarcinoma of the apocrine glands of the anal sacs. *Am J Pathol* **108:** 366–370, 1982.

Nelson, R. W., and Feldman, E. C. Hypercalcemia in the dog. *Mod Vet Pract* **62:** 359–365, 1981.

Schmidt, R. E. *et al.* Dietary induction of renal mineralization in dogs. *Can J Comp Med* **44:** 459–465, 1980.

Weller, R. E., Theilen, G. H., and Madewell, B. R. Chemotherapeutic responses in dogs with lymphosarcoma and hypercalcemia. *J Am Vet Med Assoc* **181:** 891–893, 1982.

Renal Pigmentation

Altman, N. H., Grossman, I. W., and Jernigan, N. B. Caprine cloisonne renal lesions. Clinicopathological observations. *Cornell Vet* **60:** 83–90, 1970.

Giddens, W. E. *et al.* Feline congenital erythropoietic porphyria associated with severe anemia and renal disease. *Am J Pathol* **80:** 367–386, 1975.

Grossman, I. W., and Altman, N. H. Caprine cloisonné renal lesion. Ultrastructure of the thickened proximal convoluted tubular basement membrane. *Arch Pathol* **88:** 609–612, 1969.

Light, F. W. Pigmented thickening of the basement membranes of the renal tubules of the goat ("cloisonné kidney"). *Lab Invest* **9:** 228–238, 1960.

Marcato, P. S., and Simoni, P. Pigmentation of renal cortical tubules in horses. *Vet Pathol* **19:** 572–573, 1982.

Svenkerud, R. Melanosis renum bovis. *Acta Vet Scand* **1:** 161–187, 1960.

Thompson, S. W., Bogdon, T. R., and Yost, D. H. Some histochemical studies of "cloisonné kidney" in the male Angora goat. *Am J Vet Res* **22:** 757–763, 1961.

Winter, H. "Black kidneys" in cattle—a lipofuscinosis. *J Pathol Bacteriol* **86:** 253–258, 1963.

Zahawi, S. Symmetrical cortical siderosis of the kidneys in goats. *Am J Vet Res* **18:** 861–867, 1957.

Parasites

Alstad, A. D., Berg, I. E., and Samuel, C. Disseminated *Micronema deletrix* infection in the horse. *J Am Vet Med Assoc* **174:** 264–266, 1979.

Austin, R. J., and Dies, K. H. *Klossiella equi* in the kidneys of a horse. *Can Vet J* **22:** 159–161, 1981.

Bartsch, R. C., and Van Wyk, J. A. Studies on schistosomiasis. 9. Pathology of the bovine urinary tract. *Onderstepoort J Vet Res* **44:** 73–94, 1977.

Batte, E. G., Harkema, R., and Osborne, J. C. Observations on the life cycle and pathogenicity of the swine kidney worm (*Stephanurus dentatus*). *J Am Vet Med Assoc* **136:** 622–625, 1960.

Batte, E. G., Moncol, D. J., and Barber, C. W. Prenatal infection with the swine kidney worm (*Stephanurus dentatus*) and associated lesions. *J Am Vet Med Assoc* **149:** 758–765, 1966.

Celerin, A. J., and McMullen, M. E. Giant kidney worm in a dog. *J Am Vet Med Assoc* **179:** 245–246, 1981.

Clunies Ross, I., and Kauzal, G. The life cycle of *Stephanurus dentatus* Deising, 1839: the kidney worm of pigs, with observations on its ecnomic importance in Australia and suggestions for its control. *Bull C S I R O (Aust)* **58:** 1–80, 1932.

Hallberg, C. W. *Dioctophyma renale* (Goeze, 1782). A study of the migration routes to the kidneys of mammals and resultant pathology. *Trans Am Microsc Soc* **72:** 351–363, 1953.

Mace, T. F., and Anderson, R. C. Development of the giant kidney worm, *Dioctophyma renale* (Goeze, 1782) (Nematoda: Dioctophymatoidea). *Can J Zool* **53:** 1552–1568, 1975.

McNeil, C. W. Pathological changes in the kidney of mink due to infection with *Dioctophyma renale* (Goeze, 1782), the giant kidney worm of mammals. *Trans Am Microsc Soc* **67:** 257–261, 1948.

Newberne, J. W., Robinson, V. B., and Bowen, N. E. Histological aspects of *Klossiella equi* in the kidney of a zebra. *Am J Vet Res* **19:** 304–307, 1958.

Osborne, C. A. *et al. Dioctophyma renale* in the dog. *J Am Vet Med Assoc* **155:** 605–620, 1969.

Rubin, H. L., and Woodard, J. C. Equine infection with *Micronema deletrix*. *J Am Vet Med Assoc* **165:** 256–258, 1974.

Sasaki, N., and Ishitani, R. Supplementary studies on the histopathology of swine kidney worm (*Stephanurus dentatus*) disease. *Rep Tokyo Gov Exp Stn Anim Hyg* **25:** 121–129, 1952.

Schmid, F. Ueber Parasiten und parasitäre Veränderungen der Harnorgane bei Silberfüchsen. *Berl Muench Tieraerztl Wochenschr* **50:** 33–36, 1934.

Schwartz, B., and Price, E. W. Infection of pigs through the skin with the larvae of the swine kidney worm, *Stephanurus dentatus*. *J Am Vet Med Assoc* **79:** 359–375, 1931.

Schwartz, B., and Price, E. W. Infection of pigs and other animals with kidney worms, *Stephanurus dentatus*, following ingestion of larva. *J Am Vet Med Assoc* **81:** 325–347, 1932.

Senior, D. F. *et al. Capillaria plica* infection in dogs. *J Am Vet Med Assoc* **176:** 901–905, 1980.

Taylor, J. L. *et al. Klossiella* parasites of animals: a literature review. *Vet Parasitol* **5:** 137–144, 1979.

Vetterling, J. M., and Thompson, D. E. *Klossiella equi* Baumann, 1946 (Sporozoa: Eucoccidia: Adeleina) from equids. *J Parasitol* **58**: 589–594, 1972.

Waddell, A. H. Further observations on *Capillaria feliscati* infections in the cat. *Aust Vet J* **44**: 33–34, 1968.

Waddell, A. H. The parasitic life cycle of the swine kidney worm *Stephanurus dentatus* Diesing. *Aust J Zool* **17**: 607–618, 1969.

Renal Tumors

Baskin, G. B., and De Paoli, A. Primary renal neoplasms of the dog. *Vet Pathol* **14**: 591–605, 1977.

Drew, R. A., Done, S. H., and Robins, G. M. Canine embryonal nephroma: a case report. *J Small Anim Pract* **13**: 27–39, 1972.

Haschek, W. M., King, J. M., and Tennant, B. C. Primary renal cell carcinoma in two horses. *J Am Vet Med Assoc* **179**: 992–994, 1981.

Hayes, H. M., and Fraumeni, J. F. Epidemiological features of canine renal neoplasms. *Cancer Res* **37**: 2553–2556, 1977.

Kirkbride, C. A., and Bicknell, E. J. Nephroblastoma in a bovine fetus. *Vet Pathol* **9**: 96–98, 1972.

Lucke, V. M., and Kelly, D. F. Renal carcinoma in the dog. *Vet Pathol* **13**: 264–276, 1976.

Marsden, H. B., and Lawler, W. Wilms' tumor and renal dysplasia: an hypothesis. *J Clin Pathol* **35**: 1069–1073, 1982.

Migaki, G., Nelson, L. W., and Todd, G. C. Prevalence of embryonal nephroma in slaughtered swine. *J Am Vet Med Assoc* **159**: 441–442, 1971.

Nielsen, S. W., Mackey, L. J., and Misdorp, W. Tumours of the kidney. *Bull WHO* **53**: 237–240, 1976.

Osborne, C. A. *et al.* Renal lymphoma in the dog and cat. *J Am Vet Med Assoc* **158**: 2058–2070, 1971.

Sandison, A. T., and Anderson, L. J. Tumors of the kidney in cattle, sheep and pigs. *Cancer* **21**: 727–742, 1968.

Splitter, G. A., Rawlings, C. A., and Casey, H. W. Renal hamartoma in a dog. *Am J Vet Res* **33**: 273–275, 1972.

Sullivan, D. J., and Anderson, W. A. Embryonal nephroma in swine. *Am J Vet Res* **20**: 324–332, 1959.

Vitovec, J. Carcinomas of the renal pelvis in slaughter animals. *J Comp Pathol* **87**: 129–134, 1977.

Lower Urinary Tract

General Considerations and Anomalies

Benko, L. Cases of bilateral and unilateral duplication of ureters in the pig. *Vet Rec* **84**: 139–140, 1969.

Bentley, P. J. The vertebrate urinary bladder: osmoregulatory and other uses. *Yale J Biol Med* **52**: 563–568, 1979.

Constantinou, C. E., and Hrynczuk, J. R. Urodynamics of the upper urinary tract. *Invest Urol* **14**: 233–240, 1976.

Constantinou, C. E., Silvert, M. A., and Gosling, J. Pacemaker system in the control of ureteral peristaltic rate in the multicalyceal kidney of the pig. *Invest Urol* **14**: 440–441, 1977.

Djurhuus, J. C. Dynamics of upper urinary tract. III. The activity of renal pelvis during pressure variations. *Invest Urol* **14**: 475–477, 1977.

Gleason, D. M., Bottaccini, M. R., and Drach, G. W. Urodynamics. *J Urol* **115**: 356–361, 1976.

Goss, R. J. *et al.* The physiological basis of urinary bladder hypertrophy. *Proc Soc Exp Biol Med* **142**: 1332–1335, 1973.

Hayes, H. M. Ectopic ureter in dogs: epidemiologic features. *Teratology* **10**: 129–132, 1974.

Holt, P. E., Gibbs, C., and Pearson, H. Canine ectopic ureter—a review of twenty-nine cases. *J Small Anim Pract* **23**: 195–208, 1982.

Hoskins, J. D., Abdelbaki, Y. Z., and Root, C. D. Urinary bladder duplication in a dog. *J Am Vet Med Assoc* **181**: 603–604, 1982.

Osborne, C. A. *et al.* Congenital urethrorectal fistula in two dogs. *J Am Vet Med Assoc* **166**: 999–1002, 1975.

Owen, R. ap R. Canine ureteral ectopia—a review. I. Embryology and aetiology. 2. Incidence, diagnosis and treatment. *J Small Anim Pract* **14**: 407–417 and 419–427, 1973.

Perlman, M., Williams, J., and Ornoy, A. Familial ureteric bud anomalies. *J Med Genet* **13**: 161–163, 1976.

Pollock, S., and Schoen, S. S. Urinary incontinence associated with congenital ureteral valves in a bitch. *J Am Vet Med Assoc* **159**: 332–335, 1971.

Rawlings, C. A., and Capps, W. F. Rectovaginal fistula and imperforate anus in a dog. *J Am Vet Med Assoc* **159**: 320–326, 1971.

Weaver, M. E. Persistent urachus—an observation in miniature swine. *Anat Rec* **154**: 701–704, 1966.

Degenerative and Inflammatory Lesions

Brobst, D. F., Cottrell, R., and Delez, A. Mucinous degeneration of the epithelium of the urinary tract of swine. *Vet Pathol* **8**: 485–489, 1971.

Crow, S. E. *et al.* Cyclophosphamide-induced cystitis in the dog and cat. *J Am Vet Med Assoc* **171**: 259–262, 1977.

Hooper, P. T. Epizootic cystitis in horses. *Aust Vet J* **44**: 11–14, 1968.

Johnston, S. D., Osborne, C. A., and Stevens, J. B. Canine polypoid cystitis. *J Am Vet Med Assoc* **166**: 1155–1160, 1975.

Lees, G. E., and Osborne, C. A. Antibacterial properties of urine: a comparative review. *J Am Anim Hosp Assoc* **15**: 125–132, 1979.

McKenzie, R. A., and McMicking, L. I. Ataxia and urinary incontinence in cattle grazing sorghum. *Aust Vet J* **53**: 496–497, 1977.

Middleton, D. J., and Lomas, G. R. Emphysematous cystitis due to *Clostridium perfringens* in a non-diabetic dog. *J Small Anim Pract* **20**: 433–438, 1979.

Mulholland, S. G. Lower urinary tract antibacterial defense mechanisms. *Invest Urol* **17**: 93–97, 1979.

Orikasa, S., and Hinman, F. Reaction of the vesical wall to bacterial penetration. Resistance to attachment, desquamation, and leukocytic activity. *Invest Urol* **15**: 185–193, 1977.

Parson, C. L., and Mulholland, S. G. Bladder surface mucin. Its antibacterial effect against various bacterial species. *Am J Pathol* **93**: 423–432, 1978.

Richardson, D. W., and Kohn, C. W. Uroperitoneum in the foal. *J Am Vet Med Assoc* **182**: 267–271, 1983.

Rooney, J. R. Rupture of the urinary bladder in the foal. *Vet Pathol* **8**: 445–451, 1971.

Root, C. R., and Scott, R. C. Emphysematous cystitis and other radiographic manifestations of diabetes millitus in dogs and cats. *J Am Vet Med Assoc* **158**: 721–728, 1971.

Tanagho, E. A. Mechanisms of ureteral dilatation. *Can J Surg* **15**: 4–14, 1972.

Wellington, J. K. M. Bladder defects in newborn foals. *Aust Vet J* **48**: 426, 1972.

Zachary, J. F. Cystitis cystica, cystitis glandularis, and Brunn's nests in a feline urinary bladder. *Vet Pathol* **18**: 113–116, 1981.

Urolithiasis

Bailey, C. B. Silica metabolism and silica urolithiasis in ruminants: a review. *Can J Anim Sci* **61**: 219–235, 1981.

Briggs, O. M., Rodgers, A. L., and Harley, E. H. Uric acid urolithiasis in a Dalmatian coach hound. *J S Afr Vet Assoc* **53**: 205–208, 1982.

Briggs, O. M., and Sperling, O. Uric acid metabolism in the Dalmatian coach hound. *J S Afr Vet Assoc* **53**: 201–204, 1982.

Brown, N. O., Parks, J. L., and Greene, R. W. Canine urolithiasis: retrospective analysis of 438 cases. *J Am Vet Med Assoc* **170:** 414–418, 1977.

Bunce, G. E., and King, G. A. Isolation and partial characterization of kidney stone matrix induced by magnesium deficiency in the rat. *Exp Mol Pathol* **28:** 322–329, 1978.

Bushman, D. H., Emerick, R. J., and Embry, L. B. Experimentally induced ovine phosphatic urolithiasis: relationships involving dietary calcium, phosphorus and magnesium. *J Nutr* **87:** 499–504, 1965.

Cornelius, C. E. Studies on ovine urinary biocolloids and phosphatic calculosis. *Ann NY Acad Sci* **104:** 638–657, 1963.

Crookshank, H. R., Robbins, J. D., and Kunkel, H. O. Relationship of dietary mineral intake to serum mineral level and the incidence of urinary calculi in lambs. *J Anim Sci* **26:** 1179–1185, 1967.

Dutt, B., Majumbar, B. N., and Kehar, N. D. Vitamin A deficiency and urinary calculi in goats. *Br Vet J* **115:** 63–66, 1959.

Dyer, R., and Nordin, B. E. C. Urinary crystals and their relation to stone formation. *Nature* **215:** 751–752, 1967.

Easterfield, T. H. *et al.* A widespread occurrence of xanthine calculi in sheep. *Vet J* **86:** 251–265, 1930.

Finlayson, B. Physiochemical aspects of urolithiasis. *Kidney Int* **13:** 344–360, 1978.

Fleisch, H. Inhibitors and promoters of stone formation. *Kidney Int* **13:** 361–371, 1978.

Lewis, L. D. *et al.* Effect of various dietary mineral concentrations on the occurrence of feline urolithiasis. *J Am Vet Med Assoc* **172:** 559–563, 1978.

McIntosh, G. H. Urolithiasis in animals. *Aust Vet J* **54:** 267–271, 1978.

Marretta, S. M. *et al.* Urinary calculi associated with portosystemic shunts in six dogs. *Am J Vet Res* **178:** 133–137, 1981.

Momotani, E. *et al.* Pathological changes of xanthinurolithiasis in calves. *Natl Inst Anim Health Q (Tokyo)* **19:** 65–71, 1979.

Oliver, J. *et al.* The renal lesions of electrolyte imbalance. IV. The intranephronic calculosis of experimental magnesium depletion. *J Exp. Med* **124:** 263–278, 1966.

Osborne, C. A. *et al.* Canine struvite urolithiasis: problems and their dissolution. *J Am Vet Med Assoc* **179:** 239–244, 1981.

Osborne, C. A., Hammer, R. F., and Klausner, J. S. Canine silica urolithiasis. *J Am Vet Med Assoc* **178:** 809–813, 1981.

Osborne, C. A., and Klausner, J. S. War on canine urolithiasis: problems and solutions. *Proc 45th Annu Meet Am Anim Hosp Assoc* pp. 569–620, 1978.

Ottosen, H. E. A case of renal sulfathiazole concretions and nephrosis in a calf. *Nord Vet Med* **1:** 410–415, 1949.

Packett, L. V., and Coburn, S. P. Urine proteins in nutritionally induced ovine urolithiasis. *Am J Vet Res* **26:** 112–119, 1965.

Pope, G. S. Isolation of two benzocoumarins from "clover stone," a type of renal calculus found in sheep. *Biochem. J* **93:** 474–477, 1964.

Porter, P. Urinary calculi in the dog. II. Urate stones and purine metabolism. *J Comp Pathol* **73:** 119–135, 1963.

Porter, P. Chromatographic studies of the urinary colloids of dog and man with the identification of components derived from the serum. *J Comp Pathol* **76:** 197–206, 1966.

Porter, P. Colloidal properties of urates in relation to calculus formation. *Res Vet Sci* **7:** 128–137, 1966.

Randall, A. The origin and growth of renal calculi. Ann Surg **105:** 1009–1027, 1937.

Rich, L. J., and Norcross, N. L. Feline urethral obstruction: immunologic identification of a unique protein. *Am J Vet Res* **30:** 1001–1005, 1969.

Roch-Ramel, F. Renal excretion of uric acid in mammals. *Clin Nephrol* **12:** 1–6, 1979.

Rosenstein, I., Hamilton-Miller, J. M. T., and Brumfitt, W. Infection stones and the role of bacterial urease. *J Infect* **2:** 211–214, 1980.

Schneeberger, E. E., and Morrison, A. B. The nephropathy of experimental magnesium deficiency. *Lab Invest* **14:** 674–686, 1965.

Schneeberger, E. E., and Morrison, A. B. Increased susceptibility of magnesium-deficient rats to a phosphate-induced nephropathy. *Am J Pathol* **50:** 549–558, 1967.

Senior, B. W., Bradford, N. C., and Simpson, D. S. The ureases of *Proteus* strains in relation to virulence for the urinary tract. *J Med Microbiol* **13:** 507–512, 1980.

Swingle, K. F., and Marsh, H. Vitamin A deficiency and urolithiasis in range cattle. *Am J Vet Res* **17:** 415–424, 1956.

Treacher, R. J. The amino-aciduria of canine cystine-stone disease. *Res Vet Sci* **4:** 556–567, 1963.

Treacher, R. J. The aetiology of canine cystinuria. *Biochem J* **90:** 494–498, 1964.

Treacher, R. J. Quantitative studies on the excretion of the basic amino acids in canine cystinuria. *Br Vet J* **120:** 178–185, 1964.

Treacher, R. J. Intestinal absorption of lysine in cystinuric dogs. *J Comp Pathol* **75:** 309–322, 1965.

Treacher, R. J. Urolithiasis in the dog. II. Biochemical aspects. *J Small Anim Pract* **7:** 537–547, 1966.

Trotter, G. W., Bennett, D. G., and Behm, R. J. Urethral calculi in five horses. *Vet Surg* **10:** 159–162, 1981.

Udall, R. H., and Chow, F. H. C. The etiology and control of urolithiasis. *Adv Vet Sci Comp Med* **13:** 29–57, 1969.

Udall, R. H., and Jensen, R. Studies on urolithiasis. 2. The occurrence in feedlot lambs following implantation of diethylstilbestrol. *J Am Vet Med Assoc* **133:** 514–516, 1958.

Vermeulen, C. W. *et al.* The renal papilla and calculogenesis. *J Urol* **97:** 573–582, 1967.

Walker, A. D. *et al.* An epidemiological survey of the feline urological syndrome. *J Small Anim Pract* **18:** 283–301, 1977.

Waltner-Toews, D., and Meadows, D. H. Urolithiasis in a herd of beef cattle associated with oxalate ingestion. *Can Vet J* **21:** 61–62, 1980.

Weaver, A. D., and Pillinger, R. Relationship of bacterial infection in urine and calculi to canine urolithiasis. *Vet Rec* **97:** 48–50, 1975.

White, E. G. Symposium on urolithiasis in the dog. I. Introduction and incidence. *J Small Anim Pract* **7:** 529–535, 1966.

Willeberg, P. Interaction effects of epidemiologic factors in the feline urological syndrome. *Nord Vet Med* **28:** 193–200, 1976.

Bovine Enzootic Hematuria

Clark, I. A., and Dimmock, C. K. The toxicity of *Cheilanthes sieberi* to cattle and sheep. *Aust Vet J* **47:** 149–152, 1971.

Evans, I. A. *et al.* The carcinogenic, mutagenic and teratogenic toxicity of bracken. *Proc R Soc Edinburgh* [*Biol Sci*] **81:** 65–77, 1982.

Evans, W. C. Bracken thiaminase-mediated neurotoxic syndromes. *Bot J Linn Soc* **73:** 113–131, 1976.

McKenzie, R. A. Bovine enzootic haematuria in Queensland. *Aust Vet J* **54:** 61–64, 1978.

Page, C. N. The taxonomy and phytogeography of bracken—a review. *Bot J Linn Soc* **73:** 1–34, 1976.

Pamukcu, A. M. Tumors of the urinary bladder in cattle, with special reference to etiology and histogenesis. *Acta Unio Int Cancrum* **18:** 625–638, 1962.

Pamukcu, A. M. Tumors of the urinary bladder. *Bull WHO* **50:** 43–52, 1974.

Pamukcu, A. M., Price, J. M., and Bryan, G. T. Naturally occurring and bracken-fern-induced bovine urinary bladder tumors. Clinical and morphological characteristics. *Vet Pathol* **13:** 110–122, 1976.

Tumors

Bourne, C. W., and May, J. E. Urachal remnants: benign or malignant? *J Urol* **118:** 743–747, 1977.

Bryan, G. T. The role of urinary tryptophan metabolites in the etiology of bladder cancer. *Am J Clin Nutr* **24:** 841–847, 1971.

Bryan, G. T. The pathogenesis of experimental bladder cancer. *Cancer Res* **37:** 2813–2816, 1977.

Friedell, G. H. Carcinoma, carcinoma *in situ,* and "early lesions" of the uterine cervix and the urinary bladder: introduction and definitions. *Cancer Res* **36:** 2482–2484, 1976.

Hayes, H. M. Canine bladder cancer: epidemiologic features. *Am J Epidemiol* **104:** 673–677, 1976.

Hicks, R. M., and Chowaniec, J. Experimental induction, histology and ultrastructure of hyperplasia and neoplasia of the urinary bladder epithelium. *Int Rev Exp Pathol* **18:** 199–280, 1978.

Kelly, D. F. Rhabdomyosarcoma of the urinary bladder in dogs. *Vet Pathol* **10:** 375–384, 1973.

McKenzie, R. A. An abattoir survey of bovine urinary bladder pathology. *Aust Vet J* **54:** 41, 1978.

Melicow, M. M. Tumors of the bladder: a multifaceted problem. *J Urol* **112:** 467–478, 1974.

Murphy, W. M., and Soloway, M. S. Urothelial dysplasia. *J Urol* **127:** 849–854, 1982.

Osborne, C. A. *et al.* Neoplasms of the canine and feline urinary bladder: incidence, etiologic factors, occurrence and pathologic features. *Am J Vet Res* **29:** 2041–2055, 1968.

Seely, J. C., Cosenza, S. F., and Montgomery, C. A. Leiomyosarcoma of the canine urinary bladder, with metastases. *J Am Vet Med Assoc* **172:** 1427–1429, 1978.

Strafuss, A. C., and Dean, M. J. Neoplasms of the canine urinary bladder. *J Am Vet Med Assoc* **166:** 1161–1163, 1975.

Tarvin, G., Patnaik, A., and Greene, R. Primary urethral tumors in dogs. *J Am Vet Med Assoc* **172:** 931–933, 1978.

Vitovec, J. Carcinomas of the renal pelvis in slaughter animals. *J Comp Pathol* **87:** 129–134, 1977.

Ward, A. M. Glandular neoplasia within the urinary tract. The aetiology of adenocarcinoma of the urothelium with a review of the literature. I. Introduction: the origin of glandular epithelium in the renal pelvis, and ureter and bladder. *Virchows Arch [Pathol Anat]* **352:** 296–311, 1971.

Weller, R. E., Wolf, S. M., and Oyejide, A. Transitional cell carcinoma of the bladder associated with cyclophosphamide therapy in a dog. *J Am Anim Hosp Assoc* **15:** 733–736, 1979.

Wilson, G. P., Hayes, H. M., and Casey, H. W. Canine urethral cancer. *J Am Anim Hosp Assoc* **15:** 741–744, 1979.

Wimberley, H. C., and Lewis, R. M. Transitional cell carcinoma in the domestic cat. *Vet Pathol* **16:** 223–228, 1979.

CHAPTER 6

The Respiratory System

D. L. DUNGWORTH
University of California, Davis

413

General Considerations

The responses of the respiratory tract to injury, and the resulting patterns of disease, are determined largely by the structural and functional complexity of the system. Most of the diseases of the respiratory system are caused by damaging agents arriving by either the airborne (aerogenous) or blood-borne (hematogenous) routes, each with its own special pathogenetic considerations.

There is constant exposure of the respiratory system to potentially harmful agents in the ambient air. The defenses of the respiratory tract against **aerogenous injury** are remarkably effective but are not always successful. Airborne infectious agents commonly cause respiratory diseases, and in some intensive systems of animal management they constitute the most important cause of morbidity and mortality. Each instance represents a breach of pulmonary defenses. An understanding of the pathogenesis of the diseases requires knowledge of the defensive mechanisms and the factors leading to their being overcome. A variety of inhaled noninfectious agents cause disease less frequently, notably organic allergens, caustic gases, fumes and chemicals, and inorganic dusts. The respiratory tract can also serve as a portal of entry of infectious agents that do not primarily affect the respiratory system.

Respiratory defenses serve principally to protect the delicate alveolar parenchyma of the lung from damage. This is accomplished by removing harmful agents as much as possible in the nasal passages and conducting airways. Alveolar mechanisms form a second level of defense. The upper respiratory tract functions to warm and humidify inspired air and to remove larger particles and water-soluble gases by means of the mucous lining. Warming and humidifying principally occurs during passage of air through the nose. It is facilitated by the extensive surface area and the rich, readily engorged vascular plexus in the submucosa, particularly of the turbinates, and nasal septum. Many particles in inspired air are first deposited on the mucous lining of nasal passages and conducting airways and are then cleared by movement of the mucociliary blanket. The larger the particles, the more efficient their removal in the upper airways. Deposition on

surfaces is mainly by inertial impaction, gravitational sedimentation, diffusion, or a combination of these. Inertial impaction is chiefly in the nasal passages and pharynx and at points of branching of airways, where the airstream changes its direction and where turbulence occurs. The efficiency of nasopharyngeal trapping depends on the anatomic complexity of the nasal passages, especially with regard to the turbinates, and on the pattern of respiration. The gravitational settlement of particles is directly proportional to their size and density and is favored in the relatively still air of deeper parts of the respiratory system. Diffusion of particles is due to molecular collision and affects only the very smallest of them, that is, particles of less than ~ 0.3 μm in size. Since displacement velocity by diffusion is low, deposition by this method is effective only in the alveoli, where movement of gases is also by diffusion rather than linear flow.

Deposition of particles greater than ~ 10 μm aerodynamic diameter is virtually complete above the larynx. With decreasing particle size, an increasing proportion of inhaled particles pass into the deep lung, although many are subsequently exhaled. The critical feature, from the point of view of pulmonary homeostasis, is that droplet nuclei and other irritant or infectious particles around $1-2$ μm in diameter mostly deposit at the bronchiolar–alveolar junction. This is because the total cross-sectional area of airspaces increases suddenly, linear velocity of the airstream falls to zero, and there is time for the particles to deposit by gravitational settling. As will be discussed later, this is one of the reasons for the vulnerability of the bronchiolar–alveolar junction to damage by inhaled irritants.

Statements on relationship between particle size and deposition are relative rather than absolute. Sizes quoted for mathematical modeling of particle deposition are in terms of equivalent cross-sectional diameters of unit-density spheres (aerodynamic diameter). The most obvious exception to the generalization that particles greater than 10 μm in diameter do not penetrate beyond the larynx is that fine fibers up to 100 μm or longer, notably of asbestos, do reach alveolar parenchyma. Additionally, there might be opportunity for redistribution of particles deposited in the proximal respiratory tract by reflux of excess secretions or aspiration of fluid.

Once particles are deposited on the mucus of airways, clearance by normally functioning mucociliary transport is highly efficient. Most particles are removed from central airways within a few hours, and even from distal airways within 24 hr. The mucociliary blanket consists of cilia bathed in a watery sol on top of which lies mucus with physical properties of a viscoelastic gel. Whether the mucus usually forms a patchy or continuous surface layer is still debated, but it will probably prove to be continuous in healthy individuals. In any event, the cilia beat mostly in the watery hypophase, except during the active forward stroke when their tips contact the overlying mucus. The net effect of a ciliary frequency of around 1000 beats a minute is to propel the mucus toward the pharynx at a linear velocity of the order of 10 mm/min. The greater density of ciliated cells in proximal airways, the more rapid ciliary beat, and possibly, absorption of a portion of the aqueous periciliary fluid are believed to prevent swamping of these airways, especially the trachea, by fluid collected from the large number of distal airways.

Most of the mucous secretions of the respiratory tract, and the particulate matter they carry, reach the pharynx and are swallowed. The concentration of material into the nasopharynx coincides with well-developed diffuse and focal lymphoid tissue of the tonsillar region and dorsal nasopharynx. This enhances the efficiency of development of immune responses but also makes the region vulnerable to primary infections by organisms such as *Brucella* spp. and *Mycobacterium paratuberculosis*. Swallowing of material originating in the lungs also serves as a mode of spread of diseases such as tuberculosis and as part of the migratory pathway of helminth eggs and larvae.

The specific roles and controlling influences of mucous cells, serous cells, and other secretory cells in surface epithelium and submucosal glands, and the differences among species, are still poorly understood. In addition to the physical aspects of the sol and gel phases of the secretion, however, a variety of other components with defensive capabilities are recognized. The major immunoglobulin is locally synthesized IgA, although IgE, IgG, and other classes are present. Immunoglobulin A is produced by plasma cells resident in the lamina propria of the respiratory mucosa and secreted through epithelial serous cells. A major function of organized lymphoid tissue in the walls of the nasal passages, nasopharynx, and airways is believed to be to populate, through the circulation, the respiratory mucosa with precursors of IgA-secreting plasma cells. This includes bronchus-associated lymphoid tissue. The principal functions of IgA are thought to be viral neutralization, aggregation of macromolecular antigens to impede their mucosal absorption, and inhibition of bacterial colonization. Important nonspecific humoral components of the secretions are interferon, which helps limit viral infection in nonimmune hosts, and lysozyme (muramidase) and lactoferrin, which have selective antibacterial activity. The normal bacterial flora of the nose and nasopharynx are important in that by specific adherence of their specialized surface structures (pili) to receptors on cilia and surfaces of epithelial cells, they prevent adherence and colonization by more pathogenic flora. Most current investigations of bacterial interference are on flora of the alimentary tract and skin of

humans. By analogy, however, the phenomenon is undoubtedly important in the upper respiratory tract of animals.

The physical and humoral defenses of the mucociliary blanket, which are constantly in operation, are boosted by cellular and humoral mechanisms recruited from blood at the onset of inflammation, and by sneezing, coughing, and bronchoconstriction provoked by irritation of airway receptors. Normal mucociliary function depends on structurally and functionally intact ciliated epithelium as well as normal viscous properties and quantity of secretions. Interference with any one or more of these predisposes to infection, and is considered under Bronchopneumonia.

Alveolar defense against small-sized particles depends heavily on phagocytosis by alveolar macrophages. Phagocytosis of readily ingested particles, for instance, opsonized bacteria, is largely complete by 4 hr after alveolar deposition. Actual physical removal of particulates from alveoli is inefficient, in contrast to their removal when deposited on the mucociliary blanket. Fifty per cent clearance of particles deposited in alveoli takes from several days to months or longer, depending on their physical nature and irritant capability. Most particles are therefore phagocytosed by macrophages and either inactivated or sequestered. The alveolar macrophages move toward the bronchioles and hence eventually onto the mucociliary blanket. Reasons for their centripetal movement are not known, but the surface-lining liquid in alveoli is also believed to move centripetally, possibly because of its continual secretion and a "milking" action of respiratory movements. Alternative fates of particles in alveoli are clearance in the lining liquid without phagocytosis, or penetration into the pulmonary interstitium. The latter becomes of increasing importance as the particulate load increases. Although not completely proven, it appears that most particles reach the interstitium by endocytosis across the alveolar type I epithelial cells. Once in the interstitial space, particles move with the flow of lymph and are phagocytosed by interstitial macrophages. Particle-laden macrophages associated with lymphatics occur in peribronchiolar and perivascular clusters, and some eventually find their way to the local lymph nodes. Overloading the alveolar macrophage system favors accumulation of particles in the interstitium, as occurs in the pneumoconioses.

Sterility of alveoli is thus maintained largely by the ability of macrophages to kill ingested bacteria and to secrete interferon. These activities are enhanced by immunoglobulin, particularly through the opsonizing effect of IgG, which is the predominant immunoglobulin in the alveolar lining liquid. Alveolar macrophages are also capable of initiating a variety of amplification mechanisms, particularly by their recruitment of neutrophils and sensitized T lymphocytes. The latter in turn can cause macrophage activation. Macrophage factors are also important in the pathogenesis of emphysema and pulmonary fibrosis, as mentioned in the sections on those diseases.

Lysozyme, lactoferrin, and complement are also present in alveolar lining liquid. Humoral components capable of inhibiting inflammatory mediators or destructive enzymes are now recognized to be of great importance. The components of most active study are superoxide dysmutase, which helps protect against injury by reactive oxygen radicals, and α_1-protease inhibitor, which is important in protection against the development of alveolar emphysema.

Just as factors interfering with mucociliary defense mechanisms of airways predispose to bronchopneumonia, so will factors depressing alveolar defenses, especially the alveolar macrophage (see Bronchopneumonia).

The entire output of the right ventricle flows through the low-pressure pulmonary circulation. The densely anastomosing network of capillaries in alveolar septa provides the equivalent of "sheet" flow when they are all patent. This arrangement both provides for easy trapping of emboli in the pulmonary vascular bed and for minimizing the deleterious effects of blockage. Effects of blockage are minimized further by the dual pulmonary and bronchial arterial blood supplies to the lung. Nevertheless, emboli carry a risk and are associated with a variety of lesions, according to the nature of the emboli. The types of emboli vary greatly. Unusual ones are epidermal fragments and hair inadvertently introduced into the blood at the time of injection, or fragments of nucleus pulposus from intervertebral disks. More commonly they are bacteria, fungi, protozoa, endogenous fat, normal cells (which may be represented by megakaryocytes), or abnormal cells (which are principally neoplastic). They can also be fragments of bland or septic thrombi, helminth parasites for which the respiratory system is a natural or accidental habitat, or even parasitic ova, as required by *Pneumostrongylus tenuis* of deer for the continuation of its life cycle. In general, the benefit of the lung acting as a blood filter is the prevention of emboli reaching the systemic circulation and the protection of organs such as the brain, heart, and kidneys against infarction. The detriments are spread of infection, metastasis of tumors, and pulmonary thromboembolism causing shock. The last named is rare in animals.

The lung is also prone to injury by a variety of blood-borne toxic agents, both exogenous and endogenous, and can be affected by certain metabolic abnormalities. These will be considered further under Interstitial Pneumonia. The reasons for the special vulnerability of the lung are only now emerging. Pulmonary capillary endothelium as a whole forms a highly metabolic organ, particularly with respect to vasoactive substances and the blood-clotting, fibrinolytic, and arachidonic acid cascades. For reasons still unclear, in conditions such as shock and septicemia there is a tendency in pulmonary capillaries for activation of Hageman factor, release of prostaglandins and leukotrienes, and aggregation of platelets and neutrophils. This causes the acute pulmonary injury seen in these conditions.

Patterns of Respiratory Tract Disease

Respiratory diseases can be caused by a large variety of infectious or noninfectious agents. The site of damage in the respiratory tract is determined by the interplay of portal of entry of the agent, the nature and concentration of the agent, and the relative susceptibility of the tissues exposed to the agent. The portal of entry is the major determinant.

Aerogenous insult, as would be expected, usually leads to damage centered on airways. Nasal passages and upper airways are mostly affected by irritants contained in large particles, by highly soluble gases, or by infectious agents whose cell receptors are most numerous or more readily accessible in upper respiratory epithelium. Distal airways are more affected by fine particles, weakly soluble gases, and infectious agents with affinity for bronchiolar or alveolar epithelium. The greater vulnerability of the bronchiolar–alveolar junction to damage is also an extremely important determinant at this level (see Bronchopneumonia).

Hematogenous insult usually affects the lungs and is manifest, depending on the cause, as diffuse, patchy, or discrete focal lesions without orientation on airways. An important exception to the generalization that blood-borne agents affect alveolar septa and pulmonary interstitium more than airways is where a toxin specifically damages bronchiolar epithelium. The best example of this for present purposes is the necrosis of nonciliated bronchiolar epithelial (Clara) cells of the horse caused experimentally by 3-methylindole. Localization of damage to Clara cells in the horse is because that is where cellular binding of 3-methylindole and metabolism to the toxic intermediate by the cytoplasmic microsomal monooxygenase (mixed-function oxidase) system occur in this species.

Other, less common types of injury to the respiratory tract are traumatic, as by penetration of a foreign body, or by extension of lesions along fascial planes and lymphatics from adjacent tissues or cavities.

Differences in patterns of lesions among species of animals are well recognized, but few have been formally studied. An obvious example is the complete lobular septation and absence of collateral ventilation (low interdependence) in the bovine lung, which predisposes it to poor resolution of bronchopneumonia and to the development of acute interstitial emphysema under conditions of excessively labored breathing. Another example is the acute pulmonary congestion and edema almost invariably found in sheep dying as a result of any acute disease process. More precise mechanistic reasons for differences in species response are coming to light as more is learned about the interspecies variations in specific cell types and their metabolic capabilities. One example already alluded to is that the selectivity of damage caused by some pneumotoxins depends on the distribution of enzymes capable of metabolizing them. This is the basis for 3-methylindole's causing mostly nonciliated bronchiolar cell necrosis in the horse, in contrast to extensive pulmonary endothelial and alveolar epithelial damage in the cow.

Nasal Cavity and Sinuses

Congenital Anomalies

Congenital anomalies of the nasal region are rare but occur in all species. They are usually part of more extensive craniofacial defects in which they accompany various combinations of malformations of mouth and eyes. Animals with absent, underdeveloped, or severely distorted nasal regions are usually stillborn or die immediately after birth, often because of an imperforate buccopharyngeal membrane (choanal atresia). The milder defect of cleft palate is compatible with life, but affected animals generally die because of aspiration pneumonia.

A variety of localized, developmentally related defects, which take time to become apparent, can affect the nasal region, particularly those of tooth germ origin. Maxillary cysts in foals or young adult horses can distort the profile of the maxillary bone sufficiently to cause obstruction of the ipsilateral nasal passage, destruction of the nasal turbinates, and deviation of the nasal septum.

Metabolic Disturbances

Deposits of amyloid sometimes occur in the nasal submucosa of horses. The deposition is not part of a generalized amyloidosis, and the cause is unknown. The nasal vestibule and anterior portions of the septum and turbinates are involved. The amyloid might be in nodules of various sizes or occur as a diffuse deposition. Resulting stenosis can be severe enough to cause clinical signs of nasal obstruction. The nodules or diffuse thickenings have a smooth surface and the usual waxy sheen of amyloid on the cut surface. The amyloid is deposited in the walls of submucosal vessels and the basement membrane of mucosal glands as well as in the connective tissues. There might be mild inflammatory changes in the mucous membrane.

Circulatory Disturbances

The arteries, veins, and capillaries of the nasal mucosa are capable of remarkable adaptive changes in the content of blood. Vascular engorgement occurs by relaxation of the arteries and contraction of the thick tunica media of the veins. This lability of the vessels is responsible for the frequency of hyperemia and edema. Active hyperemia is part of the acute stage of inflammation. Passive congestion is the result of local or general circulatory failure.

Of rather more concern is nasal hemorrhage, which is known as **epistaxis**. The term epistaxis is used in a general sense to refer to hemorrhage from the nose, but this does not necessarily mean that the source of bleeding is within the nasal passages or sinuses. The hemorrhage might be from the nasopharynx or from deep within the respiratory tract. This distinction is particularly important in horses, where in epistaxis associated with heavy exercise the blood originates from the lung. The condition is more appropriately termed exercise-induced pulmonary hemorrhage and will be described under Pulmonary Hemorrhage. Bloodstained foam is frequently present in and issues from the nose of cadavers, especially sheep. This is an indication of terminal pulmonary congestion, edema, and hemorrhage.

Hemorrhage originating within the nasal region is most commonly caused by traumatic, inflammatory, or neoplastic breakdown of vessels. It might also be part of any of the hemorrhagic diatheses (see the Hematopoietic System, Volume 3). In some of the hemorrhagic diatheses, such as those of thrombocytopenic origin, the bleeding might be copious. Hemorrhage in rhinitis is associated with mucosal ulceration, a frequent happening in acute inflammation, and in some specific types of chronic inflammation. In most inflammatory hemorrhages, the extravasation is initially submucosal. Mycotic infections of the guttural pouches can cause epistaxis in horses. Rarely, nasal hemorrhage might be the result of hypertension or vascular aneurysms.

Inflammation of the Nasal Cavity

Rhinitis

The nasopharyngeal mucous membrane has a normal resident microbial flora, established by specific adherence between the bacterial pili and sugar-containing surface binding sites on epithelial cells. An important role of the normal flora is to exclude adherence and subsequent colonization of the mucosa by more pathogenic organisms, particularly Gram-negative ones. Injury to the mucosal surface can lead to pathogenic activity by certain of the normal flora or, more importantly, affect surface binding sites such that adherence and colonization by pathogenic microorganisms can occur. Similar changes can occur because of systemic immunodeficiency states or nonspecific stress situations, such as occur postoperatively. The frequency of fungal and other opportunistic infections following prolonged antibiotic therapy probably has the same basis, that is, removal of the normal ''blocking'' bacterial flora.

Primary injurious agents are usually viruses. Allergens are probably important in cattle and, to a lesser extent, in dogs and cats. Irritant volatile gases, dust, and excessive dryness of the atmosphere are occasional causes of injury to the nasal epithelium. In summary, rhinitis is usually related to the interaction between viruses, or other devitalizing influences, and bacteria or fungi.

Rhinitis can be differentiated, according to its course, as acute or chronic. It can be differentiated morphologically, according to the nature of the response, into serous, catarrhal, purulent, ulcerative, pseudomembranous, hemorrhagic, or granulomatous inflammation. Most acute cases of rhinitis begin with a serous exudation, which changes in the course of the disease to a catarrhal and then purulent inflammation. Pseudomembranous, ulcerative, or hemorrhagic rhinitis is a sign of very severe damage. Chronic rhinitis is most commonly manifested by proliferative changes, but occasionally it causes atrophy.

During the initial **serous** stages of rhinitis, whether viral, allergic, or nonspecific, the mucosa is swollen and gray to red, depending on the degree of hyperemia. Histologically, the epithelial cells show hydropic degeneration and loss of cilia. There is hyperactivity of the goblet cells and submucosal glands. The secretion is a thin, clear seromucin that contains a few leukocytes and epithelial cells. The underlying lamina propria is edematous and sparsely infiltrated by inflammatory cells. The swelling of the mucous membrane tends to cause mild respiratory discomfort and the familiar sneezing and snuffling.

Within hours or a few days, serous rhinitis is modified partly by changes in glandular secretion and partly by bacterial infection. The hyperemia, edema, and swelling are then aggravated and the discharge becomes catarrhal (mucous) or frankly purulent because of the emigration of large numbers of leukocytes and desquamation of epithelial cells. Erosion and regenerative hyperplasia of the epithelium occur, and in purulent rhinitis extensive ulcerations might be evident.

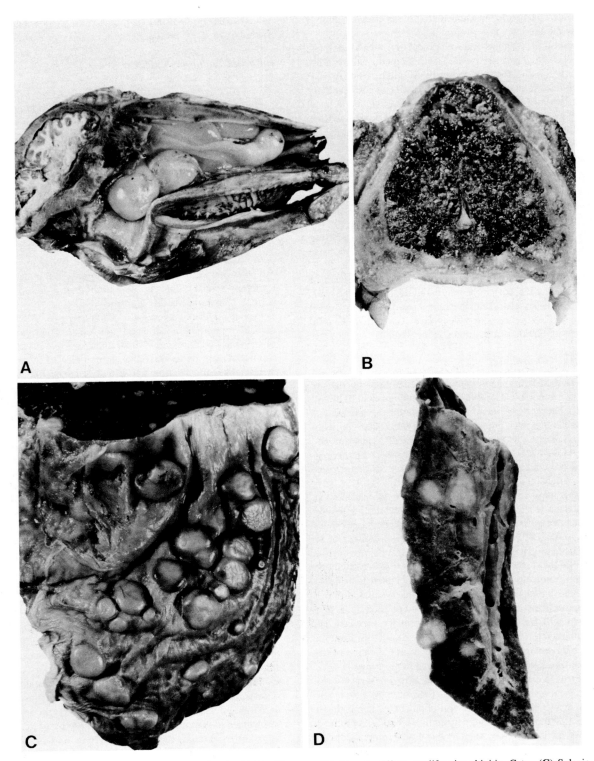

Fig. 6.1.   **(A)** Myxomatous polyps in chronic rhinitis. Sheep.   **(B)** Chronic diffuse, proliferative rhinitis. Cat.   **(C)** Splenic abscessation in melioidosis. Sheep.   **(D)** Chronic pulmonary abscessation in melioidosis. Sheep. (**C** and **D** courtesy of W. T. Hall and the Queensland Department of Agriculture.)

In subacute to chronic rhinitis, diffuse or localized polypous thickenings of the mucosa develop (Fig. 6.1A). The polyps are initially sessile but can, when larger, become pedunculated. They consist of a core of edematous stroma resembling myxoma tissue and a covering epithelium that is variously hyperplastic, squamous, or ulcerated. Chronic **catarrhal** or **suppurative rhinitis** causes progressive fibrosis of the lamina propria with atrophy of the glands and atrophy with focal squamous metaplasia of nasal epithelium. The atrophic epithelium is dry and shiny.

Pseudomembranous rhinitis may be fibrinous or fibrinonecrotic (diphtheritic), but it is usually the former, and the membranes can be peeled off without leaving gross underlying defects. The deeper, fibrinonecrotic inflammations are associated with severe bacterial infections and frequently have a dry, yellowish quality that indicates infection with *Fusobacterium necrophorum*. The fibrinonecrotic membrane is firmly adherent to the underlying tissue and when removed leaves a raw, ulcerated surface.

Granulomatous rhinitis is a typical lesion in some specific diseases. The lesions are nodular and polypoid or become large, space-occupying masses. The smaller ones are more firm, the larger ones more friable or gelatinous. The histologic structure is specific for the disease.

Rhinitis occurs commonly as part of a more generalized disease process. Important specific entities in which rhinitis is the sole or a major lesion will be covered subsequently. A chronic nonspecific rhinitis is an important condition in the dog, and to a lesser extent in the cat. There is a chronic unilateral or bilateral mucopurulent discharge, and the inflammatory proliferation leads to diffuse or polypoid thickening of the nasal mucosa and obstruction of nasal passages (Fig. 6.1B). The glandular elements are hyperplastic, the epithelium is variously ulcerated, hyperplastic, and metaplastic (squamous), and the edematous, fibrotic stroma is heavily infiltrated by lymphocytes and plasma cells. There is no sign of foreign bodies, at least in the chronic lesion, and bacterial cultures do not reveal significant organisms. The pathogenesis is unclear, but following initial damage that is no longer detectable there is probably a vicious cycle involving impaired local defenses, further infection and damage by normally nonpathogenic flora, and self-sustaining inflammation by release of mediators from the large numbers of inflammatory cells. Pooling of exudate in obstructed portions of the lumen and compromised venous and lymphatic drainage in the hyperplastic mucosa are also likely to be factors leading to progression of the lesion.

Rhinitis of itself can have unfortunate sequelae. Aspiration of nasal exudate might lead to bronchopneumonia. The potentiality for reflex flow in the valveless veins of the head explains the occurrence of intracranial thrombophlebitis, abscess, or meningitis; these are, however, rare. Sinusitis probably is the sequel most common to rhinitis.

Sinusitis

Inflammation of the paranasal sinuses often goes undetected unless it has caused facial deformity or a fistula in the overlying skin. Sinusitis is very common in sheep as a response to larvae of *Oestrus ovis*. It also follows penetration of infection in dehorning wounds, fractures, and periodontitis. Seromucinous sinusitis of little significance occurs in viral infections of the upper respiratory tract. In acute catarrhal or purulent rhinitis, the mucosal swelling tends to occlude the orifices of the sinuses. The secretions and exudates then accumulate and render chronic purulent sinusitis almost inevitable. The histologic features of sinusitis are the same as those of rhinitis. The accumulation of seromucinous secretion is referred to as mucocele, and the accumulation of purulent exudate is referred to as empyema of the sinus. Purulent inflammations of the sinuses are more significant than rhinitis because of proximity to the brain. They are also less liable to spontaneous drainage and resolution. Therefore, they are more likely to cause epithelial atrophy and metaplasia, and distortion of the bony walls of the sinuses by pressure or osteomyelitis.

Rhinitis in Specific Diseases

In addition to the specific diseases to be discussed below, rhinitis is a prominent feature of a variety of respiratory or more generalized infectious diseases. The nature, cause, and specificity of the various forms of rhinitis differ according to species. Examples are canine distemper, the feline respiratory disease complex, bovine virus diarrhea, rinderpest and malignant catarrhal fever of cattle, bluetongue of sheep, and equine influenza, equine rhinopneumonitis, and equine viral arteritis.

INCLUSION-BODY RHINITIS OF SWINE. Inclusion-body rhinitis is widespread in Europe, but its prevalence in the United States and other major pig-raising areas of the world is unknown. It is caused by a cytomegalovirus that characteristically produces large, basophilic intranuclear inclusions in swollen glandular epithelia of the nasal cavity.

Inclusion-body rhinitis is an acute to subacute disease of suckling piglets about 1–5 weeks of age. The signs are those usual for rhinitis with modest fever. The early discharge is seromucinous, but it might become catarrhal or purulent if the course is prolonged, probably owing to secondary bacterial infection. The morbidity is high, but the mortality in the absence of suppurative complications is low; the complications include sinusitis, otitis media, and pneumonia.

The uncomplicated histologic changes in the mucosa are those of a nonsuppurative rhinitis, with a tendency to squamous metaplasia, and the presence of specific basophilic inclusions in the epithelial cells of the glands and their ducts (Fig. 6.2C). The inclusions are large and readily visible at low magnification. Affected glands occur in irregular clusters, and all their epithelial cells tend to contain inclusions. The inclusion bodies can persist for a month but become less numerous as the course of the disease advances.

As the inclusion develops, the nucleus and cytoplasm of the affected cell expand. The cytoplasm becomes clear and finely granular, and cell borders become indistinct. The inclusion body fills the nucleus, except for small peripheral indentations in which minute neutrophilic or acidophilic bodies may be found. The affected nuclei continue to swell and the nuclear membrane loses its distinctiveness; by this time the inclusion bodies resemble bluish gray smears among degenerating cytoplasm. Sloughing of the epithelium is followed by liquefaction and the accumulation of leukocytic debris. The necrotic glands are obliterated by collapse of the lamina propria and infiltration by

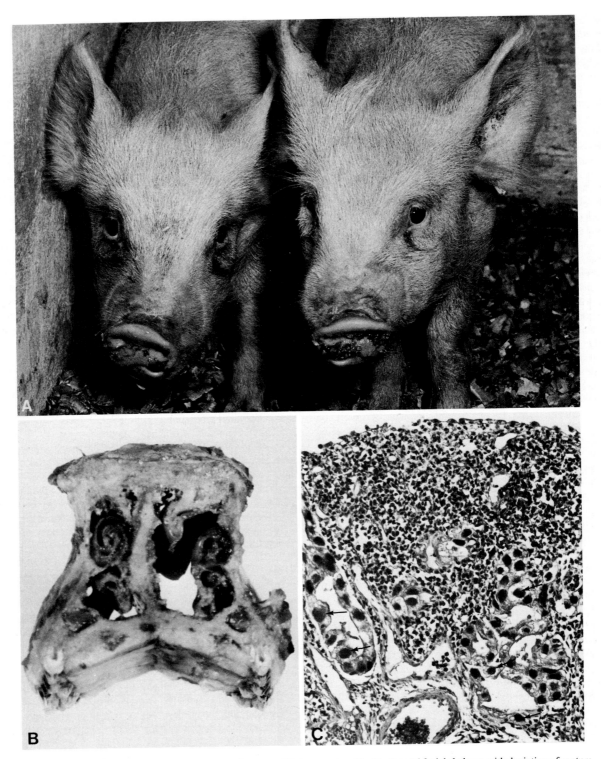

Fig. 6.2. (**A**) Atrophic rhinitis with deviation of snout. (**B**) Asymmetry of turbinates and facial skeleton with deviation of septum in atrophic rhinitis. Pig. (**C**) Large, basophilic intranuclear inclusions (arrows) in inclusion-body rhinitis. Pig.

lymphocytes. There is slight vascular reaction in this disease. The infiltrating cells are predominantly lymphocytes, and although distributed diffusely, they tend to form more dense aggregates in the superficial layers of the lamina propria. Regeneration of glands may take place by downgrowth and differentiation from the superficial epithelium.

Occasionally, in addition to rhinitis, there is severe generalized cytomegalovirus infection, with focal necrotizing lesions associated with intranuclear inclusions in adrenal, liver, kidney, lung, and central nervous system. Although further substantiation is needed, it appears likely that cytomegalovirus infection is one of the factors that may lead to persistent infection with *Bordetella bronchiseptica* or *Pasteurella multocida* and subsequent development of atrophic rhinitis.

ATROPHIC RHINITIS OF SWINE. Atrophic rhinitis of swine is a disease of uncertain cause characterized by atrophy of the nasal turbinates (conchae). Less constant features are irregular atrophy of the nasal bones and plates of paranasal sinuses, and with variation from case to case, there is also irregular hypertrophy of facial bones and remnants of turbinates. On clinical and experimental grounds, the disease is generally regarded as being principally of infectious origin, but the proportional involvement of the various agents that have been incriminated and the role of enhancing factors have to be clarified. A variety of inflammatory stimuli can cause atrophy of turbinates, often of a temporary nature. The morphologic features of atrophic rhinitis are therefore not particularly specific. There is growing evidence that the naturally occurring disease is mainly the result of adherence and persistent colonization of nasal mucosa by virulent strains of *Bordetella bronchiseptica, Pasteurella multocida,* or perhaps more importantly, both organisms. Other bacteria found on the nasal mucosa, such as *Haemophilus parasuis,* probably play a lesser role. Factors known to be capable of enhancing the severity of the clinical disease, for instance, cytomegalovirus infection (inclusion-body rhinitis) or adverse environmental and nutritional circumstances, probably act by facilitating the colonization and persistence of the pathogenic bacteria. Nutritional defects, particularly those involving calcium and phosphorus, can also interfere with metabolism of bone at the time when rapid growth and remodeling of turbinates in young pigs make them most susceptible to the effects of the infectious agents. Nutritional deficiencies alone, however, do not cause atrophic rhinitis. The precise proportional mix of factors resulting in chronic, irreversible atrophy undoubtedly varies according to local geographic influences. The mechanism by which *B. bronchiseptica* or *P. multocida* cause the atrophy of turbinates is uncertain. The basic abnormality, as will be described, appears to be defective osteoblast function, leading to osteoporosis and hypoplasia of the turbinate bone. Studies with *B. bronchiseptica* implicate diffusible toxin, although in one experimental study, bacteria believed to be *B. bronchiseptica* were detected ultrastructurally within the cytoplasm of degenerating osteoblasts and extracellularly in the vicinity of the surface of bone.

Atrophic rhinitis occurs with high incidence in most of the major pig-raising areas of the world. It is an important cause of economic loss because in young pigs it causes decreased rate of growth and reduced efficiency of feed conversion. The endemic disease is insidious in onset and progression, but there can be acute episodes when a herd first becomes affected.

Acute signs are observed in young piglets and consist of rhinitis with sneezing, coughing, and a serous or mucopurulent nasal discharge. Large or small flecks of blood may be expelled by sneezing when damage is severe, and occasionally the hemorrhage is profuse. There is not a constant association between clinical signs of acute rhinitis and atrophic changes. Rhinitis occasionally is found not to have resulted in atrophy, at least of a permanent nature, and in some herds a high incidence of atrophy of the turbinates might be present in slaughtered pigs without there having been at any time clinical signs of rhinitis or facial deformity.

Facial deformity, which is an expression of severe disease in the rapidly growing young pig, is seldom evident before the fifth or sixth week of age. It consists of shortening and distortion of the snout and facial bones (Fig. 6.2A). As a result of the shortening, the overlying skin forms thick transverse folds. Asymmetry of the disease process causes deviation of the snout toward the more severely affected side; when the intranasal lesions are symmetric, the nose may be shortened and turned upward. Characteristically, there is often patchy encrustation of dried tears and dirt just below the medial canthus of the eye; this is usually attributed to lacrimal spillage caused by obstruction of the nasolacrimal duct, but increased lacrimation might also play a role.

The lesions of atrophic rhinitis range from indefinite to severe, and as is often the case, no clear dividing line separates the normal from the diseased. The lesions are most severe anterior to the nasofrontal suture. When mild, they may be detectable only in the ventral scroll of the ventral turbinate, but with increasing severity gross changes become detectable in the entire ventral turbinate, in the dorsal turbinate, and further back in the nasal cavity until even the ethmoids are involved. The nasal mucosa usually has less gross changes. It might be edematous and covered by a thin seromucinous exudate on the anterior portions and thick purulent exudate in posterior recesses and cells of the ethmoid, or it might be pale and dry.

The grossly detectable changes in the conformation of bones are always of the same type, but there are wide variations in the extent of the lesions. In the least affected specimens, the ventral scrolls of the ventral turbinates are reduced in size and are pliable and soft. The width of the ventral meatus is increased. This is often accompanied by slight bulging of the nasal septum toward the less affected side. With progression of the lesions in the turbinates, there is loss of both scrolls of the ventral turbinate and then of the dorsal turbinate (Fig. 6.2B). In extreme cases, nothing remains of the turbinates save for folds of mucosa on the lateral aspect of the empty nasal chamber. The bones surrounding the nasal cavity are frequently thinned. In some animals, especially those whose general health is not significantly affected by the disease and who continue to grow, hypertrophic changes frequently coexist with atrophic changes in the facial bones and rarely with hypertrophic changes in the turbinates. Combined hypertrophic and atrophic changes in the turbinates produce a series of longitudinal folds. Hypertrophy of the facial bones affects chiefly the dorsal part of the nasal bones so that the conformation is broad and flat rather than narrow and convex.

The alveolar processes may also be thickened, although the lateral plates of the maxillae tend to be attenuated.

Microscopically, the turbinate atrophy is associated with loss of cancellous bone in the core of the turbinates. Histologic and ultrastructural observations support the concept that the basic defect is decreased osteoid synthesis by severely damaged, differentiated osteoblasts. The disappearance of turbinates appears to be due more to defective osteogenesis during a period of rapid growth and remodeling of the nasal region than the result of excessive osteoclastic activity.

Histologically, there is hypoplasia of the cancellous bone of the turbinates and reduction or absence of the osteoid layer normally present between osteoblasts and the surface of the bone. The periosteum in some instances has increased cellularity of the proliferative (osteoprogenitor) cell layer, and in other instances is narrowed and composed mainly of fibroblast-like cells. Osteoclasts are not significantly changed in number or structure.

Ultrastructurally, degeneration of osteoblasts is associated with irregular folding of nuclear and plasma membranes, loss of the Golgi apparatus, and dilatation of cisternae of the endoplasmic reticulum. The types of mitochondrial and cytoplasmic changes preceding atrophy and death of the cells are less certain. Osteocytes are similarly but less severely affected. Although pigs with atrophic rhinitis sometimes have more widespread skeletal abnormalities, there is no clear evidence that they have the same cause.

The inflammatory lesions in the nasal mucous membranes are usually nonspecific and vary according to the stage of the disease. In early stages, there is loss of ciliated and goblet cells and proliferation of cuboidal cells to form layers one to several cells deep. Submucosal glands become hyperactive and distended with mucus. Neutrophils infiltrate the superficial and glandular epithelium and occasionally form microabscesses. Subsequently, there is infiltration of the lamina propria by lymphocytes and plasma cells. The only indication of a specific acute infection occurs in piglets from herds where cytomegalovirus infection is prevalent. There is no direct correlation between severity of the acute rhinitis and the later development of permanent atrophy of the turbinates. In established cases of atrophic rhinitis, there is chronic nonspecific mucosal inflammation with variation from epithelial ulceration to squamous metaplasia, and atrophy or cystic dilation of the glands within a fibrotic lamina propria.

STRANGLES IN HORSES.   Strangles is an acute contagious disease of horses characterized by inflammation of the upper respiratory tract and abscessation in the regional lymph nodes. It is caused by *Streptococcus equi*. This organism is an obligate parasite on upper respiratory mucous membranes of Equidae. Other hemolytic streptococci of Lancefield's group C are frequent commensals in the upper respiratory tract of horses. The main species are *S. zooepidemicus* and *S. equisimilis*. The former is much more commonly pathogenic and can be isolated from a variety of suppurative processes such as wound infections, sinusitis, and pneumonia secondary to respiratory viral infection. It can cause endometritis and abortion in mares, and umbilical infection, septicemia, and polyarthritis in newborn foals. *Streptococcus zooepidemicus* and, rarely, *S. equisimilis* are causes of respiratory catarrh in horses that might on other than bacteriologic grounds be indistinguishable from strangles. This is especially true for mild cases of the latter in which lymphadenitis is absent or is mild and nonsuppurative.

Streptococcus equi in exudates is very resistant to the external environment and can survive for many months in stables. The initial source of infection, however, is usually a carrier animal or one with active but not necessarily clinically obvious disease. Outbreaks of the disease occur mainly in young animals under crowded conditions. Carrier horses are difficult to detect because shedding of organisms is intermittent and the site of recovery can shift between nasal and pharyngeal regions in a single animal. The distribution of *S. equi* in populations of horses is roughly parallel to the incidence of strangles in such populations.

The incubation period of strangles is 3 or 4 days, although it might be as short as 2 or as long as 15 days; the onset is indicated by fever, slight cough, and nasal discharge. The nasal discharge is bilateral, and in a few days it changes from serous to catarrhal and then purulent. Coincidentally, there is catarrhal conjunctivitis and, in cases that pursue a typical course, inflammatory swelling of the lymph nodes of the head and neck. The submandibular and retropharyngeal nodes are the first and usually the most severely affected. The acute inflammatory swelling is firm, but the nodes begin to fluctuate as liquefaction and suppuration develop. The typical and favorable outcome of the lymphadenitis is for the abscesses to rupture onto the skin 1–3 weeks after onset of infection. Rupture is preceded by depilation and oozing of serum. The discharged pus is copious, creamy, and yellow-white. Abscessation of lymph nodes is not an invariable feature of strangles, but the diagnosis is seldom made in its absence.

The nasal lesions are those of a purulent rhinitis but are otherwise nonspecific. Large amounts of creamy, yellow pus collect in the folds of the turbinates and may produce temporary distortion. The mucosa is edematous, hyperemic, and occasionally ulcerated.

In the typical course of strangles described above, the outcome is favorable. The course, however, may be either milder or more severe and with an unfavorable outcome. In older horses, the course tends to be milder and confined to catarrhal rhinitis and pharyngitis without nodal abscessation, or the nodal abscesses may become sterile and encapsulated. When the course is severe, infection may spread to the paranasal sinuses and by way of the Eustachian tubes to the guttural pouches to cause chronic empyema of these cavities. Extensive cellulitis might develop in the connective tissues of nose, pharynx, or throat. Retropharyngeal abscesses might discharge into the pharynx, allowing pus to be aspirated into the lungs. Metastatic abscesses ("bastard strangles") occasionally form in the liver, kidneys, synovial structures, and brain. The internal organs most frequently affected, however, are the mediastinal and mesenteric lymph nodes. In each of these locations, the abscessations tend to be very large, and although frank rupture is unusual, the suppurative process can permeate to the respective serous membranes and cause a purulent pleuritis or peritonitis. Two other important sequelae are purpura hemorrhagica and local damage to cranial nerves, resulting in laryngeal paralysis (roaring), facial nerve paralysis, or Horner's syndrome.

Glanders

Glanders is an infectious disease caused by a Gram-negative bacillus, *Pseudomonas mallei*. It is mainly an equine infection, but it does occur occasionally in humans and it can be acquired naturally by carnivorous animals that eat diseased flesh of horses. Goats are susceptible to contact infection, but cattle, sheep, and pigs are not. A variety of other generic names have been used for the organism, most commonly, *Loefflerella, Pfeifferella, Malleomyces,* and *Actinobacillus.* The disease in horses is characterized by nodular lesions in the lungs, and ulcerative and nodular lesions of the skin and respiratory mucosa. "Farcy" is the term often applied to the cutaneous lesions.

Glanders is, historically, a very old disease and flourished especially among cavalry horses. Since the advent of motorized vehicles and accurate serologic diagnostic procedures, it has virtually or completely disappeared from many countries. It still exists, however, in some parts of eastern Europe and Asia.

Pseudomonas mallei is sensitive to the external environment, and infection is acquired directly or indirectly from excretions and discharges of affected animals. In horses, the disease is usually chronic and the organisms confined to the lesions and discharges, especially those of the skin and nasal mucosa. In the acute disease, which occurs in some horses and is the usual form in donkeys, the organism is distributed in most tissues and may be excreted in feces, urine, saliva, and tears. Although the most common form of the disease in horses is respiratory, the route of infection is probably oral because this is the only experimental way to produce the typical chronic respiratory disease; intranasal or intratracheal inoculation reproduces the acute disease. Percutaneous infection can occur, but this is unusual.

In the absence of definitive information it is assumed that the organisms traverse the pharyngeal mucosa, and perhaps the intestinal mucosa, and are conveyed to the lungs, where lesions almost always occur. From there, hematogenous spread is believed to result in the nasal, cutaneous, and nodal lesions. This sequence of events is speculative, however, and not entirely satisfying. The chronic syndrome of glanders is frequently divided into nasal, pulmonary, and cutaneous varieties. The division is convenient for description, but the varieties are not distinct, emphasis may at any time change from one to the other, and the same animal may suffer the three varieties at the same time. Involvement of all three sites is common in acute glanders as it is seen in donkeys and in exacerbations of the chronic disease in horses.

Rhinitis in glanders usually commences as a unilateral nasal catarrh, but the inflammation might be bilateral and also involve the pharynx and larynx. The nasal excretion is copious, purulent, and greenish yellow. It is frequently flecked with blood and fragments of desquamated epithelium. The typical nasal lesions are multiple small nodules lying in the submucosa and surrounded by a narrow hyperemic halo. Each nodule consists of a focus of intense cellular infiltration with an inner core of neutrophils and a periphery of macrophages. The core liquefies, and

the overlying mucosa might slough. The nodules might be isolated or semiconfluent, with suppurative cores separated by granulation tissue. A discrete slough of the necrotic tissue over individual nodules can occur, leaving a crateriform ulcer with a sharp margin and smooth base. The ulcers sometimes perforate the septum in severe cases. New generations of nodules develop, ulcerate, and heal irregularly; it is usual to find nodules, ulcers, and white stellate scars mixed together in an affected horse. There is variation from case to case in the number of lesions that can be found. In the milder cases, a few discrete foci are present in the posterior portions of the nasal cavity, and the anterior portions show only hyperemia and catarrh. Lymphadenitis of the submaxillary and retropharyngeal nodes is regularly present. Depending on the age and activity, nodules or scars might be found. When lesions occur on the larynx, they are of the same type as those in the nose. Lesions in the tracheal mucosa are usually ulcerative but are occasionally pyogranulomatous nodules.

Lesions of glanders can be found in lungs in all but a very small percentage of cases. The typical lesion is the nodule, but in some acute cases there may be a more diffuse pneumonia. The nodules have a miliary distribution throughout the lungs, but most of them are detected beneath the pleura. They are basically pyogranulomatous lesions, but the relative proportion of exudative and proliferative components varies. The more exudative foci typically have necrotic centers composed of karyorrhectic neutrophils. In acute stages, they have hemorrhagic and fibrinous exudation. In more mature lesions, liquefied or caseonecrotic centers are surrounded by epithelioid cells, occasional giant cells, and lymphocytes, which blend with an outer layer of granulation tissue (Fig. 6.3C). The core may be gritty because of dystrophic calcification, but the salts are deposited irregularly and incompletely. In old lesions, the capsule is thin and fibrous (Fig. 6.3D). The more proliferative nodules develop a grayish semitranslucent core of granulomatous tissue consisting of epithelioid and giant cells with an admixture of leukocytes in a fibroblastic stroma. The more diffuse lobular pneumonia has the same range of components as the nodules but extends without clear demarcations other than those provided by interlobular septa.

Lesions of glanders in the alimentary tract are rare, although they do occur in experimental infections in which large doses of the organism are given by mouth. Hematogenous metastases are common in the spleen and less common in other viscera or in locomotor organs. Metastatic lesions are similar in structure to the pulmonary nodules.

In equine "farcy," the cutaneous lesions of glanders, the cordlike thickening of the subcutaneous lymphatics has caused them to be referred to as "farcy pipes." Chains of nodules ("buds") that tend to ulcerate are distributed along the corded lymphatics (Fig. 6.3A,B), and the regional nodes are enlarged. The lymphangitis is purulent and remarkable only for the unusual degree of leukocyte necrosis.

Melioidosis

Melioidosis is occasionally known as "pseudoglanders." The causative organism is *Pseudomonas (Malleomyces) pseudomallei,* which is closely related to *P. mallei.* Melioidosis is

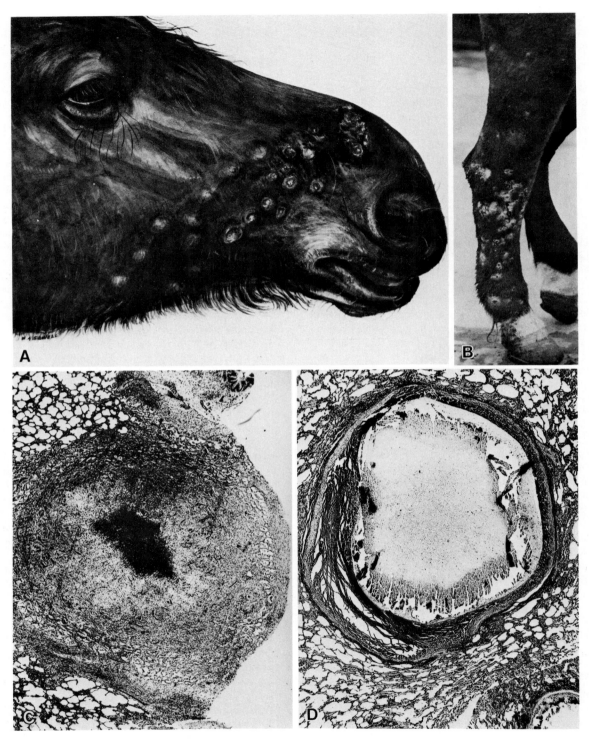

Fig. 6.3. Glanders. Horse.   (**A**) Ulcers and farcy buds along facial lymphatics.   (**B**) Cutaneous glanders with nonulcerated buds. (**A** and **B** from W. Hunting, *Glanders,* H. and W. Brown and Co., London, 1908.)   (**C**) Pyogranulomatous pulmonary nodule with central necrosis.   (**D**) Chronic pulmonary nodules with irregular calcification and thin fibrous capsules.

primarily a disease of rodents, but is occasionally a highly fatal disease of humans. All domestic species have been reported as occasionally infected, sometimes in small outbreaks in regions where the infection is endemic. The principal occurrence has been in Southeast Asia, but it is also present in parts of western Europe, the Caribbean, and Australia. Rats have been regarded as the usual source of infection, but since the organism can be found in soil and water of endemic areas, it is probably an accidental pathogen. Infection can occur through cutaneous wounds, and it can be transmitted by insects. Ingestion is probably the most important natural route of infection.

The usual course following clinical infection is pyemia followed by localization of the organism and abscessation in a wide variety of tissues, particularly lymph nodes, spleen, lung, liver, joints, and central nervous system. Depending on the severity of the process, there might be an acute disease associated with fulminating suppuration, or a more indolent one associated with chronic abscessation. Melioidosis in dogs can also cause dermal abscesses and epididymitis. In cattle, acute fatal infection, pneumonia, placentitis, and endometritis are important lesions.

Outbreaks of melioidosis, as well as isolated cases, occur in sheep, goats, and pigs, and the infection can be transmitted to these species more regularly than to other domestic animals. Pneumonia and arthritis are common in the clinical course of the disease, which otherwise is nonspecific. Goats may develop a chronic infection or recover. The lesions are those of a pyemia with multiple abscesses in the lungs, regional lymph nodes, spleen, and less often in other viscera and joints. The splenic abscesses are less than a centimeter in diameter, and they project from the surface of the organ (Fig. 6.1C). Larger purulent cavities, as well as multiple small abscesses, occur in the lungs and are associated with focal adhesive pleuritis (Fig. 6.1D). The abscesses are encapsulated and contain a creamy or caseous, yellow-green pus. In some cases, there is a purulent exudation in the bronchi. Except for the lamination that occurs in old lesions of caseous lymphadenitis caused by *Corynebacterium pseudotuberculosis*, there is nothing in the morphology of the lesions to distinguish the two diseases in sheep and goats. Experimental infections in sheep can produce, in addition to the lesions of the natural disease, microabscesses in the brain and lesions in the nasal mucosa similar to those of glanders.

INFECTIOUS BOVINE RHINOTRACHEITIS.   This is an acute contagious disease of cattle caused by bovine herpesvirus-1 characterized by inflammatory lesions in the upper respiratory tract and trachea. The virus also can cause a wide variety of other syndromes, notably conjunctivitis, infectious pustular vulvovaginitis or balanoposthitis, abortion, and meningoencephalitis, enteritis, or more generalized infection in young calves. Although other members of the herpesvirus family collectively share similar tissue tropisms, bovine herpesvirus-1 is unusual in the wide variety of the disease syndromes it can cause. It is not certain to what extent different manifestations of disease are due to differences in strains of the virus or to epidemiologic factors such as density of susceptible populations, route of transmission, and management practices.

On clinical and virologic evidence the disease is widely distributed in the world, and on serologic evidence the infection is more widespread than is any clinical evidence of it. As rhinotracheitis, the disease occurs chiefly where cattle are crowded, and most outbreaks occur among animals kept in feedlots or indoor fattening pens. The disease in dairy cattle is usually milder. The onset in feed lots is usually preceded by introduction of animals from an outside source, and from there on, the pattern is typically that of an epidemic maintained by the continual movement of cattle into and out of the feedlots. The morbidity is high, and many cases are mild and unrecognized. The fatality rate is usually low, but it can be more than 30% in exceptional outbreaks.

The clinical course is characterized by fever, increased respiratory rate, coughing, and serous nasal discharge. Lacrimation sometimes occurs. If the course is prolonged, the nasal discharge becomes mucopurulent and inspiratory dyspnea develops. The lesions in typical and uncomplicated cases are those of seromucinous rhinotracheitis and possibly conjunctivitis. In cases of greater severity, and those with bacterial complications, there is a glairy or mucopurulent exudate with acute diffuse inflammation and focal hemorrhages, erosions, and ulcerations. In the most severe cases, and especially in fatal ones, there are widespread fibrinopurulent or fibrinonecrotic membranes on nasopharyngeal, laryngeal, and tracheal surfaces (Fig. 6.4A). The region of most severe damage varies, but in field outbreaks the necrotizing and diphtheritic inflammation is often most dramatic in the larynx and adjacent pharynx and trachea (Fig. 6.4C). Bacteria contribute to the severity of these lesions, particularly *Pasteurella* spp., *Mycoplasma* spp., and *Fusobacterium necrophorum*.

The histologic changes can be anticipated from the gross appearance of the lesions. In mild cases, there are the expected features of serous to mucopurulent inflammation with minor amounts of epithelial necrosis. In fatal cases, the emphasis is on extensive epithelial necrosis and formation of a surface layer of admixed fibrin and necrotic debris (Fig. 6.4B). There is an intense vascular, neutrophilic, and mononuclear response in the underlying viable tissue. Acidophilic intranuclear viral inclusion bodies, best demonstrated after use of acid fixatives, can sometimes be found in infected cells. Because they usually appear for a transient period around 2 or 3 days after infection, they are mostly seen in experimental situations. They can rarely be detected in autopsy samples from field cases, although they occasionally persist long enough to be found in bronchial or alveolar epithelium. They are of little practical diagnostic value.

Assessment of the role of bovine herpesvirus-1 in causing pneumonia is complicated because in most descriptions of both the experimental and naturally occurring respiratory form of the disease it is impossible to distinguish between the effect of the virus itself, its role in predisposing to severe secondary bacterial pneumonia, or even the confounding effect of preexisting pneumonic lesions, which are common in calves or feedlot animals. Currently, it seems fairly safe to conclude that the lung is not significantly affected in the mild viral disease. At the other end of the disease spectrum, severe viral infection seriously impairs pulmonary defenses and leads to the extensive secondary bacterial pneumonia usually present in fatal cases. *Pasteurella* species are usually involved in such instances. The appearance of lungs is commonly that of severe fibrinous pneumonia with or

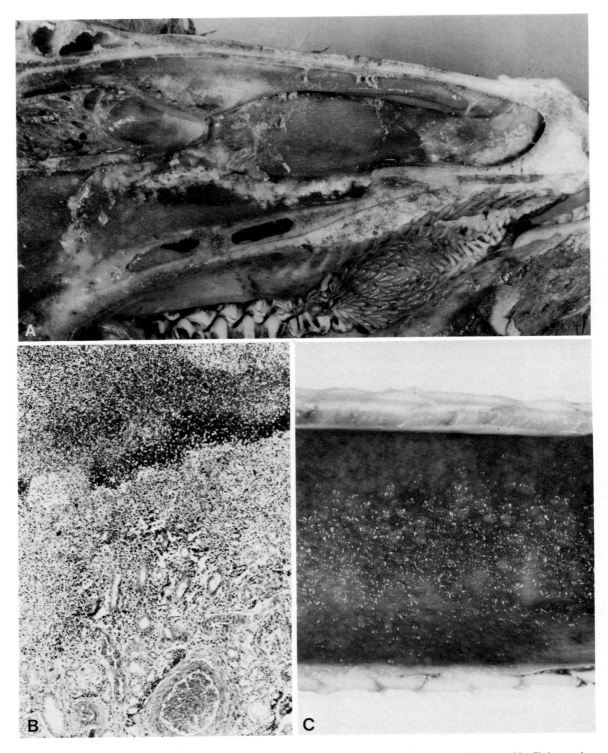

Fig. 6.4. Infectious bovine rhinotracheitis. (A) Inflamed mucous membranes of nasal cavity partially covered by fibrinopurulent exudate. (B) Acute rhinitis with ulceration and fibrinonecrotic covering. (C) Granular surface of ulcerated tracheal mucosa.

without pleuritis, as described under Pasteurellosis. An additional feature is interstitial emphysema, which frequently follows the labored respiration caused by upper and lower airway obstruction. The most severe viral lesion, in which secondary organisms might not play a significant role, is in fulminating infections. In these instances there is a severe necrotizing bronchitis and bronchiolitis, and there is extensive serofibrinous flooding of alveoli.

The pattern of generalized disease in newborn calves is rare but spectacular. Affected calves are young, less than ~1 month of age, and part of a herd in which infectious bovine rhinotracheitis affects all age groups. They are febrile and have serous ocular and nasal discharge, inspiratory difficulty, anorexia, and depression, and sometimes a laryngeal stertor suggesting laryngeal necrobacillosis. There is acute rhinitis and erosive pharyngitis, with intense hyperemia under the eroded areas and yellowish pellicles of epithelium at the margin. The epiglottis might be similarly involved, but the more distal parts of the respiratory tract remain unaffected. The most prominent changes are in the epithelium of the esophagus and forestomachs, which appear as if plastered with clumps of curdled milk. This caseous material is adherent epithelial debris. The necrosis involves the epithelium to its full depth, with intense neutrophil infiltration. Surviving epithelial cells and those at the margins of the lesions contain inclusion bodies in their vesicular nuclei. Additional lesions of systemic viral action include acute lymphadenitis with focal cortical necrosis, especially in nodes draining the upper respiratory tract. Necrotic foci can also be seen in the kidney, spleen, and liver. Miliary white necrotic foci 1–2 mm in diameter are particularly prominent in the liver. They are either uniformly distributed or concentrated in the right lobe.

The pathogenesis of meningoencephalitis, which mostly occurs in calves, is not fully understood. The virus apparently can travel to the brain from the mouth and nasopharynx by way of cranial nerves, and it can persist for long periods in the trigeminal ganglion. On the other hand, calves are also susceptible to viremic infection, so this is a possible alternative route. The lesions are those of a nonsuppurative meningoencephalitis in which granular acidophilic intranuclear inclusions are present in astrocytes and degenerating neurons.

When abortion is caused by the virus, the fetuses are edematous, and advanced autolysis indicates death of the fetus perhaps 2 days before abortion. There are no characteristic gross lesions, but microscopic lesions occur in many parenchymatous organs and lymph nodes as well as in the placenta. These lesions take the form of foci of intense necrosis and leukocytic infiltration. They are most prominent and consistent in the liver and could be confused with listeriosis. Specific inclusion bodies might not be found in autolyzed fetuses. Vaccinal strains of virus, prepared for this purpose in tissue culture, are as effective as field virus in causing abortion, and the natural infections may not be preceded or accompanied by signs of rhinitis or other illness. Thus far, it appears that cows pregnant less than ~5 months are less likely to abort following exposure to bovine herpesvirus-1.

FELINE VIRAL RHINOTRACHEITIS. Feline viral rhinotracheitis is principally an upper respiratory disease caused by feline her-

pesvirus-1 and is one of the major components of the feline respiratory disease complex. The other major component is feline calicivirus infection. Feline reovirus and the feline-adapted strain of *Chlamydia psittaci* (feline pneumonitis agent) are minor causes. *Mycoplasma felis* is probably relegated to the role of an opportunist capable of causing mucopurulent conjunctivitis, usually in association with viral or chlamydial infection.

Feline viral rhinotracheitis is characterized by fever, sneezing, salivation, oral respiration, coughing, and serous to mucopurulent nasal and conjunctival discharges. Most cats recover in 7 to 14 days, but mortality can be high in young kittens or debilitated animals, including those whose immune system is depressed by feline leukemia virus infection.

The distribution of gross lesions corresponds to the predilection sites for viral replication, namely, the epithelium of nasal passages, pharynx, soft palate, conjunctivae, tonsils, and to a lesser extent, trachea. The initial serous inflammation becomes mucopurulent or fibrinous within a few days. Lethal cases usually have the more extensive fibrinous rhinotracheitis, possibly with extension to an acute viral or secondary bacterial pneumonia. Tonsils are enlarged and often petechiated. The regional lymph nodes are also usually enlarged, reddened, and edematous. Ulcerations of the tongue are only rarely seen, and then only in severely affected cats. This contrasts with the frequent finding of vesicular to ulcerative lesions on tongue, hard palate, or nostrils of cats with calicivirus infection. The ocular involvement is usually limited to purulent conjunctivitis, but it can progress to an ulcerative keratitis.

Microscopically, the respiratory and conjunctival lesions are associated with intranuclear viral replication causing epithelial cell death and the multifocal necrosis characteristic of active herpesvirus infection. The virus is pathogenic enough in its own right to cause extensive lesions, but mixed secondary bacterial infection by organisms such as *Pasteurella multocida, Bordetella bronchiseptica, Streptococcus* spp., and *Mycoplasma felis* enhance the suppurative response. Most active viral replication and cell necrosis occur from 2 to 7 days after infection, and during this period herpesvirus inclusions are present in the nuclei of affected cells. They are typically large, acidophilic, and surrounded by a clear halo (Cowdry type A). Fixation in acid fixative such as Bouin's solution is best for their demonstration. They might be found in lesions from cats dying of the disease, but they are rarely detected beyond 7 days after infection and cannot be relied upon for diagnosis. Cells bearing inclusion bodies become large and pale, with a perinuclear clear zone, or ballooned and granular, with loss of epithelial organization. The disrupted epithelium is soon eroded or ulcerated, and there is an acute inflammatory reaction with exudation of fibrin and many neutrophils. Focal necrosis accompanied by acute inflammation might be found in tonsils and local lymph nodes. Necrosis and resorption of turbinates have also been described.

Pulmonary involvement is uncommon except in fatal cases. In fulminating cases of viral infection, there is widespread multifocal necrotizing bronchitis, bronchiolitis, and interstitial pneumonia, with extensive serofibrinous flooding of airspaces. In other instances, there is a secondary bacterial bronchopneumonia.

Naturally occurring infection by feline herpesvirus-1 rarely causes manifestation of the wider tissue tropisms seen with other members of the family, such as bovine herpesvirus, but they occur occasionally. The virus is suspected of being a cause of abortion, but this has been difficult to prove in natural outbreaks. Experimentally, it has been possible to produce abortion and generalized neonatal infection by intravenous or intravaginal inoculation of the virus into pregnant cats. Necrosis accompanied by inclusion bodies has also been found in sites of osteogenesis in a wide variety of bones of kittens after intravenous inoculation. Degeneration of olfactory nerve fibers and focal lymphocytic infiltration of the olfactory bulbs has occurred in experimentally infected, germ-free cats, but the extent of lesions in the brain has not been properly documented.

Feline **calicivirus** infection is the other main component of the feline respiratory disease complex. Although clinical signs overlap with those of feline herpesvirus infection, and occasionally both viruses occur together, the caliciviruses have more affinity for epithelium of the mouth and lung than for that of the upper respiratory tract and conjunctiva. The tendency of virulent strains of calicivirus to affect lungs is discussed under Calicivirus Infections.

The cat-adapted strain of *Chlamydia psittaci* (*C. felis*) is mostly a cause of persistent conjunctivitis more analogous to trachoma in humans. The disease is misleadingly called feline pneumonitis, although there might be a mild or inapparent bronchointerstitial pneumonia.

Allergic Rhinitis

Sporadic instances of what probably is an allergic rhinitis are observed occasionally in dogs and less commonly in cats. The disease, clinically and in response to treatment, resembles hay fever in humans, but the immunologic basis has not been adequately established. Frequently in cattle, and occasionally in sheep, there is a rhinitis that in its clinicopathologic features is consistent with an allergic pathogenesis, but here also rigorous proof is lacking. The disease has been mainly reported from Australia, but it does occur elsewhere. It is more common in Channel Island breeds. It occurs chiefly in the summertime, when the pastures are in bloom, and affects individuals or most of a herd or flock. The nasal mucosa is pale and thick from edema fluid, and mucosal erosions might be visible in the anterior nares. The exudate is at first serous but later becomes mucopurulent or contains floccules of detritus and mucus. Eosinophils are a prominent component of the exudate.

Histologically, the surviving nasal epithelium is hyperplastic or eroded and is infiltrated by eosinophils. The glandular epithelium can be hypertrophied, and mucus is produced in excess; if the orifices of excretory ducts are occluded by the superficial reaction, the mucus accumulates in the ducts and eventually lifts off the debris on the surface. In more severe cases, in which there is extensive superficial diphtheresis, many of the small mucosal vessels show fibrinoid necrosis.

Nasal "granuloma" is considered to be generally a more chronic form of allergic rhinitis. The affected mucosa is mainly in the posterior portion of the nasal vestibule and the anterior region of the nasal septum and ventral meatus. The hyperplastic epithelium is granular or has multiple nodular projections covered by intact epithelium (Fig. 6.5A). Histologically, the nod-

ules typically consist of hyperplastic and metaplastic epithelium covering a superficial edematous lamina propria with a central core of inflammatory granulation tissue (Fig. 6.5B). Nonkeratinizing squamous epithelium usually covers the surface of the nodules, and goblet-cell hyperplasia is more pronounced in the terminal portions of nasal gland ducts, which often form the lateral boundaries of the nodules. Active lesions have prominent eosinophil infiltration of the superficial lamina propria and epithelium. They are associated with increased numbers of submucosal mast cells. Vascular proliferation, fibroplasia, and accumulation of mostly lymphocytes and plasma cells in the cores of nodules are features of chronicity. Correlation of acute inflammatory events with degranulation of mast cells and accumulation of eosinophils is strong evidence that an immediate (type I) hypersensitivity is involved. Further support for this hypothesis has been provided by experimental production of closely similar lesions by repeated intranasal exposure of cattle to powdered ovalbumin. In view of the varied components of chronic lesions, however, it is probable that other classes of hypersensitivity (types III and IV) also play some role. It is believed that the condition is due to hypersensitivity to a variety of plant pollen grains or fungal spores. Because there appears to be a familial predisposition in Jersey cattle, the existence of susceptible "atopic" animals has been proposed. The condition is therefore sometimes referred to as atopic rhinitis.

Less commonly, nasal granulomas in cattle are attributable to fungal infection. They also occur mostly in the anterior portion of the nasal cavity but tend to be larger polypoid masses. They frequently have yellow-green cores associated with massive eosinophil accumulation. Histologically, components of the lesions are similar to those described for the chronic allergic "granulomas," but hyphae and chlamydospores of fungi surrounded by macrophages, giant cells, and eosinophils are present. Various fungi normally saprophytic on plants have been isolated. It is tempting to speculate that the mycotic granulomas represent the small proportion of the more nonspecific allergic granulomas in which the causative allergen is able to vegetate.

Granulomatous Rhinitis

Local damage to nasal mucosa or reduced defenses because of depressed immune response or other systemic influence make the nasal cavity prey to occasional opportunistic fungal or yeast infections. The range of fungi varies with species of animal affected.

Aspergillus fumigatus is the commonest cause in the dog, but it is rare in other species. The usual lesion is a chronic necrotizing to granulomatous lesion causing large amounts of friable exudate that often consists mainly of necrotic fungal hyphae. Viable surface hyphae can sometimes be seen grossly as a blue-green mat. The lesion is slowly aggressive and causes destruction of turbinates and sometimes the nasal septum, but it rarely erodes through the nasal, maxillary, or palatine bones. Similar lesions can be caused by *Penicillium* spp.

Cryptococcus neoformans is the most frequent cause of granulomatous rhinitis in cats and also occurs in horses and dogs (in descending order of frequency). The lesion in cats is more gelatinous than granulomatous, since it consists mainly of massed organisms with their abundant mucopolysaccharide capsular

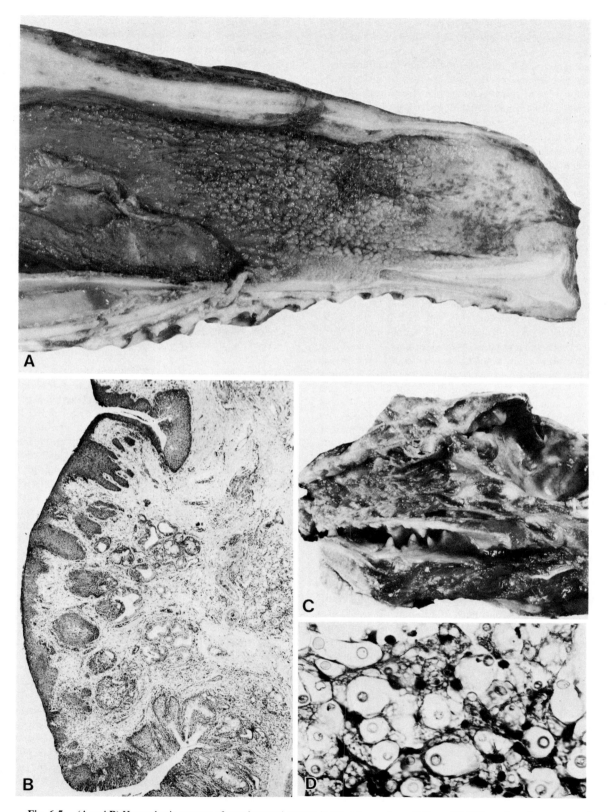

Fig. 6.5. (**A** and **B**) Hyperplastic mucosa of anterior nasal septum in ''nasal granuloma.'' Ox.   (**C**) Filling of nasal passages and obliteration of turbinates in nasal cryptococcosis. Cat.   (**D**) *Cryptococcus neoformans* surrounded by clear zones of unstained capsular material.

material (Fig. 6.5C,D). Reaction by macrophages, epithelioid cells, and lymphocytes is usually minor. Impaired immune responsiveness and weak antigenicity of the capsular mucopolysaccharide are possible reasons for the lack of inflammatory response. The lesions are polypoid nodules or more widely space-occupying and slowly destructive masses. In cats, there is often facial swelling. Extension through the bony boundaries of the nasal cavity can involve skin and, possibly, oral mucosa. Local extension occurs to eyes or brain, and occasionally there is wider dissemination to local lymph nodes and lung or a variety of visceral organs (see Pulmonary Mycoses).

Actinomycosis and actinobacillosis, the latter in sheep especially, sometimes involve or are limited to the nasal cavities.

Rhinosporidiosis

Rhinosporidiosis in animals is a chronic polypous rhinitis caused by *Rhinosporidium seeberi*. The disease occurs in horses, cattle, and to a lesser extent, dogs, goats, and waterfowl. It also occurs in humans, sometimes in a more generalized form. The disease is endemic in India and Sri Lanka, and it is sporadic in some other tropical and subtropical countries.

Rhinosporidium seeberi has resisted cultivation *in vitro*. Its mode of transmission is unknown, and the sketchy knowledge of its life cycle is based on studies of tissue sections. The definitive stage is the sporangium, which has a diameter of 100 to 300 μm and is visible to the naked eye as a white spot in the lesions or squash preparations. The sporangia have thick, double-contoured, chitinous walls and contain numerous spherical endospores ~2 μm in diameter. The mature sporangium releases the endospores into tissue or into the nasal discharge, and these in turn form new sporangia to complete the cycle.

The source of the organism is unknown; the only recognized association is with proximity to water. Initiation of the disease is thought to be influenced by local trauma to the nasal mucosa; an association has been observed between rhinosporidiosis and the nasal lesions produced by *Schistosoma nasalis,* as well as with punctures of the nasal septum for nose leads in draft oxen.

The lesion is a polyp, usually single and unilateral. The polyps range from sessile to pedunculated and cauliflower-like. They vary in size up to a diameter of 2 to 3 cm. They are soft, pink, and bleed easily because of their insubstantial myxomatous nature. On section, the sporangia may be visible grossly. Histologically, the bulk of the polyp consists of a stroma of fibrous or fibromyxoid tissue covered by usually intact epithelium. The organisms are present in the stromal tissues as spherical bodies of various sizes. There is scant reaction to them except when sporangia rupture. Then there is a granulomatous and occasionally a neutrophilic response.

Parasitic Diseases of the Nasal Cavity and Sinuses

Myiasis

The larvae of a number of flies of the family Oestridae are parasites of nasal cavities of domestic animals. *Cephalopina titillator* deposits its larvae in the nasal passages of camels. Species of the genus *Cephenomyia* are the "head bots" of deer. *Rhinoestrus purpureus*, the Russian gadfly, is parasitic in

horses; its larvae can also be found in the conjunctival sac. The life cycles and effects of each of these parasites are similar to those of their most ubiquitous relative, the nasal bot of sheep, *Oestrus ovis*.

The first-stage larvae of *Oestrus ovis* are deposited by the flies on the nares and molt twice as they migrate through the nasal passages. Larvae that find their way through small openings into sinuses or recesses of turbinates are unable to leave after they have grown, so they remain and eventually die there. Development in the nasal passages can take up to 10 months, although larvae deposited early in summer are able to mature in that season. Pupation occurs on the ground.

The larvae attach themselves to the mucous membrane by their mouthparts. They produce mucosal defects at the points of attachment and, since the cuticle is spinous, a more general irritation as they move about. Affected sheep develop a catarrhal rhinitis, with a discharge that may be copious. Irritation of the mucosa of the sinuses, especially the frontal, can cause a gelatinous hypertrophy of the mucous membrane that may almost obliterate the sinus. Apart from persistent annoyance, and the debility that this may cause, there are seldom untoward effects of the parasitism. Sometimes larvae penetrate the cranial cavity, and secondary bacterial infections spread from the olfactory mucosa to the meninges; such complications are rare.

Linguatulosis

The cause of linguatulosis is *Linguatula serrata*, a tongue-shaped, degenerate arthropod 1–2 cm in length and of cosmopolitan distribution. The definitive hosts are carnivorous animals, but in aberrant parasitisms, herbivores and humans might be host to the final stage. Herbivorous animals are the intermediate hosts, and the nymphs can be detected in their mesenteric lymph nodes. Carnivores are infected by eating the infected viscera of herbivores, and the nymphs migrate to the nasal passages and mature. The parasites may be found anywhere in the nasal cavity, and occasionally they find their way into the paranasal sinuses or pass via the Eustachian tube to the inner ear. They lie on the surface of the nasal mucosa and produce, at most, a mild catarrh.

The gravid females discharge a large number of eggs, which are removed by sneezing. The larvae develop in the alimentary tract of the intermediate host and migrate to the mesenteric nodes and other organs, where they encyst and develop into the infective nymphs. The cysts are common in mesenteric nodes of cattle and sheep in some countries. They appear as brownish, fluid-containing foci 2–3 mm in diameter; older lesions may calcify and resemble tubercles.

Miscellaneous Parasitisms

Schistosoma nasalis, which is a cause of granulomatous rhinitis in cattle, goats, and horses in India, is described with other species of the genus under the Cardiovascular System (Volume 3). The only other trematode parasitic in the upper respiratory tract of animals is *Troglotrema acutum*, a European parasite of mink, skunks, and foxes. The first and second intermediate hosts are snails and frogs, respectively. The adult parasites occur in the paranasal sinuses. In foxes, they are attached to the mucous membrane. In mink and skunks, however, they lie in cysts beneath the mucosa. The cysts, which also contain the eggs, are formed by suppurative granulation tissue. The reaction extends to cause a local rarefying osteomyelitis, which might eventually perforate and release purulent discharge into the cranial cavity, nasal cavity, or to the exterior.

The larvae of the genus *Habronema* may be deposited by flies in the anterior nares to burrow through the skin and produce granulomas similar to those of cutaneous habronemiasis. *Capillaria aerophila*, whose final habitat is the tracheobronchial system of carnivores, is found occasionally in the nasal passages and frontal sinuses. The leeches *Limnatis nilotica* and *L. africana* are taken in while drinking and attach to the mucosa of the pharynx and nasopharynx. They suck large quantities of blood, but the emergency caused by their presence depends on the development of large, edematous swellings in the affected areas, leading to dyspnea and, in severe cases, asphyxiation. The nematode *Syngamus nasicola* is found in the nasal passages of ruminants in tropical countries.

The mite *Pneumonyssoides* (*Pneumonyssus*) *caninum* is occasionally found in the nasal passages and sinuses of dogs. It is usually an incidental finding not associated with clinical signs or the development of lesions, but there are occasional reports of the mites causing mild rhinitis and sinusitis, and one in which they were associated with bronchitis.

Nasal Polyps

Polyps tend to be a sequel to focal chronic inflammation in the nasal mucosa. The ease with which the nasal lamina propria becomes engorged and edematous, plus the tendency of protruberances into the nasal meatus to compromise venous and lymphatic drainage because of constriction in their basal regions, are probable factors in the persistence or progression of inflammatory polyps. They occur occasionally in horses, less commonly in other species. Polyps are soft, pink-gray, irregularly nodular, pedunculated, or sessile masses. They have a chronically inflamed edematous core covered by variously hyperplastic, metaplastic, or ulcerated epithelium. Old polyps can become more fibrous.

Two special types of polyp deserve mention. One is the **hemorrhagic nasal polyp** (progressive hematoma) arising from the ethmoid region of the horse. This is a unilateral hemorrhagic mass, which can extend to the nostril or choanae. It tends to enlarge progressively and might recur after surgical excision. Histologically, it consists mostly of organizing hemorrhages of various ages, with extensive siderosis and calcification of connective tissue fibers. The extent to which capillary angiomatous changes are the forerunner of hemorrhage and hematoma formation is uncertain. The other special form of polyp affecting the region is the **nasopharyngeal polyp** of **cats**, which arises in the middle ear or Eustachian tube.

Neoplastic Diseases of the Nasal Cavity

With the exception of endemic ethmoidal tumors to be described subsequently, primary nasal and paranasal tumors are uncommon. They occur frequently enough, however, to be an important entity in dogs and, to a lesser extent, cats and horses. There is no clear relationship between frequency of nasal tumors

in various breeds of dogs and length of their noses. The breeds with significantly increased risk, such as collie and German shepherd, do have long noses, however, and this has led to the mistaken generalization that dolichocephalic breeds as a whole are at greater risk. Origin from the nasal cavity is usual in dogs and cats, but in horses, tumors of the paranasal sinuses arise almost as frequently as those from the nasal cavity. Any of the tissues forming the lining or present in the boundaries of the nasal cavity and sinuses can give rise to either benign or malignant tumors. In general, most are carcinomas (Fig. 6.6A,B,D), followed in decreasing frequency by sarcomas of cartilage (Fig. 6.6C), fibrous tissue, and bone. The precise mix of types varies according to species.

Epithelial tumors of the nasal cavity and sinuses are classified as follows:

> Papilloma
> Adenoma
> Squamous-cell (epidermoid) carcinoma
>   Spindle-cell variant
> Transitional carcinoma
> Adenocarcinoma
> Undifferentiated (anaplastic) carcinoma

Squamous-cell carcinomas predominate in the cat and horse. In the cat, a large proportion originates from the nasal vestibule, whereas in the horse, the maxillary sinus is a common site (Fig. 6.6A). It is speculated that the latter might arise from the epithelium of dental alveoli. Transitional carcinomas and adenocarcinomas are the most common in dogs. Transitional carcinomas are so called because they assume the characteristics of transitional epithelium. They typically consist of thick, stratified layers of dysplastic surface epithelial cells with a distinct basement membrane (Fig. 6.6D). Large transitional carcinomas have complex infolding or pleating of the thick epithelial sheets, with the basement membranes usually separated by inconspicuous stroma. Small, acinar-like spaces often appear within the epithelial sheets, frequently by swelling and necrosis of cells, and can cause difficulty in separation between transitional carcinomas and adenocarcinomas. Adenocarcinomas have a more obvious glandular pattern, however, with numerous acini lined by cells usually only one or two layers deep.

The tendency of the stroma of large, more rapidly growing tumors to become edematous can result in difficulty in distinguishing between the more undifferentiated carcinomas and sarcomas. Regardless of histogenic type, malignant nasal tumors tend to be soft, pale and fleshy to friable masses that slowly invade and destroy adjacent structures but rarely metastasize.

Tumors arising from the ethmoturbinate region have been reported to be endemic in a variety of species. They have the most widespread geographic distribution in sheep; cattle are affected less often. Whether endemic tumors occur at present in horses or pigs is uncertain. The tumors in sheep are adenopapillomas or locally invasive adenocarcinomas that arise from olfactory mucosa of the ethmoid region. Ultrastructural evidence indicates their origin from sustentacular cells of olfactory mucosa or the dark cells of Bowman's glands. Epidemiologic evidence does not differentiate between genetic, environmental, or infectious influences in causing the clusters of

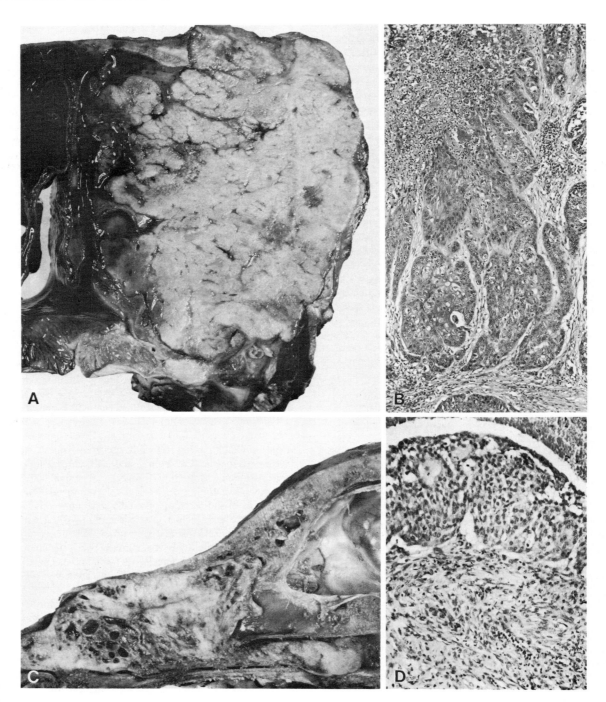

Fig. 6.6. (**A**) Squamous-cell carcinoma of maxillary sinus. Horse.   (**B**) Squamous-cell carcinoma of nasal cavity. Dog. (**C**) Chondrosarcoma filling nasal cavity and extending into caudal nares. Dog.   (**D**) Transitional carcinoma of nasal cavity with chronic inflammation and fibroplasia of lamina propria. Dog.

affected animals. Transmission experiments have had inconsistent results. The occasional ultrastructural finding of viral particles structurally resembling retroviruses (type C particles) led to the suggestion that a slow virus of the maedi–visna type might be responsible. In view of the fact that *jaagsiekte* (pulmonary adenomatosis) in sheep is now known to be caused by a retrovirus, this too becomes a candidate. Both carcinomatous and sarcomatous ethmoidal tumors have been found in cattle. There is one report of viral particles being detected ultrastructurally, but it has also been suggested that carcinogenic mycotoxins such as aflatoxin might play a causative role.

Pharynx and Guttural Pouches

The pharynx, being common to upper respiratory and alimentary systems, shares the misfortunes of both. Because of the complicated organogenesis of the region, various congenital malformations are occasionally encountered. Most attention is drawn to defects in the dog and horse. In the dog, the excess of soft tissue over skeletal framework that occurs in brachycephalic breeds leads to a variety of conditions of which excessive length of the soft palate, eversion of laryngeal saccules, and laryngeal collapse are most common. In the horse, complications are signaled by exercise intolerance and associated noisy respiration. Subepiglottic cysts believed to arise from thyroglossal duct remnants and entrapment of the epiglottis appear to be most frequent. Entrapment of the epiglottis below the aryepiglottic fold in horses is usually associated with congenital hypoplasia of the epiglottis or acquired shortening or distortion of the structure. A short epiglottis also predisposes to dorsal displacement of the soft palate, and sometimes epiglottal entrapment and dorsal displacement of the palate occur together.

A posterior diverticulum of the pharynx lies immediately dorsal to the esophagus in pigs. In young pigs, awns of barley and similar foreign materials occasionally lodge in the diverticulum and cause inflammation. The local reaction may cause dysphagia and death from starvation. In some cases, the pharyngeal wall is perforated and an ultimately fatal cellulitis spreads down the fascial planes of the neck. Perforation of the posterior–dorsal wall of the pharynx by drenching guns also occurs in sheep and is usually fatal.

Pharyngeal inflammation is a part of inflammatory diseases affecting the upper respiratory system, upper alimentary system, or both. These have been covered elsewhere. An entity deserving of brief mention here is **equine chronic pharyngitis** with **lymphoid hyperplasia**. It is detected mostly by endoscopy in thoroughbred racehorses less than 5 years of age. In its most severe manifestation, there are polypoid projections in the dorsolateral boundaries of the pharynx, with prominent white plaques or nodules representing lymphoid aggregates. The extent of lymphoid hyperplasia found in biopsies sometimes raises the suspicion of neoplastic proliferation, except for the follicular structure and predominance of mature lymphocytes. Although presumed due to persistent lymphoproliferative stimulus by an infective agent or combination of agents, possibly aided by excessive drying or other factors leading to reduced local defenses, nothing definite is known about the cause and pathogenesis. It is the equine analog of adenoids in children.

The guttural pouches of Equidae are ventral diverticula of the Eustachian tubes. They tend to become involved in inflammatory processes in analogous fashion to the paranasal sinuses. Complications differ, however, because severe guttural pouch inflammation can extend to involve nearby cranial nerves (VII, IX, X, XI, XII), vessels, and the cranial sympathetic trunk or even spread to adjacent bones, middle ear, brain, or atlanto-occipital joint. Suppurative inflammation leading to empyema occurs mostly after upper respiratory infections, particularly *Streptococcus equi* or other streptococcal infection. Fibrinous or fibrinonecrotic (diphtheritic) inflammation is usually associated with fungal infection, generally *Aspergillus* spp., and hence is commonly referred to as guttural pouch mycosis. The lesion is highly suggestive of, but not pathognomonic for, fungal infection. Because the fibrinonecrotic inflammation extends deeply, and fungi when present can frequently invade vessels and other structures, complications such as rupture of the internal carotid artery with epistaxis, ischemic lesions, or osteitis are much more likely to follow than is the case from guttural pouch empyema. A less common condition is guttural pouch tympany. This is seen mostly in young animals, where the accumulation of air is presumed to be due to valvular action of the nasopharyngeal orifice of the Eustachian tube. Tumors of the guttural pouches are rare but when encountered are most likely to be squamous-cell carcinomas. Pharyngeal tumors are discussed with neoplasia of the mouth (in the Alimentary System, this volume).

Larynx and Trachea

Laryngeal Paralysis

Unilateral or bilateral paralysis of the larynx is the most common cause of abnormal respiratory noise (roaring) in horses. The condition is almost always a left-sided hemiplegia and is due to degeneration of the left recurrent laryngeal nerve. Resulting denervation atrophy affects all intrinsic laryngeal muscles supplied by this nerve, but not all are affected equally. The most obvious atrophy occurs in the cricoarytenoid muscle, which may be reduced to fascial remnants. Atrophy of the other muscles, which is less severe, is indicated by pallor and a reduction in size. The cricothyroid muscle, which is supplied by the cranial laryngeal nerve, is the only intrinsic muscle not affected. The cricoarytenoid muscle is the main abductor of the larynx. As a result of its paresis and atrophy, the left arytenoid cartilage droops into the lumen, thus interfering with airflow, particularly during the inspiration associated with severe exercise.

In cases detected clinically, microscopic examination reveals severe loss of myelinated fibers in middle and distal portions of the left recurrent laryngeal nerve. Less obvious loss occurs in subclinical cases. Ultrastructural features indicate progressive loss of fibers in the left recurrent nerve, accompanied by chronic demyelination, remyelination, and abortive regenerative attempts. Similar but milder changes can be detected electron microscopically in the distal right recurrent nerve. The reasons for the axonal disease are still disputed. The axons in the left recurrent laryngeal nerve are much longer than those in the right recurrent nerve, and this presumably makes them more susceptible to damage. The extent to which damage is caused by traumatic interruption of axoplasmic flow, neuritis by extension from guttural pouch disease, vitamin deficiency, or neurotoxins has still to be established. It is unlikely that there is a single cause, as evidenced by the circumstantial implication of delayed neurotoxicity by oral haloxon administration as a cause in Arabian foals. Another organophosphate, trichlorfon, also is linked circumstantially with an incident of left recurrent laryngeal nerve degeneration in horses.

Neurogenic atrophy of laryngeal muscles occurs occasionally in large breeds of dogs. It is usually bilateral and associated with lesions in the recurrent laryngeal nerves or, rarely, occurs as part of generalized degeneration of the nervous system. The condition appears to follow an autosomal dominant hereditary pattern in Bouviers. Laryngeal paralysis occurs rarely in the cat.

Congenital Anomalies

Congenital anomalies of the larynx are rare. Hypoplasia of the epiglottis has been observed in horses and swine. Partial or complete agenesis of the trachea is a rare finding. Tracheal hypoplasia characterized by reduction in the luminal diameter of the entire trachea, sometimes associated with bronchial hypoplasia, occurs in dogs. The higher frequency in English bulldogs indicates the possibility of an inherited basis. Malformations of the cross-sectional shape are important in the dog and to a lesser extent in the horse. The condition in dogs referred to as tracheal collapse occurs principally in miniature breeds. The trachea becomes flattened dorsoventrally. The cartilages form shallow arcs, and the dorsal tracheal membrane is widened and flaccid. The membrane is thin in uncomplicated cases but becomes thickened when there is chronic or periodic acute tracheitis. These are frequent complications of the mechanical obstruction. The nature of the basic defect is still unclear. The major feature appears to be slowly progressive loss of cartilage in tracheal rings, but the extent to which there is a congenital cartilaginous defect or how else the process might be related to miniaturization in the affected breeds is not known.

In horses, lateral compression of the trachea produces the so-called scabbard trachea. In this species also, a scroll-like curling affects the ends of the cartilages.

Acquired malformations of the trachea are caused by external pressure, in most cases from enlarged thyroid or regional lymph nodes, or inflammatory or neoplastic lesions within the wall.

Circulatory Disturbances

Active hyperemia occurs in acute inflammation, which is common. Laryngeal hemorrhages particularly affect the mucous membrane on the dorsal surface of the epiglottis and occur in many septicemic diseases. They are of some diagnostic significance in salmonellosis of swine and hog cholera. The hemorrhagic speckling of the tracheal mucosa in slaughtered cattle is produced by small extravasations in the submucosal lymphoid follicles. In cattle that die with severe dyspnea, and to a lesser extent in sheep, these follicular hemorrhages spread in a linear form. In severe cases the whole mucosa is red-black. The hemorrhages are reflected in the regional lymph nodes, which are also red-black, firm, and enlarged.

Edema of the larynx is usually inflammatory and part of acute

respiratory infections, or caused by inhalation of irritant materials or by local trauma or inflammation (Fig. 6.7A). Mild edema of the glottis is occasionally observed in edema disease of swine. Edema occurs in cattle with acute interstitial pneumonia. It is also observed in cattle as part of a rapidly developing edema of the face and throat; this latter syndrome is probably of allergic origin and responds well to antihistamines. If neglected, it leads to asphyxiation. It can also be part of the localized anaphylactic response to insect stings in most species. Edema of the fauces and larynx occurs in equine purpura hemorrhagica and in the same species as a response to the leech *Limnatis nilotica* or lead poisoning.

The amount of edema varies but in any case is most severe in the region of the epiglottis, the aryepiglottic folds, and the ventricles. Severe cases are obvious; mild cases show a soft swelling of the mucosa. The edema fluid is usually bloodstained when associated with acute inflammation, and clear or pale yellow at other times. The fluid might disappear postmortem, but wrinkling of the mucous membrane remains to indicate the prior presence of fluid.

Severe mucosal and submucosal edema of the dorsal region of the distal half of the trachea occasionally causes death by asphyxiation in feedlot cattle. The loud inspiratory noise made by severely affected cows has given rise to the clinical term "honker" syndrome. There is correlation with increased respiratory movements brought about by exercise or hot weather, usually in heavy cattle, but it is not known whether the condition is triggered by trauma, tracheal compression, inhalation of dusts, toxins in feed, or a combination of these.

Laryngitis and Tracheitis

The location of the larynx and trachea is such that frequently they become inflamed as part of inflammatory diseases of either the upper or lower parts of the respiratory tract. Their involvement in major upper respiratory tract diseases has already been covered. Tracheitis frequently accompanies bronchitis and is sometimes a minor component of pneumonias that do not arise by extension from severe upper respiratory disease. Laryngitis can, however, occur without wider involvement of the respiratory tract (Fig. 6.7B). Laryngitis can occur as a part of oral necrobacillosis (calf diphtheria) caused by *Fusobacterium necrophorum* in calves and swine, or it might occur without lesions elsewhere. Ulcers or scarred sites of previous ulceration are found in a small proportion of larynges in slaughtered feedlot cattle. They occur mainly at points of apposition of vocal processes and medial angles of arytenoid cartilages. It is speculated that mucosal damage by the repeated trauma of laryngeal closure is the main predisposing cause of ulceration. It has also been suggested that *Haemophilus somnus* infection may sometimes be a factor. Lesions of acute or chronic diphtheria (*F. necrophorum*) and papillomatosis occur occasionally at the same sites and are believed to develop secondarily to mucosal ulceration.

Small foci of mineralization, often with accompanying granulomatous inflammation, occur in the lamina propria of dorsal trachea and ventral turbinate of adult pigs, particularly males. A causal association with inhalation of dusty, mineral-containing feed has been suggested, but this is unlikely. More widespread

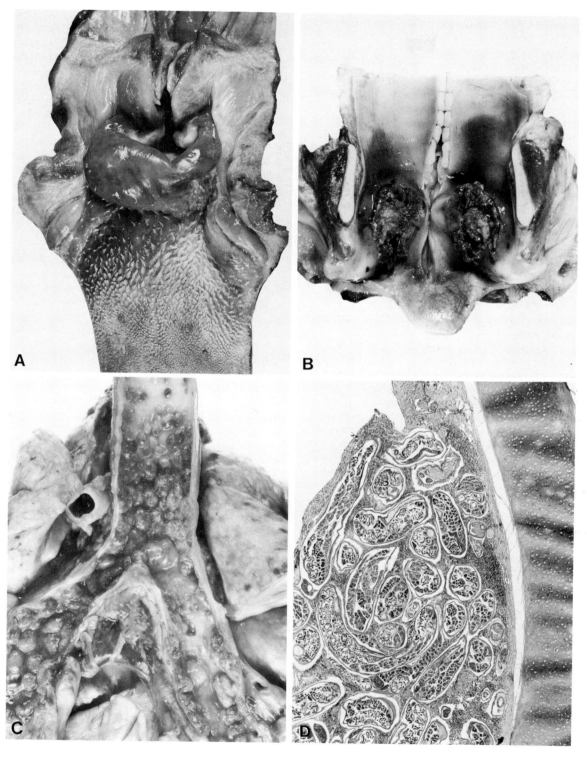

Fig. 6.7. (A) Inflammatory edema of epiglottis associated with abscess in base of tongue. Dog. (B) Necrotic laryngitis. Calf. (C) Parasitic tracheobronchitis. Nodules contain coiled *Filaroides osleri*. Dog. (D) Histologic section of nodule in (C), showing cross sections of worms and mononuclear-cell reaction.

mineralization is frequently also present in severely affected pigs.

Corynebacterium pyogenes is responsible for sporadic cases of laryngeal abscessation in calves and sheep and for local endemics in sheep grazing on mature dry grass. Recovery from the infection results in scarring and deformity; the latter is most prominent when inflammatory necrosis of the cartilage occurs. A diphtheritic laryngotracheitis caused by untyped streptococci is occasionally observed in litters of piglets.

A chronic and diffuse tracheitis can develop following tracheotomy. The reaction is most severe adjacent to the wound; the mucosa is swollen and, in the late stages, heavily scarred. Foci of chronic polypoid tracheitis are occasionally observed in dogs and cats. The thickening may be sufficient to cause significant stenosis and dyspnea. The cause is unknown, but the various pathogenetic factors involved are probably similar to those responsible for nasal polyps. Squamous metaplasia of tracheal epithelium is a feature of vitamin A deficiency and severe iodide toxicosis.

Parasitic Diseases of the Larynx and Trachea

Syngamus laryngeus occurs in the larynx of cattle in tropical Asia and South America.

Capillaria aerophila (*Eucoleus aerophilus*), a relative of *Trichuris*, parasitizes the trachea and bronchi of dogs, foxes, and occasionally, cats. They are slender worms, 4–6 cm long and of a faint greenish tinge. The eggs are operculate and not distinguishable from those of *T. vulpis* of the intestine or *C. plica* of the urinary bladder. The eggs are laid in the airways, move with mucus to the pharynx, are swallowed, and passed in the feces. The larvae develop to the infective stage within the egg and remain there until the egg is swallowed by a suitable host. Hatching occurs in the intestine. The larvae reach the lungs in ∼1 week and are mature in the trachea in ∼6 weeks.

The effects of *Capillaria aerophila* depend on the numbers present. Mild infestations are asymptomatic and provoke nothing more than a mild catarrhal inflammation. Heavy infestations cause more severe irritation as well as some obstruction to the lumen of the airways. Chronic coughing and intermittent dyspnea may then be observed, and secondary bacterial bronchopneumonia might occur.

Filaroides (*Oslerus*) *osleri* is an ovoviviparous, filiform worm 0.5–1.5 cm long, parasitizing the dog and related species. The typical lesions are protruding submucosal nodules in the region of the tracheal bifurcation (Fig. 6.7C). The parasite has a wide geographic distribution but is uncommon and seldom seen. Pups are infected by larvae in the saliva or feces of their mother. Larvae migrate from gut to lung through the blood. Efficient transmission depends on pups being licked by the dam and also on the habit of disgorgement of food by the adults to feed the young.

The lesions vary in size from nodules that are barely visible to larger nodules or plaques that project 1.0 cm or more into the lumen of the trachea (Fig. 6.7C). The larger masses are oval, with the long axis parallel to that of the trachea. The parasites do not typically incite acute bronchitis or tracheitis, although they can provoke paroxysmal coughing and dyspnea. The nodules are gray or whitish in color, and the worms are visible through the intact overlying mucosa.

The small nodules contain immature worms, and the larger ones a mass of tightly coiled adults (Fig. 6.7D). The worms lie in tissue spaces between the cartilage rings of the trachea and large bronchi, and in the adventitia and lymphatics. The live worms provoke a minimal reaction consisting of a thin capsule and an infiltration of the lamina propria by lymphocytes and plasma cells. Superficially, the nodules are covered by intact epithelium, except for small pores through which female worms protrude their tails to lay eggs. Dead worms provoke a foreign-body reaction with neutrophils and a few giant cells. Immature worms without significant tissue reaction may be found in the pulmonary lymphatics and occasionally in the alveoli. These immature worms are probably still migrating toward the trachea.

Spirocerca lupi occasionally forms nodules in the trachea or bronchi, examples of aberrant localization.

Neoplastic Diseases of the Larynx and Trachea

Neoplasms of the larynx and trachea are rare, and the information is therefore fragmentary. Any tissue in or adjacent to the wall of these structures can give rise to tumors, so a variety of epithelial and mesenchymal tumors have been found. Epithelial tumors are most likely to be papillomas or squamous-cell carcinomas. Adenocarcinomas are exceedingly rare. Leiomyomas and rhabdomyosarcomas can arise in or close to the wall. Chondromas or osteochondromas occasionally originate from the laryngeal or tracheal cartilages. The osteochondromas are usually cartilaginous nodules with central endochondral ossification. They are derived from perichondrial proliferation of developmental, inflammatory, or neoplastic basis. It is difficult or impossible to decide what the basic process is in any one tumor. Although it has been argued that the lesions should be classified as osteochondral dysplasias, the term osteochondroma is well established and can be understood to embrace the full range of pathogenetic possibilities. Chondrosarcomas and osteosarcomas are also rare findings. Mucosal involvement in lymphosarcoma or malignant mast-cell tumor is an uncommon occurrence in cats and dogs, and possible deformation or invasion by adjacent neoplasms in the thyroid or lymph nodes has already been mentioned.

Oncocytomas have been reported as rare, benign tumors arising as solitary projecting nodules in or close to the lateral ventricle of the canine larynx. They consist of lobular masses of pleomorphic cells with abundant, deeply eosinophilic, granular or foamy cytoplasm. Ultrastructurally, there is an excessive number of mitochondria and intermitochondrial glycogen granules. Oncocytes (oxyphil cells) occur in a variety of endocrine glands and epithelial tissues of humans, where they occasionally give rise to tumors. Evidence indicates that they are atypical neuroendocrine cells, hence oncocytomas are related to carcinoid tumors.

Bronchi

Major bronchi form the conducting zone between the upper and lower respiratory tract and therefore tend to be involved either as an extension of severe upper respiratory tract diseases on the one hand, or as part of pulmonary diseases on the other. Distal orders of bronchi and the bronchioles are mostly involved as part of pulmonary diseases, to be addressed later in this chapter. There are important acquired conditions, however, in which the bronchi are the principal sites of abnormality, and these will be presented here. Congenital malformations are included under Congenital Abnormalities (of the Lungs), and tumors arising in bronchi are considered under Neoplastic Diseases (of the Lungs).

Bronchitis

In postmortem situations, **acute bronchitis** is usually overshadowed by more severe upper respiratory lesions or by pneumonia. The same range of inflammation described for upper airways can be encountered. Catarrhal, mucopurulent, fibrinous, fibrinopurulent, or purulent exudates are most common. Lesions in the inflamed bronchial tree depend to some extent on the causes; for instance, eosinophils are present in immediate hypersensitivity reactions, and inclusion bodies may be found at certain stages of some viral infections, but to a large degree the lesions are not specific and reflect the severity and duration of injury more than its cause.

Catarrhal bronchitis is the simplest form of inflammation. Acute mild irritation of the bronchial mucosa causes discharge of secretion from goblet and serous cells and from such seromucinous glands as are present. Since the types, relative numbers of epithelial secretory cells, and density of the glands differ from species to species, fine details of the response vary accordingly. Hyperemia and edema of the lamina propria accompany the secretory discharge. Ciliated epithelial cells are most sensitive to injury; they lose their cilia, become necrotic, and slough. The usual traffic of leukocytes through the epithelium becomes exaggerated. If the inflammation is transient, the integrity of the epithelium is rapidly restored by proliferation of residual basal and intermediate cells. Peripheral surviving secretory cells can also proliferate to play a part in the regenerative phase if the defect is large.

The course of bronchitis after the initial catarrhal phase depends on the nature of the irritant and the duration of exposure. In common bacterial infections, **purulent bronchitis** occurs, and the exudate in the bronchi becomes characteristically yellowish and viscid. The exuded dead and dying neutrophils collect in the lumen together with mucus and sloughed epithelial cells. **Ulcerative bronchitis**, in which large areas of epithelium are destroyed and the lamina propria directly involved, is usually an extension of prolonged purulent bronchitis. **Fibrinous** or **fibrinonecrotic bronchitis** is characterized by a thick, yellow membrane firmly attached to many points. Reactions of this severity usually also involve the larynx, trachea, and cranioventral portions of the lungs. This form of bronchitis is seldom observed. Primary bacterial infections might sometimes be responsible, but the masses of organisms seen in the membrane are probably mostly superimposed on a primary viral lesion, such as in malignant catarrhal fever or infectious bovine rhinotracheitis. A necrotizing **putrid bronchitis** can occur in bronchiectasis or as a result of aspiration of foreign materials. In such lesions, the microflora is mixed, and the greenish or brown putrid debris is characteristic. Gangrene might supervene.

Inflammation of large bronchi often heals without trace, which indicates that although the surface epithelium of bronchi might be severely damaged, there is seldom significant damage to the deeper structures of the wall. Polyps of granulation tissue

are rare. Inflammation of small bronchioles, on the other hand, frequently leads to bronchopneumonia.

Bronchiolitis fibrosa obliterans or organizing bronchiolitis is a nonspecific response to a variety of severe forms of damage to bronchioles and adjacent alveoli. It can follow viral infections such as influenza, inhalation of toxic gases (including 100% oxygen), or damage by lungworms or pneumotoxins such as those associated with acute interstitial pneumonia in cattle. Prerequisites are necrosis of epithelium at the bronchiolar–alveolar junction and the presence of a fibrin-rich exudate that stimulates the infiltration and maturation of fibroblast precursors. The lesion is typically a polypoid projection of fibroblastic tissue partially or completely obliterating the bronchiolar lumen (Fig. 6.15,A,B). Different stages of fibroblastic organization of exudate composed of fibrin and necrotic cell debris can usually be seen in any one lung. In species with well-developed respiratory bronchioles, for instance, the dog, organization of exudate is often seen to be taking place from septa of alveoli situated at intervals along the length of the bronchioles. Organization of exudate into cellular granulation tissue can take place in as few as 7 to 10 days after onset of severe damage, and regeneration of epithelium over its surface can occur in the same time period.

The major causes of bronchitis, as alluded to earlier, are those already mentioned as causes of upper respiratory disease or those to be given later as causes of bronchopneumonia. Although bronchitis most commonly results from an aerogeneous portal of injury, an ascending route of involvement can be of importance. This applies to the verminous pneumonias and to several granulomatous infections. Thus metastatic tubercles frequently erode into the airways to produce tuberculous bronchitis, with subsequent spread as tuberculous bronchopneumonia, and pulmonary abscesses of caseous lymphadenitis might be evacuated into bronchi, resulting in persistent caseous bronchitis.

The consequences of inflammation limited to larger bronchi are much less serious than the consequences of inflammation of small bronchi and especially of bronchioles. The larger bronchi lie in interstitial tissue outside the pulmonary lobules. The epithelium is pseudostratified and well supplied with secretory and ciliated cells. The peribronchial connective tissue is mature and relatively abundant. The lumen is large enough to remain patent even in the presence of copious exudate, and the exudate is so placed as to be expelled by an effective cough reflex. In contrast, the small bronchi and bronchioles lie within the parenchyma. There is a paucity of peribronchial connective tissue. The epithelium is simple, and under normal circumstances the ciliated and mucus-secreting cells dwindle and disappear from the smallest branches. The walls are thin, and the small lumen is easily occluded by exudate that may be too far distal for the cough reflex to be properly effective, especially in lungs with little collateral ventilation. It follows that while inflammation of larger bronchi might not have significant consequences for the lung, inflammation of bronchioles frequently leads to parenchymal damage. Bronchopneumonia, atelectasis, or emphysema are the most important forms of damage.

From the previous discussion, it will be evident that limited bronchitis or tracheobronchitis rarely causes death and is observed mainly as a clinical problem for which detailed pathologic (necropsy) information on the naturally occurring disease is seldom available. This should change as data obtained from bronchial biopsies accumulate. A good example of this situation is the **infectious tracheobronchitis** causing "**kennel cough**" in dogs. The disease is characterized clinically by a hard, persistent, and usually nonproductive cough that can become paroxysmal. Affected dogs usually recover, although signs can persist for 3 weeks or longer. Available evidence indicates that clinical signs are accompanied either by no significant gross lesions or, with about equal frequency, by catarrhal or mucopurulent tracheobronchitis. There is sometimes extension to a cranioventral bronchopneumonia, and occasionally, serous to mucopurulent rhinitis. Palatine tonsils and tracheobronchial and retropharyngeal lymph nodes are usually enlarged and reddened. Microscopically, various degrees of tracheobronchitis and bronchiolitis are usually present. These range from a focal, superficially necrotizing tracheobronchitis and bronchiolitis to a more severe process characterized by mucopurulent inflammation. There is epithelial degeneration and necrosis, with disorganization of the normal pseudostratified pattern in the necrotizing lesions. The response in the underlying lamina propria is limited. The necrosis is associated mainly with viral infection, particularly canine parainfluenza type 2 virus. Extensive infiltration of neutrophils characteristic of mucopurulent tracheobronchitis is associated with *Bordetella bronchiseptica* infection, and the bacteria can be found by electron microscopy to be attached to cilia by fibrillar material (pili). Bacteria might be in sufficient numbers to be visible by light microscopy after staining for Gram-negative bacteria. The etiology of the disease in dogs is complex, as is that of many respiratory conditions. The most important agent appears to be *B. bronchiseptica,* often acting in concert with canine parainfluenza type 2 virus or canine adenovirus-2. All possible variations of these organisms, singly or mixed, have been recovered at one time or another, however. Mixed infection with canine distemper virus also occurs occasionally. The role of agents such as reovirus, *Mycoplasma, Pasteurella multocida,* and other Gram-negative bacteria is unclear but probably not large.

Acute bronchitis of presumed allergic cause is part of the condition referred to clinically as "asthma" or **allergic bronchitis**. Since cases are frequently episodic or chronic and what little information available on the lesions relates to the longer-standing cases, allergic manifestations are considered in more detail under the next heading.

Chronic Bronchitis

Chronic bronchitis is usually of infectious, parasitic, or presumed allergic cause. The relative importance of these causes varies according to species. Chronic catarrhal or mucopurulent bronchitis is of most importance in dogs, where bronchial irritation and hypersecretion of mucus causes a chronic intractable cough. The condition is seen mostly in small breeds, particularly in obese animals.

At postmortem examination the major finding is excess mucus or mucopus in the tracheobronchial tree. This ranges from pooling of turbid, viscous fluid at the tracheobronchial junction to large amounts of tenacious, white or green to brown exudate in all airways. Sometimes the exudate is profuse enough to cause terminal foamy filling of the airways. The bronchial mucosa is thickened, often hyperemic and edematous. Occasional polypoid projections into the lumen can be seen grossly in advanced cases, as can pale foci representing lymphoid nodules. Microscopically, the mucosal thickening and folding are caused mostly by increase in number and size of the mucosal glands and extensive infiltration of the lamina propria by lymphocytes, plasma cells, and occasional macrophages and neutrophils (Fig. 6.8C). The superficial epithelium has prominent hyperplasia of goblet cells and usually has foci of ulceration or squamous metaplasia. Histochemical techniques reveal a shift in the character of secretions from sulfomucins to more viscous sialomucins. The intraluminal mucus is commonly mixed with abundant neutrophils.

The amount of fibrosis, hyperemia, and edema in the bronchial wall depends on the age and severity of the lesion and whether there has been recent acute exacerbation. The airway involvement usually extends to involve bronchioles, and in ~25% of cases, there is extension to a usually minor degree of bronchopneumonia. Hypertrophy of the smooth muscle in the wall of medium- and small-sized pulmonary arteries accompanies severe chronic bronchitis. The resulting pulmonary hypertension causes the cor pulmonale occasionally detected clinically. Significant lesions of emphysema are not associated with chronic bronchitis in the dog, although there is often exaggeration of the marginal emphysema commonly found along the sharp ventral borders of the lungs in older dogs. A more frequent complication is alveolar atelectasis and bronchiectasis.

The pathogenesis of the disease in dogs is uncertain, as it is in humans. The multiple factors believed to be involved in the development of chronic bronchitis in humans are episodes of viral bronchitis, particularly in childhood, continued damage by cigarette smoking or, to lesser extent, air pollution, and superimposed bacterial infection. In dogs, it is likely that chronic bronchitis occurs mostly in those dogs that fail to recover from a syndrome similar to that described above as infectious tracheobronchitis (kennel cough). Whatever reasons there are for initial failure of the acute episode to resolve, eventually there occurs a vicious cycle of disruption of normal defense mechanisms and persistent interaction of bacteria and leukocytes capable of mediating continued inflammation. The most important infectious agent in dogs is *Bordetella bronchiseptica.*

Chronic suppurative bronchitis is a frequent sequel to bronchopneumonia in cattle and is usually associated with bronchiectasis. The greater frequency with which bronchopneumonia fails to resolve in cattle compared to other species is presumably due, at least in part, to the complete lobular separation in this species. A variety of bacteria can be isolated from the suppurative lesions, of which *Corynebacterium pyogenes* and *Pasteurella* spp. are the most important.

Although circumstantially there is evidence that allergens can be an important cause of bronchitis, rigorous proof is lacking in most instances. The role of allergens in causing the chronic bronchiolitis–emphysema complex in the horse and the airway lesions associated with hypersensitivity pneumonitis are dealt with later. There remains a broad clinical syndrome, mostly in cats and dogs, commonly referred to as **asthma, allergic bronchitis**, or **allergic pneumonia**. Diagnosis is usually made on the

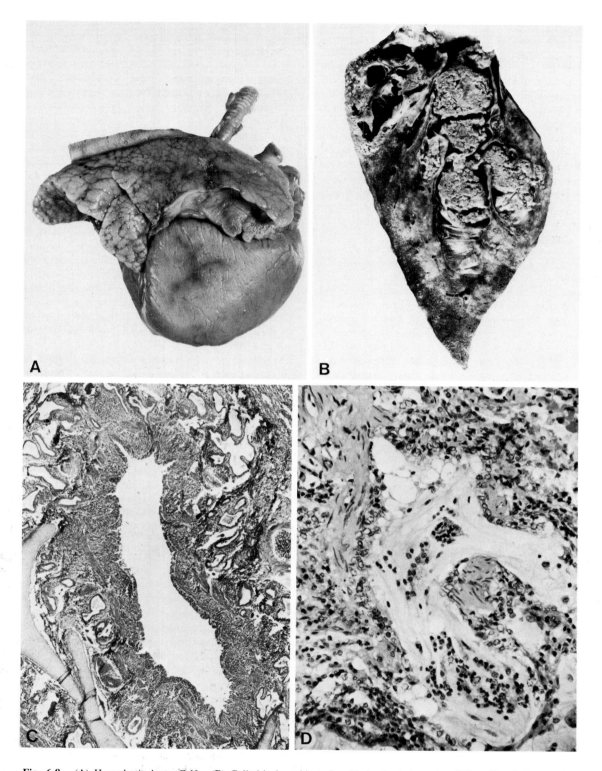

Fig. 6.8. (A) Hypoplastic lung. Calf. (B) Cylindric bronchiectasis with inspissated exudate filling dilated airways. Dog. (C) Chronic bronchitis. Dog. (D) Chronic bronchiolitis of presumed allergic origin with smooth muscle hypertrophy, mucus plugging, and eosinophils. Cat.

basis of coughing, wheezing, respiratory distress, eosinophilia in blood or tracheobronchial lavage fluid, and alleviation of signs by sympathomimetic drugs and corticosteroids. There have been no definitive studies of the lesions associated with the clinical syndrome. Bronchial biopsies indicate an edematous and hyperemic lamina propria, with infiltration of eosinophils and fewer plasma cells and lymphocytes. The epithelium is highly susceptible to sloughing, which is exaggerated by sampling and processing artifacts. The lesions found postmortem usually are in an animal that has had repeated episodes or chronic involvement and therefore have features of a chronic bronchitis in which eosinophils are the predominant inflammatory cell. In the cat, for instance, there is narrowing of bronchial lumens because of prominent hyperplasia of mucosal glands. The epithelial goblet cells are also hyperplastic. Numerous eosinophils infiltrate the epithelium and the edematous hyperemic lamina propria. Plasma cells and lymphocytes are usually less conspicuous. Bronchial lumina are filled with mucus and sloughed cells mixed with many eosinophils. Eosinophils, plasma cells, and lymphocytes form an irregular collar in the adventitia of the bronchi, and small numbers of these cells infiltrate between the glandular acini. Hypertrophy of bronchial smooth muscle is common but not always present. Bronchioles are affected in severe cases (Fig. 6.8D). Occasionally the lesion extends into peribronchiolar alveoli. Since lesions seen at postmortem are usually from an animal dying as a result of acute exacerbation, there is also a widespread patchy alveolar and interstitial edema. In other instances, particularly in the dog, the numbers of eosinophils may be low relative to the other inflammatory cells of a chronic bronchitis, making the assumption of an allergic mechanism more tenuous.

Bronchiectasis

Bronchiectasis is dilation of bronchi. Rarely it is a congenital malformation. More commonly it is an acquired lesion secondary to some form of bronchitis. There are two main anatomic varieties of bronchiectasis, saccular and cylindric. **Saccular bronchiectasis** is less common and consists of thin-walled, circumscribed outpouchings of bronchial or bronchiolar walls. It is much more easily detected in lungs fixed by intratracheal infusion of fixative under pressure. This type of bronchiectasis can result from focal necrotizing bronchitis and bronchiolitis and occurs occasionally in sheep and cattle. It can also be found to a mild degree in the small airways of horses with the bronchiolitis–emphysema complex to be described later (Fig. 6.10C).

Cylindric bronchiectasis affects bronchi partially or along their entire lengths (Fig. 6.8B). In cattle it is almost always a sequel to chronic suppurative bronchitis, which is a frequent aftermath of bronchopneumonia. It therefore affects airways in cranioventral portions of the lung where bronchopneumonia occurs. Although the mechanism of bronchiectasis has never been formally investigated, two main requirements appear to be necessary. One is accumulation of exudate in the lumen, and inflammatory weakening of the bronchial wall. The other is extensive atelectasis of alveolar parenchyma supplied by the affected airways. The loss of alveolar volume leads to traction on the walls of the airways, especially during inspiration. Since the

airways have weak walls and are ventilated during breathing, they expand to accommodate for the lost parenchymal volume. The complete lobular septation and lack of collateral ventilation in the cow both lessens the effectiveness of resolution of bronchopneumonia and leads to more extensive atelectasis because of airway blockage. On both accounts, therefore, bronchiectasis is particularly likely to follow bronchopneumonia in this species.

Affected lungs have irregularly dilated bronchi in cranioventral regions. They are filled with viscous to caseous, yellow-green pus. The intervening parenchyma is atelectatic and sometimes fibrotic. In the anterior lobes the atelectasis tends to be complete, but in the caudal lobe there is often a mixture of areas of bronchopneumonia, hyperinflated lung and atelectasis. In the bovine lung, in which the demarcation of lobules is distinct, dilation of the central bronchiole and alveolar collapse make a small "hillock" of each lobule, resembling the surface of a pineapple (Fig. 6.9A). The superficial appearance is often obscured by fibrous pleural adhesions, so the induration of the parenchyma and the dilated, thin-walled bronchi filled with exudate are best appreciated when the lobe is sliced so that the bronchi are sectioned transversely. In severe cases, the dilated bronchi give a honeycombed or cystic appearance to the lobe (Fig. 6.9B).

Microscopically, depending on the severity and chronicity of the lesion, there are various degrees of reconstruction of the wall of the bronchus by granulation tissue. The lumen contains mucus, detritus, large collections of inflammatory cells, and frequently some blood. The mucosa might be destroyed by ulceration almost to the muscularis, or it might show a combination of ulcerative, atrophic, metaplastic, and hyperplastic changes. The bronchial walls are densely infiltrated with all types of leukocytes, and the lamina propria takes on the histologic properties of granulation tissue with progressive fibrosis. When the necrotizing process extends more deeply than the mucosa and involves the full width of the wall and some of the adjacent alveolar tissue, the lesion is equivalent to a lung abscess.

Cylindric bronchiectasis in the dog (Fig. 6.8B) arises against the background of severe chronic bronchitis, but in contrast to the cow, it is not as consistent a sequel. A major determinant is probably the extent to which alveolar atelectasis occurs in the dog. Since there is very effective collateral ventilation in dogs, atelectasis is less likely to follow airway obstruction. This could be the reason bronchitis is less prone to cause bronchiectasis in this species. In addition to generalized bronchiectasis associated with severe, diffuse, chronic, mucopurulent bronchitis, the condition sometimes is limited to only one or two lobes, more often the middle lobes. Whether localized or generalized, the greatly dilated bronchi often contain casts of either crumbly or tenacious and rubbery, partially dehydrated exudate.

Chronic mucopurulent bronchitis with bronchiectasis and bronchiolectasis is rare in cats. A case in which there was accompanying miliary broncholithiasis has been recorded. In pigs, sheep, and goats, bronchiectasis is usually associated with severe parasitic bronchitis. Occasionally in all species, localized bronchiectasis follows obstruction by a foreign body, granuloma, or tumor.

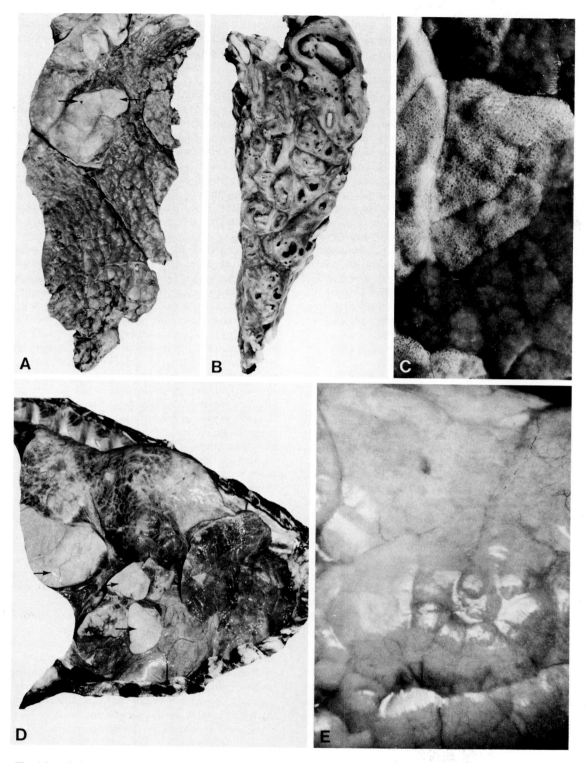

Fig. 6.9. (**A**) Bronchiectasis in cranial lobe. Air trapping in lobules above (arrows). Ox.   (**B**) Cut surface of (**A**).   (**C**) Hyperinflation (compensatory emphysema) in lobules bordering areas of consolidation. Note the relative smallness of the consolidated lobules and mottling produced by peribronchial infiltrates. Ox.   (**D**) Chronic bronchopneumonia. Cranial bronchiectasis, widespread lobular consolidation, interstitial bulla protruding in caudal lobe, and a few pale lobules caused by air trapping (arrows). Calf.   (**E**) Pale, puffy emphysematous lung associated with chronic obstructive bronchiolitis. Horse.

The course of bronchiectasis is chronic and unfavorable. Complications, other than bronchopneumonia, include bronchopleural fistula, septic thrombosis and hemorrhage or production of septic emboli with metastatic abscessation, and secondary amyloidosis.

Kartagener's syndrome was the eponym applied to a congenital and often familial disorder in infants in which there was coexisting situs inversus, sinusitis, and bronchiectasis. Investigations have revealed that Kartagener's syndrome is a subset of various abnormalities now referred to collectively as the immotile cilia syndrome or primary ciliary dyskinesia. Abnormalities are referable to improper function of ciliated cells, particularly of respiratory and reproductive organs. The basic defect in each case is now known to be one of several ultrastructural or metabolic abnormalities of cilia throughout the body. The most common defect is absence of one or both of the inner and outer dynein arms attached to the peripheral doublets of microtubules in the cilia. Several isolated cases with features resembling Kartagener's syndrome have been recorded for the dog. The condition has been found in three littermates in which abnormal dynein arms and excessive ciliary rotation were detected. A deliberate father–daughter mating produced an affected male without situs inversus and indicated a possible autosomal recessive pattern of inheritance.

Lungs

Congenital Anomalies

Congenital anomalies are rare. Various forms have been recorded, more for calves than for other species. Major malformations are incompatible with life but are extremely rare. Accessory lungs are the most common finding. These are edematous, lobulated masses and can be found within the abdominal or thoracic cavities or subcutaneously. The main histologic features are dilated bronchiolar structures, hypoplastic bronchi, and various degrees of development of alveolar ducts and alveoli. Bronchial hypoplasia also appears to be the basic defect in what is usually referred to as congenital adenomatoid malformation or adenomatoid hamartoma. This is where one or more lobes of the normal lung are replaced by swollen, spongy or cystic, lobulated tissue. Histologically, as in accessory lungs, there are dilated bronchioles, which sometimes are large enough to be noted grossly as cystic spaces. Bronchi are hypoplastic and lack cartilage and smooth muscle in their walls. Alveolar structures appear more normal.

Pulmonary hypoplasia (Fig. 6.8A) is particularly likely to accompany congenital diaphragmatic hernia. Congenital cysts and congenital bronchiectasis are localized variations on the same theme. Other rare findings are pulmonary agenesis, usually accompanying other major developmental defects, and ectopic lungs. Congenital alveolar dysplasia has been observed in pups. The gross form of the lungs is regular, but they retain a fetal appearance and become poorly aerated and poorly crepitant. The distribution, size, and shape of the alveoli are uneven, they are reduced in number, and there is too much interstitial tissue. Many dilated capillaries are present in the interstitial tissue. The formed alveoli are lined by mature alveolar epithelium. In such cases it is difficult or impossible to determine whether infection of the fetal lung played a pathogenetic role.

Abnormal lobulations and fissures are quite common and are found incidentally at postmortem examination.

Atelectasis

Atelectasis means incomplete expansion of the lung and was originally applied to defective aeration of fetal lung at the time of birth. It is now also applied to collapse of previously air-filled pulmonary parenchyma. Atelectasis is therefore divided into congenital and acquired forms.

In **congenital (neonatal) atelectasis** the lungs range from those of the stillborn animal, which have never been aerated (**fetal atelectasis**), to minor degrees of incomplete expansion. In fetal atelectasis the lungs appear as in the fetus but are dark reddish blue because of dilation of alveolar capillaries. They are of fleshy consistency and do not float. The alveoli are partially distended with fluid, and the epithelial cells are rounded. Sloughed epithelial cells (squames) from the oronasal regions and amniotic fluid are usually present in the alveolar fluid, possibly with bright yellow particles of meconium. These materials are aspirated during the exaggerated respiratory movements of the asphyxiated fetus *in utero*. Patchy congenital atelectasis due to incomplete expansion is usually due to weak respiratory movements caused by general debilitation or damage to respiratory centers in the brain stem. Laryngeal dysfunction, obstruction of airways, and abnormalities of the lung or related thoracic structures are other possible causes. In the neonatal period it is often not possible to distinguish between atelectasis of incomplete expansion and acquired atelectasis of briefly aerated lung. The atelectasis is frequently seen affecting groups of lobules or occasionally more widespread regions during the first week of life. The larger zones are more likely to occur in weak, recumbent animals and mostly affect the lowermost region of the down side (Fig. 6.12A). The atelectic lobules are distinct because they are dark red, depressed below the surface of the surrounding aerated lung, and in contrast to pneumonic lung, have a flabby consistency. The sectioned surface is homogeneous and dark red, and free blood is easily expressed from it. Microscopically, the alveolar walls are in close apposition. Only small amounts of fluid, epithelial debris (including "squames" from the upper oronasal regions or amniotic fluid), and alveolar macrophages are present.

Extensive neonatal atelectasis is a feature of neonatal hyaline membrane disease (neonatal respiratory distress syndrome). This is a common disease in human infants, particularly in premature babies and those born to diabetic mothers. A similar condition in animals is best recognized in foals, but it has been reported in lambs, pigs, puppies, and a calf. Foals and pigs have been called "barkers" because of the doglike sound made during forced expiration. Foals that show evidence of presumed hypoxic brain damage are sometimes referred to as "wanderers." Affected lungs are extensively atelectatic, although the borders of the lobes might be spared. They are heavy, fleshy, and often edematous. Cream-colored or bloodstained foam frequently exudes from cut surfaces and is present in large airways. The lungs sink or almost submerge in fixative. The main microscopic abnormalities are alveolar septal congestion, variably collapsed or edema-containing alveoli, and presence of acidophilic hyaline membranes lining alveolar ducts and distal portions of bronchioles. Focal hemorrhages and interstitial edema are common.

There is general agreement that lack of normal surface-tension-reducing capacity of the alveolar-lining liquid plays the central pathogenetic role. This in turn is linked to defective production by alveolar type II epithelial cells of the phospholipid surfactant material, which consists mainly of dipalmitoylphosphatidylcholine. There is still debate, however, about the extent to which decreased surfactant activity is due to immaturity of type II cells or to a more specific metabolic derangement of their surfactant synthesis. Fetal hypothyroidism and, possibly, hypoadrenocorticism also play a role in the condition in piglets by being responsible for delayed maturation of type II cells. Other pathogenetic factors are fetal asphyxia, reduction in pulmonary arteriolar blood flow, and inhibition of surfactant by fibrinogen or other serum constituents in edema fluid.

Acquired atelectasis and **alveolar collapse** are used synonymously. Acquired atelectasis is most commonly the **obstructive** type, caused by complete airway obstruction. Whether atelectasis follows obstruction depends on the size of the airway obstructed and the degree of collateral ventilation. Complete blockage of lobar or segmental bronchi is necessary for atelectasis in the dog and cat, where collateral ventilation is extensive. Blockage of small bronchi or even bronchioles can result in atelectasis in bovine lungs, where there is insignificant collateral ventilation. Lungs of sheep are also prone to atelectasis, pigs less so, and the horse is intermediate between ruminants and dogs. Atelectasis is more likely to develop in dependent lung regions, where alveoli are smallest and airways most easily compressed. Atelectatic lung caused by obstruction has the appearance of other forms of atelectasis. It is sunken relative to aerated lung, homogeneously dark red, and flabby. Evidence of bronchial obstruction by exudate, parasites, aspirated foreign material, granulomas, or tumors can often be seen grossly. Resorption of oxygen from nonventilated lung occurs quickly, but nitrogen is resorbed very slowly. Obstruction of airways by aspirated material or foamy exudate shortly before death does not, therefore, produce atelectasis in animals breathing air.

Microscopically, simple atelectasis appears as slightly congested alveolar walls lying in close apposition with slitlike residual lumina having sharp angular ends (Fig. 6.12E). Atelectasis, which is sometimes seen preceding the development of bronchopneumonia or during the final phase of its resolution, is usually associated with small amounts of edema fluid and excess alveolar macrophages in the alveolar lumina. The edema accompanying large zones of atelectasis is due partly to leakage because of hypoxic damage and partly to the hypoxic vasoconstriction of vessels in the affected region. Reduced surfactant activity also plays a role. Microatelectasis of small groups of alveoli is often an artifact of immersion fixation, and the apparent blending of several alveolar septa is easily mistaken for interstitial pneumonia.

Acquired atelectasis of **compression** type is caused by pleural or intrapulmonary space-occupying lesions. Examples are hydrothorax, hemothorax, exudative pleuritis, and mediastinal and pulmonary tumors. In large animals, the atelectasis

caused by pleural effusions often occurs below a sharply demarcated fluid line. Abdominal distension, as in severe ascites and ruminal tympany, may cause partial atelectasis, typically in the cranial regions, where ventilatory movements are most easily compromised by intraabdominal pressure.

What might be termed *hypostatic atelectasis* occurs in the lowermost zone of the lung of the down side in recumbent large animals. This is a hazard of prolonged anesthesia or of weakened animals, particularly if there is a condition causing chest pain. The contributing factors are shallow amplitude of respiration (causing impaired ventilation of dependent lung), gradual loss of surfactant activity, and pooling of secretions in the lower airways.

Sharp-bordered, ribbon-shaped or lobular zones of atelectasis are present to some extent in the cranioventral regions of the lungs of slaughtered sheep. Although many of these are associated with blockage of bronchioles and small bronchi with purulent exudate, some have no detectable blockage of airways, and the reason for the atelectasis is not known.

Massive atelectasis is seen mostly as a sequel to pneumothorax. What appears to be total atelectasis is seen in animals, usually dogs and cats, that die during the course of breathing 80–100% oxygen as part of intensive care. Because of the speed with which the oxygen is resorbed into the tissues, the lungs are usually completely degassed by the time they are examined postmortem. They are uniformly shrunken, dark red, and flabby and ooze blood on cut section.

Emphysema of the Lungs

Emphysema in its widest sense refers to tissue puffed up by air or other gas. In the lung there are two major forms. **Alveolar (vesicular) emphysema** is excessive amounts of air within airspaces of the lung. **Interstitial emphysema** is the presence of air within interlobular, subpleural, and other major interstitial zones of the lung. **Emphysema**, unless otherwise qualified, should only be used for alveolar emphysema. The most widely accepted definition of human emphysema is abnormal enlargement of airspaces distal to the terminal bronchioles, with evidence of loss or destruction of their walls. Some broaden the definition to include abnormal enlargement of airspaces, with or without evidence of destruction. The advantages of requiring evidence of destruction of walls of the airspaces is that it enables more precise recognition of an irreversible, functionally significant lesion. Simple enlargement, or hyperinflation, can be a temporary and relatively insignificant lesion. An example of this is the so-called compensatory emphysema, which occurs along the margin of a consolidated lung (Fig. 6.9C). What appear to be emphysematous lesions in lungs removed postmortem are often not significant antemortem changes but mostly result from failure of the lung to deflate normally (Fig. 6.9A,D). This is caused by air trapping, usually by blockage or spasm of airways. Accurate assessment of emphysema therefore can only be obtained in lungs inflated with fixative to a volume approximating the *in vivo* state. In the following discussion, *emphysema* will refer to abnormal enlargement of airspaces distal to terminal bronchioles with evidence of destruction of their walls.

Several morphologic types of emphysema are recognized in human lungs, according to the distribution of the enlarged air-

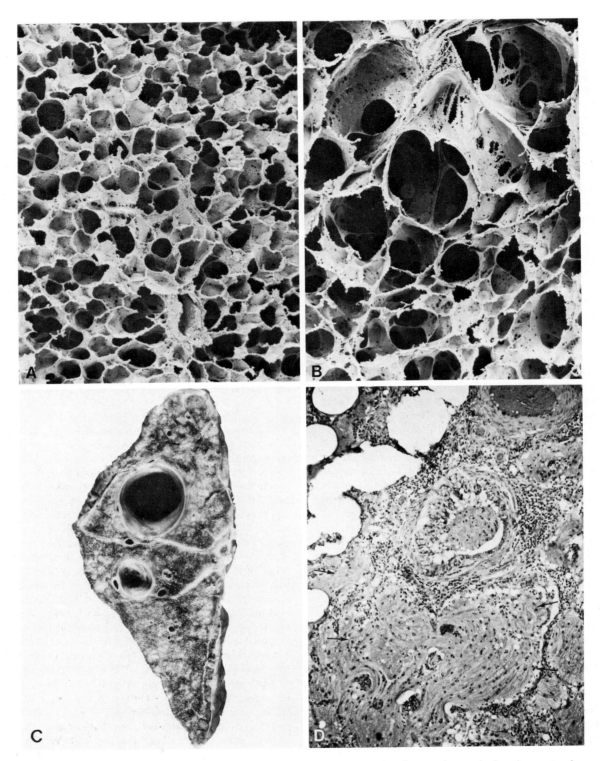

Fig. 6.10. (A) Scanning electron micrograph of normal lung. Horse.   (B) Scanning electron micrograph of emphysematous lung. Same magnification as (A). Horse. Note alveolar enlargement and alveolar wall destruction.   (C) Saccular bronchiectasis in chronic obstructive bronchiolitis. Horse.   (D) Histologic detail of bronchiolitis in (C). Note mucous plugging of bronchiole and mucus reflux into adjacent alveoli (arrows).

spaces. **Centriacinar (centrilobular) emphysema** principally affects respiratory bronchioles and adjacent central portions of the respiratory acini. **Panacinar (panlobular) emphysema** more uniformly involves all portions of acini. An acinus is defined as the terminal unit of lung supplied by a single terminal (nonrespiratory) bronchiole. These two major anatomic types of emphysema in humans also differ with regard to other clinicopathologic features. Less important forms of emphysema are **paraseptal emphysema**, which affects distal alveoli bordering interlobular septa or pleura, and **irregular** or **paracicatricial emphysema**, which results from distortion of airspaces by adjacent contracted scar tissue.

Regardless of distribution, severely emphysematous lung is grossly voluminous, pale, and puffy. When the lesion is diffuse, the lungs fill the thoracic cavity even after the chest has been opened, and they might bear imprints of the ribs. The enlarged airspaces are often visible as small vesicles, and in severe cases coalescence of airspaces can produce large, air-filled bullae one to several centimeters in diameter. Enlargement and coalescence of airspace in inflation-fixed lungs can readily be detected in moderate to severe cases. Scanning electron microscopy, which dramatically reveals the moth-eaten appearance (Fig. 6.10A,B), is best for visualization of early lesions.

With the exception of the chronic bronchiolitis–emphysema complex in the horse, which is to be addressed later, naturally occurring emphysema is rarely of significance in animals. It can be found postmortem in the apices and along the sharp ventral border of the lungs of old animals and is therefore seen mostly in dogs (Fig. 6.11A,B), cats, and horses. Emphysematous bullae also occasionally occur in these regions, and in rare instances rupture to cause fatal pneumothorax. Even where not noted grossly, subpleural airspaces, particularly along cranioventral margins of the lung, are often noted to be larger than more central ones on microscopic examination.

In contrast to animals, emphysema is an extremely important condition in humans, where it frequently coexists with chronic bronchitis and bronchiolitis in causing chronic obstructive pulmonary disease. Most of what is known about the pathogenesis of emphysema is therefore derived from the human condition or, more recently, from experimental animal models. With regard to pathogenetic factors in emphysema, there has been considerable speculation over the years concerning the relative importance of genetic factors, inflammatory alveolar destruction, atrophy of alveolar septa due to ischemic or unknown cause, and mechanical factors leading to widening and rupture of airspaces. Two important findings led to convergence of these ideas. One was the discovery that persons deficient in α_1-antitrypsin (now referred to as α_1-protease inhibitor) have increased incidence and earlier onset of emphysema. The other was that intratracheal injection of papain in hamsters produced an emphysematous lesion. Further developments led to the current basic hypothesis that emphysema is caused by excessive proteolysis in the lung because of protease–antiprotease imbalance. The critical structural component undergoing lysis is elastin, because experimentally the development of emphysema is only correlated well with elastolytic activity and evidence of elastin breakdown. In homozygous α_1-protease-inhibitor deficiency, the emphysema is pan-

acinar in distribution, and the protease–antiprotease imbalance is presumed to be due mainly to the reduction in the antiprotease. In centriacinar emphysema, such as associated with cigarette smoking, there is a slowly smoldering inflammation at the bronchiolar–alveolar junctions, where the emphysema develops. This inflammation is associated with release of elastases by neutrophils and macrophages acting in concert.

Chronic bronchiolitis–emphysema complex in the **horse** has long been associated with the lay terms "heaves" or "broken wind," and more recently with the pathophysiologic term "chronic obstructive pulmonary disease." The term chronic bronchiolitis–emphysema complex is used here because it emphasizes the lesions, which tend to coexist, and the fact that the causes and pathogenesis are both complex and poorly understood. The most consistent finding in horses with clinical signs of chronic obstructive pulmonary disease is a generalized chronic bronchiolitis. Emphysema, as defined by enlargement and destruction of airspaces, is less common (Fig. 6.9E and 6.10B), although in excised lungs the alveoli might appear hyperinflated because of air trapping. Rarely, emphysema is present without significant bronchiolitis. The emphysema is mostly in cranial regions, even when it accompanies a more generalized bronchiolitis.

Constant features of the chronic bronchiolitis are epithelial hyperplasia, goblet-cell metaplasia, and peribronchiolar fibrosis and infiltration by lymphocytes and plasma cells. Lumina of bronchioles are narrowed by accumulation of exudate and the peribronchiolar fibrosis. Mucus is usually a major component of the exudate and sometimes occurs in such large quantities that reflux into adjacent alveolar ducts and alveoli occurs (Fig. 6.10D). The major variable component of the bronchiolitis is the eosinophil. This is sometimes the most obvious feature, both of the intraluminal exudate and within the epithelial and peribronchiolar sites. At other times, relatively few eosinophils are scattered within the mucus and the bronchiolar wall. There often seems to be an inverse relationship between the amount of mucus and the number of eosinophils. There are usually increased numbers of mast cells surrounding the bronchioles. Neutrophils are less common than eosinophils, but sometimes the lesion has the characteristics of a mucopurulent bronchiolitis.

The relative importance of allergy, infection, and toxicity in causing the bronchiolitis is not established; it almost certainly can differ across a series of cases. The frequent presence of eosinophils, circumstantial evidence of clinical exacerbation on exposure to moldy hay, bedding, or stable dust, and limited information from aerosol challenges using suspect fungal antigens all indicate that an allergic response to inhaled allergens is an important mechanism. Infection probably plays some part in a proportion of cases. Experimental evidence that blood-borne toxins, specifically 3-methylindole in the horse, can selectively damage bronchiolar epithelium introduces a further possible set of causes. From the point of view of the characteristic goblet-cell metaplasia and mucus hypersecretion, there is evidence that histamine, prostaglandins, and leukotrienes released during type I allergic responses (anaphylaxis) have a stimulatory effect on mucus secretion. This could explain the association of goblet-

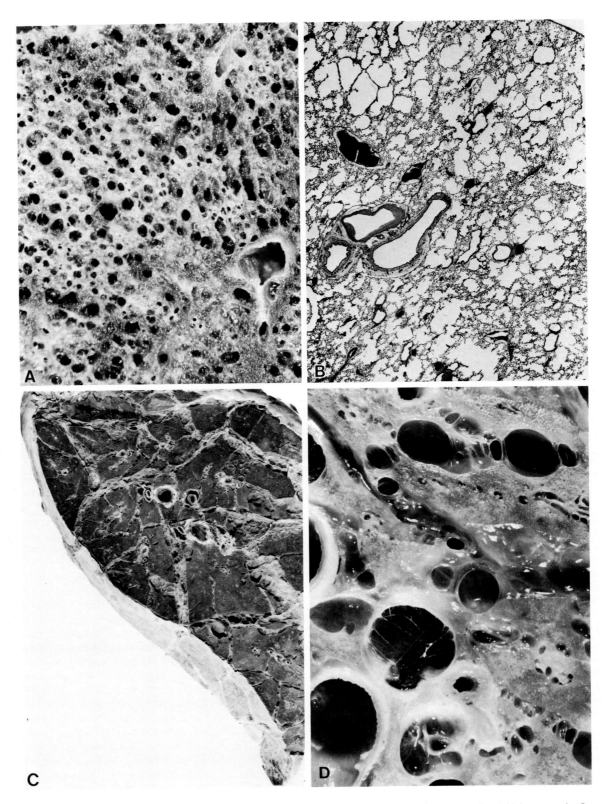

Fig. 6.11.   (**A** and **B**) Emphysema. Lung. Dog.   (**C** and **D**) Interstitial emphysema secondary to acute interstitial pneumonia. Ox. Note bubbles of air in interstitial tissues and lymphatics of interlobular septa.

cell increases, mucus hypersecretion, eosinophils, and mast cells. As indicated previously, asthma and chronic allergic bronchitis and bronchiolitis are not clearly separable in animals.

Interstitial emphysema is distinguished from alveolar emphysema by the presence of air in the connective tissues and lymphatics of the lung, chiefly the interlobular septa but also beneath the pleura and around vessels and airways (Fig. 6.11C,D). Interstitial emphysema occurs mainly in lungs with well-developed interlobular septa. Lungs of the cow, sheep, and pig have this feature, but only the cow is readily susceptible to the lesion. Any condition causing forced expiratory maneuvers, even agonally, can cause the condition in the cow. It is common in slaughtered cattle. It occurs in most dramatic form as a prominent feature of acute interstitial pneumonia in cattle (acute bovine pulmonary emphysema and edema). A point to be emphasized most strongly is that there is no connection whatsoever between the pathogenesis of alveolar emphysema, as described previously, and interstitial emphysema in the cow. Although there is as yet no proof, it is presumed that air is forced into the complete but delicate interlobular septa because bronchioles are collapsed during forced expiration. For this to occur, there has to be a lack of collateral ventilation and highly uneven deflation among neighboring lobules. In cows surviving sufficient length of time with severe interstitial emphysema, the air can extend along lymphatics to the bronchial and mediastinal lymph nodes, or along fascial planes of the mediastinum to beneath the skin of the back.

Circulatory Disturbances of the Lungs

The lungs are affected by a large variety of circulatory disturbances. They are caused by abnormalities principally involving the pulmonary vessels and heart, or by vascular changes secondary to pulmonary disease. The most important functional consequence is hypoxemia due to mismatching of ventilation and perfusion or shunting of blood through nonventilated regions of lung.

Pulmonary **ischemia** occurs following emphysematous or fibrotic attenuation of alveolar capillaries and can be associated with severe reduction in blood volume. Because of the dual blood supply from pulmonary and bronchial arteries, and the extensive collateral circulation, congestion rather than ischemia is the usual sequel to arterial obstruction. Active **hyperemia** is part of the acute inflammatory response and is a feature of acute pulmonary injury of many types. Pulmonary **congestion** is most commonly caused by left-sided or bilateral cardiac failure. It can also be due to changes in vascular tone causing shifting of blood from the systemic to the pulmonary circulation. Such shifts can be caused by autonomic disturbances, such as those produced by traumatic or other acutely damaging lesions in the hypothalamic region of the brain. The main importance of pulmonary congestion is that it leads to pulmonary edema, as explained below.

Pulmonary Edema

Starling's equation for flow of liquid across a capillary membrane applies in general to pulmonary capillaries; that is, flow is dependent on the permeability characteristics of the vascular wall and the balance of hydrostatic and osmotic pressures be-

tween the intravascular and interstitial compartments. The situation is more complicated in the lung, however, because the set of factors involved in the pathogenesis of alveolar edema also includes the permeability of the alveolar epithelium, air pressure and surface tension acting on the alveolar surfaces, and preferential drainage of liquid through the pulmonary interstitium. Uncertainty still exists about the exact magnitude of some of the factors and the routes by which water, solutes, and macromolecular substances cross endothelial and epithelial boundaries.

Despite the low capillary hydrostatic pressure in the pulmonary circulation, there is a slow but steady flow of liquid from the alveolar interstitium into pulmonary lymphatics. Two factors are important in ensuring that alveoli do not become flooded under normal circumstances. One is that alveolar epithelium and its intercellular junctions are much less permeable than endothelial structures and therefore effectively seal off the alveolar lumen. The other is that the interstitial space is at lower pressure than intraalveolar pressure. The interstitial pressure in the loose fascia surrounding vessels and airways where lymphatics are situated becomes increasingly subatmospheric ("negative") toward the pulmonary hilus. The net effect is that liquid is drained from alveolar interstitium to lymphatics and thence to the hilus of the lung. The bronchovascular interstitium and lymphatics therefore constitute a highly compliant sump. Providing the alveolar epithelium remains undamaged, alveolar edema does not occur until the capacity of the sump is overwhelmed. In slowly developing cardiogenic edema, the volume of interstitial liquid can be increased severalfold before alveolar flooding occurs. This explains why the first morphologic evidence of edema due to cardiac insufficiency is excess liquid in interstitium and lymphatics, particularly in the more compliant hilar regions. The increased capillary hydrostatic pressure and higher interstitial pressures caused by gravitational effects in dependent regions of the lungs predispose these sites to edema in large animals.

Physiologic studies indicating different rates of movement of water and molecules of various size ranges and polarity have led to the development of mathematical models postulating the presence of pores of differing size ranges in the air–blood barrier. There is as yet no good correlation between the mathematical pore concept and ultrastructural evidence for sites of the pores. Probably, water and small solutes pass through the endothelium by a transcellular route, and larger solutes by way of intercellular junctions. Macromolecules appear to be largely transported by pinocytotic vesicles. Under some circumstances, water and protein are also actively transported across the alveolar epithelium. It is usually assumed that alveolar edema occurs by passage of edema fluid locally from interstitium to lumen. This is unquestionably the case for edema associated with increased capillary and type I epithelial permeability. It is not necessarily true for edema caused by increased capillary hydrostatic pressure (cardiogenic edema). There is the possibility that in this form of edema, excess fluid accumulates in the perivascular and peribronchiolar interstitium before overflowing into the alveoli through an as yet unidentified pathway close to the bronchiolar–alveolar junction. Although there is experimental evidence supporting this mechanism, its importance in naturally occurring, clinically significant cardiogenic edema remains to be established.

Pulmonary edema is a frequent complication of many diseases and is therefore one of the most commonly encountered pulmonary abnormalities. Most causes of edema act by increasing capillary hydrostatic pressure or by increasing permeability of the air–blood barrier. Decreased plasma oncotic pressure, such as occurs in hypoalbuminemia, and lymphatic obstruction caused, for instance, by widespread tumor infiltration of lymphatics and pulmonary lymph nodes, are less important.

Edema due to increased capillary hydrostatic pressure is usually the result of increased left atrial pressure in left-sided or bilateral cardiac failure and is commonly referred to as **cardiogenic edema**. The congestion and edema are important parts of the pulmonary complications of congestive heart failure (see the Cardiovascular System, Volume 3). Increased capillary hydrostatic pressure is also the basis for the edema of hypervolemia developing in some cases of excessive fluid transfusion, and the systemic vasoconstriction induced by autonomic discharge following acute brain injury (''**neurogenic**'' edema).

Many agents cause pulmonary edema by damaging alveolar type I epithelium and capillary endothelium. The increase in permeability leads to edema of more rapid onset and of higher protein concentration than in cardiogenic forms. Inhaled corrosive gases (including 80–100% oxygen), systemic toxins, anaphylaxis in certain species (e.g., cow and horse), endotoxins, and shocklike states all can cause acute pulmonary edema. As in edema elsewhere, there is no clear dividing line between these ''inflammatory'' edemas and serous exudates. Many of the toxic or shocklike states causing the edema accompanying acute pulmonary injury may be sufficiently severe to cause acute interstitial pneumonia. They will be considered further under Interstitial Pneumonia. Loss or inhibition of phospholipid-rich surfactant in the alveolar lining layer can enhance edema formation because high surface tension at the air–liquid interface tends to draw fluid into the alveolus. This is probably not of primary importance except in neonatal hyaline membrane disease (respiratory distress syndrome) and perhaps in loss of surfactant activity accompanying prolonged shallow respiration.

Clinically evident pulmonary edema is a sign of serious underlying disturbance. Cardiogenic edema is not fatal if the cardiac insufficiency can be controlled, but pulmonary edema is often the cause of death from sudden cardiac decompensation. Whether other forms of pulmonary edema cause death depends on the severity and speed of onset of the underlying disease process and the edema it produces. Alveolar edema prevents ventilation of flooded alveoli. In the presence of surfactant material, it becomes stable foam by mixing with air in small airways, and the foam further compromises ventilation. Edema fluid can be removed slowly from alveoli if the animal survives, but the details of the mechanisms are not established.

Edematous lungs are wet, heavy, and do not collapse completely when the thorax is opened. Frequently there is excess fluid in the thoracic cavity. Subpleural and interstitial tissues are edematous, and in lungs with well-developed interlobular septa, there is an accentuated pattern because the septa become distended by edema fluid (Fig. 6.12C). Air can be mixed with edema in the bovine lung and distended, tortuous, and beaded lymphatics become visible grossly. Foam is discharged from the nostrils in severe cases, and foam variously mixed with fluid is often present in trachea (Fig. 6.12D) and intrapulmonary airways. Presence of foam indicates edema of at least moderate severity and the presence of alveolar surfactant not inhibited by fibrinogen or other high molecular weight constituents of serum. Fluid oozes from cut surfaces of edematous lungs.

The color of edema fluid and foam depends on the amount of hemorrhage. If absent, the interstitial edema is clear, colorless, to slightly yellow, and the foam is white. Various amounts of hemorrhage cause corresponding degrees of bloodstaining of fluid and foam. The pulmonary parenchyma varies from dark pink to reddish black, according to the amount of congestion or hyperemia. When severe, the distinction between acute pulmonary edema and peracute pneumonia is not possible grossly and can be blurred even on microscopic examination.

Histologically, edema fluid is acidophilic, homogeneous or faintly granular material filling alveoli, except for occasional discrete holes that represent trapped air bubbles. The same material is usually present in interstitial tissue and lymphatics around vessels and airways, and in interlobular septa and subpleural zones in those species where these are well developed. The amount of protein present in cardiogenic edema is small enough, particularly in dogs and cats, that it does not stain well after the leaching that occurs in formalin fixative. It can therefore easily be overlooked. Noting the presence of foam or fluid at gross examination, and distension of interstitial tissue and lymphatics microscopically, then takes on added importance. Coagulant fixatives containing mercury are best for demonstration of protein in edema fluid. Edema due to permeability defects stains more acidophilic than cardiogenic edema, even after formalin fixation, and frequently contains strands or clumps of fibrin. The postmortem seepage of fluid into the alveoli of animals killed by barbiturate euthanasia solutions can easily be mistaken for edema. This artifact usually prevents detection of any antemortem edema unless the latter is revealed by dilatation of interstitial lymphatics.

When the lungs are congested, the capillaries are distended and intraalveolar hemorrhages are common. Alveolar macrophages containing erythrocytes or hemosiderin are present and increase in number with duration of the congestion. These cells are known as ''heart failure'' cells (Fig. 6.12B). They are not usually a prominent feature of congestive heart failure in animals, however. This is at least partly because of the shorter time animals with severe failure are kept alive compared to humans. A more usual feature accompanying the pulmonary hypertension of chronic cardiogenic edema, as in the dog and cat, is hypertrophy of the muscular walls of small pulmonary vessels and thickening of pulmonary capillary walls by fibrous tissue (Fig. 6.12B). Occasionally in terminal cardiac failure in the dog and cat, there is accumulation of leukocytes in pulmonary capillaries, severe damage to endothelium and alveolar type I epithelium, and filling of alveoli with fibrin-rich fluid. The cause is not established, but the morphologic evidence indicates acute pulmonary injury of shocklike antecedents, described under Interstitial Pneumonia.

Pulmonary Hemorrhage

Hemorrhages occur frequently in the lung and beneath the pleura in the hemorrhagic diatheses, septicemias, and severe

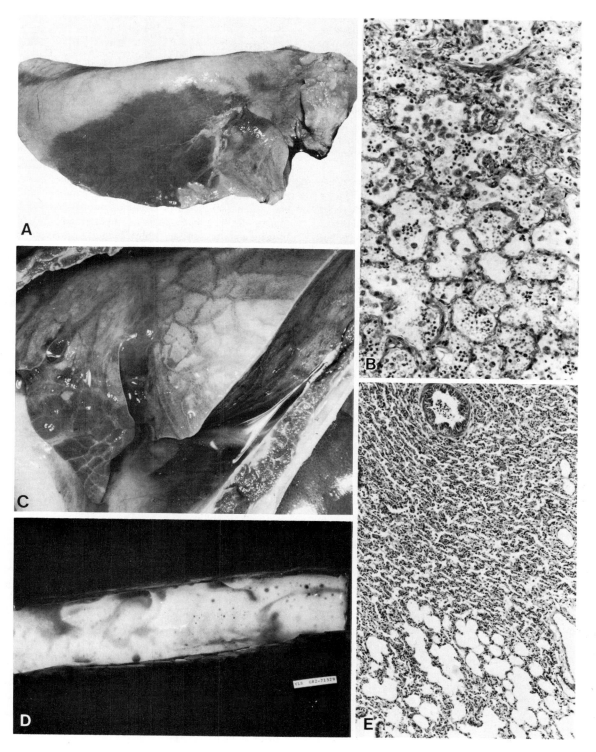

Fig. 6.12. (A) Atelectasis of lateral aspect of right caudal lobe. Lamb. (B) Chronic pulmonary congestion due to heart failure. Dog. (C) Pulmonary edema and hydrothorax. Ox. Interstitial accumulation of fluid accentuates the lobular pattern. (D) Tracheal foam due to severe terminal pulmonary edema. Horse. (E) Atelectasis. Lamb.

congestion. They can also be caused by infarction, ruptured aneurysms, and trauma. Hemorrhages vary from petechiation to massive filling of large regions by blood. Aspiration of blood is frequent at slaughter. It has a characteristic pattern of multiple, small, bright red foci with feathery or indistinct borders. Massive hemorrhage sufficient to cause hemoptysis or epistaxis is occasionally observed in cattle. It is caused by erosion of a large vessel and rupture into a bronchus. It can be a complication of a bronchogenic abscess but is more often the sequel to septic thromboembolism and arteritis, usually caused by embolism from a septic thrombus in a large hepatic vein or the posterior vena cava.

Exercise-induced pulmonary hemorrhage is the term currently used for hemorrhage occurring in horses during racing or training. It used to be referred to as epistaxis, but with endoscopic examination it has been shown that close to 50% of horses examined soon after racing have detectable hemorrhage, but only 1% or fewer have blood at the nostrils. The frequency of the exercise-induced hemorrhage increases with age and severity of exertion. The exact locations and cause, or more likely, contributory causes, of the hemorrhage are not known. The main debate is whether pulmonary hypertension and mechanical stressing of normal pulmonary tissue during severe exertion is sufficient to cause hemorrhage, or whether preexisting pulmonary lesions are necessary. Since few, if any, lungs of horses are structurally perfect, this is a difficult matter to address. The argument that hypertension alone is unlikely to be the cause because there is no accompanying edema is, however, a forceful one. It appears likely that localized, partial obstruction of small airways or pulmonary scars will be found to play an important part. This is in accord with the hypothesis that distending pressures applied to poorly ventilated regions of lung during inflation of adjacent normal parenchyma are sufficient either to tear lung tissue or produce capillary transmural pressures high enough to cause rupture of the capillary walls. The critical feature is that the transmural pressure of the capillary is the difference between the blood pressure in the capillary and the intraalveolar pressure. Since the intraalveolar pressure becomes reduced well below atmospheric pressure in regions of limited mobility during inspiration, the capillary transmural pressure could become large enough to cause rupture.

Embolism, Thrombosis, and Infarction

The lungs are strategically situated to catch emboli carried in venous blood. In accordance with the general pathology of **embolism**, the outcome will depend on the nature of the embolic material and on the features of the pulmonary circulation. Because the lung is supplied by both pulmonary and bronchial arteries and has extensive collateral channels, infarction usually does not follow embolism and thrombosis unless the pulmonary circulation is already compromised. It is possible, for instance, to find a major pulmonary artery occluded by large, pale, friable thromboembolic material without gross abnormality of the pulmonary parenchyma. Bacterial emboli are associated with fulminating septicemias and cause acute pulmonary edema or interstitial pneumonia. Septic emboli arising from infected thrombi cause thromboembolism, arteritis, usually multiple abscessation, and possibly more extensive chronic suppurative

pneumonia. The tendency for aneurysms to occur and be a source of fatal hemorrhage has already been mentioned. In the cow, septic emboli arise mainly from thrombosis of the posterior vena cava due to local spread of a hepatic abscess. They can also originate in uterine and pelvic veins. They arise mainly from mesenteric veins in horses; they can originate from vegetative endocarditis in any species.

Tumor emboli vary in number from a few widely separated foci to extensive showering of capillaries and larger vessels with neoplastic cells. The latter is more common with highly invasive anaplastic carcinomas, such as sometimes occur with mammary carcinomas in bitches. An unusual form of embolism occurs where carcinoma cells lodge and proliferate within vessels, producing multiple discrete foci surrounded by smooth muscle and collagen. In some foci there is thrombosis, which stimulates organization by granulation tissue and frequently leads to death of the neoplastic cells and obliteration of the vascular lumen. Malignant cells usually proliferate more in perivascular lymphatics than in the vessels themselves.

Fat embolism is only occasionally important in animals. The fat can originate from bone marrow at sites of fracture and from severe hepatic lipidosis. The emboli lodge in alveolar capillaries and produce sausage-shaped distensions that are empty in routine paraffin sections. Megakaryocytes are frequently found in pulmonary capillaries, particularly in dogs. A small number of megakaryocytes derived from bone marrow are present in circulating blood and lodge in the lungs, where they continue to produce platelets. This is a normal occurrence, but might be accentuated when there is compensatory extramedullary hematopoiesis.

Pulmonary thrombosis can be triggered, as elsewhere, when there is hypercoagulability, stasis of blood, or vascular endothelial damage. Embolism and endarteritis as causes have been mentioned already. There is an association between pulmonary thrombosis and renal amyloidosis in dogs. The endarteritis caused by *Dirofilaria immitis* or *Angiostrongylus vasorum* is also a cause of thrombosis in dogs; less commonly thrombosis is secondary to ulceration of intimal atherosclerotic plaques. Disseminated intravascular coagulation in septicemic, toxic, and advanced neoplastic states is also an important cause of pulmonary thrombosis (see the Cardiovascular System, Volume 3). Pulmonary thrombosis of unexplained cause is found occasionally in any species.

Pulmonary infarction is an unlikely event unless the pulmonary circulation is already compromised. Thrombosis of large vessels is more likely to lead to congestion, edema, and atelectasis of the affected regions. Most infarctions occur in lungs that have generalized passive congestion. Thrombi occurring in conditions associated with general circulatory collapse, such as disseminated intravascular coagulation, are therefore particularly likely to cause infarction.

All recent infarcts are hemorrhagic. They occur most frequently in the caudal lobes. They usually extend to the pleura and are particularly prone to affect the sharp costophrenic borders of the lung. At the costophrenic margin they are wedge-shaped, with the broad base toward the hilus of the lung. When they involve only one pleural surface they are cone-shaped, with the base at the pleura. The shape is difficult to appreciate when they are small because their margins blend laterally with adjacent congested parenchyma. Infarcted areas bulge on the pleural aspect and are red-blue to black. They are firm, and the overlying pleura becomes roughened, opaque, and covered by blood-stained exudate if the infarct is more than a few hours old. When the infarct is large, the occluded vessel can usually be detected at or near its apex. Histologically, an early infarct has extensive hemorrhage against a background of necrotic parenchyma. If the animal survives, there is lysis of red cells, and a border of neutrophils and macrophages appears within 1 or 2 days. Organization by peripheral encroachment of granulation tissue occurs subsequently and eventually results in scar formation. The sequelae to septic infarction consist of the more severe changes described previously for septic thromboembolism.

Pulmonary Hypertension

Pulmonary hypertension can be initiated by high-pressure flow of blood from the right heart, such as occurs in congenital ventricular septal defect, or by increased resistance in the pulmonary vascular system. The increased resistance to flow may be the result of left-sided heart failure, luminal narrowing of vessels by arteriosclerotic changes, or hypoxic vasoconstriction, as seen in high-altitude disease of cattle (see the Cardiovascular System, Volume 3). Regardless of initial cause, there occurs a vicious cycle of hypertension, causing arteriosclerosis, which in turn leads to more hypertension.

Any subacute or chronic lesion causing narrowing or obliteration of pulmonary vessels can cause pulmonary hypertension. Thromboembolic situations mentioned previously may therefore produce hypertension and "cor pulmonale." Widespread fibrosis in chronic interstitial pneumonias can also cause pulmonary hypertension by occluding small vessels. Chronic bronchitis and bronchiolitis stimulate muscular hypertrophy in the walls of small arteries, and this too can result in cor pulmonale. The effects of hypertension alone are mainly in the small muscular arteries, where there is proliferation of myointimal and medial smooth muscle cells, and in arterioles, which develop prominent muscle coats by proliferation of pericytes. Severe hypertension causes endothelial degeneration and intimal and adventitial fibroplasia. Eventually, leakage of plasma protein into the degenerating muscular and collagenous components of the wall can produce fibrinoid necrosis.

Inflammation of the Lungs

Pneumonia is the usual term for inflammation of the lungs involving alveolar parenchyma. There has been a tendency to use the term **pneumonia** for the more acute and exudative inflammations and **pneumonitis** for the more chronic, proliferative lesions. Since proliferative components are mostly within or become incorporated into the interstitium of the lung, pneumonitis and chronic interstitial pneumonia are largely synonymous terms. Separate and sometimes conflicting use of pneumonia and pneumonitis has more potential for confusion than clarification, however, so the term pneumonia will be in general use for pulmonary inflammation throughout this chapter. Salient morphologic and pathogenetic features of the various

types of pneumonia are conveyed by additional descriptive terms.

Alveolar Response to Injury

Alveoli are completely lined by a mosaic of two types of epithelial cells. The **type I cell** (**membranous pneumonocyte**) has a flattened nucleus and thin cytoplasmic extensions covering large areas of alveolar wall. Its thin cytoplasmic layer provides a minimal barrier for diffusion of oxygen, but the presence of few organelles and high surface-to-volume ratio makes the cell's plasma membrane, and hence the cell itself, extremely vulnerable to injury. The **type II cell** (**granular** or **secretory pneumonocyte**), in contrast, is more numerous than the type I cell, but because of its compactness it covers far less of the alveolar wall. It has a cuboidal shape, surface microvilli, a rich complement of organelles, and the specific osmiophilic lamellar inclusions that are the sites of surfactant storage prior to its release into the alveoli. In addition to its secretory activity, the type II cell's other main function is that of epithelial renewal and repair, as described below. A third cell type, the brush cell, has been found rarely in the alveoli of various species of animals. Its function is unknown.

The type I epithelial cell, having little reparative capacity and no regenerative capability, is highly susceptible to acute injury. The opposite is true for the type II cell. The usual pattern of alveolar response is for necrosis and sloughing of type I cells, accompanied by the acute exudative phase of inflammation. Providing the severity of the process is not sufficient to cause necrosis of type II cells and other components of the alveolar septa, the type II cells begin to proliferate within 24 hr and eventually completely line the previously denuded alveolar wall. Histologically, small clusters of alveolar cells can be detected 2 or 3 days after loss of type I cells, and by 6 days there can be complete lining of alveoli by cuboidal type II cells. This is the appearance commonly referred to as epithelialization. During the active proliferation of type II cells, it is common to see small syncytial clusters and individual atypical cells with increased nuclear and cytoplasmic volumes, abnormal shape, and increased basophilia. Atypical cells are particularly likely to be seen in canine lungs. This active proliferation is sometimes erroneously interpreted as a neoplastic process. The complete lining of alveoli by type II cells, which is a common response to injury, has also misleadingly been referred to as "adenomatosis." Proliferation of type II cells marks the shift from the exudative to the proliferative stage of pneumonia and is usually accompanied by an alveolar exudate increasingly composed of macrophages and other mononuclear cells. Resolution of the epithelial lesion, once inflammation has subsided and provided there has not been scarring of the alveolar wall, is accomplished by transformation of type II cells into type I epithelium. An important aspect of the proliferative response of type II cells is their increased susceptibility to the toxic effects of 60 to 100% oxygen during this phase.

The character of alveolar exudate depends on its cause. In general, it changes with time from serous fluid (inflammatory edema) containing various quantities of fibrin, through a neutrophil phase that predominates in most bacterial infections, to an accumulation mostly consisting of alveolar macrophages.

Both the dominant features and the rate of change vary according to cause of the inflammation. The quantity of fibrin in alveolar exudate is an index of the amount of damage to the alveolar–capillary membrane because it reveals leakage of its precursor fibrinogen. Fibrin forms, together with other serum constituents and cell debris, the hyaline membranes found in conditions involving severe damage to the alveolar wall. The amount of fibrin is an important determinant of fibrosis. When alveolar epithelium is denuded, fibrinous membranes or plugs are infiltrated by fibroblast precursors from the alveolar wall, and collagen-containing fibrous tissue can be detected as early as 7 days after initial fibrinous exudation. There is usually an associated defect in fibrinolytic systems in such instances. The prominence of fibrin in acute alveolar injury in cattle is related to the high fibrinogen content of bovine blood, a low level of plasminogen (precursor of plasmin, a major fibrinolytic enzyme), and a high concentration of a plasmin inhibitor in pulmonary tissue.

Alveolar macrophages are derived mainly from the interstitial compartment in normal lungs, but in inflammatory conditions they come mostly from blood monocytes. Local proliferation can also play a role as evidenced by the occasional finding of mitotic figures in macrophages within alveolar lumina. Once inflammation supervenes, they take their place in an intricate interplay of amplifying and inhibitory processes. Among the more important are chemotactic attraction and stimulation of neutrophils and lymphocytes, increased phagocytic and bactericidal activity in the activated state, release of lysosomal hydrolases, and enhancement of fibrinolysis by activation of plasminogen. They are also involved in pulmonary fibrosis by the secretion, under certain conditions, of fibroblast-stimulating factors. Acute damage to alveolar septa is also accompanied by the usual vascular components of acute inflammation, with accumulation of inflammatory fluid and leukocytes in the interstitium as well as in the alveoli. The inflammatory fluid in the interstitium, as in edema, is mostly accommodated in the compliant fascia and lymphatics surrounding airways and vessels, and in interlobular septa and subpleural tissue. It is most pronounced in those species having more complete interlobular septa, particularly ruminants and pigs. Cellular accumulation in alveolar walls can become pronounced in acute processes involving cell-mediated immune mechanisms, such as influenza virus infection, but they are more often associated with chronic conditions.

Chronic inflammation of the alveolar septa is the major feature of chronic interstitial pneumonias and will be discussed more fully under Interstitial Pneumonia. Chronic bronchopneumonia, on the other hand, is much more likely to lead to destruction of alveolar walls and abscessation because of persistent suppuration caused by pyogenic bacteria. An aspect of the response of alveolar type II cells to **chronic injury** deserving of mention is their potential for undergoing metaplasia to squamous, ciliated or fetal-type, glycogen-containing cells. One of the most important general features to emerge concerning the response of pulmonary epithelial cells to both acute and chronic injury is the extent to which transdifferentiation (metaplasia of one cell type to another) can occur in airways and alveoli. Persistent irritation or disruption of the normal epithelial interaction with basement membrane and alveolar stroma, as in scarring,

leads to persistence of atypical alveolar type II cells and the possibility that they might occasionally give rise to bronchioloalveolar tumors. This seems to be the case with "scar cancers" of humans and some bronchioloalveolar tumors of dogs and rodents.

Anatomic Patterns of Pneumonia

The pulmonary inflammatory response varies according to the nature of the causative agents, their distribution (particularly the route by which they reach the lung), and their persistence. Pneumonia can be classified on a temporal basis as acute, subacute, or chronic, on an etiologic basis by major categories of causative agent, or according to morphologic features. Morphologically, there are two approaches. One approach is to classify according to the type of inflammation. Here there are two main subcategories: **exudative** pneumonias, in which the emphasis is on filling of alveoli by exudate with predominant **catarrhal**, **fibrinous**, **suppurative**, **hemorrhagic**, or **necrotizing** characteristics; and **proliferative** pneumonias, in which the emphasis is on proliferation of alveolar type II cells, fibroblasts, macrophages, and possibly additional elements. The second, and more useful, morphologic approach is to classify pneumonias according to initial site of involvement and the pattern of spread of the lesion. On this basis, most pneumonias fall into three main categories: **bronchopneumonia**, **lobar pneumonia**, and **interstitial pneumonia**. The importance of this form of classification lies in its providing the most important clues regarding pathogenesis and possible cause of pneumonia.

There is often a good link between the various classifications. For example, acute pneumonias are commonly of infectious cause, exudative in nature, and of bronchopneumonic pattern. Chronic pneumonias are of highly varied cause, proliferative in nature, and often of interstitial pattern. Other correlations, and exceptions to these generalizations, will become evident.

Bronchopneumonia

The hallmark of bronchopneumonia is the originating of inflammation in the bronchiolar–alveolar junction, as the name implies. This is correlated with an aerogenous portal of entry of the causative agents, involvement usually of cranioventral regions of the lungs, and a patchy or variegated gross appearance. The irregular lobular involvement is reflected in the older term **lobular pneumonia**.

The defenses of the healthy lung are remarkably effective. Whether or not inflammation results from the constant bombardment of the lung by inhaled irritants depends on the balance between the intensity of the insult and the effectiveness of local defense mechanisms at each structural level of airways and parenchyma. The bronchiolar–alveolar junctions are the loci of greatest vulnerability to damage by many types of inhaled particles and vapors, including droplet nuclei carrying infectious agents. There are three main reasons for the vulnerability of these regions. First, they are the major site of deposition of small particles (0.5–3.0 μm in diameter) capable of reaching deep lung. Second, the epithelium of bronchioles is probably susceptible to damage because it is not protected by the mucous blanket of larger airways nor an effective alveolar macrophage system. Third, the cellular (mostly macrophage) and noncellular material cleared from large volumes of alveolar parenchyma has to pass through the narrow lumen of its parent bronchiole, an easily plugged "funnel" or "bottleneck," especially where lack of collateral ventilation hampers expulsion of material.

Epidemiologic and experimental evidence indicates that the important infectious bronchopneumonias of animals usually develop only when the balance is tipped in favor of disease by an increase in number of pathogenic microorganisms reaching vulnerable bronchiolar–alveolar regions of the lung or when pulmonary defenses are impaired. In most situations, both of these circumstances are present. Increased exposure to pathogenic microorganisms is particularly likely to occur in crowding of animals collected from a variety of sources. This is often associated with lack of specific immunity to the organisms involved. Lack of nonspecific defense mechanisms occurs in congenital or acquired immunodeficiency states or is caused by a variety of factors impairing one or both of the mucociliary blanket and alveolar macrophage defensive systems. Dehydration, extreme chilling, viral infection, inhalation of toxic gases and particles, certain anesthetics, and ciliary abnormalities inhibit mucociliary clearance and can predispose to bacterial colonization. Functions of alveolar macrophages are impaired by severe chilling, starvation, viral infection, toxic gases, metabolic disorders such as uremia and acidosis, and immunosuppressants such as corticosteroids. Chronic diseases of heart or lungs also reduce pulmonary defensive capability.

Various combinations of the factors just mentioned exist in circumstances recognized as predisposing to a high risk of bronchopneumonia. The same holds true for the more aggressive lobar pneumonias. Most outbreaks are in young, intensively managed animals, especially soon after stresses associated with shipping. Mixing of animals with different microbial floras and levels of acquired immunity is often involved as well. Sporadic cases of bronchopneumonia in individual animals are likely to be associated with interactive predisposing causes such as debility, immunodeficiency, preexisting cardiopulmonary disease, and prolonged anesthesia or recumbency of illness. Aspiration of foreign material can cause bronchopneumonia but because of its severity more commonly has the distribution of a lobar pneumonia.

The characteristic cranioventral distribution of infectious bronchopneumonias in animals indicates that in these regions the balance between insult and defense is most precarious. This is supported by the fact that pneumonia caused by inhalation of acutely irritant particles or gases does not have a cranioventral distribution. All the reasons for the cranioventral involvement have not been determined. It is reasonable to hypothesize that there is increased deposition of infectious particles in these regions, that defenses are more easily compromised, or both. There is slightly increased deposition of particles in cranial regions. This is believed to be due to the shorter and more abruptly branching airways. Gravitational influences impeding clearance of cranioventral regions, and possibly leading to pooling or reflux of secretions, are probably more important contributory factors. The smaller size of ventral airspaces and their greater vulnerability to collapse or blockage may also be a factor.

Bacteria are the main causes of clinically significant bronchopneumonia, most commonly after pulmonary defenses have been lowered by viral infection, severe stress, or other predisposing factors. Many species of bacteria are involved, the particular set of agents varying with species and sometimes geographic location. In sheep and cattle, *Pasteurella* spp. and *Corynebacterium pyogenes* are common. In swine, *P. multocida*, *Haemophilus* spp., *C. pyogenes*, *Bordetella bronchiseptica*, and *Salmonella choleraesuis* are often involved. In horses, the chief offenders are *Streptococcus* spp. and *C. equi*. In dogs, *B. bronchiseptica*, *Klebsiella* spp., *Streptococcus* spp., *Staphylococcus* spp., and *Escherichia coli* are important. In cats, in which the disease is less common, *P. multocida* and a variety of other Gram-negative organisms are found. Bacteria generally tend to cause a suppurative pneumonia. Exceptions, such as the fulminating fibrinonecrotic pneumonias that can be caused by *Pasteurella* and *Haemophilus*, will be addressed later in the chapter. The involvement of viruses, mycoplasmas, and chlamydiae will also be considered further under specific pneumonias, as will their roles in causing the enzootic pneumonias of cattle, sheep, and swine.

The typical gross appearance of bronchopneumonia is of irregular consolidation in cranioventral regions. The cranial and middle lobes are most often affected in those species having well-defined lobation. Consolidated lung varies from dark red, through gray-pink, to more gray, depending on the age and nature of the process. Palpable firmness (consolidation) of the tissue is the single most important gross criterion of pneumonia. The extent to which there is a lobular or sublobular mosaic of consolidated, atelectatic, congested, and more normal lung tissue depends partly on the severity and rate of spread of the pneumonia and partly on the degree of septation. It is most common in relatively slow-spreading bronchopneumonias of ruminants and swine, which have well-developed septation. (Fig. 6.13C). The more uniform and rapidly spreading the pneumonia, the more homogeneous and extensive the consolidation. Even where complete lobes become involved, however, the bronchopneumonic pattern can often be detected on careful gross examination by the presence of multiple, small, evenly spaced, gray-white, bulging foci separated by narrow, deep red zones. The bulging pale foci denote areas of exudation centered on bronchioles, and the deeper red zones represent more congested, edematous, and atelectatic alveolar parenchyma in peripheral acinar regions. This gross pattern is more usual in bronchopneumonia of dogs and cats, which have rudimentary interlobular septa, and in the "enzootic" bronchopneumonias of ruminants and swine (Fig. 6.36A). The pleura overlying mild to moderately inflamed pulmonary parenchyma usually has its normal smooth, glistening sheen. Where the inflammatory process is severe, however, it extends to produce reddening, roughening, and superficial accumulation of yellow-gray fibrinous or fibrinopurulent exudate, indicating pleuritis (Fig. 6.28A). The cut surface of affected lung reflects the variability of involvement seen on the pleural surface. In catarrhal or suppurative bronchopneumonias, the section of consolidated lobules is moist; mucopurulent or purulent material can be expressed from small airways and can be seen in fluid or foamy state in the large airways. Frank abscesses can be present in severe suppurative inflammation (Fig. 6.14C). The cut surface of fibrinous inflammation, in contrast, has a dull, dryish appearance (Fig. 6.16B).

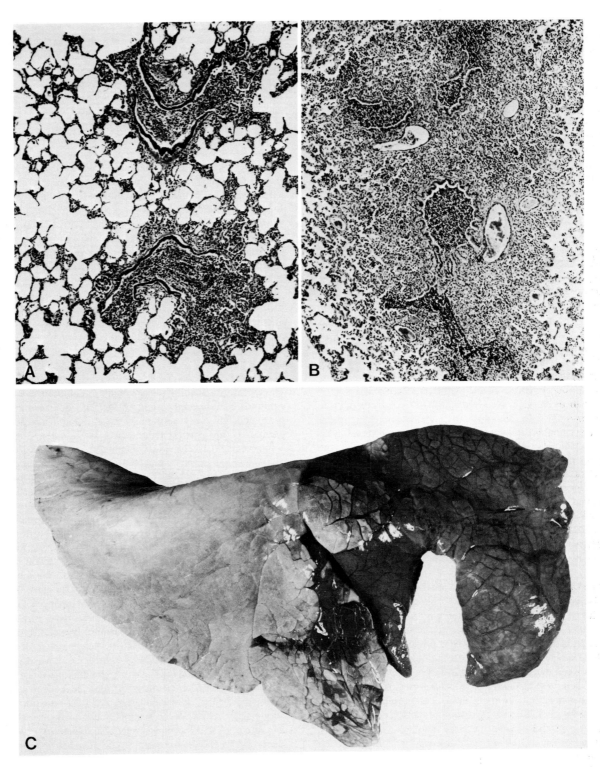

Fig. 6.13. Bronchopneumonia.   (**A**) Initial lesion of bronchopneumonia at bronchioloalveolar junction. Dog.   (**B**) Later stage of bronchopneumonia. Dog.   (**C**) Acute bronchopneumonia. Calf. Lobulation is emphasized in dark areas of consolidation by interlobular edema. Note focal pattern within affected lobules.

Histologically, the nidus of inflammation in bronchopneumonia is in the bronchiolar–alveolar junctions (Fig. 6.13A,B). In early bronchopneumonia, bronchioles and immediately adjacent alveoli are filled with neutrophils, and sometimes an admixture of various amounts of cell debris, mucus, fibrin, and macrophages. The bronchiolar epithelium varies from necrotic to hyperplastic, depending on the nature and pathogenicity of causative agents, and there is a mild acute inflammation in the peribronchiolar connective tissue. Bronchi often show similar but usually less severe changes. Necrotizing (Fig. 6.14A) or proliferative lesions indicating the possibility of prior viral infection may be present (see specific viral infections), but pathognomonic inclusion bodies can be found only occasionally in clinical material. Adenovirus inclusion bodies are the exception, and these inclusion bodies can be found readily in infection caused by this virus. Care must be taken not to interpret the apparently thickened epithelium of collapsed airways as evidence of epithelial hyperplasia. Alveoli peripheral to the severely inflamed bronchiolar regions are partially atelectatic and contain various amounts of edema or serofibrinous exudate, erythrocytes, macrophages, and a sprinkling of leukocytes. Vessels in the early acute stage are engorged and are responsible for the predominant red color of the lung noted macroscopically. Edematous or serofibrinous fluid can be found in interstitial sites but is not an important feature of this early mild to moderate form of catarrhal bronchopneumonia.

The spread of infection after its initial foothold in the bronchiolar–alveolar regions is mostly by airways, both proximally through bronchioles and bronchi and distally through alveolar ducts and alveoli within a respiratory acinus (Fig. 6.14B). The rate and extent of spread depends mainly on the balance between virulence of the causative agent and host defense. Rapid bacterial proliferation leads to severe suppurative pneumonias if pyogens (e.g., streptococci) are involved, and fibrinous through hemorrhagic and necrotizing pneumonias if highly toxigenic bacteria such as *Pasteurella haemolytica* and *Haemophilus pleuropneumoniae* are the cause. In the latter instances, the pneumonia is likely to take on the lobar characteristics; spread of infection through edematous interlobular septa can become important in these cases.

The time sequence of inflammatory events obviously varies with the severity and speed of onset, which in turn depend on the balance between the virulence of the agent and host defense. The red stage of consolidation is present for only 2 or 3 days in a typical bacterial pneumonia. The increasing amount of leukocytic or fibrinous exudation reduces capillary volume and results in an gray appearance within 5 to 7 days. Proliferation of alveolar type II cells can also occur during this period unless there is severe purulent or fibrinonecrotic inflammation. Variations on this theme will be dealt with under the headings of the special types of pneumonia or under those on the specific etiologic agents.

Just as the rate at which bronchopneumonia reaches maturity and the type of inflammation attained vary greatly, so the rate and degree of resolution vary. A catarrhal or mild purulent bronchopneumonia can begin to resolve within 7 to 10 days and the lung return to normal within 3 to 4 weeks. Once the agent has been overcome by the cellular and humoral defenses, mac-

rophages become the predominant cell. They phagocytose debris and aid in lysis of fibrin. The macrophages and extracellular debris are mostly cleared through the airways with the aid of coughing and collateral ventilation (if present). Treatment facilitates this process. This milder inflammation is not associated with significant damage to alveolar basement membranes or capillaries, and resolution can occur without recognizable trace. In these cases, there is a stage as the inflammation begins to wane when the alveoli are lined by alveolar type II cells. Transformation to type I cells occurs as the inflammatory exudate is cleared. A transitory stage of partial atelectasis is usually present between clearance of exudate and regeneration of the pulmonary parenchyma. If there is a residual bronchiolitis or bronchitis, however, and especially if the lack of collateral ventilation impedes expulsion of exudate from small airways, the atelectasis, bronchiolitis, and bronchitis persist. This probably explains why resolution of bronchopneumonia is frequently incomplete in ruminants and swine, and why cattle in particular are prone to develop chronic suppurative bronchiectasis and bronchopneumonia.

Severe bronchopneumonia causes death mostly by a combination of hypoxemia and toxemia. Complete resolution can occur but requires integrity of alveolar basement membranes, readily cleared exudate, and rapid killing of the infectious agent. Necrosis of alveolar septa, intractable exudate, or persistence of the agent therefore preclude complete resolution, even if the animal survives. Often all three conditions occur together. The resulting complications range from healing with scarring, through atelectasis, chronic bronchopneumonia, and bronchiectasis, to abscessation or necrosis with sequestration.

Atelectasis is both a prelude and a sequel to bronchopneumonia. As a complication of bronchopneumonia it follows resolution of parenchymal inflammation with persistence of obstructive bronchiolitis and bronchitis. Obstructive bronchiolitis can occur in three ways. In the simplest form there is a chronic bronchiolitis, with persistent plugging of the lumen by exudate. The second form occurs when there is necrosis of bronchiolar epithelium, presence of fibrin-rich exudate, and development of plugs or polypoid projections of granulation tissue (Fig. 6.15A). These can cause complete obliteration of the bronchiole if epithelial necrosis is total. An alternative finding is that reepithelialization of incompletely obliterating granulation tissue can occur to produce multiple, small, rudimentary lumina analagous to a recanalized thrombus (Fig. 6.15B). These bronchiolar lesions are referred to as bronchiolitis fibrosa obliterans. The third form of bronchiolar obstruction is by compression or constriction of peribronchiolar origin. This can be caused by constricting fibrous tissue, in which case it denotes a preceding severe acute inflammation and usually occurs with obliterative bronchiolitis, or by lymphoid proliferations, such as occur in *Mycoplasma* pneumonias.

Bronchopneumonia may become chronic. This is seen most commonly in cattle and, to a lesser extent, sheep and swine. It is reasonable to associate the tendency for poor resolution of bronchopneumonia with complete lobular septation and lack of collateral ventilation. The extent to which this is true is not known. The pathogenicity of the bacteria involved also undoubtedly plays some part. The lesions of chronic bronchopneumonia are

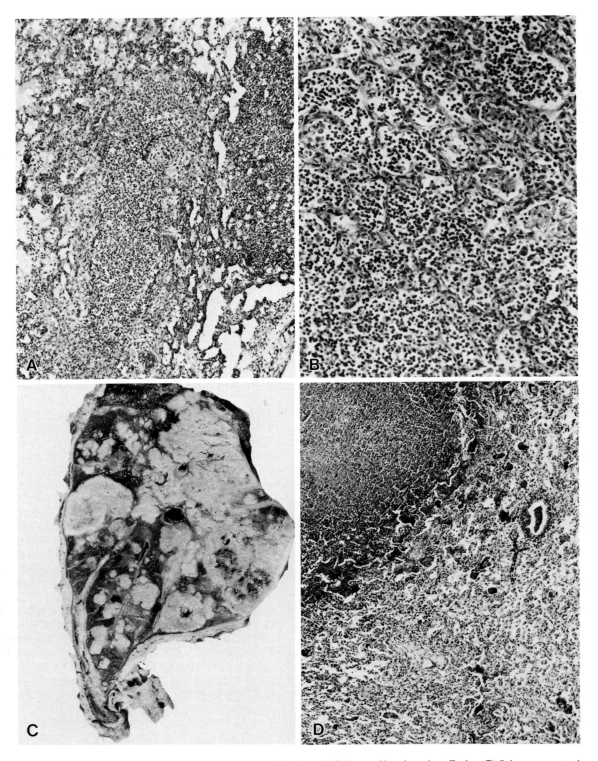

Fig. 6.14. (A) Acute bronchopneumonia based on necrotizing bronchiolitis caused by adenovirus. Foal. (B) Subacute suppurative bronchopneumonia. Pig. (C) Suppurative bronchopneumonia with abscessation and fibrinous pleuritis caused by streptococci. Horse. (D) Periphery of abscess in (C).

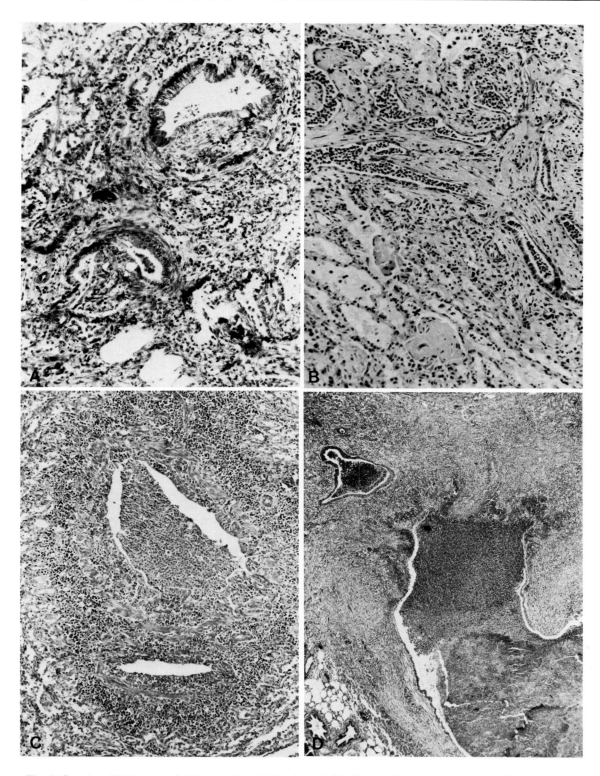

Fig. 6.15. (**A** and **B**) Patterns of obliterative bronchiolitis (bronchiolitis fibrosa obliterans). Calf. (**C** and **D**) Development of bronchogenic abscess in chronic suppurative bronchopneumonia. Sheep.

those of chronic suppuration with fibrosis. The suppurative lesions in ruminants and swine tend to involve mostly the airways (Fig. 6.15C,D), and in cattle especially, there is bronchiectasis and abscessation (see Bronchiectasis). Alveolar parenchyma is mainly atelectatic and fibrotic. Severe acute exudative pneumonias cause prominent widening of interlobular, subpleural, and peribronchial zones by accumulation of serofibrinous or fibrinopurulent exudate in the loose fascia and lymphatics. This becomes organized and visible as broad seams of moist fibrous tissue. It is mostly seen as an aftermath of lobar pneumonias in ruminants and swine and will be mentioned again under Lobar Pneumonia. It also affects the subpleural region and irregular interlobular septa of the horse as a sequel to severe exudative pneumonia. Organization of fibrin-containing pleural exudate often produces pleural adhesions.

Severe suppuration and abscessation of pulmonary parenchyma can be caused by pyogenic organisms. Suppuration is common in dogs when the pneumonia is caused by *Bordetella bronchiseptica*. The exudate has a grayish yellow, slimy quality. Bronchopneumonia in the horse commonly causes abscessation because the organisms are usually pyogenic streptococci (Fig. 6.14C,D). The suppuration usually begins deep in the consolidated areas. The alveolar tissues undergo necrosis in volumes large enough to be visible as many gray nodules, around each of which is a narrow hyperemic zone. These nodules coalesce, and most of the lobe might be converted into a fragile mass of dull gray detritus. Some of this can liquefy and be discharged into a bronchus so that a cavity remains. With *C. pyogenes,* typical abscesses occur in sheep, cattle, and swine. The abscesses might develop first in the alveolar tissue, or they might be associated with chronic suppurative bronchitis, bronchiolitis, and bronchiectasis. The abscesses can be numerous and very large. The reaction usually extends to the pleura to produce dense, adhesive pleuritis, or abscesses may fistulate to produce pleural empyema. Metastatic abscessation can occur in other organs. Erosion of a blood vessel might lead to severe fatal pulmonary hemorrhage. A variety of other bacteria can occasionally cause abscesses, the set of possible agents varying according to species of animal affected.

Lobar Pneumonia

Lobar pneumonia, as the term implies, is one in which entire pulmonary lobes, or major portions of lobes, are diffusely and uniformly consolidated. Pathogenetically, lobar pneumonias are rapidly confluent, fulminating bronchopneumonias in which gross evidence of bronchiolar orientation and spread is not evident. Since lobar pneumonias have this close relationship to bronchopneumonias, it is not surprising that separation between the two is difficult, often arbitrary, and prone to cause confusion. This is further complicated by the fact that even though large areas of uniform consolidation might be seen on gross examination, microscopic evidence often reveals orientation of the inflammation about bronchioles, and hence basically a bronchopneumonic pathogenesis. The term *lobar* is entrenched, however, and is useful to indicate a fulminating or highly aggressive bronchopneumonia. To use this term with as little confusion as possible, it is best applied as a gross designation of

extensive pneumonic consolidation in which the parenchymal involvement appears uniform (Fig. 6.16A). Exceptions to the uniform appearance are the necrotic foci that can develop, as in pneumonic pasteurellosis of cattle or contagious bovine pleuropneumonia (Fig. 6.16B,C), and the exudative distension of interlobular septa in ruminants and swine.

Since lobar pneumonia can be regarded as a fulminating bronchopneumonia, it follows that similar pathogenetic factors are involved. Lobar pneumonia is the result of overwhelming spread of the inflammatory process and is usually caused by the action of a virulent organism in an animal with severely impaired pulmonary defense. The prototype in animals is lobar pneumonia caused by *Pasteurella haemolytica* in cattle that have recently been stressed by transportation and that frequently have a predisposing respiratory viral infection. A strong correlation exists between a fulminating pulmonary inflammation and production of a profuse fibrinous exudate, as exemplified by the condition in cattle. Therefore, a tendency has arisen to use the terms lobar and fibrinous interchangeably. This is unwarranted, however, because although there is considerable overlap, not all lobar pneumonias are fibrinous and vice versa. Other than overwhelming *Pasteurella* infection, *Haemophilus* species sometimes cause lobar pneumonia in ruminants and swine. *Mycoplasma mycoides* is an etiologic agent in cattle and goats. Lobar pneumonia can occasionally be caused by *P. multocida* in cats. In horses, massive proliferation of streptococci or, occasionally, *Corynebacterium equi* can be responsible. Another cause in all species is the aspiration of foreign fluids or gastric contents.

Infectious lobar pneumonias diffusely affect large portions of cranioventral lung (Fig. 6.16A). Those caused by aspiration affect portions of lung lowermost at the time of aspiration, and therefore in a recumbent animal might involve the lateral zones of the caudal lobe of one side or the dorsal zones of both sides. As would be expected from their peracute or acute nature, lobar pneumonias are hemorrhagic, fibrinous, fibrinopurulent or necrotizing, and sometimes gangrenous (usually caused by aspiration). The gross appearance therefore varies with age of the lesion from reddish black through deep red, to reddish brown or gray. In all but the peracute hemorrhagic cases, there is usually roughening of the overlying pleura and a coating of fibrin. Two additional features are often seen in ruminants, swine, and to a lesser extent, horses. One is the prominent distension of interlobular septa by serofibrinous exudate, and the other is the development of irregular, discrete zones of necrosis with swollen pale borders (Fig. 6.16B). The cut surface in early cases exudes bloody fluid and, later, in the fibrinous lobar pneumonias, becomes grayish brown, finely granular, dry, and friable. Necrotic areas might become crumbly and cavitated.

The intial stage of red consolidation (hepatization) is characterized by hyperemia of alveolar capillaries and flooding of alveoli with serofibrinous exudate admixed with various amounts of hemorrhage, small numbers of alveolar macrophages, and neutrophils (Fig. 6.17A). The amount of fibrin precipitated in alveoli as dense, pink, fibrillar or more homogeneous clumps rapidly increases. It is accompanied by neutrophils, which predominate in some regions. The capillaries are compressed by

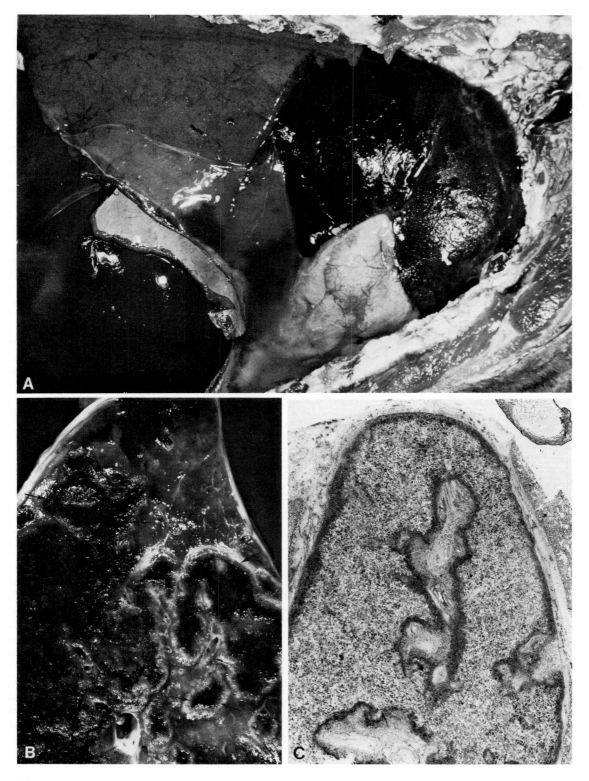

Fig. 6.16. (A) Acute, fibrinous, lobar pneumonia and serofibrinous pleuritis of pneumonic pasteurellosis. Lamb. (B) Areas of necrosis (arrows) in lobar pneumonia. Cow. (C) Necrotic lobule in contagious bovine pleuropneumonia. Connective tissues of septa and surrounding bronchioles and blood vessels are viable and separated from necrotic parenchyma by zones of leukocytes.

pressure of exudate, and many become occluded by thrombi. This is the stage of red-brown or gray consolidation, depending on the degree of ischemia and extent of hemorrhage and lysis of extravasated red cells. During this time, the interlobular septa (when present) and perivascular, peribronchial, and subpleural sheaths become widely distended by serofibrinous or fibrinous exudate within the loose connective tissue, and especially in the lymphatics. The latter often become greatly distended by fibrin thrombi (Fig. 6.17B). Small airways in affected regions are filled either with a purulent exudate or more fibrinous exudate similar to that filling alveoli. Arteries and especially veins passing through severely inflamed regions can develop vasculitis by local extension across their walls, and occasionally thrombi are formed. There is a tendency for leukocytic aggregates in alveoli to become condensed or spindle-shaped (oat-shaped) under the influence of toxins from Gram-negative bacteria such as *Pasteurella* (Fig. 6.17C) and to the development of necrotic foci (Fig. 6.17D). A feature common to most lobar pneumonias is massive proliferation of bacteria, which can be readily detected even in sections stained by hematoxylin and eosin. They are especially prominent within developing necrotic foci and tend to be concentrated close to the leukocytic boundary zones.

This description of lobar pneumonia has drawn heavily on the fibrinous lobar pneumonias, best exemplified by pneumonic pasteurellosis in cattle. However, the features of predominantly fibrinous pneumonia in a series of affected cattle often present a mix of lobar and bronchopneumonic patterns. This should be expected as the difference between lobar and bronchopneumonia is mostly a matter of degree.

The **complications** of lobar pneumonia are obviously more frequent and serious than those of the less severe bronchopneumonias. Death is frequent, usually with accompanying pleuritis, and sometimes with pericarditis. If the animal survives, resolution without some degree of scarring is well nigh impossible. Extensive organization by granulation tissue leading to fleshy fibrous tissue (carnification) is likely, as is chronic abscessation. Peritonitis may arise by hematogenous spread of the infection or direct extension from the pleura through the diaphragmatic lymphatics. Additional complications include toxemic degeneration of parenchymatous organs, endocarditis, fibrinous polyarthritis, meningitis, and hemolytic icterus. A late complication might be empyema of the pleural cavity, following rupture of an abscess peripherally. Erosion and rupture of an abscess into a bronchus can cause a rapid onset of purulent bronchopneumonia, or hemorrhage if an artery is affected.

Interstitial Pneumonia

Diffuse or patchy damage to alveolar septa is the essential feature of interstitial pneumonia. It can be caused by many forms of pulmonary injury. The lack of a completely satisfactory morphologic designation embracing the variants of interstitial pulmonary disease has led to a confusing array of terms. Two terms are most commonly used: **interstitial pneumonia** and **diffuse fibrosing alveolitis**. The former is preferred because it more appropriately covers the necessarily broad range of morphologic, etiologic, and pathogenetic aspects. Other relevant

terms, with emphasis on more chronic diseases, are chronic diffuse infiltrative lung disease and diffuse interstitial pulmonary fibrosis.

Interstitial pneumonias have been thought of as chronic inflammatory conditions in which there is predominantly a proliferative response involving alveolar walls and supporting stroma. However, increasing attention has been drawn to a variety of circumstances in which there is acute diffuse damage of alveolar walls. This causes an early intraalveolar exudative phase, which can be quickly followed by proliferative and fibrotic responses. The acute pulmonary injury can be caused by, or associated with, a wide variety of conditions, such as severe viral pneumonia, chemical lung injury, acute pancreatitis, shock, and septicemia. Often there is superimposed toxicity caused by the high concentrations of oxygen used therapeutically. In human medicine, a variety of terms were used that referred to the various circumstances under which acute damage occurred, for instance, "shock lung," "respirator lung," and "traumatic wet lung." Clinically, however, the common feature is acute respiratory distress, and so the collective term "adult respiratory distress syndrome" has come into increasing usage. The syndrome was originally called acute respiratory distress syndrome in adults, to distinguish it from neonatal respiratory distress syndrome in human infants. For veterinary medicine, it is more apt to refer to acute respiratory distress syndrome because there is no established need to distinguish between the adult form and the less often encountered neonatal form. The clinician evaluating a patient with acute respiratory distress and the pathologist interpreting an acute interstitial pneumonia (alveolitis) are both dealing with acute pulmonary injury and therefore need to consider the same set of differential diagnoses.

Most of the literature on interstitial pneumonia and related entities refers to human diseases or experimental animal models of human diseases. There has been preoccupation in veterinary medicine with the common and economically important infectious lobar and bronchopneumonias. Interstitial pneumonias do comprise a significant proportion of veterinary diseases, however, particularly those of infectious, toxic, or allergic cause.

Pathogenetically, interstitial pneumonia results from diffuse or patchy damage to alveolar septa. The absence of obvious orientation of the lesions around small airways differentiates interstitial pneumonia from bronchopneumonia. Grossly, the lesions are distributed widely throughout the lungs, often with greater involvement of dorsocaudal regions (Figs. 6.18A,C and 6.20A,B). This pattern is in sharp contrast to the cranioventral distribution of affected regions in the common infectious lobar and bronchopneumonias.

The alveolar septal damage is caused by a blood-borne insult in most instances. This accounts for the widespread or random distribution of lesions within affected acini, as opposed to the centriacinar localization of damage caused by most inhaled irritants. There are two notable exceptions to this generalization. One is that certain blood-borne chemicals exert their toxic effect only after they are metabolized to reactive intermediates by microsomal enzyme systems, particularly monooxygenases (mixed-function oxidases). Depending on the chemical and the species of animal affected, damage can be limited to nonciliated

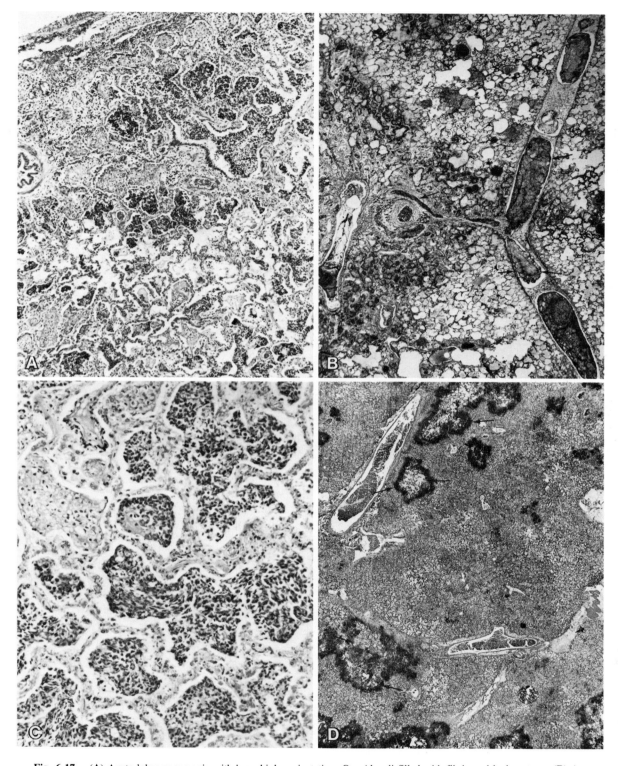

Fig. 6.17. **(A)** Acute lobar pneumonia with bronchiolar orientation. Ox. Alveoli filled with fibrin and leukocytes. **(B)** Acute fibrinous lobar pneumonia. Ox. Fibrin clots in septal and perivascular lymphatics (arrows). **(C)** Streaming, oat-shaped leukocytes. Pneumonic pasteurellosis. Ox. **(D)** Necrotic foci (arrows) in acute fibrinous pneumonia of pasteurellosis. Pig. Necrotic tissue surrounded by dark-staining zones of leukocytes.

bronchiolar epithelial (Clara) cells, sparing the pulmonary alveolar parenchyma, even though the parent chemical is in the blood. The effect of 3-methylindole in the horse is the best known example in domestic animals. The second exception to the generalization is that inhalation of irritants that become widely distributed in the lung causes sufficiently diffuse damage to present as interstitial pneumonia. Severe, acute diffuse damage is associated with inhalation of high concentrations of toxic gases or fumes because there is not an appreciable concentration gradient of the toxic substance between small airways and distal portions of the pulmonary acini. Inhalation of 100% oxygen is the best example. The pneumoconioses, on the other hand, are chronic progressive lesions caused by inhalation of inorganic dusts. Here, although there might initially be a greater tendency for the granulomatous or fibrotic foci to be located close to terminal airways, this often becomes obscured by the time the lesions progress to the point of causing clinical pulmonary dysfunction. There is no precise information explaining why interstitial pneumonias, whether of hematogenous or aerogenous origin, tend to be more severe in dorsocaudal regions of the lung.

Histologically, the interstitial pneumonias as defined here can range from acute to chronic. Although the term implies that the inflammatory response takes place predominantly within the alveolar walls and the interstitial tissues of the lung, interstitial pneumonias of acute onset have an initial phase in which the most obvious feature is exudate into alveolar lumina. The interstitial components soon come to predominate, however, if the animal survives. The apparent paradox that some interstitial pneumonias can have an acute exudative phase is the principal reason for the alternative term "diffuse alveolitis." It was also the reason for the initial designation of acute interstitial pneumonia in cattle as "atypical" interstitial pneumonia.

As in other organs, the morphologic responses following damage by a large variety of agents have many features in common. The lesions therefore frequently lack etiologic specificity. Acute injury, whether of toxic, metabolic, or infectious origin, causes damage principally to alveolar–capillary endothelial cells and type I epithelial cells. Whether the endothelium or epithelium is damaged first depends on the nature, portal of entry, intensity of the insult, and to some extent, the species affected. Usually, however, the alveolar type I cells eventually suffer most damage because of their poor reparative capacity and inability to regenerate. During this acute phase, the most dramatic features of the lesion are flooding of alveoli with serofibrinous exudate, and congestion and edema of alveolar walls. Fibrin, other serum proteins, and cell debris frequently condense to form hyaline membranes lining airspaces, or aggregates plugging their lumina (Fig. 6.18B). There is usually some admixture of leukocytes and erythrocytes in the alveolar exudate, and an initial accumulation of mixed leukocytes within the alveolar interstitium that tends to become mostly mononuclear cells if the inflammation persists. Replacement of necrotic type I epithelium takes place on intact basement membranes by proliferation of type II epithelium, as described under Alveolar Response to Injury. The resulting lining of alveoli by cuboidal cells (epithelialization) is a common feature of subacute to chronic interstitial pneumonias (Figs. 6.18D and 6.19A–C). Once the

inflammation has subsided, and if there is not severe scarring of the alveolar wall, complete resolution can be effected by differentiation of type II cells into type I epithelium.

Proliferation of alveolar type II cells marks the shift from the exudative to the proliferative stage of interstitial pneumonia. Onset of fibrosis is a critical feature of the proliferative phase because it is irreversible, at least in its mature form. Fibroblast proliferation can occur as early as 72 hr after severe alveolar damage. It is most evident when alveoli are filled with fibrinous exudate. Immature or "pro-" fibroblasts can appear within alveoli in the lungs by 3 days after severe fibrinous exudation, such as caused by paraquat toxicity. Mature fibroblasts can be seen by 4 days, and collagen fibers can be detected histologically by 5 to 7 days. Interstitial fibrosis also occurs in such instances, though not to such a dramatic degree. It occurs more rapidly when there is considerable interstitial edema or serofibrinous exudation. Both intra- and interalveolar (interstitial) fibrosis, therefore, are sequelae to severe exudative lesions and can be a striking feature by 14 days after onset. If the animal survives and residual scarring is present, it is no longer possible to determine the relative contributions of intra- and interalveolar fibrosis (Fig. 6.19C). Chronic, smoldering lesions in which there are prominent interstitial cellular accumulations, mostly of mononuclear cells, cause fibrosis within the alveolar walls.

The rate of fibrosis is therefore heavily dependent on the intensity of inflammation. Studies on mechanisms underlying fibrosis focus on two major areas. One is the biochemistry of collagen; the other the nature of factors influencing collagen synthesis and degradation. A relative increase of type I collagen (dense fibers of high tensile strength) over type III (reticulin-type fibers) occurs wherever active fibroplasia can be recognized histologically or where there is extensive scarring. There might be an early, transient increase in type III collagen in conditions where the rate of accumulation of fibrous tissue is slow.

Factors influencing the balance of synthesis and degradation of collagen are extremely complex. Potentially any of the cellular and biochemical alterations in an inflammatory site might have an influence, and presumably most of them do. Biochemical mediators, disruptions between cells and their normal extracellular matrices, and cell-to-cell interactions are presumed to be involved.

If the animal survives, most acute interstitial pneumonias of animals resolve with various amounts of residual scarring (Fig. 6.19C). Chronic, progressive inflammation is not ofen encountered in animals. The chronic inflammation, where a specific cause can be identified, is usually associated with persistence of, or repeated exposure to, the causative agent (e.g., dusts, drugs, or infectious agents). Often, immunologic processes are known or suspected to be at least partly involved in the pathogenetic mechanisms. In those instances where a specific cause cannot be identified, immunologic mechanisms are also often incriminated.

The central features of chronic interstitial pneumonia are intraalveolar accumulation of various mononuclear cells (mostly macrophages), proliferation and persistence of alveolar type II cells, and interstitial thickening by accumulations of lymphoid cells and fibrous tissue. Granulomatous interstitial pneumonia is

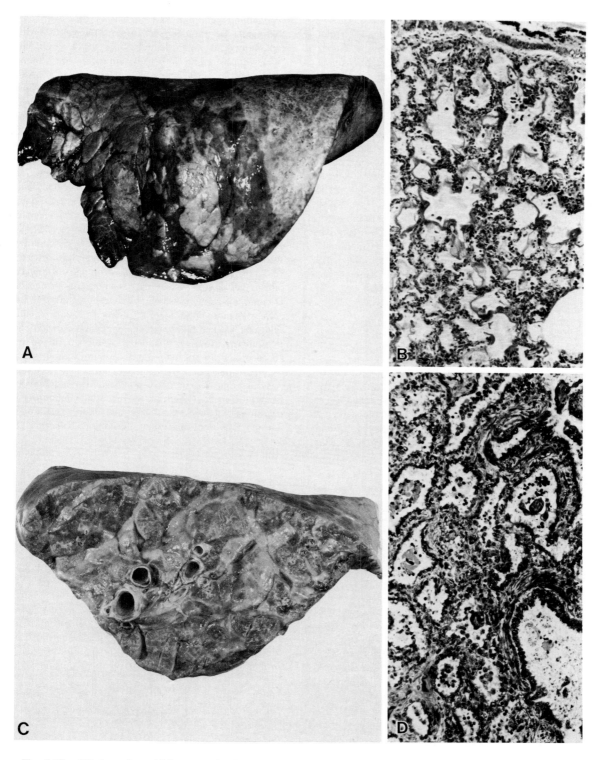

Fig. 6.18. (**A**) Acute interstitial pneumonia. Ox. The lung has failed to collapse. Subpleural and interstitial emphysema is present. (**B**) Acute interstitial pneumonia caused by *Zieria arborescens* poisoning. Ox. Diffuse alveolar wall damage, with edema and hyaline membrane formation. (**C**) Acute interstitial pneumonia. Ox. Cross section of caudal lobe. Emphysema and edema in interlobular septa and around vessels and airways. (**D**) Acute interstitial pneumonia. Ox. Note prominent epithelialization of thickened alveolar walls.

probably the most common chronic form (Fig. 6.20). Hyperplasia of smooth muscle and distortion of airspaces ("honeycombing") are sometimes present in more advanced cases, not necessarily in proportion to one another. Hyperplasia of smooth muscle, for instance, is a prominent feature of chronic progressive pneumonia (maedi) in sheep (Fig. 6.27C).

A large variety of agents representing all major etiologic categories of disease can cause interstitial pneumonia. The list of recognized causes or associations is much larger for humans than for animals. Most of the recognized interstitial pneumonias in animals are caused either by infectious or parasitic agents or by toxins entering via the digestive tract. Hypersensitivity pneumonitis (extrinsic allergic alveolitis) and pneumoconiosis occur occasionally, as described later. Occupational exposure to dusts, gases, fumes, and vapors, which are the largest groups of causative agents in humans, are essentially lacking in animals for obvious reasons. Other important categories of interstitial pneumonia in humans for which there is little or no specific information concerning analogous conditions in animals are those caused by adverse drug reactions and those associated with collagen–vascular disorders such as systemic lupus erythematosus and rheumatoid arthritis.

Most interstitial pneumonias in animals are infectious in origin and are caused by viral, bacterial, fungal, or parasitic diseases (Table 6.1). Many different agents are involved; most produce pulmonary lesions as the result of systemic or blood-borne infection, for example, toxoplasmosis (Fig. 6.21A,B).

Most **inhaled viruses**, particularly myxoviruses, can infect both airway and alveolar epithelium. When uncomplicated viral pneumonia occurs, the lesion is centered on bronchioles and

adjacent alveolar parenchyma and is therefore a bronchopneumonia by pathogenetic pattern. Because interstitial accumulation of leukocytes rapidly becomes the dominant feature of the lesions, these viral pneumonias are often termed "interstitial." Since the interstitial response in most instances is clearly associated with bronchioles and adjacent alveoli, such cases can be distinguished from the more characteristic interstitial pneumonias not orientated on bronchioles. For these viral bronchopneumonias a combined morphologic designation of **bronchointerstitial pneumonia** is preferable.

The pattern of viral pneumonia resulting from aerogenous exposure is affected by the extent to which viral proliferation is limited by the immune system and by the cell tropism of the virus. With influenza virus infection in mice, for instance, limitation of viral proliferation to airways is an important determinant in minimizing the severity of the disease. Cell tropism is important in pneumonia such as that caused by certain virulent strains of feline calicivirus, in which type I alveolar epithelial cells are principally affected following aerosol infection. Although early lesions are in regions adjacent to bronchioles, this orientation becomes obscured by 4 days postinfection, when the damage is more widespread.

Severe diffuse pulmonary parenchymal damage caused by inhaled gases, fumes, or vapors is rarely encountered in animals because they do not have the occupational exposures that are usually responsible in humans. Occasional poisoning of cattle, pigs, and chickens by nitrogen dioxide generated in corn silos has been suspected but never proven. Acute pulmonary injury is occasionally seen in animals trapped in burning buildings. When asphyxiation is not immediate, the combined chemical and heat

TABLE 6.1

Causes of Interstitial Pneumonia in Animals

Acute	Chronic
Infections	Infections
Principally systemic viral, bacterial, or parasitic involvement, e.g., canine distemper, feline infectious peritonitis, septicemic salmonellosis in calves and pigs, toxoplasmosis, and acute parasitism by lungworm or migrating ascarid larvae	Principally systemic viral, bacterial, fungal, or parasitic involvement, e.g., ovine progressive pneumonia, chronic African swine fever, tuberculosis, pneumocystosis, histoplasmosis, and some verminous pneumonias
Inhaled chemicals	Inhaled inorganic dusts (pneumoconioses)
Oxygen (>50% concentration)	Silicosis in horses
Smoke	Ingested toxins or precursors
Ingested toxins or precursors	Pyrrolizidine alkaloids in horses, pigs, cattle, and sheep; Crofton weed toxicity in horses
L-Tryptophan, *Perilla* mint ketone, and furanoterpenoid from moldy sweet potatoes in cattle; paraquat and kerosene in dogs	Hypersensitivity
Adverse drug reactions	Hypersensitivity pneumonitis in cattle and horses; microfilariae of *Dirofilaria immitis* in dogs
Uncertain	Irradiation
Hypersensitivity	Experimental studies in dogs and other laboratory animals
Acute hypersensitivity pneumonitis	Collagen–vascular disorders
Endogenous metabolic/toxic conditions	Uncertain
Shock (particularly endotoxic)	Possibly canine systemic lupus erythematosus
Disseminated intravascular coagulation	Unknown
Uremia, pancreatitis	Occasionally in all species
Unknown	Diffuse fibrosing alveolitis in cattle
Acute/subacute interstitial pneumonia in a variety of species, particularly dogs	

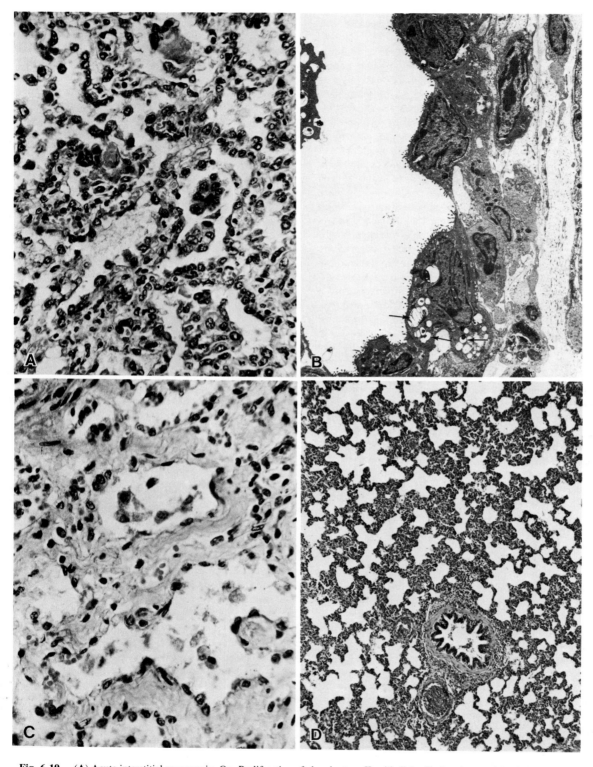

Fig. 6.19. (**A**) Acute interstitial pneumonia. Ox. Proliferation of alveolar type II epithelial cells forming partial cuboidal lining of alveoli 4 or 5 days after onset of damage. (**B**) Ultrastructure of (**A**), showing lining of alveolus by type II cells, some of which contain characteristic lamellar inclusions (arrows). (**C**) Aftermath of acute interstitial pneumonia. Ox. Fibrosis of alveolar walls and persistence of type II cells. (**D**) Acute interstitial pneumonia in salmonellosis. Pig. Thickening of alveolar walls by leukocytes.

effect of smoke can cause widespread epithelial necrosis and exudation, and death within a few days.

With the advent of increased attention to intensive care units in veterinary hospitals, oxygen toxicity is emerging as an important form of inhaled chemical injury in animals. Most cases of oxygen toxicity are superimposed on the preexisting pulmonary abnormality, which necessitates oxygen therapy in the first instance. Susceptibility to oxygen toxicity varies with species, previous exposure history, metabolic state, and the severity of preexisting pulmonary damage, if any. Concentrations over 50%, particularly in the range 80–100%, can produce damage in already compromised lungs after 2 or 3 days of exposure. The lesion is nonspecific, consisting of damage to alveolar–capillary endothelium, necrosis of bronchiolar epithelium and of alveolar type I cells, and serofibrinous exudation. The relative proportion of these changes also varies with species. Reactive oxygen radicals (superoxide, hydroxyl, and excited singlet oxygen) are favored as the active metabolites. These are believed, in turn, to damage cell membranes by lipid peroxidation, to inactivate sulfhydryl-containing enzymes, and to damage a variety of macromolecules, including DNA. The enhanced toxic effect of oxygen in the period shortly after acute pulmonary injury of some other cause has important implications for therapeutic use of high oxygen concentrations. It also raises the possibility that alveolar epithelial cells exert some controlling influence on proliferating fibroblasts.

Ingested toxins or precursors are second in importance to infections as causes of interstitial pneumonia in animals generally. In cattle, they are probably the most important cause. Several plant or feed-related substances can cause a nonspecific **acute interstitial pneumonia in cattle.** L-Tryptophan and 3-methylindole are implicated in causing the pasture-related form in cattle (commonly referred to as "acute bovine pulmonary emphysema and edema" or "fog fever"). Similar pulmonary damage in cattle is caused by *Perilla* mint, moldy sweet potato, and stinkwood (*Zieria arborescens*) poisoning. Pulmonary lesions are also produced in horses, pigs, sheep, and cattle by pyrrolizidine alkaloids from a variety of plants (mostly *Crotalaria, Trichodesma,* and *Senecio*). Crofton weed (*Eupatorium adenophorum*) is another poisonous plant that produces chronic interstitial pneumonia in horses. Toxicity is associated with ingestion of the flowering plant, but the nature of the toxin is not known. The lungs have a multifocal chronic interstitial pneumonia in which proliferation and metaplasia of alveolar epithelial cells and fibroplasia are the prominent features.

Pneumotoxins produce different patterns of pulmonary response according to the specific toxin and the species of animal affected. This appears to be due at least in part to the distribution of monooxygenase enzymes among pulmonary cells potentially at risk, because the actual damage often requires production of reactive metabolites from parent toxins by the action of the monooxygenase system.

Poisoning of dogs and cats by the herbicide paraquat is another common toxic cause of acute interstitial pneumonia in animals. As with most other pneumotoxins, paraquat produces a nonspecific, acute to subacute lesion. Cases of malicious poisoning are more likely to cause fulminating pulmonary edema and hemorrhage because of the high dosage, whereas in acciden-

tal poisonings there is more often time for hyperplasia of alveolar type II cells and fibroplasia to be superimposed on the earlier exudative changes. Affected animals are often placed on oxygen therapy, but it is difficult or impossible to determine whether oxygen might have exacerbated the lesions because of the severity of the preexisting damage caused by paraquat. Poisoning by the rodenticide α-naphthylthiourea (ANTU) also causes respiratory distress, but it causes pulmonary edema and pleural effusion without the tendency to epithelial hyperplasia and fibroplasia if the animal survives. There is insufficient damage to components of the alveolar wall for it to be included in the interstitial pneumonias as defined here.

Little is known concerning pulmonary damage caused by therapeutic use of drugs in animals. Development of acute pulmonary edema as part of the anaphylactic or anaphylactoid shock caused by drugs such as penicillin is widely recognized but not well documented.

Inhaled inorganic dusts (pneumoconioses) are uncommon in animals because they lack occupational exposures to dusts, which are the basis for pneumoconioses in humans. There are old reports of asbestosis in animals with industrially related exposure. A very mild form of pneumoconiosis was found in ponies used in coal mines. There were multiple compact aggregates of coal dust, particularly around small vessels adjacent to terminal and respiratory bronchioles. The amount of fibrosis was minimal. More recently, there have been reports of silicate pneumoconiosis or diatomaceous pneumoconiosis in animals kept in zoos. The minimal to mild, clinically insignificant lesions mostly consist of focal dust granulomas associated with lymphatics in perivascular, peribronchiolar, and other interstitial sites. Similar foci can be seen in the lungs of many animals living in a dusty environment, but the amount of dust retention appears to be greater in birds.

Silicate pneumoconiosis in horses is the only reported clinically important pneumoconiosis in animals. Multifocal granulomatous interstitial pneumonia with interstitial fibrosis (Fig. 6.21C) is associated with exercise intolerance of various degrees. Necrosis and mineralization are frequently present in the centers of granulomas in the most severely affected lungs (Fig. 6.21D). Small crystalline particles are difficult to detect in the macrophages by light microscopy but are plentiful when examined electron microscopically. The type of silicate responsible is cristobalite, one of the highly fibrogenic species.

In its most specific sense, **hypersensitivity pneumonitis (extrinsic allergic alveolitis)** refers to pulmonary disease caused by inhalation of organic antigens. Naturally occurring hypersensitivity pneumonitis in animals occurs in cattle and, to a lesser extent, horses. Lesions are those of a lymphocytic interstitial pneumonia. Noncaseating granulomas can be found in the farmer's lung analog in cattle, caused by spores of thermophilic actinomycetes (especially *Micropolyspora faeni*) from moldy hay. A lymphocytic and plasmacytic bronchitis and bronchiolitis is frequently a prominent feature of the disease in cattle and horses.

There is probably some degree of mixed immediate and delayed-type hypersensitivity in many infectious and parasitic conditions. An example of the latter is the interstitial pneumonia associated with microfilaria of *Dirofilaria immitis* in dogs with

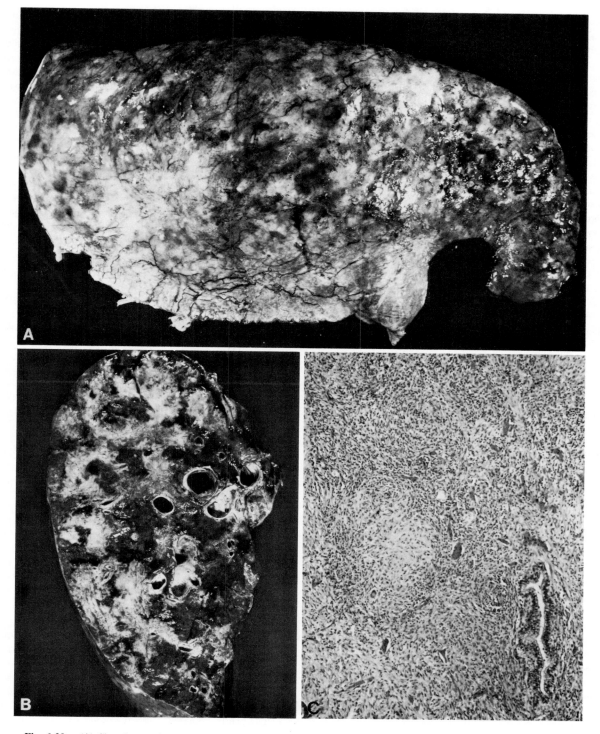

Fig. 6.20. (A) Chronic granulomatous interstitial pneumonia of undetermined cause. Horse. (B) Section of caudal lobe of (A), showing multiple, confluent foci of consolidation. (A and B courtesy of T. E. Dorr.) (C) Effacement of pulmonary parenchyma by granulomatous inflammation.

both occult and nonoccult heartworm disease. Immunologic mechanisms will undoubtedly be found to play some part in the pathogenesis of virtually all chronic interstitial pneumonias.

This is a convenient place to consider **eosinophilic syndromes** involving the lung. As would be expected of any set of diseases grouped on the basis of the presence of a particular inflammatory cell, these represent an ill-defined, poorly understood mixture. Little is known of the range of eosinophilic involvement of animal lungs, though their presence in helminth infections and presumed allergic bronchitis is well recognized. The term ''pulmonary infiltrates with eosinophilia'' has come into use to include all cases in which, as the name implies, there is radiologic evidence of interstitial pulmonary infiltrates together with a blood eosinophilia. Eosinophils may be present in bronchoalveolar lavage fluid, with or without the blood eosinophilia. Since affected animals usually recover with corticosteroid treatment, the precise nature of the pulmonary lesion and the etiology often remain uncertain. The best known causes of pulmonary infiltrates with eosinophilia are dirofilariasis in dogs and migrating helminth larvae in many species. Involvement in hypersensitivity pneumonitis, allergic bronchitis, and ''asthmatic'' states is more often suggested than clearly proven. Whether pulmonary infiltrates with eosinophilia can be part of adverse drug responses or immune-mediated disorders can only be determined by extensive, careful studies. ''Pulmonary infiltrates with eosinophilia'' is not a diagnosis, and there should be concerted efforts to make the term redundant by identification of the specific disease responsible in each case.

A variety of **endogenous metabolic** and **toxic conditions** can cause acute pulmonary injury leading to inflammatory edema or more severe alveolar wall damage and serofibrinous exudation, as described for acute interstitial pneumonia. Acute uremia frequently causes severe pulmonary edema. Acute pancreatitis in dogs is occasionally associated with radiologic evidence of pulmonary edema. Shocklike states, massive burns and trauma, and prolonged surgery can also produce acute pulmonary injury, and these are also a major cause of the acute respiratory distress syndrome in humans. Endotoxin is suspected to play an important role in many instances, for example, shock associated with severe enteric diseases in horses. But the situation is extremely complex because essentially all mediators implicated in any form of acute inflammation have to be considered. Involvement of clotting factors starting with activation of Hageman factor, the alternate pathway of complement activation, and arachidonic acid metabolites are all likely, but most attention is on derivatives of the arachidonic acid cascade. A summary of current understanding of the endotoxin-induced pulmonary injury is that there is an early transient severe pulmonary hypertension followed several hours later by an increased vascular and alveolar-wall permeability phase lasting up to 36 hr. The initial hypertension appears to be due mainly to release of thromboxane and prostaglandin $F_{2\alpha}$, which are derived from the cyclooxygenase pathway of arachidonic acid metabolism. Their effect is to some extent counteracted by prostacyclin, another endoperoxide derived from the cyclooxygenase pathway. The subsequent increased permeability phase is associated with aggregation of leukocytes, mostly neutrophils, in pulmonary capillaries. Exactly how this is brought about is less clear, but hydroperox-

ides (hydroperoxyeicosatetraenoic acids, hydroxyeicosatetraenoic acids, and leukotrienes) derived from the lipoxygenase pathway of arachidonic acid metabolism appear to be involved.

Acute and chronic interstitial pneumonias of unknown cause are encountered in all species, but the sporadic reports do not enable assessment of their prevalence. Since the clinicopathologic picture of interstitial pneumonias is often nonspecific, many are not identified by a specific cause and go unreported. In cattle, acute interstitial pneumonia occurs in calves and feedlot cattle. Chronic interstitial pneumonia (diffuse fibrosing alveolitis) of adult cattle has been described. In pet animals, particularly dogs, acute interstitial pneumonia is occasionally seen where there is no evidence of access to a pneumotoxin such as paraquat. There seems sometimes to be an association with cardiac insufficiency. An acute shocklike pulmonary injury occurs in terminal cardiovascular collapse. Similar lesions, often with superimposed oxygen toxicity, are seen in animals that have been treated in intensive care units.

Acute Respiratory Distress Syndrome

Acute respiratory distress syndrome is a term used to refer to the clinical signs associated with acute pulmonary injury of diverse causes. Clinically, there is acute onset of respiratory distress, with rapid death, or there might be temporary recovery followed by progressive worsening of respiratory function and death in one to several weeks. Functionally, there is hypoxemia caused by intrapulmonary shunting of blood or mismatching of ventilation and perfusion. There are also reduced compliance and decreased functional residual capacity. Radiographically, there are widespread alveolar infiltrates or mixed alveolar and interstitial patterns. Lesions in affected lungs are usually of a nonspecific, acute to subacute interstitial pneumonia. The causes of acute respiratory distress are the following:

Acute viral and bacterial pneumonias
Septicemia and endotoxemia
Shock, massive burns or trauma, and prolonged surgery
Aspiration of liquids
Chemical or drug toxicity
Uremia and pancreatitis
Disseminated intravascular coagulation
Oxygen toxicity

Bronchointerstitial Pneumonia

The most important attribute of a classification scheme in pathology is that it provides an effective framework for diagnosing, interpreting, and conveying information about disease processes. From this point of view the designation of certain pneumonias as bronchointerstitial is justified. As referred to previously under Interstitial Pneumonia, bronchointerstitial pneumonia is caused commonly by aerogenous viral infections, particularly myxoviruses. The essential features of the lesion are that it is centered on bronchioles and that interstitial accumulation of lymphocytes is a prominent feature. Sequential studies reveal that the early lesion is one of bronchiolar epithelial necrosis and accumulation of acute inflammatory components in the bronchioles and adjacent alveoli. Pathogenetically, the lesion is therefore a bronchopneumonia. Because of the mainly cell-me-

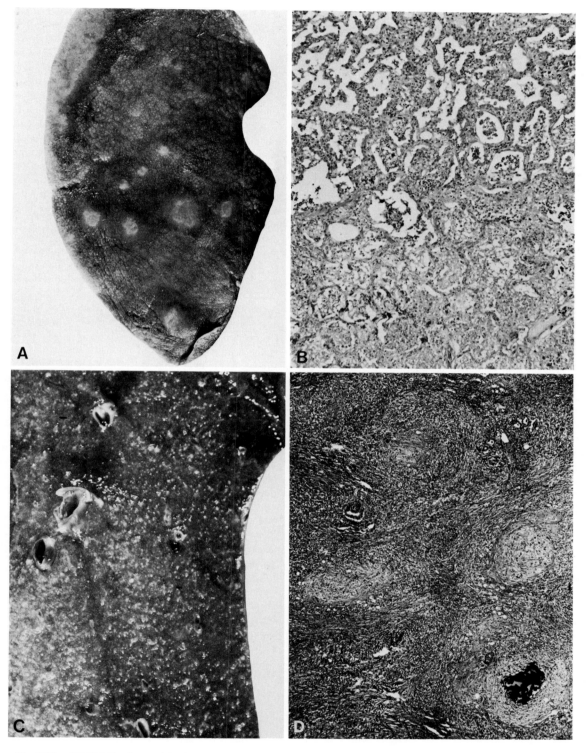

Fig. 6.21. (**A**) Multifocal necrotizing interstitial pneumonia. Toxoplasmosis. Cat. (**B**) Histology of periphery of a necrotic focus in (**A**). (**C**) Multifocal granulomatous pneumonia of silicate pneumoconiosis. Horse. (**D**) Details of granulomas in (**C**). Some have central necrosis or mineralization.

diated immune responses that develop, however, accumulation of lymphocytes in the peribronchiolar and adjacent alveolar interstitium becomes the dominant feature (Fig. 6.22A). This has resulted in the lesions being referred to as interstitial pneumonia. It is important, however, from the standpoint of pattern recognition and interpretation, that this type of response, which is orientated on bronchioles, be differentiated from the interstitial pneumonias that do not have a bronchiolar orientation. Hence the special designation bronchointerstitial pneumonia. This is not merely an academic exercise, because careful analysis of whether parenchymal abnormalities are centered on bronchioles is one of the most important criteria in the histologic diagnosis and interpretation of pneumonias. In ruminants and swine, *Mycoplasma* infection is the most common cause of bronchointerstitial pneumonia (Fig. 6.22B).

Abscesses of the Lung and Embolic Pneumonia

Pulmonary abscesses usually arise either from foci of severe, suppurative lobar or bronchopneumonia, or from septic emboli lodging in the pulmonary vascular bed (Fig. 6.22C). Cranioventral location and associated scarring or bronchiectasis are evidence of origin from a suppurative pneumonia. Multiple, widely distributed abscesses indicate hematogenous origin and are usually associated with an obvious source of septic emboli elsewhere in the body, for example, septic thrombosis of the posterior vena cava in cattle. Isolated abscesses in dorsocaudal regions are more likely to have arisen from septic emboli, but in the absence of a pattern of abscesses in other organs, the origin remains uncertain. Difficulty is encountered in interpreting the pathogenesis of pulmonary abscesses in horses; they are relatively frequent and can arise by either major route. It is often impossible to determine with certainty the pathogenesis of isolated old abscesses.

Two less common causes of pulmonary abscesses are aspirated foreign bodies, such as plant awns, or direct traumatic penetration of the lung. Complications of abscessation include pleural fistulation and empyema, hemorrhage from a ruptured blood vessel, and fulminating suppurative bronchopneumonia subsequent to rupture into a bronchus.

The term embolic pneumonia could be extended to include pneumonias caused by any circulating particulates, including bacteria and parasites, but it is preferable to consider pneumonia caused by hematogenous infectious agents under the general heading Interstitial Pneumonia. Embolic pneumonias can be considered as a special category of interstitial pneumonia in which there are focally discrete lesions. In addition to the abscesses caused by septic emboli mentioned previously, other examples are the hematogenous abscesses, which are an integral part of specific diseases such as caseous lymphadenitis and melioidosis.

Special Forms of Pneumonia

Gangrenous Pneumonia

Gangrene can be a complication of other forms of pneumonia in which there is extensive necrosis of pulmonary parenchyma. It is occasionally seen in cattle as a result of penetration of a foreign body from the reticulum, but mostly it

is a result of aspiration of foreign material and associated saprophytic, putrefactive bacteria. The yellowish to greenish black color and foul odor are characteristic. Extensive ragged cavitation rapidly develops. If a gangrenous cavity extends to the pleura, a foul empyema results, with putrefactive pneumothorax.

Aspiration Pneumonia

Aspiration pneumonia refers to pneumonia caused by large amounts of foreign material, often in liquid form, reaching the lungs through the airways. This distinguishes it from pneumonias caused by inhalation of small respirable particles, which includes the bulk of aerogenous pneumonias. The response to the aspirated material depends on three factors: the nature of the material, the bacteria carried with it, and the distribution of the material in the lungs.

Widespread distribution of inhaled milk or combination of milk and gruel is observed occasionally in pail-fed calves. The course of the disease in these cases can be as short as 1 day. The gross appearance is not characteristic. The lungs remain inflated; they are hyperemic, and small amounts of exudate can be expressed from the small airways. Histologically, there is an acute bronchiolitis with various degrees of acute alveolar inflammation. Lipids, and sometimes plant material, can be seen in the lesions. Aspiration of ruminal contents can produce a similar picture in recumbent cattle, but in these cases the aspirated material is usually obvious, and there is hemorrhagic tracheobronchitis.

When the distribution of foreign material is more localized, either discrete foreign-body granulomas, bronchopneumonia (Fig. 6.22D), lobar pneumonia, or gangrene of the lungs occurs. Cattle and lambs frequently aspirate inflammatory exudate from necrobacillary laryngitis. Lambs with nutritional myopathy affecting the muscles of deglutition aspirate milk and plant material, including whole grain. Pigs in dry, dusty environments can aspirate starch granules and particles of plants from the feed. Any cause of dysphagia, pharyngeal paralysis in particular, is likely to lead to aspiration pneumonia. It is also a hazard of anesthesia. Aspiration of vomitus and medications occurs in all species. The aspiration of vomitus in a simple-stomached animal is often rapidly disastrous, and death can occur from laryngeal spasm or acute pulmonary edema before there is time for much inflammation to develop. The possibility of aspirated material's being responsible must always be considered in any case of fulminating lobar or bronchopneumonia, especially one with a history of one of tbe predisposing conditions just mentioned. Careful search will usually reveal evidence of foreign material, but this is not the case when the material is largely or entirely liquid.

Lipid (Lipoid) Pneumonia

Lipid (lipoid) pneumonia is a special form of aspiration pneumonia in which large droplets of oil are inhaled. It used to be fairly common in cats but occurs in all species in which animals are subjected to the forced administration of mineral oil (liquid paraffin), as a laxative, or cod-liver oil, for its antirachitic properties. The reaction is typically macrophagic and proliferative, with some qualitative differences depending on the nature of the

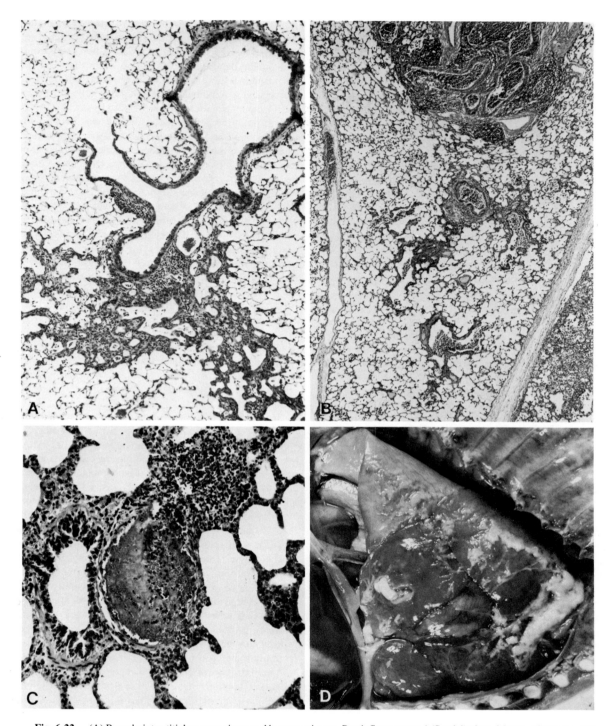

Fig. 6.22. (A) Bronchointerstitial pneumonia caused by myxoviruses. Parainfluenza type 1 (Sendai) virus. Mouse. (Courtesy of D. G. Brownstein). (B) Bronchointerstitial pneumonia of mycoplasmosis. Calf. (C) Thromboembolic suppurative pneumonia. Ox. Early lesion associated with septic thrombus. (D) Aspiration pneumonia. Cat. There is confluent bronchopneumonia and fibrinopurulent pleuritis.

oil. In general, vegetable oils, such as olive oil, are not irritating, and they are eventually resorbed with little reaction or fibrosis. Oils of animal origin are irritants and provoke an early exudation of serofibrinous fluid and leukocytes. This is replaced later principally by macrophges, among which giant cells can be numerous. Foamy macrophages fill the alveoli, and the alveolar walls are thickened by infiltrated mononuclear cells and fibrosis. The oil is ultimately resorbed. The purest cellular response occurs to mineral oil, which is the usual offender in animals. The nature of the oil can be distinguished by its permanence and its failure to stain with osmic acid. The lipid is both extracellular and intracellular. Lipid-laden macrophages tend to fill the alveoli, and in time they accumulate in the lymphatics that surround the bronchi and blood vessels (Fig. 6.23B). Fibrosis of alveolar walls and proliferation of alveolar type II epithelial cells are conspicuous, and the foamy macrophages tend to be incorporated into the alveolar septa by extension of the fibroplasia. Unless complicated by secondary bacterial infection, the lesions have a characteristic yellowish, homogeneous or finely mottled appearance (Fig. 6.23A). They vary from multiple small nodules to complete consolidation of a lobe. Involvement is usually bilateral and tends to be in ventral regions. The bronchial lymph nodes are grossly normal, but histologically often contain droplets of oil.

Pneumonias caused by aspiration of foreign (exogenous) lipid must be differentiated from the so-called endogenous-lipid pneumonias, described below. Accumulation of lipid-filled macrophages and various amounts of interstitial response are common to both conditions. The most important distinguishing feature is that in lipid-aspiration pneumonias there are large, discrete extracellular globules of lipid. In paraffin-embedded sections these appear as clear, spherical spaces with distinct borders formed by the compressed cytoplasm of macrophages and giant cells.

Uremic Pneumonopathy

Severe uremia causes increased permeability of the alveolar air–blood barrier and is therefore a cause of pulmonary edema. The usual form of uremic pneumonopathy occurs in dogs with chronic uremia, where the principal lesion is degeneration and calcification of smooth muscle and connective tissue fibers (see the Urinary System, this volume). This occurs mainly in the walls of respiratory bronchioles and alveolar ducts in mild cases. Severe involvement results in extensive mineralization of alveolar septa, which can be recognized grossly by the gritty, porous texture of the lung. Inflammatory cell components are not usually a significant feature of uremic pneumonopathy in dogs, and although the condition is sometimes referred to as uremic pneumonitis, this is not appropriate.

Alveolar Filling Disorders

Alveolar filling disorders is a convenient term for lumping together an ill-defined group of conditions with overlapping morphologic features. They are usually found as incidental lesions in which alveoli are filled by one or more of the following: collections of large, foamy, lipid-filled macrophages with lipofuscin pigment and, possibly, cholesterol crystals (endogenous-lipid pneumonia); amorphous acidophilic material (al-

veolar lipoproteinosis); or clusters of macrophages and giant cells containing hyaline or faintly laminated material (pulmonary hyalinosis). The amount of inflammation varies from minimal to mild, depending on the variety of the disorder. The central feature in these conditions is accumulation of lipid-filled macrophages. Accumulation can be caused by one or more of three factors: their clearance is impeded by obstructed airways, they are produced in excess, or metabolic abnormalities interfere with their mobility. More than one of these circumstances may coexist. These conditions could be regarded as forms of lipidosis rather than pneumonia in the usual sense. They are included here because some do have an inflammatory component, especially the so-called endogenous-lipid pneumonia. The various conditions are grouped for convenience because of overlapping morphologic features. Clarification of the range of causes and pathogenic mechanisms will eventually enable more precise and useful classification.

Endogenous-lipid pneumonia (foam-cell pneumonia, cholesterol pneumonia) is characterized by large, focal accumulations of foamy macrophages. The disease is encountered mostly in laboratory rodents and furbearing animals. It is seen occasionally in cats, rarely in dogs. Grossly, the lungs have irregularly distributed, yellowish white, firm foci. Most of the foci are subpleural and appear as sharply defined small flecks or bulging nodules up to a centimeter or more in width (Fig. 6.23C). The overlying pleura is often thickened, and the adjacent lymphatics may be prominent because of accumulations of macrophages and lipid.

Histologically, the bulk of the lesion in many instances is composed of distended alveoli filled with foamy macrophages (Fig. 6.23D). There is a small amount of interstitial fibrosis and accumulation of lymphocytes and plasma cells. In more severe cases, there are intracellular and extracellular cholesterol crystals, more severe interstitial fibrosis and mononuclear-cell accumulation, and regions of alveolar type II cell proliferation. The large cholesterol crystals stimulate development of giant cells and intraalveolar fibroplasia. Extensive fibrosis is accompanied by obliterative periarteritis and endarteritis.

The causes of endogenous lipid pneumonia are not clearly defined. In some instances, the accumulation of alveolar macrophages is associated with localized bronchitis and bronchiolitis and is therefore attributed to obstruction of alveolar clearance. In other instances, there is no evident obstruction of clearance pathways. Excessive production of macrophages and reduction of their mobility by ingested surfactant or serum-derived lipids are probable causes of accumulation in such cases.

Alveolar lipoproteinosis is characterized by accumulation of acellular acidophilic material within alveoli. The predominantly mucopolysaccharide–lipid complex is homogeneous or granular by light microscopy and is strongly PAS (periodic acid–Schiff) positive. Ultrastructurally, the material consists mostly of lamellar and tubular arrays of surfactant phospholipid. Because of the predominance of lipid, the condition is also referred to as pulmonary lipidosis. Alveoli are lined by type II epithelial cells, but inflammatory and fibrotic changes in alveolar walls are usually minimal. Alveolar lipoproteinosis has been produced experimentally in animals by exposing them intratracheally to massive concentrations of silica or coal dust, or by parenteral

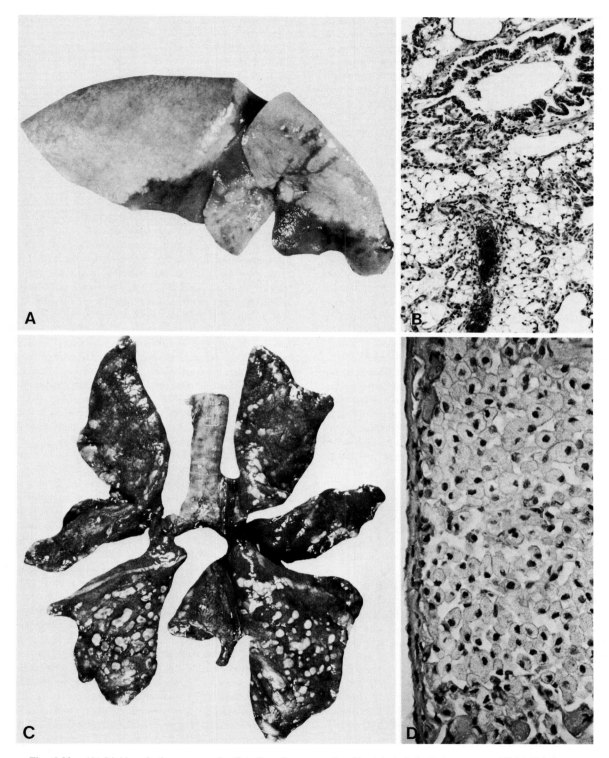

Fig. 6.23. **(A)** Lipid aspiration pneumonia. Cat. Bronchopneumonia with atelectasis in darker areas. **(B)** Lipid-laden macrophages in alveoli and perivascular lymphatics of **(A)**. **(C)** Endogenous lipid pneumonia. Cat. Multiple, discrete, pale subpleural nodules. **(D)** Histology of **(C)**, showing accumulations of foamy macrophages.

administration of amphiphilic drugs such as chlorphentermine. It has not been recognized as a naturally occurring entity in domestic animals other than in association with chronic interstitial pneumonia in goats, such as is caused by the caprine arthritis–encephalitis virus. The relative roles of alveolar type II cells and macrophages in producing the acellular debris are still in dispute, but most evidence indicates alveolar type II cells are more important.

Pulmonary hyalinosis, which consists of multifocal accumulations of macrophages and giant cells containing hyaline or laminated material, is seen in the lungs of dogs. Grossly detectable foci occur mainly subpleurally, especially at the narrow ventral margins of the lungs. They are grayish white to tan, nodular or confluent, and firm to gritty. Histologically, the cytoplasm of macrophages and giant cells is greatly distended and disrupted by amorphous or sometimes laminated material. The material is amphophilic, often staining with a pronounced bluish tinge with hematoxylin and eosin. It is strongly PAS-positive, and limited ultrastructural observations have shown that it consists of packed segments of cytoplasmic membranes. Plasma cells, lymphocytes, and small amounts of fibrous tissue usually surround individual or clustered giant cells and macrophages.

The lesions can be found occasionally as incidental findings in the lungs of old dogs. They have been referred to as pulmonary granulomas with PAS-positive bodies and are reported to occur mostly in brachycephalic breeds, particularly boxers. They are usually found accompanying chronic pulmonary injury such as pneumoconiosis or experimental radiation pneumonitis. Although the lesions described as pulmonary hyalinosis in dogs have some differences from pulmonary corpora amylacea of humans, the extent to which they represent clearly separable responses remains to be established.

Granulomatous Pneumonia

Granulomatous or pyogranulomatous pneumonia may occasionally be caused by *Actinobacillus, Actinomyces,* or *Nocardia.* In these cases there is usually local damage to pulmonary tissue, such as by trauma or aspirated foreign body, or suspicion of systemic immunodeficiency. An example of the latter is the occasional finding of systemic nocardiosis, including multifocal pulmonary pyogranulomas, in dogs with distemper or in Arabian foals with combined immunodeficiency. More important granulomatous pneumonias are tuberculosis and fungal infections of the lung (pneumonomycoses), which are described under the appropriate headings.

The Specific Infectious Pneumonias

Naturally occurring infectious pneumonias of clinical significance usually have complex causes. Interaction of two or more organisms is commonly involved, and often there are predisposing environmental factors. The relatively nonspecific nature of many pneumonic lesions compounds the difficulty of attributing them to specific causes. In the following discussion, features of pneumonias caused by, or strongly associated with, individual infectious agents will be presented first. The variety of agents implicated in causing conditions grouped under epidemiologic terms such as ''enzootic pneumonia'' will be summarized afterward.

Viral Diseases

Myxovirus Infections

Myxoviruses typically cause inapparent to mild infections, mainly of the upper respiratory tract, unless they are unusually virulent or the affected animals unduly susceptible. This is the pattern of human influenza. Where severe disease does occur, it is mostly due to the viral infection's predisposing to secondary bacterial involvement.

SWINE INFLUENZA. Swine influenza is an acute contagious disease caused by a type A influenza virus, which is closely related to human type A strains. The disease was first recognized in swine at the time of the human pandemic in 1918, and there is circumstantial evidence that pigs acquired the virus from humans and have remained as permanent hosts since then. More recently, limited outbreaks or sporadic cases of influenza in humans have been caused by the swine virus. The disease occurs regularly in parts of the United States, and sporadically in Canada and Europe. Typically it appears suddenly in swine herds in fall and early winter. The epidemiology is incompletely understood, but outbreaks are usually associated with stress of climatic changes or management procedures. Once a few cases in a herd are triggered, the disease spreads rapidly by the airborne route. The reservoir of infection between seasonal outbreaks appears to be either carrier swine or lungworm larvae and earthworms. The classical work of Shope showed that earthworms that ingested lungworm larvae from influenza-infected pigs could harbor the virus for long periods. Subsequent feeding of the earthworms to susceptible pigs reproduced the disease, but only if the virus was ''activated'' by a provoking factor, such as repeated intramuscular injection of killed *Haemophilus* organisms. Migrating ascarid larvae can also precipitate the disease. Lungworm larvae and earthworms are not important under most current management practices, but predisposing factors are necessary for infection to cause clinical disease.

Affected herds have sudden onset of coughing and high fever, which rapidly spreads to pigs of all ages. There is stiffness, weakness, and serous oculonasal discharge. The virus itself causes a mild illness lasting no more than a week; more severe illness and deaths are usually because of secondary bacterial pneumonia.

Uncomplicated viral infection rarely causes death, and the lesions have been mostly studied in experimental situations. Grossly, there is evidence of acute tracheobronchitis with reddened, swollen mucosa and filling of the airways by tenacious mucus, particularly in cranioventral regions. Because of the airway obstruction there is alveolar atelectasis. This is seen as groups of clearly defined, plum-colored lobules in the cranioventral lung regions. The overall extent of the atelectasis depends on the severity of the viral bronchitis and bronchiolitis. In fatal cases, in addition to atelectasis, there is diffuse hyperemia and edema of the lungs, and the interlobular septa are widened by edema fluid. The airways contain bloodstained foam as well as thick mucus, and as a result there can be terminal air trapping in nonatelectatic regions of the lung. Tbe pleura is normal or covered by a small amount of serous or serofibrinous exudate, and there is excess fluid in the pleural cavity. The pulmonary lymph nodes are enlarged by hyperemia and edema. There is usually a nonspecific severe congestion of the gastric mucosa along the greater curvature. In the more common instances where pigs die of secondary bacterial pneumonia, usually involving *Haemophilus, Pasteurella multocida,* or both, the lesions are characteristic of an acute bacterial bronchopneumonia.

Microscopically, there is patchy, acute inflammation of oculonasal membranes and mucosa of the tracheobronchial tree. The severity of infection is correlated with the extent of involvement of the respiratory tract. In mild cases, viral replication and the lesions it causes are limited to the upper respiratory tract. In severe infection, viral involvement extends to the bronchioles and alveolar parenchyma. Viral replication begins in epithelial cells by 2 hr after infection, and by 8 hr there is loss of cilia, extrusion of mucus, and vacuolar degeneration of epithelial cells. Within 24 hr there is epithelial necrosis and sloughing with emigration of leukocytes, chiefly neutrophils, into the airway lumen. The net effect in severe infections is an acute bronchiolitis and bronchitis in which plugs of neutrophilic exudate are responsible for alveolar atelectasis. Extension of virus infection to alveolar epithelial cells causes alveolar flooding by serofibrinous exudate and neutrophils. The response after the first 24 to 48 hr becomes increasingly mononuclear. There is extensive infiltration of lymphocytes and smaller numbers of other leukocytes into the walls of airways and into the peribronchiolar and adjacent alveolar interstitium. Macrophages become the predominant cell in alveolar lumina. Epithelial proliferation and repair are easily detected histologically by the third to fourth days and lead to hyperplastic cells, which by light microscopy have an undifferentiated appearance. Return to ciliated and secretory cells occurs more slowly. The bronchial and bronchiolar epithelium frequently consists of several layers of stratified cells, with the superficial ones degenerating and desquamating into the residual luminal exudate.

The lesion likely to be seen in the few animals dying primarily of the pure viral infection is one in which there is severe involvement of the bronchiolar–alveolar regions. The acute inflammatory exudate and associated interstitial accumulation of mononuclear cells gives the characteristic bronchointerstitial pattern of pneumonia defined earlier. In pigs dying of secondary bacterial infection, the exudative bacterial pneumonia obscures the earlier viral lesion. In addition to the constitutional signs associated with severe infection, swine influenza in pregnant sows may cause abortion or weakness of the newborn.

EQUINE INFLUENZA.   Equine influenza is caused by either of two strains of type A virus (A/Equi–1/Prague and A/Equi–2/Miami). A role for type B virus is unconfirmed. The clinical syndrome caused by the influenza viruses overlaps those caused by equine herpes (rhinopneumonitis) virus, equine arteritis virus (see the Cardiovascular System, Volume 3), and perhaps equine parainfluenza type 3 virus, rhinovirus, and reovirus. Only virologic techniques establish the diagnosis with certainty.

In common with other influenza infections, the disease spreads rapidly among susceptible horses. All ages in a previously unexposed population are susceptible, but the disease is seen most often in young animals brought together or mixed with older animals. Main clinical signs are cough, serous to purulent oculonasal discharge, fever, and weakness. Most horses have a mild illness that resolves within 1 to 2 weeks, but death can occur either from secondary bacterial bronchopneumonia or from severe viral infection involving damage to heart, gastrointestinal tract, kidney, and other parenchymal organs, as well as severe ocular and pulmonary lesions. Edematous swelling of subcutaneous tissues of legs and, less commonly, ventral trunk might also be present.

Respiratory lesions are those of hyperemia, edema, exudation, desquamation, and focal erosions in the upper respiratory tract. In severe cases there is an acute bronchointerstitial pneumonia accompanied by more widespread pulmonary edema, as described for swine influenza, and a tendency for secondary bronchopneumonia caused mostly by streptococci, but occasionally by *Escherichia coli, Pasteurella multocida,* or various other organisms normally resident on the nasopharyngeal mucosa.

Parainfluenza Virus Infections

Parainfluenza viruses are best established as a cause of pneumonia in cattle. They can cause pneumonia by themselves but more commonly are part of the etiologic complex of enzootic pneumonia in calves or more acute episodes of the "shipping fever" type. Uncomplicated **parainfluenza-3 virus** infection in **cattle** has been studied mainly in natural or experimental infections of calves. The disease is either clinically inapparent or causes coughing, moderate fever, tachypnea, and slight mucoid or mucopurulent nasal discharge. Signs are most evident from about 4 to 12 days after infection. Disease caused by the virus alone is more likely to be encountered in calves from 2 weeks to a few months of age, depending on management practices. Uncomplicated infection does not appear to be an important cause of death.

Lesions caused by the virus are basically similar to those caused by influenza viruses, that is to say, the pattern is of a bronchointerstitial pneumonia. Grossly, there is usually evidence of mild mucopurulent inflammation of nasal passages and upper airways. Early macroscopic lung lesions are limited to irregular lobular foci of atelectasis or slightly consolidated purple-red foci in cranioventral regions. In more developed lesions, some 4 to 12 days after experimental infection, there is more confluent consolidation. Thereafter, affected regions are less frequent and more atelectatic as they undergo resolution.

Histologically, in the more severe viral infections there is initially an acute bronchitis and a more obvious bronchiolitis, with extension to adjacent alveoli. The bronchiolar and alveolar exudate is predominantly neutrophilic, although edema and hemorrhage might be present in the alveoli. From about 2 to 4 days after infection, bronchiolar epithelium is variously hyperplastic or vacuolated and necrotic. Acidophilic intracytoplasmic inclusions can be found at this stage in vacuolated bronchiolar epithelium and, to a lesser extent, bronchial epithelium. They are usually in a basal location relative to the nucleus. Intranuclear inclusions are rare. Intracytoplasmic inclusions are present infrequently in alveolar epithelial cells. The exudate in bronchioles and alveoli contains macrophages and lymphocytes mixed with neutrophils. Many alveoli are atelectatic because of bronchiolar obstruction. Lymphocytes and plasma cells also accumulate around vessels, bronchioles, and within alveolar septa. Lesions are of maximum cellularity somewhere between 6 and 12 days after infection and are dominated by hyperplasia of bronchiolar epithelium and alveolar type II epithelial cells. Squamous metaplasia may be present. Many alveoli are "epithelialized." Occasional binucleate or multinucleate cells are present. Exudate in bronchioles and alveoli is mixed cell debris, macrophages, and serofibrinous exudate. Intracytoplasmic inclusions are seldom found after 7 days, which is the height of the epithelial proliferative response. Early obliterative bronchiolitis (bronchiolitis fibrosa obliterans) can be seen in severely affected bronchioles at the peak of the pneumonic involvement but is more prominent in later, incompletely resolved lesions.

Several points need emphasizing relative to the range of lesions reported in naturally occurring or experimental disease. The severity of alveolar damage depends on the extent to which virus reaches the alveolar epithelium and replicates, thus causing necrosis. This in turn is governed by the virulence of the strain of virus, the mode of infection, and the resistance of the calf. In general, experimental infections deliver more virus to deep regions of the lung and hence cause more alveolar damage. In natural infection, viral replication seems usually to be limited more to airways and hence is characterized more by bronchiolitis than pneumonia. In severe experimental infections, the amount of alveolar epithelial damage can be pronounced. The degree of alveolar exudation and subsequent proliferation of alveolar type II epithelial cells (epithelialization) is correspondingly more dramatic. The extent to which syncytial or multinucleated giant cells are seen on the alveolar walls or in the bronchiolar epithelium varies. They are not usually a notable feature. Occasional multinucleated cells are seen in the active proliferative phase of alveolar and bronchiolar epithelium following severe damage by a wide variety of infectious and noninfectious agents, particularly in cattle. It therefore appears that no specificity can be attributed to occasional giant cells in the absence of viral inclusions or ultrastructural or immunochemical demonstration of virus. The same holds true for occasional macrophage-derived giant cells. Finally, although intracytoplasmic inclusion bodies tend to be present as the viral lesion approaches its peak, they are rarely encountered in calves that die, because secondary bacterial damage usually obscures possible earlier viral lesions or causes death after the stage at which inclusion bodies are detectable.

The role of parainfluenza-3 virus in **sheep** is similar to its role in cattle in that it acts mostly to pave the way for severe pasteurella pneumonia. The experimental lesions in lambs are essentially the same as those produced in calves. The situation in goats might well be the same, but there has been less study in this species. The pathogenic role of the equine parainfluenza 3 virus is also uncertain.

Parainfluenza-2 virus infection in dogs, formerly referred to as parainfluenza SV-5, has been discussed in its role as one of the causative agents of infectious tracheobronchitis. Lesions are those of a mild tracheobronchitis and bronchiolitis.

CANINE DISTEMPER. Canine distemper is the most ubiquitous and serious of the diseases of dogs. In spite of the development of effective vaccines, the disease remains endemic in most parts of the world. All members of the Canidae (e.g., dog, dingo, fox, coyote, wolf, jackal), Procyonidae (e.g., raccoon, coati, kinkajou, panda), and Mustelidae (e.g., ferret, mink, badger, weasel, otter) are thought to be susceptible, but cases have not been proven in some species of these families. The ferret is remarkably susceptible and for this reason was used extensively in investigation of the disease. Carré first demonstrated that the causative agent is a filterable virus. This virus is now identified as a paramyxovirus, a large RNA virus closely related to measles virus of humans and to rinderpest virus of cattle. Various isolates of the virus cannot be distinguished serologically, but they differ in the type and severity of the disease they produce.

Infection by canine distemper virus is pantropic, and the manifestations protean. The disease is described here because respiratory signs and lesions, although variable in severity, are relatively constant in occurrence. Effective antibacterial therapy has greatly reduced the incidence of secondary bronchopneumonia, but it is still frequently seen in neglected cases. Intestinal disease is also common in dogs with distemper.

The disease is a summation of the effects of the virus and of secondary infections with other organisms. These secondary infections are particularly important in this disease because one of the primary sites of action of the virus is the lymphoid tissue. This causes suppression of immune function. Secondary bacterial infections in the alimentary tract are nonspecific, but in the respiratory tract, *Bordetella bronchiseptica* is frequently associated with suppurative bronchopneumonia. Activated toxoplasmosis develops in dogs whose immune systems have been damaged by the distemper virus, and in fact, toxoplasmosis as a clinical disease seldom occurs in dogs other than in association with canine distemper or other diseases that cause immunodeficiency.

The virus is shed in all the excretions from infected animals during the systemic phase of the infection, and natural transmission is usually by inhalation. The pathogenesis of the infection has been followed in dogs, and the distribution of the virus monitored by the use of immunofluorescence. After aerosol exposure, the virus appears in macrophages of the bronchial lymph nodes and tonsils during the first 24 hr. The virus proliferates in the bronchial lymph nodes, and 2 to 5 days after exposure is distributed throughout the lymphatic tissue, including bone marrow, thymus, and spleen. The animals become febrile and viremic at this stage, and cells of the buffy coat contain virus. The infection is primarily confined to the lymphoid tissues until 8 or 9 days after exposure. In some infections, the virus spreads no further, and the disease is mild or inapparent. The control of the infection at this stage is correlated with the development of neutralizing antibody. If protective titers develop within the first 2 weeks of infection, spread of virus does not occur, and virus disappears from lymphatic tissues. If protective levels of antibody are not reached, the infection persists in lymphatic tissues and spreads to the epithelium of the alimentary, respiratory, and urogenital tracts as well as to the skin and endocrine glands and may reach the brain. In the central nervous system, the virus appears first in perivascular and meningeal macrophages, but infection of the choroid plexus epithelium occurs early, and the cerebrospinal fluid contains large amounts of virus. The critical timing involved in the rise of neutralizing antibody titer, and its role in influencing the pattern of disease, appears to offer a partial explanation for the variability in the severity of the disease produced by the canine distemper virus. The disease is more severe in young animals, in which the immune system is less well developed, but even among littermates infected by the same strain of virus, the disease is unpredictable in severity.

The incubation period of canine distemper, as indicated by the onset of acute fever, is rather constant at ~5 days. The febrile reaction is typically diphasic, with a second peak occurring at ~11 days, but this diphasic response is seldom observed clinically. The fever is continuous for the course of the systemic infection, which may be some weeks. The clinical signs are variable in their severity and in their emphasis on particular systems. A syndrome consisting of catarrhal oculonasal discharge, pharyngitis, and bronchitis is common but may be so mild as to be missed. Signs of pulmonary involvement accompany moderate to severe damage, whether purely viral with edema and interstitial inflammation, or mainly bacterial with bronchopneumonia. The alimentary disturbance is usually expressed as diarrhea, which becomes more severe as the disease advances. The feces become semifluid, slimy, foul, and occasionally streaked with blood. The animals lose weight, and dehydration results. Vesicles and pustules develop in the skin in some cases. These cutaneous lesions are confined to the epidermis beginning in the deeper layers and are particularly to be found on the thin skin of the abdomen and inner aspects of the thighs. They are bacterial complications usually produced by staphylococci and streptococci. Cutaneous hyper- and parakeratosis also occur, but these never reach the degree of development seen in ferrets and mink, except on the footpads (Fig. 6.24A) and nose. In dogs, there is at most a generalized scurfiness of the skin. Small zones of moist alopecia are common on the palpebral margins and oral commissures.

Blindness, or some loss of vision, is common. Keratitis developing as an extension of conjunctivitis is rare. Few if any dogs, however, escape completely from a retinitis if the disease becomes generalized, and in many there are degenerative and inflammatory changes in the optic nerves and pathways. There may be complete or focal retinal degeneration, patchy edema of the retina with focal detachments, and retinal ischemia with pallor and contraction of the papilla that can be recognized ophthalmoscopically. Proliferations of the pigmented epithelium are visible in the tapetal fundus.

The onset of neurologic signs is usually sudden and follows the systemic signs by 1 to 5 weeks, but it can be longer, and in some cases only neurologic signs are recognized. Certain patterns of signs can be identified: generalized convulsions of cerebral cortical origin; ataxia, the result of cerebellar or vestibular dysfunction; and posterior paralysis due to cord damage. But the neurologic signs of distemper are usually progressive and the result of multifocal damage. Convulsions, depression, paralysis, and rhythmic motor movements (myoclonus) are the most common. Myoclonus may persist as a residual sign of the diseases in animals that recover from the infection.

The gross lesions seen in canine distemper will depend on the phase of the disease when the animal dies or is killed. When death occurs early in the course of the disease and systemic effects are still prominent, as is usual in pups, gross lesions can be expected. But in the majority of cases, which die or are killed because of the encephalitic effect of the virus, there may be little to be seen grossly.

Visceral lesions of canine distemper are common in the respiratory system, but they may be subtle. Inflammation of the nasopharynx is serous in initial stages, and in the course of 3 or more weeks becomes catarrhal and sometimes purulent. The mucosal vessels of the larynx and trachea are congested. The bronchi contain a small amount of foamy, serous fluid from the edematous lungs, and they may contain a mucopurulent exudate in complicating bacterial pneumonia. The lungs are edematous, and when this is severe, there is also serous effusion in the pleural sacs. The specific lesion is an interstitial pneumonia (see Anatomic Patterns of Pneumonia). To a variable extent, the lungs may reveal the smooth, liver-like appearance associated with extensive serofibrinous filling of alveoli, but the more usual lesions are reddish tan patches immediately beneath the pleura, and grayish zones of firmer consistency along the sharp margins of the lobes. Deflation is incomplete in such lungs.

Lesions are regularly present in the lymphoid organs, but except for the thymus, these changes are difficult to recognize grossly. If the animal dies or is killed during the acute systemic phase of the disease, the lymph nodes may be variable in size. Some are large and edematous, others small and atrophic. In the large, edematous nodes, cortical and medullary distinction may be lost. The thymuses of affected animals at this stage are greatly reduced and in some cases are difficult to identify. Later in the course of the disease, lymphoid tissue of lymph nodes and thymuses can regenerate and may be of normal size in animals dying in the chronic neurologic phase of the disease.

Many animals dying of canine distemper are severely emaciated and their muscles wasted. The lobular pattern of the liver is sometimes prominent because of mild fatty change and centrilobular congestion. Large, irregular, whitish areas of necrosis and mineralization are often seen in the myocardium of very young suckling pups, which are most apt to die during the acute early phase of the disease.

The histologic changes in canine distemper, when present, are fairly specific; specificity depends on the demonstration of the viral inclusion bodies or, better yet, detection of viral antigen by immunofluorescence.

The number and distribution of inclusion bodies vary from case to case and with the phase of the disease. Their appearance coincides with, or follows shortly after, the appearance of systemic signs of illness. This is from about 10 to 14 days after infection. By about the fifth or sixth week, their numbers diminish rapidly in most tissues and disappear. Of the nonneural tissues, they persist longest in the lung. Inclusion bodies can be found in the central nervous system before changes of encephalomyelitis are present, and they persist in the neural tissue when they have disappeared from all extraneural sites, provided that infection of the brain has occurred.

The inclusion bodies are acidophilic and occur in either the nucleus or cytoplasm, or both, depending on the tissue. They are

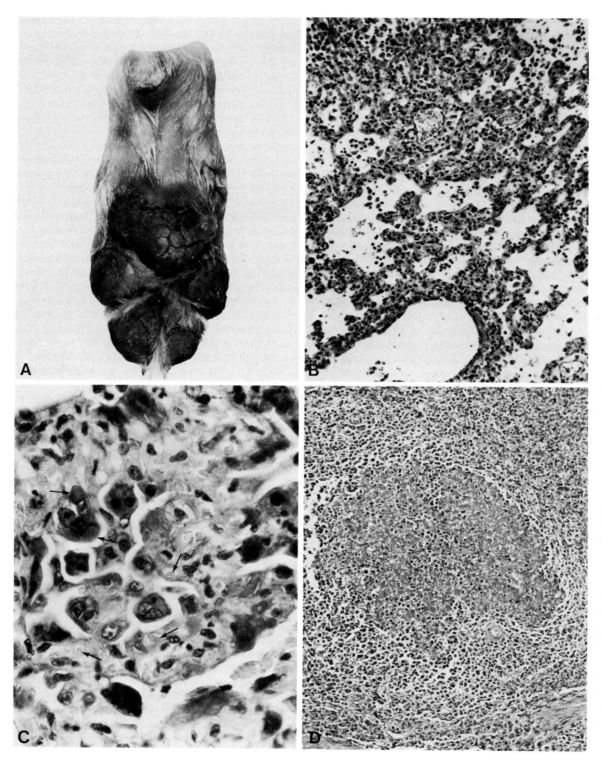

Fig. 6.24.   Canine distemper.   (**A**) Hyperkeratosis of foot pads.   (**B**) Acute interstitial pneumonia with predominance of mono-nuclear cells in alveolar walls.   (**C**) Giant cells in alveoli with intracytoplasmic inclusions (arrows).   (**D**) Necrotic focus. Spleen.

usually easier to find and recognize with confidence in brain and epithelial tissues. In lymph nodes they can be very easily confused with eosinophilic debris unless their specificity can be proven by fluorescent antibody.

The earliest lesions of canine distemper are those affecting the lymphatic tissues. These are rarely seen in clinical cases, as dogs only rarely die during this period, but in experimental series it has been shown that as early as the sixth day after exposure there is a depletion of lymphocytes in the cortical zone of the lymph nodes. By the ninth day the lymph nodes are largely depleted of lymphocytes, and the cortical zones are reduced to thin rims. Individual lymphocytes undergo necrosis, and the sinusoids and cords are infiltrated by neutrophils. Similar lesions develop in the spleen, and small foci of necrosis may be scattered throughout the white pulp (Fig. 6.24D). Large multinucleated syncytial cells form in the nodes; often these cells contain acidophilic inclusion bodies. Approximately 2 weeks after exposure, hyperplasia of the reticulum cells develops, focally at first, and later as diffuse sheets of cells. In some fatally infected animals, the nodes are not repopulated by lymphocytes. The nodes are of normal size but filled only with proliferating large mononuclear cells when the animal dies 25–35 days after infection. Repopulation of the node by both B and T cells can occur in convalescent dogs. The recovery is not complete in some of these dogs, and some die with neurologic signs. The thymus also undergoes a severe lymphocytic depletion in parallel with the lymph nodes. The thymic atrophy is due to loss of cortical thymocytes as well as great reduction in the medulla. In some animals that die, the thymuses show no tendency to regenerate, but regeneration, if it is to occur, commences at the same time as it does in the nodes.

Severe leukopenia is a characteristic feature of canine distemper. It is due chiefly to a lymphopenia. The lymphopenia develops at the time the initial necrosis of lymphatic tissue occurs and is most likely the result of viral multiplication and destruction of the lymphoid tissues. The lymphopenia persists in the acute disease until death or recovery, but some animals die of encephalitis after the circulating lymphocyte levels have returned to normal. Lymphopenia coincides with the onset of the leukocyte-associated viremia but persists long after viral antigen can no longer be demonstrated in the buffy coat.

The characteristic changes in the lung produced by the virus of canine distemper are those of interstitial pneumonia, as described above (Fig. 6.24B), but the lesion found at autopsy may be complicated by secondary bacterial bronchopneumonia. The change is diffuse in the lungs, although more severe in some areas than in others. Syncytial giant cells formed by alveolar type II epithelial cells are a characteristic feature of the interstitial pneumonia caused by the virus. Many contain the acidophilic intracytoplasmic viral inclusions (Fig. 6.24C). As the systemic phase is overcome in the chronic disease, residual changes tend to persist in patches beneath the pleura and about venules and small bronchioles as areas of thickened alveolar septa with epithelialization or accumulation of alveolar macrophages. Specific inclusion bodies can sometimes still be found in the cytoplasm of altered alveolar epithelium and in the bronchial mucosa. Among nonneural tissues, they are most likely to be found in the alveolar epithelium because they persist longest

in these cells in terms of the disease process, and these cells are not as subject to postmortem lysis and sloughing as most epithelial cells.

Intracytoplasmic inclusion bodies are regularly found in the transitional epithelium of the urinary tract in the acute systemic disease. Intranuclear inclusions are less common. In some cases, inclusions are found in the epithelium of the collecting tubules. The epithelial cells are often swollen and hydropic, and in the absence of these degenerative changes, inclusion bodies are unlikely to be found. Mild interstitial epididymitis and orchitis are common in canine distemper; inclusion bodies are found in the epididymal epithelium, and the interstitium is mildly infiltrated with mononuclear cells. Inclusion bodies can occasionally be found in the epithelium of the biliary and pancreatic ducts, and in the pancreatic exocrine tissue. Inclusions are common in the gastric epithelium but uncommon in the intestine. In the stomach, they are found in superficial epithelium as well as in chief and parietal cells. The latter frequently show acute degenerative changes.

Necrosis and cystic degeneration of ameloblastic epithelium of the developing tooth give rise to the defective enamel seen in animals that have recovered from infection. The defects may consist of small, focal depressions to large areas lacking enamel. The boundaries of the defects are discrete.

Intraocular lesions occur in most cases of canine distemper. Ulcerative keratitis may complicate a purulent conjunctivitis, but this is uncommon, and otherwise the anterior segment is not significantly changed, except for leukocytic infiltrations in the ciliary body. Distinctive retinal lesions of variable severity and extent are present, and nuclear and cytoplasmic inclusions may be found in the retinal ganglion cells and glia, as well as in glia of the optic nerve. The retinal changes may be predominantly exudative in the acute cases, but in those of longer duration they are predominantly degenerative (Fig. 6.25A); in all cases, there is prominent proliferation of the pigmented epithelium. The earliest changes include severe degeneration of the retinal ganglion cells, revealed as dispersion of the Nissl substance and migration of the nucleus to the margin of the cell. The degenerative changes in the ganglion cells are diffuse, but these cells tend to persist until the layered organization of the retina is lost. In acute retinitis, there is congestion and cuffing of the blood vessels in the optic nerve and ganglion cell layers. Patchy edema often separates the fibers of the optic nerve layer and the reticular layers and produces focal retinal detachments. Atrophy of the retina may be patchy, or spare none of it. In some cases, the atrophy is limited to the layer of rods and cones, the outer limbs of which shorten and disappear concurrently with pyknosis of the nuclei. In other foci or cases, the atrophy results in disorganization of the layers, and when the ganglion cell layer disappears also, the retina in such areas consists of disorganized remnants of the layer of bipolar cells. Swelling and proliferation of the cells of the pigment epithelium are common and more marked in the ventral than in the tapetal fundus. It is also common in the pars ciliaris retinae. Associated with the reactive changes in the pigmented epithelium is a migration of pigment into the retina. Pigmentation of the retina is rather common in old dogs, but in these it tends to be restricted to the periphery of the retina and is not obviously associated with reactive changes

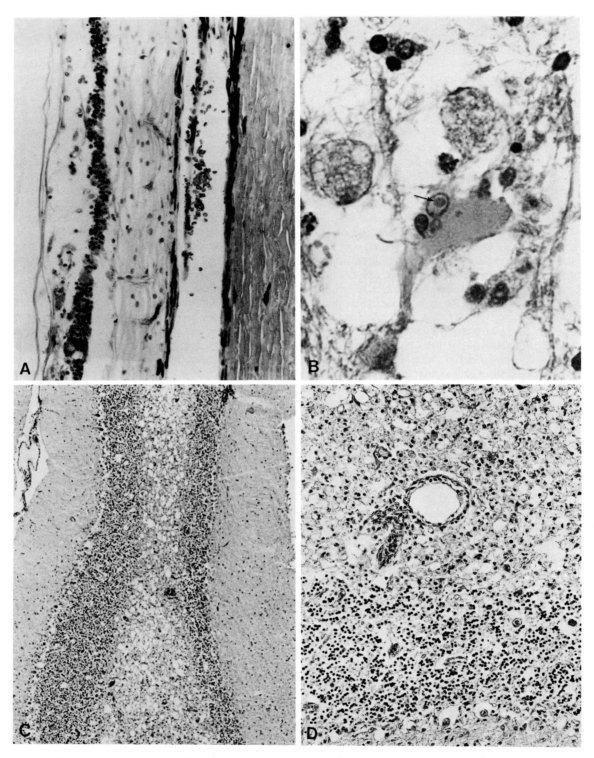

Fig. 6.25.   Canine distemper.   (**A**) Severe retinal degeneration. Only a few ganglion cells and remnants of outer nuclear layer persist.   (**B**) Myelin vacuoles, *Gitter* cells, and one swollen astrocyte containing an intranuclear inclusion body (arrow).   (**C**) De-myelination in cerebellar folium.   (**D**) Perivascular cuffing and demyelination in cerebellar folium.

in the epithelium. In canine distemper, the pigmentation occurs centrally as well as peripherally, and activity of the epithelium may be sufficient to cause focal detachments of the retina. Changes in the optic nerve are not constantly present, but papilledema may be observed in acute cases, and gliosis of the nerve head or demyelinating neuritis in chronic ones.

Demyelination is the salient feature of the encephalomyelitis of distemper. The lesions are widespread, but correlation with the clinical signs is often not apparent. The lesions have a pattern of development with regional differences in quality and severity. They are most severe and obvious in the cerebellum (Fig. 6.25C,D), surrounding the fourth ventricle and in the optic tracts. Meningitis is always present but is usually mild and consists of accumulation of mononuclear cells, mainly lymphocytes, most obvious on the ventral surface of the brain. Inclusion bodies can be demonstrated in meningeal macrophages in both nuclei and cytoplasm.

Acute degenerative changes in the neurons occur extensively in the brain but are modest in the spinal cord. Experimental studies, both immunofluorescent and ultrastructural, associate this degeneration with viral infection of the neurons. The cells most susceptible to this viral-induced injury are the small pyramidal cells of the motor cortex and Purkinje cells of the cerebellum. More widespread neuronal degeneration occurs in subacute or chronic cases, particularly in the pyriform cortex, Ammon's horn, and deep structures in the temporal lobes. The degenerating neurons have eosinophilic, granular cytoplasm and are often shrunken. The nuclei are pyknotic and may be eccentric. The surrounding neuropil is edematous, and the endothelial cells of the capillaries are swollen and proliferating. The malacic lesion remains viral associated in these cases, and inclusion bodies can be seen in the neurons and astrocytes, but the neuronal injury may be indirect and caused by immune mechanisms, ischemia, or anoxia.

Patchy demyelination is very common in dogs that come to autopsy. Early in the course of the cerebral involvement (this may be difficult to judge in clinical material because of the great variation in the onset in neurologic signs) there is vacuolation of the white matter. This vacuolation may be widely spaced or in foci, giving the lesion a spongy appearance. In some foci there is only a reduction in the intensity of myelin staining, which can be best demonstrated by myelin stains. At this stage there is no perivascular infiltration and little or no astrocytic reaction, although viral inclusion bodies can be frequently seen in their nuclei. There appears to be no special affinity of the demyelinating process for particular tracts, but it is usually more severe in some locations than others. The commonly involved sites are the anterior medullary velum, the cerebellar peduncles and arbor vitae, and the periphery of the optic chiasm and tracts. Demyelination is also common in subpial areas of the brain stem, either patchily or encircling it completely. Large foci of acute demyelination are uncommon in other parts of the brain.

Later stages of demyelination are characterized by reactive changes of astrocytes, consisting of diffuse proliferations of astrocytes and some microglia. Occasionally, proliferating astrocytes form multinucleated syncytial cells. Inclusion bodies can be found in both types of astrocytes. The demyelination becomes more obvious, but it is usual for the original framework

of the tissue to remain and produce a lacelike appearance. Occasionally, especially in the folia of the cerebellum, there are foci of colliquative necrosis in which nothing remains except a few vessels and cells surrounded by fluid. These colliquative foci in the cerebellum may involve the granular layer but, as is usual for the lesions of canine distemper, spare the molecular layer. The demyelination reaction can progress to this stage with only very minor perivascular cuffing developing.

In canine distemper, perivascular cuffing is a late development and follows the demyelination. At the margins of larger foci in the chronic stage of the demyelination, thick perivascular cuffs of mononuclear cells form. At this stage the lesions have a distinctly "moth-eaten" appearance. Macrophages are prominent in the lesion, and astrocytic proliferation and fusion continue. The astroglia have abundant, glassy cytoplasm and plump processes. Viral inclusion bodies in the astrocytic nuclei may be common (Fig 6.25B). Animals that survive the encephalomyelitis of canine distemper may be left with old sclerotic astrocytic foci and myelin loss.

The role of the canine distemper virus in old-dog encephalitis remains unclear. **Old-dog encephalitis** (see the Nervous System, Volume 1) is a disease of mature dogs, characterized clinically by progressive motor and mental deterioration and pathologically by encephalitis with widely scattered perivascular infiltrations of lymphocytes and plasma cells and by intranuclear inclusions in the astrocytes and neurons. The inclusion bodies have been shown to contain paramyxovirus nucleocapsids and the viral antigen of canine distemper, but most investigators have been unable to recover the distemper virus from affected dogs or to transmit the disease to either dogs or distemper-susceptible ferrets. The nature of the lesions and the localization are distinct between old-dog encephalitis and the demyelinating encephalitis of canine distemper. The cerebellum, which is regularly involved in canine distemper encephalitis, is usually spared in old-dog encephalitis, and clinical signs of the two entities are different. If the canine distemper virus is the cause of old-dog encephalitis, the pathogenetic mechanisms must differ from those that operate to produce the conventional disease.

BOVINE RESPIRATORY SYNCYTIAL VIRUS INFECTION. Bovine respiratory syncytial virus belongs to the genus *Pneumovirus* of the Paramyxoviridae. Although serologic evidence of widespread infection in cattle populations has been recognized since 1975, only more recently has the virus been widely accepted as an important respiratory pathogen. Current evidence indicates that virulent strains of the virus are one of the synergistic agents involved in bovine respiratory disease, but they are also capable of causing outbreaks of respiratory disease and occasional deaths independently, most often in animals less than 1 year of age. Outbreaks usually occur in fall or early winter, generally within a few weeks of the animals' being housed. Late-weaned calves seem to be most susceptible to the disease. Prominent clinical signs are coughing and tachypnea, and in the most severely affected animals there is respiratory distress with open-mouthed breathing and forced, grunting expiration.

Gross lesions in animals dying of the naturally occurring disease are irregular lobular or confluent regions of atelectasis and consolidation in cranioventral portions of the lungs. Interstitial emphysema is frequently present and is particularly evident in more caudal regions, where there sometimes are large bullae within interlobular septa. There is often mucopus within bronchi of pneumonic and atelectatic regions. The exudate may be foamy in major bronchi. Histologically, as with other myxoviruses, an acute bronchiolitis is a major component of the disease. A special characteristic of the bronchiolar response is the frequent prominance of syncytial giant cells formed by proliferating bronchiolar epithelial cells, some of which may contain acidophilic intracytoplasmic inclusion bodies. Alveoli are either atelectatic, because of bronchiolar obstruction, or contain a mixed cellular exudate in their lumina and mononuclear thickening of their septa. When alveoli are directly involved, alveolar epithelial proliferation with a tendency to form large syncytial giant cells is even more prominent than in bronchioles, and here also acidophilic intracytoplasmic inclusion bodies are sometimes seen. There is moderate accumulation of lymphocytes and plasma cells in the peribronchiolar and associated connective tissues.

Experimental infections with virulent strains produce a bronchointerstitial pneumonia with peak involvement about 5–8 days after infection. Syncytial giant cells of bronchiolar and alveolar epithelium are an outstanding feature during this period, and many contain intracytoplasmic inclusions. Both natural and experimental infections can lead to obliterative bronchiolitis in surviving animals.

In comparing bovine respiratory syncytial virus and parainfluenza-3 infections, it appears that bovine respiratory syncytial virus is more likely to cause severe respiratory disease by itself and that in fatal cases there is a reasonable chance of finding intracytoplasmic inclusion bodies in the exaggerated syncytial giant-cell formations. Once the giant-cell and inclusion-body stage has passed, it is not possible to distinguish the lesions.

A feature of the respiratory syncytial virus infection that has not been fully explained is its association with lesions of acute (atypical) interstitial pneumonia. This usually occurs during the fall in newly weaned, well-fed calves. After signs of an initial viral infection there is sometimes a period of 2 or 3 days during which partial recovery takes place, and then some of the calves develop severe respiratory distress, which often leads to death. In such cases, the most dramatic findings are those of widespread interstitial edema and emphysema accompanying acute interstitial pneumonia. Lesions of cranioventral bronchopneumonia may also be detected. The role played by the syncytial virus in causing the diffuse alveolar damage and its sequelae is not known. The diffuse damage has not been produced experimentally. It has been suggested that a hypersensitivity mechanism is involved, such as is believed to occur in children with antibodies to human respiratory syncytial virus who are reinfected with the virus, but there is no supporting evidence. Other alternatives are that the viral infection predisposes the calves to acute interstitial pneumonia of dietary or other origin, or that in some cases the infection is merely coincidental.

Antibodies to bovine respiratory syncytial virus have been detected in sheep, and mild pulmonary disease has been produced experimentally in young, colostrum-deprived lambs using a bovine strain.

Picornavirus Infections

Two serotypes of rhinovirus are widespread among cattle populations. **Bovine rhinovirus** is generally believed to be of minor importance as a cause of respiratory disease in cattle. Viral isolation and serologic responses occasionally provide circumstantial evidence that it is involved in causing upper respiratory disease. Experimental production of disease is inconsistent, but there have not been recent attempts to confirm earlier indications that the virus might be able to produce a bronchointerstitial pneumonia. It seems most probable that the viral replication and damage are limited to the upper respiratory tract in natural infections. The same holds true for **equine rhinovirus**, which is incriminated as a minor cause of acute upper respiratory disease in horses.

Calicivirus Infections

Caliciviruses are closely related to picornaviruses, and originally, feline caliciviruses, which are the important members of the genus causing respiratory disease, were considered feline picornaviruses. **Feline calicivirus** infection is commonly manifest as an upper respiratory tract disease (see Rhinitis). Feline caliciviruses can replicate in a variety of tissues, but their pathogenic effects are usually limited to the oral and respiratory mucosa and, to a lesser extent, the conjunctiva. Clinical signs are principally fever, oral ulceration, rhinitis, conjunctivitis, and possibly pneumonia. The range and severity of lesions depends on the virulence and tropism of the particular strain of calicivirus and on the mode of infection. Ulceration of oral epithelium is a common finding in both natural and experimental infections and reveals the close relationship of feline caliciviruses to vesicular exanthema virus of swine. The ulcers, which occasionally are detected in the earlier transient vesicular stage, are most often present on the dorsal surface or lateral margins of the tongue and on the hard palate and external nares. Serous or mucous rhinitis and conjunctivitis are less consistent findings but are more common in natural infections, or in experimental infections if the virus is administered intranasally rather than by aerosol exposure. Clinical signs of pneumonia may be present in natural infections, but affected cats usually recover within 7 to 10 days unless bacterial complications ensue.

Most information on the pneumonia caused by feline caliciviruses is derived from experiments using heavy exposure to aerosolized pneumotropic strains. This produces an exaggerated picture of lung lesions compared to natural infections. Nevertheless, certain strains of the virus have a strong tropism for alveolar type I epithelial cells. The resulting lesion is an acute to subacute interstitial pneumonia with little of the bronchiolitis produced by the viral infections described previously. Grossly, the pneumonia involves cranioventral margins of the lungs, and possibly irregular foci elsewhere. Early lesions are bright red and become gray-red at the peak of consolidation (7–10 days) and thereafter become gray-tan as resolution occurs. Histologically, the lesion is an interstitial pneumonia initiated by virus-induced necrosis of alveolar type I epithelial cells. The epithelial necrosis is extensive from $\frac{1}{2}$ day to 4 days after infection and is accompanied by exudation of serofibrinous fluid and large numbers of neutrophils. Hyaline membranes may be present. As the viral replication, necrosis and acute inflammation subside, type II epithelial cells proliferate to line denuded alveolar walls, and the inflammatory cells become increasingly mononuclear. Between 7 and 10 days after infection, alveoli are epithelialized by type II cells; lumina contain mostly macrophages, and alveolar septa are thickened by accumulation of lymphocytes, plasma cells, and sometimes, fibroblasts. Few residual lesions are present after 30 days, other than scarring as the result of necrosis of alveolar walls and hemorrhage that occurred during the acute phase. The upper respiratory tract involvement in feline herpesvirus infections compared to the oral and pulmonary distribution of lesions in calicivirus infections are useful differential features, especially so in cats reaching the pathologist. Specific diagnosis, however, requires demonstration of virus in tissues by immunofluorescence.

Adenovirus Infections

Adenoviruses have been isolated from most species of animals. They have differing virulence and tissue tropisms, but more often cause respiratory and enteric disease than other manifestations. The most pronounced feature of the pneumotropic strains is a necrotizing and proliferative bronchiolitis. Severe, naturally occurring disease usually requires an immunodeficiency state.

Canine adenovirus type 1 is the cause of **infectious canine hepatitis** and is described with diseases of the liver (in the Liver and Biliary System, this volume). **Canine adenovirus-2** is more strictly associated with respiratory disease, but strain differences within both serotypes makes the distinction between them not as clear-cut as once thought. Naturally occurring respiratory disease caused by adenovirus in dogs is mostly found in conjunction with canine distemper or other conditions causing immunologic impairment. The salient features are necrotizing bronchiolitis and the presence of large, amphophilic, intranuclear inclusions in swollen nuclei of degenerating bronchiolar epithelial cells. Intranuclear inclusions are usually less common in alveolar and bronchial epithelial cells and alveolar macrophages. The inclusions either fill the nuclei or are separated by a narrow clear zone from the thickened nuclear membrane (Cowdry type A inclusion). Affected bronchioles are filled with debris of sloughed epithelium and neutrophils. When viral infection of alveolar cells is extensive, there is an accompanying exudate of serofibrinous material, neutrophils, erythrocytes, and macrophages. Alveolar epithelialization can be prominent after viral replication has peaked (~10 days). Interstitial thickening by mononuclear cells and neutrophils occurs but is not an impressive feature.

Equine adenovirus infection is widespread in horses but mainly causes disease in young Arabian foals with congenital, combined or selective immunodeficiency disease. Pulmonary lesions are a combination of coalesced atelectatic and consolidated lobules in cranioventral regions; large amounts of lung may be affected. Mucopurulent exudate is frequently present in the airways. Histologically, the main lesion is a severe bronchiolitis, which varies from necrotizing to proliferative, depending on the age of the lesions and the proportion of epithelial cells infected with virus. In the early stage of severe infection, there is extensive necrosis and sloughing of bronchiolar epithelium (Fig. 6.26A). Later, bronchiolar epithelium is hyperplastic, and swollen superficial epithelial cells contain amphophilic intra-

nuclear inclusion bodies. Large, indistinct, blue inclusions are present in nuclei of dead cells that have been sloughed into the lumen (Fig. 6.26B). The combination of sloughed or hyperplastic epithelium and luminal filling by cell debris and neutrophils causes bronchiolar obstruction, which is responsible for the widespread alveolar atelectasis. The uncomplicated adenoviral lesion is sometimes limited to airways, without direct alveolar involvement. In other instances there are intranuclear inclusions in alveolar epithelial cells and an alveolitis mainly characterized by accumulations of macrophages and a variety of leukocytes. Epithelial lesions and inclusions may also be present in conjunctival and upper respiratory epithelium during the height of the disease. They can also occur in epithelium of the renal pelvis, ureters, urinary bladder, urethra, lacrimal and salivary glands, and pancreas. The viral bronchiolitis or bronchopneumonia and the associated immunodeficiency state may combine to lead to secondary bacterial pneumonia or pneumocystis pneumonia (Fig. 6.26C,D).

A variety of epitheliotropic and endotheliotropic **bovine** and **ovine adenoviruses** has been isolated from ruminants. Circumstantial evidence indicates that certain serotypes can cause mild respiratory or enteric disease or a combination of both. They are not generally considered to be important pathogens, however. Experimental infection of calves with epitheliotropic strains can cause necrotizing and proliferative bronchiolitis, with intranuclear inclusions similar to the lesions occurring in foals. Only rarely are the characteristic lesions found in naturally occurring disease, usually in very young calves that lack colostral antibody or in which environmental stress or intercurrent diseases have impaired immune responses. A similar situation seems to exist in sheep. A noteworthy feature of the lesions caused by at least one strain of adenovirus from sheep is the exaggerated enlargement of both nucleus and cytoplasm of inclusion-bearing bronchiolar and alveolar epithelial cells. The pronounced cytomegaly can cause confusion with the cellular enlargement associated with cytomegalovirus infections.

Porcine adenoviruses studied so far appear to have less affinity for pulmonary epithelium than those from the species already mentioned. Limited experimental information indicates that pulmonary lesions are probably more of a true interstitial pneumonia, with alveolar septa thickened by proliferation of alveolar epithelial cells and accumulation of macrophages, lymphocytes, and plasma cells. Cells within alveolar septa, some possibly capillary endothelial cells, contain bluish intranuclear inclusions. Bronchiolar epithelial necrosis or hyperplasia is not a significant feature. Porcine adenoviruses have been associated with field cases of encephalitis or diarrhea but have not been established as an important cause of respiratory disease.

Herpesvirus Infections

Members of the family Herpesviridae are important causes of respiratory disease. Three of them are discussed under Rhinitis: inclusion-body rhinitis of swine, infectious bovine rhinotracheitis, and feline viral rhinotracheitis. Another described elsewhere is malignant catarrhal fever (see the Alimentary System, this volume). Pseudorabies (Aujeszky's disease) mainly causes disease of the nervous system (see the Nervous System, Volume 1), but certain strains of the virus can also cause rhinitis

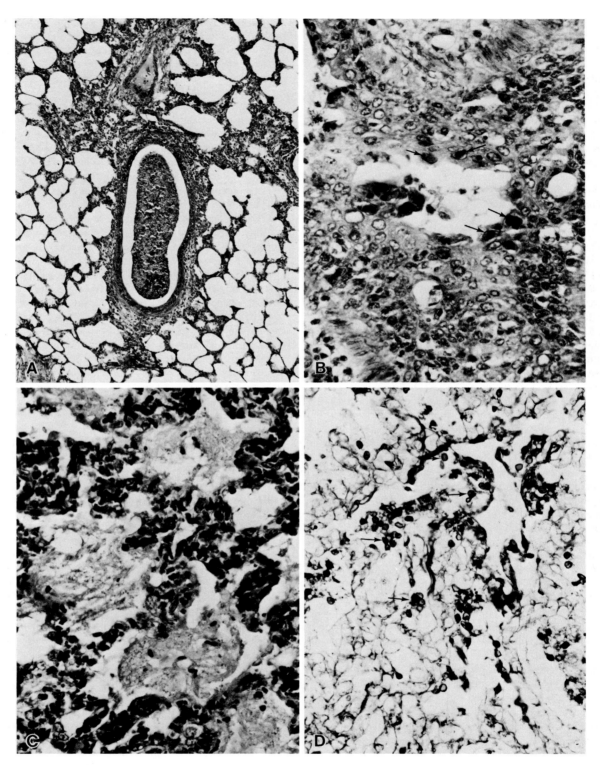

Fig. 6.26. Adenovirus infection in Arabian foal with combined immunodeficiency. (**A**) Acute necrotizing bronchiolitis.
(**B**) Intranuclear inclusions (arrows) in superficial hyperplastic bronchiolar epithelium.   (**C**) Pneumocystis pneumonia complicating
adenovirus infection. Alveoli contain abundant foamy and granular acidophilic material.   (**D**) *Pneumocystis carinii* organisms revealed
by methenamine–silver stain (arrows).

and pneumonia in swine. The severe acute lesion is hemorrhagic consolidation of cranioventral regions of the lung, which histologically has necrotizing lesions in bronchioles and adjacent alveoli as the principal features. Acidophilic or amphophilic intranuclear inclusions might be found in bronchiolar and alveolar epithelial cells early in the infection.

Canine herpesvirus is most important as a cause of fatal, generalized infection in neonatal puppies (see the Female Genital System, Volume 3). It can occasionally be associated with usually nonfatal respiratory infection in older animals, either alone or with other infectious agents. The respiratory lesions are those to be expected from herpesviruses, namely, a necrotizing rhinotracheitis and, possibly, bronchopneumonia. Acidophilic intranuclear inclusions can sometimes be found in epithelial cells in early lesions, more commonly in nasal and turbinate mucosa.

Equine herpesvirus (rhinopneumonitis virus) is an important respiratory tract pathogen, and even when herpesviruses cause abortion, they appear to affect mostly full-term foals and cause predominantly pulmonary lesions. The respiratory disease often occurs independently of abortions, and it appears likely that different strains of equine herpesvirus are specifically associated with each syndrome. Currently, strains causing rhinopneumonitis and abortion are grouped together as equine herpesvirus-1, but eventually they will probably be separated. For the role of equine herpesviruses in causing genital lesions and abortion, see the Female Genital System (Volume 3). A syndrome of paresis or ataxia is occasionally seen in mares (see the Nervous System, Volume 1).

The clinical respiratory disease is seen mostly in weanling foals during the fall. It is characterized by slight fever, and serous or catarrhal rhinitis and conjunctivitis. Rarely, there is diarrhea and edema of the extremities. Recovery occurs in ~1 week but may be delayed when secondary bacterial infections supervene and cause mucopurulent or suppurative rhinitis and pharyngitis, or possibly pneumonia. The uncomplicated viral infection is not fatal, even when severe, as it can be in young horses crowded in stockyards or stables. When fatalities occur, they are usually due to secondary suppurative bacterial bronchopneumonias. Intranuclear inclusions are extremely rare in postnatal respiratory infections.

Parvovirus Infections

Canine parvovirus is mainly a cause of enteritis and myocardial necrosis [see the Alimentary (this volume) and Cardiovascular (Volume 3) Systems]. Pulmonary lesions are usually those of severe acute to subacute pulmonary congestion and edema, secondary to the myocardial damage. A true viral interstitial pneumonia is generally limited to very young pups (<2 weeks of age) in which there is generalized parvovirus infection. In such cases, basophilic intranuclear inclusions can be found in the vascular endothelium of many organs, including the lung. In the lung, viral infection of capillary endothelium, and perhaps alveolar epithelium, causes necrosis and accumulation of mixed inflammatory cells, mostly lymphocytes and monocytes. Alveolar edema is partly the result of local alveolar septal inflammation, and partly cardiac failure.

Reovirus Infections

Of the three serotypes of reovirus, one or more have been isolated from cattle, horses, dogs, and cats. They are associated with inapparent infection or a mild upper respiratory disease. Their role as significant causes of, or predisposers to, pneumonia is not established.

Retrovirus Infections

OVINE PROGRESSIVE PNEUMONIA. Chronic progressive pneumonia of sheep (maedi) is a slow virus infection of the ovine lung, characterized by a gradually progressive interstitial pneumonia. It is caused by identical or very closely related strains of maedi–visna virus. Maedi–visna virus belongs to the lentivirus subfamily of retroviruses and therefore resembles the type C oncornaviruses and the virus causing pulmonary adenomatosis (*jaagsiekte*) of sheep (see Neoplastic Diseases of the Lungs). The name of the maedi–visna virus is derived from the fact that investigators in Iceland were the first to isolate the virus and demonstrate that the progressive pneumonia they referred to clinically as maedi (''shortness of breath'') and the meningoencephalitis they designated clinically as visna (''wasting'') were different manifestations of the same slow virus infection. For descriptions of visna, see the Nervous System (Volume 1).

The pulmonary disease caused by the maedi–visna virus occurs widely throughout Europe, North America, Africa, and Asia, and until the development and use of serologic tests for detecting infected animals, was being spread further by importation of affected sheep. In addition to the terms ovine progressive pneumonia and maedi, the condition is known as **Graaff–Reinet disease** in the Republic of South Africa, *zwoegerziekete* in the Netherlands, and *la bouhite* in France.

The virus is spread by close contact among sheep, and in milk from ewe to lamb. *In utero* infection can also occur. Infection of sheep is common in regions where the disease is endemic, but many go to slaughter without developing clinical signs. Because of the slow rate of progression of pulmonary lesions, clinical signs are uncommon until sheep reach 2 years of age. Evidence of disease is most frequent among sheep 5 to 10 years of age. The early signs are loss of weight and increased respiratory rate on exertion. Once signs begin, death usually occurs within about 6 to 8 months because of continuing deterioration in condition and increasing respiratory difficulty.

The specific lesions of ovine progressive pneumonia occur in the lungs and their associated lymph nodes. Grossly, the lungs of severely affected sheep do not collapse fully when the thorax is opened, and sometimes the impressions of the ribs are retained. In cases uncomplicated by bronchopneumonia or abscessation, the lungs are mottled gray to grayish tan, and the pleura is smooth and glistening (Fig. 6.27A). Lungs are much heavier than usual, often two or more times the normal weight. Close examination of the lung reveals that although the lesions are widespread, there is relative sparing of the cranioventral regions in the absence of secondary bronchopneumonia. Least involved regions have an irregular grayish speckling against a light tan background. More involvement results in a reticular pattern, and in most severely affected regions there is homogeneous grayish consolidation. The lungs have a soft rubbery consistency or are

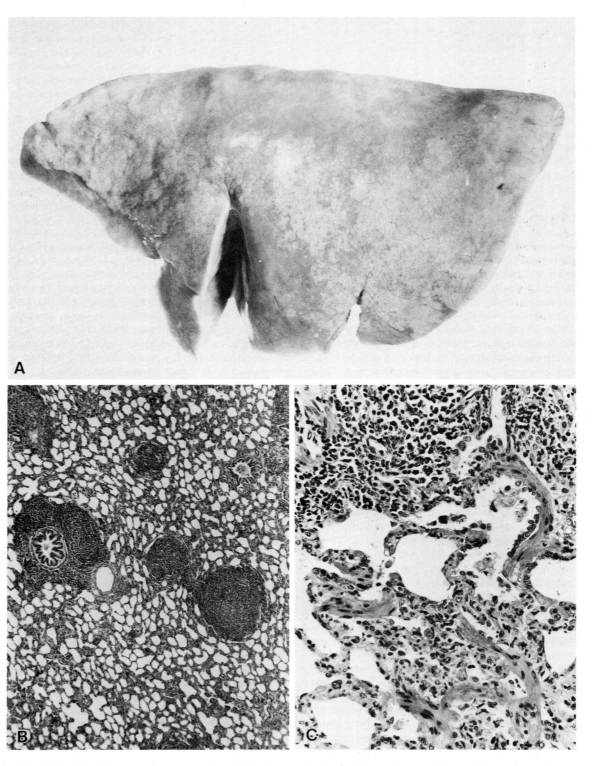

Fig. 6.27. Chronic progressive pneumonia (maedi). Sheep. (**A**) Lungs fail to collapse and have widespread, grayish mottling. (**B**) Diffuse thickening of alveolar walls and lymphofollicular accumulations around vessels and airways. (**C**) Hyperplasia of smooth muscle of terminal bronchioles and alveolar ducts, with adjacent interstitial accumulation of lymphoid cells.

moderately firm, depending on the degree of confluence of the lesions. The cut surface is moist, but without oozing of free fluid. When complicated by bronchopneumonia, there are the typical cranioventral consolidations, with pus-filled airways. There can also be coexistent lungworm lesions. A consistent gross finding in ovine progressive pneumonia is enlargement of bronchial and mediastinal lymph nodes, with soft, grayish white, homogeneous thickening of cortical regions on cut section.

Histologically, the most characteristic feature of ovine progressive pneumonia is the extensive lymphofollicular proliferations that occur predominantly in the perivascular, peribronchial, and peribronchiolar sheaths in association with the pulmonary lymphatics. The most consistent association is with pulmonary veins. Many of the lymphoid follicles contain germinal centers (Fig. 6.27B). The next most striking feature is hyperplasia of smooth muscle, which is most evident in the walls of terminal bronchioles and alveolar ducts but also extends into the walls of neighboring alveoli (Fig. 6.27C). Alveolar septa are thickened by infiltrations of lymphocytes and macrophages, especially at the peripheries of the lymphoid nodules. The amount of interstitial fibrosis is usually slight but tends to be exaggerated by collapse of small clusters of alveoli and apposition of their walls (microatelectasis). Hyperplasia of alveolar type II epithelial cells is not a prominent feature of ovine progressive pneumonia, in striking contrast to ovine pulmonary adenomatosis (see Neoplastic Diseases of the lungs). Partial or complete lining of alveoli by cuboidal type II cells does occur, but usually only in alveoli adjacent to the large interstitial lymphoid follicles or occasionally lining large, cystlike spaces. Bronchiolar epithelial hyperplasia is also not a prominent feature of uncomplicated ovine progressive pneumonia, although collapsed airways have pleated epithelium that can be mistaken for hyperplasia or that leads to exaggerated interpretation of it. The alveolar exudate in the uncomplicated disease is usually sparse and consists mainly of alveolar macrophages and small amounts of debris. Multinucleated macrophages are a variable feature. Suppurative lesions oriented around bronchioles indicate a secondary bacterial bronchopneumonia. Bronchial and mediastinal lymph nodes have a chronic hyperplastic lymphadenitis in which the main feature is pronounced follicular hyperplasia.

In infected flocks, there is usually serologic evidence of infection of many animals, and the maedi–visna virus can be isolated from both normal and diseased lungs. The diagnosis of ovine progressive pneumonia depends mainly on the presence of the characteristic lymphofollicular interstitial pneumonia.

Progressive pneumonia is the most common manifestation of disease in sheep infected by the maedi–visna virus. Meningoencephalitis (visna) is less common and occurs separately or, occasionally, in the same sheep. It is now recognized that the virus also causes a chronic proliferative arthritis about as frequently as the meningoencephalitis. Lymphofollicular lesions sometimes occur in mammary glands of infected sheep. In these respects, the range of lesions caused by maedi–visna virus closely resembles those produced by the caprine arthritis–encephalitis virus described below. The extensive lymphoid proliferations in ovine progressive pneumonia and the similarities of the maedi–visna virus to the oncornaviruses have given rise to the speculation that

the proliferations are neoplastic in nature. The proliferative lymphoid elements do not resemble any of the forms of lymphoma, however, and the cells do not exhibit malignant cytologic or behavioral characteristics.

Caprine arthritis–encephalitis is a disease complex in goats caused by a retrovirus antigenically related to the maedi–visna virus but separable on the basis of the large differences in nucleic acid sequences. The caprine virus has mainly been studied in reference to its ability to cause encephalitis and arthritis, as the name indicates (see the Nervous System, and Bones and Joints, Volume 1). An alternative term for the disease is viral leukoencephalomyelitis–arthritis. There are brief descriptions of a chronic interstitial pneumonia produced by the virus, but there has not been a detailed study of the pulmonary lesions. Naturally occurring chronic pneumonia in older goats often has two prominent features lacking in ovine progressive pneumonia. One is extensive alveolar filling mainly by a dense, acidophilic, proteinaceous (lipoproteinaceous) material. The other is widespread lining of alveolar septa by alveolar type II epithelial cells. The pathogenesis of these components and their relationship to infection with the caprine arthritis–encephalitis virus remain to be determined.

Other Virus Infections

A variety of viruses, particularly those of enteric origin, such as enteroviruses, coronaviruses, and bovine virus diarrhea virus, have occasionally been isolated from cases of respiratory disease. Significant primary roles have not been established for such agents, although the immunosuppressive effects of viruses like bovine virus diarrhea virus could be important in predisposing infected cattle to respiratory infection.

Bacterial Diseases

Pasteurellosis

The pasteurellae are strict parasites of animals, their usual habitat the mucous membranes of the nasopharyngeal and oral regions. The type species is *Pasteurella multocida*. The other species of major importance for respiratory disease in domestic animals is *P. haemolytica*. A third, *P. pneumotropica*, can frequently be isolated from the pharynx of cats and may contaminate bite wounds made by cats.

The collective term pasteurellosis will be used here for infections by either *Pasteurella multocida* or *P. haemolytica*. Pasteurellosis may be manifested as a peracute or acute septicemia, or be slightly less acute and cause signs according to the organ in which the infection is localized. Thus, in the various species, pasteurellosis can take a variety of forms. It may be a primary infection, a contaminant of cutaneous or mucosal injuries, or a secondary infection, especially following viral disease of the respiratory tract.

Pasteurella multocida can be isolated from pathologic conditions in cattle, sheep, buffalo, deer, pigs, rabbits, and other animals, and from a variety of birds in which it causes fowl cholera. The different strains had been named for the species of host in which they were found, but it is current practice to regard these as types of the one species *P. multocida*. Mammalian isolates of *P. multocida* are typed by biologic characteristics (biotype), and serologically (serotype). The important strains form smooth colonies and are assigned on the basis of capsular antigens to one of four serotypes: A, B, D, and E. Further characterization can be made on the basis of somatic O antigens. Types B and E are the cause of epidemic pasteurellosis, the classical hemorrhagic septicemia of cattle, sheep, goats, deer, and buffalos. Type B is widespread in tropical Asia and Africa and in southern Europe. Type E occurs mainly in central Africa. Type A is ubiquitous and responsible for sporadic infections in many species; strains of this serotype are the ones usually isolated from pneumonia of cattle and fowl cholera and are sometimes found in pneumonia of swine. Type D is ubiquitous but has been found particularly in association with atrophic rhinitis and pneumonia in swine. It is also occasionally isolated from pneumonia in sheep.

Strains of *Pasteurella haemolytica* are also classified by biotype and serotype. The organism is weakly hemolytic, and as a rule is nonpathogenic for rodents. The two main biotypes are A (arabinose fermenters) and T (trehalose fermenters). There are 15 currently recognized serotypes based on analysis of capsular antigens. Of these, 3, 4, 10, and 15 belong to biotype T, and the remainder to biotype A. Type A1 is the usual cause of severe pneumonic pasteurellosis ("shipping fever") of cattle. Type A strains are associated with pneumonia in sheep and septicemia in lambs before weaning. Type T strains cause septicemia in lambs past weaning age.

Pasteurella multocida and *P. haemolytica* are both members of the bacterial flora of normal nasopharyngeal and oral mucous membranes, with the former usually predominating. Outbreaks of disease caused by the organisms occur when local and systemic defense mechanisms are impaired and virulent strains of pasteurellae undergo massive proliferation prior to invading the nasopharyngeal mucosa or being inhaled in large numbers into the lung. Predisposing factors, such as the stress induced by shipping, crowding, climatic changes, and poor management, or the damaging effects of respiratory viral infections, were mentioned previously (see Bronchopneumonia). Many of the effects of stress are mediated by adrenocorticosteroid release.

CATTLE. The major pasteurelloses of cattle are hemorrhagic septicemia and pneumonic pasteurellosis. Two other forms of pasteurellosis, meningitis in calves and mastitis in cows, occasionally are important in local situations. Meningeal pasteurellosis of calves is caused by *Pasteurella multocida,* and it is usually a disease of housed calves 2–4 months of age. The reaction is fibrinopurulent and is sometimes accompanied by polyarthritis of the same type. Bovine mastitis is caused by either *P. multocida* or *P. haemolytica.* Sporadic, peracute, fatal mammary infections occur that are caused by *P. haemolytica;* these infections are characterized by severe hemorrhagic inflammation of the parenchyma and a fibrinous and necrotizing inflammation of the ducts, quite similar to the peracute inflammation produced by coliform organisms. The pathway of infection is via the duct system. *Pasteurella multocida* can be responsible for outbreaks of mastitis in a herd. If the mastitis is acute, it may be progressive and result in fibrosis and atrophy. The route of infection is assumed to be through the ducts, and the source of

infection, in some cases at least, is assumed to be the suckling calf. *Pasteurella haemolytica* is sometimes responsible for outbreaks of abortion in cattle in which there are no premonitory signs.

The classical form of bovine pasteurellosis is **hemorrhagic septicemia**, which is caused by *Pasteurella multocida* types B or E. This disease was originally recognized in western Europe in the last century as a severe epidemic in deer that later spread to cattle, wild and domestic pigs, and horses. It has been observed as an epidemic disease of cattle, sheep, and horses in Argentina, in bison in the western United States, and it is the disease known as *el guedda* of Syrian camels, and *barbone* of Italian buffalo. Hemorrhagic septicemia is now limited largely to tropical lands from Egypt to the Philippine Islands and in these regions is primarily a disease of buffalo.

The most detailed descriptions are of the disease as it occurs in Asia. There outbreaks occur particularly during the rainy season. In intervening periods, the organism is apparently maintained in the nasopharyngeal regions of carrier cattle or buffalo. The start of an outbreak depends on some stress disturbing the balance in a carrier animal. This results in extensive proliferation and dissemination of the organisms to susceptible contact animals.

Approximately 10% of animals survive subclinical infections and become immune, but once the infection is established clinically, the mortality is 100%, even though the bacteria may be killed by chemotherapy. This, together with the immense proliferation of organisms in the clinical disease, indicates that toxins, particularly endotoxins, are important in causing the fatal outcome.

Hemorrhagic septicemia is almost by definition a peracute disease, with death often so early that few signs are observed. When observed clinically, there is high fever and rapid prostration, with profuse salivation. The saliva and feces contain large numbers of pasteurellae. The postmortem picture is characterized by petechial hemorrhages on the serous membranes and in the various organs, especially the lungs and muscles. Severe endotoxemia may cause an acute fibrinohemorrhagic interstitial pneumonia. The lymph nodes are swollen and hemorrhagic, and there may be bloodstained fluid in the serous cavities. Acute gastroenteritis, which can be hemorrhagic, is often present. The spleen is not greatly enlarged, which is a point of differentiation from anthrax.

There is an edematous form of hemorrhagic septicemia, which may also be peracute. Actually, edema of the throat is a regular part of hemorrhagic septicemia, but in some cases it can be unusually pronounced. It is characterized by extensive swelling of the subcutaneous tissues, especially of the throat, but it might affect the whole head, the tongue, or some other part of the body, such as the brisket or a limb. The swellings are produced by a copious, clotted, straw-colored exudate. The additional lesions in this form of pasteurellosis are those of hemorrhagic septicemia, although death may be caused by asphyxiation.

Pneumonic pasteurellosis refers to forms of pneumonia in which the predominant pulmonary damage is caused by pasteurellae. The most important form is the fulminating fibrinous lobar pneumonia caused, usually, by *Pasteurella haemolytica.* The frequent occurrence of this form of the disease in the period soon after shipping and crowding of beef cattle led to the widespread use of the term "shipping fever." This term emphasizes the major circumstances under which pneumonic pasteurellosis occurs but cannot be used with precision as a synonym. Acute fibrinous lobar pneumonia can also occur in very young calves, in older calves as an infection superimposed on enzootic pneumonia, and sporadically in cattle of any age. The fulminating fibrinous pneumonia is principally the result of rapid and massive proliferation of organisms. Although this is mostly associated with pathogenic strains of *P. haemolytica* in animals whose pulmonary defense has been compromised by various environmental stresses, and often a predisposing viral infection, it can also be caused by *P. multocida*. Occasionally, *Haemophilus somnus* causes an indistinguishable lesion. Of the various viruses that have been incriminated as predisposing to the severe *Pasteurella* pneumonia, parainfluenza-3 virus appears to be the most common. It has also been the virus used in most of the successful attempts to reproduce the characteristic pneumonia. When specific-pathogen-free calves or lambs are exposed to parainfluenza-3 virus, and 4–7 days later to aerosolized pathogenic strains of *P. haemolytica,* a severe pneumonia can be produced. Infectious bovine rhinotracheitis virus and, possibly, bovine respiratory syncytial virus and others appear to play a similar role.

The general features of fibrinous lobar pneumonia are described under Lobar Pneumonia. In addition to the extensive reddish black to grayish brown cranioventral regions of consolidation with prominent gelatinous thickening of interlobular septa and fibrinous pleuritis, areas of coagulation necrosis are a characteristic feature. At their most prominent, they appear as irregular but sharply demarcated regions with thick, white boundaries and sunken, deep red, central zones. Histologically, the necrotic regions are frequently seen to supervene in previously pneumonic tissue. They usually contain very large numbers of bacteria, particularly at their peripheries adjacent to the compacted debris of inflammatory cells that form the white boundary zones seen grossly. The cause of the necrosis is not fully determined. Although it has been attributed to thrombosis (infarction), the occurrence of thrombosed vessels is not consistent enough to be a satisfctory explanation, nor would it account for the necrosis sometimes cutting across interlobular septa into neighboring lobules (Fig. 6.29A). In view of the massive numbers of bacteria present, it is much more likely that the necrosis is caused by the necrotizing effect of the large amounts of bacterial endotoxins and cytotoxins released locally and by the associated capillary thrombosis. Another characteristic histologic feature is the presence of clustered inflammatory cells with elongated or streaming nuclei. These are commonly referred to as "oat cells." They seem to be an effect of bacterial toxins on leukocytes accumulating within inflamed alveoli. The extent to which they are derived from blood monocytes or neutrophils is not firmly established.

Also properly included in the general term "pneumonic pasteurellosis" is the less fulminating, fibrinous or fibrinopurulent bronchopneumonia (Fig. 6.28). This is more commonly caused by *Pasteurella multocida* but can be caused by *P. haemolytica.* The nature of the pneumonia caused by pasteurellae depends on the rate and extent of bacterial proliferation and the amount of toxins released, which in turn depend on the virulence of the strain of organism and the degree to which the defenses of the host are impaired. Although there is a tendency for *P. haemolytica* to be the cause of fulminating fibrinous lobar pneumonias, and *P. multocida* the cause of fibrinopurulent bronchopneumonias, this can change with local circumstances, and intermediate lesions (Fig. 6.29B) may be found among cases in the same outbreak.

SHEEP.   There are several syndromes in sheep associated with *Pasteurella haemolytica* or *P. multocida*. Mastitis in ewes caused by *Pasteurella* spp. is discussed with the Female Genital System (Volume 3). The principal forms of pasteurellosis in sheep are septicemia caused by *P. haemolytica,* and sporadic or enzootic pneumonia, which is associated more often with *P. haemolytica* than *P. multocida.*

Septicemia caused by *Pasteurella haemolytica,* biotype T, occurs mainly in weaned lambs during the fall months, but it can occur in other age groups and at other times of the year. Deaths, which seldom exceed 5% of the sheep at risk, usually follow within a few days of changes in pasture, feed, or other management practices.

The clinical syndrome is not specific. Signs of illness are vague, and the usual course is short, with sudden death reminiscent of clostridial enterotoxemia. At necropsy, petechial and ecchymotic hemorrhages are usually present but sometimes difficult to detect. They occur in subcutaneous tissues, particularly of the neck and thorax, in intermuscular fascia, and in the pleura, epicardium, and mesentery. The lymph nodes are mainly affected in the throat and mesenteric regions, where they are hemorrhagic and edematous. Yellow plaques of necrotizing pharyngitis are common, especially around tonsillar crypts, and ulcers may involve the esophageal mucosa. The abomasal and colonic mucosae sometimes have shallow ulcers. The lungs have diffuse, severe congestion and edema with abundant white or bloodstained foam in the airways. Discrete hemorrhagic foci (infarcts) can sometimes be seen scattered throughout the lungs. The liver is usually congested, and in some cases there are many yellowish necrotic foci disseminated through the parenchyma. These are usually of miliary size but can be up to 1.0 cm in diameter and surrounded by a narrow red border. Occasionally there is inflammation of many joints, the pericardium, meninges, and choroid plexus, but the development of these lesions requires that the course be a little longer than it normally is. These additional lesions are observed more frequently in the experimental disease, which is less fulminating than the natural one.

Microscopic examination of tissues reveals a widespread bacterial embolism. The pale hepatic foci consist of colonies of bacteria with a surrounding ischemic zone. There may be thrombosis of the adjacent tributaries of the portal vein, and small amounts of parenchymal necrosis, but generally there is little or no leukocytic response. This is probably related to the short course of the disease, and partly the effects of bacterial toxin on the leukocytes. The pulmonary lesions are a combination of the effect of multiple bacterial emboli and the severe diffuse pulmonary congestion and edema found in sheep dying suddenly of

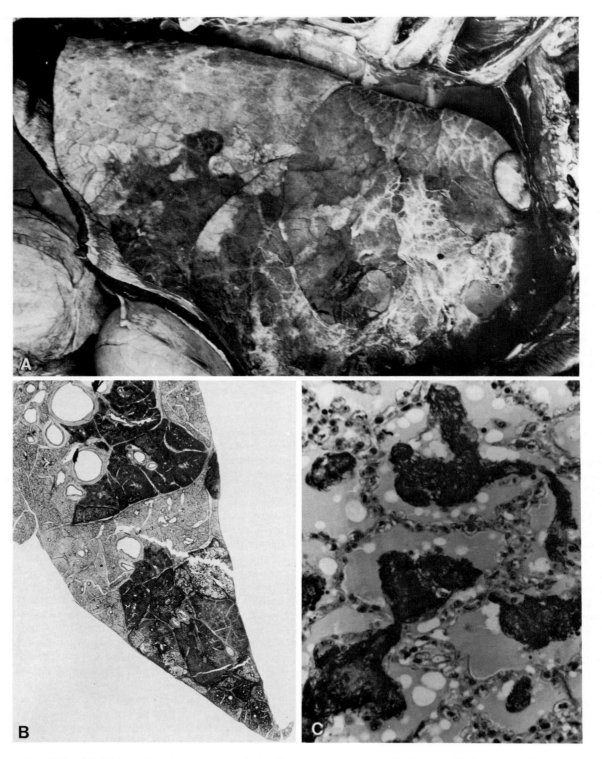

Fig. 6.28. (**A**) Fibrinous bronchopneumonia and pleuritis of pneumonic pasteurellosis. Ox. (**B**) Section of middle lobe in pasteurellosis. Ox. Irregular lobular involvement. (**C**) Intraalveolar fibrin clumps connecting through pores of Kohn in alveolar septa. Fibrinous pneumonia. Ox.

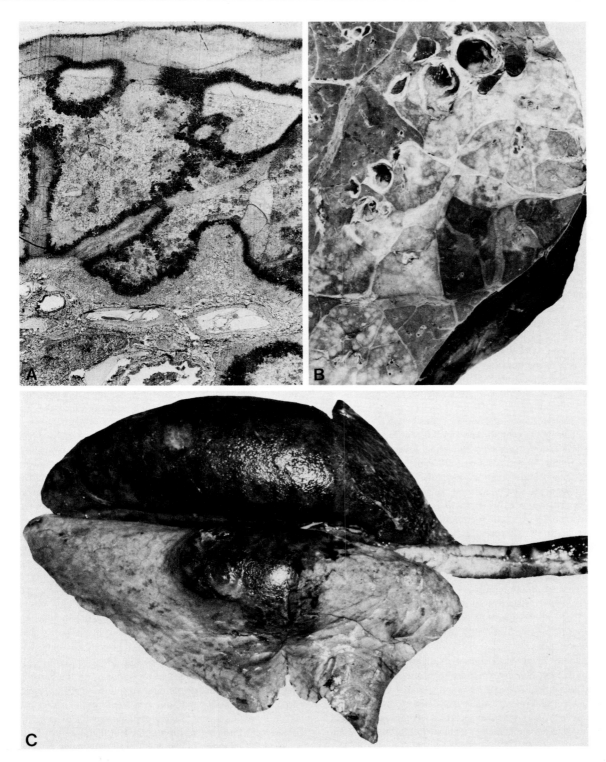

Fig. 6.29. (**A** and **B**) Fibrinonecrotic pneumonia of pneumonic pasteurellosis. Ox. (**A**) Large areas of pneumonic lung are necrotic and marginated by densely packed leukocytes. (**B**) ''Marbled'' pattern produced by differing degrees and stages of consolidation. (**C**) Porcine contagious pleuropneumonia (*Haemophilus pleuropneumoniae*). Hemorrhagic consolidation and necrosis in dorsal and hilar regions with fibrinous pleuritis. (Courtesy of B. W. Fenwick.)

almost any cause. In the focal hemorrhagic lesions, masses of bacteria occluding capillaries are accompanied by hemorrhagic and fibrinous exudate into the alveoli and sometimes with a peripheral zone of necrosis and degenerating, spindle-shaped leukocytes. Occlusive bacterial emboli are regularly found in the spleen and adrenals, and occasionally kidney, but are rare in other organs. Masses of bacteria adhere to the surface of the pharyngeal ulcerations and occlude underlying blood vessels and lymphatics. Peripheral and intermediate sinuses of the local lymph nodes also contain huge numbers of bacteria within the hemorrhagic and edematous exudate. The principal site of bacterial proliferation and subsequent systemic invasion is believed to be the pharyngeal lesion.

Pneumonic pasteurellosis in sheep is usually caused by *Pasteurella haemolytica,* biotype A. The same biotype can also cause septicemia in the absence of pneumonia in lambs less than 2 months of age. The generalizations regarding circumstances giving rise to pneumonic pasteurellosis in cattle hold true for sheep. Most outbreaks occur in lambs during late spring and early summer. Sudden climatic changes, gathering, and handling are the most commonly recognized predisposing situations. Viral infection, particularly by parainfluenza-3 virus, is also believed to play a role. The lesions tend to be those of acute hemorrhagic or fibrinonecrotic lobar pneumonia and serofibrinous pleuritis in acute cases, and fibrinopurulent bronchopneumonia leading to abscessation and fibrous pleural adhesions in subacute to chronic cases.

SWINE. Pasteurellosis of swine is caused by *Pasteurella multocida.* The most common and important infections by *P. multocida* are usually those complicating mycoplasmal (enzootic) pneumonia, which produce a chronic suppurative bronchopneumonia with abscessation. Pleuritis frequently accompanies the pneumonia, and sometimes pericarditis also occurs. Septicemic pasteurellosis due to *P. multocida* is occasionally observed in neonatal pigs, and meningitis can also be present in the same age group. *Pasteurella haemolytica* rarely affects swine but has been recovered from aborted fetuses.

Septicemic disease without localization or distinctive lesions is seen in adult pigs, especially those that are specific pathogen free. The disease in these animals is peracute, and *Pasteurella multocida* can be recovered from all organs in large numbers. The only recent report of a "hemorrhagic septicemia" type of pasteurellosis in pigs is from India, from which *P. multocida* type B was isolated.

Severe, acute, fibrinous pneumonias analogous to the more fulminating *Pasteurella* pneumonias in cattle and sheep are sometimes caused by *P. multocida* in pigs. As in cattle and sheep, stressing factors are usually suspected to be important. These are usually poor management, and perhaps intercurrent infection by viruses such as swine influenza or hog cholera (swine fever).

The acute fibrinous or fibrinonecrotic pneumonia is similar in many respects to the lesion in cattle. The extensive gelatinous thickening of interlobular and subpleural tissues and the severe serofibrinous pleuritis lead to the term "pleuropneumonia" being used on occasion. In this connection, although epidemiologic patterns indicate that most severe pneumonias of the

"pleuropneumonia" variety are caused by *Haemophilus pleuropneumoniae (H. parahaemolyticus)*, there is no clear separation between the severe pneumonia caused by the two organisms. Massive proliferation of a Gram-negative organism releasing abundant endotoxins and cytotoxins is common to both infections, hence a common pulmonary response.

In addition to the severe thoracic lesions in pneumonic pasteurellosis, there is often acute pharyngitis and inflammatory edema of the throat, and yellow, jaundice-like discoloration of the carcass of unknown cause. Severe pharyngitis can be necrotizing and ulcerative. A fibrinohemorrhagic polyarthritis may be present, and there is intense congestion of the gastric and intestinal mucosa. Complete recovery from pneumonic pasteurellosis seldom occurs in pigs. Animals that survive the acute disease tend to develop chronic lesions that are usually fatal in due course. In these, most obvious findings are polyarthritis, adhesive pericarditis and pleuritis, and extensive areas of fibrotic lung which contain numerous abscesses or fibrous capsules enclosing sequestra or caseous detritus. As usual in the fibrinous pneumonias caused by *Pasteurella* spp., the bacterium can often be cultured from the blood and other organs as well as the lung. The septicemic or bacteremic nature of the infection is revealed also by the recovery of the bacterium from aborted fetuses from pregnant sows that survive the acute disease.

OTHER SPECIES. *Pasteurella multocida* has been reported in fatal infections in horses, and this species was included in the earliest reports of "hemorrhagic septicemia" from Europe. Pasteurellae may be found along with other bacteria in the fibrinous pneumonias that complicate infections of the upper respiratory tract in horses.

Pasteurella species are common inhabitants of the oral cavity of cats and dogs. They are important as infections in bite wounds. Pulmonary infections with pasteurellae are uncommon in dogs, and when present are usually found with other bacteria as complications of canine distemper and aspiration pneumonia. *Pasteurella multocida* causes meningitis and otitis media in cats. It is also commonly associated with pyothorax, often together with other bacteria, and probably results in many instances from penetration of the pleural cavity by a foreign body.

Haemophilus Infections

The most important *Haemophilus* infection is porcine contagious pleuropneumonia, which is caused by *H. pleuropneumoniae (H. parahaemolyticus)*. This disease has increased dramatically in major swine-raising areas of the world. The characteristic lesion is a severe fibrinonecrotic and hemorrhagic pneumonia with accompanying fibrinous pleuritis, hence the designation pleuropneumonia. *Haemophilus pleuropneumoniae* is highly pathogenic and often appears capable of invading and rapidly proliferating within the lung in the absence of obvious predisposing factors. All aspects of pathogenesis of field outbreaks of the disease, however, are not understood.

Contagious pleuropneumonia can affect pigs of any age but is more common from about 6 weeks to 6 months of age. The severe form of the disease occurs mostly in later stages of fattening with a mortality rate of 20 to 80%. Peracute, acute, and subacute to chronic forms are recognized. Deaths in the peracute and acute forms occur suddenly or after a short period of depression, fever, and possibly, hemorrhage from nose and mouth. The main gross lesions are bloody nasal discharge, bloodstained foam in trachea and bronchi, and large regions of hemorrhagic or fibrinonecrotic pneumonia accompanied by fibrinous pleuritis. Since the tissue damage is caused by massive bacterial proliferation and release of toxins, the essential features are those already described for fulminating pneumonic pasteurellosis in cattle. There is less tendency for the pneumonic foci caused by *Haemophilus pleuropneumoniae* to be limited to the cranioventral lung regions, however, presumably because of the greater virulence of the organism. Irregular, well-circumscribed regions of hemorrhagic consolidation or necrosis are commonly found in more dorsocaudal regions, especially surrounding major bronchi near the hilus of the lung (Fig. 6.29C). The foci of consolidation are also particularly prone to undergo sequestration, with the result that in subacute cases there may be large foci of caseous or cavitating yellow-gray or tan necrotic debris surrounded by fibroblastic zones. Many of these can subsequently become abscesses through secondary contamination by *Corynebacterium pyogenes, Pasteurella multocida, Bordetella bronchiseptica,* Gram-negative enteric organisms, streptococci, or others. The end result can be a severely scarred, abscessed lung tightly bound to the thoracic wall by fibrous adhesions.

Extrapulmonary vascular lesions sometimes occur in acutely affected pigs, particularly in the kidneys. Hyaline thrombosis and fibrinoid necrosis of glomerular capillaries, afferent arterioles, and interlobular arteries indicate the probable effect of severe endotoxemia.

Other *Haemophilus* species can cause lung lesions. *Haemophilus parasuis* is a common synergistic infection with swine influenza virus. It causes a nonspecific suppurative bronchopneumonia. For its involvement in polyserositis and arthritis of swine, see Bones and Joints (Volume 1). *Haemophilus somnus* is discussed with diseases of the Nervous System (Volume 1). Its occasional production in cattle of a severe lesion indistinguishable from the fibrinous lobar pneumonia of pneumonic pasteurellosis was mentioned earlier.

Bordetellosis

Bordetella bronchiseptica is an obligate parasite of the upper respiratory tract of rodents, dogs, and pigs and can occasionally be found in various other species. In dogs, it is involved in the causation of kennel cough and chronic bronchitis, as discussed previously. It is also frequently associated with the development of suppurative bronchopneumonia in dogs with interstitial pneumonia caused by the distemper virus. *Bordetella bronchiseptica* can also cause secondary bronchopneumonia in association with other diseases leading to reduced pulmonary defenses.

In swine, the role of *Bordetella bronchiseptica* in the production of atrophic rhinitis has been dealt with under Atrophic Rhinitis of Swine. As a pulmonary pathogen, *B. bronchiseptica* is most important as the occasional cause of septicemia or severe bronchopneumonia in suckling pigs usually less than 3 weeks of age. Mortality can be high in these outbreaks. The bronchopneumonia is predominantly suppurative. Typically, it is associated with acute arteritis and rapid onset of fibrosis, most evident in peribronchiolar sites. Fibrosis may extend to other interstitial

regions when the amount of inflammation and exudation is severe. *Bordetella bronchiseptica* may also be a cause of suppurative bronchopneumonia in older pigs, mostly as a complication of mycoplasmal pneumonia in fattening animals.

Bordetella bronchiseptica has also been recorded as an occasional cause of suppurative bronchopneumonia in cats and foals.

Tuberculosis

Tuberculosis is typically a chronic infectious disease caused by bacteria of the genus *Mycobacterium*. Various forms of the disease have many features in common, but the exact pattern differs according to the species of *Mycobacterium* involved and the species of animal affected.

Tuberculosis is an ancient disease and is still widespread in some parts of the world. In many areas, however, the incidence of classical tuberculosis in humans and animals has been reduced to the point where mycobacterial disease is more often caused by atypical (nonmammalian) acid-fast bacilli. Infection and disease caused by these atypical mycobacteria are probably more widely recognized because they are no longer overshadowed by the classical disease and have been revealed for more detailed investigation. Changing environments and a susceptible population no longer provided with the cross-protection afforded by infection with the classical mycobacteria probably also play some role. The emergence of a wide range of mycobacteria as agents capable of causing disease has resulted in both diagnostic and taxonomic confusion. This is compounded by the large number of saprophytic mycobacteria now recognized and the lack of clear-cut separation between saprophytic and potentially pathogenic species. Assessment of the etiologic role of a mycobacterium isolated or identified in a particular case therefore needs to be made on the basis of specific evidence available for that case rather than on the basis of generalizations.

Mycobacteria are widely distributed in nature. Many are saprophytes, and some of these are opportunistic pathogens. Others, as far as known, are strictly parasitic. Some of the pathogenic types cannot be cultivated *in vitro,* and those that can be cultivated generally grow slowly. For these reasons taxonomic classification has been difficult. Currently, a variety of cultural and biologic characteristics, including serotyping, lipoprotein analyses, and phage typing, are used in numerical classification schemes. More than 100 properties of new isolates can be subjected to computer analysis. A high degree of matching (>80% of characteristics) is used to group organisms together as the same species. Mycobacterial classification is still incomplete, however, so in the meantime the following categorization puts the organisms into useful perspective. The listing is incomplete, and not all are of known veterinary significance.

The classical tubercle bacilli are *Mycobacterium tuberculosis* (human), *M. bovis* (bovine), and *M. avium* (avian). *Mycobacterium tuberculosis* and *M. bovis* are the principal, closely related mammalian pathogens. Two other closely related species are *M. microti* from voles and *M. africanum*. Differing strains of *M. avium* are now commonly included with strains of the very closely related *M. intracellulare* as the *M. avium–intracellulare* complex. To avoid confusion surrounding the term ''tuberculosis,'' a convention that has been adopted is to limit it to diseases caused by *M. tuberculosis* or *M. bovis*. Other conditions are referred to as **mycobacteriosis**, qualified with the specific agent where known (e.g., avian mycobacteriosis when caused by *M. avium*). Atypical mycobacteriosis is sometimes used as a general term to cover all the diseases other than those caused by *M. tuberculosis* and *M. bovis*. In most veterinary literature, however, disease caused by *M. avium* is still included as one of the classical forms of tuberculosis, and this usage will be continued in this chapter.

Mycobacteria, which can have an independent saprophytic existence in nature, are widespread in soil and water, on vegetation, and in mucous membranes of the oropharynx. There are a large number of species whose taxonomic status is not fully established. When these organisms cause disease, it is usually in immunologically compromised hosts, and the manifestations are either cervical lymphadenitis, pulmonary lesions similar to tuberculosis, or cutaneous lesions associated with local penetration of organisms through wounds or abrasions of the skin. An example is *Mycobacterium marinum*, which is abundant in pools in regions with temperate climates and causes tuberculous disease in fish and cutaneous ulcers in humans. This organism is grouped with the photochromogens (Runyon's group I) together with *M. kansasii*. The latter produces cervical lymphadenitis and pulmonary disease in humans, and has been isolated from cow's milk and from cattle in the United States and the Republic of South Africa. Scotochromagens produce pigment without photoactivation (Runyon's group II) and include *M. scrofulaceum*, which is closely related to the *M. avium–intracellulare* complex. These organisms have been isolated from disease in cattle and tuberculous-type lesions in dogs. Another member of the group, *M. aquae*, has been isolated from nodular lesions on the teats of cows. Nonphotochromagens (Runyon's group III) have organisms in the *M. avium–intracellulare* complex as the most important members. Organisms belonging to this complex have been isolated from tuberculin-sensitive cattle and pigs, and their pathogenicity has been assessed experimentally in calves and pigs. Some strains are virtually nonpathogenic, and others produce generalized disease.

Mycobacteria of group IV are rapid growers at room temperature, are usually nonpigmented, and include many saprophytes. Within this group, *Mycobacterium smegmatis* is one of the organisms isolated from tubercle-like lesions in lymph nodes of swine. *Mycobacterium smegmatis* has also been associated with development of bovine mastitis following its injection into the udder in oily infusions of penicillin. Another member, *M. fortuitum*, was initially isolated from lesions in bovine lymph nodes and is an occasional cause of mastitis in cattle. Members of this group, particularly *M. fortuitum* and *M. chelonei*, are the usual causes of cutaneous mycobacteriosis in cats and dogs. Further discussion of cutaneous lesions caused by mycobacteria, including those associated with *M. lepraemurium*, will be found with bacterial diseases of the skin (in the Skin and Appendages, Volume 1).

Other important distinct species of mycobacteria are *Mycobacterium leprae* (human leprosy), *M. lepraemurium* (rat leprosy), and *M. paratuberculosis* (*M. johnei*). The last named causes Johne's disease in ruminants (see the Alimentary System, this volume).

It will be evident that the pathogenic mycobacteria present a wide range of specializations, from saprophytes to the extremes of parasitism represented by *Mycobacterium leprae*, and from a wide host range to infectivity for only specific hosts. As parasites, they are principally intracellular. They are mostly within macrophages in an association that does not necessarily cause their death or the death of the host cell. The lesions produced tend to be similar and of granulomatous type, characterized by collections of macrophages, epithelioid cells, and giant cells. Additional components of inflammation and necrosis depend on the degree of cell-mediated response of the host against living bacilli, with the corresponding production of lymphokines and other inflammatory mediators. The phenomena of chronicity and latency are common to the mycobacterial infections. Both are related to the resistance of the organisms to phagocytic killing, to the slow growth of the organisms, and to the complex interactions between the organisms and the host's cellular immune system.

The three main species of tubercle bacilli (*Mycobacterium tuberculosis*, *M. bovis*, and *M. avium*) occur most frequently in their respective hosts, but cross-infections do occur, and various other species of animals are affected. Under natural conditions, the bovine type of the bacillus causes disease chiefly in cattle, humans, swine, and occasionally, horses, dogs, cats, and sheep; the avian type causes disease chiefly in birds and occasionally is found in cattle, swine, horses, sheep, and captive monkeys; the human-type bacillus is chiefly responsible for tuberculosis in humans and occasionally infects pigs, captive monkeys, dogs, cats, cattle, and psittacine birds. The expression of tuberculosis in the different hosts usually differs somewhat according to the type of bacilli involved as well as other factors. Although the human and bovine bacilli can produce disease in a wide range of species under conditions of special exposure, they are each naturally maintained in only one species, the human bacillus in people and the bovine in cattle. Thus, in the absence of infection from cattle, the bovine type disappears from the human and porcine populations. The situation with the *M. avium–intracellulare* complex is not so clear because of saprophytic members.

In addition to the hosts just mentioned, others of almost unlimited variety can be infected experimentally with one or more species of the tubercle bacilli. The differential pathogenicity of the organisms for guinea pigs, rabbits, and fowls was the original basis of the biologic classification of organisms as to type in diagnostic laboratories. Fowls are highly susceptible to the avian types, but highly resistant to the mammalian types. The avian type will, with the usual test doses, produce progressive infection in rabbits, but only localized lesions in guinea pigs. For the differentiation of mammalian strains, the rabbit is usually used. In rabbits, the bovine bacillus, in the standard dose for the test, produces progressive infection that is fatal in up to 3 months; the human type does not kill rabbits, although isolated tubercles can be found in various organs. The guinea pig is highly susceptible to both mammalian types and therefore useful for isolating the organisms.

The mycobacteria are nonmotile, non-spore-forming pleomorphic coccobacilli. They are Gram-positive but almost unstainable by the simpler bacterial stains because of their high content of lipids. They are routinely stained with hot carbol dyes, usually carbolfuchsin, and then resist decoloration by inorganic acids. This property of acid fastness, or acid–alcohol fastness, of the stained bacilli depends on the amount and spatial arrangement of mycolic acids in the bacterial wall. Sometimes, in cultures or in old lesions, the organisms have a beaded or granulated appearance. This beading is partly caused by presence of lipid droplets within the bacteria and is an indication of an unfavorable environment for organisms in the postexponential growth phase. Staining of the bacilli can be facilitated by incorporating a surface-active wetting agent, such as Tween 80, in the dyes. They are also demonstrable by fluorescence microscopy when stained by a fluorescent dye such as auramine.

Much attention has been given to the chemical composition of the mycobacteria, particularly the cell walls, in the interests of clarifying the pathogenesis of the lesions, perfecting diagnostic techniques, and developing vaccines. The chemical composition of the cell wall is dominated by complex lipids, which include glycolipids, peptidoglycolipids, lipopolysaccharides, lipoproteins, and waxes. The mycolic acids, on which acid fastness depends, are among them. The precise role of the various lipids in contributing to the virulence and immunogenicity of the organisms is still unclear. The waxes, which are themselves composed of various proportions of lipids, glycolipids, and peptidoglycolipids, depending on the species of *Mycobacterium,* are important in the initial ''foreign body'' type of macrophage response. Waxes, together with peptidoglycan (muramyl dipeptide) and various glycolipids, are responsible for most of the adjuvant activity of mycobacteria. Attraction of antigen-processing cells (macrophages) and presentation of antigen in appropriate surface configuration are major attributes of adjuvant activity. The relative importance of purified components is still under investigation. Increased glycolipid content of mycobacterial cell walls is associated with increased virulence. A close parallel is with the amount of ''cord factor'' (virulent mycobacteria form cordlike aggregates when trehalose dimycolate is in the culture medium). This correlates with the fact that, in general, the more acid fast strains are more virulent. Other glycolipids (mycosides) appear to form a barrier against lysosomal digestion and partly explain the ability of the organisms to survive after phagocytosis by macrophages. Intracellular survival is also facilitated by the bacteria preventing fusion of phagosomes and lysosomes, possibly by secretion of cyclic AMP. The differing effectiveness of such mechanisms determines the relative ability of various mycobacteria to resist intracellular degradation.

Tuberculoproteins are the other major category of immunoreactive substances in mycobacteria. They provide most of the antigenic determinants, but in order for an animal to produce an immunologic response to these determinants, the adjuvant activity of the lipids and polysaccharides in the mycobacterial cell wall is needed. Purified protein derivatives from mycobacteria are capable of eliciting the delayed type of hypersensitivity once the animal is sensitized, however, and this is the basis of tuberculin testing. Both tuberculoproteins and the adjuvant lipids are present in infection, and the result is the development of both humoral and cell-mediated immune responses. The humoral antibodies can be demonstrated by serologic techniques but do not participate in the pathogenesis of the characteristic lesions or in the production of immunity. Cell-mediated responses are responsible for both aspects of the disease.

Cell-mediated immunity and delayed-type hypersensitivity are expressions of immune responses mediated by lymphocytes, mostly T cells. Both manifestations usually develop simultaneously. They do not have identical mechanisms, however, because sometimes one is present without the other, and there is no quantitative relationship between them when both are present. Since both are mediated by T lymphocytes, the dissociation between the two responses will perhaps eventually be explained on the basis of involvement by different subpopulations of T cells.

Cell-mediated immunity is effected by the enhanced ability of activated macrophages to phagocytose and kill bacilli. Macrophages are activated by lymphokines secreted by specifically sensitized T lymphocytes, which respond to processed antigens released by previously infected macrophages. Most activated macrophages are derived from blood monocytes. Immunity to tuberculosis therefore is principally determined by the ability of macrophages to inhibit the growth of intracellular bacilli. Both innate (genetic) and acquired resistance are involved. Macrophages, for unexplained reasons, can also respond differently in organs such as the liver and kidney in the same animal. Since the balance between the virulence of the myobacteria and the ability of macrophages to kill them is often a precarious one, any compromise of the host's immune system is prone to precipitate or exacerbate the disease. This is revealed by the frequent clinical association of tuberculosis with immunosuppression caused by diseases, drugs, hormones, or malnutrition.

Delayed-type hypersensitivity is also mediated by lymphokines released mainly from sensitized T cells in response to antigenic materials from the tubercle bacilli. The lymphokines cause further accumulation of macrophages and lymphocytes. Release of cytotoxic lymphokines and hydrolytic enzymes from macrophages is principally responsible for the caseation necrosis characteristic of many tuberculous lesions.

Functionally heterogeneous populations of lymphocytes and macrophages are present in tuberculous lesions. Relative numbers of the various subpopulations of these cells partly determine whether activation of macrophages and inhibition of bacterial growth (cell-mediated immunity) or a severe, delayed-type hypersensitivity response is the dominant feature.

The importance of hypersensitivity in the pathogenesis of lesions of tuberculosis was first demonstrated by Koch in what is now known as the Koch phenomenon. If a normal guinea pig is inoculated subcutaneously with a culture of tubercle bacilli, generalization of the infection causes death in 2 to 3 months. At the site of inoculation, a hard nodule, or tubercle, develops in 10 to 14 days. This nodule soon breaks down to form an ulcer that persists until the animal dies. If the inoculation is made into a tuberculous guinea pig, however, the events are quite different. An acute response characterized by exudation and necrosis develops at the site of inoculation. The necrotic tissue soon sloughs, the lesion heals permanently and quickly, and the infection is not disseminated from it, even to the regional lymph node. The injected organisms that provoke the hypersensitivity reaction in the skin are fairly rapidly destroyed, but those in the primary lesions of the disease are not destroyed, and their persistence and proliferation might eventually kill the animal. Whether the hypersensitivity reaction is beneficial or harmful to the host depends on the circumstances. In common with most complex inflammatory conditions, there is a balance between inhibitory and amplifying factors. On the one hand, hypersensitivity to relatively small numbers of bacilli causes accelerated tubercle formation, which enhances the killing of the organisms and helps prevent reinfection or dissemination from the initial site of infection. On the other hand, the hypersensitivity response to large amounts of mycobacterial antigen causes extensive cell necrosis and tissue destruction, which is seriously detrimental. Liquefaction, which is brought about by hydrolytic enzymes of macrophages, and possibly neutrophils, is the most harmful response. The bacilli multiply extracellularly in the liquefied material and are available in large numbers for dissemination through cavities, vessels, and airways. In summary, the final determinants of the nature and intensity of lesions are the mass of bacterial antigen presented to specifically reactive lymphocytes and the modifying influences of the structure of the tissue involved.

The lesions of tuberculosis are the prototype of a granulomatous inflammation. The tuberculous granuloma (tubercle) is mainly cellular, and its development is frequently designated as ''productive'' or ''proliferative'' in contrast to the more exudative type of lesion it occasionally causes.

When tubercle bacilli are initially implanted in tissue, they behave as relatively bland, lipid-rich foreign particles would be expected to do and incite a ''foreign body'' macrophage response. Bacilli are phagocytosed by macrophages, and if the resistance of the macrophages is adequate, the bacilli are eventually killed. If the balance tips the other way, however, the bacilli proliferate and are released from killed macrophages together with antigenic materials that sensitize attracted T lymphocytes. By the tenth day or so after exposure, by which time hypersensitivity is developing, many bacilli are present, and the tempo of events begins to quicken. Lymphokines secreted by the sensitized T lymphocytes cause the attraction, proliferation, and activation of macrophages, which are derived mostly from blood monocytes. In the infected foci, macrophages assume a distinctive appearance, causing them to be designated as epithelioid cells because of a vague histologic similarity to sheets of large epithelial cells. The epithelioid cells have large, vesicular nuclei, and extensive pale cytoplasm with ill-defined borders. The epithelioid cells ultrastructurally are characterized by abundant organelles and extensive interdigitations of their plasma membranes. They contain ingested bacilli within their cytoplasm, and the structural changes indicate a heightened bactericidal activity. Mixed in with the epithelioid cells are variable numbers of giant cells of the Langhans type (Fig. 6.30B). These are large cells with several eccentric nuclei and are formed by the fusion of macrophages. This admixture of epithelioid and giant cells forms the center of young tubercles. At the periphery is a narrow

zone of lymphocytes, plasma cells, and unaltered monocytes. As the lesion progresses, the classical tubercle develops peripheral fibroplasia and central necrosis (Fig. 6.31C). These two features are not present in all tuberculous infections; there are both species and individual variations. Encapsulating fibroplasia is more conspicuous in those individuals that have considerable powers of resistance, and it might, as tuberculous granulation tissue, overgrow and dominate the lesions. It is the development of central necrosis that gives the tubercle its high degree of histologic specificity. The necrosis is a product of the cell-mediated hypersensitivity and is of caseous character. The necrotic material is most commonly inspissated into a yellowish, cheesy mass, but may liquefy or calcify. Calcification is a characteristic development in some species of animals, but seldom observed in others.

The exudative type of lesion in tuberculosis usually develops acutely. The exudate is relatively voluminous and consists of fibrin and neutrophils as well as the usual mononuclear cells. Eventually, the exudate clots, and it too caseates. A combination of factors is usually regarded as responsible for the exudative lesions. Chief among them are rapid bacterial proliferation, presence of abundant reactive lymphocytes, and a site of localization in easily distensible or space-lining tissues.

There are various portals of entry available to the tubercle bacilli. Infection can occur congenitally by way of the umbilical veins, or postnatally through alimentary, respiratory, genital, or cutaneous routes. Growth of the original tubercle takes place by centrifugal expansion and by the development of satellite tubercles formed by spread of bacilli from the initial focus. The new tubercles may coalesce to produce large lesions. In a susceptible, unsensitized animal, the bacilli spread rapidly, either free or in macrophages, along the lymphatics (Fig. 6.30C) to the regional lymph nodes, where further tubercles develop. The combination of lesions in the initial focus and in the regional lymph node is known as the *primary complex* of Ranke. It is always present with first infection in animals, but both components may not be detectable, because when infection occurs across a mucous membrane, such as of the pharynx or intestine, the initial lesion in the membrane might not be visible when the nodal lesions are present. The decision as to which lesions in a case of generalized tuberculosis constitute the primary complex is often impossible to make. The relative age of the lesions is an indication, as is their localization, because the site must be intimately related to one of the portals of entry.

As lesions develop in the regional lymph node, the infection passes successively from one node to another, and can eventually reach the blood, for potential widespread dissemination. Extensive hematogenous dissemination, however, is most frequently the result of breakdown of a blood vessel by an expanding, caseating tubercle or cavitating lesion. The number of bacilli then released into the blood can be very large, and when these are removed by phagocytes in the various organs, a large number of small tubercles develop. The course of the disease after massive generalization is short, and the disease is then referred to as miliary tuberculosis because of the large number of tubercles the size of millet seeds observed. Hematogenous dissemination is, however, not always massive; the

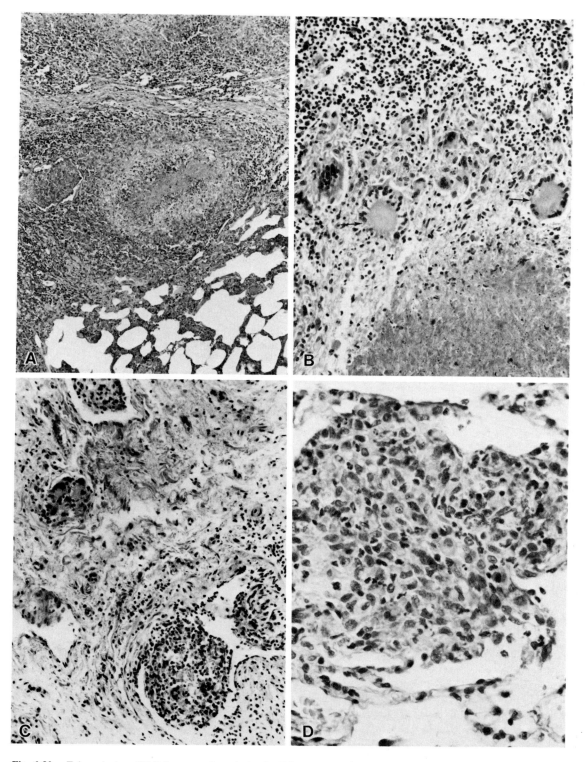

Fig. 6.30. Tuberculosis. (**A**) Pulmonary tuberculosis. Ox. Effacement of pulmonary tissue by granulomas. (Courtesy of D. M. Gillette.) (**B**) Periphery of tubercle with Langhans' giant cells (arrows) and epithelioid cells bordering caseation necrosis. Ox. (**C**) Tuberculous lymphangitis. Liver. Pig. (**D**) Nonspecific appearance of pulmonary granuloma in disseminated (miliary) tuberculosis. Dog.

course then is much longer, and the metastatic foci are large and few or solitary. Some organs, such as muscle, thyroid, and pancreas, seldom develop lesions of hematogenous origin.

Spread can occur via natural passages. Common examples are spread from the kidney along the ureter to the bladder, from one bronchus to another by coughing and aspiration, or from the lungs to the intestine when infected sputum is swallowed. Rapid spread is possible in cavities such as the meningeal space and serous cavities of the trunk. Involvement of a serous membrane is usually by direct extension from an underlying lymph node or viscus. When the bacilli are freed on the serous surfaces, they are readily distributed by movements such as respiration and peristalsis.

CATTLE. Bovine tuberculosis has been, and in some areas remains, one of the most important diseases of cattle. In areas where the incidence is high, the disease is caused almost exclusively by *Mycobacterium bovis*. But when bovine tuberculosis is brought under control by eradication programs, the patterns of infection change, and the proportion of infections caused by the *M. avium–intracellulare* complex increases. Infections with *M. avium* usually have a benign, self-limiting course. Often no lesions are detectable. If lesions develop, they are usually found in the mesenteric and retropharyngeal lymph nodes and are seldom larger than 2 cm in diameter. They are usually caseous and encapsulated and might be either calcified or liquefied. There is commonly no spread from these sites, but sometimes initial lesions in intestinal mucosa are detected as focal thickenings. When extension of the avian type infection occurs in cattle, the serous surfaces are most often involved. Occasionally, lesions may be found in the udder, lungs, liver, kidney, and spleen. The uterus is the most frequently involved organ in pregnant cows and abortion or congenital disseminated tuberculosis in newborn calves can result. Large numbers of epithelioid cells are a regular feature of the histologic response and pleomorphic acid-fast bacilli are abundant. The human bacilli, at most, cause small nonprogressive lesions in the lymph nodes of the pharynx, thorax, and mesentery.

The usual routes of infection by *Mycobacterium bovis* are respiratory and alimentary. The unusual routes, which will be considered first, are cutaneous, congenital, and genital. Infection via the **skin** is rather rare. It requires that other primary cutaneous lesions be contaminated with the tubercle bacillus. The infection is limited to the initial site or may spread to the local lymph node. In **congenital tuberculosis**, the infection spreads via the umbilical vessels to the fetus. This route of infection is of some importance where the disease is common in cattle, and where as many as 0.5% of newborn calves have been found to have tuberculosis. This route is of little significance in other species, because only in cows is tuberculous endometritis common. When the primary complex is present in congenital infection of calves, it is in the liver and portal lymph nodes. But, as elsewhere, the complex might be apparently incomplete, and the lesions are found only in the nodes. In a fetus or calf of a few days of age, lesions in the portal node are assumed to be evidence of congenital infection; this is not necessarily the case in older calves because the portal node is also the regional node of

the duodenum. Congenital tuberculosis in calves progresses quite rapidly, and the animals usually die in a few weeks or months. By that time, the disease has generalized, and lesions can be found especially in the lungs and regional lymph nodes, and in the spleen. Tuberculous lesions rarely occur in the spleen of adult cattle, and when present, irrespective of the age of the animal, they are regarded as indicative of congenital infection. For congenital tuberculosis to occur, infection must be present in the uterus. Small tubercles can be found in the endometrium. Typical placental lesions are a slimy exudate separating the placenta from the endometrium, and caseonecrotic foci in the cotyledons. Extensive areas of tuberculosis in the uterus result in repeated abortions. **Genital infection** occurs in cattle but is not common; its development requires that the sexual organs of either the female (usually uterus) or male (usually epididymis) be tuberculous. Mammary infusions used in the treatment of mastitis and contaminated with tubercle bacilli are responsible for occasional, but epidemiologically important, cases of tuberculosis of mammary gland.

Most bovine tuberculosis is acquired by inhalation or ingestion. Management factors and age at which the disease is contracted are major determinants of which route is the more probable. Search for whether the primary complex is alimentary or respiratory can be helpful, but the evidence is sometimes not clear.

The incidence of respiratory versus alimentary infection in postnatal calves is difficult to determine precisely, especially in very young calves, because it depends on whether involvement of the portal nodes, in the absence of intestinal or hepatic lesions, is taken to indicate alimentary or congenital infection. Primary complexes in the intestine are common in calves, particularly those that have been allowed to suck tuberculous udders or that have been given tuberculous milk to drink. Pulmonary complexes are also common in calves more than a few weeks of age. Pulmonary infections may well be more important than alimentary infections under crowded conditions. Tuberculosis of the anterior cervical nodes occurs with both aerogenous and alimentary routes of infection and is not, therefore, an indication of the route of infection.

Most cattle obtain their infections when they are older than 6 months. In these adult infections, the majority of lesions are in the retropharyngeal, mediastinal, and bronchial lymph nodes. When the lesions are limited to the retropharyngeal nodes, infection could be by either oral or nasal routes. Lesions have seldom been found in the lungs with a frequency equal to their occurrence in the thoracic lymph nodes. This is probably because primary lesions in the pulmonary parenchyma can be very small and difficult to detect. In the very few series in which the examination has been thorough, the preponderance of primary complexes in the lung has been revealed. Intestinal infections do occur, and lesions in the mesenteric lymph nodes are common; a significant proportion of these, perhaps most, are secondary infections, which are established when sputum is swallowed.

In adult cattle, therefore, primary infection is usually in the lungs and is caused by inhalation of infected droplet nuclei. The primary lesions may be single or multiple and may occur in any lobe, but they occur predominantly in a subpleural location in

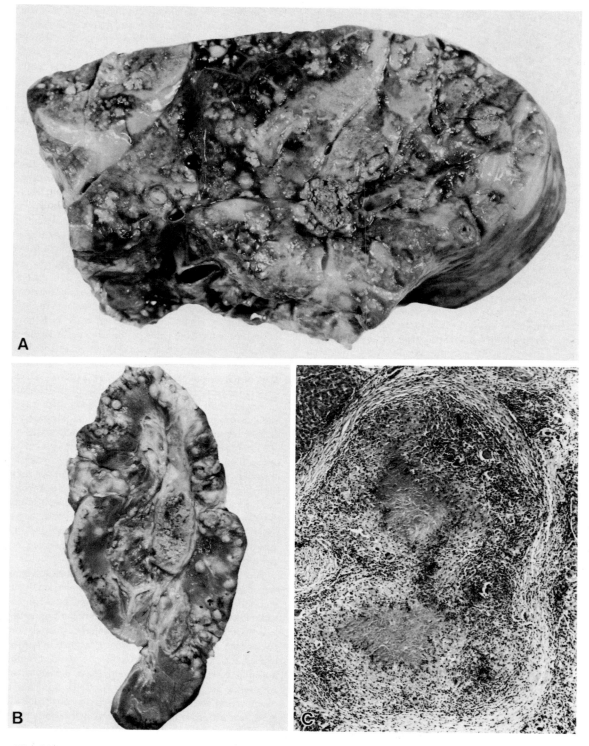

Fig. 6.31. Tuberculosis.   (**A**) Tuberculous bronchopneumonia. Ox. Larger granulomas (tubercles) have crumbly caseonecrotic centers (arrows).   (**B**) Tuberculous lymphadenitis. Ox.   (**C**) Caseous tubercles with encapsulation. Liver. Sheep.

the dorsocaudal portions of the caudal lobes. There are almost always lesions in the regional lymph nodes, but they might be absent in some cases of chronic tuberculous pneumonia.

The **tuberculous pulmonary process** usually starts at the bronchiolar–alveolar junction and extends into the alveoli, so that it is initially sublobular or lobular. The histologic structure is typically tuberculous (Fig. 6.30A). There may be more than one focus within a lobule, giving a cloverleaf appearance, and more than one lobule can be involved (Fig. 6.31A).

The initial lesions and their secondaries in the lymph nodes can heal completely, persist without progression, or progress. It is generally believed, on good but not certain grounds, that bovine tuberculosis most often progresses, with acquired cellular resistance slowing the progress considerably but not halting it.

The appearance of the pulmonary lesions varies with their age and rate of progress. The earliest lesions are not encapsulated but are small and surrounded by condensed alveolar tissue. Even in these early lesions, the yellowish caseation and the calcification so characteristic of bovine tubercles can be seen. Caseated lesions can be encapsulated and heavily calcified. The capsules are not necessarily evidence of successful containment because many such nodules communicate with an airway and allow local dissemination. Multiple initial foci can coalesce to form large regions of caseating bronchopneumonia (Fig. 6.31A), which in due course are usually encapsulated and calcified. Cavitations may form in any of these lesions, but they are never large because of the limitations imposed by the interlobular septa.

Dissemination of the infection within the lung can be by way of an intrapulmonary tuberculous lymphangitis but is mainly through the airways. The bronchogenic extension may be by direct contiguity, or it might be by aspiration of exudates, but in either case what is initially a lobular type of lesion comes to involve much or all of a bronchopulmonary segment, or even most of a lobe. The reaction is the same as that in the primary lesion, although often more severely caseating. Depending on the rapidity and extent of spread, the lesions form a pattern of irregular caseous bronchopneumonia or more confluent caseous lobar pneumonia.

In association with chronic progressive pulmonary tuberculosis, it is common to find ulcers in the trachea and bronchi. These can arise by implantation of bacilli coughed up in the sputum or by progression of tuberculous lymphangitis. They begin as typical tubercles in the mucous membrane, especially near the bifurcation of the trachea, and are followed shortly by ulceration. Similar ulcers develop on the larynx by implantation of bacilli.

A feature of tuberculosis in cattle is the tendency to spread to the serous membranes (Fig. 6.32A). This can take place by direct expansion of the original lesion, by lymphogenous extension from the lungs, by direct hematogenous dissemination, or by local expansion from a hematogenous focus in an adjacent organ. Once the tuberculous process breaches the serosa, the bacilli are distributed by respiratory movements and may be widely implanted. **Pleural tuberculosis** may be largely nodular, diffusely caseous, or with transitions between the two. The affected areas of pleura, both visceral and parietal, are thickened by fibrous granulation tissue, and as a rule the tuberculous pro-

cess does not invade the underlying tissue. The characteristic lesions are nodular, and these tend to occur in clusters. They may be sessile or pedunculated, and frequently coalesce to form cauliflower-like masses. In the early stages, they consist of reddish tags of granulation tissue containing typical tubercles and may be soft. Later, heavy calcification is usual and largely responsible for the term "pearl disease." Caseous tuberculous pleuritis consists of large plaques of caseous exudate beneath which the pleura is uniformly thickened. Fibrin may be deposited on and between the plaques.

Generalization of the infection (dissemination to other organs) can occur early in the course of the disease (postprimary generalization) or late in the course of the disease (late generalization). In late generalization, it is assumed that the immunity the animal has acquired has broken down, thereby permitting wide spread. Generalization might be sudden and massive, when large numbers of the bacilli enter the bloodstream (miliary tuberculosis), or it may be more protracted, with fewer bacilli entering the circulation. The latter, whether early or late, is the more usual, and the lesions are larger and often of different ages.

In the respiratory pattern being described, the bacilli can enter the bloodstream in the lungs when the caseating process erodes a vessel, usually a small vein, or they might pass through the lymphatics and lymph nodes to the vena cava. In either event, the hematogenous metastases occur more frequently in the lung than elsewhere. Hematogenous metastases can also occur in most of the major organs and in lymph nodes, skeleton, and serous membranes, including the peritoneum, pericardium, and meninges. Organs such as salivary glands, pancreas, spleen, brain, and muscles, including myocardium, are rarely affected by hematogenous metastases in postnatal infections.

Miliary lesions in the lungs are associated with a fulminating course of the disease. The lesions are typical, small, grayish tubercles, translucent at first but soon becoming caseous and centrally calcified. Hematogenous tubercles are diffusely scattered in both lungs, although there is a tendency for them to be more numerous in the cranial portions. In slow or protracted generalization, which is the more usual type, the metastatic tubercles tend to be few in number, large, caseated and calcified, and often surrounded by a heavy capsule.

Tuberculosis of the **peritoneum** is less common than that of the pleura. It can arise in a number of ways. Peritonitis surrounding the liver is common in the congenital infection and is regarded as being of local and lymphatic spread. Peritonitis might also be hematogenous in the congenital disease as well as in postprimary and late generalization. Ulcerative intestinal tuberculosis that extends to the serosa is an important route of peritoneal infection in postnatal life. In adults, the intestinal lesions are usually secondary to respiratory lesions. Spread to the peritoneum from the uterus via the uterine tubes no doubt occurs, but the reverse is probably more common. The peritoneal lesions are similar to those of the pleura but are usually not so clearly nodular or "pearly." They tend to be softer and more diffuse and to consist of extensive granulation tissue in which the tubercles are embedded (Fig. 6.32A).

Hepatic lesions are hematogenous in origin. Infection arrives either through umbilical veins, as in congenital infections, through arteries as part of hematogenous dissemination, or

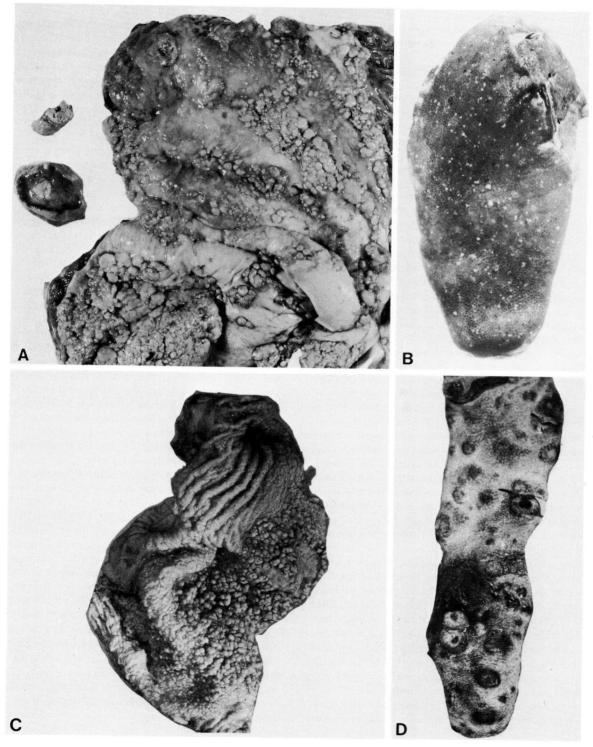

Fig. 6.32. Tuberculosis. **(A)** Tuberculous peritonitis. Ox. **(B)** Miliary tuberculosis of avian type in liver. Pig. **(C)** Hypertrophic tuberculous gastritis caused by *Mycobacterium bovis*. Pig. **(D)** Multiple tuberculous granulomas caused by *M. bovis* in spleen. Pig.

through portal veins when lesions are present in the intestine. The hepatic foci might be miliary, but as elsewhere, it is more usual for the coarse, nodular type of lesion to be present, sometimes only in one lobe. The portal lymph nodes are affected. The coarse, nodular types of lesion occur in varying numbers and can be quite small or up to 10 cm in diameter. They tend to be rounded and often project hemispherically above the surface. When sectioned, the nodules are seen to be enclosed by a heavy capsule, and the contents are bright yellow and caseous; the exudate might be inspissated and calcified or, sometimes, liquefied.

The **renal lesions** resemble in structure and type those of the liver. Miliary lesions are limited to the cortex, the initial development of the tubercles occurring in the interstitial tissue. The coarse, nodular lesions might be multiple, but often they are limited to one or two adjacent lobules of the kidney. The caseating tubercles can be very large and might erode into the pelvis to cause a descending infection of the urinary tract. Frequently, the renal lymph nodes are concurrently involved.

Tuberculosis of the **skeleton** is usually hematogenous and occurs mainly in young animals. Its distribution is governed by the usual factors in hematogenous osteomyelitis. The lesions are most frequently in the vertebrae, ribs, and flat bones of the pelvis—all bones that are spongy and highly vascular. The epiphyseal–metaphyseal regions of long bones are also predilection sites. The osteomyelitis is in the form of miliary tubercles or large granulomas. Caseation is extensive in the granulomas, and there is a tendency to liquefaction, resulting in the formation of tuberculous abscesses. The liquefied lesions especially tend to be progressive. They erode and fistulate through the cortex and erode the articular cartilages to produce tuberculous arthritis. Regenerative osteophyte formation is not prominent in tuberculosis, as it is, for example, in actinomycosis. The predominantly erosive type of process is referred to as ''caries.'' Through the cortical fistulae the infection spreads to the adjacent connective tissues and muscle. This is the usual pathogenesis of tuberculous myositis.

Tuberculosis in the **central nervous system** begins mainly as a meningitis and is more common in the cerebral than in the spinal meninges. Involvement of the spinal meninges may be direct from a vertebral osteomyelitis, or hematogenous. Involvement of the cranial meninges is hematogenous, the initial lesions occurring usually in the basilar meninges and extending from there in the arachnoid spaces between the hemispheres and cerebellum, to the choroid plexuses and, to a limited extent, into the Virchow–Robin spaces and the brain itself. The meningeal lesions are similar to those of the serous membranes but are generally more exudative and necrotizing. Miliary or conglomerate tubercles are an uncommon development.

Tuberculous lesions, either small nodules or craterous ulcers, are occasionally found in the epithelium of the upper alimentary tract and abomasum. Whether primary or as endogenous secondaries, however, lesions in the alimentary lining membranes are uncommon. In contrast, the regional nodes, particularly of the retropharynx (Fig. 6.31B) and mesentery, are often severely involved. In young calves, round or oval ulcers of small size may be found, especially in the ileum. These probably begin as small tubercles in the Peyer's patches or solitary lymphoid nodules. Tubercles and ulcers can be found in the small intestine and cecum in adults, in which they frequently represent reinfection from the lungs. The ulcers vary in size and are either rounded or elongate in the axis of the intestine. The margins of the ulcers are distinct, firm, and raised. The bases are firm granulation tissue speckled with tiny hemorrhages and usually covered with dry, caseous exudate. Granulomas might be visible in the draining lymphatics.

HORSES.   Horses apparently possess a high innate resistance to tubercle bacilli, and the disease is rare in them. Most infections involve *Mycobacterium bovis,* but both *M. avium* and *M. tuberculosis* can produce localized or generalized disease. Many of the bovine strains recovered from horses are of lowered virulence when tested in laboratory animals.

The route of infection is almost exclusively alimentary. The primary complex is often incomplete, with large lesions in the retropharyngeal or mesenteric nodes, but without an obvious primary focus in the related mucosa. In some cases, primary ulcers are present in the intestine. Bacilli of the *Mycobacterium avium–intracellulare* complex sometimes produce a proliferative enteritis closely resembling Johne's disease of cattle. Lesions might be limited to the alimentary tract, but in fatal cases there is generalization with either miliary tubercles or scattered coarse, nodular lesions. Secondary lesions have been described in the lungs, liver, spleen, serous membranes, mammary gland, and skin. They are unusual in the last two sites. Tuberculous changes in cervical vertebrae are repeatedly cited as being common in the disease in the horse, but this has not been thoroughly explored. If lesions occur in the central nervous system or genitalia, they are rare.

The lesions of tuberculosis in the horse often differ from those in cattle. Whereas extensive caseation and calcification are typical of bovine tubercles, the equine tubercles more commonly have a uniform, gray, smooth (lardaceous) appearance, grossly resembling a sarcoma.

Caseation does occur sometimes in the center of a lesion, but it is of minor degree, and calcification is rarely observable by the naked eye. Histologically, the early lesion is a tubercle consisting of macrophages, epithelioid cells, and few or many giant cells, without a peripheral zone of lymphocytes. As the lesion progresses, it develops more and more proliferative fibrous tissue in which ill-defined tubercles are scattered. It is sometimes very difficult to find bacilli in these lesions, but the occasional tubercle that liquefies contains very large numbers. Pulmonary tuberculosis in horses is usually hematogenous and might be miliary or coarsely nodular. Usually there are miliary foci, which appear like glassy dewdrops but are very firm. The coarse, nodular lesions, which grossly resemble sarcomas, are fewer and larger. Progression is by expansion of the lesion. Intrabronchial spread, which is so important in cattle, is of no significance in horses. The bronchial lymph nodes are invariably involved when the lung is; their appearance is that of a firm sarcoma, and corticomedullary distinction is lost.

When the primary lesions are found in the intestine, they take the form of tuberculous ulcers, which are more common in the large than in the small intestine. Tubercles in the liver and spleen are usually nodular rather than miliary. They can be extremely large, and the organs correspondingly so; the spleen is more frequently affected than the liver. The lesions are of the usual lardaceous type. The serosal lesions, which are relatively common, are nodular and sometimes accompanied by much effusion into the cavity.

SHEEP AND GOATS.   Sheep and goats appear not to have any special resistance to tubercle bacilli, except possibly the human type, but tuberculosis in them is rare. It is usually caused by either *Mycobacterium bovis* or *M. avium*. The main route of infection in goats, and possibly in sheep, is thought to be respiratory, because lesions are more common in the thorax than elsewhere. In general, tuberculosis in the small ruminants is similar in most respects to the disease in cattle.

SWINE.   Pigs are susceptible to all three major species of mycobacteria. The incidence of a particular species in any population of pigs depends largely on the species to which they are exposed and is, therefore, a reflection of the incidence of tuberculosis in associated cattle, poultry, or humans. *Mycobacterium bovis* is more capable of producing generalized disease than the *M. avium–intracellulare* complex. *Mycobacterium tuberculosis* rarely spreads past the nodes local to the point of entry. Tuberculosis is seldom observed in pigs except at meat inspection, and because these animals are usually young, a local lymphadenitis is the extent of the disease usually observed.

Tuberculous infections of wounds, castration wounds especially, occur in swine, and occasionally the primary infection is respiratory. As a general rule, however, the route of infection is alimentary (Fig. 6.32C). The primary complex in swine is seldom complete by gross inspection, but tubercles can usually be found microscopically in the mucosa of the pharynx or small intestine when gross lesions are present in the retropharyngeal, portal, or mesenteric nodes. Ulceration of a primary focus in a mucous membrane is rare.

There are certain differences between the lesions produced by the bovine and avian types of bacilli. The bovine bacilli produce caseocalcareous tubercles similar to those that occur in cattle, and the lesions are often surrounded by a fibrous capsule. In the liver, there is a tendency for the caseous centers to liquefy. The avian bacilli produce lesions that are proliferative in nature and consist of tuberculous granulation tissue resembling the lardaceous or sarcomatous lesions described in equine tuberculosis. Caseation is not a feature of these lesions, although it might occur as minute foci, especially in the hepatic tubercles. There is little tendency for these caseous foci either to calcify or to liquefy, or for the lesions to be encapsulated. Affected lymph nodes are only slightly enlarged, and on cut surface they have a lardaceous appearance. The histologic appearance is of diffuse accumulations of macrophages, epithelioid cells, and Langhans' giant cells accompanied by extensive fibroplasia. The bacilli are numerous in these lesions, and they may also be recovered from nodes that appear grossly to be normal.

Pulmonary tuberculosis in swine is hematogenous and usually of the miliary pattern. In some infections with the bovine bacillus, there is extensive consolidation of the cranial lobes, resembling grossly the caseous bronchopneumonia of cattle, but

histologically seen to be a confluence of numerous hematogenous tubercles. In this form of the pulmonary disease, there might be a tuberculous tracheitis. Miliary lesions in the lungs produced by the avian bacilli resemble dewdrops, and there appears to be a characteristic tendency for these to spread along the subpleural and septal lymphatics, which are beaded by small tubercles.

The hepatic lesions produced by the bovine bacilli take the form of miliary or, more usually, coarse nodules. Those produced in the liver by the avian bacilli (Fig. 6.32B) are quite different. The early lesions are scattered and miliary and are not discrete but blend peripherally with the interlobular septa. The later lesions are merely an extension of this and, although softer, closely resemble the lesions of parasitic hepatitis produced by *Ascaris suum* and *Stephanurus dentatus*. Hepatic tuberculosis of avian type also cannot be distinguished grossly from the infiltrates of myeloid or lymphoid leukemia. Tuberculous granulation tissue spreads along the portal triads, surrounding and obliterating lobules, and at the periphery unites with the expansions of adjacent lesions. Typical tubercles do not occur.

Splenic lesions regularly occur in the generalized disease (Fig. 6.32D). They project hemispherically above the surface, and their appearance, as indicated above, depends on the type of bacilli present. Tuberculosis of the serous membranes is seldom observed in swine. Skeletal lesions, often confined to individual bones of the axial skeleton, are common. Tuberculous meningitis, primarily basilar in location, is relatively frequent in generalized infections by the bovine bacilli. The meningeal lesions in swine are more nodular than those in cattle, in which there tends to be diffuse exudation. Tubercles may also be found in the genital organs, skin, and eye.

CATS AND DOGS.   Cats appear to be more susceptible to *Mycobacterium bovis* than to *M. tuberculosis* or *M. avium*. The route of infection in cats is usually by ingestion of contaminated milk or, possibly, diseased wildlife. Dogs are susceptible to *M. bovis* and *M. tuberculosis,* and less so to *M. avium*. Dogs are more prone than cats to contract tuberculosis, usually by inhalation, in households with tuberculous persons. Exposure of dogs to tuberculous cattle usually results in the alimentary form of the disease, by ingestion of milk or other contaminated food.

The lesions of tuberculosis in carnivores differ from those in other species. Typical tubercles are not as common, and when they occur, caseation necrosis is not a prominent gross feature. More often there is a nonspecific granulation tissue in which macrophages are scattered at random and giant cells are rare (Fig. 6.30D). The discrete tuberculous granulomas that do occur are composed principally of epithelioid cells surrounded by narrow zones of fibrous tissue in which are scattered small collections of lymphocytes and plasma cells. Necrosis is often present in the centers of larger granulomas. Giant cells are rare or absent. The presence of central necrosis and fairly small numbers of acid-fast bacilli in lesions of cats helps to distinguish lesions of tuberculosis from those of feline leprosy.

The frequently sarcomatous gross appearance of the lesions can easily lead to misdiagnosis. This is particularly the case in cats. The pattern of pale homogeneous tissue causing enlargement and effacement of lymph nodes, and present as diffuse or nodular lesions in the intestine and possibly other viscera, can readily be mistaken grossly for lymphoma.

The primary foci in the lungs of dogs develop in most cases in the dorsal part of the caudal lobes. They appear as firm, pale, bulging nodules about 1–3 cm in size. The cut surface can be uniform, but frequently there is central liquefaction and a tendency to fistulation onto the pleura to produce serofibrinous or serohemorrhagic pleuritis. Metastatic nodules in the lung are usually few in number, with an appearance similar to that of the primary foci. The bronchial lymph nodes are regularly involved. They might be only moderately enlarged with softened necrotic areas on cut surfaces, or they might be very large and centrally liquefied. Dissemination within the lungs occurs quite rapidly and is predominantly intrabronchial, with the production of a tuberculous bronchitis and bronchiolitis rather than a bronchopneumonia. The granulation tissue involves and destroys segments of the bronchial walls, and cavitation occurs by liquefaction and evacuation of exudate.

Pleuritis is particularly common in tuberculosis of dogs, and ascites is also likely to be present when the abdominal viscera are affected. The serosal lesions are not at all like those in cattle. Instead, there is diffuse or finely nodular pleural thickening by nonspecific granulation tissue. A large amount of serofibrinous exudate accumulates in the pleural cavity; this is often bloodstained. The pleural lesions may be unilateral or bilateral. Peritoneal tuberculosis accompanies lesions in the mesenteric nodes and liver and is accompanied by ascites. Large or small nodules of granulation tissue or a diffuse thickening occur on the visceral layers especially, and the omentum is often converted to a partially necrotic, ropy mass in which there are very large numbers of bacilli. Tuberculous processes are seldom found in other organs, although involvement of the meninges, uveal tract of the eye, genitalia, bones, and skin have all been reported. Hypertrophic osteopathy is a possible sequel to pulmonary tuberculosis (see Bones and Joints, Volume 1).

CORYNEBACTERIUM EQUI INFECTION. *Corynebacterium (Rhodococcus) equi* is an important cause of pneumonia in foals. It can also cause intestinal lesions, and occasionally produce more widespread involvement. Bacteria of the genera *Corynebacterium, Mycobacterium,* and *Nocardia* share the property of having cell walls containing complex lipids. *Corynebacterium equi* therefore has pathogenic features resembling those of mycobacteria. It is a facultative intracellular parasite of macrophages and causes a predominantly pyogranulomatous response characterized by abundant caseation necrosis. *Corynebacterium equi* is an inhabitant of both soil and the equine intestinal tract. Whether it is a true soil saprophyte is still uncertain. Buildup of organisms in soil and dust occurs principally in association with the presence of carrier horses. This emphasizes the importance of its commensal status in the horse.

Pneumonia caused by *Corynebacterium equi* generally causes clinical signs in foals 2–6 months of age, but the subacute to chronic nature of the lesion indicates that infection occurs well before clinical signs in most cases. Signs of the disease are fever, cough, nasal discharge, and increased respiratory rate. Because lesions are usually well advanced by the time the pneumonia is clinically apparent, mortality is commonly 40–80%.

Characteristic gross lesions are multiple firm nodules of various sizes separated by congested and partly atelectatic lung. A typical feature is the very large size of many of the foci. Evidence of their origin by coalescence of clustered small nodules is sometimes evident. There is a tendency for more rapidly progressive lesions to be distributed widely throughout the lungs, and occasionally an acute clinical form in foals is associated with miliary pyogranulomatous foci. Lesions of slower, more insidious onset occupy cranioventral regions of the lungs, usually bilaterally, and therefore have the distribution pattern of a bronchopneumonia (Fig. 6.33A). The nodular lesions are often referred to as abscesses if circumscribed, or as areas of suppurative bronchopneumonia if irregular and less well defined. They are, in fact, usually regions of caseation necrosis with either a slimy, homogeneous texture or a moist crumbly consistency with fluidfilled fissures. In most instances there is no distinct fibrous tissue capsule surrounding the necrotic tissue (Fig. 6.33B).

Histologically, the lesions produced by *Corynebacterium equi* are predominantly pyogranulomatous. Alveoli are filled with masses of macrophages containing many organisms (Fig. 6.33D). Giant cells containing organisms are common; neutrophils are less numerous. Lymphocytes and plasma cells are present in moderate numbers, mostly in alveolar septa and other interstitial zones. Necrosis of bacteria-laden macrophages and other cells involves local alveolar septa. Necrosis spreads gradually to affect large amounts of pulmonary parenchyma and produce the caseonecrotic foci seen macroscopically.

The bronchial lymph nodes are swollen and edematous. Sometimes they contain soft caseonecrotic foci. Histologically there is a pyogranulomatous lymphadenitis, with components similar to the pneumonia. Pleuritis is uncommon, even when pulmonary involvement is extensive.

After the lungs, the next most frequent sites of lesions caused by *Corynebacterium equi* in foals are the intestinal tract and mesenteric lymph nodes. These sites can be affected with or without accompanying lung lesions. The intestinal lesion is an ulcerative enterocolitis (Fig. 6.33C) that mainly involves the cecum and colon. The mucosa has numerous irregular but well-defined ulcers with fibrinonecrotic surfaces, red bases, and raised borders. They can be recognized as based on lymphoid tissues, Peyer's patches in the ileum, and solitary nodules of the large intestine. Mesenteric lymph nodes are swollen and edematous. Those of the large intestine frequently contain caseonecrotic foci. Histologically, the main intestinal lesions are pyogranulomatous inflammation of lymphoid tissue and fibrinonecrotic ulceration of the overlying epithelium. Inflammatory cellular components are the same as those in the pulmonary lesions.

More widespread dissemination of infection in foals can occasionally give rise to suppurative arthritis, hepatic or splenic "abscesses," vertebral abscesses, and hypopyon. *Corynebacterium equi* may also be a cause of ulcerative lymphangitis.

The pathogenesis of *Corynebacterium equi* infection in foals is incompletely understood. The abundance of the organism in dusty environments where foals contract pneumonia, together with the predominant bronchopneumonic pattern of the disease, indicate that aerosol infection is the usual route of pulmonary involvement. It also appears that the alimentary route of infec-

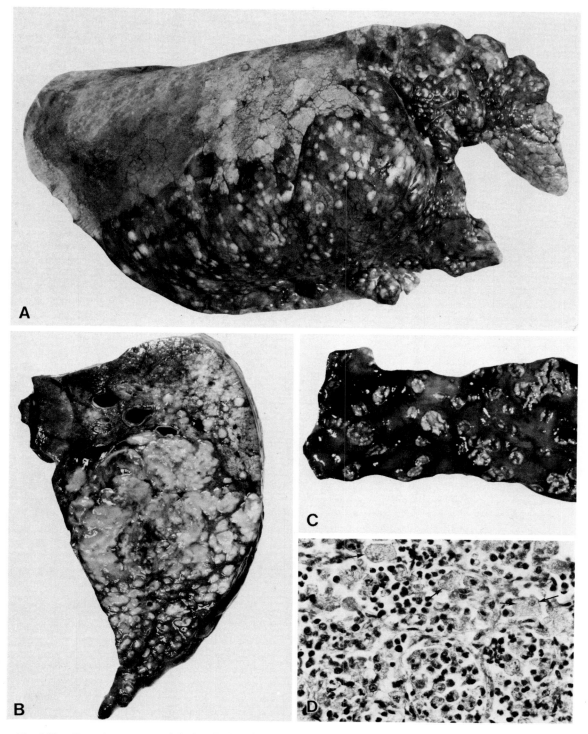

Fig. 6.33. *Corynebacterium equi* infection. Foal. (**A**) Extensive bronchopneumonia with multiple pyogranulomatous foci (''abscesses''). (**B**) Cross section of (**A**), showing variation in size and consistency of foci and absence of distinct capsules. (**C**) Multiple discrete ulcers in colon (Courtesy of J. A. Johnson and *Veterinary Pathology*.) (**D**) Alveoli filled by macrophages, which contain large numbers of *C. equi* (arrows).

tion is the usual one for the intestinal form of the disease. Isolated pyogranulomatous foci can develop in the lung by spread from intestinal lesions. Infection of foals *in utero,* during birth, or through neonatal umbilical contamination is probably unimportant.

Corynebacterium equi has also been associated with metritis and abortion in mares, metritis in cows, pneumonia in calves, and tubercle-like lesions in lymph nodes of pigs and cattle. Its etiologic role in some of these instances is still questionable.

Other Bacterial Infections

A large variety of Gram-positive and Gram-negative bacteria can cause pneumonia, either singly or in mixed infections. They mostly cause a suppurative bronchopneumonia in lungs damaged by a preceding disease process such as a viral or mycoplasmal infection, or when pulmonary defenses are impaired for reasons outlined previously. There is considerable overlap among the bacteria found in the different species of animals, but the sets of organisms most commonly involved, and their relative importance, vary according to the species of animals affected. There is also some variation according to geographic location. Since the pneumonic lesions are relatively nonspecific, identification of causative agents must be by bacteriologic means. But because bacteria can be opportunistic invaders of pneumonic tissue, isolation of an organism by culture does not necessarily indicate a causal role. The presence of large numbers of a bacterial species in pure culture, or as the predominant agent, provides presumptive evidence of its importance in causing the pneumonic process. Difficulty in fulfilling Koch's postulates often leaves a measure of uncertainty even after considerable study. This was formerly the case for pneumonic pasteurellosis and still holds true for many of the mycoplasmal infections, as will be discussed later. A further example of a bacterium whose pathogenic capability is not fully established is *Streptobacillus (Bacillus) actinoides* in calves.

Pyogenic organisms, especially streptococci, staphylococci, *Corynebacterium pyogenes, Pseudomonas aeruginosa,* and *Klebsiella pneumoniae,* are usually associated with suppurative bronchopneumonias that may progress to abscessation. Either more virulent organisms or more severely compromised host defenses can lead to fibrinonecrotic or hemorrhagic pneumonias, such as the pneumonia caused by *Salmonella choleraesuis* in swine. This pneumonia can have the same appearance as pneumonic pasteurellosis in swine. In contrast, *S. typhisuis* characteristically causes a chronic suppurative bronchopneumonia in which, grossly, there are large, confluent regions of swollen, creamy tan consolidation. On cut section these appear smooth and homogeneous, except where there are granular or friable foci of necrosis.

In addition to the bronchopneumonias, various bacteria cause interstitial pneumonia as part of a pyemia or septicemia. These are usually in very young animals and are most commonly caused by streptococci, *Escherichia coli,* and in foals and pigs, by *Actinobacillus* spp. *Actinobacillus (Shigella) equuli* in foals is typically associated with multifocal purulonecrotic foci, often recognizably involving small vessels. Fulminating systemic bacterial infections causing septicemias may be accompanied by little evidence of direct pulmonary involvement, or there may be a severe, diffuse, acute interstitial pneumonia with intravascular

leukocyte sequestration, foci of alveolar wall necrosis, and widespread fibrinohemorrhagic exudation into alveoli. The acute interstitial pneumonia is particularly likely to be associated with the endotoxemias and septicemias caused by Gram-negative organisms like *Salmonella* spp. and *E. coli.*

Finally, it is convenient to mention here that bacteria resembling *Pseudomonas mallei* and *Pasteurella* spp. have been isolated from multifocal interstitial pneumonia in several cats, a dog, and a tiger cub, representing regions as far apart as California, Australia, and Northern Ireland. The bacteria are of uncertain taxonomic status and are currently referred to as Eugonic Fermenter-4. These organisms are present in the oral and nasopharyngeal flora of dogs and cats, and have been isolated from infected bite wounds in humans and animals. The pulmonary lesions are numerous, firm, cream-colored or light tan nodules up to 1 cm in diameter scattered throughout the pulmonary parenchyma. Histologically, they are foci of massive accumulations of neutrophils, monocytes, and macrophages that efface alveolar architecture and contain numerous bacterial colonies interspersed among them. Necrosis of inflammatory cells and alveolar walls occurs in foci of intense inflammation. The distribution of the lesions indicates a probable hematogenous origin, but the site of bacterial invasion of the bloodstream has not been identified to provide supporting evidence for this speculation.

Mycoplasmal Diseases

Mycoplasmas are the smallest, free-living prokaryotes. They are placed in a class separate from other bacteria, mainly on the basis of their lacking the genetic capability to synthesize a cell wall (class Mollicutes, "soft skinned"). Lack of a cell wall results in extreme pleomorphism of the organisms. The taxonomic type of *Mycoplasma* is *M. mycoides* subsp. *mycoides.* This organism was isolated from contagious bovine pleuropneumonia and therefore gave rise to the former designation of mycoplasmas as pleuropneumonia-like organisms (PPLOs).

It is difficult to prove a definite pathogenic role in the production of pneumonia for many infectious organisms. This is especially true for the mycoplasmas. They are ubiquitous inhabitants of moist mucosal surfaces, particularly of the respiratory tract, and are common opportunistic inhabitants of pneumonic lung. Proving the etiologic role of mycoplasmas isolated from pneumonic lung is complicated by several factors. Species of mycoplasmas vary in pathogenicity, and there is a tendency for the more pathogenic strains to be the most difficult to culture. This can divert attention to relatively nonpathogenic species. When a mycoplasma suspected of having a causal role is cultured, Koch's postulates are hard to fulfill because enhancing factors are usually involved in development of the naturally occurring disease. Simultaneous evaluation of the role of the mycoplasma and the nature and importance of enhancing factors, whether they are additional damaging agents or act by reducing pulmonary defenses in other ways, causes difficulty in designing experimental protocols that can convincingly demonstrate the mycoplasma's pathogenic importance. The degree of uncertainty regarding the significance of a species or strain of *Mycoplasma* is inversely proportional to its pathogenicity. Since establishment of a relatively highly pathogenic organism, *M. mycoides* subsp. *mycoides,* as the causal agent of contagious bovine pleuropneumonia was difficult, it is easy to understand why considerable uncertainty still exists concerning the importance of many much less virulent species. A further source of uncertainty is the lack of understanding of the mechanisms by which mycoplasmas cause injury to tissues. The relative importance of a direct effect on cilia, toxic effects on ciliated and other cells, macrophage–neutrophil interactions, and various immune-mediated responses are under investigation. The set of pathogenetic mechanisms appears to vary from one species of *Mycoplasma* to another.

Respiratory Mycoplasmosis of Cattle

There are two types of pneumonia associated with mycoplasmal infection in cattle. One is contagious bovine pleuropneumonia. The other is mycoplasmal bronchitis, bronchiolitis, and pneumonia of calves, which is an important component of enzootic pneumonia.

CONTAGIOUS BOVINE PLEUROPNEUMONIA. Contagious bovine pleuropneumonia is caused by *Mycoplasma mycoides* subsp. *mycoides* (small-colony type). The small-colony designation is currently used to distinguish the organism causing bovine pleuropneumonia from *M. mycoides* subsp. *mycoides* (large-colony type), which is a cause of disease in goats. Contagious bovine pleuropneumonia is characterized by a fibrinonecrotic pneumonia (Fig. 6.34C,D) with abundant serofibrinous pleuritis. Presence of necrotic material sequestered by fibrous capsules is a usual finding in subacute or chronic cases (Fig. 6.34A,B). The pattern of pneumonia is usually that of a lobar or bronchopneumonia (see Anatomic Patterns of Pneumonia). The lungs of cattle dying in the more acute stages of the disease typically have a "marbled" appearance in which relatively normal lobules are intermixed with lobules showing red or gray consolidation or necrosis. The marbled effect is heightened by the distension of interlobular septa, and interstitium surrounding vessels and airways by broad bands of fibrinous exudate. It is also enhanced by the dense, yellow-gray zones of packed inflammatory cells surrounding the necrotic areas. The fibrinonecrotic pneumonia and accompanying pleuritis of contagious bovine pleuropneumonia have features similar to the fibrinonecrotic pneumonia of acute pneumonic pasteurellosis. The marbled effect is more pronounced in contagious bovine pleuropneumonia, however, and the lesions are more prone to involve the caudal lobes. There is also a much greater frequency of development of sequestra in the mycoplasmal disease.

It appears that the disease originated in central Europe and remained endemic there until spread by the movement of cattle during the Napoleonic wars, and later by the growth in international commerce. Toward the end of the nineteenth century it had become almost worldwide in distribution. It was eradicated from North America and much of Europe before the turn of the century, and more recently appears to have been eradicated from Australia. It now occurs mostly in portions of Asia, central Africa, Spain, and Portugal. Enormous losses were reported from this disease in the last century, and in endemic areas the mortality rate among indigenous breeds of cattle is reported still to be more than 40%; in improved European breeds, the mortality in an unrestricted outbreak is not expected to exceed 10%

of the animals. Species such as the buffalo, reindeer, and yak are susceptible to the disease but are seldom affected. Sheep and goats do not contract the natural disease caused by *Mycoplasma mycoides* subsp. *mycoides* (small-colony type) and do not appear to develop the pulmonary disease after experimental infection, but they do develop a severe local reaction and septicemia if the organism is inoculated.

The transmission of infection requires close contact between infected and susceptible animals. It seems probable that the disease is transmitted by the inhalation of infected droplets exhaled by affected animals, because the most reliable means of reproducing the disease experimentally is by endobronchial or aerosol exposure of susceptible cattle with suspensions of infected lung or organisms obtained from early subcultures. Factors other than the administration of the organism are evidently involved in determining whether cattle develop the disease, but exactly what these are is not known. Variations in innate susceptibility, interaction with other microorganisms or preexisting pneumonic lesions, and the state of pulmonary defenses have all been suggested as being important. It appears necessary for the organisms to reach the alveolar parenchyma, but the subsequent chain of pathogenetic events is still uncertain. It has been suggested that the acute vasculitis, fibrinous exudation, thrombosis, and necrosis are due in part to an Arthus-type or mixed hypersensitivity in animals with circulating antibodies capable of reacting with surface antigens on the mycoplasmas. Whatever the pathogenesis of the vasculitis, the thrombosis it can cause is to a large extent responsible for the infarction and sequestrum formation.

The disease that can be produced in a percentage of animals following the aerosolization or endobronchial instillation of cultured organisms is similar to the natural disease, but the lesions are frequently small and multifocal and are not as likely to cause confluent consolidation of large regions of lung, such as occurs in field outbreaks. Use of a suspension of infected lung is a more reliable method of reproducing the disease. Transmission experiments have confirmed that in an exposed population, 10–30% of the animals are refractory to infection. This resistance is native and not acquired by prior exposure to the organism. The natural incubation period is quite variable, but usually it is longer than 1 month. The clinical signs are those of a febrile pleuropneumonia, with a course of 2 to 8 weeks, ending in death or slow recovery. Peracute cases that die in less than 1 week do occur. On the other hand, there are mild cases, and some that are subclinical. Mortality can range from 10 to 70% in outbreaks. Slaughter of affected herds of cattle on occasion reveals frequency of pulmonary lesions approaching 90% even though clinical signs might be obvious in only 30% of the animals at the time killing starts. There is no particular age distribution. Evidence of extrapulmonary localization may be observed in young calves as a polyarthritis, and in pregnant cows as abortion. Up to a third of cases that recover from the acute disease harbor residual infection in pulmonary sequestra. The organisms may remain viable in a sequestrum for several years. Cattle with sequestra that break down and discharge liquefied or caseous debris containing viable mycoplasmas into the airways are frequently the source of new outbreaks of the disease.

MYCOPLASMAL BRONCHIOLITIS AND PNEUMONIA OF CALVES. Mycoplasmal bronchitis and bronchiolitis or bronchointerstitial

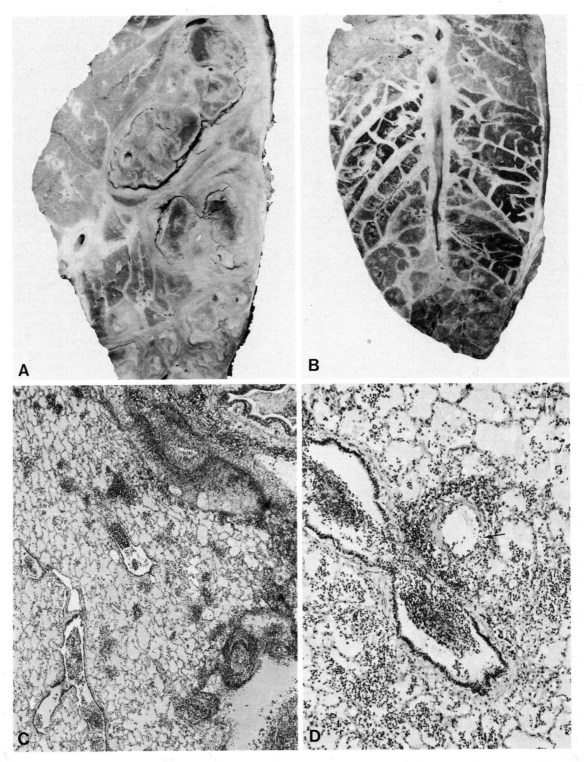

Fig. 6.34. Contagious bovine pleuropneumonia.   **(A)** Encapsulation of necrotic tissue (sequestra).   **(B)** Scarring of distended interlobular septa in chronic disease.   **(C)** Acute fibrinonecrotic pneumonia with inflammation and necrosis within interlobular septa and peribronchial interstitium.   **(D)** Acute arteritis (arrow) affecting portion of the wall of peribronchial artery.

pneumonia is an important component of enzootic pneumonia of calves, involving synergistic action of several infectious agents. Enzootic pneumonia will be discussed subsequently, but the pulmonary lesions attributable to mycoplasmas will be considered here. More than a dozen species of mycoplasmas can be isolated from bovine lungs. The difficulties in proving pathogenetic significance for mycoplasmas recovered from pneumonic lung was referred to earlier. Nevertheless, on the basis of both field and experimental studies, *Mycoplasma dispar*, *M. bovis*, and *Ureaplasma* spp. are generally accepted as being capable of producing subclinical bronchiolitis or pneumonia. A fourth species, *M. bovigenitalium*, is experimentally pathogenic for lung but is rarely isolated from the respiratory tract. *Mycoplasma dispar* appears to be the most important mycoplasmal pathogen in lungs of calves.

The mycoplasmas colonize the upper respiratory tract of calves soon after birth and extend to various depths of airways. They attach to the ciliated epithelial cells, and when present in large numbers can be seen by electron microscopy to be packed two or three layers deep on and between the microvilli and base of the cilia. Their characteristic effect is to cause a chronic catarrhal bronchitis and bronchiolitis that over the course of several months leads to the development of prominent lymphofollicular sheaths around the airways. The term ''cuffing pneumonia'' is sometimes applied to lungs in which this is the predominant finding (Fig. 6.35C).

The uncomplicated mycoplasmal lesion is usually inconspicuous. Grossly, there are patchy, purple-red atelectatic foci in cranioventral regions of the lungs (Fig. 6.35A). More confluent, meaty consolidation is an indication of probable involvement by additional organisms. Microscopically, the lesion for the first several weeks after infection is a catarrhal bronchitis and bronchiolitis. There are accumulations of neutrophils and mucus in the lumina of the airways, and increased prominence of bronchial submucosal glands and epithelial goblet cells. There are moderate accumulations of lymphocytes and lesser numbers of plasma cells in the walls of the airways and around accompanying blood vessels. There is loss of cilia, and many ciliated cells have degenerative changes. Inflammation of alveoli adjacent to terminal bronchioles occurs in heavy experimental infections in colostrum-deprived, specific-pathogen-free calves and can probably occur in heavy natural infection. The alveolitis is nonspecific. There is a mixed intraluminal accumulation of neutrophils and alveolar macrophages, with occasional plasma cells and giant cells. The alveolar septa appear thickened. This is partly because of accumulation of mononuclear cells within the septa but often has a large artifactual component because of microatelectasis. Hyperplasia of alveolar type II cells can occur but is usually minimal in uncomplicated infections. More commonly, alveolar regions distal to occluded bronchioles are atelectatic rather than directly inflamed, and this correlates with the usual gross finding of atelectasis. The composite picture is of a bronchointerstitial pneumonia and partial atelectasis (Fig. 6.35B).

Widespread lymphofollicular accumulations containing germinal centers develop slowly and are not usually present in calves less than 3 months of age. The follicular or ensheathing collars of lymphocytes extend into the lamina propria, often

obliterate the bronchiolar smooth muscle, and cause narrowing of the bronchiolar lumina. This is the hallmark of cuffing pneumonia (Fig. 6.35C). There is associated epithelial hyperplasia, including goblet cells in bronchi and large bronchioles, and hypertrophy of bronchial submucosal glands. Alveolar regions are principally atelectatic because of bronchiolar occlusion by lymphofollicular accumulations and intraluminal exudate, but might have an alveolitis as described for the earlier stages. The epithelium covering large lymphofollicular nodules in the submucosa of bronchi tends to assume the flattened appearance characteristic of lymphoepithelium.

Because the uncomplicated mycoplasmal lesion is rarely lethal, if ever, it is usually detected as a cuffing type of pneumonia in slaughtered veal calves or in calves dying for other reasons. It can also be a component of other pneumonias of calves. Other than the designation cuffing pneumonia, various morphologic terms have been used. The most appropriate one for the airway lesion is chronic catarrhal bronchitis and bronchiolitis with lymphofollicular cuffing. When the inflammation extends to peribronchiolar alveoli, the general term bronchointerstitial pneumonia is applicable. Although the lesion is a chronic one, examination of the lungs of cattle older than 9 to 12 months of age indicates that it does gradually regress in most instances.

Respiratory Mycoplasmosis of Goats

Mycoplasmas are an important cause of disease in goats. A variety of species are responsible for pneumonia, mastitis, polyarthritis, keratoconjunctivitis, or a combination of these. Septicemic forms can also occur, mostly in young kids. Manifestations of mycoplasmosis vary according to prevalence of the various species and strains of *Mycoplasma*, the husbandry practices, and the presence of environmental influences or intercurrent diseases that act as predisposing factors.

CONTAGIOUS CAPRINE PLEUROPNEUMONIA. Contagious caprine pleuropneumonia is the most important form of respiratory mycoplasmosis in goats. The disease occurs mainly in Africa, the Middle East, and western Asia. The prominent lesions are a severe fibrinous or fibrinonecrotic pneumonia and a profuse serofibrinous pleuritis. Fibrinous pericarditis is also common. Three taxa of *Mycoplasma* are associated with severe outbreaks of caprine pleuropneumonia: *M. mycoides* subsp. *capri*, *M. mycoides* subsp. *mycoides* (large-colony type), and an unclassified organism referred to as strain F38. The relative importance of these organisms in the various geographic regions is not clearly established. Strain F38, which was isolated in Kenya, has been reported to be the cause of a pleuropneumonia most resembling the classical caprine contagious pleuropneumonia reported from South Africa at the end of the nineteenth century. The points of resemblance are a high degree of contagiousness for goats but not sheep or cattle, a fibrinous pleuropneumonia lacking conspicuous serofibrinous widening of interlobular septa, and absence of local inflammation when the organism is inoculated subcutaneously. *Mycoplasma mycoides* subsp. *capri* and *M. mycoides* subsp. *mycoides* (large-colony type) appear to cause a form of caprine pleuropneumonia resembling the disease in cattle in that there is often extensive widening of interlobular septa and peribronchial interstitium by serofibrinous exudate. They

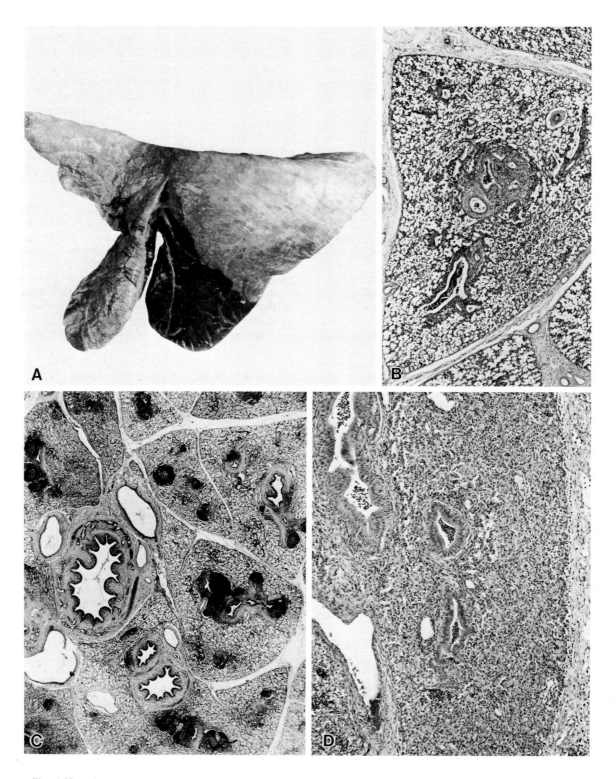

Fig. 6.35. (**A**) Atelectasis and consolidation of enzootic pneumonia. Calf. (**B**) Bronchointerstitial pneumonia and atelectasis associated with *Mycoplasma* infection. Calf. (Courtesy of M. L. Anderson.) (**C**) Prominent lymphofollicular sheaths around bronchioles and vessels in chronic enzootic (''cuffing'') pneumonia. Calf. (**D**) Bronchointerstitial pneumonia caused by *Chlamydia psittaci*, with epithelial hyperplasia of bronchioles and increased cellularity of atelectatic alveoli. Goat.

also seem to be less readily transmitted from goat to goat by contact. Necrotic sequestra are present in chronic stages of disease caused by all three mycoplasmas but are not as conspicuous a feature as in contagious bovine pleuropneumonia. The distinction between the pleuropneumonia caused by F38 and related strains on the one hand and *M. mycoides* subsp. *capri* or *M. mycoides* subsp. *mycoides* (large-colony type) on the other is not firmly established. There is a positive correlation, however, between the profuse interstitial pulmonary exudation produced by the *M. mycoides* subspecies and their ability to cause an intense local reaction when inoculated subcutaneously.

Mycoplasma mycoides subsp. *capri* and *M. mycoides* subsp. *mycoides* (large-colony type) are also found in areas of the world where explosive outbreaks of caprine contagious pleuropneumonia do not occur. Both organisms have been isolated in Australia, and *M. mycoides* subsp. *mycoides* (large-colony type) is widespread in North America. Syndromes caused by *M. mycoides* subsp. *mycoides* (large-colony type) vary. In North America and France, it causes severe disease with high mortality in kids. The predominant lesion is fibrinopurulent polyarthritis, but fibrinous pleuritis and pericarditis, acute interstitial pneumonia, and meningitis frequently accompany the severe mycoplasmemia. In older goats, less fulminating cases of mastitis, pneumonia, or arthritis are more usual. Peritonitis and abortion are occasional complications.

Various other mycoplasmas have been isolated from the lung. *Mycoplasma capricolum* is principally a cause of fibrinopurulent polyarthritis in kids. A mild, acute interstitial pneumonia, such as occurs in other septicemias, occurs in the septicemia associated with acute polyarthritis in young kids. Mastitis can occur in milking females.

Other mycoplasmas, particularly *Mycoplasma ovipneumoniae* and *M. bovis,* have been isolated from pneumonic lungs of goats. Their significance is uncertain. It is probable that they play a role similar to that of *M. bovis* in calves and *M. ovipneumoniae* in sheep by causing a mild, subacute to chronic catarrhal bronchiolitis or bronchointerstitial pneumonia and perhaps acting synergistically with other infectious agents to produce an enzootic type of pneumonia.

Respiratory Mycoplasmosis of Sheep

The mycoplasma most frequently isolated from lungs of sheep is *Mycoplasma ovipneumoniae*. Most of the evidence indicates that it is one of the combined etiologic factors causing enzootic pneumonia of sheep, usually in association with *Pasteurella haemolytica*. Experimental studies using *M. ovipneumoniae* alone have been inconsistent and often difficult to interpret. There is sufficient evidence, however, to show that at least some strains of the organism can cause mild, subclinical lesions in some infected sheep. Lesions are principally chronic catarrhal bronchitis and bronchiolitis, with development of lymphofollicular collars around the airways. The affected alveoli are mostly atelectatic because of bronchiolar obstruction, although a mild chronic alveolitis might be present. The role of *M. ovipneumoniae* therefore appears to be analogous to that of *M. dispar* in calves.

Mycoplasma mycoides subspecies of caprine origin experimentally cause fibrinous pneumonia and pleuritis in sheep. They

are isolated only on rare occasions from naturally occurring outbreaks of pneumonia in sheep, and even in these instances their etiologic importance is open to question because of the presence of *Pasteurella haemolytica*.

Respiratory Mycoplasmosis of Swine

Mycoplasmas are by far the most important cause of enzootic pneumonia of pigs. In the absence of other proven etiologic agents, there is a tendency to regard mycoplasmas as the sole cause. It remains to be determined whether this is too sweeping a generalization. It is safe to say, however, that mycoplasmal pneumonia is the overwhelmingly preponderant form of enzootic pneumonia in pigs. Now that mycoplasmas are established as the main causative agents, the term **mycoplasmal pneumonia** replaces the earlier one, virus pneumonia of pigs (enzootic virus pneumonia).

Mycoplasma hyopneumoniae (*M. suipneumoniae*) and *M. hyorhinis* are both established respiratory pathogens, *M. hyopneumoniae* the more important. A variety of other mycoplasmas, such as *M. flocculare* and *Ureaplasma* spp., can also be isolated occasionally from enzootic pneumonia. Their relative importance in causing the disease is still under investigation.

ENZOOTIC MYCOPLASMAL PNEUMONIA OF SWINE. Enzootic mycoplasmal pneumonia is a chronic, usually nonfatal disease of young pigs. It is widespread throughout the world, and in its most severe form can affect from 70 to 100% of pigs in a herd. Clinical expressions of the uncomplicated disease are coughing, unthriftiness, poor weight gain, and reduced food conversion ratio. Because there is usually low mortality associated with mycoplasmal pneumonia, the lesions are generally seen in slaughtered animals or those dying from other diseases. When deaths do occur because of pneumonia, it is due mainly to superimposed bacterial infections. *Pasteurella multocida* is the most common secondary invader, but *Corynebacterium pyogenes, Haemophilus* spp., streptococci, staphylococci, *Klebsiella* spp., and *Bordetella bronchiseptica* can be involved singly or in combination.

The characteristic gross feature of mycoplasmal pneumonia is confluent consolidation of cranioventral regions of the lungs (Fig. 6.36A). When the amount of consolidation is small, it tends to affect portions of the right middle and right cranial lobes and the caudal portion of the left cranial lobe, but frequently there is bilateral involvement of more than 50% of cranial and middle lobes together with the accessory lobe and cranioventral portions of caudal lobes. The consolidated lung ranges from dark red through grayish pink to more homogeneous gray, according to the age of the lesion. This change occurs over the several-month course of disease. Even though there is often extensive confluent consolidation, careful examination reveals a regular pattern of small grayish nodules against a red background. This denotes the bronchiolar orientation of the inflammation. The cut surface of consolidated lung is moist and meaty, and mucopus is present in the airways. Minor mycoplasmal lesions are less characteristic and have a mosaic pattern of intermixed consolidated, atelectatic, hyperinflated, and more normal lobules. Occasional atelectatic lobules represent the minimal

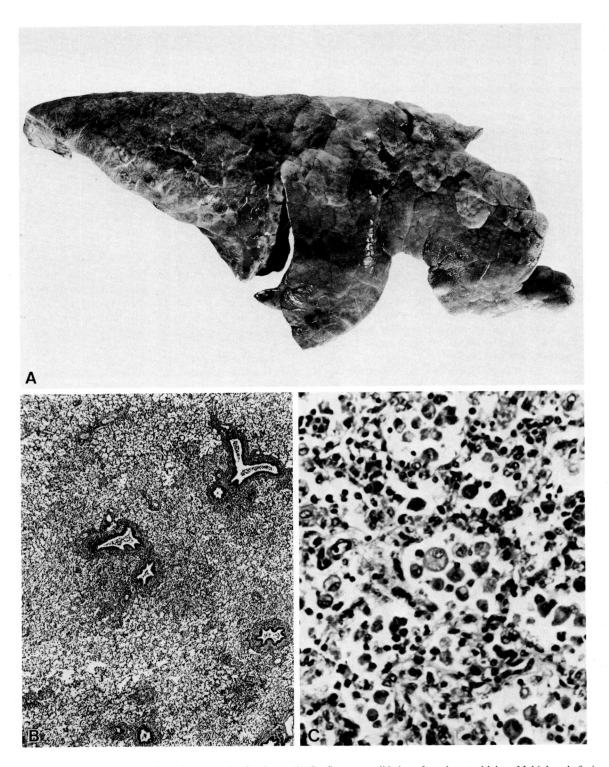

Fig. 6.36. Enzootic mycoplasmal pneumonia of swine.   (**A**) Confluent consolidation of cranioventral lobes. Multiple pale foci within affected lobules, indicating bronchiolar orientation of the pneumonia.   (**B**) Bronchointerstitial pattern of early lesion. (**C**) Peribronchiolar alveoli in (**B**), showing thickening of septa by lymphoid cells and macrophages within lumina.

gross lesion. Sometimes, pale nodules indicating the presence of peribronchiolar lymphoid tissue can be detected in the centers of atelectatic lobules. Lesions of severe exudative bronchopneumonia or lobar pneumonia, especially with necrosis or abscessation, indicate secondary bacterial infection.

Mycoplasma hyopneumoniae can cause fibrinous or serofibrinous pleuritis and inflammation of other serous surfaces. When pleuritis is present, however, it is more probably associated with *M. hyorhinis* or infections complicated by *Pasteurella multocida* or *Haemophilus* spp. Pulmonary lymph nodes are enlarged by nonspecific hyperplastic lymphadenitis to a degree corresponding to the extent and activity of pulmonary consolidation. On cut surface they are moist, usually bulging, and sometimes hyperemic.

Histologically, mycoplasmal pneumonia in swine has the morphologic pattern of a catarrhal bronchointerstitial pneumonia (Fig. 6.36B), with development of prominent peribronchial and peribronchiolar accumulations of lymphoid tissue in the chronic stages. Thus there is a resemblance to the lesions caused by mycoplasmas associated with enzootic pneumonias in calves and lambs. The mycoplasmas of swine appear to be much more capable of eliciting chronic inflammation of the alveolar parenchyma without the assistance of other organisms, however, even though they mainly colonize the surface of ciliated cells in the airways, as do the mycoplasmas of calves and lambs.

In the fully developed mycoplasmal pneumonia, there is extensive lymphoid hyperplasia around airways and their associated vessels. In severe cases, the lymphoid nodules or sheaths efface the muscularis mucosae and cause narrowing of the lumina of airways. Germinal centers may be present. The epithelium over prominent nodules is often degenerated or ulcerated. Elsewhere, there is epithelial hyperplasia, particularly in bronchioles. Cilia are absent from many surface regions. There is hyperplasia of goblet cells in the bronchi and larger bronchioles, and the bronchial submucosal glands are increased in size and number. The increased activity of mucus-secreting cells is responsible for the presence of large amounts of mucus or mucopus. The alveolitis component of the bronchointerstitial pneumonia consists of wide thickening of the septa of alveoli adjacent to bronchioles, and accumulation of exudate in their lumina. The alveolar septa are thickened by accumulations of various-sized lymphocytes and small numbers of plasma cells. The intraalveolar exudate consists predominantly of macrophages (Fig. 6.36C), but plasma cells, lymphocytes, and neutrophils are present to various degrees. There is hyperplasia of type II alveolar epithelial cells of inflamed alveoli in established lesions. This can be difficult to detect histologically when alveolar architecture is obscured by absence of detectable demarcation between thickened alveolar septa and atelectatic or exudate-filled lumina.

Experimental studies of the pathogenesis of mycoplasmal pneumonia indicate that typical gross lesions do not occur until 2 to 4 weeks after infection. The rate of development of lesions is dependent on factors relating to the dose and strain of *Mycoplasma,* method of administration, and susceptibility of the pigs exposed. Inoculation of suspensions of lung containing mycoplasmas is a more reliable way of reproducing the disease,

as is also the case with experimental production of respiratory mycoplasmosis in cattle, sheep, and goats. Young pigs naturally exposed to infectious aerosols soon after birth can also develop lesions by the time they are 3–5 weeks of age. Initial lesions caused by the mycoplasma, that is, within a week after infection, are a neutrophilic bronchitis and bronchiolitis, and a mixed neutrophil and macrophage accumulation in adjacent alveoli. The numbers of neutrophils diminish, and the lymphoid cells increase over the subsequent several weeks to reach the fully developed stage of consolidation described earlier. There is conflicting evidence concerning persistence of the pneumonia after it has reached its peak some 5–6 weeks after infection. Estimations range from essentially complete resolution of uncomplicated mycoplasmal pneumonia within 2 months to no appreciable reduction in its extent even after 3 months. In view of the large number of variables in experimental and especially in field situations, the wide range in persistence is to be expected.

Respiratory Mycoplasmosis of Horses

Although several mycoplasmas have been isolated from the respiratory tract of horses, particularly *Mycoplasma equirhinis* and *M. felis,* there have been no studies to determine whether any of them is capable of causing a subclinical bronchiolitis or bronchointerstitial pneumonia. *Mycoplasma felis* has been implicated as a possible cause of pleuritis in the horse.

Respiratory Mycoplasmosis of Dogs and Cats

Of the various mycoplasmas isolated from canine pneumonia, *Mycoplasma cynos* experimentally is capable of causing a mild bronchointerstitial pneumonia similar to that produced by mycoplasmas in other species. *Mycoplasma bovigenitalium* is also pathogenic, but to a lesser extent. The clinical significance of these mycoplasmas is doubtful, however, because they are usually isolated from severe exudative lesions in which pathogenic bacteria are also present, often in dogs with distemper.

Mycoplasma felis is an opportunistic pathogen of the conjunctiva in cats. Neither it nor the other mycoplasmas isolated from the respiratory tract of cats are recognized as significant respiratory tract pathogens.

Chlamydial Diseases

Indigenous strains of *Chlamydia psittaci* have been associated with respiratory disease in cats, cattle, sheep, goats, and horses. Feline *C. psittaci* was the first agent isolated from cats with conjunctivitis and respiratory disease, and therefore became known rather misleadingly as the feline pneumonitis agent. It is now recognized to be mainly a cause of chronic conjunctivitis, although it can cause transient rhinitis and subclinical bronchointerstitial pneumonia. Strains of *C. psittaci* can occasionally be isolated from pneumonia in cattle, sheep, and goats. The pneumonias are usually of the enzootic type and are sometimes accompanied by enteritis. Since the intestine is a major carrier site for chlamydiae, and they can readily be isolated from feces of ruminants, inhalation of dust contaminated with feces is assumed to be a source of respiratory infection.

In all the domestic animals studied, experimental pulmonary infection by indigenous strains of *Chlamydia psittaci* causes a mild, acute bronchointerstitial pneumonia that resolves within 3 to 4 weeks unless secondary bacterial invasion occurs. The extent of the pneumonia varies according to the amount of inoculum and whether it is delivered by aerosol, intranasal, or intratracheal routes, but the course of the disease remains the same. There is an initial neutrophilic bronchiolitis and alveolitis, but by 5 days after infection there is predominance of macrophages in the alveolar exudate and extensive hyperplasia of alveolar type II epithelial cells. Moderate-sized cuffs of lymphoid cells are present around bronchioles and small blood vessels at the height of the lesion, and alveolar septa are thickened by a mixed infiltrate of mononuclear cells with a few neutrophils. A similar lesion, in which chlamydiae can be detected by immunofluorescence, is occasionally encountered in naturally occurring pneumonia in ruminants (Fig. 6.35D). The chlamydiae are mostly destroyed during the acute phase of inflammation, which then subsides and resolution can be complete within 3 to 4 weeks after experimental infection.

In assessing the importance of chlamydial infections in ruminants, it is important to note that they are usually only capable of inducing a transient inflammation. This is in contrast to mycoplasmas, which tend to persist on ciliated epithelium and cause chronic lesions. The part chlamydiae play in contributing to the cause of chronic enzootic pneumonia is therefore probably a relatively minor one.

Rickettsial Diseases

Several rickettsial diseases can cause interstitial pneumonia as one of the manifestations of their systemic involvement. This is particularly true for rickettsias affecting vascular endothelium. The important organism of this type in animals is *Cowdria ruminantium,* which causes heartwater in cattle, sheep, and goats (see the Cardiovascular System, Volume 3). A mild interstitial pneumonia can be present in salmon poisoning of dogs caused by *Neorickettsia helminthoeca* (see the Alimentary System, this volume).

Pulmonary Mycoses

Aspergillosis

Fungi of the genus *Aspergillus* are ubiquitous, and exposure to the spores is an everyday matter. Nonetheless, established infections that produce disease are uncommon in mammals, although of great importance in birds. *Aspergillus fumigatus* is responsible for most infections in mammals, birds, and humans. Other species, including *A. flavus, A. niger,* and *A. nidulans,* occasionally act as pathogens.

Aspergillosis in animals is most often a respiratory infection initiated by inhaled spores. Moldy litter and feeds, especially hay and grain that have been damp and heated during storage, support an enormous growth of fungi among which *Aspergillus fumigatus* can predominate. In view of the high rate of exposure that takes place among housed animals, it is perhaps surprising that more progressive infections are not detected. Very little is known concerning the pathogenesis of aspergillosis. Questions concerning the susceptibility of hosts, the number of spores necessary to initiate infection, toxigenicity of the organisms, and the role of immunity and hypersensitivity still have to be resolved.

Aspergillosis can be a respiratory or placental disease in animals. Infections of either the upper or lower respiratory tract are sporadic in all species, but thus far infection of the pregnant uterus and fetus has been found mainly in cattle. The latter, which is described with diseases of the pregnant uterus (in the Female Genital System, Volume 3), is the more economically important of the two.

Aspergillosis of the respiratory tract appears often to be a complication of some other debilitating disease, but there are cases in which no clear predisposition can be found. The infection may develop as an implantation on the mucous membrane of the nasal cavity, sinuses, guttural pouches, and tracheobronchial airways, or it may be in the form of a nodular bronchopneumonia. Secondary intestinal infections have been observed in cattle. When the fungi grow on a mucous membrane, they may be visible to the naked eye, first as a whitish growth and later as a powdery, feltlike growth with a typical blue-green color produced by the conidia. These superficial colonies may develop after death, and the presence of colonies of the fungus on a mucosa is not significant unless there is a tissue reaction. The usual reaction is caseating necrosis surrounded by a zone of hemorrhagic inflammation. Breakdown of these lesions in the walls of bronchi can result in bronchiectatic cavities.

The pulmonary lesions typically occur as one or many discrete gray-white nodules about 1–10 mm in diameter, with a narrow hyperemic rim. They may be obscured, especially in young animals, by severe pulmonary congestion. The nodules develop around fungal colonies that proliferate in the terminal bronchioles (Fig. 6.37B) and adjacent alveoli. The fungal colony consists of long, branching, septate hyphae (Fig. 6.37A) and is surrounded by a zone of neutrophils, macrophages, and debris. The focus expands and compresses adjacent alveoli. The affected bronchioles contain plugs of purulent exudate. As is common in invasive fungal lesions of this type, occasional blood vessels are invaded, inflamed, and thrombosed. The nodules may become cavitated if they evacuate into airways. Chronic lesions are granulomatous. Macrophages and epithelioid cells predominate in the nodules and extensively infiltrate the septal tissues, and encapsulating fibroplasia is evident. Giant cells are not a significant part of the lesion, although they may be present later when the focus is being obliterated by fibrosis. Perhaps as an indication of host resistance, the form of the colonies changes in chronic infection. Instead of stretching out freely as long hyphae in all directions, as they do in early and progressive infections, the colonies become composed of shorter, radiating hyphae that branch freely near their outer ends—the so-called actinomycotic forms of the fungus. Sometimes "asteroid" bodies can be found in the nodules being obliterated. These consist of small tangled remnants of the colony, surrounded by radiating acidophilic clubs quite similar to those of the granules of actinomycosis (Fig. 6.37C). Dissemination of the infection from the pulmonary lesions can occur. Of the many organs in which metastases develop, including the meninges, the kidney seems to be the most prone.

Mortierellosis

Acute fatal mycotic pneumonia may be associated with placental infection by *Mortierella wolfii,* the most important cause of mycotic abortion of cattle in New Zealand. An acute fibrino-

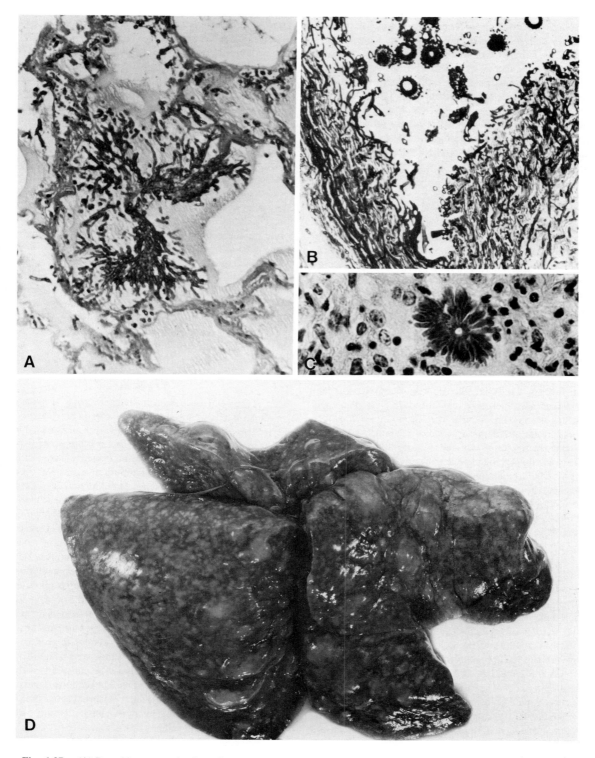

Fig. 6.37. (**A**) Branching septate hyphae of *Aspergillus fumigatus* in lung. Ox.   (**B**) Mycelium invading bronchiolar wall and fruiting bodies in lumen. Pulmonary aspergillosis. Ox.   (**C**) Chronic pulmonary aspergillosis. Ox. Clubs surrounding fungus in epithelioid-cell granuloma.   (**D**) Disseminated granulomatous foci of severe pulmonary blastomycosis. Dog.

necrotic pneumonia can occur in infected cows at or within a few days of abortion or parturition. There is apparently extensive hematogenous dissemination of fungal elements when the placenta separates. This is followed by widespread vegetation of hyphae in pulmonary capillaries and larger vessels, with resulting inflammation, thrombosis, and necrosis. Less severe pulmonary involvement leads to chronic, focal, granulomatous lesions.

Other fungi within the class Phycomycetes, such as *Mucor* and *Rhizopus,* are occasional opportunistic invaders of lung and are usually associated with the nodular caseonecrotic or granulomatous lesions.

Blastomycosis

Blastomycosis is a disseminated or localized mycotic infection caused by *Blastomyces dermatitidis.* It is chiefly a disease of humans and dogs in North America and Africa. It is sometimes referred to as North American blastomycosis, to distinguish it from South American blastomycosis (*B. brasiliensis*) and European "blastomycosis" (*Cryptococcus neoformans*). The lesions are typically granulomatous or pyogranulomatous.

Blastomyces dermatitidis is a dimorphic fungus; in cultures at room temperature it produces a mycelial growth, whereas in tissues or culture at 37°C it is yeastlike, 8–25 μm in diameter with a thick, double-contoured wall, and reproduces by budding. The epidemiology of blastomycosis is obscure. The infection appears not to be contagious from animal to animal or animal to human. The available evidence suggests that the source of infection is the soil or related site. In North America, most cases of the disease occur in the Mississippi–Ohio river basins and the central Atlantic states of the United States, and near the northern border of Ontario and Manitoba in Canada.

The disease in dogs is found predominantly in young males of large breeds. The lung is the most frequent site of primary involvement, but primary cutaneous infections are also found. Systemic dissemination often occurs and is particularly prone to cause clinical signs associated with lesions in lymph nodes, eyes, skin, subcutaneous tissue, bones and joints, and the urogenital tract. The pulmonary form of the disease is insidious in onset and has a chronic course that may last many months. The usual syndrome is one of a chronic debilitating disease with cough, exercise intolerance, and terminal respiratory distress. The other clinical signs depend on the pattern of dissemination.

The pulmonary lesions of fatal blastomycosis are multiple, gray-white nodules of various sizes distributed throughout all lobes (Fig. 6.37D). Superficial nodules produce elevations of the pleura, but it is exceptional for there to be pleuritis. When this does occur, it is because of fistulation from a mycotic abscess. Most pulmonary nodules are of firm granulomatous tissue, but some undergo central abscessation or caseation and then may fistulate into a bronchus or onto the pleura. Calcification is minimal or absent. Microscopically, the high frequency with which small lesions affect bronchioles and adjacent alveoli can be taken as evidence of aerogenous infection, although intrabronchial spread of organisms confuses the picture. The regional lymph nodes are consistently involved and contain granulomas, abscesses, or caseous foci. It is usual for the pulmonary nodules to be more or less of equivalent age, but it is sometimes possible to locate larger, older caseous lesions in the lung and lymph node, which together are probably comparable to the primary complex of tuberculosis.

Disseminated lesions take the same form as those in the lungs and have been observed in peripheral lymph nodes, eyes, skin, subcutaneous tissues, bones, and joints. Testes, prostate, brain, heart, liver, spleen, kidneys, intestines, and other organs are less commonly affected. The lesions are either typical granulomas with abundant epithelioid and giant cells, or pyogranulomatous foci with central accumulation and necrosis of neutrophils and macrophages. The yeastlike fungi are plentiful and readily detected in the lesions, either free or in the cytoplasm of macrophages and giant cells. Identification of the organism, and its characteristically broadbased, single-budding forms, is aided by use of PAS or methenamine–silver stains.

The cutaneous lesions begin as papules, which soon develop into small abscesses with a surrounding inflammatory reaction. The lesions expand, with new small abscesses forming in the expanding margin of the papules while the central areas undergo some cicatrization.

Microscopically, the abscesses and granulomas found within the skin and subcutis are structurally similar to the pulmonary lesions.

Pulmonary, cutaneous, or systemic blastomycosis occasionally occurs in cats, particularly in the Siamese breed. It has also been found in other species.

Cryptococcosis

Cryptococcosis (European "blastomycosis") is a subacute or chronic mycosis caused by *Cryptococcus neoformans* (*Torula histolytica*). *Cryptococcus neoformans* is monomorphic, yeastlike, reproduces by single buds, and is approximately 5–10 μm in diameter, not including the large amount of capsular material. The disease has worldwide distribution. It may be a localized or disseminated disease, but it has a predilection for the respiratory system, particularly the nasal region, and for the central nervous system. All species of animals appear to be affected occasionally. Most attention has been focused on the disease in cats.

There are several species in the genus, but only one, *Cryptococcus neoformans,* is a pathogen. It is distinguished from the nonpathogens by producing disease in experimental mice. The yeast is surrounded by a wide capsule composed of mucopolysaccharides, and although cultivation of the organism is necessary for proper identification, a confident diagnosis can be made on pathologic material by identification of the capsule. The capsular material is sometimes copious enough to give the lesions a grossly mucinous texture, and it stains well with mucicarmine, the PAS reaction, or Alcian blue. The capsule is wider in hydrated than in dehydrated sections. The organisms in wet mounts are not easily distinguished from erythrocytes or lymphocytes, but they are clearly evident by negative staining of the wide capsular zones with India ink or nigrosin.

The source of infection is generally believed to be soil, especially when enriched with pigeon or other bird droppings. Cases are sporadic, and as usually true for the deep mycoses, the infection is not contagious. Cryptococci are natural saprophytes and only accidentally act as pathogens in animals with impaired local or systemic immunity. Debility, malnutrition, prolonged

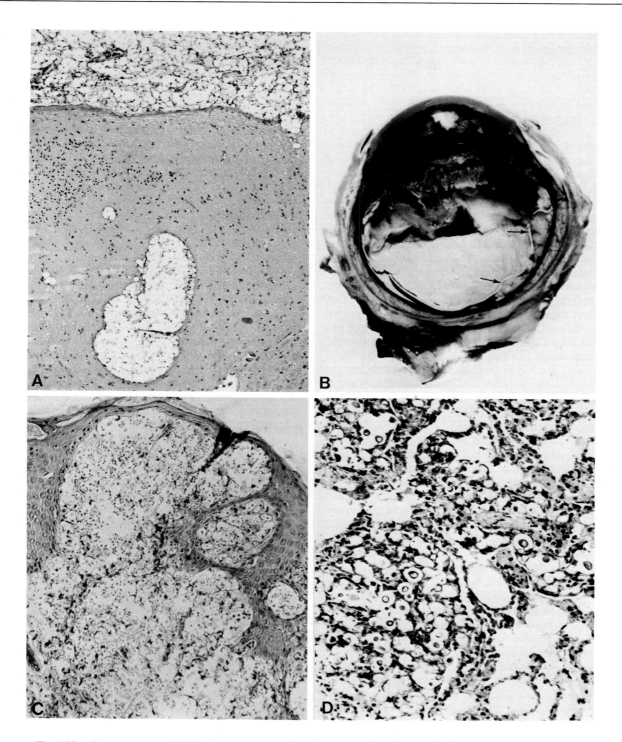

Fig. 6.38. Cryptococcosis. (A) Granulomatous meningitis with extension along Virchow–Robin space of penetrating vessel. Cat. Note characteristic "soap bubble" appearance. (B) Cryptococcal choroiditis with exudative detachment of retina (arrows). Dog. (C) Cutaneous lesion. Dog. (D) Yeastlike *Cryptococcus neoformans* in pulmonary alveoli. Dog.

use of corticosteroids, and feline leukemia virus infection are some of the conditions suspected of predisposing cats to cryptococcosis. Infection is acquired in most instances by inhalation of contaminated dust. The respiratory tract is the usual site of primary infection, with the nasal cavity more often affected than the lungs. The lungs are often stated to be the usual site for systemic dissemination of cryptococcal organisms, but the nasal region is probably the more important because its involvement leads much more frequently to dissemination to the central nervous system, eyes, lymph nodes, skin, and other organs than does pulmonary involvement. There is also the possibility of local spread to the meninges and brain from nasal lesions. Local inoculation of the organism does not appear to be of general significance, although it has resulted in outbreaks of cryptococcal mastitis in cows (see the Female Genital System, Volume 3). The cutaneous lesions, which are observed occasionally, may be primary or metastases following hematogenous dissemination from respiratory infection. The infection has a predilection for the central nervous system (Fig. 6.38A). Lesions can occur there without being grossly apparent in any other organ, but it is usual in the disseminated infection to find gross or microscopic lesions in some combination of the respiratory tract and other organs. Intraocular metastases may occur (Fig. 6.38B).

The cutaneous lesions of cryptococcosis take the form of firm small nodules (Fig. 6.38C) that tend to ulcerate, discharge a small amount of serous exudate, and may then heal. In cats, the skin of the head is most commonly affected, but sometimes the lesions are distributed widely over the body. Nasal involvement was described earlier with granulomatous rhinitis. In the parenchymatous organs, the lesions are discrete, whitish, gelatinous foci and may not be more than a few millimeters in diameter. Lesions in the meninges, brain, and spinal cord also have a discrete, gelatinous character when they are visible, but often there are no significant gross changes. There may be some gelatinous areas in arachnoid spaces, especially around the larger vessels and in the cisterns, but the opacity of bacterial meningitis is seldom observed. The parenchymal lesions are chiefly in the peripheral gray matter and probably develop by extension of the lesions along the Virchow–Robin spaces (Fig. 6.38A).

The usual cryptococcal lesions are characterized histologically as having a "soap bubble" appearance because of the unstained capsules of massed organisms. A profound cellular reaction is not typical, in contrast to other mycotic infections, and usually consists of a few macrophages, lymphocytes, and plasma cells (Fig. 6.38D). Vacuolated and degenerating macrophages may occasionally dominate the picture. Sometimes, particularly in lungs, the lesions become more typically granulomatous, with numerous epithelioid and some giant cells. The changes in organisms and cell-mediated responses that modulate the differences in host response are not understood. Caseation may occur in lesions in lymph nodes, but otherwise necrosis is not part of the reaction to these organisms.

When examined in sections stained by hematoxylin and eosin, the fungi appear as typical yeasts surrounded by a clear halo produced by unstained capsular substance. The capsular substance immediately around the organism is often condensed into an acidophilic rim. The free-lying organisms may calcify and stain intensely with hematoxylin.

Coccidioidomycosis

Coccidioidomycosis, which is caused by *Coccidioides immitis*, is important in humans but also occurs in animals in areas in which the infection is endemic. Most cases of coccidioidomycosis occur in the endemic area of the United States, which includes the arid parts of California, Arizona, and Texas. The disease is also endemic in portions of South and Central America. In arid regions there is an association between the feces of desert rodents and high concentrations of the fungus. It is not clear to what extent numbers of organisms are increased by spherules excreted in the feces of the rodents, as compared to the fecal matter's enhancing vegetative growth of the organism in the soil. Vegetative growth of the fungus occurs in soil after rains, and subsequently large numbers of infective arthroconidia (spores) are disseminated widely in windblown dust after the soil dries. It is estimated that most animals living in endemic areas eventually become infected, but relatively few become clinically diseased.

The fungus is dimorphic. In tissues, the distinctive form is a spherule (sporangium) measuring about 10–70 μm in diameter, with a thick, double-contoured wall (Fig. 6.39B). It is called a sporangium because reproduction in tissues is by endosporulation; the endospores are globose, 2–5 μm in diameter, and are released into the tissues in large numbers when a spherule ruptures. Mycelia are rare in animal tissues. On most artificial media, however, growth is mycelial. Reproduction in mycelial growth is by arthroconidia, produced in very large numbers along the hyphae. These arthroconidia are highly infective and easily detached from the mycelial growth.

Coccidioidomycosis is a primary respiratory infection. Local traumatic inoculation can occur and result in a fluctuating abscess, but dissemination from such a focus is unusual. The high susceptibility of the lungs to the establishment of infection can be demonstrated experimentally by intranasal insufflation of spores. The great majority of respiratory infections are benign and nonprogressive. This form in humans is known as San Joaquin Valley fever. A small percentage of the infections disseminate from the lung, and the generalized disease is known as coccidioidal granuloma, with secondary lesions anywhere in the body. Among domestic animals, the disseminated disease has been observed mostly in dogs, and occasionally in horses, sheep, and cats. In these species, the lesions may be limited to the lungs and associated lymph nodes. In cattle and swine, lesions have so far only been observed in the lungs and their lymph nodes. The disease is common in cattle in endemic areas. As many as 20% of slaughtered cattle from feedlots in Arizona have lesions of the disease, but they are observed only in slaughtered animals. There is either a complete pulmonary complex, or an incomplete complex with lesions only in the bronchial and mediastinal lymph nodes.

Dissemination is common only in dogs, and in this species there is reported to be a predisposition for boxers and Doberman pinschers. The clinical signs frequently lack specificity and depend on the sites of active lesions. Persistent fever with one or more of respiratory abnormalities, shifting lameness, and the development of cutaneous nodules suggest the diagnosis in chronically ill dogs in endemic areas. The lameness is ephemeral

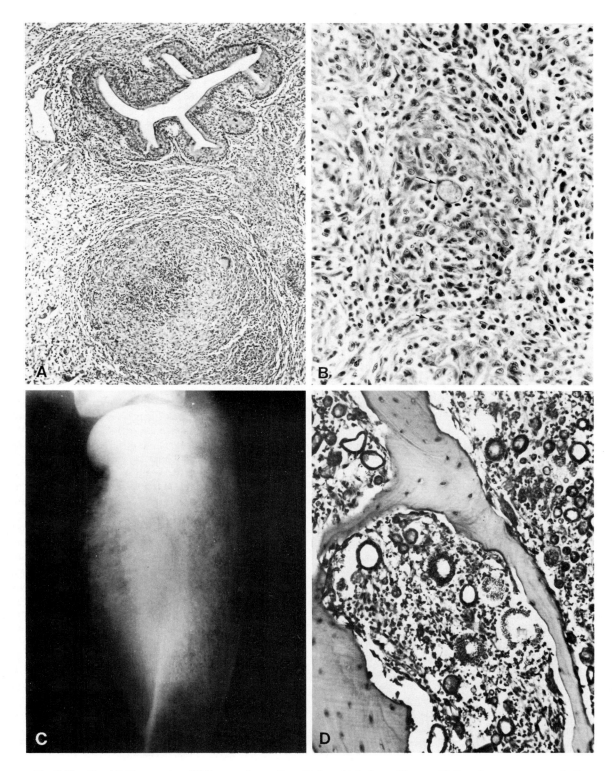

Fig. 6.39. Coccidioidomycosis. (A) Pyogranuloma adjacent to bronchiole. Lung. Horse. (B) Granulomatous pneumonia. Dog. Spherule (arrow) in center of small granuloma. (C) Radiograph of coccidioidal osteomyelitis. Dog. (D) Granulomatous osteomyelitis from (C). There are spherules in various stages of their developmental cycle.

when first seen, and radiographic evidence of the underlying osteomyelitis (Fig. 6.39C,D) is obvious only late in the course of disease. Usually the progressive debility leads to cachexia and eventual death, although recoveries do occur.

The lesions of coccidioidomycosis are granulomas or pyogranulomas (Fig. 6.39A,B). The granulomas are grayish white and usually nodular. There may be central caseation necrosis or liquefaction, but calcification is unusual. A common finding, particularly in the dog, is that large granulomatous nodules are composed of collections of discretely unitized small granulomas separated by fibrous tissue (Fig. 6.39B). The cellular reaction on the part of the host depends on the phase of the organism against which it is directed. Spores, whether endospores or the initial arthroconidia, provoke an acute exudative reaction in which neutrophils predominate. The larger spherules are usually surrounded by a wide zone of epithelioid cells mixed with a few giant cells, lymphocytes, and neutrophils. Because the organisms in any large focus are often in different phases of growth, there can be variations in the proportions of suppurative and granulomatous responses. In contained infections, however, the granulomatous response predominates, and it may then be difficult to find organisms. In such cases they are most likely to be found in the cytoplasm of giant cells as large spherules that are either evacuated and crenated or contain endospores. Often in cattle, and occasionally in other species, the spherules become surrounded by a corona of acidophilic clubs similar to those that form around colonies of *Actinomyces bovis* and some other microorganisms. This is an indication of high host resistance.

A variety of other fungal diseases can affect the lung, the most important being histoplasmosis (see the Hematopoietic System, Volume 3). Among the occasional opportunistic infections are sporotrichosis (*Sporothrix schenkii*), adiaspiromycosis (*Emmonsia* spp.), and geotrichosis (*Geotrichum candidum*).

Parasitic Diseases of the Lungs

The lungs are at the crossroads of parasitic migrations, and the many parasites that pass through them cause various degrees of damage according to the nature and intensity of the host–parasite interaction. Usually the lesions produced by transient parasites are of slight significance and are resolvable. There are exceptions, however. Severe and possibly fatal pulmonary lesions may develop if the migrating parasites are large in number, or large in size, or especially when the host has a hypersensitivity reaction to them. Hypersensitivity occurs because of previous exposure of a natural host or because of infection of an unnatural host. *Ascaris suum,* because of its tremendous biotic potential, may migrate in huge numbers and sometimes kill pigs, which are its natural hosts. It can also cause death of cattle, which are its frequent unnatural hosts. The lesion is an acute, diffuse, eosinophilic, interstitial pneumonia associated with the presence of large numbers of larvae. The trematodes *Fasciola gigantica* and *F. hepatica* invade the lungs accidentally from the liver. Since they are large parasites that wander extensively, a small number of them in the lungs can produce extensive cavitations. In other instances, lesions caused by parasites may be of some importance for differential diagnosis even though not of much clinical significance. In this category are the ''worm nod-

ules,'' such as those caused by migrating *Parascaris equorum* larvae in horses. Although distinctive when young by virtue of the mass of eosinophils present, when scarified and calcified they need to be differentiated from residual lesions of small abscesses or infectious granulomas, such as occur in glanders.

The transient parasites with principal habitats in other organs are discussed elsewhere. Here we are mainly concerned with ''lungworms,'' whose final habitat is the airways or, less commonly, the parenchyma of the lungs.

Dictyocaulus

Dictyocaulus contains the most important lungworms. There are three species: *D. filaria* is parasitic in sheep, goats, and other small ruminants; *D. viviparus* is parasitic in cattle; and *D. arnfieldi* is parasitic in the horse and its relatives. The three species are similar morphologically and in the details of their life cycles. *Dictyocaulus filaria* will serve as the type for discussion.

Dictyocaulus filaria, the large lungworm of sheep and goats, is a slender, whitish worm 3–10 cm long. The adults live mainly in the small bronchi. The life cycle is direct. The eggs are embryonated when laid, and some of them hatch in the lungs. The eggs and larvae are expelled from the lung by coughing; most are subsequently swallowed. The eggs that have not hatched in the air passages hatch in the alimentary canal, and first-stage larvae are passed in the feces. Further development occurs on the ground and requires moisture and moderate to low temperatures. This explains why verminous pneumonia is predominantly a disease of cool, moist climates. The larvae can develop at temperatures as low as 5°C, and their viability is prolonged at these temperatures. The combination of long survival at low temperatures and long patent periods in the host endow these worms with the ability to persist in northern, cold latitudes.

The larvae undergo two molts on pasture in ~1 week. The third stage is infective, and infestation can occur only if the third-stage larvae are ingested by the final host. The infective larvae penetrate the wall of the intestine and migrate via the lymphatics to the lungs. In the abdominal nodes, they undergo the third molt. Some larvae accidentally take the portal route and are destroyed in the liver. Some, on reaching the lungs, continue into the systemic circulation and are lost, except for those rare ones that pass the placenta and produce intrauterine infections in the fetus. The worms take ~1 month to reach maturity, and it is then that clinical signs are most common because of the development of parasitic bronchitis. Adult worms persist for ~3 months.

The life cycle of *Dictyocaulus viviparus* in cattle is a little shorter than that of *D. filaria* but is otherwise comparable. Adult worms can continue to lay eggs for 6 months, but most are expelled within 3 months. *Dictyocaulus arnfieldi* is mostly a patent infection in donkeys, but the worms can develop to maturity if horses or ponies are infected as young foals.

The lesions produced by *Dictyocaulus* depend on the susceptibility of the host and on the number of invading larvae. Cattle and sheep are most susceptible to infection when they are first exposed to contaminated pastures, and therefore severe lesions and the clinical disease they cause are most commonly seen in animals less than a year of age where infection is endemic. Minor reaction occurs along the pathway of larval migration, but the important lesions are found in the lungs. The lesions in the pulmonary tissues can be considered in two main phases, the first when the larvae reach the lung and break out into the alveoli, and the second when the mature parasites are located in the bronchi. In natural infections, these two phases overlap and are associated with hyperplastic lymphadenitis in the related nodes. The larvae arrive in the lungs from about 5 to 7 days after ingestion. Where they emerge from pulmonary capillaries, they cause microscopic foci of necrosis or rupture of alveolar walls with an infiltrate of eosinophils, neutrophils, macrophages, and a few giant cells. With more severe larval invasion, these foci become more numerous and larger. Mononuclear cells thicken the alveolar walls, and there is focal exudation of fibrin into alveoli together with the inflammatory cells. Eosinophils are a prominent feature of the reaction. Various degrees of hyperplasia of alveolar type II epithelial cells also occur. The larvae, some of them dead, can be found in the alveoli. When the number of larvae is large, the foci of acute interstitial pneumonia may be visible grossly as small, lobular or sublobular areas, slightly depressed, purplish, and distributed widely throughout the lungs.

By about the tenth day, many of the larvae have gained the terminal bronchioles. Frothy fluid is present in the bronchi, and in very heavy infestations there is often edema and emphysema of the interlobular septa. Eosinophils invade the septal tissues in large numbers and follow the larvae into the bronchioles. Most of the bronchioles contain plugs of exudate composed largely of eosinophils. Neutrophils, lymphocytes, and macrophages are present in smaller numbers in both the lumina and walls of the bronchioles. The early bronchiolar epithelial response is of degeneration and sloughing, but subsequently hyperplasia and metaplasia also occur. As the worms reach maturity, beginning ~4 weeks after infection, emphasis shifts to the bronchial lesion, and some resolution of the initial alveolar lesion occurs. The mature, threadlike worms in the bronchi and perhaps caudal trachea are easy to see in moderate to severe infections. Although the early development of lungworms takes place in all lobules, the mature worms are most numerous in the dorsocaudal bronchi of the caudal lobes, and in light infections may be found only in these regions. The worms are usually bathed in mucinous, foamy bronchial exudate. In some cases there may be no superficial indications of the worms, except for failure of the lungs to collapse. It is usual for gross lesions to be present in patent infections, however. Typically, there are large, wedge-shaped areas of dark red or grayish consolidated lung at the posterior border of the caudal lobes (Fig. 6.40A). These consolidated areas have firm consistency and are slightly depressed below the surface of surrounding inflated or sometimes hyperinflated lung. The patchy consolidations may also occur in other dorsocaudal regions, and with severe involvement they can be found on cut section to occupy much of the pulmonary tissue surrounding larger bronchi. There is no pleuritis.

The adult worms cause chronic catarrhal bronchitis and bronchiolitis, with a large component of eosinophils. The epithelium of bronchi is thickened and hyperplastic. Increase in the proportion of mucus-producing cells is a prominent feature. Elsewhere there might be ulceration or, occasionally, squamous metaplasia. The epithelium and lamina propria are infiltrated by mixed leukocytes, with a preponderance of eosinophils, and there is hyperplastic bronchus-associated lymphoid tissue. The lumina contain adult worms, plugs of mucus, numerous leukocytes, eggs, and larvae. Components of the verminous bronchiolitis are similar, but there is also a tendency for obliterative bronchiolitis to occur. The hyperplasia of bronchiolar smooth muscle, the increase in peribronchiolar fibrous tissue, and proliferation of lymphoid cells in bronchiolar walls also assume relatively greater prominence (Fig. 6.41A).

The parenchymal lesions that accompany the bronchitis caused by the adult worms are compounded mostly of atelectasis secondary to the bronchiolitis, and of pneumonia, which is provoked by aspirated eggs and newly hatched larvae. It is complicated in some cases by bacteria. Granulomas are frequently present around fragments of discarded cuticle, eggs, or dead larvae. The alveoli, which are partially collapsed, contain many giant cells and vacuolated macrophages. Their walls are thickened by cellular infiltration and slight fibroplasia and may be more or less completely covered by low cuboidal epithelium. Toward the end of the patent period the alveolar reaction subsides and resolution begins, especially in the periphery of the lobules. Around the bronchioles, however, many of the alveoli are permanently obliterated by the organizing peribronchiolar reaction. The lymphoid nodules that develop in the walls of bronchi and bronchioles are not generally as conspicuous as those occurring in chronic mycoplasmal infection. In resolving lesions, however, when worms are no longer present, there is no clear morphologic distinction. A useful clue to separate these two major causes of lymphoid proliferation is that the airways mainly affected by mycoplasmas are in cranioventral regions, whereas those affected by lungworms in ruminants are dorsocaudal.

Two features of the lesions caused by *Dictyocaulus viviparus* in cattle deserve special mention. The first is that extremely severe damage is associated with pulmonary edema and interstitial emphysema. In fatal cases, these may be the most obvious gross finding and therefore lead to confusion with the edema and interstitial emphysema accompanying acute interstitial pneumonia of toxic origin. This is particularly likely where the pulmonary damage is caused by massive invasion of larvae, and mature worms are not yet present for gross detection. Microscopic detection of larvae and immature worms usually provides the diagnosis. The second feature is the presence in the lungs of older animals of scattered lymphocytic nodules 2–4 mm in diameter. The nodules are homogeneously gray, or gray with a greenish center. The gray tissue represents dense accumulations of lymphocytes, and the greenish center the degenerating larval or adult worm surrounded by eosinophils. The nodules are an indication of reinfection of an immune animal, vaccination with X-irradiated larvae, or anthelmintic treatment.

Dictyocaulus arnfieldi is mainly a lungworm of donkeys and survives for long periods without causing undue clinical signs. The gross lesions are scattered, discrete foci of hyperinflated pulmonary parenchyma, mostly in caudal lobes. In the center of the lesions are small bronchi packed with coiled adult worms. Histologically, the worms are associated with a chronic catarrhal bronchitis. Goblet-cell hyperplasia and extensive lymphoid-cell infiltration of the walls are the main features. Adult worms cause

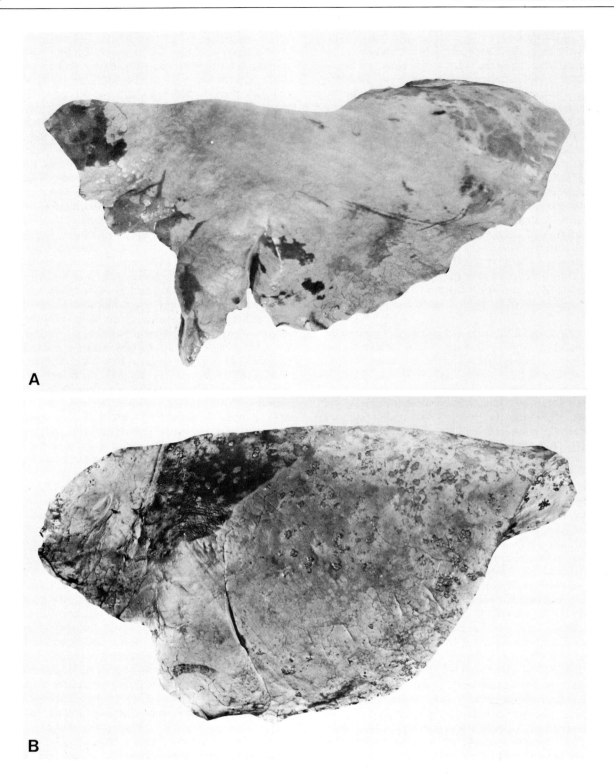

Fig. 6.40.   Verminous pneumonia.   (**A**) Bronchopneumonia caused by *Dictyocaulus filaria* in dorsocaudal region of caudal lobe. Unrelated areas of atelectasis and enzootic pneumonia in cranioventral regions. Sheep.   (**B**) Multifocal subpleural nodules of interstitial pneumonia produced by *Muellerius capillaris*. Sheep.

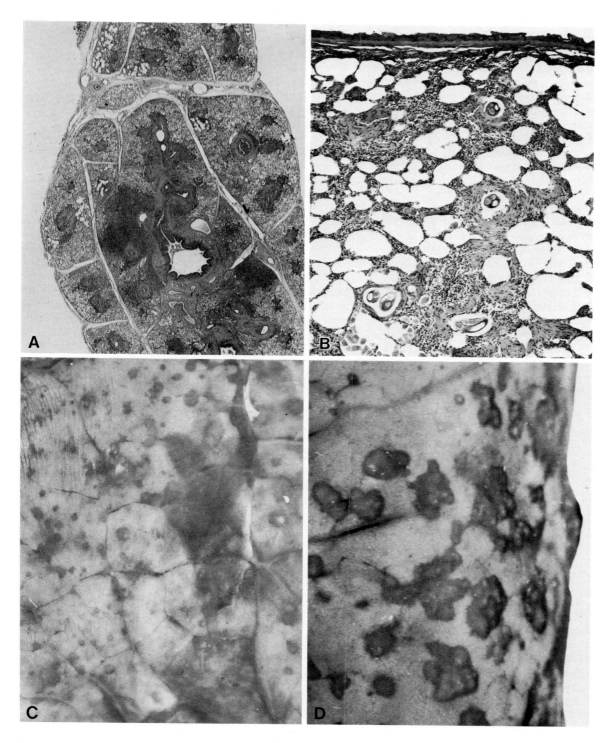

Fig. 6.41. Verminous pneumonia. (**A**) Residual lesions caused by *Dictyocaulus filaria*. Sheep. Note the obliterative bronchiolitis and prominent hyperplasia of bronchiolar smooth muscle with lymphofollicular cuffing. (**B**) Moderate reactions to *Muellerius capillaris*. Sheep. Adults lie in bronchioles and alveolar ducts and are associated with muscular hyperplasia. Eggs and first-stage larvae have provoked a chronic interstitial pneumonia. (**C**) Multiple subpleural nodules produced by *Metastrongylus* sp. Pig. (**D**) Subpleural nodules produced by *M. capillaris*. Sheep.

relatively little luminal response, whereas first-stage larvae stimulate an intense mucopurulent reaction. There is also a chronic catarrhal and eosinophilic bronchiolitis of bronchioles distal to affected bronchi. Alveoli are reported to be hyperinflated, but it is uncertain to what extent this reflects true *in vivo* hyperinflation as opposed to air trapping and failure to collapse when the lungs are examined after death. Infection of adult horses with *D. arnfieldi* usually results in failure of the worm to develop to sexual maturity. The lesions are similar to those described for the donkey and are occasionally associated with chronic coughing and abnormal sounds on auscultation.

Protostrongylus

The most common and important member of *Protostrongylus* is *P. rufescens*. Whereas *Dictyocaulus* species have direct life cycles, *P. rufescens* and the other worms to be discussed below have indirect life cycles.

Protostrongylus rufescens is parasitic in sheep, goats, and deer. The adults are smaller than *Dictyocaulus filaria*, being 16–35 mm in length. They are reddish and mainly inhabit the bronchioles. The lesions that accompany the infection are similar to those produced by *D. filaria* but are quantitatively less, lobular in size, and located chiefly in the periphery of the caudal lobes. The lesions are not readily distinguished grossly from those produced by *Muellerius capillaris*. The first-stage larvae are passed in the feces and enter the intermediate hosts, which are various genera of land snails, by boring through the foot. Two molts occur in the snail, and the infective third-stage larvae develop in 2 weeks. Sheep and goats obtain the parasites by eating the snails.

Neostrongylus linearis is a species comparable to *Protostrongylus rufescens*. It is common in western Europe and probably elsewhere but is confused with other small lungworms of sheep.

Muellerius and Cystocaulus

Cystocaulus ocreatus (*C. nigrescens*) is little studied, but it is stated to resemble *Muellerius* in the details of life cycle and pathogenicity.

Muellerius capillaris, which is parasitic in sheep and goats, is the most common and ubiquitous of the lungworms. The species is sometimes referred to as the nodular lungworm because the adults live in the alveolar parenchyma and almost always provoke an enveloping, granulomatous response. The adult worms are found on rare occasions in the bronchioles. There is usually no clinical evidence of respiratory disease in sheep, even when the number of nodules is large. Sometimes they become confluent. Diminished weight gains have been recorded in heavily infested lambs, and it has been postulated that the worms might predispose to pulmonary bacterial and viral infections.

The eggs are laid and hatch in the nodules. This requires that the sexes be paired in the nodules. Often this does not occur, and therefore the examination of feces for larvae may give no indication of the degree of pulmonary parasitism. The first-stage larvae break out of tissues into the airways and are eventually passed with feces or mucus. The intermediate hosts are various slugs and snails. The infective stage is reached after two molts in the intermediate host, and the life cycle is completed when sheep

and goats swallow the intermediate hosts. The larvae migrate to the lungs, presumably via the lymphatic pathway, and break out into the alveoli. As a consequence of this type of life cycle, infections are acquired gradually, and large worm burdens are seldom observed in animals less than 6 months of age. On the other hand, heavy infections are not common in old sheep and goats.

The nodules produced by these parasites represent lesions of multifocal interstitial pneumonia. They may occur anywhere in the lung, but most of them are located beneath the pleura of the dorsal region of the caudal lobes (Figs. 6.40B and 6.41D), so the severity of infestation can be assessed quite accurately by superficial inspection. Why there should be this predilection for the subpleural tissues is not known. The nodules range in size from 1 mm to several centimeters. They are soft and hemorrhagic early in an infection. Later they are greenish gray and project above the pleural surface of adjacent lung at necropsy. Some of them become calcified. Similar nodules are present in various numbers in the bronchial and mesenteric lymph nodes. Sheep are rather tolerant of initial exposure and readily develop patent infections. With repeated exposure, sheep become resistant and inhibit fourth-stage larval migration or development. Immature adults may have their development checked, or mature worms may cease reproduction in a resistant animal. The cellular reaction reflects the stage of the parasite present and resistance of the host. The earliest form of nodule is produced by the fourth-stage larvae when they enter the lungs, and usually consists of little more than groups of alveoli that are mechanically disrupted. There may be little cellular reaction to these larvae of the first infestation, but an eosinophilic infiltration may accompany later ones. The adult worms also disrupt the alveolar septa. The eggs and first-stage larvae lie in the alveolar spaces and provoke little inflammatory response, although there is a mild fibrous thickening of the alveolar septa with infiltrated lymphocytes in the septa and around the blood vessels and bronchioles. In older animals, presumably as a result of a developing resistance, the cellular reaction is more marked, especially to the first-stage larvae and the adults (Fig. 6.41B). There are intense foci of infiltrated eosinophils around the larvae; the alveolar spaces become crowded with macrophages and some giant cells, and the distorted alveolar walls are thickened by fibrous tissue. The larvae that escape into small bronchioles are enclosed in plugs of mucus and cellular debris. The epithelium of the bronchioles is hyperplastic, and the muscularis much thickened. When the larvae leave the nodules, the cellular reaction subsides, but the thickening of the alveolar septa persists because of patchy or diffuse fibromuscular hyperplasia. An intense reaction also occurs to the adult worms. There are large numbers of eosinophils, a narrow zone of epithelioid and giant cells, and a periphery of fibroblastic tissue. The cellular debris becomes calcified, particularly when the worms die, and these calcified nodules persist indefinitely as spherical masses of calcium salts surrounded by a fibrous capsule. Not all the calcification, however, occurs about adult worms. Some is precipitated in the inspissated mucus that collects in obstructed bronchial glands, and some in mucus and debris that accumulate in the bronchioles.

An extensive diffuse interstitial pneumonia has been reported to be associated with *Muellerius* infection in goats, but in such cases it is often impossible to assess the possible role of concurrent infection with *Mycoplasma* or the caprine arthritis–encephalomyelitis virus.

Metastrongylus

There are three important species of *Metastrongylus*, *M. elongatus* (*M. apri*), *M. pudendotectus*, and *M. salmi*, and they are all parasitic in the bronchi and bronchioles of pigs. They are believed to be responsible for the occasional transmission of the virus of swine influenza. The adult worms are white, threadlike, and 14–60 mm in length, depending on species and sex. In heavy infections, which are mostly in young pigs, they may be found in all lobes of the lung. But when there are fewer worms, particularly as occurs in older animals, the worms may be restricted to airways along the ventrocaudal borders of the caudal lobes. These apparently are areas of predilection or residual infestation. The eggs are laid in the bronchi, and a few of them hatch there, but most hatch after passing to the exterior in the feces. The first-stage larvae are inactive and are capable of prolonged survival in moist conditions. Their further development depends on ingestion by earthworms, which are the intermediate hosts. The larvae develop to the third, infective stage in ~10 days and then remain quiescent unless the earthworm is eaten by a pig. The larvae may survive for as long as 18 months in the earthworms, and by that time, some thousands of them may be accumulated by a single worm without doing it any harm. Migration within the pig is through the lymphatics from the intestine to the lungs. Some larvae pass through the liver and produce a focal hepatitis for which the larvae of *Ascaris suum* are, however, more usually responsible.

Even with heavy adult infestations, gross lesions are inconspicuous and seldom as extensive as those produced in ruminants by *Dictyocaulus*. In light infections the worms live in the smallest airways, and on superficial examination of the lungs the presence of the parasites frequently is indicated only by grayish nodules 1–3 mm in diameter, and by hyperinflated lobules along the ventrocaudal margins of the caudal lobes (Fig. 6.41C).

Histologically, the lesions are basically the same as those produced by *Dictyocaulus*. The initial lesions are multiple foci of intense accumulations of eosinophils surrounding larvae in alveoli. Subsequently, when reproduction is active, a granulomatous alveolar response occurs to the eggs and larvae. The prepatent period for *Metastrongylus* is ~25 days, after which the rate of egg production rapidly reaches a peak and then subsides to a low level. At this later stage, the adults persist mainly in the bronchioles and small bronchi and provoke a chronic catarrhal and eosinophilic bronchiolitis and bronchitis with the features as described for *Dictyocaulus* infection in ruminants. Large, lymphofollicular nodules are mainly responsible for the grayish nodules visible grossly (Fig. 6.41C).

CRENOSOMA VULPIS. *Crenosoma vulpis* is a common lungworm of foxes, but it also occurs in other Canidae. It is occasionally found in dogs that have access to the snails and slugs that are intermediate hosts. The adult worms live in bronchioles and small bronchi. The gross lesions usually observed in dogs are grayish consolidations in dorsal regions of the caudal lobes. Histologically, the lesions caused by adult worms are catarrhal,

eosinophilic bronchitis and bronchiolitis closely resembling those caused by *Dictyocaulus* in ruminants.

FILAROIDES ROSTRATUS. *Filaroides (Anafilaroides) rostratus* is a parasite of cats that appears to have very limited distribution since it has been recorded mainly from Sri Lanka. In that its final habitat is the walls of large airways it resembles *F. osleri* of dogs (see Parasitic Diseases of the Larynx and Trachea). It does not form nodules, however, but causes sinuous thickenings of the bronchial walls. When the infective larvae invade the bronchial walls, they provoke only slight cellular response. The adults develop in cystic spaces that are probably dilated lymphatics and that cause displacement of the surrounding tissues. The worms are viviparous, and the larvae escape to the bronchiolar lumen where they provoke a catarrhal bronchitis. The adults remain alive for ~1 year, and possibly for much longer. When they die, they provoke an intense infiltration of neutrophils and may calcify. There is residual fibrosis in the bronchial wall. The larvae are passed in the feces and develop to the infective stage in a variety of molluscs. They can probably survive for a long time in the intermediate hosts, and the capacity for survival and dissemination is increased by the fortuitous use of transport hosts, such as mice and chickens.

There are other species of lungworms in cats, which are probably similar to *Filaroides rostratus*, but virtually the only details concerning them are taxonomic. *Vogeloides massinoi (Osleroides massinoi)* lives in the bronchial wall. *Vogeloides ramanujacharii* occurs in cats in India. *Troglostrongylus brevior* occurs in cats in the Middle East and is known to use snails as intermediate hosts.

FILAROIDES HIRTHI. Two similar filarid worms have been recorded as inhabiting the pulmonary parenchyma of dogs, *Filaroides hirthi* and *F. milksi*. Original reports were of *F. milksi*, but more recent descriptions have been of a worm that, although it closely resembles *F. milksi*, has been assigned to a separate species, *F. hirthi*. This description summarizes the current knowledge concerning *F. hirthi*, leaving the taxonomic and pathogenic uncertainties surrounding *F. milksi* for resolution in the future.

Adult *Filaroides hirthi* worms, which are 6–10 mm in length, live in alveoli and respiratory bronchioles. Clinical signs of infection are rare, and evidence of the worms' presence is usually limited to the incidental finding at necropsy of tan, green, or gray subpleural nodules 1–5 mm in diameter. The nodules are widely scattered over subpleural regions, the numbers varying with the severity of infection. Histologically, there is little response to living adult worms (Fig. 6.42A), but a severe granulomatous response featuring many eosinophils occurs around dead or degenerating worms (Fig. 6.42B). Larvae provoke a more acute neutrophilic reaction. Foci of granulomatous interstitial pneumonia can often be found in which worm remnants may no longer be identified. Killing the worms with anthelmintic is particularly prone to cause the severe response.

Filaroides hirthi has a direct life cycle, like *F. osleri*. Infective first-stage larvae are passed in the feces, and usually the infection is passed from dam to pups. Infection is reported to occur mostly in colonies of beagles reared for experimental stud-

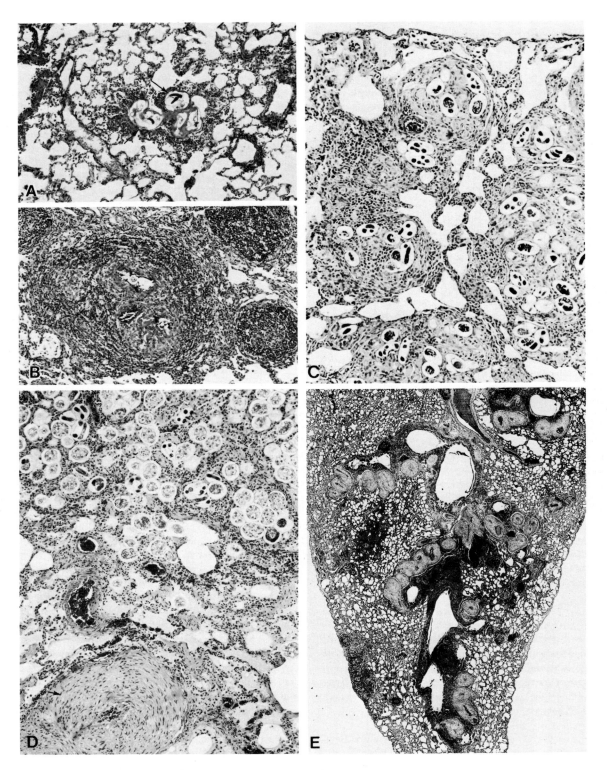

Fig. 6.42. Verminous pneumonia. (**A**) Eosinophilic and lymphocytic interstitial reaction to adult *Filaroides hirthi* (arrow). Dog. (**B**) Severe granulomatous response surrounding dead *F. hirthi*. Dog. (**C**) Chronic interstitial pneumonia with prominent fibrosis surrounding eggs and larvae of *Angiostrongylus vasorum*. Dog. (**D**) Granulomatous interstitial pneumonia provoked by eggs and larvae of *Aelurostrongylus abstrusus*. Cat. Note hyperplasia of smooth muscle of pulmonary artery (arrow). (**E**) Residual lesions of *Aelurostrongylus abstrusus*. Tortuous hypertrophied arteries have infiltration of walls by eosinophils. Cat.

ies in which lungs are routinely given thorough examinations. The incidence of *F. hirthi* in the canine population at large is not known. There are a few single-case reports of dogs with lethal infection, however, so it is probably more widespread than realized. The fatalities have been caused by severe miliary granulomatous pneumonia with a superimposed acute exudative component associated with huge numbers of worms and larvae. This type of hyperinfection and probable autoinfection seems to occur in dogs with drug or disease-induced immunosuppression.

AELUROSTRONGYLUS ABSTRUSUS. *Aelurostrongylus abstrusus* is a widespread lungworm of the cat. The adults live in the respiratory bronchioles and alveolar ducts. The eggs form nodular deposits in alveoli and hatch to give first-stage larvae that reach the airways and are eventually passed in the feces. The indirect life cycle involves various snails and slugs as intermediate hosts, and birds, rodents, frogs, and lizards as transport hosts. The life cycle can be completed if a cat eats either an intermediate host or a transport host.

The extent to which infective larvae reach the lungs in the blood or by migration through peritoneal and pleural cavities is not certain. Worms reach maturity about 5–6 weeks after ingestion of the third-stage larvae. The pulmonary lesions are quite characteristic, usually being in the form of nodules 1–10 mm in diameter that represent nests of eggs and larvae (Fig. 6.42D). These nodules, which are yellowish and firm, are scattered throughout the parenchyma but are more common in the peripheral parts of the lungs and usually project from the surface of the deflated lung. A small amount of creamy exudate containing numerous eggs and larvae can be expressed from the cut surface of incised nodules. Severe, confluent consolidation caused by heavy infections of *Aelurostrongylus abstrusus* can produce clinical signs of chronic coughing, and perhaps progressive loss of weight. Occasionally, death occurs when there is secondary infection.

Microscopically, the eggs and larvae are visible in the alveolar spaces, with some disruption of alveolar septa. They are surrounded by dense collections of mixed mononuclear cells with some giant cells. The latter are more numerous around dead or disintegrating larvae. Eosinophils and neutrophils are mostly a feature of early infection. Lymphocytic nodules form around vessels and airways (Fig. 6.42E). Necrosis and calcification seldom occur. In older lesions from which eggs and larvae have disappeared, the alveoli remain epithelialized for a time and the septa are persistently thickened by fibrous tissue and smooth muscle. This fibromuscular hyperplasia is often focal and barely appreciable, but in some cases is diffuse and rigid enough to produce a rubbery consistency.

Hypertrophy and hyperplasia of the smooth muscle in the walls of the bronchioles and alveolar ducts occur early in the course of the infestation and are progressive, but are not so well developed as the increase in smooth muscle in the media of small pulmonary arteries and arterioles. The presence of one or more of adult worms, eggs, or larvae in the bronchioles is associated with a chronic catarrhal and eosinophilic bronchiolitis similar to that caused by *Dictyocaulus* in ruminants. A prominent component is the hyperplasia of submucosal glands, which is a usual but generally inconspicuous feature of small airways of cats.

The most active phase of the parasite is 6–12 weeks after infection, and this is associated with the peak pulmonary response. Adult worms can persist up to 9 months. Although the granulomatous alveolitis and catarrhal bronchiolitis gradually regress, the hypertrophy and hyperplasia of smooth muscle in arteries, bronchioles, and alveolar ducts persist. The association between *Aelurostrongylus* infection and the dramatic muscular thickening of the walls of pulmonary arteries has been the subject of controversy. The current evidence indicates that hyperplasia and hypertrophy of smooth muscle in pulmonary arteries are a common finding in cats of all ages for reasons that are obscure. Infection with *Aelurostrongylus abstrusus* appears to be the major recognized cause of enhancement of this inherent tendency.

ANGIOSTRONGYLUS VASORUM. *Angiostrongylus vasorum* is a parasite of the pulmonary arteries and the right ventricle of dogs and foxes. The adult worms are 15–25 mm in length. They cause a proliferative endarteritis, but the more severe damage is caused by eggs that lodge in arterioles and capillaries. They and the larvae that hatch from them provoke a chronic inflammation in which fibroplasia predominates (Fig. 6.42C). The larvae break into the alveoli, migrate in the respiratory passages, and are eliminated in the feces. Various snails and slugs serve as intermediate hosts.

In the acute form of the disease, with heavy infestations of larvae in alveoli, the fatal outcome is in large part attributable to pulmonary edema and pneumonia. The chronic expression of the disease is largely one of congestive cardiac failure secondary to obliterative and thrombotic vasculitis, organizing infarcts, and progressive granulomatous response to eggs and larvae. Inflammation and scarring of alveolar walls leads to distortion and enlargement of remaining airspaces, which can result in a "foam rubber" appearance. This is sometimes referred to as emphysema but is more a form of "honeycombing" than emphysema in the conventional sense.

Because of their similar location, there is overlap in the types of abnormalities caused by *Angiostrongylus vasorum* and *Dirofilaria immitis* (see the Cardiovascular System, Volume 3).

PARAGONIMUS. Of the trematodes, the only genus that has its final habitat in the lungs is *Paragonimus*. A number of species have been described for the genus. The important ones are *P. westermanii* (the oriental lung fluke) in the Far East, and *P. kellicotti* in America. For the latter species, mink and other fish-eating carnivores are regarded as the usual hosts. The fluke is not selective in its final hosts, however, and has also been found in humans, swine, and ruminants. Among domestic animals, it is most commonly found in cats. Its natural habitat is the lung, but aberrant localizations have included the nervous system.

The life cycle of the parasite is typical of the cycles of the trematodes. The first intermediate hosts are small aquatic snails. The second intermediate host is a freshwater crab or crayfish. When the crayfish is eaten by the final host, the metacercariae are liberated in the intestine and migrate across the peritoneal and pleural cavities to the lungs. Their passage through the pleura is marked by multiple small hemorrhages and foci of eosinophilic and fibrinous pleuritis, which heal as small umbilicate scars (Fig. 6.43A). The adult flukes are ovoid, reddish brown, and up to 7 mm in length. They are found, usually in pairs, in inflammatory cysts in the pulmonary parenchyma (Fig. 6.43B) and, occasionally, the bronchi. The cysts are more common in the caudal lobes, particularly the right side. They are spherical, approximately 10–15 mm in diameter, and dark red-brown. Their size and the fact that surrounding lung is frequently atelectatic give them a distinctive appearance. The cysts frequently communicate with bronchioles. Rupture of cysts on the pleural surface and resulting pneumothorax is a rare complication. The cysts become progressively surrounded by fibrous tissue and partially lined by bronchiolar epithelium. Eosinophilic granulomatous pneumonia develops around degenerating eggs adjacent to the cysts containing flukes (Fig. 6.43C). There is also a chronic catarrhal eosinophilic bronchiolitis with smooth muscle hyperplasia. Clusters of eggs, which occasionally are visible grossly as yellowish brown streaks, occur in subpleural and mediastinal lymphatics and cause a granulomatous pleuritis and lymphangitis. The large operculate eggs are quite distinctive (Fig. 6.43C); in old lesions only fractured shells may remain.

PNEUMOCYSTIS CARINII. *Pneumocystis carinii* is an organism of uncertain taxonomic status that is widespread as a latent infection in the lungs of animals. It has been considered in the past to be either a fungus in the class Ascomycetes or a protozoan. Currently it is generally held to be a form of protozoan, possibly within the class Sporozoa.

Pneumocystis carinii is an important cause of pneumonia in various forms of congenital or acquired immunodeficiency states in humans. Latent infection in rats can be regularly converted to the active disease by administration of corticosteroids. *Pneumocystis* pneumonia has been recorded occasionally in young dogs, foals, goats, and pigs as well as in laboratory animals. In horses, it appears mainly in Arabian foals with known or suspect congenital immunodeficiency, sometimes as a complication of adenovirus or other infectious pneumonia. Most of the reported canine cases have been in miniature dachshunds ranging from about 8 to 24 months in age. Clinical signs are gradually increasing exercise intolerance, respiratory difficulties, and progressive loss of weight. The unusual frequency of involvement of miniature dachshunds raises the possibility of a heritable immunodeficiency in this breed.

Gross lesions associated with pneumocystis pneumonia are diffuse or patchy, red to yellow-brown regions of rubbery firmness or consolidation. The appearance may be modified by coexisting viral or bacterial pneumonia. Histologically, *Pneumocystis carinii* causes a diffuse interstitial pneumonia in which the characteristic feature is prominent filling of alveoli by a foamy, pale, acidophilic material (Fig. 6.26C). The amount of interstitial inflammation varies from minimal to moderate accumulation of lymphocytes, plasma cells, and macrophages. There are various degrees of hyperplasia of alveolar type II epithelial cells (epithelialization), and accumulation of macrophages within alveolar lumina. Fibrosis accompanies intense cellular inflammation within alveolar septa.

Pneumocystis carinii stains poorly with hematoxylin and eosin and is therefore easily overlooked. Its presence should be suspected when alveoli contain abundant, foamy, pale,

eosinophilic material. This is particularly important in young animals where there might be congenital, drug-induced, or disease-induced immunodeficiency. The foamy acidophilic material consists mainly of trophozoite and cyst forms of the organism. These might be seen as indistinct outlines of erythrocyte-sized structures, possibly with the presence of pale, basophilic dots. The organism is best demonstrated histologically by methenamine–silver staining. This reveals the argyrophilic capsules of the cysts as round, distorted, or crescentic structures from 3 to 8 μm in width (Fig. 6.26D). The PAS stain is not as satisfactory for demonstration of the organism.

Current evidence indicates that *Pneumocystis carinii* is mainly kept in check by alveolar macrophages in normal animals, but that this process fails in immunodeficient states. Progressive colonization of alveolar type I epithelial cells by *P. carinii* causes their necrosis and replacement by type II cells, with eventual filling of alveoli by the organisms and acellular material rich in alveolar surfactant lipid.

Various protozoa are capable of causing interstitial pneumonia, most notably *Toxoplasma gondii* (see the Alimentary System, this volume). *Sarcocystis* species also produce a multifocal interstitial pneumonia as part of the widespread multiplication of tachyzoites in vascular endothelium during acute sarcocystosis in herbivores (see Muscles and Tendons, Volume 1).

Enzootic Pneumonia

Enzootic pneumonia refers to pneumonia prevalent in groups of young animals maintained in close contact. It is mainly of importance in calves, lambs, and young pigs. Since it is an epidemiologic term, it allows considerable latitude in the morphologic and etiologic types of pneumonia it embraces. Both acute exudative bronchopneumonias and more chronic bronchointerstitial pneumonias have been included under the general designation enzootic pneumonia, but the emphasis has differed according to the species of animal concerned, as will be evident from the following discussion.

Enzootic pneumonia of **calves** is a disease complex in intensively managed calves, caused by the synergistic action of two or more of a wide variety of viruses, mycoplasmas, and bacteria. The morphologic appearance of the pneumonia varies according to the mix of agents and the age of lesions encountered. The disease mainly affects calves less than 6 months of age and is of most importance as a cause of unthriftiness. Mortality is low unless there is a coincidence of highly pathogenic agents and predisposing factors associated with poor husbandry and, possibly, intercurrent disease.

Evidence to date indicates that the acute pneumonia is usually initiated by viral infection. More than one species of virus may be involved in an outbreak or even in a single calf. The relative importance of the 10 or so candidate viruses varies geographically to some extent. In general, respiratory syncytial and parainfluenza-3 viruses are considered to be most important. Infectious bovine rhinotracheitis virus, adenovirus, and the bovine virus diarrhea virus are the next most commonly mentioned. The lesions caused by those and the other viral respiratory pathogens were described earlier in this chapter. Although calves can die because of acute, uncomplicated viral lesions, most fatal cases have a superimposed acute bacterial bronchopneumonia or lobar pneumonia. These have the acute fibrinonecrotic to suppurative

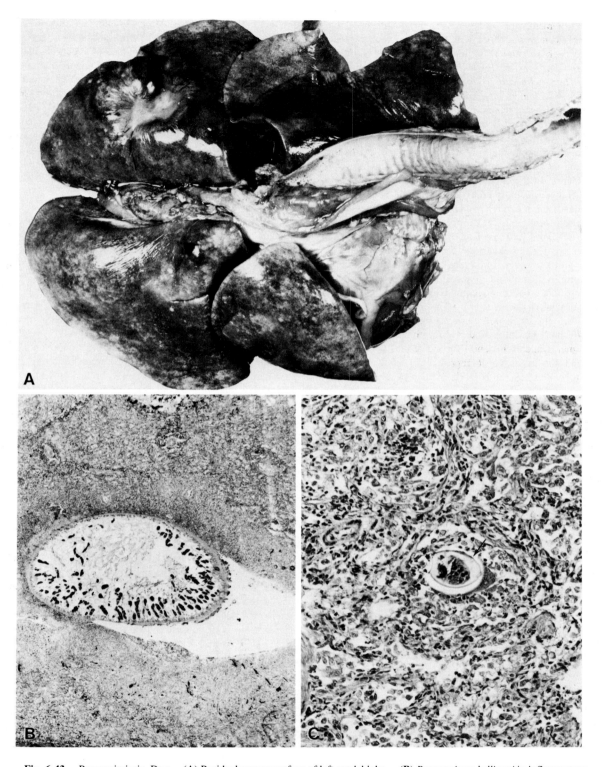

Fig. 6.43. Paragonimiasis. Dog. (**A**) Residual scar on surface of left caudal lobe. (**B**) *Paragonimus kellicotti* in inflammatory cyst in pulmonary parenchyma. (**C**) Granulomatous pneumonia surrounding distinctive operculate egg (arrow).

exudation characteristic of severe bacterial infection, particularly by *Pasteurella*. More than 20 different species of bacteria have been isolated at various times however, often in mixed infection. Next to *Pasteurella*, the most common are *Streptobacillus actinoides*, *Corynebacterium pyogenes*, and *Escherichia coli*. Chlamydiae may also be involved occasionally. Since most fatal pneumonias are predominantly the result of bacterial activity, clearly establishing the initial role of viral infection can be difficult and requires attempts to isolate viruses by culture, demonstrate their presence by immunofluorescence and electron microscopy, and obtain serologic evidence of an active infection in the affected groups. Histologic search for inclusion bodies is usually unrewarding in fatal field cases but pays dividends often enough to make the attempt necessary.

Mycoplasmas, especially *Mycoplasma dispar*, *Ureaplasma* spp., and *M. bovis*, are implicated in helping cause the acute form of enzootic pneumonias together with viruses and bacteria. They are probably more important, however, in causing the chronic form of enzootic pneumonia. This is the grayish pink, meaty consolidation of cranioventral regions of the lung found in slaughtered veal calves or calves dying because of other diseases. Histologically, it is a chronic bronchointerstitial pneumonia with both exudative and proliferative components (see Mycoplasmal Bronchiolitis and Pneumonia of Calves).

This type of lesion appears to represent persistent infection by both the mycoplasmas and bacteria of species similar to those found in more acute lesions. The usual course of chronic enzootic pneumonia is that of a low-grade inflammatory lesion that resolves in several months to a year. The term "cuffing pneumonia" has been used for chronic enzootic pneumonia in which a dramatic feature is sheathing of small airways by lymphofollicular proliferations. Acute exudative bacterial pneumonia can supervene at any time and cause severe clinical disease or death if the calf's pulmonary defenses are impaired or there is additional infection by virulent pathogens. An alternative sequel is chronic abscessation and scarring.

Enzootic pneumonia of **lambs** has many similarities to enzootic pneumonia of calves. The acute form is manifest as pneumonic pasteurellosis and has been described under Pasteurellosis. The chronic, enzootic bronchointerstitial pneumonia (Fig. 6.44) has features essentially the same as in enzootic mycoplasmal pneumonia of swine mentioned previously. Because the term enzootic pneumonia was used initially only for acute pneumonic pasteurellosis in sheep, various descriptive terms have been used for the chronic form. The most frequent ones are proliferative interstitial, proliferative exudative, atypical, and chronic nonprogressive. To avoid confusion, however, the chronic bronchointerstitial pneumonia of lambs should also be referred to as an enzootic pneumonia, just as it is in calves and pigs.

The causes of chronic enzootic pneumonia in lambs are not completely established. The disease can be regularly produced by intratracheal inoculation of a suspension of pneumonic lung. Attempts to produce the disease using various combinations of cultured microorganisms isolated from pneumonic lung have indicated that intratracheal or endobronchial inoculation of mixed strains of *Mycoplasma ovipneumoniae* and *Pasteurella haemolytica* is the most successful.

It therefore seems that most cases of chronic enzootic pneu-

monia in lambs involve the synergistic action of *Mycoplasma ovipneumoniae* and *Pasteurella haemolytica*. Either of these agents alone or in combination with other infectious agents may occasionally be responsible. The active pneumonic consolidation persists for about 3 to 12 weeks after infection and largely resolves within a few months unless acute bacterial exacerbations occur. Since the disease is not usually fatal, the characteristic cranioventral consolidations (Fig. 6.44A) are mostly seen in slaughtered lambs or those dying of other diseases.

Enzootic pneumonia of **swine** is generally held to be synonymous with enzootic mycoplasmal pneumonia (see Respiratory Mycoplasmosis of Swine).

Interstitial Pneumonia of Cattle

The general features and wide range of causes of interstitial pneumonia were discussed under Interstitial Pneumonia. The condition in cattle is deserving of further mention, however, because of its frequency and the confusion concerning its causes.

Acute interstitial pneumonia is the result of acute diffuse damage to alveolar septa. Characteristic features in cattle are pulmonary hyperemia, alveolar edema and hyaline membrane formation, hyperplasia of alveolar type II epithelial cells, and interstitial emphysema and edema. Other components may be present, such as larvae and eosinophils when migrating helminth larvae are the cause, but in general the lesion is nonspecific. Extensive interstitial emphysema and edema are usually only found in cows dying after a bout of severe, labored respiration. When this is prolonged, the interstitial emphysema can dissect through the mediastinum and reach subcutaneous regions of the back. Since the structure of the bovine lung predisposes it to the development of interstitial emphysema when there is severe pulmonary insufficiency and labored respiration for any cause, the diagnosis of acute interstitial pneumonia cannot be made solely on the basis of air in the pulmonary interstitium.

Various terms have been used for acute interstitial pneumonia in cattle, the most general one being "atypical" interstitial pneumonia, in recognition of the acute exudative nature of the process. Other terms have been used in certain geographic regions and have emphasized epidemiologic or morphologic features, the latter usually misleadingly. Examples of common usage are "fog fever" and "acute bovine pulmonary emphysema and edema" for the pasture-associated acute interstitial pneumonia in Britain and the United States, respectively.

The pasture-associated condition usually occurs in adult, beef-type cattle soon after a change from sparse summer range or pasture to relatively lush pastures containing regrowth following removal of a crop for hay or silage. Cows dying of the disease have gross lesions dominated by interstitial emphysema and edema. Major airways contain abundant white foam. The pulmonary parenchyma is purplish to brownish red, depending on the acuteness of the disease, and affected lobules have a homogeneous, moist cut section and a soft, rubbery texture (Fig. 6.18A,C). Irregular lobular or sublobular distribution of the lesions occurs to some extent. There is a tendency for most diffuse involvement to be found in dorsocaudal regions of the lungs. Histologically, the main features are as outlined previously, but hyperplasia of alveolar type II epithelial cells is not a pronounced feature until 4 to 6 days after the onset of the

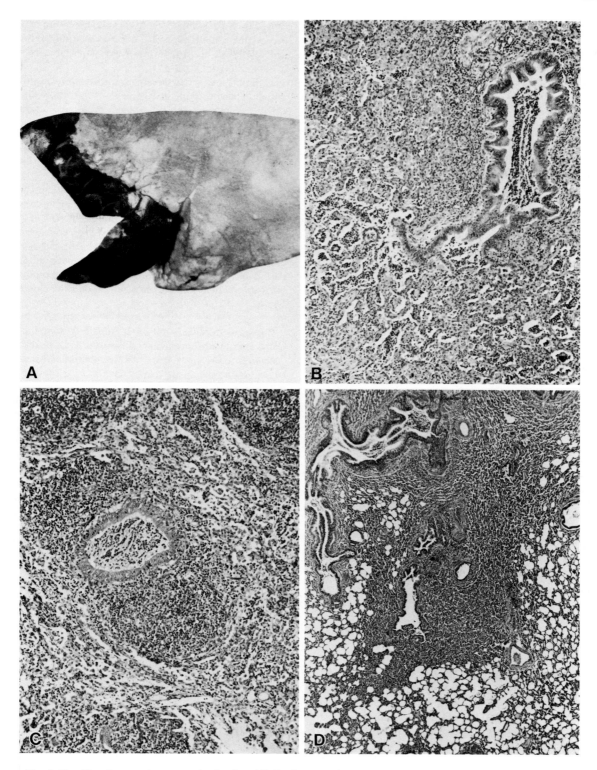

Fig. 6.44. Chronic enzootic pneumonia. Lamb. (**A**) Confluent cranioventral consolidation. (**B**) Histology of (**A**), showing bronchointerstitial pneumonia with mixed exudative and proliferative components. (**C**) Prominent peribronchiolar lymphofollicular nodules in chronic lesion. (**D**) Residual atelectasis in resolving pneumonia.

alveolar damage (Fig. 6.18B,D). Cows that survive the acute episode usually have residual interstitial fibrosis and some persistence of alveolar type II epithelial cells (Fig. 6.19C).

Current evidence indicates that the pasture-associated form of acute interstitial pneumonia is related to increased amounts of L-tryptophan in the ingested feed; the quantity of L-tryptophan can be sufficient to provide toxic levels of 3-methylindole under the special conditions of rumen fermentation occurring at the time of change in pasture. Acute interstitial pneumonia can also be caused by the pneumotoxic activity of 4-ipomeanol and related furanoterpenoids from moldy sweet potatoes, *Perilla* ketone from purple mint (*P. frutescens*), and an unidentified toxin from stinkwood (*Zieria arborescens*). Apart from chemical toxins, a similar lesion can be caused by massive invasion of the lungs by larvae of *Dictyocaulus viviparus* or, less commonly, *Ascaris suum* (see Parasitic Diseases of the Lungs).

Acute interstitial pneumonia also occurs occasionally in housed or feedlot cattle. There is frequently an associated, more chronic, cranioventral bronchopneumonia. The factor or factors involved in the pathogenesis of the acute interstitial pneumonia occurring under these circumstances are not understood, however. The association of severe infection with bovine respiratory syncytial virus and acute interstitial pneumonia, particularly in newly weaned calves in the fall, has given rise to the suggestion that the respiratory syncytial virus alone can cause the interstitial pneumonia under certain circumstances. This is not proven (see Bovine Respiratory Syncytial Virus Infection). An acute interstitial pneumonia also occurs in weanling foals in the early fall. Affected foals are usually those in best condition that eat more of the feed supplementation. The relative roles of dietary-related toxic factors and infection have not been explored.

Chronic interstitial pneumonia in cattle occurs chiefly as a manifestation of **hypersensitivity pneumonitis**. This condition is also referred to as bovine farmer's lung or extrinsic allergic alveolitis and is caused by inhalation of dust from moldy hay that contains spores of *Micropolyspora faeni* and other thermophilic actinomycetes. The disease is primarily one that develops in the winter in housed dairy animals. Death does not usually result from lesions occurring early in the disease. If lungs are available for examination, careful search reveals multiple, small, gray, subpleural foci and many pulmonary lobules with slightly pale, hyperinflated peripheral zones. Characteristic histologic lesions are a lymphocytic and plasmacytic bronchitis and bronchiolitis, often with severe obliterative bronchiolitis, the presence of scattered granulomas composed of epithelioid and giant cells, and thickening of alveolar septa by infiltration of lymphocytes, plasma cells, and macrophages. Eosinophils, globule leukocytes, and increased mast cells are usually present. Cattle are more likely to die as the result of severe, chronic disease. Additional features of severe interstitial fibrosis, accumulation of alveolar macrophages, and hyperplasia of alveolar type II epithelial cells are present in such cases. There can also be metaplasia of type II cells to ciliated or mucus-secreting cells. Vascular compromise can lead to pulmonary hypertension and cor pulmonale in a small proportion of cases. In these advanced cases, epithelioid granulomas are inconspicuous or absent. The lungs grossly are pale and heavy. Most severely affected lobules are yellow-white and fibrous or may show evidence of distortion and enlargement of airspaces by the scarring ("honeycombing"). "Asteroids"

caused by *Aspergillus* spp. may also be present in these lungs because the conditions leading to heavy exposure to dusts containing *M. faeni* are also those in which large numbers of spores of *Aspergillus* are present.

A chronic interstitial pneumonia (diffuse fibrosing alveolitis) similar to that occurring in dairy cattle with advanced hypersensitivity pneumonitis is sometimes seen in pastured beef cattle. Its cause remains undetermined.

Neoplastic Diseases of the Lungs

Primary pulmonary tumors are rare in domestic animals. Metastatic lesions are relatively common, however, because of the vulnerability of the lungs to tumor emboli. In view of the much greater frequency of metastatic tumors, and because their gross and microscopic patterns can sometimes be difficult or impossible to distinguish from those of a primary tumor, an important part of the diagnosis of a primary lung tumor is thorough examination to exclude possible primary sites elsewhere in the body.

Primary Tumors

The rarity of primary pulmonary tumors in domestic animals is in contrast to their frequency in humans. This can probably be accounted for by the lack of carcinogenic stimuli from cigarette smoke or occupationally related chemicals in animals, and by the absence of large numbers of aged individuals. Primary tumors are encountered more often in dogs and cats than in other species. Reported incidence for the dog is about 4 or 5 per 100,000 animals in the population per year. The frequency based on postmortem examination varies with the population sampled, but up to 1% of dogs necropsied have been recorded as having primary tumors of the lung. Comparable statistics for the cat indicate a frequency approximately half that for the dog.

Neoplasms can arise from any of the tissues present in the lung, but with few exceptions the significant ones arise from pulmonary epithelium. Classification of epithelial tumors of the lung is complicated by the recognition that what were once looked on as specific cell types can undergo metaplasia (transdifferentiation) in both inflammatory and neoplastic lesions. The histologic appearance of cells in a tumor is therefore not certain evidence of histogenetic origin. Thus there can be no absolutely rigid histogenetic classification. With this in mind, the following classification provides a useful working basis for categorization:

Primary Epithelial Tumors of the Lung

Bronchial papilloma
Bronchial gland adenoma
Bronchogenic carcinoma
  Squamous-cell (epidermoid) carcinoma
  Adenocarcinoma
  Adenosquamous carcinoma
  Undifferentiated (anaplastic) carcinoma
    Small-cell type
    Large-cell type
Bronchioloalveolar tumor
  Adenoma
  Carcinoma
Carcinoid

Most pulmonary tumors in animals are adenocarcinomas of bronchogenic or bronchioloalveolar origin. Squamous-cell carcinomas are occasionally found, mostly in the dog, and the other varieties are extremely rare. Affected animals are usually middle-aged to old, with the mean age in dogs and cats around 10 to 12 years.

Bronchogenic carcinomas are conventionally subdivided into squamous-cell (epidermoid), adenocarcinoma, and undifferentiated forms. There is a strong tendency, however, for both glandular and squamous components to occur in the same tumor (Fig. 6.45B). Sometimes these are mixed with more anaplastic regions. It is more useful to classify these pleomorphic tumors according to the predominant invasive and destructive component, rather than to put them in the adenosquamous category. Squamous-cell and undifferentiated carcinomas are especially prone to arise from major airways and therefore have a more central (hilar) location in the lung. The bronchogenic carcinoma is typically a large, irregular, pale, fleshy mass with ill-defined border and, possibly, satellite nodules. More distant intrapulmonary metastasis can occur in the same or opposite lung. Consistency ranges from firm to soft and friable. Mucinous, cystic, or hemorrhagic and necrotic regions are sometimes present in the center of large, bulky masses. Occasionally, highly malignant infiltrative tumors cause more diffuse, discolored, rubbery, or solid regions that cannot be distinguished grossly from pneumonia. Squamous-cell carcinomas have a preponderance of large cells with vesicular nuclei and abundant faintly granular acidophilic cytoplasm. Intercellular bridges can often be detected, but keratinization is usually limited to individual cells with intracytoplasmic clumps of keratin. Bronchogenic adenocarcinomas are invasive and destructive. They have disordered acinar, papillary, solid, or mixed patterns (Fig. 6.45A), and intermixed squamous components are frequently present (Fig. 6.45B). Differentiation from metastatic adenocarcinomas is often difficult.

Undifferentiated (anaplastic) carcinomas are the rarest variety in animals. Those recorded have mainly been of the small-cell type. This type can be further subdivided into round (oat cell), fusiform, and polygonal forms, according to the appearance of the component cells. The so-called oat-cell carcinoma has ill-defined clusters of small, round or oval cells resembling lymphocytes because of their hyperchromatic nuclei and small amounts of cytoplasm. In humans, the small-cell anaplastic tumors mostly arise from solitary neuroendocrine cells or organized neuroepithelial bodies, as do carcinoids. They are therefore particularly likely to be associated with paraneoplastic syndromes caused by secretion of polypeptide hormones (e.g., adrenocorticotropin, antidiuretic hormone, calcitonin) or biogenic amines (e.g., serotonin). Paraneoplastic syndromes accompanying primary pulmonary tumors do not appear to have been identified in animals.

In general, squamous-cell and undifferentiated carcinomas are more malignant than adenocarcinomas, but all have a strong predilection for spread through intrapulmonary lymphatics. Dissemination through airways to alveoli also occurs. Metastasis can also take place to thoracic lymph nodes, abdominal nodes and kidneys, liver, brain, heart and bones.

Bronchioloalveolar tumors originate from either secretory bronchiolar (Clara) cells or alveolar type II epithelial cells. Be-cause of the close phenotypic relationship between these two cell types, it is not surprising that histologic and ultrastructural examination sometimes reveals both cell types in the same tumor. Bronchioloalveolar tumors are found most often in dogs, occasionally as an incidental finding at necropsy. They comprise over half the tumors found in some surveys of primary pulmonary tumors of dogs. Typically, they occur as solitary nodules in the periphery of the lung (Fig. 6.46B). Occasionally there are multiple nodules. The more benign tumors (adenomas) grow slowly by peripheral expansion and compression of surrounding parenchyma. Centers of large nodules frequently become necrotic. Other tumors, in which the neoplastic cells spread peripherally over alveolar walls, have the characteristics of low-grade adenocarcinomas. Less frequently, there is a rapidly spreading diffuse or disseminated multifocal type (Fig. 6.46A). Histologically, the special feature of bronchioloalveolar tumors is the regular alveolar pattern and preservation of pulmonary architecture (Fig. 6.46C). The preexisting alveolar stroma becomes lined by cuboidal or columnar epithelium, often with small, papillary projections into the alveolar lumina. As with many tumors, there is difficulty in clearly separating benign and malignant bronchioloalveolar tumors. Because there seems to be potential for eventual development of malignant behavior, there is often no attempt to categorize them as adenomas or carcinomas, but to regard them all as low-grade carcinomas unless there is clear evidence of highly aggressive behavior.

There are two major pitfalls in the diagnosis of bronchioloalveolar tumors. One is that the hyperplasia of bronchiolar and alveolar type II epithelial cells frequently caused by chronic inflammation of the bronchioloalveolar junction can be mistaken for neoplastic proliferation. The other is that rapidly invasive spread of neoplastic cells from either a bronchogenic adenocarcinoma or a metastasis from elsewhere in the body can sometimes mimic the regular pattern of a bronchioloalveolar carcinoma. Exclusion of alternative primary sites is therefore an integral part of the diagnosis of bronchioloalveolar tumors, especially the multinodular or diffuse varieties.

PULMONARY ADENOMATOSIS. Pulmonary adenomatosis (*jaagsiekte*) of sheep is an infectious form of bronchioloalveolar tumor that has the behavioral characteristic of a low-grade carcinoma. For this reason it is sometimes referred to as pulmonary carcinoma. The cause is now established as a retrovirus, probably type B or D. The term *jaagsiekte* appeared in original descriptions of the disease from South Africa, *jaagsiekte* being the Afrikaans word for "driving sickness."

Pulmonary adenomatosis occurs in many sheep-raising areas of the world. It is most important under conditions of intensive management, which favor aerosol transmission of the causative virus. The disease is less common where populations of sheep are dispersed, and it can escape detection for a time, as happened in the United States. The condition belongs in the category of slow virus diseases. Lesions develop slowly, with the result that the disease has an insidious onset. Clinical signs are not apparent for several months to several years and therefore are seen only in adult sheep. Early signs of the disease are coughing and exercise intolerance. Later there are also crackles and wheezes associated with the production of abundant watery exudate. The exudate is

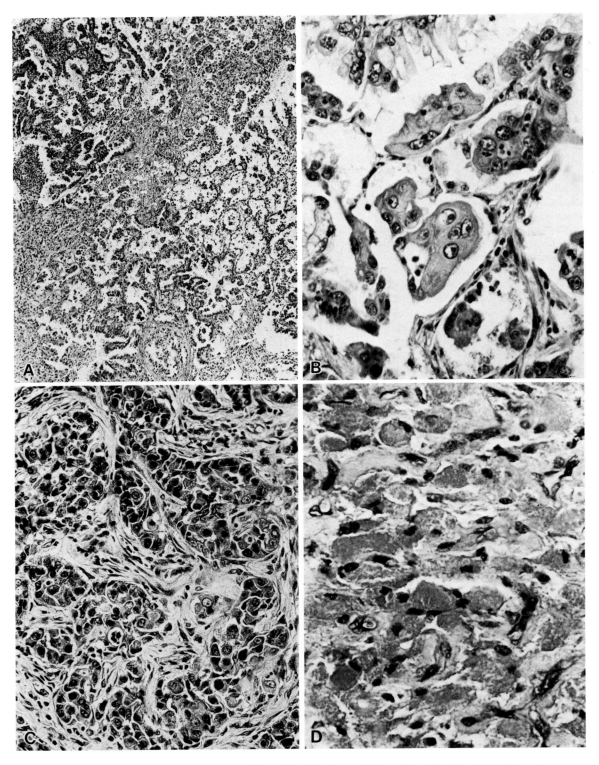

Fig. 6.45. (**A**) Invasive and destructive pattern of bronchogenic adenocarcinoma. Cat. (**B**) Mixed glandular and squamous elements in bronchogenic carcinoma. Dog. (**C**) Granular-cell tumor of the lung. Horse. (**D**) Higher magnification of (**C**), showing cells with abundant acidophilic granular cytoplasm.

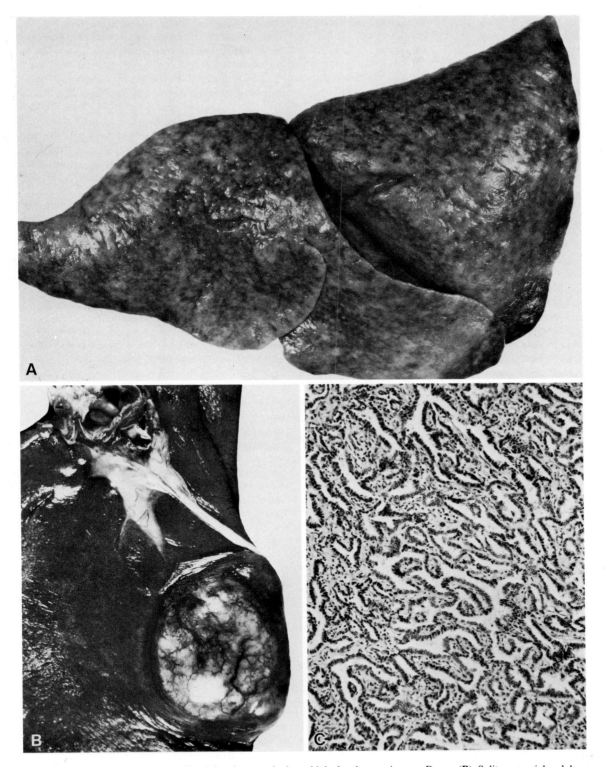

Fig. 6.46. (A) Widespread multifocal involvement in bronchioloalveolar carcinoma. Dog. (B) Solitary, peripheral bronchioloalveolar tumor. Dog. (Courtesy of S. W. Nielsen.) (C) Histology of bronchioloalveolar tumor, showing regular pattern of spaces lined by cuboidal to low columnar epithelium. Dog.

discharged from the nose, especially when the head is lowered, and is an important diagnostic clinical feature.

Early gross lesions are scattered, small gray-white nodules, sometimes with surrounding hyperinflated zones (Fig. 6.47A). Sheep with clinical signs have extensive nodular and confluent firm gray lesions affecting much of the pulmonary tissue. The lungs are heavy and fail to collapse. The cut surface is moist and reveals the basic nodularity of the lesion, even in regions where they coalesce. The centers of advanced lesions lose their friability and become fibrotic. There can be coexisting bronchopneumonia, verminous pneumonia, chronic progressive pneumonia (maedi), or combinations of these. This has been a source of considerable confusion in the past, particularly where the viruses causing chronic progressive pneumonia and pulmonary adenomatosis were both present in the same flock. The lesions of chronic progressive pneumonia and pulmonary adenomatosis are quite different histologically.

The characteristic histologic lesion of pulmonary adenomatosis consists of multiple proliferative foci of cuboidal or columnar cells that line alveoli and form papillary projections into their lumina (Fig. 6.47B,C). Continued proliferation obscures this pattern, and fibroplasia often occurs in more disorganized and degenerative regions. Early and uncomplicated proliferative lesions are not associated with significant accumulations of inflammatory cells, although there is usually some aggregation of macrophages in alveolar lumina. The papillary proliferation of cuboidal or columnar epithelium in the absence of significant interstitial inflammation is in marked contrast to the lymphofollicular interstitial pneumonia of chronic progressive pneumonia (maedi), in which alveolar epithelial hyperplasia is an inconstant and relatively minor feature.

The papillary proliferations involve both alveoli and bronchioles in many nodules. Ultrastructurally, the cuboidal cells usually have lamellar bodies characteristic of alveolar type II cells, whereas the columnar cells have secretory granules and glycogen compatible with origin from secretory bronchiolar epithelial (Clara) cells. The potentially carcinomatous nature of the lesions of pulmonary adenomatosis is confirmed by the occasional finding of metastatic foci in the bronchial or mediastinal lymph nodes.

Carcinoids have been reported to occur in lungs of animals but have not yet been adequately documented. Carcinoids in humans originate from neuroendocrine components of major airways. They have an endocrine pattern of nests or ribbons of uniform cells separated by well-vascularized stroma. The cells are round to polygonal. They have relatively small nuclei and abundant, pale, acidophilic cytoplasm. Ultrastructurally, their neuroendocrine derivation is revealed by large numbers of small, dense, secretory granules. It is probable that carcinoids occur in animals, albeit extremely rarely.

GRANULAR-CELL TUMORS. Granular-cell tumors (myoblastomas) are the only neoplasm of mesenchymal origin deserving of special mention. These are tumors that were originally thought to be derived from myoblasts but are now believed to originate from a fibroblast-like cell related to the progenitor of Schwann cells. Although granular-cell tumors can occur in various tissues, there is a difference in predilection sites among

species. All granular-cell tumors found to date in the lungs of animals have been in horses, and in fact this has become the most frequently reported primary pulmonary tumor of the horse. The tumors have occurred in older horses and were either associated with coughing and pulmonary insufficiency or were found as incidental lesions at slaughter. Gross lesions are usually multiple discrete or semiconfluent nodules that have a tendency to be associated with major bronchi and cause obstruction by bulging into their lumina. The lesions are limited to one lung in most instances, more often the right one. The main histologic feature of the tumor is lobular aggregation of large, round to polyhedral cells with abundant acidophilic granular cytoplasm (Fig. 6.45C,D). The lobules are surrounded and dissected by fibrovascular stroma. The cytoplasmic granules in the tumor cells are PAS-positive and have characteristic ultrastructural features.

LYMPHOMATOID GRANULOMATOSIS. Lymphomatoid granulomatosis refers to a rare condition of dogs in which there is extensive infiltration of one or more lobes of the lung by accumulations of mixed atypical lymphoreticular cells. The cells have a pronounced tendency to invade the walls of vessels (Fig. 6.47D) and airways. The few reported cases have been in young dogs. Cells comprising the neoplasm are of various types. Large histocytic and plasmacytoid forms predominate (Fig. 6.47E), but binucleate cells, eosinophils, lymphocytes, and plasma cells are often also present. A network of fibrous stroma runs throughout the tumor. Mitotic figures are plentiful.

The exact nature of the condition is not known, and too few cases have been described for a clear pattern to emerge. It might represent primary pulmonary involvement by a form of polymorphous lymphoma similar to that occasionally found affecting other viscera or the skin of the dog. It is important, however, not to use this diagnosis for generally unclassifiable tumors of the lung or for those typical forms of lymphoma in which there is extensive invasion of perivascular and peribronchial regions of the lung by the neoplastic lymphoids cells.

Metastatic Tumors

Many types of malignant tumors can metastasize to the lungs. Among the most frequent are mammary carcinomas in dogs and cats, uterine adenocarcinomas in cattle (Fig. 6.48B), and malignant melanoma in the horse. Carcinomas originating in endocrine gland or skin are also a common source. Osteosarcomas, hemangiosarcomas, and fibrosarcomas are frequent varieties of sarcoma. The most easily recognizable pattern of metastatic tumors is of multiple nodules scattered throughout the pulmonary parenchyma, without great variation in size range (Fig. 6.48A). The presence of a few gross lesions, especially if there is great discrepancy in size, requires careful analysis of all gross and microscopic findings to provide the best chance of making an unequivocal distinction between metastatic foci and primary pulmonary tumor. The probability of neoplastic foci in the lungs being metastases is increased if the animal is a young one. Sometimes, microscopic examination is needed to differentiate between neoplastic nodules and multifocal granulomas.

Microscopically, metastatic tumors usually resemble the primary lesions, although they may be either better or less differentiated. Presence of tumor cells within arteries is an important

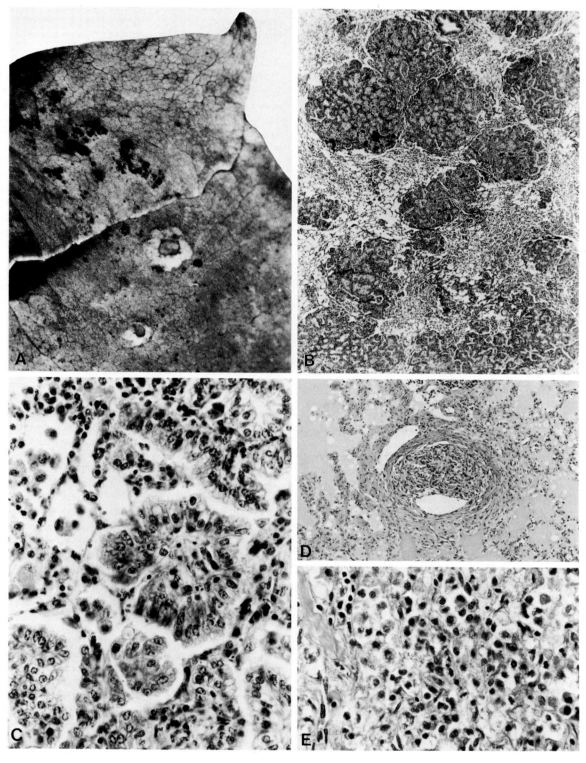

Fig. 6.47. (**A**) Isolated subpleural nodules present in early case of pulmonary adenomatosis (*jaagsiekte*). Sheep. (**B**) Multiple discrete tumor nodules with acinar and papillary patterns in pulmonary adenomatosis. Sheep. (**C**) Higher magnification of (**B**), showing columnar cells lining alveolar walls and forming papillae within lumina. (**B** and **C** courtesy of K. Perk and *Advances in Veterinary Science*.) (**D**) Eccentric invasion of intima of small artery in lymphomatoid granulomatosis. Dog. (**E**) Predominance of histiocytic and plasmacytoid cells in lymphomatoid granulomatosis. Dog.

indicator of metastatic origin, although this can be difficult to identify in some instances. This is particularly so where scirrhous response around invaded lymphatics gives them a superficial resemblance to thick-walled blood vessels.

In some cases where there is fulminating metastasis, there is no gross evidence of solid neoplastic infiltrations, merely tan discoloration of the lung and slightly increased firmness. Microscopically, however, widespread vascular embolization by anaplastic cells is seen (Fig. 6.48C), with early invasion of alveoli and lymphatics. Regardless of source or initial pattern of pulmonary involvement, highly malignant tumors have a predilection for widespread dissemination through intrapulmonary lymphatics.

Pleura and Mediastinum

Pleural abnormalities are usually secondary to lesions in tissues or organs forming the pleural cavity, especially the lung, or are part of more generalized disorders.

Congenital anomalies of the pleura and mediastinum are of little significance unless associated with a condition such as congenital diaphragmatic hernia. Congenital cysts may occasionally be found in the anterior mediastinum, mostly of brachycephalic dogs, and are presumed to be vestiges of the branchial pouches. Usually they are detected microscopically as cystic spaces lined by a single layer of cuboidal epithelium, often in close association with thymic tissues. Cysts of ~1 cm or more in diameter can be seen grossly as thin-walled structures containing clear, light yellow fluid. Air- or fluid-filled cysts in the caudal mediastinum are more likely to be of bronchogenic origin and can be large enough to cause pulmonary insufficiency.

Degenerative changes in the pleura occur in some cases of uremia in dogs (see the Urinary System, this volume). They are most evident in parietal pleura of the intercostal spaces, particularly the second, third, and fourth. Calcification centered on degenerated subpleural elastin and collagen fibers is visible as white horizontal striations.

Pneumothorax refers to the presence of air or gas in the pleural cavities. Air in the cavities allows the lungs to collapse to a degree proportional to the amount of air present. A normal subatmospheric pressure can be assumed to have been present at necropsy if the diaphragm moves caudally when the thorax is pierced and air allowed to enter. In small animals, pneumothorax can be detected by opening the chest under water and observing the escape of air bubbles.

Pneumothorax can be spontaneous or traumatic. Spontaneous pneumothorax is rare. It may complicate any pulmonary disease that leads to rupture of pulmonary parenchyma at the pleural surface. It is most often associated with rupture of emphysematous bullae. Less commonly it follows rupture of a parasitic cyst such as can occur in paragonimiasis. Traumatic pneumothorax is usually the result of accidental perforation of the thoracic wall or rupture of lung and visceral pleura. Air that tracks through the pulmonary interstitium to the mediastinum (pneumomediastinum) does not usually escape into the pleural cavities unless there is traumatic rupture of the mediastinum.

Traumatic pneumothorax can also be a complication of cardiac resuscitation or biopsy of the lung. Whatever the cause of pneumothorax, if entry of air stops before there is critical reduction of pulmonary function, the air is slowly resorbed.

Noninflammatory Pleural Effusions

Hydrothorax is the accumulation of edema fluid in the thoracic cavities. It is usually bilateral and has the same wide range of causes as edema of the lung or elsewhere. The fluid is clear, watery, and ranges from almost colorless to light yellow. Large amounts of it are present when there is widespread neoplastic involvement of pleural surfaces or when lymphatic drainage is impeded by neoplastic enlargement of the thymus or cranial mediastinal lymph nodes.

Hydrothorax may be present in cases of congestive heart failure, particularly in dogs, cats, and cattle. It is also present in severe anemias or in hypoproteinemias associated with the nephrotic syndrome, hepatopathy, protein-losing enteropathy, or malnutrition. Hydrothorax is also a feature of disease syndromes such as mulberry-heart disease in swine, black disease in sheep, African horsesickness, and ANTU poisoning. Chronic hydrothorax causes pleural opacity because of reactive hyperplasia of mesothelial cells and fibrous thickening of the underlying pleural connective tissue.

Chylothorax refers to the accumulation of milky fluid in the thorax (Fig. 6.49B). The fluid is lipid-rich lymph, which can be distinguished from other turbid effusions by extraction of the fat with ether or by staining the droplets with a Sudanophilic dye. Occasionally the source of the chylothorax is traced to rupture of the thoracic or right lymphatic duct. This is presumed to be the case in the many instances where the origin is not found. The most common association of chylothorax is with a traumatic event, bouts of severe coughing, or tumors in the cranial mediastinum.

Hemothorax is the presence of blood in the pleural cavities. It is most often the result of traumatic rupture of blood vessels, but it can also be caused by erosion of the wall of a vessel by an inflammatory or neoplastic process. Less common causes are diseases in which there is a clotting disorder. Hemorrhage may also arise from highly vascularized tumors (e.g., hemangiosarcoma) or inflammatory processes, such as pleural tuberculosis in dogs. Chronic hydrothorax may lead to the development of well-vascularized papillae on the pleura, and rupture of these might cause the effusion to resemble blood.

Pleuritis

Inflammation of the pleura (pleuritis) is the most commonly encountered abnormality. It is usually secondary to pneumonia (see Anatomic Patterns of Pneumonia). Other pathways by which inflammatory agents reach the pleura are the bloodstream, lymphatic permeation from the peritoneal cavity, traumatic penetration from outside the chest or from the esophagus or abdominal viscus (such as the bovine reticulum), or direct extension from a mediastinal abscess or esophagitis. The agents causing pleuritis as part of blood-borne infections vary with species of animal affected. *Haemophilus* species are commonly the cause in swine, as are mycoplasmas in swine and goats. *Chlamydia psittaci* is occasionally involved in ruminants. The virus of feline infectious peritonitis is the most common cause in

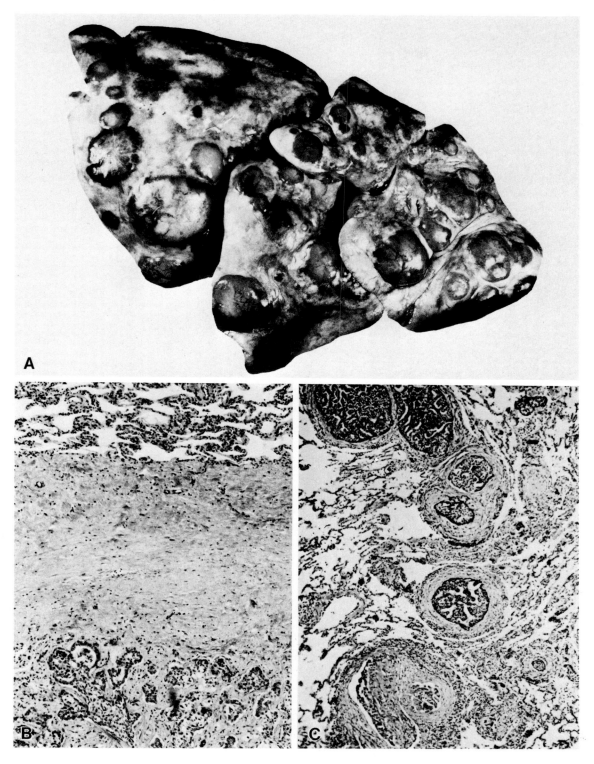

Fig. 6.48. (A) Metastatic nodules of mammary adenocarcinoma. Dog.   (B) Metastatic uterine adenocarcinoma with extensive scirrhous response. Cow.   (C) Multiple foci of malignant mammary adenocarcinoma resulting from neoplastic embolization of pulmonary vessels. Dog.

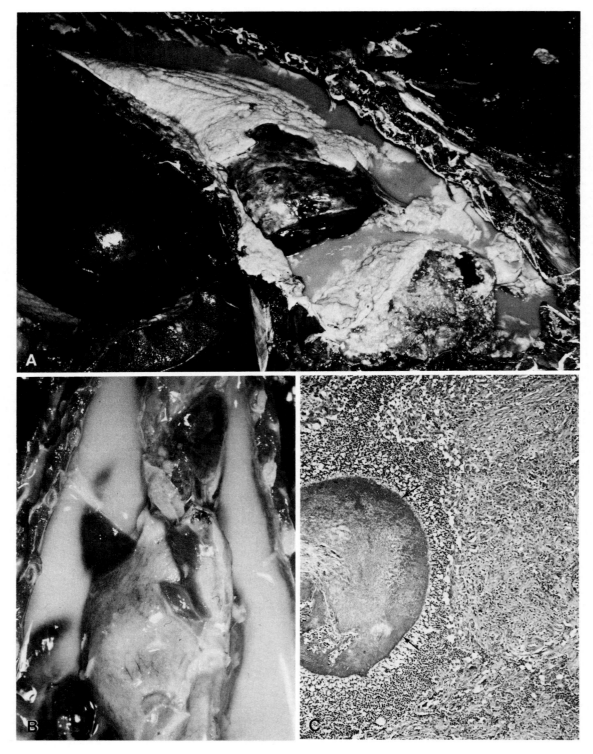

Fig. 6.49. (**A**) Severe fibrinopurulent pleuritis and pyothorax. Horse. (**B**) Chylothorax. Cat. (**C**) Pyogranulomatous pleuritis caused by *Actinomyces* sp. Dog. Note the large bacterial colony (arrows).

cats. Pleural defenses against microorganisms are much less effective than those of the lung. Even a few organisms reaching the pleural surfaces are therefore apt to have serious consequences in contrast to the result of a similar exposure in the lungs. The reactions of the pleura to inflammation are the same as those of the pericardium (see the Cardiovascular System, Volume 3).

Abundant purulent effusion into the pleural sacs is designated as **pyothorax** or **thoracic empyema**. The condition can occur in any animal but is of most clinical significance in horses, dogs, and cats. It can be caused by pyogenic organisms reaching the pleural cavities by any of the pathways mentioned previously, but the relative importance of the pathways and the mix of organisms involved varies with the species of animal. The majority of cases of serofibrinous effusion or pyothorax in the horse are secondary to either pneumonia or pulmonary abscessation. The exudate is usually thin and dirty yellow in color (Fig. 6.49A) and may be either unilateral or bilateral. Streptococci are the organisms most consistently isolated, sometimes in mixed infections with *Escherichia coli*, *Klebsiella*, *Pasteurella*, *Pseudomonas*, or staphylococci. *Pasteurella*, staphylococci, and *Bacteroides* are isolated in pure culture on occasion. *Mycoplasma felis* has been added to the list of possible agents. There is failure to culture organisms from the pleural effusion in as many as 50% of cases, however. In horses, exudative pleuritis occurs most often in racehorses and in many cases the onset is associated with stress of traveling, training, or racing.

Pyothorax unassociated with significant pneumonia occurs in dogs, mostly in sporting breeds with access to rural environments. It particularly affects dogs used for hunting or those in training. The exudate is unilateral or bilateral, more commonly the latter. It is usually bloodstained and viscous or flocculent, but may be creamy or darkly serofibrinous. Yellowish "sulfur granules" may be present in the bloodstained pus. The pleural surfaces are thickened and velvety red or grayish yellow and fibrotic, depending on age and nature of the lesion. The cranial mediastinum is the main site of thickening. *Actinomyces*, *Nocardia*, and *Bacteroides* are the most frequently recovered organisms, and these are commonly associated with the presence of sulfur granules and a characteristic pyogranulomatous pleuritis and mediastinitis (Fig. 6.49C). Mixed infections are common, however, and a variety of other organisms can be present, including *Corynebacterium*, *Pasteurella*, *E. coli*, *Fusobacterium necrophorum*, *Pseudomonas*, and streptococci. The pathogenesis of the lesion is uncertain, but the circumstantial evidence supports the belief that infection reaches the pleural cavity in most instances by way of migrating grass awns or florets. It is next to impossible to find plant material in the copious pleural exudate, but there is sometimes an association with subcutaneous abscesses or fistulous tracts compatible with migration of grass awns, and affected dogs are those with greatest exposure to the species of grasses responsible for invasion of bodily orifices and subcutis. The damage caused by the migrating grass awns also seems particularly favorable for growth of the actinomycetes. Pyothorax is fairly common in cats. The pus is usually creamy yellow or a grayish brown. As in dogs, it is more often bilateral than unilateral. A variety of bacteria are responsible, often in mixed infection. *Pasteurella multocida*,

various Gram-negative enteric bacteria, streptococci, and staphylococci have been isolated. *Actinomyces*, *Nocardia*, and *Bacteroides* are recovered on occasion, but much less consistently than in dogs. There are few pointers regarding the pathogenesis of the condition in cats. Although it is speculated that infection could gain access by penetration of a foreign body from the external surface or esophagus, or by a penetrating bite wound, there are few concrete data available.

Neoplastic Diseases of the Pleura

Primary pleural tumors are rare. The specific type is the pleural mesothelioma, which has been found in the cow, dog, cat, horse, and goat. Mesotheliomas arise from the pericardial and peritoneal surfaces as well as from the pleura; details of their appearance are given with diseases of the peritoneum (in the Peritoneum, Retroperitoneum, and Mesentery, this volume). There is one report of ferruginous bodies being present in significantly large numbers in the lungs of a small series of dogs with mesotheliomas. Ferruginous bodies are fine fibers irregularly coated by ferritin and amorphous protein. The cores are most commonly asbestos fibers, and therefore the numbers of ferruginous bodies are usually accepted as an index of exposure to asbestos. The finding of large numbers in the lungs of dogs with mesotheliomas suggests that inhalation of asbestos fibers could be related to the development of mesotheliomas in this species, as it is in humans.

Primary tumors can also arise from the chest wall and mediastinal tissues. Tumors of bone and cartilage, nerve sheaths, thymus, lymph nodes, and ectopic glandular tissue are discussed elsewhere.

Secondary tumors of the pleura are also uncommon, but transpleural dissemination of carcinomas and sarcomas occasionally occurs by extension from the lungs, chest wall, or mediastinum. Carcinomas from the abdominal cavity can reach the pleura by penetrating diaphragmatic lymphatics.

ACKNOWLEDGMENTS

We are deeply indebted to Laurie Noe and Mary Whitehill for assistance with bibliographic searches, and to Jody Wall for perseverance in typing successive versions of the manuscript. Much of the credit for the quality of the photographic plates belongs to Andrej T. Mariassy.

BIBLIOGRAPHY

General

Adamson, I. Y. R., and Bowden, D. H. The type 2 cell as progenitor of alveolar epithelial regeneration. A cytodynamic study in mice after exposure to oxygen. *Lab Invest* **30:** 35–42, 1974.

Adamson, I. Y. R., and Bowden, D. H. Bleomycin-induced injury and metaplasia of alveolar type 2 cells. *Am J Pathol* **96:** 531–544, 1979.

Adrian, R. W. Segmental anatomy of the cat's lung. *Am J Vet Res* **25:** 1724–1733, 1964.

Astrup, T., Glas, P., and Kok, P. Thromboplastic and fibrinolytic activity in lungs of some mammals. *Lab Invest* **22:** 381–386, 1970.

Bang, F. B. Mucociliary function as protective mechanism in upper respiratory tract. *Bacteriol Rev* **25A:** 228–236, 1961.

Billups, L. H. *et al.* Pulmonary granulomas associated with PAS-positive bodies in brachycephalic dogs. *Vet Pathol* **9:** 294–300, 1972.

Bowden, D. H., and Adamson, I. Y. R. The alveolar macrophage delivery system. Kinetic studies in cultured explants of murine lung. *Am J Pathol* **83:** 123–134, 1976.

Boyden, E. A., and Thompsett, D. H. The postnatal growth of the lung in the dog. *Acta Anat (Basel)* **47:** 185–215, 1961.

Brain, J. D., and Valberg, P. A. Deposition of aerosol in the respiratory tract. *Am Rev Respir Dis* **120:** 1325–1373, 1979.

Breeze, R. G., and Wheeldon, E. B. The cells of the pulmonary airways. *Am Rev Respir Dis* **116:** 705–777, 1977.

Evans, M. J. *et al.* Renewal of the terminal bronchiolar epithelium in the rat following exposure to NO_2 or O_3. *Lab Invest* **35:** 246–257, 1976.

Fishman, A. P., and Pietra, G. G. Handling of bioactive materials by the lung. *N Engl J Med* **291:** 884–890, and 953–959, 1974.

Gail, D. B., and Lenfant, C. J. M. Cells of the lung: biology and clinical implications. *Am Rev Respir Dis* **127:** 366–387, 1983.

Goetzl, E. J., Derian, C., and Valone, F. H. The extracellular and intracellular roles of hydroxy-eicosatetraenoic acids in the modulation of polymorphonuclear leukocyte and macrophage function. *J Reticuloendothel Soc* **28:** 105S–111S, 1980.

Green, G. M. *et al.* Defense mechanisms of the respiratory membrane. *Am Rev Respir Dis* **115:** 479–514, 1977.

Gross, P., Pfitzer, E. A., and Hatch, T. F. Alveolar clearance: its relation to the lesions of the respiratory bronchiole. *Am Rev. Respir Dis* **94:** 10–19, 1966.

Gross, P., Westrick, M. L., and McNerney, J. M. The pulmonary response to certain chronic irritants. *Arch Pathol* **68:** 252–261, 1959.

Hance, A. J., and Crystal, R. G. The connective tissue of the lung. *Am Rev Respir Dis* **112:** 657–711, 1975.

Hare, W. C. D. The broncho-pulmonary segments in the sheep. *J Anat (Basel)* **89:** 387–402, 1955.

Hawkey, C. M. Fibrinolysis in animals. *In* "The Haemostatic Mechanism in Man and Other Animals," R. G. MacFarlane (ed.). London, Academic Press, 1970.

Heppleston, A. G., and Young, A. E. Alveolar lipo-proteinosis: an ultra-structural comparison of the experimental and human forms. *J Pathol* **107:** 107–117, 1972.

Heppleston, A. G., and Young, A. E. Uptake of inert particulate matter by alveolar cells: an ultrastructural study. *J Pathol* **111:** 159–164, 1973.

Jakab, G. J. Viral–bacterial interactions in pulmonary infection. *Adv Vet Sci Comp Med* **26:** 155–172, 1982.

Kadowitz, P. J. *et al.* Pulmonary vascular responses to prostaglandins. *Fed Proc* **40:** 1991–1996, 1981.

Kapanci, Y. *et al.* "Contractile interstitial cells" in pulmonary alveolar septa: a possible regulator of ventilation/perfusion ratio? Ultrastructural, immunofluorescence and *in vitro* studies. *J Cell Biol* **60:** 375–392, 1974.

Lauweryns, J. M., and Baert, J. H. Alveolar clearance and the role of the pulmonary lymphatics. *Am Rev. Respir Dis* **115:** 625–683, 1977.

McLaughlin, R. F., Tyler, W. S., and Canada, R. O. A study of the subgross pulmonary anatomy in various mammals. *Am J Anat* **108:** 149–166, 1961.

Mauderly, J. L., and Hahn, F. F. The effects of age on lung function and structure of adult animals. *Adv Vet Sci Comp Med* **26:** 35–78, 1982.

Newhouse, M., Sanchis, J., and Bienenstock, J. Lung defense mechanisms. *N Engl J Med* **295:** 990–998 and 1045–1052, 1976.

Pearlstein, E., Gold, L. I., and Garcia-Pardo, A. Fibronectin: a review of its structure and biological activity. *Mol Cell Biochem* **29:** 103–128, 1980.

Pickrell, J. A. "Lung Connective Tissue: Location, Metabolism and Response to Injury." Boca Raton, Florida, CRC Press, 1981.

Proctor, D. F. The upper airways. I. Nasal physiology and defense of the lungs. *Am Rev Respir Dis* **115:** 97–129, 1977.

Reid, L. Secretory cells. *Fed Proc* **36:** 2703–2707, 1977.

Robinson, N. E. Some functional consequences of species differences in lung anatomy. *Adv Vet Sci Comp Med* **26:** 2–34, 1982.

Rungger-Brandle, E., and Gabbiani, G. The role of cytoskeletal and cytocontractile elements in pathologic processes. *Am J Pathol* **110:** 361–392, 1983.

Ryan, J. W., and Ryan, U. S. Metabolic functions of the pulmonary vascular endothelium. *Adv Vet Sci Comp Med* **26:** 79–98, 1982.

Slauson, D. O., The mediation of pulmonary inflammatory injury. *Adv Vet Sci Comp Med* **26:** 99–144, 1982.

Sorokin, S. P., and Brain, J. D. Pathways of clearance in mouse lungs exposed to iron oxide aerosols. *Anat Rec* **181:** 581–626, 1975.

Sprunt, K., and Leidy, G. Prevention and conversion to normal of bacterial overgrowth in the pharynx. *In* "Bacterial Interference," R. Aly and H. R. Shinefield (eds.). Boca Raton, Florida, CRC Press, 1982.

Thomson, R. G., and Gilka, F. A brief review of pulmonary clearance of bacterial aerosols emphasizing aspects of particular relevance to veterinary medicine. *Can Vet J* **15:** 99–107, 1974.

Tyler, W. S., Coalson, J. J., and Stripp, B. (eds.) The comparative biology of the lung. *Am Rev Respir Dis* **128:** S1–S91, 1983.

Unanue, E. R. Secretory function of mononuclear phagocytes. A review. *Am J Pathol* **83:** 396–418, 1976.

Veit, H. P., Farrell, R. L., and Troutt, H. F. Pulmonary clearance of *Serratia marcescens* in calves. *Am J Vet Res* **39:** 1646–1650, 1978.

Vijeyaratnam, G. S., and Corrin, B. Fine structural alterations in the lungs of iprindole-treated rats. *J Pathol* **114:** 233–240, 1974.

Volkman, A. Disparity in origin of mononuclear phagocyte populations. *J Reticuloendothel Soc* **19:** 249–268, 1976.

Wanner, A. Clinical aspects of mucociliary transport. *Am Rev Respir Dis* **116:** 73–125, 1977.

Weibel, E. R. Morphological basis of alveolar–capillary gas exchange. *Physiol Rev* **53:** 419–495, 1973.

West, J. B. "Respiratory Physiology—The Essentials." Baltimore, Williams & Wilkins, 1974.

Wheat, L. J., Kohler, R. B., and White, A. Bacterial interference in the nose. *In* "Bacterial Interference," R. Aly and H. R. Shinefield (eds.). Boca Raton, Florida, CRC Press, 1982.

Witschi, H. Proliferation of type II alveolar cells: a review of common responses in toxic lung injury. *Toxicology* **5:** 267–277, 1976.

Wright, G. W. Structure and function of respiratory tract in relation to infection. *Bacteriol Rev* **25:** 219–227, 1961.

Nasal Cavity and Sinuses

Allan, E. M., Gibbs, H. A., and Wiseman, A. Pathological features of bovine nasal granuloma (atopic rhinitis). *Vet Rec* **112:** 222–223, 1983.

Bazeley, P. L. Studies with equine streptococci. *Aust Vet J* **18:** 141–155 and 189–194, 1942; **19:** 62–85, 1943.

Bedford, P. G. C. Origin of the nasopharyngeal polyp in the cat. *Vet Rec* **110:** 541–542, 1982.

Bryans, J. T., Doll, E. R., and Shephard, B. P. The etiology of strangles. *Cornell Vet* **54:** 198–205, 1964.

Carbonell, P. L. Bovine nasal granuloma: gross and microscopic lesions. *Vet Pathol* **16:** 60–73, 1979.

Cook, W. R., and Littlewort, M. C. G. Progressive haematoma of the ethmoid region in the horse. *Equine Vet J* **6:** 101–108, 1974.

Creech, G. T., and Miller, F. W. Nasal granuloma in cattle. *Vet Med* **28:** 279–284, 1933.

Delmage, D. A. Some conditions of the nasal chambers of the dog and cat. *Vet Rec* **92**: 437–442, 1973.

George, J. L. *et al.* Identification of carriers of *Streptococcus equi* in a naturally infected herd. *J Am Vet Med Assoc* **183**: 80–84, 1983.

Hjarre, A., and Nordlund, I. Om atypisk amyloidos hos djuren. (Atypical amyloidosis in animals.) *Skand Vet Tidskr* **32**: 385–441, 1942.

Lane, J. G. *et al.* Nasopharyngeal polyps arising in the middle ear of the cat. *J Small Anim Pract* **22**: 511–522, 1981.

Negus, V. "The Comparative Anatomy and Physiology of the Nose and Paranasal Sinuses." Edinburgh and London, Livingstone, 1958.

Pemberton, D. H., and White, W. E. Bovine nasal granuloma in Victoria. 2. Histopathology of nasal, ocular and oral lesions *Aust Vet J* **50**: 89–97, 1974.

Pemberton, D. H., White, W. E., and Hore, D. E. Bovine nasal granuloma (atopic rhinitis) in Victoria, experimental reproduction by the production of immediate type hypersensitivity in the nasal mucosa. *Aust Vet J* **53**: 201–207, 1977.

Platt, H. Haemorrhagic nasal polyps of the horse. *J Pathol* **115**: 51–55, 1975.

Robinson, V. B. Nasal granuloma—a report of two cases in cattle. *Am J Vet Res* **12**: 85–89, 1951.

Wisecup, W. G., Schroder, C., and Page, N. P. Isolation of *Streptococcus equi* from burros. *J Am Vet Med Assoc* **150**: 303–306, 1967.

Rhinitis of Swine

Booth, J. C., Goodwin, R. F. W., and Whittlestone, P. Inclusion-body rhinitis of pigs: attempts to grow the causal agent in tissue cultures. *Res Vet Sci* **8**: 338–345, 1967.

Corner, A. H. *et al.* A generalized disease in piglets associated with the presence of cytomegalic inclusions. *J Comp Pathol* **74**: 192–199, 1964.

Done, J. T. An "inclusion-body" rhinitis of pigs (preliminary report). *Vet Rec* **67**: 525–527, 1955.

Drummond, J. G. *et al.* Effects of atmospheric ammonia on young pigs experimentally infected with *Bordetella bronchiseptica*. *Am J Vet Res* **42**: 963–968, 1981.

Duncan, J. R. *et al.* Pathology of experimental *Bordetella bronchiseptica* infection in swine: atrophic rhinitis. *Am J Vet Res* **27**: 457–472, 1966.

Duncan, J. R., Ramsey, F. K., and Switzer, W. P. Electron microscopy of cytomegalic inclusion disease of swine (inclusion body rhinitis). *Am J Vet Res* **26**: 939–947, 1965.

Fetter, A. W., Switzer, W. P., and Capen, C. C. Electron microscopic evaluation of bone cells in pigs with experimentally induced *Bordetella* rhinitis (turbinate osteoporosis). *Am J Vet Res* **36**: 15–22, 1975.

Giles, C. J. *et al.* Clinical, bacteriological and epidemiological observations on infectious atrophic rhinitis of pigs in southern England. *Vet Rec* **106**: 25–28, 1980.

Goodwin, R. F. W., and Whittlestone, P. Inclusion-body rhinitis of pigs: an experimental study of some factors that affect the incidence of inclusion bodies in the nasal mucosa. *Res Vet Sci* **8**: 346–352, 1967.

Hanada, M. *et al.* Production of lesions similar to naturally occurring swine atrophic rhinitis by cell-free sonicated extract of *Bordetella bronchiseptica*. *Jpn J Vet Sci* **41**: 1–8, 1979.

Obel, A.-L, Über Lungenveranderungen bei "Inclusion-body rhinitis" des Schweines. *Zentralbl Veterinaermed* **8**: 509–522, 1961.

Plowright, W., Edington, N., and Watt, R. G. The behaviour of porcine cytomegalovirus in commercial pig herds. *J Hyg (Lond)* **76**: 125–135, 1976.

Runnels, L. J. Infectious atrophic rhinitis of swine. *Vet Clin North Am (Large Anim Pract)* **4**(2): 301–319, 1982.

Rutter, J. M., and Rojas, X. Atrophic rhinitis in gnotobiotic piglets: differences in the pathogenicity of *Pasteurella multocida* in combined infections with *Bordetella bronchiseptica*. *Vet Rec* **110**: 531–535, 1982.

Silveira, D., Edington, N., and Smith, I. M. Ultrastructural changes in the nasal turbinate bones of pigs in early infection with *Bordetella bronchiseptica*. *Res Vet Sci* **33**: 37–42, 1982.

Switzer, W. P. Studies on infectious atrophic rhinitis. *Am J Vet Res* **17**: 478–484, 1956.

Underdahl, N. R., Socha, T. E., and Doster, A. R. Long-term effect of *Bordetella bronchiseptica* infection in neonatal pigs. *Am J Vet Res* **43**: 622–625, 1982.

Yoshikawa, T., and Hanada, T. Histopathological studies on pigs with atrophic rhinitis showing retarded growth. *Jpn J Vet Sci* **43**: 221–231, 1981.

Infectious Bovine Rhinotracheitis

Abinanti, F. R., and Plumer, G. R. The isolation of infectious bovine rhinotracheitis virus from cattle affected with conjunctivitis—observations on the experimental infection. *Am J Vet Res* **22**: 13–17, 1961.

Allan, E. M. *et al.* The pathological features of severe cases of infectious bovine rhinotracheitis. *Vet Rec* **107**: 441–445, 1980.

Crandell, R. A., Cheatham, W. J., and Maurer, F. D. Infectious bovine rhinotracheitis—the occurrence of intranuclear inclusions in experimentally infected animals. *Am J Vet Res* **20**: 505–509, 1959.

Hall, W. T. K. *et al.* The pathogenesis of encephalitis caused by the infectious bovine rhinotracheitis virus. *Aust Vet J* **42**: 229–237, 1966.

McKercher, D. G. Infectious bovine rhinotracheitis. *Adv Vet Sci* **5**: 299–328, 1959.

McKercher, D. G., Wada, E. B., and Straub, O. C. Distribution and persistence of infectious bovine rhinotracheitis virus in experimentally infected cattle. *Am J Vet Res* **24**: 510–514, 1963.

Obi, T. U. *et al.* An infectious bovine rhinotracheitis-like respiratory syndrome in young calves. *Vet Rec* **108**: 400–401, 1981.

Wiseman, A. Infectious bovine rhinotracheitis. *Vet Annu* **20**: 204–208, 1980.

Yates, W. D. G. A review of infectious bovine rhinotracheitis, shipping fever pneumonia and viral–bacterial synergism in respiratory disease of cattle. *Can J Comp Med* **46**: 225–263, 1982.

Feline Viral Rhinotracheitis

Crandell, R. A. Feline viral rhinotracheitis (FVR). *Adv Vet Sci Comp Med* **17**: 201–224, 1973.

Crandell, R. A. *et al.* Experimental feline viral rhinotracheitis. *J Am Vet Med Assoc* **138**: 191–196, 1961.

Ditchfield, J., and Grinyer, I. Feline rhinotracheitis virus: a feline herpesvirus. *Virology* **26**: 504–506, 1965.

Gaskell, R. M., and Povey, R. C. Feline viral rhinotracheitis: sites of viral replication and persistence in acutely and persistently infected cats. *Res Vet Sci* **27**: 167–174, 1979.

Kahn, D. E., and Hoover, E. A. Infectious respiratory diseases of cats. *Vet Clin North Am (Small Anim Pract)* **6**(3): 399–413, 1976.

Palmer, G. H. Feline upper respiratory disease: a review. *Vet Med Small Anim Clin* **75**: 1156–1158, 1980.

Povey, R. C. A review of feline viral rhinotracheitis (feline herpesvirus 1 infection). *Comp Immunol Microbiol Infect Dis* **2**: 373–387, 1979.

Pharynx, Larynx, and Guttural Pouches

Boles, C. L., Raker, C. W., and Wheat, J. D. Epiglottic entrapment by arytenoepiglottic folds in the horse. *J Am Vet Med Assoc* **172**: 338–342, 1978.

Cook, W. R., Campbell, R. S. F., and Dawson, C. O. The pathology and aetiology of guttural pouch mycosis in the horse. *Vet Rec* **83:** 422–428, 1968.

Duncan, I. D. *et al.* A correlation of the endoscopic and pathologic changes in subclinical pathology of the horse's larynx. *Equine Vet J* **9:** 220–225, 1977.

Duncan, I. D., Griffiths, I. R., and Madrid, R. E. A light and electron microscopic study of the neuropathy of equine idiopathic laryngeal hemiplegia. *Neuropathol Appl Neurobiol* **4:** 483–501, 1978.

Fau, D. Pathologie chirurgicale du tractus respiratoire superieur du chien. *Rev Med Vet* **132:** 651–660, 1981.

Hardie, E. M. *et al.* Laryngeal paralysis in three cats. *J Am Vet Med Assoc* **179:** 879–882, 1981.

Haynes, P. F. Persistent dorsal displacement of the soft palate associated with epiglottic shortening in two horses. *J Am Vet Med Assoc* **179:** 677–681, 1981.

Jensen, R. *et al.* Laryngeal contact ulcers in feedlot cattle. *Vet Pathol* **17:** 667–671, 1980.

Jensen, R. *et al.* Laryngeal diphtheria and papillomatosis in feedlot cattle. *Vet Pathol* **18:** 143–150, 1981.

Koch, D. B., and Tate, L. P. Pharyngeal cysts in horses. *J Am Vet Med Assoc* **173:** 860–863, 1978.

O'Brien, J. A. *et al.* Neurogenic atrophy of the laryngeal muscles of the dog. *J Small Anim Pract* **14:** 521–532, 1973.

Pass, D. A. *et al.* Canine laryngeal oncocytomas. *Vet Pathol* **17:** 672–677, 1980.

Raker, C. W., and Boles, E. L. Pharyngeal lymphoid hyperplasia in the horse. *J Equine Med Surg* **2:** 202–207, 1978.

Raphel, C. F. Endoscopic findings in the upper respiratory tract of 479 horses. *J Am Vet Med Assoc* **181:** 470–473, 1982.

Rose, R. J., Hartley, W. J., and Baker, W. Laryngeal paralysis in Arabian foals associated with oral haloxon administration. *Equine Vet J* **13:** 171–176, 1981.

Venker-van Haagen, A. J. Larynxparalyse bij Bouviers en een fokadvies ter preventie. (Laryngeal paralysis in Bouviers Belge des Flandres and breeding advice to prevent this condition.) *Tijdschr Diergeneeskd* **107:** 21–22, 1982.

Venker-van Haagen, A. J., Hartman, W., and Goedegebuure, S. A. Spontaneous laryngeal paralysis in young Bouviers. *J Am Anim Hosp Assoc* **14:** 714–720, 1978.

Wheeldon, E. B. Suter, P. R., and Jenkins, T. Neoplasia of the larynx in the dog. *J Am Vet Med Assoc* **180:** 642–647, 1982.

Trachea and Bronchi

Amis, T. C. Tracheal collapse in the dog. *Aust Vet J* **50:** 285–289, 1974.

Appel, M., and Bemis, D. A. The canine contagious respiratory disease complex (kennel cough). *Cornell Vet [Suppl]* **68:** 70–75, 1978.

Carb, A., and Halliwell, W. H. Osteochondral dysplasias of the canine trachea. *J Am Anim Hosp Assoc* **17:** 193–199, 1981.

Carrig, C. B. *et al.* Primary dextrocardia with situs inversus, associated with sinusitis and bronchitis in a dog. *J Am Vet Med Assoc* **164:** 1127–1134, 1974.

Done, S. H. Canine tracheal collapse—aetiology, pathology, diagnosis and treatment. *Vet Annu* **18:** 255–260, 1978.

Edwards, D. F. *et al.* Immotile cilia syndrome in three dogs from a litter. *J Am Vet Med Assoc* **183:** 667–672, 1983.

Gilka, F., and Sugden, E. A. Focal mineralization and nonspecific granulomatous inflammation of respiratory mucous membranes in pigs. *Vet Pathol* **18:** 541–548, 1981.

Hamerslag, K. L., Evans, S. M., and Dubielzig, R. Acquired cystic bronchiectasis in the dog: a case history report. *Vet Radiol* **23:** 64–68, 1982.

Jensen, R. *et al.* Bronchiectasis in yearling feedlot cattle. *J Am Vet Med Assoc* **169:** 511–514, 1976.

Lettow, E. *et al.* Solitäre Hohlraumbildung im bronchialsystem bei einem Hund (angeboren Bronchialzyste?). *Tieraerztl Umsch* **28:** 274–280 and 282–283, 1973.

McCandlish, I. A. P. *et al.* A study of dogs with kennel cough. *Vet Rec* **102:** 298–301, 1978.

Mangkoewidjojo, S., Sleight, S. D., and Convey, E. M. Pathologic features of iodide toxicosis in calves. *Am J Vet Res* **41:** 1057–1061, 1980.

Pirie, H. M., and Wheeldon, E. B. Chronic bronchitis in the dog. *Adv Vet Sci Comp Med* **20:** 253–276, 1976.

Pommer, A., and Walzl, H. Die chronisch-polypose Tracheitis bei Katzen. *Wein Tieraerztl Monatsschr* **44:** 129–135, 1957.

Stamp, J. T. The distribution of the bronchial tree in the bovine lung. *J Comp Pathol* **58:** 1–8, 1948.

Suter, P. F., Colgrove, D. J., and Ewing, G. O. Congenital hypoplasia of the canine trachea. *J Am Anim Hosp Assoc* **8:** 120–127, 1982.

Turk, M. A., Breeze, R. G., and Gallina, A. M. Pathologic changes in 3-methylindole-induced equine bronchiolitis. *Am J Pathol* **110:** 209–218, 1983.

Anomalies

Ball, V., and Girard, H. Kystes aeriens congénitaux du poumon chez le chien. *Rec Med Vet* **118:** 5–12, 1942.

Dennis, S. M. Congenital respiratory tract defects in lambs. *Aust Vet J* **51:** 347–350, 1975.

Dieter, R. Ueber kongenitale Lungenveränderungen. *Arch Wiss Prakt Tierheilkd* **73:** 218–231, 1938.

Joest, R. Intrathorakale Nebenlunge beim Pferde. *Tieraerztl Arch* **3:** 329–333, 1923.

Krediet, G. Over buiklongen. (Abdominal lungs.) *Tijdschr Diergeneeskd* **60:** 745–751, 1933.

Rubarth, S. On some congenital lung anomalies in animals. *Skand Vet Tidskr* **26:** 581–606, 1936.

Sjolte, I. P. and Christiansen, M. J. Zehn Falle von Nebenlungen bei Tieren. *Virchows Arch Pathol Anat Physiol* **302:** 93–117, 1938.

Thomson, R. G. Congenital bronchial hypoplasia in calves. *Pathol Vet* **3:** 89–109, 1966.

van den Ingh, T. S. G. A. M., and van der Gaag, I. A congenital adenomatoid malformation of the lungs in a calf. *Vet Pathol* **11:** 297–300, 1974.

Atelectasis and Emphysema

Bradley, R., and Wrathall, A. E. Barker (neonatal respiratory distress) syndrome in the pig: the ultrastructural pathology of the lung. *J Pathol* **122:** 145–151, 1977.

Breeze, R. G. Heaves. *Vet Clin North Am (Large Anim Pract)* **1**(1): 219–230, 1979.

Carlson, J. R. *et al.* Pulmonary edema and emphysema in cattle after intraruminal and intravenous administration of 3-methylindole. *Am J Vet Res* **36:** 1341–1347, 1975.

Cooper, J. E. Pulmonary cystic emphysema in piglets. *Vet Rec* **103:** 185–186, 1978.

Egberts, J., and Rethmeir, H. B. Hyaline membrane disease in lambs: a changing morphology. *Pathol Eur* **8:** 299–306, 1973.

Eriksson, S. Pulmonary emphysema and alpha-1-antitrypsin deficiency. *Acta Med Scand* **175:** 197–205, 1964.

Farrell, P. M., and Avery, M. E. Hyaline membrane disease. *Am Rev Respir Dis* **111:** 657–688, 1975.

Foley, F. D., and Lowell, F. C. Equine centrilobular emphysema. *Am Rev Respir Dis* **93:** 17–21, 1966.

Gillespie, J. R., and Tyler, W. S. Chronic alveolar emphysema in the horse. *Adv Vet Sci Comp Med* **13**: 59–99, 1969.

Gross, P. *et al.* Enzymatically produced pulmonary emphysema. A preliminary report. *J Occup Med* **6**: 481–484, 1964.

Howard, E. B., and Ryan, C. P. Chronic obstructive pulmonary disease in the domestic cat. *Calif Vet* **36**(6): 7–11, 1982.

Kikkawa, Y., and Smith, F. Cellular and biochemical aspects of pulmonary surfactant in health and disease. *Lab Invest* **49**: 122–139, 1983.

Lowell, F. C. Observations on heaves. An asthma-like syndrome in the horse. *J Allergy* **35**: 322–330, 1964.

Mahaffey, L. W., and Rossdale, P. D. Convulsive and allied syndromes in new-born foals. *Vet Rec* **69**: 1277–1286, 1957.

Manktelow, B. W., and Baskerville, A. Respiratory distress syndrome in newborn puppies. *J Small Anim Pract* **13**: 329–332, 1972.

Rossdale, P. D., Prattle, R. E., and Mahaffey, L. W. Respiratory distress in a newborn foal with failure to form lung lining film. *Nature* **215**: 1498–1499, 1967.

Snider, G. L. The pathogenesis of emphysema—twenty years of progress. *Am Rev Respir Dis* **124**: 321–324, 1981.

Wrathall, A. E. *et al.* Studies on the barker (neonatal respiratory distress) syndrome in the pig. *Cornell Vet* **67**: 543–598, 1977.

Circulatory Disturbances

Breeze, R. G. *et al.* Thrombosis of the posterior vena cava in cattle. *Vet Annu* **16**: 52–59, 1976.

Cook, W. R. Epistaxis in the racehorse. *Equine Vet J* **6**: 45–58, 1974.

Crandall, E. D. (ed.) Fluid balance across alveolar epithelium. *Am Rev Respir Dis* **127**: S1–S65, 1983.

Durlacher, S. H., Banfield, W. G., and Bergner, A. D. Postmortem pulmonary edema. *Yale J Biol Med* **22**: 565–572, 1950.

Krahl, V. E. The lung as a target organ in thromboembolism. *In* "Pulmonary Embolic Disease," A. A. Sasahara and M. Stein (eds.). New York, Grune & Stratton, 1965.

Lees, G. E., Suter, P. F., and Johnson, G. C. Pulmonary edema in a dog with acute pancreatitis and cardiac disease. *J Am Vet Med Assoc* **172**: 690–696, 1978.

Nimmo-Wilkie, J. S., and Feldman, E. C. Pulmonary vascular lesions associated with congenital heart defects in three dogs. *J Am Anim Hosp Assoc* **17**: 485–490, 1981.

Pascoe, J. R. *et al.* Exercise-induced pulmonary hemorrhage in racing thoroughbreds: a preliminary study. *Am J Vet Res* **42**: 703–707, 1981.

Porter, R., and O'Connor, M. (eds.) "Lung Liquids. Ciba Foundation Symposium," No. 38 (new ser). Amsterdam, Excerpta Medica, 1976.

Raphel, C. F., and Soma, L. R. Exercise-induced pulmonary hemorrhage in thoroughbreds after racing and breezing. *Am J Vet Res* **43**: 1123–1127, 1982.

Robin, E. D., Cross, C. E., and Zelis, R. Pulmonary edema. *N Engl J Med* **228**: 239–246 and 292–304, 1973.

Robinson, N. E., and Derksen, F. J. Small airway obstruction as a cause of exercise-associated pulmonary hemorrhage: an hypothesis. *Proc Am Assoc Equine Pract* **26**: 421–430, 1980.

Schneider, P., and Pappritz, G. Hairs causing pulmonary emboli. A rare complication in long-term intravenous studies in dogs. *Vet Pathol* **13**: 394–400, 1976.

Staub, N. C. Pulmonary edema. *Physiol Rev* **54**: 678–811, 1974.

Staub, N. C., Nagano, H., and Pearce, M. E. Pulmonary edema in dogs, especially the sequence of fluid accumulation in lungs. *J Appl Physiol* **22**: 227–240, 1967.

Weir, E. K. *et al.* Vascular hypertrophy in cattle susceptible to hypoxic pulmonary hypertension. *J Appl Physiol* **46**: 517–521, 1979.

Interstitial Pneumonia

Ashbaugh, D. G. *et al.* Acute respiratory distress in adults. *Lancet* **2**: 319–323, 1967.

Breeze, R. G. *et al.* The pathology of respiratory diseases of adult cattle in Britain. *Folia Vet Lat* **5**: 95–128, 1975.

Breeze, R. G., and Wheeldon, E. B. Fibrosing alveolitis. *In* "Spontaneous Animal Models of Human Disease," E. J. Andrews, B. C. Ward, and N. H. Altman (eds.). New York, Academic Press, 1979.

Carrington, C. B. Organizing interstitial pneumonia: definition of the lesion and attempts to devise an experimental model. *Yale J Biol Med* **40**: 352–363, 1968.

Carrington, C. B., and Gaensler, E. A. Clinical–pathologic approach to diffuse infiltrative lung disease. *In* "The Lung: Structure, Function and Disease," W. M. Thurlbeck and M. R. Abell (eds.). Baltimore, Williams & Wilkins, 1978.

Crystal, R. G. *et al.* Interstitial lung disease: current concepts of pathogenesis, staging and therapy. *Am J Med* **70**: 524–568, 1981.

Dungworth, D. L. Interstitial pulmonary disease. *Adv Vet Sci Comp Med* **26**: 173–200, 1982.

Haschek, W. M., and Witschi, H. P. Pulmonary fibrosis—a possible mechanism. *Toxicol Appl Pharmacol* **51**: 475–487, 1979.

Katzenstein, A. A., Bloor, C. M., and Liebow, A. A. Diffuse alveolar damage—the role of oxygen, shock and related factors. *Am J Pathol* **85**: 210–228, 1976.

Liebow, A. A. New concepts and entities in pulmonary disease. *In* "The Lung," A. A. Liebow and D. E. Smith (eds.). Baltimore, Williams & Wilkins, 1968.

Liebow, A. A. Definition and classification of interstitial pneumonias in human pathology. *Prog Respir Res* **8**: 1–33, 1975.

Pratt, P. C. Pathology of adult respiratory distress syndrome. *In* "The Lung: Structure, Function and Disease," W. M. Thurlbeck and M. R. Abell (eds.). Baltimore, Williams & Wilkins, 1978.

Scadding, J. G., and Hinson, K. F. W. Diffuse fibrosing alveolitis (diffuse interstitial fibrosis of the lungs). *Thorax* **22**: 291–304, 1967.

Snider, G. L. Interstitial pulmonary fibrosis—Which cell is the culprit? *Am Rev Respir Dis* **127**: 535–539, 1983.

Turk, J. R., Brown, C. M., and Johnson, G. C. Diffuse alveolar damage with fibrosing alveolitis in a horse. *Vet Pathol* **18**: 560–562, 1981.

Toxin- and Drug-Induced Diseases

Bedrossian, C. W. M. Pathology of drug-induced lung diseases. *Semin Respir Med* **4**: 98–106, 1983.

Boyd, M. R. Role of metabolic activation in the pathogenesis of chemically induced pulmonary disease: mechanism of action of the lung-toxic furan, 4-ipomeanol. *Environ Health Perspect* **16**: 127–138, 1976.

Breeze, R. G., and Carlson, J. R. Chemical-induced lung injury in domestic animals. *Adv Vet Sci Comp Med* **26**: 201–32, 1982.

Collis, C. H. Lung damage from cytotoxic drugs. *Cancer Chemother Pharmacol* **4**: 17–27, 1980.

Darke, P. G. G. *et al.* Acute respiratory distress in the dog associated with paraquat poisoning. *Vet Rec* **100**: 275–277, 1977.

Deneke, S. M., and Fanburg, B. L. Normobaric oxygen toxicity of the lung. *N Engl J Med* **303**: 76–86, 1980.

Dickinson, E. O., Spencer, G. R., and Gorham, J. R. Experimental induction of an acute respiratory syndrome in cattle resembling bovine pulmonary emphysema. *Vet Rec* **80**: 487–489, 1967.

Doster, A. R. *et al.* Effects of 4-ipomeanol, a product from mold-damaged sweet potatoes, on the bovine lung. *Vet Pathol* **15**: 367–375, 1978.

Frank, L., and Massaro, D. Oxygen toxicity. *Am J Med* **69**: 117–126, 1980.

Gillet, D. G., and Ford, G. T. Drug-induced lung disease. *In* "The Lung: Structure, Function and Disease," W. M. Thurlbeck and M. R. Abell (eds.). Baltimore, Williams & Wilkins, 1978.

Hammond, A. C. *et al.* 3-methylindole and naturally occuring acute bovine pulmonary edema and emphysema. *Am J Vet Res* **40:** 1398–1401, 1979.

Harding, J. D. J. *et al.* Experimental poisoning by *Senecio jacobaea* in pigs. *Pathol Vet* **1:** 204–220, 1964.

Johnson, R. P., and Huxtable, C. R. Paraquat poisoning in a dog and cat. *Vet Rec* **98:** 189–191, 1976.

Kelly, D. F. *et al.* Pathology of acute respiratory distress in the dog associated with paraquat poisoning. *J Comp Pathol* **88:** 275–294, 1978.

Logan, A. *et al.* Experimental production of diffuse pulmonary fibrosis and alveolitis in cattle: the effects of repeated dosage with 3, methylindole. *Res. Vet Sci* **34:** 97–108, 1983.

Longstaffe, J. A. *et al.* Paraquat poisoning in dogs and cats—differences between accidental and malicious poisoning. *J Small Anim Pract* **22:** 153–156, 1981.

Main, D. C., and Vass, D. E. Cambendazole toxicity in calves. *Aust Vet J* **56:** 237–238, 1980.

Moore, J. N. *et al.* Equine endotoxemia: an insight into cause and treatment. *J Am Vet Med Assoc* **179:** 473–477, 1981.

O'Sullivan, B. M. Crofton weed (*Eupatorium adenophorum*) toxicity in horses. *Aust Vet J* **55:** 19–21, 1979.

Theiler, A. Jagziekte in horses (*Crotalariosis equorum*) *In* "7th and 8th Reports of the Director of Veterinary Research, Department of Agriculture, Union of South Africa." Capetown, Government Printers, 1920.

Wilson, B. J. *et al.* Perilla ketone: a potent lung toxin from the mint plant, *Perilla frutescens* Britton. *Science* **197:** 573–574, 1977.

Pneumoconiosis

Abrabam, J. L. Recent advances in pneumoconiosis: the pathologist's role in etiologic diagnosis. *In* "The Lung: Structure, Function and Disease," W. M. Thurlbeck and M. R. Abell (eds.). Baltimore, Williams & Wilkins, 1978.

Brambilla, C. *et al.* Comparative pathology of silicate pneumoconiosis. *Am J Pathol* **96:** 149–170, 1979.

Dagle, G. E. *et al.* Pulmonary hyalinosis in dogs (from uranium ore dust). *Vet Pathol* **13:** 138–142, 1976.

Heppleston, A. G. Changes in the lungs of rabbits and ponies inhaling coal dust underground. *J Pathol Bacteriol* **67:** 349–359, 1954.

Schuster, N. H. J. Pulmonary asbestosis in a dog. *J Pathol Bacteriol* **34:** 751–757, 1931.

Schwartz, L. W. *et al.* Silicate pneumoconiosis and pulmonary fibrosis in horses from the Monterey–Carmel Peninsula. *Chest* **80:** S82–S85, 1981.

Smith, B. L., Poole, W. S. H., and Martinovich, D. Pneumoconiosis in the captive New Zealand kiwi. *Vet Pathol* **10:** 94–101, 1973.

Webster, I. Asbestosis in non-experimental animals in South Africa. *Nature* **197:** 506, 1963.

Hypersensitivity Diseases

Berkwitt L., Chew, D. J., and Rojko, J. Pulmonary granulomatosis associated with immune phenomena in a dog. *J Am Anim Hosp Assoc* **14:** 111–114, 1978.

Breeze, R. G. *et al.* The pathology of respiratory diseases of adult cattle in Britain. *Folia Vet Lat* **5:** 95–128, 1975.

Castleman, W. L., and Wong, M. M. Pulmonary ultrastructural lesions associated with retained microfilariae in canine occult dirofilariasis. *Vet Pathol* **19:** 355–364, 1982.

Confer, A. W. *et al.* Four cases of pulmonary nodular eosinophilic granulomatosis in dogs. *Cornell Vet* **73:** 41–51, 1983.

Dawson, C. O. *et al.* Studies on the incidence and titres of precipitating antibody to *Micropolyspora faeni* in sera from adult cattle. *J. Comp Pathol* **87:** 287–299, 1977.

Gershwin, M. E., and Steinberg, A. D. The pathogenetic basis of animal and human autoimmune disease. *Semin Arthritis Rheum* **6:** 125–164, 1976.

Howie, J. B., and Helyer, B. J. The immunology and pathology of NZB mice. *Adv Immunol* **9:** 215–266, 1968.

Hunningshake, G. W., and Fauci, A. S. Pulmonary involvement in the collagen vascular diseases. *Am Rev Respir Dis* **119:** 471–503, 1979.

Johnson, K. J., and Ward, P. A. New concepts in the pathogenesis of immune complex–induced tissue injury. *Lab Invest* **47:** 218–226, 1982.

Lazary, S. *et al.* Hypersensitivity in the horse with special reference to reaction in the lung. *In* "Allergology, Proceedings of the VIII International Congress of Allergology, Tokyo, 1973." Amsterdam, Excerpta Medica; New York, American Elsevier, 1974.

Lewis, R. M., Shwartz, R., and Henry, W. B. Canine systemic lupus erythematosus. *Blood* **25:** 143–160, 1965.

Liebow, A. A., and Carrington, C. B. Hypersensitivity reaction involving the lung. *Trans Stud Coll Physicians Phila* **34:** 47–70, 1966.

Liebow, A. A., and Carrington, C. B. The eosinopbilic pneumonias. *Medicine (Baltimore)* **48:** 251–285, 1969.

Lord, P. F., Schaer, M., and Tilley, L. Pulmonary infiltrates with eosinophilia in the dog. *J Am Vet Radiol Soc* **16:** 115–120, 1975.

Mansmann, R. A. *et al.* Chicken hypersensitivity pneumonitis in horses. *J Am Vet Med Assoc* **116:** 673–677, 1975.

Nicolet, J., de Haller, R., and Herzog, J. Serological investigations of a bovine respiratory disease ("Urner pneumonie") resembling farmer's lung. *Infect Immun* **6:** 38–42, 1972.

Nicolet, J., de Haller, R., and Scholar, H. J. La pneumonie d'Uri: une pneumonie allergique au foin moisi chez le bovin. *Pathol Microbiol* **34:** 252–253, 1969.

Pauli, B., Gerber, H., and Schatzmann, U. "Farmer's Lung" beim Pferd. *Pathol Microbiol* **38:** 200–214, 1972.

Pirie, H. M., and Selman, I. E. A bovine disease resembling diffuse fibrosing alveolitis. *Proc R Soc Med* **65:** 987–990, 1972.

Wilkie, B. N. Bovine allergic pneumonitis: an acute outbreak associated with mouldy hay. *Can J Comp Med* **42:** 10–15, 1978.

Wilkie, B. N. Allergic respiratory disease. *Adv Vet Sci Comp Med* **26:** 233–266, 1982.

Wiseman, A. *et al.* Bovine farmer's lung: a clinical syndrome in a herd of cattle. *Vet Rec* **93:** 410–417, 1973.

Influenza and Parainfluenza

Ahmed, M. T. Cases of purpura haemorrhagica as sequelae to equine influenza. *Indian Vet J* **15:** 213–215, 1938.

Allan, E. M. *et al.* Some characteristics of a natural infection by parainfluenza-3 virus in a group of calves. *Res Vet Sci* **24:** 339–346, 1978.

Betts, A. O. *et al.* Pneumonia in calves caused by parainfluenza virus type 3. *Vet Rec* **76:** 382–384, 1964.

Bryans, J. T. *et al.* Epizootiologic features of disease caused by myxovirus influenza A equine. *Am J Vet Res* **28:** 9–17, 1967.

Bryson, D. G. *et al.* The experimental production of pneumonia in calves by intranasal inoculation of parainfluenza type III virus. *Vet Rec* **105:** 566–573, 1979.

Cutlip, R. C., and Lehmkuhl, H. D. Experimentally induced parainfluenza type 3 virus infection in young lambs: pathologic response. *Am J Vet Res* **43:** 2101–2107, 1982.

Dawson, P. S., Darbyshire, J. H., and Lamont, P. H. The inoculation of calves with parainfluenza 3 virus. *Res Vet Sci* **6:** 108–113, 1965.

Ditchfield, J., Zbitnew, A., and Macpherson, L. W. Association of myxovirus para-influenzae 3 (RE55) with upper respiratory infection of horses. *Can Vet J* **4:** 175–180, 1963.

Gerber, H. *et al.* Influenza A/equi-2 in der Schweiz 1965. II. Epizootologie. *Zentralbl Veterinaermed [B]* **13:** 427–437, 1966.

Gerber, H., and Lohrer, J. Influenza A/equi-2 in der Schweiz 1965: III. Symptomatologie. 1. Reine Virusinfektion. *Zentralbl Veterinaermed [B]* **13:** 438–450, 1966.

Jones, T. C., and Maurer, F. D. The pathology of equine influenza. *Am J Vet Res* **4:** 15–31, 1943.

Morein, B., and Dinter, Z. Parainfluenza-3 virus in cattle: mechanisms of infection and defense of the respiratory tract. *Vet Med Nauki* **12:** 40–41, 1975.

Omar, A. R., Jennings, A. R., and Betts, A. O. The experimental disease produced in calves by the J121 strain of parainfluenza virus type 3. *Res Vet Sci* **7:** 379–388, 1966.

Wagener, J. S. *et al.* Parainfluenza type II infection in dogs: a model for viral lower respiratory tract infection in humans. *Am Rev. Respir Dis* **127:** 771–775, 1983.

Wilson, J. C., Bryans, J. T., and Doll, E. R. Recovery of influenza virus from horses in the equine influenza epizootic of 1963, *Am J Vet Res* **26:** 1466–1468, 1965.

Swine Influenza

Andrewes, C. H., Laidlaw, P. P., and Smith, W. The susceptibility of mice to the viruses of human and swine influenza. *Lancet* **2:** 859–862, 1934.

Francis, T., and Shope, R. E. Neutralization tests with sera of convalescent or immunized animals and the viruses of swine and human influenza. *J Exp Med* **63:** 645–653, 1936.

Hjarre, A., Dinter, Z., and Bakos, K. Vergleichende Untersuchungen über eine influenzaahnliche Schweinekrankheit in Schweden and Shopes Schweineinfluenza. *Nord Vet Med* **4:** 1025–1043, 1952.

Kammer, H., and Hanson, R. P. Studies on the transmission of swine influenza virus with *Metastrongylus* species in specific-pathogen-free swine. *J Infect Dis* **110:** 99–102, 1962.

Kammer, H., and Hanson, R. P. The *in vitro* association of swine influenza virus with *Metastrongylus* species. *J Infect Dis* **110:** 103–106, 1962.

Lewis, P. A., and Shope, R. E. Swine influenza. 2. A haemophilic bacillus from the respiratory tract of infected swine. *J Exp Med* **54:** 361–371, 1931.

Nayak, D. P. *et al.* Immunocytologic and histopathologic development of experimental swine influenza infection in pigs. *Am J Vet Res* **26:** 1271–1283, 1965.

Nayak, D. P., Kelley, G. W., and Underdahl, N. R. The enhancing effect of swine lungworms on swine influenza infections. *Cornell Vet* **54:** 160–175, 1964.

Shope, R. E. Swine influenza. 1. Experimental transmission and pathology. *J Exp Med* **54:** 349–359, 1931.

Shope, R. E. The swine lungworm as a reservoir and intermediate host for swine influenza virus. 4. The demonstration of masked swine influenza virus in lungworm larvae and swine under natural conditions. *J Exp Med* **77:** 127–138, 1943.

Shope, R. E. The swine lungworm as a reservoir and intermediate host for swine influenza virus. 5. Provocation of swine influenza by exposure of prepared swine to adverse weather. *J Exp Med* **102:** 567–572, 1955.

Canine Distemper

Appel, M. J. G. Pathogenesis of canine distemper. *Am J Vet Res* **30:** 1167–1182, 1969.

Appel, M. J. G. Distemper pathogenesis in dogs. *J Am Vet Med Assoc* **156:** 1681—1684, 1970.

Appel, M. J. G., and Gillespie, J. H. Canine distemper virus. *Virol Monogr* **11:** 1–96, 1972.

Carré, H. Sur la maladie des jeunes chiens. *C R Acad Sci (Paris)* **140:** 689–690 and 1489–1491, 1905.

Confer, A. W. *et al.* Biological properties of a canine distemper virus isolate associated with demyelinating encephalomyelitis. *Infect Immun* **11:** 835–844, 1975.

Cordy, D. R. Interstitial pneumonia with giant cells and inclusions. *J Am Vet Med Assoc* **114:** 21–26, 1949.

Dubielzig, R. R. The effect of canine distemper virus on the ameloblastic layer of the developing tooth. *Vet Pathol* **16:** 268–270, 1979.

Dunkin, G. W., and Laidlaw, P. P. Studies in dog distemper. *J Comp Pathol* **39:** 201–221, 1926.

Hall, W. W., Imagawa, D. T., and Choppin, P. W. Immunological evidence for the synthesis of all canine distemper virus polypeptides in chronic neurological diseases in dogs. Chronic distemper and old dog encephalitis differ from SSPE in man. *Virology* **98:** 283–287, 1979.

Higgins, R. J. *et al.* Canine distemper virus–associated cardiac necrosis in the dog. *Vet Pathol* **18:** 472–486, 1981.

Higgins, R. J. *et al.* Experimental canine distemper encephalomyelitis in neonatal gnotobiotic dogs. *Acta Neuropathol (Berl)* **57:** 287–295, 1982.

Jubb, K. V., Saunders, L. Z., and Coates, H. V. The intraocular lesions of canine distemper. *J Comp Pathol* **67:** 21–29, 1957.

Krakowka, S., Confer, A., and Koestner, A. Evidence for transplacental transmission of canine distemper virus: two case reports. *Am J Vet Res* **35:** 1251–1253, 1974.

Krakowka, S., Higgins, R. J., and Koestner, A. Canine distemper virus: review of structural and functional modulations in lymphoid tissues. *Am J Vet Res* **41:** 284–292, 1980.

Krakowka, S., and Koestner, A. Age-related susceptibility to infection with canine distemper virus in gnotobiotic dogs. *J. Infect Dis* **134:** 629–632, 1976.

Lauder, I. M. *et al.* A survey of canine distemper. 2. Pathology. *Vet Rec* **66:** 623–631, 1954.

Lincoln, S. D. *et al.* Etiologic studies of old dog encephalitis. 1. Demonstration of canine distemper viral antigen in the brain of two cases. *Vet Pathol* **8:** 1–8, 1971.

Lincoln, S. D. *et al.* Studies of old dog encephalitis. 2 Electron microscopic and immunohistologic findings. *Vet Pathol* **10:** 124–129, 1973.

Lisiak, J. A., and Vandevelde, M. Polioencephalomalacia associated in canine distemper virus infection. *Vet Pathol* **16:** 650–660, 1979.

McCullough, B., Krakowka, S., and Koestner, A. Experimental canine distemper virus–induced lymphoid depletion. *Am J Pathol* **74:** 155–166, 1974.

Summers, B. A., Greisen, H. A., and Appel, M. J. G. Early events in canine distemper demyelinating encephalomyelitis. *Acta Neuropathol (Berl)* **46:** 1–10, 1979.

Vandevelde, M. *et al.* Chronic canine distemper virus encephalitis in mature dogs. *Vet Pathol* **17:** 17–29, 1980.

Vandevelde, M. *et al.* Immunoglobulins in demyelinating lesions in canine distemper encephalitis. *Acta Neuropathol (Berl)* **54:** 31–41, 1981.

Vandevelde, M. *et al.* Immunological and pathological findings in demyelinating encephalitis associated with canine distemper virus infection. *Acta Neuropathol (Berl)* **56:** 1–8, 1982.

Vandevelde, M. *et al.* Demyelination in experimental canine distemper virus infection: immunological, pathological and immunohistological studies. *Acta Neuropathol (Berl)* **56:** 285–293, 1982.

Vandevelde, M. *et al.* Glial proteins in canine distemper virus–induced demyelination. *Acta Neuropathol (Berl)* **59:** 269–276, 1983.

Vandevelde, M., and Kristensen, B. Observations on the distribution of canine distemper virus in the central nervous system of dogs with demyelinating encephalitis. *Acta Neuropathol* **40:** 233–236, 1977.

Respiratory Syncytial Virus

Bryson, D. G. *et al.* Observations on outbreaks of respiratory disease in calves associated with parainfluenza type 3 virus and respiratory syncytial virus infection. *Vet Rec* **104:** 45–49, 1979.

Bryson, D. G. *et al.* Respiratory syncytial virus pneumonia in young calves: clinical and pathologic findings. *Am J Vet Res* **44:** 1648–1655, 1983.

Chanock, R. M. *et al.* Influence of immunological factors in respiratory syncytial virus disease. *Arch Environ Health* **21:** 347–355, 1970.

Lehmkuhl, H. D., and Cutlip, R. C. Experimentally induced respiratory syncytial viral infection in lambs. *Am J Vet Res* **40:** 512–514, 1979.

Lehmkuhl, H. D., and Cutlip, R. C. Experimentally induced respiratory syncytial viral infection in feeder-age lambs. *Am J Vet Res* **40:** 1729–1730, 1979.

Pirie, H. M. *et al.* Acute fatal pneumonia in calves due to respiratory syncytial virus. *Vet Rec* **108:** 411–416, 1981.

van den Ingh, T. S. G. A. M., Verhoef, J., and van Nieuwstadt, A. P. K. M. I. Clinical and pathological observations on spontaneous bovine respiratory syncytial virus infections in calves. *Res Vet Sci* **33:** 152–158, 1982.

Adenovirus

Belak, S. *et al.* Isolation of a pathogenic strain of ovine adenovirus type 5 and a comparison of its pathogenicity with that of another strain of the same serotype. *J Comp Pathol* **90:** 169–176, 1980.

Darbyshire, J. H. Bovine adenoviruses. *J Am Vet Med Assoc* **152:** 786–792, 1968.

Darbyshire, J. H. *et al.* Association of adenoviruses with bovine respiratory disease. *Nature* **208:** 307–308, 1965.

Darbyshire, J. H. *et al.* The pathogenesis and pathology of infection in calves with a strain of bovine adenovirus type 3. *Res. Vet Sci* **7:** 81–93, 1966.

Davies, D. H., Dungworth, D. L., and Mariassy, A. T. Experimental adenovirus infection of lambs. *Vet Microbiol* **6:** 113–128, 1981.

Ducatelle, R. *et al.* Pathology of natural canine adenovirus pneumonia. *Res Vet Sci* **31:** 207–212, 1981.

Klein, M. The relationship of two bovine adenoviruses to human adenoviruses. *Ann NY Acad Sci* **101:** 493–497, 1962.

McChesney, A. E. *et al.* Adenoviral infection in suckling Arabian foals. *Pathol Vet* **7:** 547–565, 1970.

McChesney, A. E., England, J. J., and Rich, L. J. Adenoviral infection in foals. *J Am Vet Med Assoc* **162:** 545–549, 1973.

Shadduck, J. A., Koestner, A., and Kasza, L. The lesions of porcine adenoviral infection in germfree and pathogen-free pigs. *Pathol Vet* **4:** 537–552, 1967.

Ovine Progressive Pneumonia (Maedi)

Cutlip, R. C. *et al.* Effects on ovine fetuses of exposure to ovine progressive pneumonia virus. *Am J Vet Res* **43:** 82–85, 1982.

Cutlip, R. C., Jackson, T. A., and Laird, G. A. Prevalence of ovine progressive pneumonia in a sampling of cull sheep from western and midwestern United States. *Am J Vet Res* **38:** 2091–2093, 1977.

Cutlip, R. C., Jackson, T. A., and Lehmkuhl, H. D. Lesions of ovine progressive pneumonia: interstitial pneumonitis and encephalitis. *Am J Vet Res* **40:** 1370–1374, 1979.

Georgsson, G., and Palsson, P. A. The histopathology of maedi: a slow, viral pneumonia of sheep. *Vet Pathol* **8:** 63–80, 1971.

Gudnadottir, M., and Palsson, P. A. Host–virus interaction in visna infected sheep. *J Immunol* **95:** 1116–1120, 1965.

Gudnadottir, M., and Palsson, P. A. Transmission of maedi by inoculation of a virus grown in tissue culture from maedi-affected lungs. *J Infect Dis* **117:** 1–6, 1967.

Haase, A. T. The slow infection caused by visna virus. *Curr Top Microbiol Immunol* **72:** 101–156, 1975.

Lucam, F. La "bouhite" ou "lymphomatose pulmonaire maligne du Mouton." *Rec Med Vet* **118:** 273–284, 1942.

Oliver, R. E. *et al.* Ovine progressive pneumonia: pathologic and virologic studies on the naturally occuring disease. *Am J Vet Res* **42:** 1544–1559, 1981.

Perk, K. Slow virus infection of ovine lung. *Adv Vet Sci Comp Med* **26:** 267–288, 1982.

Rajya, B. S., and Singh, C. M. The pathology of pneumonia and associated respiratory disease of sheep and goats. I. Occurrence of *jagziekte* and maedi in sheep and goats in India. *Am J Vet Res* **25:** 61–67, 1964.

Sigurdsson, B. Observations on three slow infections of sheep. *Br Vet J* **110:** 255–270, 1954.

Sigurdsson, B., Grimsson, H., and Palsson, P. A. Maedi, a chronic, progressive infection of sheep's lungs. *J Infect Dis* **90:** 233–241, 1952.

Sigurdsson, B., Palsson, P. A., and Tryggvadottir, A. Transmission experiments with maedi. *J Infect Dis* **93:** 166–175, 1953.

Miscellaneous Viral Diseases

Baskerville, A. The histopathology of pneumonia produced by aerosol infection of pigs with a strain of Aujeszky's disease virus. *Res Vet Sci* **12:** 590–592, 1971.

Baskerville, A. Ultrastructural changes in the pulmonary airways of pigs infected with a strain of Aujeszky's disease virus. *Res Vet Sci* **13:** 127–132, 1972.

Baskerville, A., McFerran, J. B., and Connor, T. The pathology of experimental infection of pigs with type 1 reovirus of porcine origin. *Res Vet Sci* **12:** 172–174, 1971.

Baskerville, A., McFerran, J. B., and Dow, C. Aujeszky's disease in pigs. *Vet Bull* **43:** 465–480, 1973.

Burki, F. Further properties of equine arteritis virus. *Arch Gesamte Virusforsch* **19:** 123–129, 1966.

Carpenter, J. L. *et al.* Intestinal and cardiopulmonary forms of parvovirus infection in a little of pups. *J Am Vet Med Assoc* **176:** 1269–1273, 1980.

Crandell, R. A. Pseudorabies (Aujeszky's disease). *Vet Clin North Am (Large Anim Pract)* **4:** 321–331, 1982.

Ditchfield, J., and Macpherson, L. W. The properties and classification of two new rhinoviruses recovered from horses in Toronto, Canada. *Cornell Vet* **55:** 181–189, 1965.

Jones, T. C., Doll, E. R., and Bryans, J. T. The lesions of equine viral arteritis. *Cornell Vet* **47:** 52–68, 1957.

Lamont, P. H. *et al.* Pathogenesis and pathology of infection in calves with strains of reovirus types 1 and 2. *J Comp Pathol* **78:** 23–33, 1968.

Langloss, J. M., Hoover, E. A., and Kahn, D. E. Diffuse alveolar damage in cats induced by nitrogen dioxide or calicivirus. *Am J Pathol* **89:** 637–648, 1977.

Langloss, J. M., Hoover, E. A., and Kahn, D. E. Ultrastructural morphogenesis of acute viral pneumonia produced by feline calicivirus. *Am J Vet Res* **39:** 1577–1583, 1978.

Lenghaus, C., and Studdert, M. J. Generalized parvovirus disease in neonatal pups. *J. Am Vet Med Assoc* **181:** 41–45, 1982.

Moll, T., and Davis, A. D. Isolation and characterization of cytopathogenic enteroviruses from cattle with respiratory disease. *Am J Vet Res* **20:** 27–32, 1959.

Ormerod, E., McCandlish, I. A. P., and Jarrett, O. Disease produced by feline calicivirus when administered to cats by aerosol or intranasal instillation. *Vet Rec* **104:** 65–69, 1979.

Phillip, J. I. H. *et al.* Pathogenesis and pathology in calves of infection by *Bedsonia* alone and *Bedsonia* and reovirus together. *J Comp Pathol* **78:** 89–99, 1968.

Plummer, G. An equine respiratory enterovirus. Some biological and physical properties. *Arch Gesamte Virusforsch* **12:** 694–700, 1963.

Robinson, W. F., Huxtable, C. R., and Pass, D. A. Canine parvoviral myocarditis: a morphological description of the natural disease. *Vet Pathol* **17:** 282–293, 1980.

Thompson, H., Wright, N. G., and Cornwell, H J. C. Canine herpesvirus respiratory infection. *Res Vet Sci* **13:** 123–126, 1972.

Wardley, R. C., and Povey, R. C. The pathology and sites of persistence associated with three different strains of feline calicivirus. *Res Vet Sci* **23:** 15–19, 1977.

Pasteurellosis

Bain, R. V. S. Haemorrhagic septicaemia of cattle: observations on some recent work. *Br Vet J* **115:** 365–369, 1959.

Bain, R. V. S. "Hemorrhagic Septicemia." Rome, Food and Agriculture Organization of the United Nations, 1963.

Biberstein, E. L., and Gills, M. G. The relation of antigenic types to the A and T types of *Pasteurella haemolytica*. *J Comp Pathol* **72:** 316–320, 1962.

Biberstein, E. L., and Kennedy, P. C. Septicemic pasteurellosis in lambs. *Am J Vet Res* **20:** 94–101, 1959.

Biberstein, E. L., and Thompson, D. A. Epidemiological studies on *Pasteurella haemolytica* in sheep. *J Comp Pathol* **76:** 83–94, 1966.

Carter, G. R. A new serological type of *Pasteurella multocida* from central Africa. *Vet Rec* **73:** 1052, 1961.

Davies, D. H. *et al.* The pathogenesis of sequential infection with parainfluenza virus type 3 and *Pasteurella haemolytica* in sheep. *Vet Microbiol* **6:** 173–182, 1981.

Davies, D. H., Herceg, M., and Thurley, D. C. Experimental infection of lambs with an adenovirus followed by *Pasteurella haemolytica*. *Vet Microbiol* **7:** 369–381, 1982.

Edwards, B. L. A note on haemorrhagic septicaemia in neonatal pigs. *Vet Rec* **71:** 208, 1959.

Friend, S. C., Thomson, R. G., and Wilkie, B. N. Pulmonary lesions induced by *Pasteurella hemolytica* in cattle. *Can J Comp Med* **41:** 219–223, 1977.

Gilmour, N. J. L. *Pasteurella haemolytica* infections in sheep. *Vet Q* **2:** 191–198, 1980.

Henning, M. W., and Brown, M. H. V. Pasteurellosis. An outbreak amongst sheep, *Onderstepoort J Vet Sci* **7:** 113–131, 1936.

Herceg, M., Thurley, D. C., and Davies, D. H. Oat cells in the pathology of ovine pneumonia–pleurisy. *NZ Vet J* **30:** 170–173, 1982.

Jericho, K. W. F. Histological changes in the respiratory tract of calves exposed to aerosols of bovine herpesvirus 1 and *Pasteurella haemolytica*. *J Comp Pathol* **93:** 73–82, 1983.

Jericho, K. W. F., Darcel, C. le Q., and Langford, E. V. Respiratory disease in calves produced with aerosols of parainfluenza-3 virus and *Pasteurella haemolytica*. *Can J Comp Med* **46:** 293–301, 1982.

Kielstein, P., Martin, J., and Janetschke, P. Experimentelle *Pasteurella-multocida*–Infektionen beim Schwein als ein Beitrag zur A^{t}iologie der enzootischen Pneumonie des Schweines. *Arch Exp Veterinaer med* **31:** 609–619, 1977.

Lopez, A., Thomson, R. G., and Savan, M. The pulmonary clearance of *Pasteurella hemolytica* in calves infected with bovine parainfluenza-3 virus. *Can J Comp Med* **40:** 385–391, 1976.

Murty, D. K., and Kaushik, R. K. Studies on outbreak of acute swine pasteurellosis due to *Pasteurella multocida* type B (Carter, 1955). *Vet Rec* **77:** 411–416, 1965.

Namioka, S., Murata, M., and Bain, R. V. S. Serological studies on *Pasteurella multocida*. V. Some epizootiological findings resulting from O antigenic analysis. *Cornell Vet* **54:** 520–534, 1964.

Pavri, K. M., and Apte, V. H. Isolation of *Pasteurella multocida* from a fatal disease of horses and donkeys in India. *Vet Rec* **80:** 437–439, 1967.

Pijoan, C., and Ochoa, G. Interaction between a hog cholera vaccine strain and *Pasteurella multocida* in the production of porcine pneumonia. *J Comp Pathol* **88:** 167–170, 1978.

Rehmtulla, A. J., and Thomson, R. G. A review of the lesions of shipping fever of cattle. *Can Vet J* **22:** 1–8, 1981.

Rushton, B. *et al.* Pathology of an experimental infection of specific pathogen–free lambs with parainfluenza virus type 3 and *Pasteurella haemolytica*. *J Comp Pathol* **89:** 321–329, 1979.

Smith, G. R. The pathogenicity of *Pasteurella haemolytica* for young lambs. *J Comp Pathol* **70:** 326–338, 1960.

Smith, G. R. The characteristics of two types of *Pasteurella haemolytica* associated with different pathological conditions in sheep. *J Pathol Bacteriol* **81:** 431–440, 1961.

Smith, G. R. Production of pneumonia in adult sheep with cultures of *Pasteurella haemolytica* type A. *J Comp Pathol* **74:** 241–249, 1964.

Smith, J. E., and Thal, E. A taxonomic study of the genus *Pasteurella* using a numerical technique. *Acta Pathol Microbiol Scand* **64:** 213–223, 1965.

Yates, W. D. G. A review of infectious bovine rhinotracheitis, shipping fever pneumonia and viral–bacterial synergism in respiratory disease of cattle. *Can J Comp Med* **46:** 225–263, 1982.

Haemophilus Infections

Hani, H. *et al.* Zur *Haemophilus*-Pleuropneumonie beim Schwein. VI. Pathogenese. *Schweiz Arch Tierheilkd* **115:** 205–212, 1973.

Martin, J. *et al.* Beitrag zur experimentellen *Haemophilus*infektion (*Haemophilus parahaemolyticus, Haemophilus parasuis*) bei SPF-Ferkeln. 2. Mitteilung: vergleichende Pathologie und Histologie. *Arch Exp Veterinaer med* **31:** 347–357, 1977.

Matthews, P. R. J., and Pattison, I. H. The identification of a *Haemophilus*-like organism associated with pneumonia and pleurisy in the pig. *J Comp Pathol* **71:** 44–52, 1961.

Nicolet, J., and Konig, H. Zur *Haemophilus*-Pleuropneumonie beim Schwein. *Pathol Microbiol* **29:** 301–306, 1966.

Nordstoga, K., and Fjolstad, M. The generalized Shwartzman reaction and *Haemophilus* infections in pigs. *Pathol Vet* **4:** 245–253, 1967.

Pattison, I. H., Howell, D. G., and Elliott, J. A *Haemophilus*-like organism isolated from pig lung and the associated pneumonic lesions. *J Comp Pathol* **67:** 320–330, 1957.

Schiefer, B. *et al.* Porcine *Hemophilus parahaemolyticus* pneumonia in Saskatchewan. I. Natural occurrence and findings. *Can J Comp Med* **35:** 99–104, 1974.

Shope, R. E. Porcine contagious pleuropneumonia. *J Exp Med* **119:** 357–375, 1964.

Watt, J. A. A. The isolation and cultural characteristics of an organism of the *Haemophilus* group in calf pneumonia. *J Comp Pathol* **62:** 102–107, 1952.

White, D. C. *et al.* Porcine contagious pleuropneumonia. *J Exp Med* **120:** 1–12, 1964.

Glanders and Melioidosis

Cottew, G. S. Melioidosis in sheep in Queensland. A description of the causal organism. *Aust J Exp Biol Med Sci* **28:** 677–683, 1950.

Cottew, G. S. Melioidosis. *Aust Vet J* **31:** 155–158, 1955.

Davie, J., and Wells, C. W. Equine melioidosis in Malaya. *Br Vet J* **108:** 161–166, 1952.

Duval, C. W., and White, P. C. The histological lesions of experimental glanders. *J Exp Med* **9:** 352–380, 1907.

Hunting, W. "Glanders, a Clinical Treatise." London, H. & W. Brown, 1908.

Ketterer, P. J., Donald, B., and Rogers, R. J. Bovine melioidosis in south-eastern Queensland. *Aust Vet J* **51:** 395–398, 1975.

M'Fadyean, J. Glanders. *J Comp Pathol* **17:** 295–317, 1904.

Olds, R. J., and Lewis, F. A. Melioidosis in goats. *Aust Vet J* **30:** 253–261, 1954.

Olds, R. J., and Lewis, F. A. Melioidosis in a pig. *Aust Vet J* **31:** 273–274, 1955.

Stedham, M. A. Histopathology of melioidosis in the dog. *Lab Invest* **36:** 358, 1977.

Sutmoller, P., Kraneveld, F. C., and van der Schaaf, A. Melioidosis (pseudomalleus) in sheep, goats and pigs on Aruba (Netherland Antilles). *J Am Vet Med Assoc* **130:** 415–417, 1957.

Tuberculosis

Amberson, J. B. A retrospect of tuberculosis: 1865–1965. *Am Rev Respir Dis* **93:** 343–351, 1966.

Armstrong, A. L., Dunbar, F. P., and Cocciatore, R. Comparative pathogenicity of *Mycobacterium avium* and Battey bacilli. *Am Rev Respir Dis* **95:** 20–32, 1967.

Bates, J. H., and Fitzhigh, J. K. Subdivision of the species *Mycobacterium tuberculosis* by mycobacteriophage typing. *Am Rev Respir Dis* **96:** 7–10, 1967.

Berthrong, M. The macrophage–tubercle bacillus relationship and resistance to tuberculosis. *Ann NY Acad Sci* **154:** 157–166, 1968.

Bull, L. B. Some comparative aspects of tuberculosis in lower animals. *Med J Aust* **2:** 827–830, 1937.

Collins, F. M., and Poulter, L. W. Effector and escape mechanisms in tuberculosis and leprosy. *In* "Immunological Aspects of Leprosy, Tuberculosis and Leishmaniasis," D. P. Humber (ed.). Amsterdam, Excerpta Medica, 1981.

Cornell, R. L., and Griffith, A. S. Types of tubercle bacilli in swine tuberculosis. *J Comp Pathol* **43:** 56–62, 1930.

Daniel, T. M. The immune spectrum in patients with pulmonary tuberculosis. *Am Rev Respir Dis* **123:** 556–559, 1981.

Draper, P., and D'Arcy Hart, P. Phagosomes, lysosomes and mycobacteria: cellular and microbial aspects. *In* "Mononuclear Phagocytes in Immunity, Infection and Pathology," R. van Furth (ed.). Oxford, Blackwell, 1975.

Feldman, W. H. Generalized tuberculosis of swine due to avian tubercle bacilli. *J Am Vet Med Assoc* **92:** 681–685, 1938.

Fourie, P. J. J., De Wet, G. J., and van Drimmelen, G. C. Tuberculosis in pigs caused by *M. tuberculosis* var. *hominis. J S Afr Vet Med Assoc* **21:** 70–73, 1950.

Francis, J. "Tuberculosis in Man and Animals." London, Cassell, 1958.

Glover, R. E. Infection of adult cattle with *M. tuberculosis avium. J. Hyg (Lond)* **41:** 290–296, 1941.

Glover, R. E. Pulmonary versus alimentary infection in tuberculosis. *Vet Rec* **53:** 746–748, 1941.

Glover, R. E., Dobson, N., and Patterson, A. B. Tuberculosis in animals other than cattle. *Vet Rec* **61:** 875–881, 1949.

Griffith, A. S. Naturally acquired tuberculosis in various animals. Some unusual cases. *J Hyg (Lond)* **36:** 156–168, 1936.

Griffith, A. S. Types of tubercle bacilli in equine tuberculosis. *J Comp Pathol* **50:** 159–172, 1937.

Gunn, F. D. *et al.* Experimental pulmonary tuberculosis in the dog. *Am Rev Tuberc* **47:** 78–96, 1943.

Gwatkin, R., and Mitchell, C. A. Avian tuberculosis infection in swine. *Can J Comp Med* **16:** 345–347, 1952.

Innes, J. R. M. The pathology and pathogenesis of tuberculosis in domesticated animals compared with man. *Vet J* **96:** 42–50 and 391–407, 1940.

Innes, J. R. M. Tuberculosis in the horse. *Br Vet J* **105:** 373–383, 1949.

Jarrett, W. F. H., and Lauder, I. A summary of the main points in tuberculosis in the dog and cat. *Vet Rec* **69:** 932–933, 1957.

Jennings, A. R. The distribution of tuberculosis lesions in the dog and cat, with reference to the pathogenesis. *Vet Rec* **61:** 380–384, 1949.

Lagrange, P. H. Tuberculosis: immunologic and clinical aspects. *In* "Immunological Aspects of Leprosy, Tuberculosis and Leishmaniasis," D. P. Humber (ed.). Amsterdam, Excerpta Medica, 1981.

Lesslie, I. W., and Birn, K. J. Tuberculosis in cattle caused by the avian type tubercle bacillus. *Vet Rec* **80:** 559–564, 1967.

Lesslie, I. W., Ford, E. J. H., and Linzell, H. L. Tuberculosis in goats caused by the avian type tubercle bacillus. *Vet Rec* **72:** 25–27, 1960.

Liu, S. K., Weitzman, I., and Johnson, G. Canine tuberculosis. *J Am Vet Med Assoc* **177:** 164–167, 1980.

Lovell, R., and White, E. G. Naturally occuring tuberculosis in dogs and some other species. 1. Tuberculosis in dogs. *Br J Tuberc* **34:** 28–40, 1941.

Lovell, R., and White, E. G. Naturally occuring tuberculosis in dogs and some other species. 2. Animals other than dogs. *Br J Tuberc* **35:** 28–40, 1941.

Luke, D. Tuberculosis in the horse, pig, sheep and goat. *Vet Rec* **70:** 529–536, 1958.

M'Fadyean, J. Equine tuberculosis. *J Comp Pathol* **4:** 383–384, 1891.

McKay, W. M. Congenital tuberculosis in bovines. *Vet J* **98:** 47–53, 1943.

Mallmann, W. L. *et al.* A study of pathogenicity of Runyon group III organisms isolated from bovine and porcine sources. *Am Rev Respir Dis* **92:** 82–84, 1965.

Mallmann, W. L., Mallmann, V. H., and Ray, J. A. Mycobacteriosis in swine caused by atypical mycobacteria. *Proc US Livestock Sanit Assoc* **66:** 180–183, 1962.

Nieberle, K. "Tuberkulose und Fleischhygiene." Jena, Fischer, 1938.

Nielsen, F. W., and Plum, N. Pulmonary tuberculosis in man as a source of infection for cattle. *Vet J* **96:** 6–18, 1940.

Orr, C. M., Kelly, D. F., and Lucke, V. M. Tuberculosis in cats: a report of two cases. *J Small Anim Pract* **21:** 247–253, 1980.

Ottosen, H. Histological studies on tuberculosis of bones in swine. *Skand Vet Tidskr* **32:** 65–77, 1942.

Plum, N. Tuberculosis abortion in cattle. *Acta Pathol Microbiol Scand [Suppl]* **37:** 438–448, 1938.

Runyon, E. H. *Mycobacterium tuberculosis, M. bovis* and *M. microti* species description. *Zentralbl Bakteriol Parasitenkd I* **204:** 415–413, 1967.

Scammon, L. A. *et al.* Nonchromogenic acid-fast bacilli isolated from tuberculous swine. Their relation to *M. avium* and the "Battey" type of unclassified mycobacteria. *Am Rev Respir Dis* **87:** 97–102, 1963.

Stamp, J. T. Tuberculosis of the bovine udder. *J Comp Pathol* **53:** 220–230, 1943.

Stamp, J. T. Bovine pulmonary tuberculosis. *J Comp Pathol* **58:** 9–23, 1948.

Wayne, L. G., Doubek, J. R., and Diaz, G. A. Classification and identification of mycobacteria. IV. Some important scotochromogens. *Am Rev Respir Dis* **96:** 88–95, 1967.

Corynebacterium equi Infection

Holtman, D. R. *Corynebacterium equi* in chronic pneumonia of the calf. *J Bacteriol* **49:** 159–162, 1945.

Johnson, J. A., Prescott, J. F., and Markham, R. J. F. The pathology of experimental *Corynebacterium equi* infection in foals following intrabronchial challenge. *Vet Pathol* **20:** 440–449, 1983.

Johnson, J. A., Prescott, J. F., and Markham, R. J. F. The pathology of experimental *Corynebacterium equi* infection in foals following intragastric challenge. *Vet Pathol* **20:** 450–459, 1983.

Martens, R. J., Fiske, R. A., and Renshaw, H. W. Experimental subacute foal pneumonia induced by aerosol administration of *Corynebacterium equi*. *Equine Vet J* **14:** 111–116, 1982.

Roberts, D. S. *Corynebacterium equi* infection in a sheep. *Aust Vet J* **33:** 21, 1957.

Smith, B. P., and Robinson, R. C. Studies of an outbreak of *Corynebacterium equi* pneumonia in foals. *Equine Vet J* **13:** 223–228, 1981.

Miscellaneous Bacterial Diseases

Baskerville, A., and Dow, C. Pathology of experimental pneumonia in pigs produced by *Salmonella cholerae-suis*. *J Comp Pathol* **83:** 207–215. 1973.

Bemis, D. A., Greisen, H. A., and Appel, M. J. G. Pathogenesis of canine bordetellosis. *J Infect Dis* **135:** 753–762, 1977.

Deem, D. A., and Harrington, D. D. *Nocardia brasiliensis* in a horse with pneumonia and pleuritis. *Cornell Vet* **70:** 321–328, 1980.

Dhanda, M. R., and Sekariah, P. C. Studies on pneumococcosis in domestic animals. 1. Isolation of *Streptococcus pneumoniae* from pneumonic lungs of sheep and goats. *Indian Vet J* **35:** 473–482, 1958.

Donald, L. G., and Mann, S. O. *Streptococcus pneumoniae* infection in calves. *Vet Rec* **62:** 257–258, 1950.

Duncan, L. G., and Mann, S. O. *Streptococcus pneumoniae* infection in calves. *Vet Rec* **62:** 257–258, 1950.

Duncan, J. R., Ramsey, F. K., and Switzer, W. P. Pathology of experimental *Bordetella bronchiseptica* infection in swine: pneumonia. *Am J Vet Res* **27:** 467–472, 1966.

Dunne, H. W., Kradel, D. C., and Dotz, R. B. *Bordetella bronchiseptica* (*Brucella bronchiseptica*) in pneumonia in young pigs. *J Am Vet Med Assoc* **139:** 897–899, 1961.

Garnett, N. L. *et al.* Hemorrhagic streptococcal pneumonia in newly procured research dogs. *J Am Vet Med Assoc* **181:** 1371–1374, 1982.

Goodnow, R. A. Biology of *Bordetella bronchiseptica*. *Microbiol Rev.* **44:** 722–738, 1980.

Gourley, R. N., Flanagan, B. F., and Wyld, S. G. *Streptobacillus actinoides (Bacillus actinoides)*: isolation from pneumonic lungs of calves and pathogenicity studies in gnotobiotic calves. *Res Vet Sci* **32:** 27–34, 1982.

Hamdy, A. H., Pounden, W. D., and Ferguson, L. C. Microbial agents associated with pneumonia in slaughtered lambs. *Am J Vet Res* **20:** 87–90, 1959.

Jang, S. S. *et al.* Focal necrotizing pneumonia in cats associated with a gram negative eugonic fermenting bacterium. *Cornell Vet* **63:** 446–454, 1973.

Koehne, G. W. *et al.* An outbreak of *Bordetella bronchiseptica* respiratory disease in foals. *Vet Med Small Anim Clin* **76:** 507–511, 1981.

L'Ecuyer, C., Roberts, E. D. and Switzer, W. P. An outbreak of *Bordetella bronchiseptica* pneumonia in swine. *Vet Med* **56:** 420–424, 1961.

McParland, P. J. *et al.* Pathological changes associated with group EF-4 bacteria in the lungs of a dog and a cat. *Vet Rec* **111:** 336–338, 1982.

Robertson, O. H., Coggeshall, L. T., and Terrell, E. E. Experimental Pneumococcus lobar pneumonia in the dog. *J Clin Invest* **12:** 433–493, 1933.

Sanford, S. E., and Tilker, A. M. E. *Streptococcus suis* type II-associated diseases in swine: observations of a one-year study. *J Am Vet Med Assoc* **181:** 673–676, 1982.

Smith, T. The etiological relation of *Bacillus actinoides* to bronchopneumonia in calves. *J Exp Med* **33:** 441–469, 1921.

Snyder, S. B. *et al.* Respiratory tract disease associated with *Bordetella bronchiseptica* infection in cats. *J Am Vet Med Assoc* **163:** 293–294, 1973.

Stevenson, R. G. *Streptococcus zooepidemicus* infection in sheep. *Can J Comp Med* **38:** 243–250, 1974.

Mycoplasmosis and Enzootic Pneumonia

Allan, E. M., and Pirie, H. M. Electron microscopical observations on mycoplasmas in pneumonic calves. *J Med Microbiol* **10:** 469–472, 1977.

Alley, M. R., and Clarke, J. K. The experimental transmission of ovine chronic non-progressive pneumonia. *NZ Vet J* **27:** 217–220, 1979.

Armstrong, C. H., and Friis, N. F. Isolation of *Mycoplasma flocculare* from swine in the U.S. *Am J Vet Res* **42:** 1030–1032, 1981.

Ball, H. J., and Bryson, D. G. Isolation of ureaplasmas from pneumonic dog lungs. *Vet Rec* **111:** 585, 1982.

Barr, J. *et al.* Enzootic pneumonia in calves. 1. The natural disease. *Vet Rec* **63:** 652–654, 1951.

Baskerville, A. Development of the early lesions in experimental enzootic pneumonia of pigs: an ultrastructural and histological study. *Res Vet Sci* **13:** 570–578, 1972.

Baskerville, A., and Wright, C. L. Ultrastructural changes in experimental enzootic pneumonia in pigs. *Res Vet Sci* **14:** 155–160, 1973.

Boidin, A. G., Cordy, D. R., and Adler, H. E. A pleuropneumonia like organism and a virus in ovine pneumonia in California. *Cornell Vet* **48:** 410–430, 1958.

Bolske, G., Nilsson, P. O., and Thunegard, E. Isolation of *Mycoplasma ovipneumoniae* from lambs with proliferative interstitial pneumonia. *Sven Veterinaertidn* **34:** 9–11, 1982.

Bryson, D. G. *et al.* Observations on outbreaks of respiratory disease in housed calves—(2) pathological and microbiological findings. *Vet Rec* **103:** 503–509, 1978.

Campbell, A. D. A preliminary note on the experimental reproduction of bovine pleuropneumonia. *J Counc Sci Ind Res Aust* **11:** 103–114, 1938.

DaMassa, A. J., Brooks, D. L., and Adler, H. E. Caprine mycoplasmosis: widespread infection in goats with *Mycoplasma mycoides* subspecies *mycoides* (large-colony type). *Am J Vet Res* **44:** 322–325, 1983.

DaMassa, A. J., Brooks, D. L., Adler, H. E., and Watt, D. E. Caprine mycoplasmosis: acute pulmonary disease in newborn kids given *Mycoplasma capricolum* orally. *Aust Vet J* **60:** 125–126, 1983.

Daubney, R. Contagious bovine pleuropneumonia. Note on experimental production and infection by contact. *J Comp Pathol* **48:** 83–96, 1935.

Davies, D. H., Jones, B. A. H., and Thurley, D. C. Infection of specific-pathogen-free lambs with parainfluenza virus type 3, *Pasteurella haemolytica* and *Mycoplasma ovipneumoniae*. *Vet Microbiol* **6:** 295–308, 1981.

Friis, N. F. *Mycoplasma dispar* as a causative agent in pneumonia of calves. *Acta Vet Scand* **21:** 34–42, 1980.

Gilmour, J. S. *et al.* Long-term pathological and microbiological progress in sheep of experimental disease resembling atypical pneumonia. *J Comp Pathol* **92:** 229–238, 1982.

Gilmour, J. S., Jones, G. E., and Rae, A. G. Experimental studies of chronic pneumonia of sheep. *Comp Immunol Microbiol Infect Dis* **1:** 285–293, 1979.

Goodwin, R. F. W., Pomeroy, A. P., and Whittlestone, P. Production of enzootic pneumonia in pigs with a mycoplasma. *Vet Rec* **77:** 1247–1249, 1965.

Goodwin, R. F. W., Pomeroy, A. P., and Whittlestone, P. Characterization of *Mycoplasma suipneumoniae*: a mycoplasma causing enzootic pneumonia of pigs. *J Hyg (Lond)* **65:** 85–96, 1967.

Goodwin, R. F. W., and Whittlestone, P. A respiratory disease of pigs (type XI) differing from enzootic pneumonia. *J Comp Pathol* **72:** 389–410, 1962.

Gourlay, R. N. *et al.* Pathogenicity of some *Mycoplasma* and

Acholeplasma species in the lungs of gnotobiotic calves. *Res Vet Sci* **27:** 233–237, 1979.

Gourlay, R. N., and Howard, C. J. Respiratory mycoplasmosis. *Adv Vet Sci Comp Med* **26:** 289–332, 1982.

Hutcheon, D. Contagious pleuro-pneumonia in Angora goats. *Vet J* **13:** 171–180, 1881.

Hutcheon, D. Contagious pleuro-pneumonia in goats at Cape Colony, South Africa. *Vet J* **29:** 299–404, 1889.

Jarrett, W. F. H. The pathology of some types of pneumonia and associated pulmonary diseases of the calf. *Br Vet J* **112:** 431–452, 1956.

Jones, G. E., Gilmour, J. S., and Rae, A. G. I. The effect of *Mycoplasma ovipneumoniae* and *Pasteurella haemolytica* on specific-pathogen-free lambs. *J Comp Pathol* **92:** 261–266, 1982.

Jones, G. E., Gilmour, J. S., and Rae, A. G. II. The effects of different strains of *Mycoplasma ovipneumoniae* on specific-pathogen-free and conventionally-reared lambs. *J Comp Pathol* **92:** 267–272, 1982.

Kaliner, G., and MacOwan, K. J. The pathology of experimental and natural contagious caprine pleuropneumonia in Kenya. *Zentralbl Veterinaermed [B]* **23:** 652–661, 1976.

Longley, E. O. Contagious pleuropneumonia of goats. *Indian J Vet Sci* **10:** 127–197, 1940.

McMartin, D. A., MacOwan, K. J., and Swift, L. L. A century of classical contagious caprine pleuropneumonia from original description to aetiology. *Br Vet J* **136:** 507–515, 1980.

Mare, C. J., and Switzer, W. P. New species: *Mycoplasma hyopneumoniae* a causative agent of virus pig pneumonia. *Vet Med Small Anim Clin* **60:** 841–846, 1965.

Mebus, C. A., and Underdahl, N. R. Scanning electron microscopy of trachea and bronchi from gnotobiotic pigs inoculated with *Mycoplasma hyopneumoniae*. *Am J Vet Res* **38:** 1249–1254, 1977.

Ojo, M. O. Caprine pneumonia. IV. Pathogenicity of *Mycoplasma mycoides* subspecies *capri* and caprine strains of *Mycoplasma mycoides* subspecies *mycoides* for goats. *J Comp Pathol* **86:** 519–529, 1976.

Ojo, M. O. Caprine pneumonia. *Vet Bull* **47:** 573–578, 1977.

Ojo, M. O., Kasali, O. B., and Ozoya, S. E. Pathogenicity of a caprine strain of *Mycoplasma mycoides* subspecies *mycoides* for cattle. *J Comp Pathol* **90:** 209–215, 1980.

Omar, A. R. The aetiology and pathology of pneumonia in calves. *Vet Bull* **36:** 259–273, 1966.

Otte, E., and Peck, E. F. Observations on an outbreak of contagious pleuropneumonia of goats in Ethiopia. *Bull Epizoot Dis Afr* **8:** 131–140, 1960.

Pattison, I. H. A histological study of a transmissible pneumonia of pigs characterized by extensive lymphoid hyperplasia. *Vet Rec* **68:** 490–494, 1956.

Roberts, E. D., Switzer, W. P., and Ramsey, F. K. Pathology of the visceral organs of swine inoculated with *Mycoplasma hyorhinis*. *Am J Vet Res* **24:** 9–18, 1963.

Rosendal, S. Canine mycoplasmas: pathogenicity of mycoplasmas associated with distemper pneumonia. *J Infect Dis* **138:** 203–210, 1978.

Rosendal, S. Experimental infection of goats, sheep and calves with the large colony type of *Mycoplasma mycoides* subspecies *mycoides*. *Vet Pathol* **18:** 71–81, 1981.

Rosendal, S., and Vinther, O. Experimental mycoplasmal pneumonia in dogs: electron microscopy of infected tissue. *Acta Pathol Microbiol Scand [B]* **85:** 462–465, 1977.

Salisbury, R. M. Enzootic pneumonia of sheep in New Zealand. *NZ Vet J* **5:** 124–127, 1957.

Shifrine, M., and Moulton, J. E. Infection of cattle with *Mycoplasma mycoides* by nasal instillation. *J Comp Pathol* **78:** 383–386, 1968.

Stamp, J. T., and Nisbet, D. I. Pneumonia of sheep. *J Comp Pathol* **73:** 319–328, 1963.

Stevenson, R. G. Proliferative interstitial pneumonia in lambs. *Can Vet J* **18:** 313–317, 1977.

Sullivan, N. D., St. George, T. D., and Horsfall, N. A proliferative interstitial pneumonia of sheep associated with *Mycoplasma* infection. I. Natural history of the disease in a flock. 2. The experimental exposure of young lambs to infection. *Aust Vet J* **49:** 57–62 and 63–68, 1973.

Thomas, L. H. *et al.* A search for new microorganisms in calf pneumonia by the inoculation of gnotobiotic calves. *Res Vet Sci* **33:** 170–182, 1982.

Underdahl, N. R., Kennedy, G. A., and Ramos, A. S., Jr. Duration of *Mycoplasma hyopneumoniae* infection in gnotobiotic pigs. *Can Vet J* **21:** 258–261, 1980.

Whittlestone, P. Enzootic pneumonia of pigs (EPP). *Adv Vet Sci Comp Med* **17:** 1–56, 1973.

Wilkinson, G. T. Mycoplasms of the cat. *Vet Annu* **20:** 145–150, 1980.

Woodhead, G. S. Some points in the morbid anatomy and histology of pleuro-pneumonia. *J Comp Pathol* **1:** 33–36, 123–133, and 339–347, 1888.

Chlamydial Infections

Dungworth, D. L., and Cordy, D. R. The pathogenesis of ovine pneumonia. *J Comp Pathol* **72:** 49–79, 1962.

Hoover, E. A., Kahn, D. E., and Langloss, J. M. Experimentally induced feline chlamydial infection (feline pneumonitis). *Am J Vet Res* **39:** 541–548, 1978.

McChesney, S. L., England, J. J., and McChesney, A. E. *Chlamydia psittaci* induced pneumonia in a horse. *Cornell Vet* **72:** 92–97, 1982.

Munro, R. *et al.* Pulmonary lesions in sheep following experimental infection by *Ehrlichia phagocytophilia* and *Chlamydia psittaci*. *J Comp Pathol* **92:** 117–129, 1982.

Omori, T., Ishii, S., and Matumoto, M. Miyagawanellosis of cattle in Japan. *Am J Vet Res* **21:** 564–573, 1960.

Ottosen, H. E. Pneumonitis in cattle. *Nord Vet Med* **9:** 569–589, 1957.

Smith, P. C., Cutlip, R. C., and Page, L. A. Pathogenicity of a strain of *Chlamydia psittaci* of bovine intestinal origin for neonatal calves. *Am J Vet Res* **34:** 615–618, 1973.

Storz, J., ànd Thornley, W. R. Serologische und aetiologische Studien über die intestinale Psittakose-lymphogranuloma–infektion der Schafe. *Zentralbl Veterinaermed [B]* **13:** 14–24, 1966.

York, C. J., and Baker, J. A. A new member of the psittacosis–lymphogranuloma group of viruses that causes infection in calves. *J Exp Med* **93:** 587–604, 1951.

Mycotic Infections

Ajello, L. Comparative ecology of respiratory mycotic disease agents. *Bacteriol Rev* **31:** 6–24, 1967.

Austwick, P. K. C., Gitter, M., and Watkins, C. V. Pulmonary aspergillosis in lambs. *Vet Rec* **72:** 19–21, 1960.

Balwant, S., Chawla, R. S., and Sanota, P. Phycomycotic pneumonia in a pig. *Indian Vet J* **53:** 818, 1976.

Barron, C. N. Cryptococcosis in animals. *J Am Vet Med Assoc* **127:** 125–132, 1955.

Benbrook, E. A., Bryant, J. B., and Saunders, L. Z. A case of blastomycosis in the horse. *J Am Vet Med Assoc* **112:** 475–478, 1948.

Bridges, C. H. Maduromycosis of bovine nasal mucosa (nasal granuloma of cattle). *Cornell Vet* **50:** 468–483, 1960.

Buchanan, C. A. Feline cryptococcosis: a case report and review. *Southwest Vet* **35:** 41–44, 1982.

Chauhan, H. V. S., and Dwivedi, P. Pneumomycosis in sheep and goats. *Vet Rec* **95:** 58–59, 1974.

Cordes, D. O., Carter, M. E., and di Menna, M. E. Mycotic pneumonia and placentitis caused by *Mortierella wolfii*. II. Pathology of experimental infection in cattle. *Vet Pathol* **9:** 190–201, 1972.

Cordes, D. O., Dodd, D. C., and O'Hara. Acute mycotic pneumonia of cattle. NZ Vet J 12: 101–104, 1964.

Finegold, S. M., Will, D., and Murray, J. F. Aspergillosis. A review and report of twelve case. Am J Med 27: 463–482, 1959.

Forbus, W. D., and Bestebreurtje, A. M. Coccidioidomycosis. A study of 95 cases of the disseminated type with special reference to the pathogenesis of the disease. Milit Surg 99: 653–719, 1946.

Harrell, E. R., and Curtis, A. C. North American blastomycosis. Am J Med 27: 750–766, 1969.

Harvey, C. E. et al. Nasal penicilliosis in six dogs. J Am Vet Med Assoc 178: 1084–1087, 1981.

Hatkin, J. M., Phillips, W. E., Jr., and Utroska, W. R. Two cases of feline blastomycosis. J Am Anim Hosp Assoc 15: 217–220, 1979.

Hilbert, B. J., Huxtable, C. R., and Pawley, S. E. Cryptococcal pneumonia in a horse. Aust Vet J 56: 391–392, 1980.

Holzworth, J., and Coffin, D. L. Cryptococcosis in a cat. Cornell Vet 43: 546–550, 1953.

Hugenholtz, P. G. et al. Experimental coccidioidomycosis in dogs. Am J Vet Res 19: 433–439, 1958.

Ivanov, X. Ustilagineous pneumonia in cattle. The spores of Ustilago maydis as a pathogenic factor. C R Acad Bulg Sci 2: 49–52, 1949.

Koller, L. D., and Helfer, D. H. Adiaspiromycosis in the lungs of a goat (associated with Pieris japonica poisoning). J Am Vet Med Assoc 173: 80–81, 1978.

Koller, L. D., Patton, N. M., and Whitsett, D. K. Adiaspiromycosis in the lungs of a dog. J Am Vet Med Assoc 169: 1316–1317, 1976.

Londero, A. T., Santos, M. N., and Freitas, C. J. B. Animal rhinosporidiosis in Brazil. Report of three additional cases. Mycopathologia 60: 171–173, 1977.

McKenzie, R. A., and Connole, M. D. Mycotic nasal granuloma in cattle. Aust Vet J 53: 268–270, 1977.

Maddy, K. T. Coccidioidomycosis in animals. Vet Med 54: 233–242, 1959.

Newberne, J. W., Neal, J. E., and Heath, M. K. Some clinical and microbiological observations in four cases of canine blastomycosis. J Am Vet Med Assoc 127: 220–223, 1955.

Nyaga, P. N. et al. Canine pulmonary geotrichosis: case report. Kenya Vet 4: 6–9, 1980.

Pappagianis, D., and Kobayashi, G. S. Approaches to the physiology of Coccidioides immitis. Ann NY Acad Sci 89: 109–120, 1960.

Ramsey, F. K., and Carter, G. R. Canine blastomycosis in the United States. J Am Vet Med Assoc 120: 93–98, 1952.

Robbins, E. S. North American blastomycosis in the dog. J Am Vet Med Assoc 125: 391–397, 1954.

Roberts, E. D., McDaniel, H. A., and Carbrey, E. A. Maduromycosis of the bovine nasal mucosa. J Am Vet Med Assoc 142: 42–48, 1963.

Roberts, M. C., Sutton, R. H., and Lovell, D. K. A protracted case of cryptococcal nasal granuloma in a stallion. Aust Vet J 57: 287–291, 1981.

Ryan, M. J., and Wyand, D. S. Cryptococcus as a cause of neonatal pneumonia and abortion in two horses. Vet Pathol 18: 270–272, 1981.

Saunders, L. Z. Systemic fungous infections in animals: a review. Cornell Vet 38: 213–238, 1948.

Sautter, J. H., Rowsell, H. C., and Holn, R. B. Actinomycosis and actinobacillosis in dogs. North Am Vet 34: 341–346, 1953.

Seibold, H. R. Systemic blastomycosis in dogs. North Am Vet 27: 162–164, 1946.

Sharma, D. N., and Dwivedi, J. N. Pulmonary mycosis of sheep and goats in India. Indian J Anim Sci 47: 808–813, 1977.

Smith, D. L. T., Fischer, J. B., and Barnum, D. A. Generalized Cryptococcus neoformans infection in a dog. Can Med Assoc J 72: 18–20, 1955.

Smith, H. A. Coccidioidomycosis in animals. Am J Pathol 24: 223–233, 1948.

Thordal-Christensen, A., and Clifford, D. H. Actinomycosis (nocardiosis) in a dog with a brief review of this disease. Am J Vet Res 14: 298–306, 1953.

Wilkinson, G. T. Feline cryptococcosis: a review and seven case reports. J Small Anim Pract 20: 749–768, 1979.

Wilkinson, G. T., Sutton, R. H., and Grono, L. R. Aspergillus spp. infection associated with orbital cellulitis and sinusitis in a cat. J Small Anim Pract 23: 127–131, 1982.

Wysmann, E. Ueber Aspergillosen beim Rind. Schweiz Arch Tierheilkd 83: 166–171, 1941.

Zontine, W. J. Coccidioidomycosis in the horse—a case report. J Am Vet Med Assoc 131: 490–492, 1958.

Pneumoncystis carinii Infection

Botha, W. S., and van Rensburg, I. B. J. Pneumocystosis: a chronic respiratory distress syndrome in the dog. J S Afr Vet Assoc 50: 173–179, 1979.

Copland, J. W. Canine pneumonia caused by Pneumocystis carinii. Aust Vet J 50: 515–518, 1974.

Farrow, B. R. H. et al. Pneumocystis pneumonia in the dog. J Comp Pathol 82: 447–453, 1972.

Lanken, P. N. et al. Alveolar response to experimental Pneumocystis carinii pneumonia in the rat. Am J Pathol 99: 561–578, 1980.

McConnell, E. E., Basson, P. A., and Pienaar, J. G. Pneumocystosis in a domestic goat. Onderstepoort J Vet Res 38: 117–126, 1971.

Seibold, H. R., and Munnell, J. F. Pneumoncystis carinii in a pig. Vet Pathol 14: 89–91, 1977.

Shively, J. N. et al. Pneumocystis carinii pneumonia in two foals. J. Am Vet Med Assoc 162: 648–652, 1973.

Shively, J. N., Moe, K. K., and Dellers, R. W. Fine structure of spontaneous Pneumocystis carinii pulmonary infection in foals. Cornell Vet 64: 72–88, 1974.

Walzer, P. D. et al. Growth characteristics and pathogenesis of experimental Pneumocystis carinii pneumonia. Infect Immun 27: 928–937, 1980.

Parasitic Diseases

Alden, C. L., Gay, S., and Adkins, A. Pulmonary trematodiasis in a cat: a case report. Vet Med Small Anim Clin 75: 612–617, 1980.

Alwar, V. S., Lalitha, C. M., and Seneviratna, P. Vogeloides ramanujacharii n. sp., a new lungworm from the domestic cat (Felis catus Linné), in India. Indian Vet J 35: 1–5, 1958.

Ameel, D. J. Paragonimus, its life history and distribution in North America and its taxonomy. Am J Hyg 19: 279–317, 1934.

Atwell, R. B., and Carlisle, C. H. The distribution of filariae, superficial lung lesions and pulmonary arterial lesions following chemotherapy in canine dirofilariasis. J Small Anim Pract 23: 667–673, 1982.

Bailey, W. S., and Williams, A. G. Verminous pneumonia in the cat. Vet Med 44: 267–269, 1949.

Beaver, P. C. Larva migrans. Exp Parasitol 5: 587–621, 1956.

Benakhla, A. Pneumonie vermineuse ovine a Muellerius capillaris ou mulleriose ovine. Ann Med Vet 125: 177–189, 1981.

Beresford-Jones, W. P. Observations on Muellerius capillaris (Müller, 1889) Cameron, 1927, III. Experimental infection of sheep. Res Vet Sci 8: 272–279, 1967.

Buckley, J. J. C. On Syngamus nasicola from sheep and cattle in the West Indies. J Helminthol 12: 47–62, 1934.

Castleman, W. L., and Wong, M. M. Light and electron micropic pulmonary lesions associated with retained microfilariae in canine occult dirofilariasis. Vet Pathol 19: 355–364, 1982.

Chu, C. C. Pathological changes of paragonimiasis: preliminary observations on 30 days. Chin J Pathol 3: 163–165, 1957.

Clayton, H. M., and Duncan, J. L. Natural infection with *Dictyocaulus arnfieldi* in pony and donkey foals. *Rev Vet Sci* **31:** 278–280, 1981.

Clayton, H. M., and Lindsay, F. E. F. *Filaroides osleri* infection in the dog. *J Small Anim Pract* **20:** 773–782, 1979.

Cohrs, P. *Paragonimus westermanii* und primares Plattenepithelkarzinom in der Lunge. *Beitr Pathol Anat* **81:** 101–120, 1928.

Craig, T. M. *et al.* Fatal *Filaroides hirthi* infection in a dog. *J Am Vet Med Assoc* **172:** 1096–1098, 1978.

Cuille, J., and Darraspen E. De la strongylose cardio-pulmonaire du chien. *Rev Gen Med Vet* **39:** 625–639, 694–710, and 753–765, 1930.

Daubney, R. The life-histories of *Dictyocaulus filaria* and *Dictyocaulus viviparus*. *J Comp Pathol* **33:** 225–266, 1920.

Davtjan, E. A. Ein neuer Nematode aus den Lungen der Hauskatze. *Osleroides massino*, nov. sp. *DTW* **41:** 372–374, 1933.

Djafar, M. I., Swanson, L. E., and Becker, R. B. Lungworm infections in calves. *J Am Vet Med Assoc* **136:** 200–204, 1960.

Dubey, J. P. *et al.* Sarcocystosis in goats: clinical signs and pathologic and hematologic findings. *J Am Vet Med Assoc* **178:** 683–699, 1981.

Dunn, D. R. The pig lungworm (*Metastrongylus* spp.). 2. Experimental infection of pigs with *M apri*. *Br Vet J* **112:** 327–337, 1956.

Dunn, D. R., Gentles, M. A., and White, E. G. Studies on the pig lungworm (*Metastrongylus* spp.). 1. Observations on natural infection in the pig in Great Britain. *Br Vet J* **111:** 271–281, 1955.

Garlick, N. L. Canine pulmonary acariasis. *Canine Pract* **4**(4): 42–47, 1977.

Hare, T. Chronic tracheo-bronchitis of the dog due to *Oslerus osleri*. *Vet Rec* **11:** 1074–1075, 1931.

Hieronymi, E. Zur Entwicklung von *Aelurostrongylus abstrusus* in der Katzenlunge. *Tieraerztl Umsch* **8:** 230–233, 1953.

Hirth, R. S., and Hottendorf, G. H. Lesions produced by a new lungworm in beagle dogs. *Vet Pathol* **10:** 385–407, 1973.

Hobmaier, A., and Hobmaier, M. Die Entwicklung des Lungenwurmes des Schafes, *Dictyocaulus filaria*, Ausserhalb und Innerhalb des Tierkorpers. *MTW* **80:** 621–625, 1929.

Hoover, E. A., and Dubey, J. P. Pathogenesis of experimental pulmonary paragonimiasis in cats. *Am J Vet Res* **39:** 1872–1882, 1978.

Jarrett, W. F. H. *et al.* Symposium on husk. 1. The disease process. *Vet Rec* **72:** 1066–1068, 1960.

Jarrett, W. F. H., McIntyre, W. I. M., and Urquhart, G. M. Recent work on husk. A preliminary report on an atypical pneumonia. *Vet Rec* **65:** 153–156, 1953.

Jarrett, W. F. H., McIntyre, W. I. M., and Urquhart, G. M. The pathology of experimental bovine parasitic bronchitis. *J Pathol Bacteriol* **73:** 183–193, 1957.

Kassai, T. Die synonymie des *Cystocaulus ocreatus*. *Acta Vet Acad Sci Hung* **7:** 157–163, 1957.

Kassai, T. Vizsgalatok a juhok gocos tudofergessegerol. 4. Resz vizsgalat a *Cystocaulus ocreatus* pathogenitasarol. (Nodular verminous pneumonia in sheep. 4. *Cystocaulus ocreatus* infestation.) *Magy Allator Lapja* **12:** 333–337, 1957.

Krishna, L., Charan, K., and Paliwal, D. P. Patbological study on the larval forms of *Linguatula serrata* infection in goats. *Indian Vet J* **50:** 317–318, 1973.

Li, P. L. A histopathologic study of small lungworm infection in sheep and goats with special reference to muscular hypertrophy of the lungs. *J Pathol Bacteriol* **58:** 373–379, 1946.

MacKenzie, A. Studies on lungworm infection of pigs. II. Lesions in experimental infections. *Vet Rec* **70:** 903–906, 1958.

Mackenzie, A. Pathological changes in lungworm infestation in two cats with special reference to changes in pulmonary arterial branches. *Res Vet Sci* **1:** 255–258, 1960.

Mackerras, M. J. Observations on the life history of the cat lungworm

Aelurostrongylus abstrusus (Railliet, 1898) (Nematoda: Metastrongylidae). *Aust J Zool* **5:** 188–195, 1957.

Mackerras, M. J., and Sandars, D. F. The life-history of the rat-lungworm, *Angiostrongylus cantonensis* (Chen) (Nematoda: Metastrongylidae). *Aust J Zool* **3:** 1–21, 1955.

McLennan, M. W., Humphris, R. B., and Rac, R. *Ascaris suum* pneumonia in cattle. *Aust Vet J* **50:** 266–268, 1974.

Michel, J. F., and Coates, G. H. D. An experimental outbreak of husk among previously parasitised cattle. *Vet Rec* **70:** 554–556, 1958.

Nicholls, J. M. *et al.* A pathological study of the lungs of foals infected experimentally with *Parascaris equorum*. *J Comp Pathol* **88:** 261–274, 1978.

Nicholls, J. M. *et al.* Lungworm (*Dictyocaulus arnfieldi*) infection in donkeys. *Vet Rec* **104:** 567–570, 1979.

Nicholls, J. M., Duncan, J. L., and Greig, W. A. Lungworm (*Dictyocaulus arnfieldi*) infection in the horse. *Vet Rec* **102:** 216–217, 1978.

Nielsen, S. W. Canine paragonimiasis. *North Am Vet* **36:** 659–662, 1955.

Nimmo, J. S. Six cases of verminous pneumonia (*Muellerius* sp.) in goats. *Can Vet J* **20:** 49–52, 1979.

Parker, G. A. *et al.* Pathogenesis of acute toxoplasmosis in specific-pathogen-free cats. *Vet Pathol* **18:** 786–803, 1981.

Patnaik, M. M. A note on bovine syngamosis. *Indian Vet J* **40** 272–274, 1963.

Pirie, H. M. The pulmonary lesions characteristic of parasitic bronchitis and the commoner pneumonias of adult cattle in Britain. *In* "Respiratory Diseases in Cattle," W. B. Martin (ed.). The Hague, The Netherlands, Martinus Nijhoff, 1978.

Prestwood, A. K. *et al.* Experimental canine angiostrongylosis. I. Pathological manifestations. *J Am Anim Hosp Assoc* **17:** 491–497, 1981.

Reardon, M. J., and Pierce, K. R. Acute experimental canine ehrlichiosis. I. Sequential reaction of the hemic and lymphoreticular systems. *Vet Pathol* **18:** 48–61, 1981.

Rose, J. H. Site of development of the lungworm *Muellerius capillaris* in experimentally infected lambs. *J Comp Pathol* **68:** 359–362, 1958.

Rose, J. H. Experimental infection of lambs with *Muellerius capillaris*. *J Comp Pathol* **69:** 414–422, 1959.

Saito, M., and Oisbi, J. Natural infection of *Paragonimus ohirai* in pigs. *Med Biol (Tokyo)* **16L** 142–145, 1950.

Schwartz, B., and Alicata, J. E. Ascaris larvae as a cause of liver and lung lesions in swine. *J Parasitol* **19:** 17–24, 1932.

Schwartz, B., and Alicata, J. E. Life history of lungworms parasitic in swine. *US Dept Agric Tech Bull* **456,** 1934.

Seneviratna, P. Parasitic bronchitis in cats due to the nematode *Anafilaroides rostratus*, Gerichter, 1949. *J Comp Pathol* **68:** 352–357, 1958.

Sharma, D. N., and Dwivedi, J. N. Pulmonary schistosomiasis in sheep and goats due to *Schistosoma indicum* in India. *J Comp Pathol* **86:** 449–454, 1976.

Sinclair, K. B. The incidence and life-cycle of *Linguatula serrata* (Frohlich 1789) in Great Britain. *J Comp Pathol* **64:** 371–383, 1954.

Soliman, K. N. Observations on the orientation of certain lungworms in the respiratory tract and on their feeding habits. *Br Vet J* **107:** 274–278, 1951.

Soliman, K. N. Migration route of *Dictyocaulus viviparus* and *D. filaria* infective larvae to the lungs. *J Comp Pathol* **63:** 75–84, 1953.

Soulsby, E. J. L. "Helminths, Arthropods and Protozoa of Domesticated Animals." Philadelphia, Lea & Febiger, 1982.

Srihakim, S., and Swerczek, T. W. Pathologic changes and pathogenesis of *Parascaris equorum* in parasite-free pony foals. *Am J Vet Res* **39:** 1155–1160, 1978.

Stockdale, P. H. G. Pulmonary pathology associated with metastrongyloid infections. *Br Vet J* **132**: 595–608, 1976.

Supperer, R. *Capillaria bohmi* sp. nov., eine neue Harrwurmart aus den Stirnhohlen des Fuchses. *Z Parasitenkd* **16**: 51–55, 1953.

Urquhart, G. M., Jarrett, W. F. H., and O'Sullivan, J. G. Canine tracheo-bronchitis due to infection with *Filaroides osleri. Vet Rec* **66**: 143–144, 1954.

Wetzel, R. Zur Biologie des Fuchslungenwurmes *Crenosoma vulpis. Arch Wiss Prakt Tierheilkd* **75**: 445–460, 1940.

Whitlock, J. H. A description of a new dog lungworm. *Wien Tieraerztl Monatsschr* **43**: 731–739, 1956.

Wirth, D. Lungenwurmkrankheit des Hundes. *Wien Tieraerztl Monatsschr* **34**: 768–771, 1947.

Tumors of the Respiratory Tract

Bradley, P. A., and Harvey, C. E. Intra-nasal tumours in the dog: an evaluation of prognosis. *J Small Anim Pract* **14**: 459–467, 1973.

Carpenter, R. H., and Hansen, J. F. Diffuse pulmonary bronchiolo-alveolar carcinoma in a cat. *Calif Vet* **36**(4): 11–14, 1982.

Cohrs, P. Infektiose Adenopapillome der Riechschleimhaut beim Schaf. *Berl Muench Tieraerztl Wochenschr* **66**: 225–228, 1953.

Confer, A. W., and DePaoli, A. Primary neoplasms of the nasal cavity, paranasal sinuses and the nasopharynx in the dog: a report of 16 cases from the files of the AFIP. *Vet Pathol* **15**: 18–30, 1978.

Ferri, A. G., and Tausk, E. Primary pulmonary carcinomas of the dog. *J Comp Pathol* **65**: 159–167, 1955.

Geisel, O. Primäre Lungensarkome beim Hund. *Berl Muench Tieraerztl Wochenschr* **93**: 174–177, 1980.

Gibbs, G., Lane, J. G., and Denny, H. R. Radiological features of intra-nasal lesions in the dog: a review of 100 cases. *J Small Anim Pract* **20**: 515–535, 1979.

Gould, V. E. *et al.* Neuroendocrine components of the bronchopulmonary tract: hyperplasias, dysplasias and neoplasms. *Lab Invest* **49**: 519–537, 1983.

Harvey, C. E. *et al.* Chronic nasal disease in the dog: its radiographic diagnosis. *Vet Radiol* **20**: 91–98, 1979.

Kuscher, A., Pommer, A., and Kment, A. Zur kasuistik bosartiger Neubildungen im Luftsack des Pferdes. *Berl Muench Tieraerztl Wochenschr/Wien Tieraerztl Monatsschr* **60**(31): 53–56, 1944.

Leyland, A., and Baker, J. R. Lesions of the nasal and paranasal sinuses of the horse causing dyspnoea. *Br Vet J* **131**: 399–346, 1975.

Lucke, V. M. *et al.* A lymphomatoid granulomatosis of the lungs in young dogs. *Vet Pathol* **16**: 405–412, 1979.

McKinnon, A. O. *et al.* Enzootic nasal adenocarcinoma of sheep in Canada. *Can Vet J* **23**: 88–94, 1982.

Madewell, B. R. *et al.* Neoplasms of the nasal passages and paranasal sinuses in domesticated animals as reported by 13 veterinary colleges. *Am J Vet Res* **37**: 851–856, 1976.

Monlux, A. W. *et al.* Adenocarcinoma of the uterus of the cow—differentiation of its pulmonary metastases from primary lung tumors. *Am J Vet Res* **17**: 45–73, 1956.

Monlux, W. S. Primary pulmonary neoplasms in domestic animals. *Southwest Vet [Suppl]*, 1–39, 1952.

Moulton, J. E., von Tscharner, C., and Schneider, R. Classification of lung carcinomas in the dog and cat. *Vet Pathol* **18**: 513–528, 1981.

Murphy, J. R., Breeze, R. G., and McPherson, E. A. Myxoma of the equine respiratory tract. *Mod Vet Pract* **59**: 529–532, 1978.

Nair, M. K. *et al.* Virus-like particles in tumors of the mucosa of the ethmoid in Indian cattle. *Acta Vet Scand* **22**: 143–145, 1981.

Nichels, F. A., Brown, C. M., and Breeze, R. G. Myoblastoma: equine granular cell tumor. *Mod Vet Pract* **61**: 593–596, 1980.

Nieberle, K. Über endemischen Krebs im Siebbein von Schafen. *Z Krebsforsch* **49**: 137–141, 1939.

Nielsen, S. W., and Horava, A. Primary pulmonary tumors of the dog, a report of sixteen cases. *Am J Vet Res* **21**: 813–830, 1969.

Njoku, C. O. *et al.* Ovine nasal adenopapilloma: incidence and clinicopathologic studies. *Am J Vet Res* **39**: 1850–1852, 1978.

Parker, G. A. *et al.* Granular cell tumour (myoblastoma) in the lung of a horse. *J Comp Pathol* **89**: 421–430, 1979.

Parodi, A. L., Tassin, P., and Rigoulet, J. Myoblastome a cellules granuleuses. Trois nouvelles observations a localisation pulmonaire chez le cheval. *Rec Med Vet* **150**: 489–494, 1974.

Pospischil, A. *et al.* Endemic ethmoidal tumour in cattle: sarcoma and carcinosarcomas: a light and electron microscopic study. *Zentralbl Veterinaermed [A]* **29**: 628–636, 1982.

Pospischil, A., Haenichen, T., and Schaeffler, H. Histological and electron microscopic studies of endemic ethmoidal carcinomas in cattle. *Vet Pathol* **16**: 180–190, 1979.

Sanford, S. E., and Bundza, A. Multicentric bronchiolo-alveolar neoplasm in a steer. *Vet Pathol* **19**: 95–97, 1982.

Sjolte, I. P. Primare miligne Tumoren der Lungen bei Tieren. *Virchows Arch Pathol Anat Physiol* **312**: 35–63, 1944.

Stunzi, H. Das epidermoide Lungenkarzinom des Hundes als Vergleichsobjekt für das Raucherkarzinom des Menschen. *Schweiz Arch Tierheilkd* **113**: 311–319, 1971.

Stunzi, H. Das anaplastische Lungenkarzinom des Hundes. *Vet Pathol* **10**: 102–113, 1973.

Stunzi, H., and Hauser, B. Tumours of the nasal cavity. *Bull WHO* **53**: 257–263, 1976.

Stunzi, H., Head, K. W., and Nielsen, S. W. Tumors of the lung. *Bull WHO* **50**: 9–20, 1974.

Theilen, G. H., and Madewell, B. R. Tumors of the respiratory tract and thorax. *In* "Veterinary Cancer Medicine," G. H. Theilen and B. R. Madewell (eds.). Philadelphia, Lea & Febiger, 1979.

Troy, M. A. Bronchogenic carcinoma in the cat. *J Am Vet Med Assoc* **126**: 410–411, 1955.

Turk, M. A. M., and Breeze, R. G. Histochemical and ultrastructural features of an equine pulmonary granular cell tumour (myoblastoma). *J Comp Pathol* **91**: 471–481, 1981.

Yonemichi, H. *et al.* Intranasal tumor of the ethmoid olfactory mucosa in sheep. *Am J Vet Res* **39**: 1599–1606, 1978.

Young, S. *et al.* Neoplasms of the olfactory mucous membrane of sheep. *Cornell Vet* **51**: 96–112, 1961.

Pulmonary Adenomatosis (*Jaagsiekte*) of Sheep

Blakemore, F., and Bosworth, T. J. The occurrence of *Jaagziekte* in England. *Vet Rec* **53**: 35–37, 1941.

Cuba-Caparo, A. La poliadenomatosis pulmonar del carnero. (Pulmonary adenomatosis in sheep.) *Bol Esc Nac Cienc Vet* **1**: 27–57, 1945.

Cutlip, R. C., and Young, S. Sheep pulmonary adenomatosis (*jaagsiekte*) in the United States. *Am J Vet Res* **43**: 2108–2113, 1982.

Dungal, N. Experiments with *jaagsiekte. Am J Pathol* **22**: 737–759, 1946.

Hod, I. *et al.* Lung carcinoma of sheep (*jaagsiekte*). III. Lymph node, blood and immunoglobulin. *JNCI* **48**: 487–507, 1972.

Hod, I., Herz, A., and Zimber, A. Pulmonary carcinoma (*jaagsiekte*) of sheep: ultrastructural study of early and advanced tumor lesions. *Am J Pathol* **86**: 545–558, 1977.

Markson, L. M., and Terlecki, S. The experimental transmission of ovine pulmonary adenomatosis. *Pathol Vet* **1**: 269–288, 1964.

Martin, W. B. *et al.* Experimental production of sheep pulmonary adenomatosis (*jaagsiekte*). *Nature* **264**: 183–184, 1976.

Nisbet, D. I. *et al.* Ultrastructure of sheep pulmonary adenomatosis (*jaagsiekte*). *J Pathol* **103**: 157–162, 1971.

Perk, K. Slow virus infections of ovine lung. *Adv Vet Sci Comp Med* **26**: 267–288, 1982.

Perk, K. *et al.* Lung carcinoma of sheep (*jaagsiekte*). II. Histogenesis of the tumor. *JNCI* **47:** 197–205, 1971.

Verwoerd, O. W., and Williamson, A. L. Preliminary characterization of newly isolated ovine retrovirus causing *jaagsikete,* a pulmonary adenomatosis. *In* "Advances in Comparative Leukemia Research 1981," D. S. Yohn and J. R. Blakeslee (eds.). New York, Elsevier Biomedical, 1982.

Pleura and Mediastinum

Creighton, S. R., and Wilkins, R. J. Thoracic effusion in the cat. Etiology and diagnostic features. *J Am Anim Hosp Assoc* **11:** 66–76, 1975.

Gruffydd-Jones, T. J., and Flecknell, P. A. The prognosis and treatment related to the gross appearance and laboratory characteristics of pathological thoracic fluids in the cat. *J Small Anim Pract* **19:** 315–328, 1978.

Harbison, M. L., and Godleski, J. J. Malignant mesothelioma in urban dogs. *Vet Pathol* **20:** 531–540, 1983.

Kramer, J. W., Nickels, F. A., and Bell, T. Cytology of diffuse mesothelioma in the thorax of a horse. *Equine Vet J* **8:** 81–83, 1976.

McCullagh, K. G., Mews, A. R., and Pinsent, P. J. N. Diffuse pleural mesothelioma in a goat. *Vet Pathol* **16:** 119–121, 1979.

Nicholson, F. R., and Horne, R. D. Grass awn penetration in the dog. *Auburn Vet* **29:** 59–65, 1973.

Prasse, K. W., and Duncan, J. R. Laboratory diagnosis of pleural and peritoneal effusions. *Vet Clin North Am (Small Anim Pract)* **6**(4): 625–636, 1976.

Quick, C. B. Chylothorax: a review. *J Am Anim Hosp Assoc* **16:** 23–29, 1980.

Raphel, C. F., and Beech, J. Pleuritis and pleural effusion of the horse. *Proc Am Assoc Equine Pract* **27:** 17–25, 1982.

Raphel, C. F., and Beech, J. Pleuritis secondary to pneumonia or lung abscessation in 90 horses. *J Am Vet Med Assoc* **181:** 808–810, 1982.

Robertson, S. A. *et al.* Thoracic empyema in the dog; a report of twenty-two cases. *J Small Anim Pract* **24:** 103–119, 1983.

Smith, B. P. Pleuritis and pleural effusion in the horse: a study of 37 cases. *J Am Vet Med Assoc* **170:** 208–211, 1977.

Straub, R. *et al.* Mesothelioma of the pleura in a horse. *Schweiz Arch Tierheilkd* **116:** 207–211, 1974.

Thrall, D. E., and Goldschmidt, M. H. Mesothelioma in the dog: six case reports. *J Am Vet Radiol Soc* **19:** 197–115, 1978.

von Recum, A. F. The mediastinum and hemothorax, pyothorax and pneumothorax in the dog. *J Am Vet Med Assoc* **171:** 531–533, 1977.

Wheeldon, E. B., Mariassy, A. T., and McSporran, K. D. The pleura: a combined light microscopic and scanning and transmission electron microscopic study in the sheep. II. Response to injury. *Exp Lung Res* **5:** 125–140, 1983.

Index